Neurological Rehabilitation

Mosby's Physical Therapy Series

Neurological Rehabilitation, ed. 2
edited by **Darcy Ann Umphred, Ph.D., R.P.T.**

Orthopaedic and Sports Physical Therapy, ed. 2
edited by **James A. Gould, III, M.S., P.T.**

Cardiopulmonary Physical Therapy, ed. 2
edited by **Scot Irwin M.S., P.T.** and **Jan Stephen Tecklin, M.S., L.P.T.**

Neurological Rehabilitation

Edited by

Darcy Ann Umphred, Ph.D., P.T.
Associate Professor, Graduate Program in Physical Therapy
University of the Pacific
Stockton, California
International Lecturer
Consultant, Private Practitioner
Carmichael, California

Second edition

with 390 *illustrations*
cover illustration by Jack Tandy

The C. V. Mosby Company

ST. LOUIS • BALTIMORE • PHILADELPHIA • TORONTO   1990

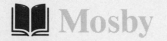

Editor: Richard A. Weimer
Developmental Editor: Kathryn H. Falk
Assistant Editor: Adrianne Cochran
Project Manager: Teri Merchant
Production Editor: Mary Stueck
Designer: Liz Fett

Second edition

Printed in the United States of America
The C.V. Mosby Company
11830 Westline Industrial Drive, St. Louis, Missouri 63146

Library of Congress Cataloging in Publication Data
Neurological rehabilitation/edited by Darcy Ann Umphred; cover
   illustration by Jack Tandy.—2nd ed.
     p. cm.
   Includes bibliographical references.
   ISBN 0-8016-5292-8
    1. Nervous system—Diseases—Patients—Rehabilitation.
  2. Exercise therapy. 3. Physical therapy. I. Umphred, Darcy Ann.
   [DNLM: 1. Nervous System Diseases—rehabilitation. WL 100
N49466]
   RC350.E85N48   1990   616.8 0462—dc20   89-14580

C/MV/MV 9 8 7 6 5 4 3

CONTRIBUTORS

C. Robert Almli, Ph.D.

Associate Professor, Department of Anatomy and Neurobiology,
Washington University School of Medicine,
St. Louis, Missouri

Marlene B. Appley, Ph.D.

Associate Professor, Department of Physical Therapy,
University of the Pacific, Stockton, California

Johnny Bonck, M.S., O.T.

Alta Bates/Herrick Hospital, Berkeley, California

Mary Jane Bouska, O.T.

Private Practitioner, Consultant, Lecturer, Practice Limited to
the Adolescent and Adult with Brain Damage, Elkins Park,
Pennsylvania

Gordon Burton, Ph.D., O.T.

Assistant Professor, Department of Occupational Therapy,
San Jose State University, San Jose, California

Sharon A. Cermak, Ed. D., O.T.

Director, Neurobehavioral Rehabilitation Research Center;
Associate Professor, Department of Occupational Therapy,
Boston University, Sargent College of Allied Health
Professionals, Boston, Massachusetts

Donna El-Din, Ph.D., P.T.

Professor and Chairman; Department of Physical Therapy,
Eastern Washington University, Cheney, Washington

Debra I. Frankel, M.S., O.T.

Special Projects Manager, Massachusetts Chapter, National
Multiple Sclerosis Society, Waltham, Massachusetts

Gertrude Freeman, M.A., P.T.

Professor, Department of Physical Therapy, School of Allied
Health Science, University of Texas Medical Branch,
Galveston, Texas

Kathryn L. Gabriel, P.T.

Physical Therapist, Area Cooperative Educational Services,
Hamden, Connecticut

Susan R. Harris, Ph.D., P.T.

Associate Professor and Coordinator, Physical Therapy
Program, University of Wisconsin at Madison,
Madison, Wisconsin

Anne Henderson, Ph.D., O.T.

Professor, Department of Occupational Therapy, Boston
University, Sargent College of Allied Health Professionals,
Boston, Massachusetts

Steven R. Huber, P.T., C.O.

Huber Associates, P.A., Physical Therapy and Orthotics,
Private Practitioner and Consultant, Auburn, Maine

Fred Humphrey, Ph.D.

Professor and Chairperson, Department of Recreation, The
University of Maryland, College Park, Maryland

Osa L. Jackson, Ph.D., P.T.

Director and Associate Professor, Program in Physical Therapy,
School of Health Sciences, Oakland University,
Rochester Hills, Michigan

Martha J. Jewell, Ph.D.

Private Consultant; Chairman, Department of Physical Therapy,
Samuel Merritt College, Oakland, California; Visiting Faculty,
Orthopedic Physical Therapy Residency Program, Kaiser
Permanente Hospital, Hayward, California

Nancy A. Kauffman

Private Practice, Consultant, Newton, Pennsylvania

Margaret Kelly-Hayes, Ed.D., R.N.

Assistant Clinical Professor of Neurology, Research Coordinator
and Investigator, Department of Neurology, Boston University
School of Medicine, Boston, Massachusetts

Steven E. Marcus, O.D.

Private Practice, King of Prussia, Pennsylvania

Anne MacRae, M.S., O.T.

Assistant Professor, Department of Occupational Therapy, San
Jose State University, San Jose, California

Guy L. McCormack, M.S., O.T.

Associate Professor, Department of Occupational Therapy, San Jose State University, San Jose, California

Marsha E. Melnick, Ph.D., P.T.

Professor and Chairman, Physical Therapy Education, University of Kansas Medical Center, Kansas City, Kansas

Linda Mirabelli, P.T. (B.S. in P.T.)

Director of Physical Therapy, Humana Hospital, Northside, St. Petersburg, Florida

Christine A. Nelson, Ph.D., O.T.

Clinical Coordinator, Department of Direct Treatment Services, Centio de Aprendizage-de-Cuernavaca, Cuernavaca, Morelos, Mexico

Roberta A. Newton, P.T., Ph.D.

Associate Professor, Department of Physical Therapy, Medical College of Virginia, Virginia Commonwealth University, Richmond, Virginia

William K. Ogard, M.A., P.T.

Associate Professor of Physical Therapy, University of the Pacific; Clinical Consultant, STAR Clinic, Stockton, California

Marilyn Pires, R.N., M.S., C.R.R.N.

Clinical Nurse Specialist, Spinal Cord Injury, Department of Nursing, Rancho Los Amigos Medical Center, Downey, California

Rebecca E. Porter, M.S., P.T.

Associate Professor and Program Director of Physical Therapy, Physical Therapy Program, Division of Allied Health Sciences, Indiana Univesity, Indianapolis, Indiana

Katharine B. Robertson, B.A., P.T.

Physical Therapist and Electroneuromyographer, Walnut Creek, California

Susan D. Ryerson, M.A., P.T.

Adjunct Assistant Professor, Program in Physical Therapy, Massachusetts General Hospital, Institute of Health Professions, Boston, Massachusetts; Partner, Making Progress, Alexandria, Virginia

Frederick J. Schneider, M.Ed., P.T.

Assistant Professor of Clinical Rehabilitation Medicine, Northwestern University Medical School; Associate Director of Education, Director of Physical Therapy Education, Education and Training Center, Physical Therapy Department, Rehabilitation Institute of Chicago, Chicago, Illinois

Jane W. Schneider, M.S., P.T.

Assistant Professor, Programs in Physical Therapy; Senior Physical Therapist, Children's Medical Hospital, Northwestern University Medical School, Chicago, Illinois

Nina Newlin Simmons, M.S., L.S.P.

Chief, Speech Pathology Department, Touro Infirmary, New Orleans, Louisiana

Laura K. Smith, Ph.D., P.T.

Institute for Rehabilitation and Research, Texas Medical Center, Houston, Texas

Susan Snyder Smith, M.S., P.T.

Assistant Professor, Department of Physical Therapy, University of Texas Health Science Center at Dallas, Dallas, Texas

Bradley W. Stockert, M.A., P.T.

Assistant Professor in Physical Therapy, University of the Pacific, Stockton, California

Marcia W. Swanson, P.T.

Lecturer, Department of Rehabilitation Medicine, Child Development and Mental Retardation Center; Clinical Training Instructor; Clinical Physical Therapist; University of Washington, Seattle, Washington

Jane K. Sweeney, Ph.D., P.T., P.C.S.

Lieutenant Colonel, Army Medical Specialist Corps, Chief, AMSC Clinical Investigation and Research, Department of Clinical Investigation, Walter Reed Army Medical Center, Washington, D.C.

Wendy L. Tada, M.A., P.T.

Physical Therapy Department Head, Clinical Training Unit, Child Development and Mental Retardation Center, University of Washington, Seattle, Washington

Darcy Ann Umphred, Ph.D., P.T.

Associate Professor, Department of Physical Therapy, University of the Pacific, Stockton, California; Private Practitioner, Consultant, International Lecturer, Partners in Learning Clinic, Carmichael, California

Nancy L. Urbscheit, Ph.D., P.T.

Associate Professor, Physical Therapy Program, Division of Allied Health, Health Sciences Center, University of Louisville, Louisville, Kentucky

Patricia A. Winkler, M.S., P.T.

President, Colorado Physical Performance Lab, Inc.; Private Practice, Englewood, Colorado

To
Gordon, Jeb, Benjamin, and **Janet,**
whose love, patience, and understanding
constantly give me strength

To
All those special people whose insights,
wisdom, guidance, and patience have
helped to give each author in this book
their unique gifts and talents, as well
as their willingness to share their
thoughts with all of you.

PREFACE

During the past decade, physical therapists have increasingly developed high-level problem-solving skills and expanded their understanding of the client as a total human being. As a result, more effective therapeutic management of client problems is being realized.

Until now there has existed no comprehensive source of information that synthesizes this practical treatment philosophy. This book was designed to provide the practitioner and advanced physical therapy student with a variety of problem-solving strategies that can be used to tailor treatment approaches to individual client needs and cognitive style.

The treatment of persons with neurological disabilities requires an integrated approach involving therapies and treatment procedures used by physical, occupational, and recreational therapists, speech pathologists, and nurses. Contributors were selected for their expertise and integrated knowledge of subject area. The result is, we hope, a blend of state of the art information about the therapeutic management of the neurologically disabled person.

This book is organized to provide the student with a comprehensive discussion of all aspects of neurological rehabilitation and to facilitate quick reference in a clinical situation. Part One, "Theoretical Foundations for Clinical Practice," comprises an overview of basic neuroanatomy, control, neurological development, and psychosocial aspects of neurological disability. Part Two, "Management of Clinical Problems," offers a clear description of the most common neurological disabilities encountered by physical and occupational therapists in general clinical practice and appropriate treatment strategies and techniques. Part Three, "Special Topics and Techniques for Therapists," is devoted to recent advances in the approach to treatment and rehabilitation, including oral speech and visual perception, electrodiagnosis, pain management, orthotics, therapeutic recreation, and health education.

Special features of all three parts are evaluation tools and illustrated demonstrations of treatment plans. A study guide has been included to direct the new student toward key concepts, procedures, and strategies presented within each chapter.

A glossary of specific physical therapy terminology should be of equal value to students and practitioners.

During the conceptualization and preparation of the original manuscript, many individuals gave time, guidance, and emotional support. To all those people I extend my sincere appreciation. My specific thanks go to:

My many teachers, but especially Martha Trotter, Sarah Semans, Nancy Watts, and my father, who taught me to reach for the impossible and realize its actuality;

The founders of the various treatment methodologies, whose conceptual ideas and flexibility created the foundation for development of an integrated problem-oriented approach to treatment;

The numerous students, colleagues, and clients who taught me how to teach them;

All the contributors who gave time, thought, and part of their lives to actualize this book;

Martha J. Jewell, Ph.D., P.T., whose support was critical during the last stage of development of the first edition;

Leinicke Design, whose original line drawings from the first edition were retained for use in the current edition.

During the reediting process of this book some additional individuals deserve special recognition.

The editorial staff at The CV Mosby Company, especially Rick Weimer, Adrianne Cochran, and Kathy Falk;

Mary Ladensack for the first edition, Debbie Crowe for the second edition, and all the secretarial staff across the country whose time was given in preparation of the manuscript;

To all those teachers who have crossed my path in the last 4 years and who helped me continually realize that before we can find answers, unknowns must be identified and acknowledged;

Special thanks to Clint Robinson who allows me both to probe his thoughts and wisdom as a friend and colleague while allowing me to grow as a student.

Special love and appreication again goes to my family. Life's complexity is constantly evolving and the demands of each person close to me grows as does our bonds. Yet, each one in my family helped me relinquish precious time to meet the requirements necessary to complete this new manuscript.

My two sons, Jeb and Benjamin, whose love and patience during the conception, gestation, and birth of this book far exceeded their age;

Last, but certainly not least, my husband Gordon, who is the only one who truly knows what demands this book has made on me and everyone around me; yet his support has never dwindled.

This book was given birth 5 years ago. It is growing with each author and each edition. We, as contributors, only hope that as the book grows, it will continually mature into a more integrated whole.

Darcy Ann Umphred

CONTENTS

Part One

THEORETICAL FOUNDATIONS FOR CLINICAL PRACTICE

Chapter 1

CONCEPTUAL MODEL
A framework for clinical problem solving

Darcy Ann Umphred

Although a physical therapist, occupational therapist, or other health professional may focus on a specific area of central nervous system (CNS) processing, a thorough understanding of the client as a total human being is critical for high-level professional performance. The purpose of this book is to orient the student and clinician to the understanding and treatment of a variety of common neurological disabilities by means of a problem-solving approach. A secondary objective is the development of a theoretical framework that justifies the use of techniques for facilitation, inhibition, and learning. Evaluation and treatment methodology incorporate all aspects of the client's CNS, including overt and nonapparent integration. The role of specific disciplines with regard to the treatment of sensory processing, gross to fine motor performance, perceptual cognitive processing, and emotional-affective growth has not been defined. In the area of neurological disabilities, the overlap of basic knowledge and practical application of treatment techniques is so great that delinea-tion of professional roles is often an administrative decision.

A problem-solving approach is used because it is logical and adaptable, and it is recommended by many professional studies.[1,4,20,31] Part One lays the foundation of knowledge necessary to understand and implement a problem-oriented approach. Part Two deals with specific clinical problems, beginning with pediatrics and ending with senescence. In Part Two each author follows the same problem-solving format to enable the reader either to focus more easily on one specific neurological problem or to address the problem from a larger perspective. Authors vary in their use of specific cognitive strategies or methods of addressing a specific neurological deficit. A variety of strategies for examining clinical problems is presented to enable the reader to see variations on the same theme and thus allow better adaptation to individual cases. Since clinicians tend to adapt learning devices to solve specific problems, many of the strategies used by one author apply to situations addressed by other authors. Readers are encouraged to use flexibility in selecting treatment with which they feel comfortable and to be creative when implementing any scheme. Part Three of the text focuses on clinical topics that might be appropriate for any one of the clinical problems discussed in Part Two.

Part Four has been added to the second edition to provide a study guide for all learners using the book. The questions were drafted by the primary author of each chapter to identify the critical components presented within that chapter. The specific way the questions were formulated was left open to present to the reader a variety of methods or problem-solving strategies used to analyze a textbook or clinical problem. Each author's task was to identify and present questions that address the critical and most important elements presented within his or her respective chapter. In no way will all aspects of the content or process of each chapter be represented within the study guide. Once mastery of the primary information has been achieved, the reader should have the knowledge and cognitive strategies available to question in greater detail the remaining information found within the book.

CONCEPTUAL MODEL FOR EVALUATING AND TREATING NEUROLOGICAL DISABILITIES
Rationale for development of a model

Traditionally, both short-term and full-semester courses, as well as literature related to treatment of clients with CNS dysfunction, have been divided into units labeled according to a technique. Often, interrelation and integration among techniques have not been explored. As a result, clinical problem solving is impeded, if not stopped, when one approach fails, because there is little integration of theories and methods achieved in the learning process. Learning is a sequential process in which the learner combines new information with previously acquired knowledge and integrates the whole.[7,19,25,26] Learning does not occur first by processing all information and then activating higher cognitive strategies. Rather processing of available information and integrating that content into higher thought processes occur in an elliptical fashion. New input is constantly being retrieved from the environment while higher thought processes are integrating the information already present. Throughout life the individual is taking in new information, processing it, and storing the content appropriately for retrieval when needed for higher cortical and integrative functioning.[8,26]

It cannot be assumed that new information (input), when presented in fragmented units, will be integrated automatically with previously acquired information to become part of a functioning whole. This is especially true when identification of how those parts are linked to the total concept has not been made. Repetitive use of the sequencing pattern is necessary for memory. If the input (content) is totally new to the individual and thus no previously stored material is available for referencing, the new content is stored in fragmented units but meaning is not applied. To assume the individual could use this fragmented content in flexible higher symbolic thought would be analogous to assuming that first graders, on initial introduction to concepts of addition, are ready for college calculus. The problem of introducing fragmented information has direct application to classroom learning and clinical performance. Clinicians may be bound to one specific treatment approach without the theoretical understanding of the step-by-step process, thus lacking the base for a change of direction when a treatment is ineffective. It is

therefore difficult to adapt alternative treatment techniques to meet the individual needs of clients. A conceptual model that allows for integration of all treatment methods is one way to avoid this problem. It permits application of a variety of techniques because it is based on thorough understanding of the rationale or higher cognitive processing behind specific actions by the clinician and reactions by the client.

Widely known and accepted theorists, with the empirical support of clinicians treating individuals with CNS damage, have identified a need for an upgraded, integrated approach to education, especially with regard to text and reference books. It is hoped that this series will provide the background for such change. The conceptual model presented here is based on principles of neurophysiology, sequential peripheral and CNS development, and human interaction and learning. Such a conceptual framework gives therapists a foundation for future growth and change. Discussions of treatment strategies are also based on neurophysiological and developmental principles. Identification of clinical problems and development of treatment programs in terms of these concepts are the two major goals of each contributor.

The clinical triad: components of the conceptual model

The majority of techniques dealing with treatment of clients with CNS damage incorporate principles of neurophysiology and normal sequential development as an evaluation and treatment tool. Both areas therefore must be included within the conceptual model. Of considerable significance also is the client-therapist interaction, which is labeled the *learning environment*. This may be the critical factor in clinical success or failure. Fig. 1-1 illustrates the model as a conceptual triad. All aspects occur simultaneously, yet each component has unique characteristics and influences the clinical performance of the therapist. Although each component is explored separately in the following pages, the reader should retain the image of the entire model. This approach should help develop a gestalt— that is, picture of the client as a total human being even though a specific aspect of therapy may be the focus. When the client is not viewed as a whole being, the therapist often misses critical response patterns, such as movement in another body part, a grimace, or an autonomic response. These responses may be the key to successful goal attainment or client-therapist rapport.

Concept of normal sequential development: a range of observable behaviors. Normal sequential development may also be referred to as normal human movement within a range of behavior. Human beings exhibit certain movement patterns that may vary in tonal characteristics, aspects of the specific movement sequences, and even the sequential nature of development. Yet the range of acceptable behavior does have limitations, and variations beyond

NORMAL HUMAN MOVEMENT
A range of observable behaviors
Constant: leads to analysis of component
parts
Foundation for
    1. Evaluation tools
    2. Treatment sequencing

LEARNING ENVIRONMENT
Deals with total person
    1. Based on input sensory systems
    2. Simultaneously active areas
        a. Motor area
        b. Affective-emotional area
        c. Perceptual-cognitive area
Personal learning differences
    1. Preferential learning styles
    2. Difficulty learning through some
       modes
Components of total clinical learning
environment
    1. The client
        a. Internal environment
        b. External environment
    2. The therapist
        a. Internal environment
        b. External environment
Dynamic: ever changing

FLEXIBILITY OF CNS CONTROL
Based on neuroanatomy/physiology
Foundation for
    1. Understanding of clinical signs
    2. Rationale for all treatment techniques
    3. Understanding of normal sequential
       development
Changing concept
    1. As knowledge base increases,
       rationale changes
    2. Content leads to new explanation for
       constant behaviors

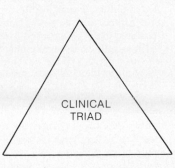

CLINICAL TRIAD

Fig. 1-1. Clinical triad.

those boundaries is recognizable by most people. A 5-year-old child may ask why a little girl walks on her toes with her legs stuck together. If questioned, that same 5-year-old may be able to break down the specific aspects of the movement that seem unacceptable. From birth a sighted individual has observed normal human movement. Because the range of behaviors identified as normal has been established, the concept behind normal human movement can be considered a constant. This concept does provide flexibility in analysis of normal movement and its sequential development. Some children choose creeping as a primary mode of horizontal movement while others may scoot. Both forms of movement are normal for a young child. In both cases each child would have had to develop normal postural function in the head and trunk to carry out the activity in a normal fashion. Thus the sequential nature of development of that function would be the constant and therefore a usable sequential treatment process for habilitation or rehabilitation. This constant also means that certain stages of development or maturation of the CNS precede others. One can feel confident that no infant will be born, jump out of the womb, walk over to the doctor and shake hands, or say 'Hi' to mom and dad.

Instead, the infant must integrate the motor plans leading to normal rolling and head control. These plans will be modified and reintegrated along with other plans to develop normal motor control in more complex movement patterns. Each pattern and movement from one pattern to another requires time and repetition for mastery and CNS maturity.

Two very important aspects of the clinical problem-solving process emerge. First, the evaluation of motor function is based on principles of sequential development. Second, rehabilitation treatment strategies become clear when the therapist observes human development from birth to aging.

Evaluation. Five categories of evaluation are used when focusing on a neurological deficit. The first four are based on development sequences (Table 1-1).

Reflex testing. Fiorentino[11] developed a reflex test that can be used on both children and adults. This form of evaluation is based on the hypothesized level of integration of reflexes and reactions within the CNS. Although the exact location of processing of many of these responses has not been identified, the behavioral aspect of the stimulus-response pattern has been recorded for decades.[24] This reflex test is easy to administer. A therapist selects a spatial position, such as supine, elicits the stimulus, and records whether the response is present or absent and the degree of obligatory behavior. Once the assessment is completed, translating the results into meaningful information often creates a barrier for clinicians. If a client has an obligatory asymmetrical tonic neck reflex (ATNR), then many activities of daily living (ADL) are severely hampered. Understanding how these reflexes and reactions assist or hinder normal activities is the key to determining whether reflex testing provides adequate evaluation data for a therapist.

Table 1-1. Categories of evaluation forms based on developmental sequencing

Type	Data recorded
Reflex testing	Presence or absence of specific reflexes and reaction related to levels of CNS integration
Gross to fine motor assessment	
Age related	Presence or absence of a variety of behaviors consistent with a specific age; often based on first 2 years of life
Sequentially based on difficulty of task	Ability of the client to hold a position, go into a position, or move in and out of a position; usually sequenced from horizontal to vertical, using functional activities such as rolling, sitting, coming to stand, and walking
Activities of daily living (ADL)	Ability of the client to carry out normal daily activities; ability to perform early test items that lay foundation for performance of more difficult tasks
Perceptual-motor assessment	
Age related	Ability of the client to carry out a variety of motor tasks related to the age norm of the test item; often items are age normed through childhood
Sequentially based on difficulty of task	Ability of the client to carry out a complex motor plan with each sequential step in a category of items based on the previous motor plan (therapist usually assuming the client can perform many items listed above under gross to fine motor assessment)

Fiorentino[12] discusses reflexes and their important clinical link to the analysis of CNS deficits in children. This link is also critical when looking at the adult CNS. Chapters 8 through 23 give more in-depth explanation in this area. The reader must remember that reflexes are only one aspect of the motor control system. This information alerts the clinician to important clinical elements affecting the motor behavior of the client. Whether the client is dominated by reflexes, has volitional control over reflexes, or has integrated the responses into refined and flexible motor plans are all critical aspects in analysis of the motor system and the client's level of function.

Motor assessment. Thousands of evaluation procedures for motor assessment are used throughout the United States. Some have been standardized, whereas others were developed to meet specific clinical needs. Although some of these evaluations may incorporate gross-motor, fine-motor, or a combination of both movement patterns, they generally focus on one of two types of developmental sequencing. The first is age related, and the second is based sequentially on the difficulty of the task. Both types focus on early movement sequences observed in humans.

AGE-RELATED MOTOR ASSESSMENT. Gesell and Amatruda[14] recorded many test items still used on age-related assessment forms. As researchers have improved their skills in assessment and children have accomplished tasks at earlier ages, the specific age norms for test items have changed;[9] yet the concept has remained stable, and its popularity as an instrument for evaluating small children still persists. As with reflex testing, problems can develop in the interpretation of test results. A combination of reflex testing and age-related behavioral responses are often used with

the neonate.[6] Understanding the tonal characteristic of in utero gestational ages seems critical when evaluating a premature or high-risk infant. This area of assessment is relatively new, and available literature is sparse. Clinicians interested in this general area are referred to Chapter 5 for additional information.

SEQUENTIAL TASK MOTOR ASSESSMENT. The second type of motor assessment based on the sequential difficulty of the task is more frequently used with older children and adults. Semans and others[29] distinctly illustrated this area of motor assessment. Their evaluation form has two sequential components. The *first* is the scoring key, which begins by having the therapist position the client in the test posture. The client is asked to hold the position and then asked to independently assume the position. If the therapist is unable to position the client in any of the test postures, the client is not asked to attempt independent positioning. The sequence of tests, starting with a totally flexed position, is based on the difficulty of holding or obtaining progressive test postures in a specific spatial plane. The nature of the test items within each spatial position gives the clinician the *second* sequential component within the evaluation form. For example, the following three items are used to evaluate supine positioning. Test position 1 is used to evaluate total flexion. Position 2 is used to evaluate flexion of one limb while the body remains extended. In posture 3 the therapist places the client's neck in flexion while the body and limbs remain extended.

The sequential nature of decreasing the amount of flexion in the supine position while asking for isolated flexor patterns has an inherent developmental base. If a client has excessive tone in the supine position, usually that tone will have a strong extensor component because of the influence of the tonic labyrinthine reflex (TLR). Taking the client out of total extension and placing the body in a total flexion pattern have strong inhibitory effects on the extension. Therefore a client can more easily comply with the request to hold a whole flexion pattern than to hold one body part in flexion while other parts remain extended.

Sequential task motor evaluation tests clients in all spatial positions. In addition to assessing motor skills, a therapist can extract important clinical information regarding the function of the client's CNS. Range of motion (ROM), reflex testing, auditory processing, sequential perceptual processing, and motor planning are but a few of the areas from which the therapist can gain vital clinical data. Results of testing also can help direct the therapist in selecting additional tests. For example, detection of persistent reflexes may suggest that a reflex test would be appropriate. On the other hand, detection of certain perceptual problems, such as auditory or temporal sequencing of a motor plan, may direct the therapist to specific perceptual tests. Many motor assessment tests also give clues to a sequential treatment plan. These methods proceed from easy to complex, often incorporating reflex integration and progression of the client from horizontal activities to vertical activities, such as kneeling and walking.

Activities of daily living tests. ADL evaluations are frequently used in adult testing, for example, following stroke or trauma. Forms for testing vary from clinic to clinic in specific tasks, number of test items, and emphasis on gross or fine motor skills required, but the formats have many consistent features. Categories are sequenced from basic motor skills, such as bed mobility, to complex motor plans, such as dressing.

The items within each category progress from simple to complex. Early ADL evaluations were designed through trial and error. Therapists realized that clients needed bed mobility skills, such as rolling, moving in bed, reaching for objects, and rising to a sitting position, before they were ready to achieve tasks such as transfers. Transfer skills normally precede walking activities. Achieving functional sitting and trunk stability is critical for addition of more complex upper-extremity and trunk skills, such as dressing and eating. Thus the sequential design of these tests developed through the success-to-failure ratio of the client's achievements.

Determining the reason a client cannot achieve bed mobility, including moving in bed, rolling, and coming to sit patterns, can be an important question. This individual might first need to modify and control some reflexes before attaining success. For example, if a client with head trauma were dominated by ATNR and TLR, then rolling over and general bed mobility would be prevented. Depending on the movement patterns the client used to come to a sitting position, the two reflexes could also prevent

that integrated motion. The ATNR would prevent the client from using a prone to crawling to side sitting to long sitting pattern because as the head turned, the arm closest to the skull would flex and be unable to support weight. The same problem would exist if a client used a side-lying, partial-rotation, coming-to-sitting pattern. The TLR would, on the other hand, stop the client from using a symmetrical supine-to-sit pattern, which requires neck and abdominal flexion in a supine position. These same and additional reflexes could hamper transfers and disrupt more complex motor plans to be used as part of the ADL assessment. In addition, rotatory and postural skills used in bed mobility are foundation skills for transfers. Without these skills more complex activities, such as transfers or dressing, are impossible. Thus ADL forms have a developmental base. Reflex testing and motor assessment data can be extracted from the results of an ADL test. Similarly, after evaluating a client with a reflex test or motor assessment, a clinician should be able to deduce the majority of test item results on an ADL checklist.

Perceptual motor assessment. Psychologists and educators have developed tests that are frequently used by therapists evaluating both children and adults.[3,13,28,33] The results not only provide data regarding gross and fine motor functioning but also focus on many specific perceptual and cognitive skills. A clear understanding of the normal development of higher-order processing and of CNS damage is vital in planning successful treatment of any client with a neurological deficit. Ayers[2] has been a principal leader in theory and implementation of perceptual-cognitive sequencing related to both physical and occupational therapy settings. Her research emphasis has been in the area of learning disabilities, but her concepts and treatment sequences have far-reaching implications. As with the other forms of evaluation, interpretation of the results in each category is the most challenging aspect. Because of the complexity of higher-order problems encountered in this form of evaluation, interpretation of the reasons why a client may not be able to perform a specific test item may be overlooked. This interpretation and integration problem is significantly influenced by the medical-model approach to evaluation, in which a clinician identifies problem areas, evaluates only those problems, and then treats them. If instead therapists evaluate systems, they can then determine what perceptual strategies are functioning when the client performs successfully on a test item. Once analysis of intact systems and their component parts has been made, specific deficits in those systems can be identified and approached.

All four categories of evaluation are based on human development. Each clinician should use whichever form or combination of forms is the most conducive to his or her learning styles. There is no "best form": each has both benefits and problems. One of the characteristics of a highly skilled therapist is the ability to extract essential information from a variety of sources. The skilled therapist looks beyond the obvious interpretations for subtle clues to CNS dysfunctions.

Motor control assessment tool. The last or fifth type of evaluation form might be labelled a motor control assessment tool. This type of form addresses the factors relating to movement function and dysfunction. As the therapeutic community integrates the research on motor control, new perspectives regarding evaluation may alter the methods and focus of assessment. The box below summarizes many aspects of motor function that the therapist may choose to identify when implementing this type of assessment tool. Motor control theory (see Chapter 3) and its clinical application have opened up an avenue for new direction in analysis. This type of evaluation incorporates the areas of reflex testing, traditional motor assessment, perceptual-motor planning abilities, and ADL information. At the same time, this tool emphasizes many additional aspects or qualities of movement, such as speed, timing, trajectory, and accuracy.

The perfect evaluation form does not and probably never will exist. Each therapist or institution must select forms that give the staff the greatest comprehension of the client's global and specific strengths and deficits. What works best for one clinician may not for the next. All assessments focus on behaviors, which reflect the sum total of all activities within the CNS. Motor output is like a hologram: any aspect should give the therapist a complete picture of the patient. Some assessments are specific and others are general, yet it is the clinician's problem-solving ability that formulates the whole.

Treatment sequences

Developmental sequence. The concept of using normal sequential development as a treatment strategy is commonly accepted by therapists treating children. The use of this approach with adults has produced conflicting results. The real controversy over developmental sequencing may

---

Factors related to movement dysfunction: types of evaluation tools or questions needing attention*

A. Range of motion—differentiate joint from muscle limitations
B. Muscle strength—types of measurements
  1. Manual muscle test: MMT
  2. Dynamometer
  3. Isokinetic testing (controlled force production)
C. State of the motor pool; presence of:
  1. Spasticity: location and extent
  2. Hypotonicity: location and extent
  3. Rigidity: location and extent
  4. Tremor (nonintentional): location and extent
D. Synergies (volitional or reflexive)
  1. What segments and in what order?
  2. Which muscles or joints does the client use to perform specific movements?
E. Postural integration
  1. Can the client hold in desired spatial positions?
  2. Can he control the proximal system or weight-bearing components while other segments are moving?
F. Balance (equilibrium)—need to determine:
  1. Sitting and standing static balance control
  2. Dynamic balance between various spatial positions, such as sitting-to-standing, walking, or higher-level activities
  3. Synergistic patterns: ankle to hip, hip to ankle
G. Speed of movement (assess quality)
  1. How fast can the patient move?
  2. What are the movement responses to speed demands?
  3. Is the rate of movement throughout the desired range appropriate for the task?

H. Timing
  1. Can the client start and stop a movement pattern appropriately, or are there delays in either initiation or stopping?
  2. Is the timing of muscle sequencing appropriate for the task?
I. Reciprocal movements
  1. Can the client change direction of a movement? If so, how easily is it performed, what rotatory components are present or absent, and are the patterns limited to only certain movement combinations?
  2. What is the turnaround delay?
    a. Does the client smoothly change direction?
    b. Does the initial pattern come to a halt before the reciprocal pattern is begun?
J. Specific pattern or trajectory of the movement
  1. How smooth or jerky is the movement?
  2. What is the specific pattern of the trajectory, velocity, and acceleration curves.
K. Accuracy
  1. How accurate is the client in placement of the body or extremity in the specific desired location?
  2. Does the accuracy change as the distance or speed of the task increases or decreases?
L. Task content
  1. Is the task a new plan or retrieval of a previously learned activity?
  2. Is the difficulty of the total plan specific to one of the previous components or a combination of factors?
  3. Does the task have an emotional component that is affecting the motor outcome?

*Adapted from a presentation by Guiliani C: Motor control theory and application, informal presentation, Harmerville, Pa, August, 1988, lecture notes.

relate more to the manner in which the activity is introduced rather than to the activity itself. If the therapist presents rolling as a childlike activity and expects the adult to get on a mat and roll like a child, the client may perceive this activity as inappropriate for his or her level of development. If instead the client is approached with an explanation of trunk rotation as critical for transfer skills and is told that one way to work on rotation is by rolling, then the activity will be better accepted.

Sequential development as a tool for treatment is enhanced as a therapeutic intervention with the realization that behavioral changes result from therapy. Once a goal or behavior has been established, the component parts necessary for attaining that goal can be identified. A thorough analysis should be made of any activity and its component parts—with the understanding that each component part may have its own developmental sequence.

Table 1-2 illustrates a developmental sequence activity testing scheme. It also provides a form for the therapist to use in recording key elements, with the first entry filled in as an example. The first activity focuses on a horizontal movement—rolling—an important component of independent bed mobility. Knowledge of developmental patterns makes us realize that humans roll by leading either with the head or the lower extremity. Therefore two alternative sites for facilitating rolling are identified, and methods for achieving head or lower extremity movement are established. The behavior is then broken into its component parts. Identifying (1) appropriate movement patterns, reflexes, and reactions that assist or prevent the desired movement and (2) perceptual concepts necessary for adequate performance of the task gives important clues to appropriate treatment strategies. Understanding the movement sequences, as well as multiple factors that may assist or prevent attaining the desired movement, allows the therapist flexibility in designing a treatment plan. Thus the therapist might work on appropriate patterns while the client is in a horizontal position or might help the client break the movement into components, approaching them from a sitting, kneeling, or half-kneeling position. Creating an environment conducive to client satisfaction and supportive of client needs can of course be considered at any time.

Introduced in Table 1-2, the second activity—coming to sitting from a supine position—is more complex than rolling. Three different patterns are presented in the order observed during normal child development. A child first rolls from a supine to a prone position. From a prone position the child pushes to a four-point position, rotates to a side-sitting position, and then to a full-sitting position. The child then progresses to a partial rotation pattern and finally into the more complex adult sitting patterns by the fifth to sixth year. Children and adults with neurological deficits may find that for them this three-stage sequence does not progress from simple to complex. Abnormal reflex activity can dominate and severely hamper successful accomplishment of one or all methods. Analysis of each of the component movements determines which pattern is most beneficial for each client. Although a developmentally higher method may be easier, each sequence of the three patterns is important for integration of more advanced motor activities and should not be neglected.

Coming to sitting requires movement patterns made up of multiple component sequences. Given the complexity of so basic a movement pattern, it is no wonder that helping a client accomplish such activities as dressing, climbing on and off a bus, or achieving wheelchair independence may be frustrating to client and to health personnel. Therefore it is important for the therapist to explain that even though a task may seem simple, it is composed of many integrated parts that may be critical for a more complex activity.

Normal sequential development as a tool for evaluation and treatment is based on visually observed behavior. The assumption is made that humans naturally develop in the most physiologically efficient manner. Thus using developmental sequencing should create an environment that not only takes into account the most socially acceptable ways to move but also those most efficient in terms of energy consumption. If an individual is allowed to use abnormal patterns of movement, then the therapist and the client must realize that integration of those patterns with higher patterns will not be viewed by others as normal. Normal movement can of course be learned if behavior patterns are changed, but normal behaviors do not sequence from abnormal ones.

If the therapist chooses to implement normal behaviors as treatment progressions, a thorough understanding of normal development from a sequential processing viewpoint and knowledge of CNS myelination are essential to effect control. A therapist who understands normal movement patterns through observation can easily detect deviations from normal and degrees of abnormality. Gross to finite aspects of abnormal patterns can be identified by components. Once identification has been made with respect to normal and abnormal behavioral responses, goals for correction of those deviations can be established and treatment begun. Treatment should be based not only on observable behavior but also on understanding of CNS function. For example, when analyzing a hemiplegic gait pattern, a therapist can identify the total movement pattern as one unit or can break down the pattern into components. Each aspect of the gait cycle—from heel strike, midstance, push off, to swing through, which consists of trunk, hip, knee, and ankle movement patterns—can be examined. If joint motion functions normally throughout the gait cycle, no intervention would be indicated. With deviations, such as the substitution of plantar flexion of the foot for dorsiflexion, treatment procedures to correct the difficulty can be selected. For example, a therapist might select a proprioceptive neuromuscular facilitation (PNF)

Table 1-2. Concept of sequential development as a treatment progression

Movement patterns	Reflex reaction to assist	Reflex reaction to prevent	Necessary perceptual concepts	Treatment sequences
Activity: horizontal movement—rolling				
1. Start at head				
a. Head flexion with rotation or head extension with rotation	Neck righting	Tonic labyrinthine reflex	Limited at this level if therapist elicits response manually	Modify reflexes preventing behavior
b. UE, trunk, and LE follow in appropriate sequential progress	Optic and labyrinthine righting	Asymmetrical tonic neck reflex	Complex if therapist expects client to perform from either auditory or visual cues	Elicit neck righting via any number of treatment techniques
				Use facilitory or inhibitory techniques when appropriate, according to desired neurophysiological response
2. Start at LE				
a. Supine to prone—LE: flexion, adduction, internal rotation, followed by trunk and head in appropriate progression				
b. Prone to supine—LE: extension, abduction, external rotation, followed by trunk and head in appropriate progression				
Activity: supine to sitting				
3. Roll to prone and push up				
a. Rolling patterns				
b. Postural tone in prone				
c. Movement patterns from prone to four-point to sitting				
d. Postural tone in sitting				
e. Balance in sitting				
4. Partial rotation				
a. Rolling patterns				
b. Head, trunk, and shoulder stability in asymmetrical pattern				
c. Balancing from side to sitting				
d. Asymmetrical patterns in LE and possibly UE				
e. Same as *d* and *e* in no. *1*				
5. Adult sitting				
a. Symmetrical head and trunk flexion, LE extension				
b. Balance from supine to sitting				
c. Same as *d* and *e* in no. *1*				

Comments: When would you facilitate neck righting versus body on body on head righting and vice versa? *Why?* When would you facilitate one coming-up-to-sitting activity versus another, and *why?*

UE, Upper extremity; LE, lower extremity.

pattern to facilitate dorsiflexion at push off, or tapping or vibrating with resistance of the dorsiflexors and evertors during swing phase. Although each joint action needs attention, the interaction of all joints during any phase of gait is even more critical. Consequently, once normal and deviant patterns have been identified, the combined responses of all muscles—and thus joint action—can be analyzed for each component of the cycle.

Combining total patterns of trunk and leg movement to correct deviations would be another important treatment protocol. Sequencing the treatment activity to a movement pattern less complex than a gait motion would be one way to recombine total patterns into normal movement sequences. For example, a client may be unable to go into dorsiflexion during stance phase, thus remaining in plantar flexion and altering the trunk, hip, and knee action. One treatment possibility is to work on half-kneel–to–stand or modified squat-to-stand over a bolster. These developmental patterns precede normal ambulation as well as maintain dorsiflexion while the hip and knee go into extension. There are many physiological reasons why this occurs. One is that because total flexion inhibits extension, the client would be initially placed in flexion. Another is that heavy joint approximation, especially down through the heel, tends to facilitate a postural weight-bearing pattern and modify the positive supporting pattern elicited by pressure on the ball of the foot. Additional treatment procedures, such as quick stretch, resistance, tapping, and prolonged stretch, when applied to the appropriate muscle groups or synergistic patterns, can further facilitate a normal combination of muscle activity. Other developmental patterns, such as rolling, might also be used to help the client relearn normal combinations of muscle groups that require interaction for normal gait to occur.

One additional link between developmental sequencing and normal movement needs mentioning. If the therapist is aware of movement combinations necessary for normal pattern responses, then those combinations can be facilitated before the client is asked to perform the higher-level activity. Using the example of the hemiplegic client stuck in plantar flexion of the foot during stance phase, the therapist should be aware of developing tonal patterns in the client's lower extremity. If, during bed mobility activities, the client develops a strong plantar flexion response everytime the lower extremity goes into an extensor pattern, the therapist should know that dorsiflexion difficulty will occur during stance. The therapist can then try to alter the movement combination before gait training, thus preventing reinforcement of an undesirable pattern and eliminating the client's frustration with walking in an abnormal fashion.

The concept of normal sequential development does not translate into a hierarchy of movement in which a patient must, for example, roll before sitting. Instead it presents the concept that all behaviors can be broken down into components. Each component may in and of itself be a separate behavior. How components combine and the number of component combinations needed in any one behavior determine the difficulty of the task. Prior learning versus new learning play significant roles in task difficulty. Familiarity with the spatial position in which the task is presented plays a key role in success. For example, eating while sitting and eating while side-lying are two totally different movement combinations, yet the task goal is the same. Side-lying may give greater support, but vertical is more familiar.

To have higher-level motor control, a person needs the schemata and plans necessary to implement the behavior. Before a client can be asked to put the whole movement together, he or she needs the components of the whole. To find the best way to develop the component parts and reintegrate them into observable movement is the goal of all therapeutic techniques. Each instructor teaching a particular approach feels that his or her way is the most viable, and because so many colleagues with so many methods seem to create positive changes in client behavior, it might seem that all methods are viable. What will best fit for each client may be client dependent and needs to be evaluated by the problem-solving clinician.

Concept of CNS control: a multicomplex control system. The concept of CNS control is based on a therapist's understanding of the CNS and how it regulates response patterns. This understanding, which requires in-depth background in neuroanatomy and neurophysiology, gives the therapist the basis for clinical application and treatment. Understanding the intricacies of neuromechanisms provides therapists with direction as to when, why, and in what order to use facilitatory and inhibitory clinical techniques. Behavioral development is based on maturation, potential, and degeneration of the CNS. Each behavior observed, sequenced, and used as a treatment protocol should be interpreted according to neurophysiological and anatomical principles. Unfortunately, our knowledge of behavioral development is ahead of our understanding of the intricate mechanism of the CNS. Thus the correlation of vital links between observed behavior and CNS processing is not always known.

Because information about the functioning of the CNS is constantly increasing, the rationale for the use of certain behavioral sequences or other treatment techniques to elicit a certain response may also change. This can create frustration among therapists who desire solutions and treatment rationales that are reliable, valid, and constant. Since it is unrealistic to expect to know all the answers, therapists should keep abreast of the literature and be open to new ideas. The following example illustrates this need.

Assume I were to learn Rood's concept of cocontraction, which is based on the intricate neuromechanism of the interaction of the Ia and II sensory receptors within the muscle spindle. Rood's theory assumes that the II receptors are polysynaptic and facilitate the antagonist of the postural muscle.[30] I then discover that some II receptors are monosynaptic,[5] which would put the validity of Rood's rationale in question. My clinical observations produce the same doubt. That is, while observing postural muscles after CNS insult in adults, I note two behaviors that contradict Rood's theory: first, a spastic postural muscle rarely facilitates antagonistic activity. Second, I note that a client who gains some voluntary control over the postural muscle, especially in the shortened range, is not necessarily able to facilitate cocontraction. In fact, the postural muscle seems to function optimally in a movement pattern but has great difficulty holding in an isometric pattern. Further, even more frustration occurs when the therapist tries to elicit dynamic-automatic cocontraction. Both clinical problems suggest that the II receptors, at a spinal level, may not be the mechanism for cocontraction. Thus I face a dilemma.

I have two recourses. First, I can decide that Rood is wrong and thus her approach invalid, and I can discard all of the treatment procedures classified under that technique. Or I could choose a second strategy; knowing that Rood's method for developing cocontraction has worked effectively on many clients, I can assume that the techniques or methods are reliable and viable treatment approaches but that the *reason* why they work can no longer be explained by Rood's theory. A new rationale might follow the assumption that postural control and dynamic cocontraction are regulated much higher in the CNS than was first thought. If the CNS needs the feedback from elements of the peripheral system—such as muscle spindles, tendons, and joint receptors—to program the function of dynamic cocontraction, then creating an environment conducive for learning that motor function would be important. First, the CNS would need to develop extreme sensitivity to the entire range of joint motion to later control and modify movement through the range. If that sensitivity developed in the shortened range, then any additional stretch or lengthening of the range would only add more input to the CNS for better control. Thus the shortened range would be the best place to begin treatment. Because the muscle's function is primarily to hold, asking the client to hold rather than move would again be consistent. To increase feedback to the CNS and develop better internal stretch and strength, resistance would also be indicated. Thus I could conclude that Rood's concept of shortened, held, resisted contraction (SHRC) as well as her sequences are still valid treatment approaches. Although this new rationale would be based on current neurophysiological concepts, in time it might also be shown to be invalid. If so, a new mechanism would be sought to take its place if the behavioral responses remain consistent.

Our understanding of the brain is still fragmented and incomplete. The more we learn, the more we are astounded and frustrated by its complexity. The problem can be likened to the technological advances of recent years. This rapid influx of knowledge, often contradicting past beliefs, creates anxiety and confusion. Thus a clinician must try to keep abreast of current scientific concepts, research, and facts by either continuing his or her education and focusing on neuroapplication, or by reading and applying advances from current textbooks. Without updated information, colleagues begin to feel that the CNS is beyond their grasp.

When a topic defies easy comprehension, people may create myths to make the complexity seem accessible. Although myths make people feel secure, they are constantly under attack. This again creates anxiety and, often, defensive behavior until a new, more acceptable myth can be established. Myths are found not only in highly technological fields; they exist in all avenues of life. One of the best-established myths within the field of physical and occupational therapy is that the various approaches to treating children or adults with neurological impairment have no similarities. A clinician often hears a colleague say, "The technique I am using is the only one that adequately treats the client according to a valid rationale." Another myth is the assumption that approaches developed to treat neurological conditions have no relevance in such specialties as orthopaedics, sports, or psychiatry. When someone attacks those beliefs, many clinicians become uncomfortable.

Before we discard the notion that commonalities may exist or that an integrated whole may be found, it might be advantageous to go back 40 or 50 years. At that time Berta Bobath, Margaret Rood, Signe Brunnstrom, Temple Fay, Margaret Knott, Dorthy Voss, Moshe Felderkrais, and others were working as clinicians trying to treat their clients with the most current techniques available. All of these colleagues were gifted in their clinical abilities. Over time they conceptualized strategies and treatment sequences, which they explained with available scientific knowledge. Their main goal was client care, not establishment of a dynasty. As these talented, intelligent pioneers tried to share their concepts with colleagues, many therapists had difficulty understanding the rationale, but they recognized that the technique worked.

It would seem at the present time that a dilemma has developed that has created havoc within the field. A clinician who is comfortable and successful with one approach and understands only its rationale (i.e., refuses to explore other approaches) reinforces the myth that his or her approach is far superior to all others or that it is the only valid one. As large numbers of colleagues begin to accept such a myth, strong lines of defense are built. Lack of communication and growth very often results, which is in direct opposition to the objectives of those who created the techniques.

Twenty years ago a large number of colleagues met to try to dissolve these barriers and again regain the momentum of growth and understanding of the whole.[23] At this meeting various treatment approaches, based on neurophysiological and orthopaedic principles, were presented. It was the intent of these colleagues to identify commonalities and develop integrated trends among the various methods. Some evidence would strongly suggest that clinicians have come closer to a gestalt approach rather than become more fragmented and territorially defensive. Farber[10] and Randolf and Heineger[27] published books emphasizing the importance of an integrated approach to client care based primarily on our understanding of the CNS. More and more courses at undergraduate and graduate levels are being offered that focus on clinical problems and alternative treatments. This is not to negate the importance of in-depth knowledge and training that may emphasize a specific philosophy toward client care. As long as clinicians strive toward a better understanding of the whole and avoid falling into the trap that one fragment is the whole, they and the professions they represent will continue to change, grow, and offer better services to the public. In this book classifications of common facilitory and inhibitory techniques, based on principles of neurophysiology, are presented to help the reader conceptualize the whole and develop an integrated treatment approach. (See Chapter 6 for additional information.)

Because this book focuses on a problem-oriented approach using a conceptualized model, a word of caution is in order. Our knowledge of the CNS is in its infancy; it is easy to identify myths from the past, but it is just as easy to create new myths. Although use of the concept of neurophysiology to explain clinical symptoms, treatment rationales, and observable behaviors is valid, details will change as our scientific knowledge grows.

Some principles regarding CNS have remained stable over time—for example, such concepts as a cephalocaudal and proximal to distal development. Myelin formation and maturational development explain many of the behaviors observed in early childhood. (Chapters 2 through 7 go into more detail regarding the links between the behavioral sciences and the neurosciences.)

Another principle that seems to flow through all techniques is the concept of duality of CNS control. Knott integrated into her treatment concepts the basic physics concept that for every action there was an equal and opposite reaction. Brunnstrom described her flexion and extension synergies. Bobath talked of posture and movement, whereas Rood referred to mobility and stability. Although at a motor response level these actions may seem to oppose each other, it is becoming clear that the intricate nature of posture and movement of synergistic-antagonistic function is highly complex and regulated by a variety of systems. It is also apparent that check and balance feedback systems exist throughout the CNS. There is something that directs one's attention to a target, and there is something that habituates that orientation. Too much of either response creates a different clinical problem. One reaction might be referred to as autistic and the other hyperactive. Both are based on imbalance within the CNS, possibly of an opposite nature. Because of the pliability of the nervous system and the multitract nature of any one response, the potential of the CNS to change seems great. All techniques are based on this assumption. If presented with an environment conducive to change, people will, theoretically, change. The importance of this principle leads us to the third concept of the model used in this book.

Concept of the learning environment. Critical to the clinical triad of our conceptual model is the concept of the learning environment. Clinicians spend a lifetime learning and teaching yet probably never intensively reflect on how they learn or how others learn from them. Awareness of and sensitivity to this learning process is vital. In each field of the health care system, there are very gifted clinicians. When these individuals are observed treating clients, it often seems as if the clients demonstrate marked improvement and show a high potential for future achievement. A sequential phenomenon can be seen even in a short time spent observing clinician with client. The observing therapist may write down step by step what the gifted therapist does with the client and may formulate it into an optimal treatment plan. Yet the therapist may attempt the plan with a client and find that it does not work—that the client is unable to function at the high level expected and may indeed be successful only with those skills already acquired. This leaves the clinician frustrated and the client at a lower level of function than desired. The question arises as to why the sequence worked effectively with one therapist on one day and not on the next with the other therapist. Many answers can be hypothesized. First, the gifted clinician has some "magic healing power." Second, the gifted clinician did not tell the observing group what was truly going on. Third, the second clinician's skills are inadequate for effective therapy. Although these explanations come quickly to mind, a more accurate explanation may be found in analyzing the learning environment.

Each clinician, as well as each client, processes millions of bits of sensory data each second. How that information is processed and how appropriate response patterns are implemented constitute a unique characteristic of each individual. When two people are interacting, as in a client-therapist relationship, each person is responding to the moment-to-moment changes occurring within the environment. At no time is that environment the same. Thus the therapist has the responsibility of interacting dynamically with the client to create an optimal situation. An analogy might be made between the therapist and a multimillion channel biofeedback system. The more skillful the therapist, the more channels he or she is able to regulate. The therapist is responsible not only for processing information within his or her CNS but also for directing appropriate input into the client's CNS. This interaction is not just a sensorimotor exchange but incorporates the entire client-therapist interaction. Thus perceptual, cognitive, and affective channels must be established, and a method of processing the data flowing through those channels must be found. Gifted therapists seem to grasp this totality and create a treatment sequence that guides the client toward optimal independence. It does not seem to be the sequential steps themselves that are the clues to successful treatment but rather the dynamic interaction of the therapist and client taking those steps. Thus a different therapist using the same sequential steps with the same client might be unsuccessful. The difference in interaction may account for the failure or success of that treatment plan.

If indeed the learning environment must be client-therapist dependent, then regimented, preestablished treatment plans would not promote optimal learning for each client because they could not take into consideration individual differences. Clients need acute care, rehabilitation, or home health services, whether they have sustained a CNS insult or a severe orthopaedic injury; they need to learn or relearn something, either a psychomotor skill or cognitive process. The individual who is relearning to walk after a stroke, a total hip replacement, or an amputation faces an environment that is different in place and time from the one in which that individual took his or her first steps. Additional problems of distorted and diminished sensory imput, processing of cognitive, perceptual, and affective data, and motor output may confound the relearning process. Seldom in a rehabilitation setting can a client be a passive participant while a clinician acts on that person. For this reason no matter what the therapist's background, knowledge, or clinical skill, both the client and the therapist are actively involved in what can be referred to as the clinical learning environment. Success within this area is dependent on the therapist's problem-solving abilities, flexibility in creating environments conducive to client growth, and sensitivity to client needs.

The concept of the learning environment is the most abstract and complex of the three concepts in the theoretical model. For that reason it is by far the hardest to present in concrete terms. Both simultaneous and successive components make up the creation and maintenance of this environment. At any one moment multitudinous input events occur simultaneously and continuously. Thus a temporal ordering of successive events plays a role in the CNS response to the environment. To comprehend the dynamics of this interaction and be able to function with optimal success, the clinician must:

1. Understand the learning process to provide an environment that promotes learning
2. Investigate the input, processing, feedback, and output system as a vital servomechanism for higher-order learning
3. Understand higher-order processing if carry-over of treatment into other environments, such as the home, is to be expected
4. Differentiate how he or she learns from how the client learns. If these learning styles conflict, then the clinician needs to teach through the client's preferential systems or learning styles
5. Be aware simultaneously of the motoric, affective, and cognitive aspects of an individual, no matter what the clinical emphasis might be at any one time

Four distinct components of the learning environment must be identified and addressed: the internal and external environments of the client and the internal and external environments of the clinician.

The client's internal environment is an obvious focus of all health care professionals. A lesion has occurred within the system and is affecting how the entire mechanism functions. If the lesion occurred before initial learning, then habilitation must take place. Although a learning style has not yet been established, the individual probably has a genetic predisposition. The therapist should test the inexperienced CNS by creating experiences consisting of a variety of input modalities as well as higher processing systems to discover optimal methods of learning best suited to that CNS. Then the therapist can focus treatment on the most effective strategies. If previous learning has occurred and preferential systems have been established, then the therapist needs to know what they are and whether they have been affected by the insult so that proper rehabilitation can be instituted. The use of preferential modes such as visual versus verbal or kinesthetic versus verbal does not mean that other modes are ineffective. Nor do all modes function optimally in any given situation.

One way to determine general preestablished preferential styles is by taking a thorough history. Leisure-time activities and job choice often give clues to learning styles. For example, a client who loved to take car engines apart or build model ships demonstrates preference to visual-spatial learning style, whereas another client, whose preference for pure enjoyment was sitting in a chair with a novel, demonstrates a probable preference toward verbal learning. Again, this does not mean both clients could not selectively use both methods, but it does illustrate preference. Both the position of the lesion and preferential learning styles can play a key role in matching the learner with a particular environment and in identifying potential. If a client has suffered massive insult to the left temporal lobe and before the trauma showed poor ability in using the right parietooccipital lobe, then spatial or verbal strategies may be ineffective in the relearning process. However, a client with the same lesion, who had high-level right parietooccipital function before the insult, will probably learn at a much faster rate if visual-kinesthetic strategies are used to promote learning.

The client's external environment is the second critical

component. All external stimuli, including noise, lighting, temperature, touch, humidity, and smell, modulate the client's internal responses. This external input can invoke negative and positive influences on the internal mechanism and alter the client's ability to manipulate his or her world. Because a therapist should make every effort to be aware of what is happening to the client externally, knowing generally what is happening within and outside the hospital is important. Any behavioral change displayed by the client, such as mood, attitude, or muscle tone change, should serve as an indicator to the therapist that a change may have occurred. Following up that observation by determining what happened can help the therapist not only in understanding but in assisting the client to deal with environmental change or in obtaining additional professional assistance.

The clinician should also be aware of personal internal and external factors that influence patient responses. Everyone has preferential styles of teaching and learning, yet many may be unaware of what they are and how they affect outlook on life and interaction with other people. A common example of a mismatch of styles is what happens when two people are arguing opposing sides of a political issue. Although both individuals may process the same data, they may also have different learning strategies and come up with very different conclusions.

The interplay of learning styles occurs continually in an academic setting. A student, asked the question, "What do you want out of this course?", would probably say, "A good grade." Getting a good grade requires doing well on course requirements, including tests. High test performance usually requires not only demonstrating knowledge of materials presented but also integration of the concepts when the student addresses teacher-formulated questions. When the clinician relates the same concepts to a client, it is important that the clinician be aware of the client's behaviors and responses and adapt to the client rather than having the client adapt to the therapist.

This external-internal interaction concept brings up another important clinical consideration. As students, most of us probably "clashed" with one or two teachers with whose learning styles we could never identify. That is, we as learners probably cannot or will not adapt to all learning styles. For that reason there may be clients whom we cannot teach and who also cannot learn through our approach. When that seems evident, a shift of therapists is most appropriate for the rehabilitation process to succeed.

The fourth component of the learning environment is the clinician's external environment. It is generally expected that personal life should never affect professional work. To accept this assumption, however, may be to deny that emotions affect behavioral patterns. When an individual is feeling unwell, emotionally upset, or under stress, response patterns vary without cognitive awareness. For example, suppose that Mr. Smith, who has a spastic condition because of a cerebrovascular accident, comes down early for therapy each morning, has a cup of coffee, and chats while you write notes. If one day you are under extreme stress and do not feel like interacting as Mr. Smith rolls his wheelchair into your office, you might say, "Mr. Smith, I'll be with you in a few minutes. Go over to the mat, lock your brakes, pick up the pedals, and we'll transfer when I get there." Mr. Smith will quickly identify a change in your behavior. He believes you are a professional and that your personal life will not affect your job. Thus he may draw a logical conclusion—that he must have done something to change your behavior. When you go to transfer him, you notice he is more spastic than usual and ask, "Is something bothering you? You are tighter than usual," and so goes the interaction. Your external environment altered your internal state and thus normal response patterns. In turn you altered Mr. Smith's external environment, changing his internal balance, and created a change of emotional tone that resulted in increased spasticity.[21] If instead of interacting with Mr. Smith as if nothing were wrong, you informed him you were upset over something unrelated to him, you might avoid creating a negative environment. First, you let Mr. Smith know that there are days you are upset and have mood changes. As he accepts your changes as normal, you help him realize he can have similar "off" days. Second, you give him an opportunity to offer his assistance to comfort or help you if he so desires. Such behavior encourages interdependence and social interaction, long-term goals for all rehabilitation clients.

Although each client is unique and thus analysis of specifics related to the learning environment is difficult, certain basic learning principles can be formulated. Six clinically significant learning concepts have been selected from many that have been established.[8,16,17] Basic learning principles relevant to clinical performance may be summarized as follows.

1. Individuals need to be able to solve problems if independence in daily living is desired.
2. Although assigned tasks must be challenging, there must be a possibility of success.
3. When tasks are difficult or unfamiliar (new problem), an individual will revert to more primitive or familiar patterns or ways to solve the problem.
4. When working on development or learning within one area of the CNS, learning is occurring simultaneously in other areas.
5. Necessary to learning are motivation to try the unknown and, simultaneously, success in learning in order to retain that motivation.
6. Clinicians need to be able to analyze an activity, to determine its components, and to use problem-solving strategies to design good individual programs. At the same time, if independence in living skills is an objective, the therapist needs to teach the

client those same problem-solving strategies rather than teaching the solution.

Although all six learning concepts seem simple, their application within the clinical setting is not always as obvious. Principles *1* and *2* are intricately linked with the appropriateness and difficulty of tasks presented to clients. If a client is asked to perform a task such as standing, rolling, relaxing, dressing, or maneuvering a wheelchair, a problem has been presented that requires a sequence of acts leading to a solution. To succeed, the client must be able to perform each of the sequential steps in the appropriate order. If steps are unmastered or if sequencing is inappropriate or absent, dependence on the clinician to solve the problem is reinforced. An alternative approach to whole-task demands is presenting the task in components that the client can probably master and then teaching strategies in areas where the client has difficulty. More specifically, a client should not be asked to perform a task unless he or she understands what is expected and can obtain the objective with some degree of success. Linked intricately with success is the challenge of the task. The greater its difficulty or complexity, the greater the challenge and consequently the greater is the satisfaction of success.

There is a subtle interplay in degree of difficulty, challenge, and success. Selecting tasks that are age appropriate, clinically relevant, and goal related is a challenge to the therapist. For the patient to be successful, the therapist must be a creative problem solver and knowledgeable of the client's needs, abilities, and goals. If the tasks are too simple or if the client considers them unimportant, boredom will ensue and progress may diminish. If the tasks are too difficult, the client may feel defeated and turn away from them. In such cases a child tends to withdraw physically, whereas an adult usually avoids the problem. Being late to therapy, having to leave early, needing to go to the bathroom, and scheduling conflicting sessions are all avoidance behaviors that may be linked to inappropriate tasks.

A third learning principle describes a behavior inherent in all people: reversal. When confronted by a problem, we revert to patterns that produce feelings of comfort and competence to solve the problem. In Fig. 1-2, a 2½-year-old child is confronted with just such a conflict. The bridge he wants to cross is unstable. Therefore the child reverts developmentally to 6-month-old behavior and thus scoots. On gaining confidence, he sequences from scooting to four-point bunny hopping, then crawling, on up to cruising, and finally to reciprocal walking. The child's developmental reversal lasted approximately 2 minutes. Although reverting to more familiar or comfortable ways of solving problems is normal, it creates constant frustration in the clinic if it is prolonged. For example, if a hemiplegic client has spent a week modifying and control-

ling a spastic upper-extremity pattern during a simple task and is now confronted with a more difficult problem, the spasticity will most likely return. If another client has successfully worked to obtain the standing position and then is asked to walk, the strong synergistic patterns that had been controlled may return. Return to lower-level patterns should be anticipated and the client prepared. Anticipating that abnormal patterns will usually return as the tasks demanded increase in complexity, the clinician can attempt to inhibit the unwanted responses. The key to comprehension of this concept is not the behavior itself; instead, it is the attitude a therapist has toward a new task presented to the client. If the clinician expects the client to be successful, the client will also expect success. If failure occurs, both parties will be disappointed and a potentially negative clinical situation will be created; however, if the client succeeds, both will have expected the result and their attitude will be neither excited or depressed. If, on the other hand, the clinician expects the client to revert to an old behavior, then he can prepare the client. If the client reverts, neither party will be disappointed; but if no reversion occurs, both will be excited, pleased, and encouraged by the higher functional skill. By understanding the concept, the clinician can maintain a very positive clinical environment without the constant negative interference of perceived failure when a client does revert.

The fourth learning principle deals with the totality of the client. Whether the area of emphasis is performance, emotional balance, or perceptual integration, all areas are affected. Therefore understanding and respect for all areas are important if optimal client function is a primary objective. This does not suggest that therapists should address each aspect of personality; however, integration of the client's physical, mental, and spiritual areas should be a responsibility of the staff. Awareness of possible adverse effects of one learned behavior on other CNS functions can help avoid potential problems. For example, if working on lower-extremity patterns creates extreme upper-extremity spasticity through associated patterns, the clinician is not dealing with the client as a whole.

The unknown creates fear as well as curiosity for most individuals, and the fifth concept points out the fact that for most clients the unknown is all-encompassing whatever the degree of prior learning. For a client whose only difficulty is a flaccid upper extremity, functional activities such as toileting, dressing, or eating will be troublesome and unfamiliar. Motivation is a critical factor for success. Fig. 1-3, *A* illustrates a child experiencing the unknown. He is walking off the bench as if the seat extended forever. He is confident, relaxed, and oblivious to the problem. Fig. 1-3, *B* and *C* shows the child's surprise, his orientation to the task, motivation to succeed, and the ability to alter his preconceived motor plans to solve the problem. Obviously, instructing clients to walk off park benches is not the point. Maintaining motivation to try while ensuring a high

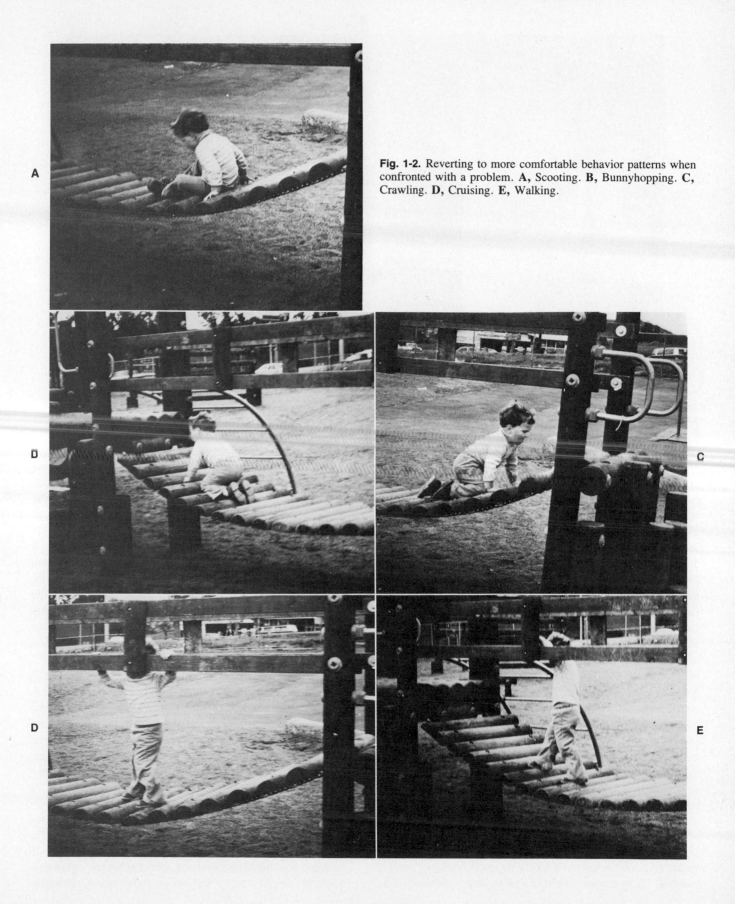

Fig. 1-2. Reverting to more comfortable behavior patterns when confronted with a problem. **A,** Scooting. **B,** Bunnyhopping. **C,** Crawling. **D,** Cruising. **E,** Walking.

A   B   C

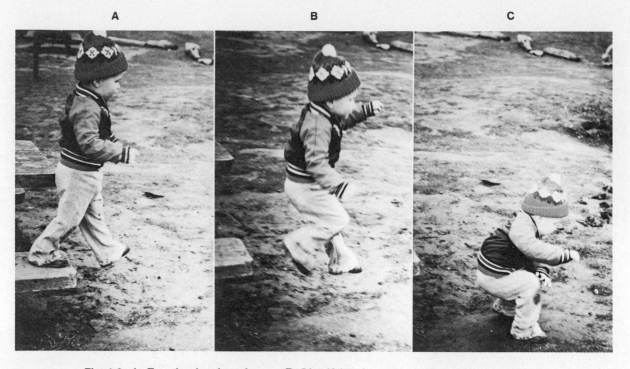

Fig. 1-3. A, Experiencing the unknown. **B,** Identifying the problem. **C,** Solving the problem.

degree of success is an important teaching strategy that tends to encourage present and future learning.

An additional comment regarding clients who lack motivation should be made. If a client wants to be totally dependent and has no need to become independent, then a therapist will probably fail at whatever task is presented. For example, Mr. Brown, a 63-year-old bank president with a wife, four children, and ten grandchildren, survives an operable brain tumor with residual right hemiparesis and minimal cognitive-affective deficits. The client's work history indicates that he was highly success oriented. Unknown to most persons is that for 63 years Mr. Brown desired to be a passive-dependent person, but circumstances never allowed him to manifest those behaviors. With the neurological insult he is in a position to actualize his needs. Until the client desires to improve, therapy will probably be ineffective. Thus, motivating the client becomes critical. This might be done in a variety of ways. Knowing that Mr. Brown values privacy, especially with respect to hygiene, that he thoroughly enjoys dancing and bird watching in the forest, and that he ascribes importance to being accepted in social situations, such as cocktail parties, helps the therapist create a learning environment that motivates this client toward independence. Being independent in hygiene requires certain combinations of motor actions, including sitting, balance, and transfer skills. Being able to bird watch deep in an unpopulated forest requires ambulation skills, tolerance to the upright position for extended periods of time, and endurance. Be-

ing socially accepted depends to a large extent not only on grooming but on normal movement patterns, especially in the upper extremity and trunk. Creating a therapeutic environment that stresses independence in the three goals identified by the client will simultaneously create further independence in other areas. Whether the client decides to return to banking and other activities in conflict with his personality will need to be addressed later. Another way to motivate Mr. Brown is to place him in an environment in which he is not satisfied, such as a nursing home or his own home with an assistant rather than his wife to help him with his needs. Dissatisfaction with the current environment will generally motivate an individual to change. Obviously, creating a positive environment for change versus a negative one would be the method of choice.

Many supplemental learning principles from the fields of education, development, and psychology can be used. It is not expected that all therapists will intuitively know how to create an environment conducive to another's optimal potential. Yet all can become better at creating a maximal learning environment by understanding how people learn. This concept, which provides the final link between behavioral and scientific theory, adds the third element in the clinical triad (see Fig. 1-1).

The sixth and last concept in this section addresses the development of sequential problem-solving strategies. The health care professions are stressing the importance of problem-solving skills, and schools are basing entire curriculum designs on problem-solving principles. Developing good problem-solving skills is paramount for high-level clinical performance. The clinician evaluates the client, establishes relevant goals, and then teaches the client the best solution to a specific problem. Unfortunately, teaching a solution to a problem can often be synonymous with teaching a splinter skill, that is, a skill that has no application to other functional activities. Thus the therapist requires other tools. For example, a therapist might identify that Janet needs to learn to perform a standing pivot transfer. They repeatedly practice the skill of transferring from a wheelchair to the toilet. The independence that Janet achieves in this activity may not carry over to other transfer activities. Therefore teaching the client to solve problems must accompany skill acquisition if that individual is to reach optimal independence.

PROBLEM SOLVING

A theoretical model that integrates the traditionally separate cognitive subject areas of behavioral development, applied neuroanatomy and neurophysiology, and learning theory has already been presented. This section deals with a specific problem-solving format that can be applied to this model. This format serves as the basis for the clinical-problem chapters within Part Two of this volume. The second topic addressed here consists of additional suggestions regarding problem-solving strategies such as development of a client profile and visual-analytical problem solving.

Problem solving format

Although cognitive strategies vary when a clinician approaches a specific clinical problem, an identifiable format is generally followed. The format has at least five areas: existence of the problem (component parts), evaluation procedures (analyzing components of the problem), goal selection (behavioral responses in terms of goals), treatment planning (choosing the best process to obtain desired goals), and specific psychological aspects and adjustment (modifying the solution to individual needs).

Before evaluating a clinical problem, an understanding of the general characteristics of the dysfunction is important. The neuroanatomical and physiological aspects of a problem and how they affect the client's general performance provide scientific understanding of the problem. Comprehension of typical clinical signs, as well as sequential stages of recovery from acute to long-term rehabilitation, also provides vital background knowledge. Pharmacological considerations and medical management during various phases of recovery or progress can change the response to and direction of a treatment sequence. All of this background information, in addition to the client's individual characteristics, helps the therapist conceptualize the nature of the problem. Although the clinician needs to remain flexible and to accept clinical signs as they occur, grasp of a total concept of the problem provides direction for evaluation, goal setting, and treatment planning. Con-

ceptualizing the clinical problem or observing the client's behavior leads the clinician to formulate questions that focus attention on both selection of evaluation procedures and direction of administration.

Once a clinical problem has been identified and questions have been formulated, evaluation procedures are selected. The selection of testing procedures may vary according to clinical preference, clinically established procedures, and client deficits, but it should be thorough and inclusive of all areas. Specific areas of evaluation have already been presented (see the discussion of the concept of normal human movement). Again, the choice of a specific evaluation form is not a critical issue. *How* the therapist extracts information from an evaluation is critical to the problem-solving strategy. Through experience clinicians learn to identify additional data not considered part of the test. For example, a therapist who is evaluating rolling and observes a strong shift in muscle tone as the head turns to the side that prevents rolling may decide that the client is incapable of rolling or cannot roll because of a strong tonal shift with head turning. However, the more observant and knowledgeable therapist might conclude that the client has an ATNR or, even more accurate, that this reflex not only prevents rolling but affects many other ADL tasks. The therapist who identifies only that the client cannot roll has answered the test questions appropriately; but the one who can pinpoint not only the observed behavior but recognize its manifest pattern and that it will affect other functional activities can extract a large amount of pertinent, additional data that can be used to reinforce other tasks. These data provide direction for further evaluation procedures, goal establishment, and possible treatment protocol. Specific suggestions regarding development of these strategies for extracting additional information is discussed in the section dealing with visual-analytical problem solving. *Caution* must be observed regarding conceptualization of a problem and evaluation procedures. Biasing findings of an evaluation to fit what is perceived as the problem is an issue all clinicians need to address. The clinician must allow the specific clinical signs of the patient to direct evaluation findings, goal setting, and treatment planning. Preconceptions based on familiarity with the medical diagnosis and general clinical problem can negate both the client's individuality and specific needs.

Although realistic goals and specific objectives are usually considered an end-product of therapeutic intervention, they need to be part of an ongoing evaluation process. Clinical signs often vary quickly. Observation of finite as well as gross changes plays a key roll in establishing and reestablishing goals. The process used to establish goals is based on the evaluation results and knowledge of the general progression the problem will take. Goals that seem appropriate for one phase of recovery or disease may need to change quickly as the phase changes. The clinician who uses high-level problem-solving strategies identifies finite clinical signs that indicate a phase change and therefore reestablishes new goals without losing precious time. For example, if a hemiplegic client has severe spasticity in the biceps and no palpable tone in the triceps, one goal might be to reduce spasticity in the biceps and facilitate triceps activity. A clinician would never isolate those two muscles without considering the rest of the client's arm, shoulder, and trunk, but for minimizing complexity, the following treatment focuses on the two identified muscle groups. Placing the biceps in extreme stretch will inhibit that muscle's action via its tendon organs (TO) (see Chapter 6). Simultaneously, the tendon organs will facilitate the triceps. Tapping and vibration of the triceps during a weight-bearing pattern should further facilitate this action. The assumption has been made that the biceps, as well as higher centers in the CNS, are inhibiting the triceps. Thus by inhibiting the biceps' function and using facilitative techniques, the therapist hopes that triceps activity will develop. However, instead of low or normal tone development in the triceps, spasticity may ensue. If that is the case, the specific goal needs to be modified as soon as excessive tone is palpated. If not, triceps spasticity may become severe, causing additional problems.

Treatment procedures are established in terms of treatment objectives. Although the problem-solving protocol seems to follow a temporal, step-by-step sequence, in reality many aspects are occurring simultaneously. The focus may be on evaluation, but treatment is also intricately intertwined, and during treatment a reevaluation is ongoing. Understanding the neurophysiological processes being facilitated or inhibited during a treatment procedure should give the clinician flexibility to alter input strategies including type, duration, and amplitude to meet the dynamic needs of the client. For example, a clinician may use quick stretch, tapping, and vibration simultaneously to facilitate a hypotonic muscle. This technique would be a temporal summation of a proprioceptive input modality. As muscle contraction begins, resistance would be applied to maintain elongation of the muscle spindle and receptor firing. As normal muscle contraction is palpated, the external input of stretch, tapping, or vibration can be removed while resistance is maintained, thus creating a normal sequence for return of muscle function. Because vibration is the least natural of the input modalities applied, removing it first would seem logical. The therapist's application of all facilitatory or inhibitory techniques should be directly correlated to the client's response to the input.

The last area generally affecting the problem environment and thus the strategies used by the therapist is specific psychosocial aspects and adjustment during various stages of recovery. An in-depth discussion of this area is presented in Chapters 4 and 7. Although most therapists focus their treatment on physical health and not on the social and adjustment aspects, the psychological state of the client affects the outcome of all other areas, including tone production.

Problem solving is continually implemented by therapists from the moment they learn they will be treating specific clients to the moment those clients leave the clinical environment. Gifted therapists are often thought to have intuition. Yet intuitive behavior is based on experience, a thorough knowledge of the area, sensitivity to the total environment, and ability to integrate the three and respond optimally. Intuitive abilities may be equated with high-level problem-solving skills.* In that respect each clinician should, with learning and practice, become more skillful and thus a better problem solver. *One very important aspect of clinical problem solving is the ability of clinicians to ask pertinent questions as they evaluate, conceptualize about, and treat their clients*. How these questions are formulated and the answers recorded varies among therapists, but the result is the development of a profile for each client.

Problem-solving strategies

The client profile. A therapist reads charts to gain background information on a client before or at the initial meeting. In the past, emphasis was to get a "feeling for" the client. Instead, time might be better spent gathering useful information about specific areas: cognition, affect, and motor. Because these three areas are interwoven, the therapist needs to focus not only on each of them but on their interaction. To optimize treatment effectiveness, clinicians should ask questions whose answers will give them valuable information regarding the client's past, present, and potential status as well as provide indicators of the most effective learning environment.

Cognitive area. Perception and cognition cannot be separated. Perception lays the foundation for higher-level cognition, but there is also spiral overlapping that cannot be overlooked. It would appear that as perception develops, it lays the foundation for cognitive development, which, along with perception, matures and sequences to higher and higher levels. Within the cognitive domain four general areas are identified: sensory input, perceptual awareness and development, preferential higher-order cognitive systems, and level of cognition. All play important roles in the optimal function of the client within the cognitive domain. The box on p. 21 (top left) summarizes pertinent questions a clinician must answer with regard to the cognitive area of the client's profile.

Affective area. The client's level of cognition is directly influenced by the affective or emotional area. Simultaneously, all other cognitive domains can be affected by or affect the emotional factor and responses of the client. When considering the affective domain at least four general areas should be explored: level of adjustment to dis-

---

*Refer to Chapter 4 for additional information on intuitive behavior.

Cognitive area questions for client profile

A. Sensory input: awareness level
 1. What sensory systems are intact?
 2. Do higher-order systems override input for lower systems?
 3. If conflict between systems is present, to which system does the client pay attention?
B. Perceptual awareness and development
 1. At which steps in various perceptual-developmental sequences does the client begin to have difficulty or failure?
 2. Do the perceptual problems relate to input distortion, processing deficits, or both? If input distortion is alleviated, is information processed appropriately?
C. Preferential higher-order cognitive system
 1. Was or is the individual's primary preferential system verbal or spatial?
 2. Is the client's preferential system different from yours? If so, can you work through the client's system?
 3. Is the client's preferential system affected by the clinical problems?
 4. Can the client adequately use nonpreferred systems?
D. Level of cognition
 1. Is the client functioning on a concrete, abstract, or fragmented level?
 2. Does the client's level of cognition change? If so, when and why?
 3. Is the client realistic? Does the client exercise judgment? If so, when? If not, when and why?
 4. Which systems or individuals are interfering with or distorting potential? (Systems within the individual and the environment around the client, such as the staff, the family, and the other patients, must be considered.)

Affective area questions for client profile

A. Level of adjustment or stage of adjustment to the disability
 1. At what level or stage of adjustment is the client with respect to the disability?
 2. At what level of adjustment is the family?
 3. Will the level of adjustment of the client or family affect treatment?
 4. If emotions are affecting treatment, what can be done to eliminate this problem?
B. Level of emotional control
 1. Can the client exercise impulse control?
 2. When does degree of emotional or impulse control vary?
 3. How did and does the client respond to stress?
 4. How did and does the client respond to perceived success and failure?
 5. What types of stresses outside of the specific physical disability are being placed on the client?
C. Attitude (attitude toward the disability is covered to some degree under level of acceptance, although additional information needs to be gathered)
 1. Before the onset of disability what was the client's attitude toward disabilities, and specifically, those related to his or her primary deficit?
 2. What is the client's attitude toward your professional domain?
 3. What is the family's attitude toward disabilities, especially those related to its family member?
 4. What is the family's attitude toward your professional domain?
D. Social adjustment
 1. At what social-developmental stage is the client's perfromance?
 2. Is the social interaction in alignment with cognitive and sensorimotor stages of development?
 3. Are the family's social interactions and expectations at the level of the client's performance?
 4. Is the client's level of social adjustment the same as the rehabilitation team's level of expectation?
 5. Is the client aware of his, her, or others' socially appropriate behavior?

---

ability, level of emotional control, attitude, and social adjustment. Questions arise within each category that indicate the client's emotional status and how it will affect a therapeutic environment (see the box at right, and for additional information refer to Chapter 7).

Sensorimotor area. Commonly used sensory, ADL, developmental, and motor assessments measure the sensorimotor area. Specific categories need to be analyzed to facilitate aggregation and use of the information that is obtained. Most therapists feel more comfortable addressing the sensorimotor area than the previous two. The therapist needs to answer questions in four identifiable categories (see the box on p. 22), although there are many additional focal areas.

Summary. Linking the cognitive, affective, and sensorimotor domains is the key to providing a productive and satisfying clinical learning environment for both the thera-

pist and the client. Identification of overlapping problems is important. The client's affective response at any one time will influence both cognitive processing and motoric performance. This affect may be extreme or mild, either positive or negative, and in many situations will need to be addressed for optimal performance. Cognitive-perceptual processing on the part of the client will often determine the learning environment to be used, the sequences for treatment, and estimated time needed for therapeutic intervention. The motoric output area is a main feedback system to the client, the family, and the clinician. Although this mo-

---

Sensorimotor area questions for client profile

A. Level of development with respect to performance
   1. Is the client's level of development or sensorimotor integration congruous with the staff's expected performance level?
   2. Is the client's level of development or sensorimotor integration congruous with the family's expected performance level?
   3. Is the client's level of development or sensorimotor integration congruous with his or her expected level of perfromance?
B. Functional skills
   1. What functional skills does the client perform in a normal fashion?
   2. What functional skills does the client perform in an abnormal manner?
   3. What functional skills has the client learned to perform that are reinforcing abnormal patterns or hindering normal movement?
   4. What functional skills does the client and family consider of primary importance? Will splintering these skills hinder normal learning?
C. Abnormal patterns
   1. What patterns are present?
   2. When are these normal and abnormal patterns observed? Do they vary according to spatial positions?
   3. Is there ever a shifting or altering in degree of these abnormal patterns? If so, under what circumstances does this variance occur?
D. Degree of cortical override
   1. Does the client need to inhibit abnormal output by intentional thought, or does he or she use automatic adjustment through normal mechanisms?
   2. What amount of energy is being used to override abnormal output?
   3. Can the client use normal mechanisms to control abnormal output?
   4. What amount of energy are you demanding the client to use when attending to the task? Are you asking the client to attend totally to the specific motoric task, or are you overloading the system to take away some cortical attending?

---

toric area can be evaluated effectively by itself, focusing on the cognitive-perceptual and the affective-emotional areas, identification of appropriate sequential treatment progressions, potential for improvement, and estimated time for therapy can be of great value to all involved.

A clinical example is used here to help the reader through the various questions posed in the client profile. Mary H. is a 22-year-old client with closed head injuries who has been admitted to Jones Rehabilitation Hospital af-

ter a 6-month stay in an acute care facility following an automobile accident. At the time of insult Mary was a senior at X University. Her major was architectural engineering, and her primary interests were sports such as tennis, skiing, and track. She was to be married after graduation. The accident, which killed her fiancé, occurred on the way home from a beer party. The doctor reported that on admission to the rehabilitation hospital, Mary was awake and verbally responded to questions, but articulation and monotone difficulties made her responses almost incomprehensible. Her volitional motor skills were limited because of extreme spasticity. Mary seemed depressed and exhibited bursts of anger at seemingly insignificant problems.

Many of the questions on the client profile cannot be answered on initial evaluation. Answers to specific questions will also change as Mary's neurological condition changes. Semans' motor assessment form[29] presented in the conceptual model section is the evaluation form used at Jones Rehabilitation Center along with an ADL assessment, range of motion (ROM) and sensory test forms, and the Southern California sensory integration battery.[2]

When the therapist addresses the cognitive profile, certain directional indicators can be identified. Mary's visual system has deficits that cause distortion in the perception of her spatial world. Her proprioceptive-vestibular system is intact, but her visual deficits override former sensory systems. Thus when sitting, Mary leans 30 degrees to the left with both head and trunk and perceives that she is in a vertical position. With her eyes closed, she still remains off vertical but can reposition herself to vertical when proprioceptive-vestibular cues are given. Knowing that one system is intact but overridden, a therapist can increase both temporal and spatial input through that modality to increase awareness. That increased awareness may help correct the deficit system. One way this might be accomplished would be asking the client to assume different positions in supine. The therapist instructs Mary to close her eyes and feel her position in space, adding approximation down through head and shoulders and quick stretch to appropriate muscle groups. Then the clinician takes Mary out of the position and asks her to reassume it. The goal would be accurate assumption of a totally symmetrical position. This would be the first step toward reorientation to verticality. It is done in a nonstressful position, thus eliminating anxiety, undue emotional tone, and conflicting input stimuli. Knowing that the client's preferential systems, based on her career choice and leisure-time activities, were visual-spatial and kinesthetic and that certain sensory systems critical to higher perceptual-cognitive performance in these areas are still intact reveals (1) which modality to use to introduce input and (2) which teaching strategies should be most beneficial to this client. That is, the client should be treated through spatial patterns rather than through verbal commands or visual demonstration of desired behavior. Thus Mary's intact systems and her preferential modes of thought are tapped. Once an accurate form of communication has been established, other forms such as visual demonstration or verbal instruction can be presented. Then additional questions posed in the profile can be addressed.

As the clinician focuses on the cognitive-perceptual area, the affective area can also be explored. Most of the questions listed under level of emotional control in the affective area outline can be answered while evaluating cognitive-perceptual performance. Many other questions can be answered by spending a few minutes with Mary's family members. Getting at least two other individual's[1] opinions of Mary's level of adjustment, emotional control, and attitude helps eliminate individual bias. Thus it might be assumed that Mary highly valued her physical status, that she was always uncomfortable around anyone with a physical disability, and that she had a quick temper and was intolerant toward failure. The therapist can assume that these values and behavior patterns have not changed drastically. In fact, the clinician might expect that these attitudes may at times be exaggerated until Mary has adjusted to her disability, or they may even be retained forever. Her temper and intolerance toward failure need to be considered if a treatment protocol is to be established. Success will be critical to motivate Mary in a rehabilitation setting, and her temper should help the therapist regulate the success-failure ratio and thus the task variation used during treatment.

Just as the affective domain influences and is influenced by the cognitive-perceptual systems, the sensorimotor area affects and is affected by the first two systems. The entire evaluation process may begin by using a motor assessment or ADL form. Answers can also be found to questions in the other areas of the profile. In actuality all areas should be addressed simultaneously while focus is placed on a specific topic, such as reflexology or level of sensorimotor integration. Perhaps Mary can be placed in total flexion when supine and can hold the position but is unable to reassume the pattern when placed in total extension. Thus she can assume aspects of the pattern but not in its entirety. If asked to position only her arms or only her legs, she succeeds. This would tell the clinician that Mary has the ability to inhibit certain reflexes, such as a dominant TLR or crossed extension reflex. The fact that Mary can remember a three-step sequence in the arms or the legs but not a six-step sequence of arms and legs together might suggest a temporal sequencing problem and that further evaluation is indicated to determine the degree of difficulty. Although this problem is perceptual-cognitive, it would severely hamper sensorimotor performance. If Mary were unable to perform a relatively simple perceptual-motor sequence as identified in the task of assuming total flexion from a supine position, the frustration she would feel when asked to do a standing pivot transfer might be enormous. This would be further exaggerated if a reflex

such as the ATNR caused tonal patterns that opposed the pivot transfer as Mary looked at the object to which she was asked to transfer. The interaction of a reflex such as the ATNR and Mary's poor temporal sequencing should limit the number of ADL tasks she would be asked to perform. Her intolerance to failure should alert the therapist to avoid test items in which there is a great likelihood Mary will fail.

Answers to questions in the sensorimotor area of the profile should direct the clinician to areas in which Mary can succeed, areas in which she will definitely fail, and areas that are still doubtful. That is, Mary may be able to perform any three- or four-step sequence in prone and supine positions but will have difficulty changing positions because of the ATNR. Sitting activities are limited as a result of the visual-perceptual distortions of verticality and their influence over muscle tone in the vertical position. Standing, ambulation, and complex ADL tasks, such as dressing, should be considered extremely difficult because of abnormal tonal patterns, that is, the ATNR in the lower extremity, the complex sequencing of the task, and the complex interaction of muscle function in all parts of the body during these high-level activities. Selection of these tasks as treatment procedure to make the client feel more normal may in reality clearly identify her disability, may cause extreme frustration and anger, and may dissolve the client-therapist rapport.

Once the therapist has a clear understanding of the client's strengths and weaknesses, specific clinical problems can be identified and treatment procedures selected that allow flexibility in treatment sessions. Many treatment suggestions for various problems can be found in Chapters 8 through 23.

VISUAL-ANALYTICAL PROBLEM SOLVING

The last section of this chapter deals with a specific type of problem-solving strategy that has definite clinical significance: the area of visual-analytical problem solving.

Problem solving has become a major issue in professional development, and the question arises as to whether all problem-solving strategies are the same. Some strategies may be more appropriate for clinical performance and others more relevant to academic achievement. The answer is still a hypothetical one, for no empirical research has been found that addresses all these specific questions. However, at least one research study was undertaken to identify a particular problem-solving strategy that seems to have important clinical application.[32] This strategy is referred to as visual-analytical problem solving (VAPS). It is defined as the ability to look at a complex array of visual stimuli, identify the critical attributes, and then use appropriate strategies to solve simple to complex problems. The solution to those problems stems from the original visual information. The following is an example of the use of VAPS. Mrs. J. sustained a closed head injury 4 months ago and has just been referred to your rehabilitation center. She was brought down in a wheelchair and placed against the wall in between two other clients (complex array of simultaneous visual stimuli). She first turns to the right to look at another client, then turns to the left (successive and simultaneous visual stimuli). You note as you are treating another client that, as Mrs. J. turns her head (critical attributes of the visual array), she has strong changes in muscle tone and that she has an obligatory bilateral ATNR. From that information you could determine many difficulties and failures that would occur if you gave an ADL test to this individual.

One problem encountered when making the transition from an academic to a clinical environment is having intellectual knowledge but being unable to associate that knowledge with the simultaneous and ongoing observation and palpation conducted in the clinic. Therefore many therapists believe that information learned in the classroom is irrelevant to the clinical environment. Another problem some students face is the frustration of working with a highly gifted therapist who cannot verbalize what is being done or why it works but can demonstrate the behavior or technique extremely well. A plausible explanation for problems of transference is that part of the high-level problem solving needed in the clinic is based on a nonverbal strategy. To communicate this nonverbal, visual-analytical model, one must translate it into verbal language, and this is very difficult because visual-analytical thought is both simultaneous and sequential. For example, a therapist who pictures a client progressing through a transfer from the wheelchair to the bathtub might visualize the activity as if observing the client from the front, the side, the back, or even from above. In fact, visualizing the movement from all directions gives additional information regarding the behavioral aspect of the client's transfer abilities. There is no rule to tell the therapist from which direction to order such visualization. The combined visualizations make up the total picture, and it is the total picture that is important. Language, on the other hand, is dominated by rules. Those rules are specific and have very clearly defined temporal sequencing. Thus translating a simultaneous process occurring internally into a temporal sequence to discuss all components changes the consistency of the thought process. Reflecting back on the original problem, a student would need to translate theoretical knowledge that has definite temporal rules into a simultaneous process observed in the clinic. The student must recognize that many gifted therapists cannot explain *verbally* what they know *spatially*. Therefore when asked to explain the treatment procedure, they translate only fragments of the whole, which is often of little help to the student.

A similar example would be taking a picture of a beautiful sunrise over a huge mountain range while the photographer sits at the mouth of a large lake that is absorbed into the mountain landscape. The photographer is engrossed with the whole experience. The totality of the multisensory, three-dimensional emotional interaction needs to be caught forever in the picture. When the picture is developed, the photographer discovers that the camera was unable to capture the whole. In fact, it recorded only a small portion of the original scene. The disappointed photographer may try to explain to friends who are looking at the picture what was really occurring, which would probably lead to frustration and a comment such as, "Well, you just had to be there."

To perceive the clinical implications of visual-analytical problem solving, understanding of its sequential steps is paramount. Although this concept tends to use a nonverbal mode of thought, it is not suggested that language is omitted from this strategy. Indeed, language may be critical in storage and retrieval of these images from memory. Development of the sequence seems to be hierachical, consisting of three general categories: visual recognition, spatial orientation, and spatial transformation.

The first step, visual recognition, implies the ability to recognize key attributes of the visual array and pull out those pieces of information necessary to begin to solve problems. Obviously, this means clinicians need to have mastery of visual information relevant to their professional responsibilities. Students often have difficulty generalizing information obtained at this level of visual recognition. An example would be a student who learns to evaluate the strength of the quadriceps muscle in a sitting position and thus assumes that this is the only position in which the strength of the muscle can be tested. Or if students study a reflex such as the ATNR and visually learn the stimulus-response pattern, they often hold the visual image of a child in the ATNR pattern. That is, they are unable to recognize the ATNR in adults who demonstrate the same reflex. The student stores the visual recognition with tremendous restrictions and thus limits clinical application of that information.

If visual content in one spatial position has been mastered, the second phase of the sequence, spatial orientation, can be addressed. This strategy requires identification of the key visual elements in various spatial planes. Take the example of an ATNR. If the clinical problem required the therapist to recognize this reflex in sitting, four-point, and standing positions, then a spatial orientation strategy would be employed. This can easily be applied in the clinic. For instance, a therapist may be giving an ADL evaluation and may ask Mrs. J. to transfer in and out of the tub to the right. She fails because she is unable to bend her hip and knee to clear the tub while she is looking at her knee or its placement in the activity. One therapist might identify only that Mrs. J. failed to transfer to the right, thus deciding that the best strategy would be to teach her to transfer to the left: a compensatory skill. A second therapist might realize that Mrs. J. failed because she has a dominant ATNR to the right. The second clinician not only identified that Mrs. J. failed but also *why* she failed. Knowing the reason gives the therapist freedom to select alternative treatment programs, such as teaching the client to modify the influence of the ATNR in tub transfer to the right, therefore eliminating the need for teaching a compensatory strategy. This would also be true in all ADL activities that require head turning, such as dressing, eating, and climbing into a car. Recognition of the ATNR in sitting position is a spatial orientation strategy because the therapist has gone beyond recognizing this reflex in supine. This second stage requires that the clinician visually recognize behavioral patterns in the three-dimensional external world. An important key to successful use of this strategy is allowing oneself the visual freedom to see what is actually present instead of preconceiving and then cognitively altering what one is seeing. Having predetermined *questions* relevant to specific clinical problems is an important aspect of problem solving. Having preconceived *answers* limits the flexibility of the clinician, decreases alternatives to treatment planning, and often limits the potential of the client.

The third stage, spatial transformation, requires a higher degree of spatial analysis. Up to this point, internalizing complex spatial or visual images was not necessary, although some imagery may have been used. That is, many people use compensatory verbal strategies to try to interpret what is being seen in the external world. Spatial visualization implies first that complex visual images are being manufactured within the mind of the observer. Then the individual must transpose one image on top of another or, while looking at one image, transform it (through the CNS), enabling the observer to view it simultaneously from a different position. For example, a woman may be looking at a picture of a lake in the mountains. If within her CNS she could form an image of that picture as if she were on the other side of the lake looking across the lake and at herself, that would be visualization transformation.

A clinical example of spatial transformation is knowing a client has an ATNR to the right from observing that individual's behavior in a sitting position and being able to transpose that behavior into a visual image of a transfer activity and determine at what point in the transfer the client would have difficulty or would fail. This could be done before confronting the client with that task. If a therapist knows a client is going to fail, there is little reason to attempt the task. Thus an evaluation could be used to maintain an environment that provides positive reinforcement.

This type of spatial thought process has to do with visually breaking down the observed environment into its component parts and then progressing visually through each component. The clinician is also confronted with a number of less complex clinical problems. If, simultaneously, a total picture of the client can be maintained, then a high-level clinical problem-solving strategy has been achieved. This manipulation of total-to-part to total-to-part is consid-

ered a highly integrated cortical function requiring both hemispheres.[21] An example is a clinician who recognizes that, as Janie walks across the floor, she is using a combination of the ATNR, symmetrical tonic neck reflex (STNR), positive supporting reactions, static postural tone, and moderate equilibrium reactions. The combination of tonal patterns creates a bizarre movement sequence that cannot be explained as a single act. Yet when the act is broken into components, the summative tonal response resulting from the combined influence of the various reflexes and reactions clearly explains the abnormal movement sequence. Treating each component problem separately and recombining the newly learned normal strategies lead to a more normalized gait pattern. That is, the whole is observed, the parts are detected and treated, and then the whole is reassembled in a new order to allow better function.

The development of visual-spatial strategies for use in visual-analytical problem solving is not specifically taught in schools. Yet these skills may provide an explanation of what is often called a therapist's intuitive gift. Academicians are beyond the point of accepting the premise that all problem-solving strategies are the same. Identifying in the next decade which problem-solving strategies lead to high-level clinical performance is a major objective for health care professionals. Learning such skills before entry into a clinical setting should ease the transition between the highly verbal environment of the classroom and the highly visual and kinesthetic environment in the clinic. How to develop this skill depends on the student's preferential learning styles and ability to change learning styles when necessary.

Some general suggestions can help all learners. The first step is to master visual content of (1) normal and abnormal stimulus-response patterns and (2) normal movement and postural patterns. Pictures or slides, where the visual stimuli can be held for extended periods of time, help the learner identify specific patterns without the demand of recognizing the pattern in a movement sequence. Next, the visual strategy should be mastered during a movement pattern. This requires recognition of key visual elements while additional simultaneous and successive visual imput are present. When this is accomplished in one spatial position, the same problems should be practiced in all spatial positions. This second strategy can be practiced by viewing videotapes or movies of individuals in a clinical setting.

The third strategy, visual transformation, requires the ability to internalize those images recognized in the first two stages. This can be practiced externally before the learner is asked to internalize two sequential images, place them on top of each other, and visualize the summative effect. Slide frames of a normal movement pattern can be taken and placed in front of the learner. A second visual input—such as the presence of a stimulus for the ATNR, as well as the response pattern—can be drawn, pictured on film, or discussed to help the learner visualize it internally. The end-product of the second stimulus-response pattern can then be overlaid on the first sequence. At some time the stimulus-response may coincide with the desired effect; at another time the stimulus for the second response may not be present in the first movement pattern. Finally, with the stimulus present, the desired response of the first pattern may conflict with that of the second, and thus the summative effect would cause deviation from normal movement. This strategy of summating externally two or more response patterns can then be practiced with internal visualization. The use of language to clarify visual images should help the learner make the transition from verbal to visual-spatial thought. Feeling and observing tonal changes in the client while visualizing what these total patterns look like should also help the learner begin to develop some of these higher-level visual-spatial strategies.

SUMMARY

This chapter has laid the foundation for an integrated problem-oriented approach to neurological disability. Three general areas were discussed: philosophy and rationale for the book; presentation of a conceptual model incorporating normal development, neurophysiology, and the learning environment; and general discussion of clinical problem solving. The concepts presented should not be taken as appropriate only for clients with CNS damage. Whenever change occurs, whether it be neurological, cardiovascular, pulmonary, or orthopaedic, a therapist's role is to structure the clinical environment in a way that promotes optimal healing and return of function for the client. Individuals with neurological damage often have orthopaedic, pulmonary, or cardiovascular problems. It has been my experience that orthopaedic patients almost always have neurological change with respect to learning or awareness of movement at the involved site. As long as clinicians can retain the concept of the total client, the integrity of the person is maintained, and the potential for that client to reach optimal function is closer to fruition.

REFERENCES

1. American Occupational Therapy Association: Standards of practice for occupational therapy in schools, Am J Occup Ther 34:900-903, 1980.
2. Ayers AJ: Sensory integration and learning disabilities, ed 1, Los Angeles, 1972, Western Psychological Services.
3. Bailey N: Manual for Bailey scales of infant development, New York, 1969, The Psychological Corp.
4. Barr J, Coordinator: Curriculum Planning Workshop, Midwinter Combined American Physical Therapy Association Sections Meeting, Washington DC, 1976.
5. Bishop B and Umphred D: Neurophysiological basis of physical therapy procedures, Workshop presented at New York University at Upstate Medical Center, in Syracuse, NY, Feb 1977.
6. Brazelton TB: Neonatal behavioral assessment scale, Philadelphia, 1973, JB Lippincott Co.
7. Bruner JS: The process of education, New York, 1968, Vintage Books.
8. Cronback LJ and Snow RE: Aptitudes and instructional methods, New York, 1977, Irvington Publishers, Inc.
9. Drillien CM and Drummond MB: Neurodevelopmental problems in early childhood: assessment and management, London, 1977, Blackwell Scientific Publications, Inc.
10. Farber S: Neurorehabilitation: a multisensory approach, Philadelphia, 1982, WB Saunders Co.
11. Fiorentino MR: Reflex testing methods for evaluating CNS development, ed 2, Springfield, Ill, 1979, Charles C Thomas, Publisher.
12. Fiorentino MR: A basis for sensorimotor development-normal and abnormal, Springfield, Ill, 1981, Charles C Thomas, Publisher.
13. Frostig M, Lefever DW, and Whittlesey J: Developmental test for visual perception, Palo Alto, Calif, 1963, Consulting Psychologists Press.
14. Gesell A and Amatruda CS: Developmental diagnosis, New York, 1947, Harper & Row, Publishers, Inc.
15. Guiliano C: Motor control theory and application. Informal presentation, Harmerville, Pa, Aug 1988, lecture notes.
16. Hunt DE: Matching models in education, Ontario Institute for Students in Education Monograph Series No 10, Toronto, Ontario, 1974.
17. Joyce B and Weil M: Models of teaching, Englewood Cliffs, NJ, 1972, Prentice-Hall, Inc.
18. Kandel ER and Schwartz JH: Principles of neural science, ed 2, New York, 1985, Elsevier Science Publishing Co.
19. Langer SK: Philosophy in a new key, Cambridge, 1942, Harvard University Press.
20. May BJ: An integrated problem-solving curriculum design for physical therapy education, Phys Ther 57:807-815, 1977.
21. Moore JC: The limbic system, Workshop presented in San Francisco, Feb 1980.
22. Moore J: Neuroanatomical structures subserving learning and memory. In Fifteenth Annual Sensorimotor Integration Symposium, San Diego, July 1987.
23. NUSTEP (Northwestern University Special Therapeutic Exercise Project): Proceedings: an exploratory and analytical survey of therapeutic exercise, Am J Phys Med 46(1), Feb 1967.
24. Peiper A: Cerebral function in infancy and childhood, New York, 1968, Consultants Bureau.
25. Piaget J: Science of education and the psychology of the child, New York, 1970, Onion Press.
26. Pribram KH: Languages of the brain: experimental paradoxes and principles in neuropsychology, Englewood Cliffs, NJ, 1971, Prentice-Hall, Inc.
27. Randolf S and Heiniger M: Neurophysiological concepts in human behavior; the tree of learning, St Louis, 1981, The CV Mosby Co.
28. Roch EG and Kephart NC: The Purdue perceptual-motor survey, Columbus, Ohio, 1966, Charles E Merrill Publishing Co.
29. Semans S and others: A cerebral palsy assessment chart: instructions for administration of the test. In The child with central nervous system deficit, Washington, DC, 1965, US Government Printing Office.
30. Stockmeyer S: Undergraduate course in advanced therapeutic exercises, Boston 1971, Boston University.
31. Umphred D: Teaching, thinking and treatment planning, Unpublished Master's Thesis, Boston, July 1971, Boston University.
32. Umphred D: Visual analytical problem solving, Unpublished doctoral dissertation, Syracuse, NY, 1978, Syracuse University.
33. Valett RE: Valett developmental survey of basic learning abilities, Palo Alto, Calif, 1966, Consulting Psychologists Press.

Chapter 2

OVERVIEW OF THE STRUCTURE AND FUNCTION OF THE CENTRAL NERVOUS SYSTEM

Martha J. Jewell

The purpose of this chapter is to provide the reader with a conceptual model of nervous system function and, based on that, with a model of nervous system dysfunction. It is hoped that the reader will be able to use this model as the initial platform from which to implement a problem-solving approach in the evaluation and treatment of the neurological patient. Additional chapters in this book (especially Chapters 3 and 4) will lend more detail to the reader's understanding of nervous system function.

NERVOUS SYSTEM FUNCTION

The function of the nervous system is to receive, assimilate, and act on information. Our model of the nervous system will be developed using the simplest structure possible. That would be a simple reflex arc consisting of an afferent neuron, interneuron, and efferent neuron, whose respective functions are reception, assimilation, and integration and action (Fig. 2-1).

This model has the advantage of being relatively simple. However, it is only a "stylized representation" and therefore may be too simplistic for some. For detailed structure and function of the central nervous system, readers are referred to the neuroscience textbooks listed in the section of additional readings.

Afferent or receptor neurons conduct impulses (carry information) to interneurons that are located within the CNS. Efferent neurons innervate glands and muscle (smooth, cardiac, or skeletal). Some efferent neurons (preganglionic autonomic neurons) innervate postganglionic autonomic neurons.

This is all the nervous system that a primitive, single-segmented organism needs. It must receive information from its internal organ(s), integrate it, and act on that information. It also needs to receive information from its external environment and to protect itself from external danger. But this primitive organism is somewhat handicapped because it can only react on one side. Therefore our model needs to include either a collateral from the single interneuron to the opposite side (Fig. 2-2) or a second interneuron that carries the information to the efferent neurons on the opposite side (Fig. 2-3). Now the organism has a commissural fiber and the ability to react on either side to a stimulus on one side.

This is still a rather primitive organism. If several seg-

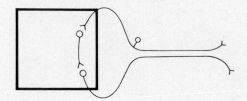

Fig. 2-1. A basic model of the nervous system.

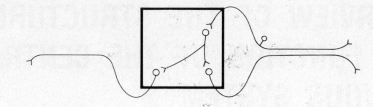

Fig. 2-2. An interneuron with a collateral to the opposite side.

Fig. 2-3. An interneuron synapses on the second interneuron, which crosses to the opposite side.

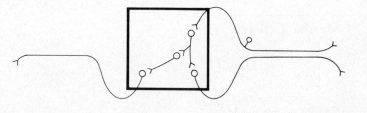

mental organisms were placed together in a stack or column, more complex functions could begin to evolve. To function as a unit, however, information received at one segment must be disseminated to the segments above and below it. This is done through two modifications of the primitive model. An afferent fiber can enter one segment and send collaterals to adjacent segments, and interneurons

can link several segments (Fig. 2-4). The latter is an example of a projection fiber. Now the organism is several segments tall, and its nervous system receives information from all segments, integrates it, and produces appropriate reactions. The appropriate reaction might require the coordinated activity of efferent neurons at multiple levels. As the complexity of the interneuronal responsibilities in-

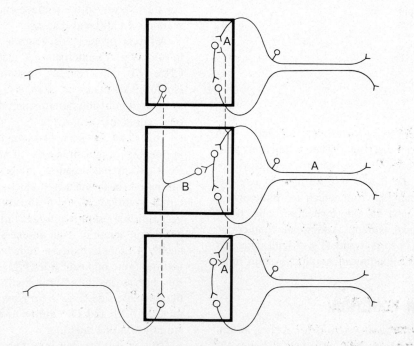

Fig. 2-4. Afferent information is disseminated to segments above and below by afferent collaterals *(A)* and interneurons *(B)*.

creases, the evolving organism needs to centralize integration of similar activities to increase efficiency and therefore survival (Fig. 2-5). For example, the model organism is now tall enough that gravity and other external forces, such as currents set up by more advanced (mobile) organisms swimming by, may tip our model organism over. And, in fact, higher centers, such as the brainstem, diencephalon, and telencephalon, can be conceptualized as interneurons that are involved in the integration of information received from various segments and in the production of an appropriate response.

Thus the nervous system consists of afferent neurons, interneurons, and efferent neurons. A few specific examples are given in Table 2-1, and many others can be found in neuroanatomy textbooks (see additional readings at the end of this chapter). The nervous system functions to receive information by way of afferent neurons to integrate and assimilate the information through a simple to extremely complex series of interneurons, and to produce appropriate responses. It is essential to realize that the appropriate response may present itself as no observable response or as the modification or cessation of a concurrent response. Therefore it is easier to generalize and say that groups of interneurons function to produce and/or regulate a response.

Nervous system function is observed clinically by noting the *result* of nervous system activity. Skeletal muscle contraction is observed most commonly. This may be as simple as a flexor withdrawal reflex or as complex as the production of speech. There are other results of nervous system activity that can be observed but that, unfortunately, are not usually considered in great detail by physical therapists. The contraction of smooth and cardiac muscle and the secretion of glands are functions that are far more important to the survival of the organism than opposition of the thumb.

CNS function may also be considered the cumulative product of evolution. The first, most primitive nervous system provided internal homeostasis. Our autonomic nervous system regulates internal homeostasis but at a much more complex, multineuronal level than seen in more primitive species. The primitive organism also needed to protect itself from its environment. To do that it needed to sense potential danger and withdraw or defend itself. The flexor withdrawal and blink reflexes are examples of protective functions. As animals became larger they were also influenced by the pull of gravity. They needed mechanisms to sense their position in relation to gravity and to sense any changes in that position. Animals also needed mechanisms to maintain their position or posture and to return them to that position if disturbed. The righting reflexes are examples of postural mechanisms.

As animals continued to evolve, they moved about in their environment, exploring and seeking food. This necessitated the production of goal-oriented movement and was dependent on sensory systems capable of providing discriminative information. Now the organism could localize the source of the stimulus more precisely and respond to it more discretely. The more discrete the information, the more precise the response necessary. Now the nervous system must process information from internal and external sources and from general and precise information, integrate all of this, and produce an appropriate response. Integration now involves processing information from several sources at different times. The nervous system must be capable of memory, learning, association and recall. The ability to generalize, to use symbols, to anticipate, predict, and plan are all CNS functions that are relatively new in evolution and that are certainly complex. Even these functions can be looked at as having afferent, interneuron, and efferent components.

Throughout the rest of this chapter we will look at four major classes of CNS function: homeostasis, posture, goal-oriented movement, and higher cortical processing, always using the afferent neuron, interneuron, and efferent neuron model to explain function and dysfunction.

But because the nervous system does not function as four separate units, we must also consider the interrelationship between the four units. All four units may access the same spinal cord circuits, but each produces different outcomes. The reader is reminded that muscle contraction

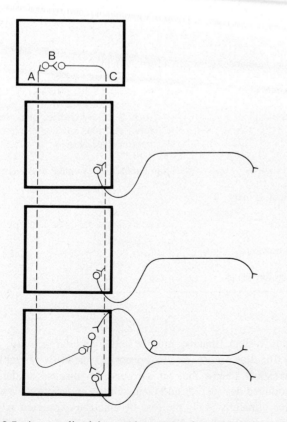

Fig. 2-5. A centralized integration center for segments. *A,* Ascending projection fibers. *B,* The integration center. *C,* The descending projection center.

Table 2-1. Examples of afferent neurons, interneurons and efferent neurons

Afferent neurons	Interneurons	Efferent neurons
Somatic		
Cutaneous		Ventral horn and cranial nerve nuclei III, IV, V, VI, VII, IX, X, XI, XII; plus visceral preganglionics (see below)
1. Receptors: touch, pain pressure, etc.	1. Synapse: dorsal horn, and trigeminal nucleus	
2. Fibers: spinal nerves and cranial nerves V, IX, X	2. Projection fibers: spinothalamic, spinoreticular, spinotectal, trigeminothalamic, and propriospinal	
Proprioceptive		Same as above plus visceral preganglionics
1. Receptors: muscle, tendon, joint	1. Synapse: dorsal horn and mesencephalic nucleus	
2. Fibers: spinal nerves and cranial nerves III, IV, V, VI, X, XI, XII	2. Projection fibers: dorsal column—medial lemniscus, spinocerebellar tracts	
Vestibulocochlear		Same as above plus visceral preganglionics
1. Receptors: labyrinth and organ of Corti	1. Synapse: vestibular nucleus, cochlear nuclei, inferior colliculus, medial geniculate	
2. Fibers: cranial nerve VIII	2. Projection fibers: lateral lemniscus, geniculotemporals (projection fibers for vestibular system not well traced at this time)	
	3. Descending tracts: vestibulospinal and tectospinal	
Visual		Same as above
1. Receptor: retina	1. Synapse: superior colliculus, pretectal nucleus, lateral geniculate	
2. Fibers: cranial nerve II	2. Projection fibers: geniculocalcarines	
	3. Descending tracts: tectospinals	
Visceral		
General		1. Preganglionics; lateral horn T1-L2,3; ventral horn S2,3,4; cranial nerve nuclei III, VII, IX, X
1. Receptors: pain, distention, pressure	1. Synapse: dorsal horn and solitary nucleus	
2. Fibers: spinal nerves, splanchnic nerves, and cranial nerves VII, IX, X	2. Projection fibers: spinoreticular, propriospinal	2. Postganglionics: collateral ganglia such as ciliary, celiac, otic, mesenteric, etc. plus somatic efferent neurons (see above)
	3. Descending tracts: reticulospinal	
Special		
1. Gustatory	1. First synapse: solitary nucleus	Same as above (somatic and visceral)
a. Receptors: tastebuds	2. Projection fibers: solitary tract	
b. Fibers: cranial nerves VII, IX, X	3. Descending tracts: reticulospinals	
2. Olfactory	1. First synapse: septal area, amygdala, insula, etc.	Same as above (somatic and visceral)
a. Receptors: olfactory epithelium	2. Projection fibers: hypothalamus, etc.	
b. Fibers: cranial nerve I	3. Descending tracts: reticulospinal	

is the final printout of the motor system and therefore the basic unit of behavior is the motor unit.[4]

NERVOUS SYSTEM DYSFUNCTION

If we agree that the function of the nervous system is to receive, assimilate, and act on information and that what is observed clinically is the efferent activity of the nervous system, that is, muscle and glandular activity, then dysfunction must be inappropriate activity. Hughlings Jackson[11] taught that nervous system disease or damage produced destruction and/or instability in function. What is seen clinically is (1) the loss of function expressed as negative signs and symptoms, such as weakness, diminished deep tendon reflexes, decreased sensation, and decreased level of consciousness, and/or (2) instability in function expressed clinically as positive signs and symptoms, such as hyperactive reflexes, seizures, hypertonicity, and involuntary movements. *Nervous system damage does not create new functions.* A lesion may prevent the expression of some functions (negative signs) and/or it may allow the inappropriate, uncoordinated, uncontrolled expression of other functions (positive signs).

Expressed in another way, nervous system damage results in too little and/or too much function. Muscle weakness is too little muscle contraction, too little movement, too little posture. Spasticity is too much posture. Athetosis is too much or inappropriate movement.

The most basic model of the nervous system shows that too little function (negative signs) will result if either the receptor, afferent neuron, efferent neuron, or muscle is damaged (see Fig. 2-1). These signs and symptoms may be typified by sensory loss and muscle weakness respectively. If the afferent neuron is from a muscle spindle, there may be decreased tendon reflexes. If it is a cutaneous afferent neuron, there may be decreased sensation and decreased cutaneous reflexes. If the efferent neuron innervates skeletal muscle, there may also be decreased tendon reflexes and weakness. Both afferent and efferent neurons are affected in many peripheral neuropathies, and skeletal-motor efferent neurons are affected in polio and Guillain-Barré syndrome. If the efferent neuron is a visceral efferent neuron, there may be decreased smooth muscle contraction. Loss of bowel and bladder control in the client with cauda equina damage demonstrates loss of afferent information as to bladder distention, loss of visceral efferent control of bladder smooth muscle, and loss of somatic motor efferents to the external sphincter to prevent urinary incontinence.

Damage to interneurons is only slightly harder to conceptualize. If the interneuron is involved in producing a function, its loss will result in negative signs, such as the flaccid weakness of a hemiplegic client or a client with a spinal cord injury. If the interneurons are involved in regulating (inhibiting, modulating) a function, their loss will result in positive signs, such as decerebrate rigidity in the client with head trauma, spasticity in the hemiplegic client, and tremor in the client with Parkinson's disease.

Perhaps the model applied to dysfunction will become clearer after a specific example of the withdrawal reflex. The afferent neuron is usually an Aδ or C fiber that conducts information from some type of nociceptor (see neuroscience textbooks for classification of receptor and fibers). Upon entering the CNS (here the spinal cord or brainstem), the afferent neuron sends collaterals to adjacent segments. Therefore there are interneurons involved at the level of entry and at several adjacent levels. These interneurons in turn synapse on other interneurons (the polysynaptic reflex). Eventually the information, which has been heavily modified by this point, reaches the effer-

ent neurons. In this example information usually reaches all three types of efferent neurons (alpha, gamma, and visceral). The usual result is contraction of the appropriate skeletal muscles to withdraw the body part and a local vasomotor response along with other autonomic responses, such as pupillary dilation and a momentary increase in heart rate. If there is a peripheral nerve lesion, there will be a decreased or absent response to the stimulus (a negative sign). The clinician will observe a decreased or absent withdrawal reflex, and the client may report a decrease in the perception of the stimulus. Thus the loss involves not only a negative sign but also the loss of afferent input, which decreases interneuron processing and flexibility of integrative responses. The astute clinician may also observe trophic skin changes secondary to changes in autonomic innervation. It is important to remember that the peripheral lesion may involve the receptor, afferent neuron, efferent neuron, or muscle. If the lesion were central, involving interneurons, the signs may be negative, positive, or both. Loss of interneurons involved in the production of the reflex results in a decreased reflex, as might be seen in syringomyelia. Loss of interneurons involved in the regulation of the reflex might result in hyperreflexia. For example, clients with spinal cord injury often demonstrate spread of withdrawal reflex to the whole limb and perhaps the whole body below the lesion. Loss of the interneurons that transmit information to higher centers results in disturbed perception of sensation and/or dissociation of somatic and visceral responses. Examples include lesions of the spinothalamic and spinoreticular tracts anywhere in the CNS.

A far more complex example will now be considered. The production of a smooth, coordinated movement such as reaching for an object and picking it up requires input from several groups of interneurons, including the cerebellum, basal ganglia, and sensory motor cortex. A motor plan is developed that is made up of small subsets or programs. The plan must include programs for control of center of mass and programs for the subsets of the movement. Not only must the sequence of muscle activity be programmed, but also speed, force, distance and how the movement is stopped. The plan is compared with a standard based on previous experience. This comparison requires sensory feedback. "How did it feel to do the movement?" The plan is executed through brainstem and spinal cord circuits, the same circuits and motor neurons that produce spinal cord and brainstem reflexes. Lesions involving this system result in motor planning disorders, involuntary movement, and uncoordinated slow, or absent movement (refer to Chapter 3 for additional information).

Any lesion of the peripheral nervous system will result in negative signs, such as weakness, decreased reflexes, and sensation. The specific signs will depend on the specific peripheral structures involved. Dermatome, myotome, and peripheral nerve charts can be referred to for specific regions of involvement. Any lesion of the CNS will result in negative signs if the interneuron is involved in producing a function, or positive signs if the interneuron is involved in regulating a function. In most CNS lesions both negative and positive signs are seen. Examples include the flaccid shoulder and spastic elbow flexors in some hemiplegic clients and the inability to produce movement (akinesia) and the tremor in the client with Parkinson's disease.

HOMEOSTASIS

As stated earlier in this chapter, homeostasis may be divided into two subfunctions: regulation of the internal milieu and protection of the organism from its environment, that is, internal and external survival.

Regulation of the internal milieu

Anatomical substrates. The afferent link of the autonomic nervous system consists of sensory fibers that carry information from the walls of blood vessels and viscera, including the entire gastrointestinal, genitourinary, and cardiopulmonary systems. This information includes tissue damage, distention, pressure, vibration, and various forms of chemical information, such as airborne (olfactory sensation) and dissolved (gustatory sensation, oxygen tension, hydrogen ion concentration) chemicals. The afferent impulses travel in both somatic and visceral efferent neurons in peripheral nerves to the limbs and body wall, in splanchnic nerves, and in cranial nerves I, VII, XI, and X. In addition, somatic afferent fibers (especially cutaneous, but also visual, auditory, and vestibular) can be involved in visceral reflexive function. The interneurons *most directly* associated with afferent visceral information are those of the dorsal horn of the spinal cord (visceral afferent nucleus), the solitary nucleus in the brainstem (which is associated with cranial nerves VII, IX and X), the cardiovascular and respiratory centers (also in the brainstem),

and the hypothalamus. Many other centers are involved in integrating visceral afferent information, including the cerebellum, thalamus, and cerebral cortex. The cell bodies of the efferent fibers in the autonomic nervous system (preganglionic visceral motor neurons) are located in the lateral and ventral horns of the spinal cord (T1 to L2 or L3, and S2 to S4 respectively) and in nuclei associated with cranial nerves III, VII, IX, and X (Edinger-Westphal, lacrimal, salivatory, and dorsal vagal nuclei respectively). Therefore preganglionic efferent fibers are found in spinal nerves T1 to L2 or L3 and S2 to S4 and in cranial nerves III, VII, IX, and X. The craniosacral outflow is the peripheral component of the parasympathetic nervous system, and the thoracolumbar outflow is the peripheral component of the sympathetic nervous system. This information is summarized in Table 2-2. Refer to gross and neuroanatomy textbooks for further details.

Dysfunction. In this discussion we will return to the basic model of nervous system function and dysfunction. If the afferent and/or efferent limb of the reflex is damaged, there is decreased or absent function (negative signs). A peripheral nerve lesion results in decreased sympathetic regulation of vascular tone in the body part innervated by that nerve. Signs might include trophic skin changes and lack of temperature regulation of the part. (The reader is encouraged to review physiology textbooks to explore smooth muscle response to denervation and circulating epinephrine.) There is also a loss of autonomic responses associated with somatic sensation from the denervated part (see the previous example of a noxious stimulus and the withdrawal reflex). Peripheral components of the autonomic nervous system are often surgically destroyed. The vagus nerve may be cut to decrease gastic acid secretion. The other functions of the vagus nerve below the lesion are also lost (gut motility, etc). Occasionally sympathetic ganglia (usually the stellate ganglion) are surgically or pharmacologically destroyed to decrease sympathetic

Table 2-2. Examples of afferent neurons, interneurons, and efferent neurons in the autonomic nervous system

Afferent neurons	Interneurons		Efferent neurons
General			
1. Aδ and C fibers carry information on stretch, pain, and pressure in spinal and splanchnic nerves	Visceral afferent nucleus; spinoreticular and propriospinal tracts		Lateral horn T1 to L2 or L3 Ventral horn S2 to S4
2. Aδ and C fibers in cranial nerves VII, IX, and X	Solitary nucleus; solitary tract; reticulospinal tract	Hypothalamus	Edinger-Westphal nucleus Lacrimal nucleus Salivatory nucleus Dorsal vagal nucleus
Special			
1. Gustatory in cranial nerves VII, IX, and X	Solitary nucleus; solitary tract; reticulospinal tract		Same as above
2. Olfactory in cranial nerve I	Septal area, amygdala, insula		Same as above

vasomotor tone. This results in decreased sympathetic function in the head and neck (Horner's syndrome) with ptosis, miosis, endophthalmos, and anhydrosis, all of which are negative signs of a peripheral sympathetic nervous system lesion.

Autonomic function may also be decreased by lesions involving the central component of the afferent or efferent limb. For example, lesions of the dorsal or ventral-lateral horn of the spinal cord or cranial nerve nuclei, where cell bodies of visceral afferent neurons are located, may also result in negative signs of an autonomic nervous system lesion. If interneurons are damaged, there may be decreased function (negative signs) and/or inappropriate function (positive signs). Spinal cord lesions result in negative signs, for example, loss of sensation, inability to voluntarily initiate emptying of bowel or bladder, and orthostatic hypotension. Reflexive voiding may be viewed as a positive sign secondary to loss of regulation of an intact reflex arc by interneurons above the level of the lesion. Taken to extremes, extensive brainstem damage may destroy cardiovascular and respiratory centers, resulting in death. Less profound brainstem lesions may result in inappropriate or uncoordinated function, such as apnea and other inappropriate breathing patterns and even cardiac arrhythmias.

The hypothalamus is an interesting grouping of interneurons in that there are areas that appear to function in direct opposition to other areas. For example, one area decreases body temperature and another increases it. Here we are presented with the first of many semantical problems. If the first area is damaged, is the client's problem inability to decrease body temperature (a negative sign) or inappropriate body warming (a positive sign)? Hyperthermia is a fairly common result of head injury.

The autonomic and somatic sensorimotor systems function together in the client and, in fact, often use the same afferent and efferent neurons. Body temperature is raised in part by shivering, which requires somatic motor neurons and skeletal muscle. Shivering may be elicited by a cool breeze on the skin. Any somatic sensorimotor act has autonomic companions. Increased muscle activity results in and is paralleled by autonomic activity: increased heart and respiratory rate, and decreased gut motility. The therapist must always be aware that these two systems do not function in isolation, but that they have profound effects on each other.

The cerebral cortex also has a profound effect on autonomic interneurons. The treatment environment, through interpretation by interneurons, can influence the autonomic nervous system. Anxiety and fear enhance sympathetic nervous system response along with somatic responses.

External survival

Anatomical substrates. For an organism to survive in a potentially hostile environment, it must be able to sense external danger. Obviously humans are capable of sensing potential danger that comes in contact with the body, but humans are also capable of seeing, hearing, smelling, and tasting potential danger. Therefore the afferent limb of this arc includes cutaneous mechanoreceptors, thermoreceptors, and nociceptors whose information is conducted over predominantly Aδ and C fibers in spinal nerves and in cranial nerves V, IX, and X. The noncutaneous information arrives by way of cranial nerves I, II, VII, VIII, IX, and X. The afferent neurons would then synapse on interneurons in the dorsal horn of the spinal cord, in the trigeminal nuclear complex and the solitary and cochlear nuclei of the medulla and pons, in the superior colliculus of the midbrain, and in the olfactory areas of the telencephalon. Through a series of interneurons, information finally reaches efferent neurons. If a person is to survive in a hostile environment, he or she must be able to withdraw from a harmful stimulus. This may necessitate withdrawing a limb from a pinprick or hot stove, blinking and ducking away from a flying object, or spitting out certain strong-tasting foods when you are rather young. The magnitude of the response may vary from a slight flinch to a full-blown startle in response to a sudden and loud noise. Therefore the efferent neurons may vary from stimulus to stimulus. In each example a somatic response was elicited; however, it must be remembered that each is also accompanied by an autonomic (usually sympathetic) response. Not only does the organism withdraw from a stimulus, but the organism also prepares internally with increased heart and respiratory rate. Some animals, including some humans, by choice or by instinct will not withdraw from certain threatening stimuli (situations); however, the autonomic response is the same. Some examples of protective reflexes are given in Table 2-3.

Dysfunction. Disturbances in the peripheral nervous system, such as a peripheral nerve lesion, may affect the afferent neuron or efferent neuron (usually both) of a protective response and result in negative signs. Loss of the blink reflex to visual or tactile stimuli, loss of a startle response, or loss of withdrawal of a body part to noxious cutaneous stimulus may result from the loss of afferent neurons (cranial nerves II, V, VIII, spinal or peripheral nerves respectively) or of efferent neurons (facial nerve or appropriate spinal and peripheral nerves respectively).

Disturbances in the CNS may result in negative and/or positive signs. Negative signs might include decreased or absent sympathetic responses, resulting from lesion of the lateral horn of the cord or involvement of the reticulospinal tract or hypothalamus. Negative signs might also include loss of awareness of the existence of the stimulus and inability to localize or identify the stimulus. It should be remembered that if the structure, path, or nucleus produces a function, a lesion in that structure, path, or nucleus will result in loss of that function. Positive signs might include spread of the reflex to the whole limb and to the opposite limb with a relatively mild stimulus. An ex-

Table 2-3. Examples of protective reflexes

Stimulus	Afferent neurons	Interneurons	Efferent neurons	Response
Pin prick to index finger	Aδ and C fibers; median nerve; brachial plexus; C6 or C7 root; dorsal horn	Spinal: Association: spread within level Commissural: to opposite side Projection: spinothalamic, spinoreticular and spinotectal; tectospinal, reticulospinal, and tectobulbar	Alpha and gamma motor neurons and adjacent levels	Withdrawal of finger and possibly whole limbs Visceral motor neurons Vasodilation
			Cranial nerve III Cranial nerves VII, X, XII	Pupillary dilation "Ouch"
Dust in eye (corneal reflex)	C fibers by way of cranial nerve V to pons	Trigeminal nucleus	Alpha motor neurons in facial nucleus (VII) Lacrimal nucleus; visceral motor fibers by way of VII	Blink Tear
Fast-moving object	Rods and cones; cranial nerve II	Superior colliculus Pretectal nucleus Lateral geniculate Tectobulbar Tectospinal	Alpha motor neurons in facial nucleus (VII) Alpha and gamma motor neurons; cervical ventral horn Visceral motor neurons; upper thoracic cord	Blink Duck head Increase heart rate

ample is the client with a spinal cord injury who reflexively goes into total body flexor withdrawal when sheets are drawn across the legs. Here interneurons responsible for regulating the reflex are damaged. Therefore positive signs include hypersensitivity or overreactivity to the stimulus, that is, some type of inappropriate response. Simplistically, tactile defensiveness is an overreaction of the protective mechanisms to cutaneous stimuli, in fact to nonthreatening stimuli. It can then be conceptualized as the result of decreased function in the interneurons that regulate protective mechanisms. When regulatory interneurons do not regulate production, interneurons tend to overproduce and/or to produce inappropriate responses to normally inadequate stimuli. One group of interneurons omitted from the previous tables is the group having to do with affective behavior (the limbic system). In addition to producing a parallel somatic and autonomic response, sensations also elicit an affective response, an emotional interpretation of the situation. This "emotional tone" has a normal resting level, just like "muscle tone." But in CNS damage, affective tone may be hyperactive and, like all other systems, it can affect all systems. In fact, it would be more practical and functional to look at sensorimotor responses as three parallel responses. They are somatic, visceral (autonomic), and affective (emotional). This "affective tone" influences somatic function dramatically, as exemplified by the client whose spasticity increases with

emotional level or the client who becomes more tactilely defensive with increased stress (refer to Chapter 4).

POSTURE
Anatomical substrates

As the size and mobility of an organism increases, so does the influence of gravity on that organism. The organism must be able to maintain itself, keeping its rostral end upright and its receptors in a position to search for food and danger. Humans attempt to keep the head upright and the eyes level. Once disturbed, humans, like other organisms, must be able to right themselves. Three sensory systems provide information regarding "uprightness" or the lack of "uprightness," that is, position in relation to gravity and to the surrounding environment. These systems are the vestibular, proprioceptive, and visual systems. The vestibular system provides information regarding the position of the head in relation to gravity and the linear and rotatory movement of the head. Proprioceptors, especially those associated with axial joints and muscles, provide information about movement of the body segments on each other. The visual system provides information about the body's position in relation to the external environment.

The interneurons in these systems are involved in the production of appropriate postures. The word *postures* tends to bring forth pictures of rigid poses. But postures produced by the intact nervous system (appropriate pos-

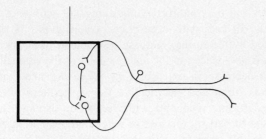

Fig. 2-6. A descending interneuron influences the motorneuron directly.

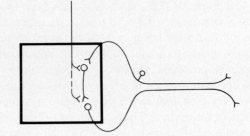

Fig. 2-7. A descending interneuron influences the motorneuron through another interneuron.

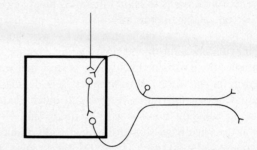

Fig. 2-8. A descending interneuron influences the motor neuron by affecting the afferent neuron.

tures) are very dynamic. They change constantly with very slight perturbations. They also change from segment to segment and limb to limb. One influences the other. Two examples may make the point clearer. First, consider the vertebral column during gait. If the subject rotates the pelvis to the left during swing, the lumbar spine will also rotate. If the upper trunk is to stay in the frontal plane and if the opposite arm swing is to occur in the sagittal plane, the thoracic spine must be stabilized on the moving lower trunk. Second, stand with your arms at your side, then lift your arms straight out in front of you. Now that your center of gravity is shifted forward you must adjust your posture to keep from falling on your outstretched arms. If you thought that those postural adjustments were made in the trunk and lower extremities, you would be correct. But adjustments are also made in the upper trunk and proximal upper-extremity musculature to provide a stable base on which the movement of the limb can occur. Again, "stable" does not mean fixed or immovable. Stability and posture are words that should be prefaced by dynamic, not static.

The terms *posture, a posture,* or *postural control* mean different things to different readers. In this chapter *posture* refers to sensorimotor activity that maintains or regains the upright position in relation to gravity. This is contrasted with sensorimotor activity, which forms a stable base for purposive movement, for example, intrinsic hand muscle activity involved in stabilizing metacarpophalangeal joints while long finger flexors and extensors produce the desired movement. Hopefully, this distinction will become clearer as we look at dysfunction in posture and movement.

If we refer back to our basic nervous system model (Fig. 2-5), we can see that it can be applied to the control of posture. The afferent neuron may be part of the visual, vestibular, or proprioceptive systems. The interneurons could be in the tectum of the midbrain, the vestibular nuclei, or the spinal cord. The efferent neurons are alpha and gamma motor neurons to muscles of the trunk and limbs. A very critical concept must be grasped at this point. There is a basic wiring diagram at the segmental level that consists of an afferent neuron, at least one interneuron, and an efferent neuron. It makes little difference what the

afferent or efferent neuron is for now. It is critical to understand that *all* systems effect output through this basic wiring diagram. The most direct route is through the alpha motor neuron (Fig. 2-6). In fact, much of vestibular control is expressed through this route. The most common way of effecting output is through one or more segmental interneurons (Fig. 2-7). Additionally, control can be exerted through the afferent neuron itself (Fig. 2-8).

A second critical concept is that the influence or effect produced may be facilitation *or* inhibition. Any synapse represented in Figs. 2-6 to 2-8 could be facilitory or inhibitory. Possibly the single most important concept in understanding neurological function is that *each event, each neuronal firing, produces an effect (facilitation or inhibition) on the postsynaptic neuron but that no single synaptic activity is adequate to fire the next neuron.* It is the *sum total of synaptic events,* both facilitory and inhibitory, at any point in time, that determines whether the next neuron will fire. In other words, what we observe clinically as a response to a stimulus—muscle contraction or the absence of muscle contraction—reflects the sum total of synaptic events on those alpha motor neurons that respond. Unfortunately this is all we can observe, record, or measure. But this is *not* to say that if there is no observable response to a stimulus, there was not effect. There was no observable effect. Only when the afferent limb of the arc is damaged is there no effect from that stimulus. Even this statement is not absolutely correct. Loss of input can have a profound effect on output. For example, cutaneous anesthesia secondary to therapeutic application of ice has been shown to effect the abnormal motor output seen in spasticity. Unilateral loss of vestibular input in acoustic neuroma patients affects their ability to produce appropriate posture.

Posture is produced ultimately through alpha motor neurons, and it most often involves alpha motor neurons to antigravity muscles such as the gastrocnemius, soleus, and quadriceps (refer again to Figs. 2-5 to 2-8). Reticulospinal and vestibulospinal tracts have both a direct (monosynaptic) and an indirect (via segmental interneuron) effect on somatic efferent neurons. All other systems involved in regulation of posture and in production of movement (except corticospinal tracts to hand intrinsics) have an indirect influence on alpha motor neurons. The monosynaptic group Ia reflex, the "quick stretch reflex," was thought to contribute to fine adjustments in standing posture when, for example, the gastrocnemius/soleus is stretched with anterior sway at the ankle. But Nashner[6] has demonstrated that the latency of this reflex response to quick ankle dorsiflexion in standing humans is 120 msec, and H-reflex studies at the knee have shown the electrically induced reflex response to be 30 msec. Therefore the Ia input probably has an "influence" but does not produce the postural response by itself. Nashner postulated that the postural response was the function of a long spinal reflex based on the latency of the response.

As we examine organisms higher and higher in the evolutionary scale, we can see that more and more functions become controlled by higher centers, especially at the level of the cerebral cortex. A spinalized cat (one whose spinal cord has been severed for experimental purposes), if suspended and stimulated properly, can be made to walk. A cat with chronic decerebrate posturing can stand if placed and may even right itself if knocked over. The basic wiring necessary to produce locomotion is present in the spinal cord. Locomotion can be triggered with limb movement in a spinalized cat that is also treated with dopamine. Then why can't a spinalized primate be made to produce locomotor movements? Primates, especially humans, are the beneficiaries and the victims of *encephalization*. The basic segmental wiring diagrams are probably the same, but the control, the "on-off" switch, is at higher centers. By control we mean the establishment of background activity in the wiring so that it can be triggered by afferent input. *Control* may be the production of a function or it may be the regulation of a function produced elsewhere. Using the vestibular system as an example, extensor or antigravity tone is produced primarily by the vestibular system and contributed to by the reticular system. Extensor tone can be modified at the spinal cord level by those joint and cutaneous afferent neurons that tend to produce flexor responses, or it can be modified by descending systems, such as the corticospinal tracts, which are capable of inhibiting extensor activity. Extensor tone can be modified from the brainstem by influencing the vestibular

nuclei and thus indirectly modifying the activity at spinal levels. In cats with decerebrate posturing this is demonstrated by the further increase in extensor tone when a lesion is also placed in the anterior lobe of the cerebellum or by a decrease in extensor tone when the intact anterior lobe is stimulated electrically. The gait pattern of the severe, chronic alcoholic with cerebellar damage may be caused in part by the loss of cerebellar regulation (inhibition in this case) of vestibular function. Also, chronic cerebellar stimulation has been used as an invasive method of modifying spasticity in humans.[8]

Another basic concept in CNS function that must be understood is Sherrington's concept of reciprocal innervation.[10] This is best explained by examples. The vestibular system, specifically the lateral vestibulospinal tract, tends to exert its facilitation on extensors or antigravity muscles. Actually this tract facilitates motor neurons to antigravity muscles and inhibits motor neurons to progravity muscles. Table 2-4 lists common examples of reciprocal innervation.

Dysfunction

Disturbances in posture occur whenever there is damage to structures whose functions are to produce, modify, or control posture. Lesions that affect structures that produce posture result in a clinical picture of too little posture, that is, negative signs such as postural hypotonicity. Referring back to the model of nervous system function, too little function, in this case too little posture, could result from damage to afferent neurons, efferent neurons or interneurons involved in the production of postural tone. Bilateral vestibulocochlear nerve damage would remove vestibular afferent neurons and result in postural hypotonicity, especially with the eyes closed. Damage to peripheral nerves to extensor muscles or to their motor neurons directly, as in Guillain-Barré syndrome or polio, results in decreased postural control. It also results in decreased movement because it does not selectively effect motor neurons to antigravity muscles. Postural hypotonia is also seen in cerebellar and central brainstem lesions.

More commonly CNS damage results in instability in function, that is, positive signs or too much posture. This is exemplified in the spasticity of antigravity muscles. Positive signs are most commonly produced when interneurons that regulate posture or that regulate other interneurons involved more directly in producing posture are damaged. Too much posture is observed when the interneurons that produce posture are not controlled by other interneurons. The example cited earlier involved the cerebellar regulation of the vestibular nuclei and therefore the control of posture indirectly. Another example is the cerebral cortex, which has a powerful inhibitor influence on brainstem and spinal postural mechanisms. The corticospinal tracts send collaterals (probably more correctly called *corticobulbar fibers*) into the brainstem reticular formation. These

Table 2-4. Examples of reciprocal innervation

System	Afferent neurons	Interneurons	Facilitates	Inhibits
Spinal cord				
Cutaneous	In skin over extensor muscle	In gray matter of cord	Underlying extensors	Antagonists
	In skin over other muscles	In gray matter of cord	Flexors	Antagonists
Proprioceptors	Joint afferents (traction)	In gray matter of cord	Flexors	Antagonists
	Muscle spindle (quick stretch)	In gray matter of cord	Motor neurons to muscle stretched	Antagonists
Brainstem				
Vestibular	Cranial nerve VIII	In vestibular nucleus, vestibulospinal tracts, gray matter of cord	Extensors, especially in stance phase of gait	Antagonists
Reticular	All types of sensory information feed into this system	In brainstem reticular nuclei, reticulospinal tracts, ascending reticular activating system	Extensors	Antagonists
Red nucleus	Receives from other CNS interneurons such as cerebellum, basal ganglia, cerebral cortex	In rubrospinal tract, gray matter of cord	Flexors, especially during swing phase of gait	Antagonists
Telencephalon				
Sensorimotor cortex	Mostly exteroceptive and proprioceptive information from cord and brainstem	In lateral corticospinal tract, gray matter of cord	Flexors or extensors	Extensors, flexors

collaterals help regulate the reticular formation's role in the production of posture. Therefore the corticospinal tracts facilitate progravity muscles and inhibit antigravity muscles directly at cord levels and indirectly at brainstem levels. Thus, when these fibers are damaged in the internal capsule, a common site of cerebrovascular accident, the combined loss of regulation of antigravity mechanisms results in a patient who has difficulty inhibiting antigravity postures and facilitating movement. Admittedly, this is stated simplistically, but treatment that uses systems that facilitate movement and inhibit posture will benefit such clients. Refer to Chapter 4 for specific examples of afferent input that could be used to increase posture in the hypotonic or decrease posture in the hypertonic client.

MOVEMENT
Anatomical substrates

Movement is the result of muscle contraction. Muscle contraction is controlled by motor neurons. Motor neurons are influenced by interneurons. Interneurons are influenced by other interneurons and by afferent neurons. Therefore movement must be produced and regulated by interneurons and afferent neurons. Although motor programs are not initiated by afferent input per se, afferent data are necessary for programming the movement, for feedback to assess the progress of the movement, and for learning new programs and developing skill.

Let us assume that there are several different groups of interneurons at different levels of the neuroaxis that are "movement generators." At the segmental level there is a generator for flexion and a reciprocal generator for extension. This generator can be triggered by an afferent neuron or by an extrasegmental interneuron. If the flexion generators of several adjacent segments are linked, a flexor pattern generator for that limb is created. If the flexor pattern generator of one limb is linked to the extensor pattern generator of the other limb, a reciprocal limb movement could be produced. If the flexor pattern generator of the lower limb were linked with the flexor pattern generator of the contralateral upper limb, reciprocal arm and leg movement could be produced. Such generators have been hypothesized based in part on Orlovsky's[7] experiments on spinalized cats. The pattern generators of upper and lower limbs could then be linked to interneurons driven by neck proprioceptors to produce tonic neck reflexes, or they could be linked to interneurons driven by labyrinthine afferent neurons to produce tonic labyrinthine reflexes.

The point is that there already exists in the spinal cord and brainstem all the wiring necessary to produce rather complex but stereotyped movements. With just the wiring in the spinal cord and brainstem, an organism could withdraw from danger, seek food, and maintain itself in relation to gravity. But evolution did not stop there. Not only are we able to protect ourselves and maintain ourselves in relation to gravity, but we are also able to explore our environment and to seek and process information. This is made possible in part by our ability to discriminatively process information. No longer is gross touch, heat, and cold adequate information. To explore our environment we need receptors that are capable of providing information in small increments, that is, two-point discrimination, and small distances between sources of reflected light. We need afferent fibers that conduct rapidly and interneurons that are capable of integrating information from multiple sources. We need interneurons capable of integrating recent and past information, that is, memory, learning, and association. And, finally, we need a sensorimotor system capable of producing more discrete, finite movements by isolating movement at distal segments.

This sensorimotor system is built on and is a refinement of preexisting wiring. It uses motor units at segmental levels to produce muscle contraction just as the withdrawal, labyrinthine, and righting reflexes do. The difference between higher-order or goal-directed movements and protective or postural movements is one of variety, flexibility, and versatility. Although a withdrawal reflex may vary in amplitude, latency, and duration, it always looks like a withdrawal reflex, and it can only be modified while in progress by amplification or damping. *What makes one movement program simple and another complex is the amount of modification made on the program while the program is in progress.* The flexor withdrawal reflex can be increased or decreased, but once initiated it is carried through to completion at an amplitude determined by events before its initiation. Simple locomotion is a fairly stereotyped movement pattern. Suprasegmental, vestibular, and rubral control is exerted by increasing the amplitude or duration of muscle activity but not the sequential relation of muscles in that phase. In other words, a locomotor pattern exists that can be increased or decreased in speed, but the program itself is not normally modified. Apparently, more complex patterns can be generated by centers above the brainstem. Grillner[3] and others have postulated something like a "central program generator" that is capable of producing both ballistic and slow movements. *Ballistic movements* are movements that are too fast to be modified while in progress. The subthalamic nucleus may play a role in the regulation of the production of ballistic movements, as evidenced by subthalamic lesions resulting in ballismus. A likely place for the central program generator is the basal ganglia.

If the central program generator exists outside the cerebral cortex, what then is the role of the cerebral cortex in movement? The motor cortex is the executor for the program generators. It carries out the orders and controls the speed and force of movements by regulating recruitment order and repetition rate. To this control the cerebellar hemispheres add order (synergy and coordination) and distance. The cerebellum controls the distance the limb traverses by regulating the time (duration) of motor unit activity. In other words, given a constant force and speed

of muscle shortening, if the muscle contacts for a longer *time,* the limb will move a greater *distance.* This, of course, is not all the cerebral cortex, cerebellum, and basal ganglia do, but it is enough to use in our model for now.

To summarize the movement model to this point, we have segmental wiring (spinal cord and brainstem) originally designed for homeostasis and modified by linking segmental generators in different patterns to produce postural responses and "whole organism" protective responses, such as the startle response or "blink and duck" reflex. We then add central program generators to this model: a cerebellum to coordinate and time movements and a motor cortex to regulate force and speed as it carries out the coordinated order of the central program generator.

These orders are carried out, not by creating new wiring at the segmental level, but by regulating, modifying, *facilitating,* or *inhibiting* the ongoing activity in existing wiring. The cerebral cortex can influence the spinal cord wiring directly through the corticospinal tract. However, only a very small percentage of that influence is expressed directly onto motor neurons. The majority of the cerebral cortex's influence is through interneurons, influencing the background activity within segmental reflex arcs. Both corticospinal and rubrospinal tracts tend to facilitate progravity muscles (movement) and inhibit antigravity muscles (posture).

Not all of the regulation of movement occurs at the segmental reflex arc. As mentioned earlier, the corticospinal tract also influences brainstem centers involved especially with regulation of posture. Therefore the cerebral cortex facilitates movement in at least two ways: by facilitating progravity muscles at the segmental level and by inhibiting brainstem level centers that facilitate antigravity muscles.

The cerebellum and the basal ganglia must be content to influence movement through the cerebral cortex. The cerebellum receives information regarding ongoing segmental activity (in part via spinocerebellar tracts) and regarding the central program generator intent via corticopontocerebellar paths. The cerebellum then monitors the program (via spinocerebellar input) to determine if the movement is according to intent regarding sequence, distance, force, etc. and signals higher centers to make adjustments if necessary.

Dysfunction

If a lesion can result in loss of function, then in this system a loss of movement or weakness should be observed. This loss of movement is different from the loss of movement seen at spinal cord levels, where, for example, a peripheral nerve injury causes weakness and loss of reflexes. Loss of function in systems that produce motor programs results in problems with planning the movement (ideation, motivation, programming) and problems in initiating the movement. Signs include akinesia, apraxia, and perseveration. Positive signs may be expressed as too much movement (athetoid or chorea-form movements). These involuntary movements appear to be parts of motor programs no longer under control of the regulatory centers. Positive signs may also be expressed as uncoordinated movement, such as past-pointing ataxia, dyssynergia or the inability to resolve conflicting sensory input.

The CNS lesion most commonly seen in older adults is ischemia secondary to cerebrovascular accident. This most often involves the white matter in the internal capsule. This includes the corticospinal and corticobulbar tracts. The resulting negative sign is an inability to perform skilled movements, especially those of distal segments. However, these clients also often have hypertonicity in the form of spasticity, that is, too much posture. So is the problem too much posture or not enough movement? It may be both. With a lesion of the corticospinal and corticobulbar fibers, there is a loss of cortical inhibition of postural mechanisms at brainstem levels as well as a loss of facilitation of progravity muscles (movement) at segmental levels, not to mention the concomitant loss of reciprocal inhibition of antigravity muscles (posture).

Studies have shown that the movement disorder in the client with spastic hemiplegia is not the result of spasticity preventing movement but of the inability to recruit motor units in the proper timing and sequence.[9,12] There is also sufficient evidence to indicate that eventually there may also be a lower motor neuron component to the weakness seen in clients with hemiplegia.[7,5,13]

In other types of CNS lesions positive signs such as involuntary movement—too much movement—are seen. In this situation there is an instability in a movement generator, there is a loss of regulation of that generator, and parts of movements are expressed without apparent purpose. Examples include athetosis, chorea, and ballismus. Tremor, although certainly an involuntary movement, may be a loss of control of the inherent oscillation within the sensorimotor system.

Because a major function of the cerebellum is the regulation or coordination (not production) of movement, cerebellar lesions manifest themselves as problems of incoordinated movement. In the case of cerebellar tremor, there may be an apparent loss of the damping of the inherent oscillation in the sensorimotor system so that there is "too much" oscillation.

As in previous sections the model can be applied to evaluation and treatment. First, it must be determined if negative signs, such as weakness, are the result of a lesion of the afferent neuron, interneuron, or efferent neuron. If afferent neurons are involved, other afferent neurons must be found to provide similar information, for example, substitute visual for proprioceptive information or use joint approximation to increase proprioceptive input. If efferent neurons are involved, other motor units must be brought in to substitute for the weak or absent functions. To recruit more motor units the clinician will use afferent input to enhance output. Biofeedback is a less obvious example of using afferent input (usually auditory) to enhance motor output.

If the interneurons are the source of the negative signs, the therapist must first attempt to determine where in the motor programming the problems lie. Is the problem ideation, motivation, generation of programs and subprograms, accessing programs, coordinating and sequencing programs, or executing programs. Then the therapist's challenge is to find alternate ways of producing motor output. Are there other ways to access the remaining programs? Is the client to learn programs as if they were new programs? Are there other strategies to perform the same task? Can the programming be augmented, facilitated, or accessed by afferent input? For example, some apraxic clients can imitate a motor task but cannot perform the task if only given verbal commands. If interneurons are the source of positive signs, such as involuntary movement and uncoordinated movement, the therapist must determine if other systems remain intact that may be used to regulate, override, or inhibit the unwanted movement programs. This is probably the most difficult task for the therapist. Control systems for movement are newer, more susceptible to damage, and fewer in number than control systems for lower-level functions. Pharmacological intervention has provided some assistance but may be more detrimental than beneficial in the long run.

HIGHER CORTICAL FUNCTIONS
Anatomical substrates

Although the integration that occurs in the cerebral hemispheres is infinitely more complex than a segmental reflex, it can still be compared to that reflex arc. Cerebral cortical activity is still based on the receipt of information from inside and outside the body. This information is carried to the CNS by way of afferent neurons—all afferent neurons (interoceptive, proprioceptive, and exteroceptive) eventually influence the cortex. Once the information reaches the CNS, it is conducted to the cortex by way of interneurons. These would include projection fibers—such as spinothalamics, the medial lemniscus, specific and diffuse thalamocortical projections, geniculocalcarine fibers (visual), and geniculotemporal fibers (auditory). Information is further processed by interneurons in the thalamus, hypothalamus, basal ganglia, and cerebral cortex. Other interneurons may carry the information from gyrus to gyrus or lobe to lobe (association fibers). Still others carry information from side to side (commissural fibers). Finally, the appropriate response must be executed. This requires descending projection fibers, such as the corticospinals and corticobulbars, to carry information to motor neurons. We now have come full circle (or arc) to our motor output. Perhaps some examples of higher cortical function will make this clearer.

Earlier in this chapter segmental reflexes in response to

cutaneous stimuli were examined. We will now examine what else happens along with that segmental reflex. If someone sticks your index finger with a pin, besides the flexor withdrawal response, possibly a brainstem-mediated "ouch," and pupillary dilation, you *perceive* the stimulus. This requires interneurons carrying the information to the cortex by way of the thalamus. The information first reaches the primary sensory cortex and then the information is carried to the sensory association cortex via association fibers (more interneurons). Now, besides knowing you were stimulated, you also know where, how much, what shape, based upon past experience, and by what object. You also have made a decision as to how threatening the stimulus was and whether or not you should flee, fight, or stay neutral. This decision involves reviewing your past experience and putting an emotional value or weight on the situation. The action you take in this situation requires descending pathways, such as the reticulospinals, for the sympathetic response (cardiovascular) and corticospinals for removing the pin with which you were stuck.

Now instead of being stuck with a pin, you are shown a picture of a sunset in the wilderness of Alaska and asked to tell about what you see. The afferent neurons are in the retina. Interneurons carry the visual information from the retinas to the visual cortex (with stops in such places as the tectum and the lateral geniculate). You see the picture. Interneurons carry information to visual association areas. You recognize the picture as a sunset in the wilderness. Your memory is searched. You do not recognize the specific picture. Interneurons carry information to the parts of the brain that have to do with emotional tone (see Chapter 4). You become apprehensive. Now you tell the person showing you the picture that you see a sunset in the woods. You begin to fidget in your chair because when you were a child you were nearly attacked by a bear while camping with your parents.

Speech is another appropriate motor response to a stimulus. It requires sequencing of motor acts (tongue, lip, larynx, diaphragm) to produce sounds that we have learned to associate with certain images, usually visual. Sequencing of motor acts requires ideation, motivation, a motor program, an executor (motor cortex), a descending pathway (corticospinals and corticobulbars), and motor neurons, such as those in cranial nerves V, VII, X, XII and in spinal nerves 3, 4, 5 (diaphragm). This is only a partial list, but it becomes clear that a signal is received, integrated, and acted on, just as we have seen at other levels. Perception involves receiving the stimulus and associating it with past experience. Speech most often is a motor response to a visual stimulus (reading) or an auditory stimulus.

Hemispheric specialization can be looked upon as a division of labor between interneurons. To be more efficient, interneurons process information differently in the two hemispheres. It is *not* that some information is processed only in one hemisphere but that each hemisphere analyzes

the afferent input for different content. In the majority of humans the left hemisphere analyzes the sequential content of an event, be it auditory, visual, tactile, or proprioceptive, and the right hemisphere analyzes the spatial content of the event. The left hemisphere counts the trees, the right hemisphere identifies it as a dense forest. Each hemisphere also contributes to the response. The left hemisphere is involved in the production of speech, a *sequence* of sounds. The right hemisphere adds the tone and rhythm of voice, the spatial content. The left hemisphere is involved in the *sequencing* of motor acts, motor planning. The right hemisphere is more involved in whole body, body in space types of integration.

Dysfunction

A lesion of the cerebral hemispheres can result in negative and/or positive signs. If, when asked what you saw in the picture, you did not answer, that is a negative sign, but is it caused by decreased afferent input? You either did not *hear* the question or you did not *see* the picture—or perhaps you heard and saw but did not understand the question, or could not formulate the answer. Or perhaps it is the result of a lesion in interneurons responsible for executing the motor command (corticospinals and corticobulbars), or is it the result of a loss of efferent neurons, motor neurons, as might be seen in bulbar polio or laryngeal nerve palsy? Is the inability to perceive a pin prick the result of a loss of afferent neurons, projection fibers, or primary sensory cortex? Or is it caused by an inability to orient to a stimulus? Hemispatial neglect appears to be an inability to orient to a stimulus rather than an agnosia, as seen in right parietal lesions. Positive signs might include inappropriate responses, such as emotional lability, hyperactive behavior, jargon speech, and perservation.

In assessing the client with hemispheric damage, the clinician may need the assistance of other members of the rehabilitation team. Does the client have an afferent lesion, that is, auditory, visual, proprioceptive, cutaneous sensation? If this is the source of the negative sign, then other sensory systems must be substituted. Does the client have an efferent lesion, that is, motor neuron loss? If so, then treatment involves recruiting functioning motor units. Does the client have an interneuronal lesion, and if so, is it production of function or regulation of function? If the interneurons produce the function, there may be few treatment alternatives since there is much less duplicity this high in the nervous system. But there is another hemisphere that does the same function with a different strategy. And if only some of the interneurons that produce the function are damaged, then appropriate afferent input can be used to enhance their function. The client with visual perceptual problems may be helped with added proprioceptive input, for example. If the dysfunction is caused by loss of regulatory interneurons, then other regulatory centers can be recruited. In some instances less is better. In the hyperactive child who cannot regulate (filter) and focus on the task at hand, decreasing afferent input by controlling the environment assists the child's nervous system to regulate function.

SUMMARY

Regardless of the systems involved and regardless of the severity of the lesion, the therapist must evaluate, identify the problems of, and treat the client with a neurological dysfunction. The evaluation procedure is testing the intactness of the afferent neuron, interneuron, efferent neuron arc. All reflex testing is based on this arc. The clinician may also wish to consider testing gait, coordination, and higher cortical functions. The clinician is attempting to determine if there is adequate and appropriate afferent information, if it is integrated appropriately, and if an appropriate response is produced. Treatment is then determined based on the same model. The clinician must find a way to provide adequate and appropriate afferent input to facilitate integration and the production of an appropriate response. In Chapter 6 categories of afferent input can be found that may be used in treating the neurological client.

For a greater in-depth analysis of the motor control and limbic systems, the reader is referred to Chapters 3 and 4, respectively. The goal of this chapter was to present an overview of the role and function of the CNS. The nervous system must be understood as a whole, for no part functions in isolation. Once a comfortable whole has been achieved, an in-depth study of or focus on one area should widen the reader's comprehension of the whole. The path to learning is exciting but complicated. As long as an understanding of the whole is maintained, the reader will always be able to find the way back to comprehension whenever he or she becomes lost.

REFERENCES

1. Aschoff JC and Kornhuber HH: Functional interpretation of somatic afferents in cerebellum, basal ganglia and motor cortex. In Kornhuber, HH, editor: The somatosensory system, Stuttgart, 1975, Thieme.
2. Chokroverty S and others: Hemiplegic amytrophy, Arch Neurol 33:104, 1976.
3. Grillner S: Locomotion in vertebrates: central mechanisms and reflex interaction, Physiol Rev 55:247, 1975.
4. Kandel ER and Schwartz JH: Principles of neural science, New York, 1985, Elsevier Publishing Co.
5. McComas AJ and others: Functional changes in motoneurons of hemiparetic patients, J Neurol Neurosurg Psychiatry 36:183, 1973.
6. Nashner LM: Fixed patterns of rapid postural responses among leg muscles during stance, Exp Brain Res 30:13, 1977.
7. Orlovsky GN: The effect of different descending systems on flexor and extensor activity during locomotion, Brain Res 40:359, 1972.
8. Penn RD and Etzel ML: Chronic cerebellar stimulation and developmental reflexes, J Neurophysiol 46:506, 1977.
9. Rosenfalck A and Andreassen S: Impaired regulation of force and firing pattern of single motor units in patients with spasticity, J Neurol Neurosurg Psychiatry 43:970, 1980.
10. Sherrington CS: The integrative action of the nervous system, New Haven, 1906, Yale University Press.
11. Walshe F: Contributions of John Hughlings Jackson to neurology: a brief introduction to his teachings, Arch Neurol 5:119, 1961.
12. Whitley DA and others: Patterns of muscle activity in the hemiplegic upper extremity, Phys Ther 62:641, 1982 (abstract).
13. Young JL and Mayer RF: Mechanical properties of single motor units in short-term hemiplegia, Neurology 29:609, 1979.

ADDITIONAL READINGS

Brooks VB: The neural basis of motor control, New York, 1986, Oxford University Press.
Bruggencate G ten: Functions of extrapyramidal systems in motor control. I. Supraspinal descending pathways, Pharmacol Ther B1:587, 1975.
Bruggencate G ten: Functions of extrapyramidal systems in motor control. II. Cortical and subcortical pathways, Pharmacol Ther B1:611, 1975.
Bruggencate G ten and Lundberg A: Facilitory interaction transmission to motoneurons from vestibulospinal fibers and contrilateral primary afferents, Exp Brain Res 19:248, 1974.
Burke D: A reassessment of the muscle spindle contribution to muscle tone in normal and spastic man. In Feldman RG and others, editors: Spasticity: disordered motor control, Chicago, 1980, Year Book Medical Publishers, Inc.
DeLong MR and Strick PL: Relation of basal ganglia, cerebellum and motor cortex units to ramp and ballistic limb movements, Brain Res 71:327, 1974.
Desmedt JE, editor: Spinal and supraspinal mechanisms of voluntary motor control and locomotion, vol 8, Progress in clinical neurophysiology, Basel, 1980, S Karger.
Desmedt JE, editor: Motor unit types, recruitment and plasticity in health and disease, vol 9, Progress in clinical neurophysiology, Basel, 1981, S Karger.
Eyzaguirre C and Fidone SS: Physiology of the nervous system, Chicago, 1975, Year Book Medical Publishers, Inc.
Feldman RG and others: Spasticity: disordered motor control, Chicago, 1980, Year Book Medical Publishers, Inc.
Grillner S: Locomotion in vertebrates: central mechanisms and reflex interaction, Physiol Rev 55:247, 1975.
Grillner S and Hongo T: Vestibulospinal relations. Vestibular influences on the lumbosacral spinal cord. In Brodal A and others, editors: Basic aspects of central vestibular mechanisms, Amsterdam, 1972, Elsevier Publishing Company.
Hongo T and others: The rubrospinal tract. II. Facilitation of interneuronal transmission in reflex paths to motoneurons, Exp Brain Res 7:365, 1969.
Kuypers HGJM: The descending pathways to the spinal cord: their anatomy and function, Prog Brain Res 11:178, 1964.
Landau WM: Spasticity: What is it? What is it not? In Feldman RG and others, editors: Spasticity: disordered motor control, Chicago, 1980, Year Book Medical Publishers, Inc.
Lundberg A and Voorhoeve P: Effects from the pyramidal tract on spinal reflex arcs, Acta Physiol Scand 56:201, 1962.
MacLeon PD: The triune brain in conflict, Psychother Psychosom 28:207, 1977.
Miller S and Scott PD: Spinal generation of movement in a single limb: functional implications of a model based on the cat. In Desmedt, JE, editor: Progress in clinical neurophysiology, vol 8, Basel, 1980, S Karger.
Sarnat HB and Netsky MG: Evolution of the nervous system, New York, 1974, Oxford University Press, Inc.
Williams PL and Warwick R: Functional neuroanatomy of man, Philadelphia, 1975, WB Saunders Co.
Willis WD and Grossman RG: Medical neurobiology, ed 3, St Louis, 1981, The CV Mosby Co.

Chapter 3

MOTOR CONTROL

Roberta A. Newton

Motor control theory has been an integral part of the base for physical and occupational therapy assessment and treatment for many years. Therapists are interested in how the brain controls movement in persons with deficits in posture and movement and also in healthy individuals. As up-to-date information about motor control becomes available, therapists reassess principles that form the basis for treatment and replace older, outmoded ideas with newer principles of motor control. The newer ideas arise from many disciplines, including neuroscience and motor learning.

This chapter has two purposes. First, it provides the reader with an understanding of models used to represent neural regulation of posture and movement. Second, it describes some deficits of motor control using these models.

A model is a schematic representation of a theory: in this case, of how the brain regulates motor behavior. Various models exist because researchers use different approaches to develop and test theories. All models have limitations and are constantly changing as researchers gain new information, and as technological advances are made. Early researchers used techniques such as visual observation and palpation to develop models of motor control. To-day researchers use techniques and tools that include film analysis, electron microscopy, and cerebral blood flow studies to develop hypotheses about motor control. Finally, models may portray only a small part of the nervous system; for example, a model of spinal cord control mechanisms would not include higher-center control processes. Other models may be more general, examining, for example, the interrelationships between various brain centers and the spinal centers. Models for motor control used as a basis for predicting motor responses during patient treatment should have a broad scope. A therapist using a spinal level reflex model, for example, may inaccurately predict motor behavior because this model may not consider motor behavior regulated by higher centers. Selecting and using a proper model is important for the analysis and treatment of individuals with posture and movement dysfunction.

MODELS FOR MOTOR CONTROL

The term motor control refers to the regulation of movement and dynamic postural adjustments. Two broad models for motor control are presented in this section: a hierarchy and a systems model.

Hierarchy

A hierarchy represents a "top-down" model for motor control. The *commander*, a higher center, plans and delegates the motor program to subordinate centers for execution. Researchers include feedback loops in contemporary models depicting a hierarchy of motor control. In these models information about the internal and external environment before and after movement is available to the commander. The commander, however, does not need to use the information during execution of movement.

Hughlings Jackson,[9] a neurologist, developed one of

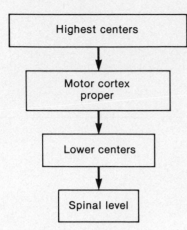

Fig. 3-1. Jackson's model of a hierarchy of motor control.

the early hierarchial models of motor control in the 1850s. Jackson was the first to state that the nervous system represented movements, and that different parts of the brain represented these movements in different combinations. The nervous system represents movements in different combinations from the lowest to highest centers. The spinal cord or cranial nuclei make up the lowest center; the motor cortex proper, the middle center; and the highest center includes the sensory cortex, the frontal motor areas, and areas responsible for consciousness.

When disease or injury damages the highest center, dissolution of the whole nervous system can occur. The more stable lower and evolutionarily older nervous centers then control function. Movements represented at the lower levels are reflexive; that is, stereotypic and not capable of modification when the external or internal environmental conditions neccessitate a change. Damage to nervous tissue in the highest centers can lead to either destruction or instability of movement. It can also lead to overreadiness of the nervous system to become active.

In this theory the highest center contains all the information necessary for movement and it may or may not use external or internal feedback to regulate movement. Fig. 3-1 illustrates this theory, which represents a limited view of motor control. The levels do not communicate with one another. Rather they serve as subordinates carrying out a series of commands generated by the highest center.

Jackson's theory for motor control represented the state of science from the middle of the nineteenth century to the early twentieth century. Although this model has limitations, it served as the basis for development of the disciplines of neurology and neurological physical therapy. Since its incorporation into physical therapy theory, researchers have developed other theories for the regulation of posture and movement. The hierarchial model is useful for examining motor activity without feedback; however, this model is of limited use when trying to understand the interrelationships of brain centers for planning and initiating motor activity.

Systems model

Components of a systems model. Researchers adopted the term *systems* from engineering terminology. They use it to describe the relationship of various brain and spinal centers working together with the use of feedback. For the purposes of this discussion, the systems model will be broken into parts. Each part, taken alone, represents a limited model for motor control. One part, the tripartate system, is a higher-center system. The central pattern generator is the spinal-level system. The other two parts of the model are a descending pathway system and feedback loops among the units (Fig. 3-2). This section will present a brief orientation to the anatomy and function of the various systems.

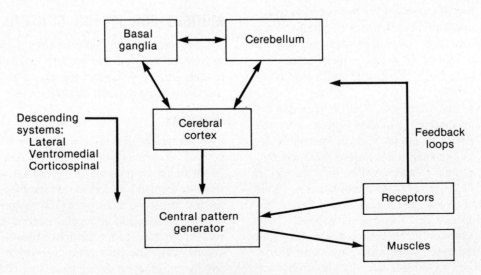

Fig. 3-2. Systems model for motor control.

The reader can find detailed descriptions of anatomy and functions of these areas in comprehensive neuroscience texts.

Tripartate system. The tripartite system includes the cerebral cortex, basal ganglia, and cerebellum. These centers function together to plan, initiate, and regulate movement. Both the cerebellum and basal ganglia communicate with the cerebral cortex. Each structure receives input from the cerebral cortex and projects information to the cortex via subcortical pathways. The cerebellum receives input from the sensorimotor cerebral cortex and sends major projections to the motor cortex (area 4). The basal ganglia receive input from the entire cortex and send major projections to the prefrontal and premotor cortical areas. Neither the cerebellum nor basal ganglia have direct projections to the spinal cord, but influence spinal level motor activity via other descending pathways. Both centers receive sensory information: the cerebellum directly from primary afferent neurons and the basal ganglia via indirect means.

Basal ganglia. In the past, researchers believed the major role of the basal ganglia was to regulate posture. However, clinical observation of patients with lesions of the basal ganglia and animal research have provided evidence that the basal ganglia also have a role in the control of movement. Patients with basal ganglia deficits show movement dysfunction, including paucity or slowness of movement and involuntary movements. They also have abnormalities of righting and equilibrium as well as changes in posture.[14]

In animal research, DeLong[5] recorded neuronal activity in certain basal ganglia cells before onset of movement. Many neurons of the putamen respond either to the direction or force of a specific movement. DeLong postulated that the basal ganglia do not participate in the initiation of the motor act. Many neuroscientists believe that the basal ganglia participate in the planning and adjustment of the motor act.

Kornhuber[10] postulated that the basal ganglia primarily regulate slow movements and the cerebellum regulates fast movements. Although intriguing, this notion has been disproven in animal studies. Recordings of neuronal activity in the basal ganglia show that some neurons are active during fast arm movements.[4]

Neuroscientists now believe that the basal ganglia, particularly the caudate nucleus, participate in cognitive functions. The caudate nucleus receives input from the prefrontal and frontal cortex. If bilateral lesions of the dorsolateral prefrontal cortex are present, the individual has a deficit in task reversal. Researchers interpret this deficit as an abnormality of spatial memory. In summary, the basal ganglia have a greater role than was previously believed in the regulation of posture and movement. They not only play an integral role in postural control, but also participate in planning motor activity. Further, researchers are continuing to explore the role of the basal ganglia in cognitive functions relative to movement.

Cerebellum. The functional roles of the cerebellum include coordination and execution of movements and motor learning. The cerebellum receives input from primary sensory neurons and the cerebral cortex. Therefore, researchers believe that one function of this center is to compare actual motor activity with intended motor activity. Clinical and research studies have shown that the cerebellum participates in regulating the relative timing, sequencing, and force generation of muscle activity.

The cerebellum also plays a major role in adaptation of motor behavior and motor learning. Adaptation is the ability to change the motor program when environmental or internal conditions change. For example, a man may lose this balance during the first few steps on an icy path. To adapt, he may use information about the condition of the support surface to change the motor program. For example, he may lower his center of gravity or widen his base of support while walking on the ice. Adaptation here is defined as improvement of the motor behavior following repeated trials. In the above example, these trials would consist in repeating the gait cycle while traversing the icy area. Motor learning occurs when adaptation creates a permanent change in motor behavior. Motor learning implies that information or experience gained from previous trials is stored and used in later motor acts.

Cerebral cortex: motor functions. Four main areas contribute to motor functions: the motor cortex, the premotor cortex, the supplementary motor area, and the posterior parietal cortex.

MOTOR CORTEX. The motor cortex (area 4) is somatotopically arranged. It regulates muscle activity via direct synaptic endings on motoneurons and indirectly via synaptic connections on spinal level interneurons. Evarts[6] noted that the pyramidal tract neurons encode the amount of muscle force needed to perform a movement. For example, if a monkey performs wrist flexion, a certain frequency of electrical activity occurs in the pyramidal tract neurons. If a monkey performs wrist flexion with a weighted wrist, an increase in neuronal activity in the pyramidal tract neurons occurs.

Researchers have also shown that the motor cortex regulates fractionation of movement, such as individualized finger movement. Monkeys with lesions of the pyramidal tracts lose the ability for finger manipulation and also lose speed and agility when performing purposeful movements.

SUPPLEMENTARY MOTOR AREA. The supplementary motor area lies rostromedial to the precentral motor area. Neuroscientists hypothesize that this area assists with the control of posture and the preparation and programming of complex sequences of movement. The sequences studied have frequently been bilateral movements involving postural adjustments and orientation of the body. The supplementary motor area also assists with regulating movements involving proximal musculature.[2]

Electrical stimulation of the supplementary motor area in both humans and monkeys produces complex, synergistic movements of the whole limb. However, removal of this area has no effect on distal movements. Researchers have examined the role of the supplementary motor area during motor activity by studying cerebral blood flow in humans. When an individual performs a simple motor task (for example, compressing a spring between the thumb and index finger), blood flow increases in both the contralateral motor and sensory cortex. However, a significant increase in blood flow in the premotor area does not occur. Researchers also examined more complex sequences of finger movements, such as repeatedly touching the thumb with each finger. In these cases they found that an increase in blood flow occurs in the contralateral motor and sensory cortical areas as well as bilaterally in the supplementary motor area. They also found that when an individual then mentally rehearses a complex sequence of hand movements, blood flow increases in the supplementary motor area but not in the motor or sensory cortex.[18]

PREMOTOR AREA. The premotor area is located rostral to the motor cortex and on the lateral surface of the cerebral hemispheres. Neuroscientists do not completely understand the role of this area, but because of its projections to the brainstem, it is believed that the premotor area controls proximal limb and axial musculature and that it may also regulate motor activity associated with orientation of the body to specific locations or targets. In this respect, the premotor area is similar to the supplementary motor area.

The premotor area exchanges information with the posterior parietal cortex. Therefore, some of the functions of these two areas are complementary. The premotor area may regulate movements associated with tactile input. For example, monkeys with lesions in the premotor area have an involuntary grasp response evoked by tactile stimulation to the palmar surface of the hand. A grasp response can also be evoked by stretching the flexor muscles of the hand.

POSTERIOR PARIETAL CORTEX. Researchers recording neuronal activity in the posterior parietal cortex in monkeys have shown that this area regulates goal-directed reaching movements, especially reaching for objects of interest. This area is also active during manipulation of objects. These manual movements depend on the motivational and attentional state of the animal. Some studies have shown activity in posterior parietal neurons during visual exploration of objects of interest. Therefore the role of this area is related to both manual and visual exploration of the environment.[15]

Lesions in this area result in both sensory and motor neglect of the contralateral side of the body. Patients with deficits in the posterior parietal cortex have trouble executing learned movements. For example, they may forget the sequence of tasks necessary for dressing (apraxia). These patients also have trouble orienting toward objects of interest. Bilateral lesions result in reduced exploratory behavior of the environment.

Descending systems. Lawrence and Kuypers[11] examined the role of descending systems in the regulation of movement. They identified three functional descending systems: ventromedial (VMS), lateral (LS), and corticospinal (CS) systems. The ventromedial system includes the lateral and medial vestibulospinal tracts, the reticulospinal tract arising from the pontine and medullary medial tegmental field and medial mesencephalic tegmentum, the interstitiospinal tract, and the tectospinal tract. These pathways end, frequently bilaterally, in the ventromedial region of the intermediate zone of the spinal cord. This region of the spinal cord contains long and intermediate propriospinal neurons. Some of the descending axons make monosynaptic connections with motoneurons innervating the axial and proximal limb musculature. Part of the VMS projects to motoneurons of the external eye muscles and facial musculature associated with the ears in the cat and monkey.

Because the terminal endings of this system are widespread, this system may help with activation of synergistic muscle patterns. Researchers have examined motor activity associated with the VMS by disrupting these tracts in the bilaterally pyramidotomized monkey. Following surgery, a flexed trunk and limb posture occurs. The monkey has elevated shoulders and adducted upper extremities. Following surgery, the monkey has a prolonged inability to right the body. When righting to a sitting position occurs, the animal assumes a forward flexed posture.

The lateral system consists of the contralateral descending rubrospinal, rubrobulbar, and pontospinal tract, which starts in the ventrolateral pontine tegmentum. The LS ends more laterally in the intermediate zone of the spinal cord. This is the region where short propriospinal neurons are located. The LS has some direct connections with motoneurons of distal musculature, and motoneurons of the perioral and periorbital muscles. This pathway is thought to be more involved with isolated than with synergistic movements. Researchers have identified the functional role of the LS by disruption of these brainstem pathways in the bilaterally pyramidotomized monkey. Following surgery, the animal can right, sit up, and climb, but monkey has deficits in the ipsilateral upper extremity (the arm hangs with slight elbow flexion and finger extension). The monkey reaches for food using a movement pattern of shoulder circumduction and slight elbow flexion and uses finger flexion to hold food. During climbing or walking, the animal's deficits are less noticable. In summary, neuroscientists believe the LS regulates movements of the extremities. Most particularly, this system aids with regulation of flexion movements of the elbow, wrist, and hand and with independent joint movements.

The third descending system described by Lawrence and Kuypers[11] includes the corticospinal and corticobulbar pathways. This system ends in the lower brainstem and in the intermediate zone of the spinal cord, including the region of the long propriospinal tracts. It ends in the same areas as the ventromedial and lateral systems. Direct monosynaptic connections occur primarily on the motoneurons of distal extremity musculature. The corticospinal system is topographically organized, represents a highly differentiated system, and provides a high degree of individualized movement.

The monkey with bilateral pyramidotomy can right, sit, and climb. The animal cannot pick up or grasp food but can climb in the cage. Following recovery, the monkey initially reaches for food, using circumduction of the whole arm, and grasp as part of the entire arm movement pattern. As recovery progresses, hand closure involves the entire hand, independent of a whole-arm pattern. Prehension never returns. The monkey with bilateral pyramidotomy can, however, perform purposeful movements. Thus the CS is not necessary for the performance of *volitional* actions. The loss of CS pathways results in a loss of prehension and individualized finger movements. The CS system also overlaps the medial and lateral systems and provides some degree of fractionization and control of speed in movements regulated by the VMS and LS.

The central pattern generator. Researchers have reinvestigated the role of spinal centers in the regulation of movement. The reflex arc or stimulus-response model was the early basis for understanding spinal-level activity. An external stimulus produces a predictable, stereotypical motor response. Grillner[7] proved the existence of central pattern generators (CPG) at the spinal level. A generator represents a group of neurons that inherently present a prearranged sequence of muscle activity, arranged both spatially and temporally. This generator can be activated without peripheral feedback. Grillner hypothesizes that the program for walking is located in a CPG. He believes CPGs for each limb are linked together to provide coordinated movement, such as walking.

Systems theory. The term *heterarchy* here means a different system of control than rule by a hierarchy. As previously discussed, a single commander assumes the role of ruler in a hierarchy. The systems model, on the other hand, is an example of a heterarchy. The following section will compare several concepts related to hierarchical and heterarchical theory of motor control.[3] Traditionally the basic spinal-level unit in a hierarchy is the reflex. If a single stimulus activates a receptor, a single stereotypical motor response results. In a heterarchy, the basic spinal-level unit is the CPG.[17] If a single stimulus activates a CPG, a series of motor responses occurs. Spontaneous activation of the neural network can also occur. For example, spontaneous activation occurs in the sinoatrial (SA) node of the heart. The SA node fibers are extremely per-

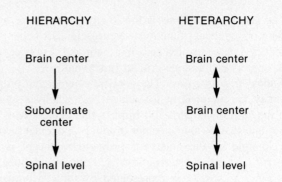

Fig. 3-3. Examples of a hierarchy with a top-down flow of information and a heterarchy with interchange of information between structures.

meable to sodium ions. When increased membrane permeability causes an influx of sodium ions into the nodal fibers, depolarization and excitation of the SA node fibers occurs. This in turn leads to excitation and contraction of atrial muscle fibers.

Reciprocity. Reciprocity means that information flows between two or more neural structures. The structures can be thought of as brain centers, for example, cerebellum and basal ganglia, or neuronal networks located within a single brain center (Fig. 3-3). Information is modified as it flows between centers. In contrast, in a hierarchy information generated by the commander flows down to structures below the commander in an unmodified form (Fig. 3-4).

Distributed function. Distributed function implies that a single center or neural network may have more than one function. Distributed function also implies that several centers may share the same function. For example, in one activity a center may serve as the coordinating unit. In another activity the center may serve as a pattern generator to continue to produce the activity. In contrast, in hierarchical theories centers serve one function. A primary commander will always assume the role of the primary commander, and a different unit will assume the role of a pattern generator. An advantage of distributing function

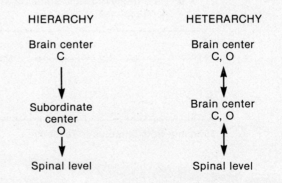

Fig. 3-4. Examples of a hierarchy with a commander and a heterarchy with a structure that serves as both a commander (C) and oscillator *(O)*.

among groups of neurons is that many centers have overlapping or redundant functions. Neuroscientists believe redundancy is a safety feature. If a neuronal lesion occurs, other centers can assume critical functional roles.

Emergent properties. The concept of emergent properties may be captured in the adage "the whole is greater than the sum of its parts." It implies that centers work together and that no single center produces movement alone. An example of the emergent properties concept is the property of continuous repetitive activity (oscillation). In Fig. 3-5 a hierarchy is represented by three neurons arranged in tandem. The last neuron ends on a responder. If a single stimulus activates this network, a single response occurs. What is the response if the neurons were arranged so that the third neuron sent a collateral branch to the first neuron in addition to the ending on the responder? In this case, a single stimulus activates neuron no. 1. Neuron no. 1 activates neuron no. 2 and no. 3, causing a response as well as reactivating neuron no. 1. This neuronal arrangement produces a series of responses rather than a single response. This function is described as endogenous activity (oscillation).

Consensus. The fourth concept associated with systems theory of motor control is command function by consensus. Instead of a single center serving the role of a commander, several centers work together as a command center. For a function to take place, a majority of neurons or centers must become active. When centers reach a critical threshold, they act. This function filters information that may not necessarily need immediate attention. If,

however, a novel stimulus enters the system it carries more *weight* and immediate action occurs.

Summary

The hierarchy and systems models are very useful when examining motor control. A hierarchy is a useful model to examine ballistic movements, where execution occurs very quickly and without the need for feedback. The hierarchy may also be a useful model when explaining the execution of well-learned or highly skilled movements not dependent on feedback. Systems theory is a proper model for understanding the role of feedback and error. To understand all aspects of motor control, the therapist should use both models.

REGULATION OF POSTURE AND MOVEMENT

A motor program is an abstract representation. Neuroscientists use the term to describe temporal and spatial aspects of muscle activity to produce coordinated motor behavior. Motor behavior is the observable outcome of the execution of a motor program. Many questions about motor programs and their relationship to motor control are still unanswered. For example, how general are motor programs? Are motor programs inherent or are they learned? Where are motor programs stored?

Some motor programs may be inherent and contain prearranged synaptic connections that specify spatial and temporal relationships among motoneurons. Grillner[7] demonstrated that central pattern generators (CPGs) for gait exist in the spinal cord of the cat. When activated, CPGs pro-

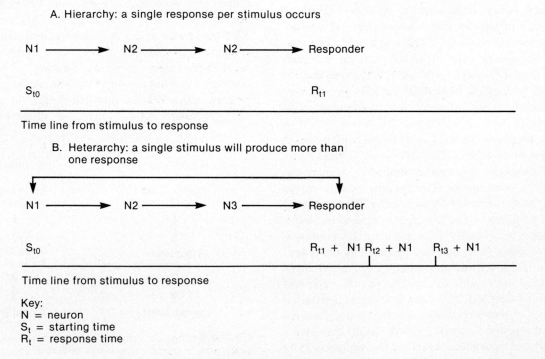

Fig. 3-5. Example of emergent properties.

duce specific sequences of muscle activity in a gait cycle. This observation would lead to the notion that specific motor programs reside in specific regions of the CNS. The following section will discuss fixed versus generalized motor programs and storage of motor programs.

Specific versus generalized motor programs

Some researchers argue that motor programs represent very specific spatial and temporal sequences involving specific muscles for a specific activity. If this is the case, then each motor program is stored separately. Because space for storage of these individualized motor programs presents a problem, most researchers believe that actions or patterns are incorporated in the motor program and not specific muscles. Selecting and sequencing of muscles would occur after motor program is selected. Researchers have examined one motor activity, handwriting, in relation to specific versus generalized motor programs.[20] If someone writes the same sentence holding a pencil in the right hand, left hand, right foot, left foot, or teeth, the sequence of letters will occur in the same order but the height of the letters and the speed of writing using the various body parts will be different. The relative smoothness of the activity using various body regions will also differ. The general shape of the letters and the order of the letters will be the same. For example, an 'r' will have an upstroke, a small arc, and then a downstroke. These elements of an "r" are located in the motor program. However, speed and amplitude are not stored as part of the motor program. If specific muscle sequences were stored for each body region, specific motor programs would exist for each body region. If, however, a generalized motor program basic to the production of the sentence exists, then muscles are selected before the motor act occurs.

The notion of general motor programs can apply to the regulation of balance abilities. Balance is the ability of the individual to maintain the body's center of mass (CM) over the base of support. Balance is also the ability of the individual to return the body's CM over the base of support following a disturbing force. Thus dynamic postural control is subdivided into anticipatory and compensatory movements. Anticipatory postural control refers to adjustments an individual makes prior to onset of a disturbing force. Compensatory postural control refers to adjustments following an unexpected disturbing force. Many researchers, including Nashner[16], Allum and Keshner[1], and Lee and Arronson,[12] have developed models for postural control. These researchers believe that a limited number of motor programs exists for balance responses. Each motor program contains a muscle sequence prearranged both temporally and spatially. Horak and Nasher[8] showed that a fixed pattern of muscle activity in the lower extremity exists. The motor program is activated to maintain dynamic balance when a person is unexpectedly displaced. When placed on a platform that suddenly moves forward or back-

ward only a few centimeters, the individual sways. An orderly pattern of muscle activity occurs to maintain upright stance. The motor program consists of a pattern for muscle activation that is sequenced in a distal to proximal order. Horak and Nashner called the resultant motor response an ankle synergy. If the individual sways backwards, a sequence of muscle activation occurs to maintain the upright position. First the anterior tibialis, then the quadriceps, and finally the abdominal muscles are activated.

If the individual stands facing perpendicular to the length of a narrow walking or balance beam and is perturbed forward or backward, a different motor response occurs. In this instance a proximal to distal sequence of muscle activation occurs. Neuroscientists call this motor behavior a hip synergy. When a person is standing on a flat surface and is suddenly pushed, a motor program will be activated. Some individuals will use a hip synergy, some will use an ankle synergy. If the push exceeds the critical limits of either synergy, a new motor program, a step, occurs or else the individual may stumble or fall. The balance response in this instance is compensatory, because the individual does not expect to be pushed. What would happen if the individual knows he will be pushed? The resultant balance response would be anticipatory. The individual might use either an ankle or hip strategy, or might take a step if the push exceeded the critical limits of either strategy.

Fixed versus relative parameters

For coordinated movement to occur, some characteristics of the motor program must be fixed. A fixed parameter is an absolute or invariant parameter. Other relative parameters are added to the program and vary with respect to the intended motor outcome. Coordinated movement is defined as an orderly sequence of muscle activity necessary to produce appropriate motor behavior. Sequence or order of muscle activation is a fixed characteristic of the motor program. For example, muscle A is activated before muscle B, and so on. The muscle sequence for maintaining standing balance and the muscle sequence for walking are examples of fixed sequences.

Neuroscientists believe duration of muscle activity is a fixed characteristic and is expressed as a ratio. For example, muscle A is active for 10% of the duration of the motor activity and muscle B is active 50% of the time. The ratio of A:B is 1:5. Grillner[7] examined both muscle sequences and timing (phasing ratios) in the gait cycle of the cat. He noted that the program contained a specific muscle sequence and specific duration ratios for muscle activity. He believes that this program resides in a central pattern generator for each limb. Fixed sequences of muscle activity with a fixed ratio of activation are also found in motor programs for dynamic balance abilities.

A third characteristic of the motor program that researchers believe is fixed is the force generated by the muscles. This characteristic is also expressed as a ratio. For example, if muscle A and muscle B have a ratio of 1:2, then muscle A will generate one half as much force as muscle B.

Parameters that can change the motor program include, for example, amplitude, speed, and selection of muscles. Application of a stimulus to the dorsum of the foot of the cat during the swing phase of gait causes an increase in limb flexion. The overall muscle sequence in the motor program remains intact. If someone writes a sentence on a piece of paper and writes the same sentence on a blackboard, the sequence of letter production will the same, but the overall amplitude or excursion of movement will increase when writing on the blackboard. However, the fixed ratio for amplitude of muscle force will remain unchanged. The amplitude of the upstroke for an "r" will be larger on the blackboard but the ratio of muscle forces will remain unchanged. The duration of movement relative to writing on a piece of paper versus writing on the blackboard will be different; however, the ratio for muscle durations will remain fixed.

These relative parameters for the motor program may be self-limiting or limited by constraints imposed by the environment or the body. For example, the amplitude of writing on the blackboard is limited by the height of the blackboard, the length of the arm, or overall height of the person stretching to make the letter larger.

As stated above, overall speed of a motor program can be increased or decreased. In gait, a person can increase speed by decreasing the stance phase and, to a lesser extent, by decreasing the swing phase. When hip extension reaches maximum excursion, the limits for the motor program for walking are reached and transition to running occurs. Each of us has experienced this phenomena when we are late to a class or a meeting. We increase speed of walking until we reach a certain speed, then we begin to run. The question remains whether specific motor programs for walking and running are available or whether there is a generalized motor program with the goal of reaching point B as quickly as possible. To determine if walking and running are specific motor programs or encompass a generalized motor program, researchers compare the fixed ratios of muscle sequencing, duration, and force. They determine whether the fixed ratios for walking and running are the same or different.

Roles of sensory information

The CNS uses sensory information in a variety of ways in the process of motor control. Before initiating movement, information about the position of the body in space, body parts to one another, and environmental conditions is obtained from sensory receptors. This information is used in selection and execution of the motor program. During movement, various brain centers use sensory information to determine if the actual motor behavior is the same as the intended motor behavior. If the actual and intended motor behavior do not match, an error signal results. The motor program is altered so that the intended motor activity can occur.

Some movements such as ballistic movements do not rely on sensory feedback loops to revise the execution of the motor program. For example, a baseball pitcher throws a fastball in a relatively short period and does not rely on feedback to control the movement during execution.

Another role of sensory information is to characterize the movement by revising existing motor programs before executing the motor programs again. It enables the performer to know what was done to produce a specific result. For example, a person is trying to stand on a balance beam with feet close together and she falls off the balance beam. An error signal occurs because the intended motor behavior and the actual motor behavior differ. If the performer knows that her feet were close together when the fall occurred, then the next time she will space her feet further apart. The information about what happened, falling or not falling, is called knowledge of results (KR). The CNS stores KR with information about foot spacing and uses its later motor programs for balancing on any narrow object, be it a balance beam or a log.

Several researchers have investigated whether peripheral feedback is necessary for the regulation of movement as it take place.[13,21] Rothwell and others[19] studied a patient with a unilateral deafferented upper extremity. The deficit was caused by a peripheral sensory neuropathy. The individual could write sentences with his eyes closed and drive a car with a manual transmission without watching the gear shift, but he had difficulty with fine-motor tasks, such as buttoning a shirt and using a knife and fork. He was also unable to sustain a muscle contraction using a pincer grasp and with his eyes closed, and he could not learn to drive a new car with a manual transmission. Based on these observations, continued peripheral feedback may not be necessary when executing a motor program. However, neuroscientists believe that peripheral feedback is necessary during the acquisition or learning of motor programs that are not inherent.

Errors in motor control

Sometimes actual motor behavior does not match the intended motor behavior. When this phenomenon happens, one or several errors working alone or in combination may be the cause of the problem. This section will discuss several kinds of errors.

One type is selecting the wrong motor program. For example, a person is unexpectedly and forcefully pushed. The individual selects a motor program, ankle strategy, to maintain upright stance. If the person falls, we can postulate that the individual selected the wrong motor program.

Although an ankle strategy is a proper program for maintaining balance, it is inappropriate for this situation because the person fell.

Selection of the wrong motor pattern can also occur when there is sensory conflict in the environment. For example, a person stopped at a red light is looking forward; peripheral vision picks up a car rolling backward. The individual slams on the brakes and sheepishly realizes that his car is not rolling. What happened? Input from peripheral vision identified movement, but information from the vestibular receptors was not used to select the response. An error in determining initial condition occurred. The resultant motor behavior is correct for the visual information, but it is not correct for the situation if both visual and vestibular information were assessed.

An individual may select an appropriate motor program but use inappropriate relative parameters. A classic example is lifting a box full of textbooks. The CNS has stored a previous experience of lifting textbooks in motor memory, and one characteristic stored is the concept that textbooks (particularly those for physical therapy) are heavy. As a result, the CNS adjusts the relative amplitude for the motor program for lifting heavy books. The person lifts the box and almost throws it in the air because it is so light. The individual used the correct motor program for lifting; however, the amplitude was inappropriate.

Errors also occur when unexpected factors disrupt the execution of the program. For example, an individual walks on a moving sidewalk. When the individual steps off the sidewalk, a disruption in walking occurs. The individual's first few steps are not smooth. The individual is still using the motor program that contains information about a moving support surface. As a result, an error occurs when the individual steps onto the stationary support surface.

Errors can occur in the selection of the program, selection of the variable parameters, or in the execution of the motor program. Errors in motor programming in patients are generally the result of a neurological deficit. An assessment of motor deficits in patients should include analysis of motor programming errors.

SUMMARY

Motor control was once thought to be a step-by-step hierachical system. Today researchers and clinicians have become increasingly aware that the systems involved in the potential motor responses available to an individual are multidimensional. Realizing that one-to-one relationships in the motor system may exist only within certain systems, clinicians now have many alternatives when analyzing motor control. This understanding also gives flexibility when evaluating and treating a client that has suffered insult.

Systems theories have enlarged the therapist's knowledge of the learning potential of both the normal and damaged motor systems. Research is continually unravelling mysteries of CNS function, recovery patterns following insult, and alternatives available to therapists when treating motor control problems. All the answers have not been found, but by improving the understanding of motor control, the scientific basis for many alternative treatment approaches can be better established. Similarly, the reasons why seemingly different approaches cause similar observable changes in motor output can be explained.

REFERENCES

1. Allum JHJ and Keshner EA: Vestibular and proprioceptive control of sway stabilization. In Bles W, editor: Disorders of posture and gait, New York, 1986, Elsevier Publishing Co.
2. Brinkman C: Supplementary motor area of the monkey's cerebral cortex: short- and long-term deficits after unilateral ablation and the effects of subsequent callosal section, J Neurosci 4:918-929, 1984.
3. Davis WJ: Organizational concepts in the central motor networks of invertebrates. In Herman RM and others, editors: Neural control of locomotion, New York, 1976, Plenum Press.
4. DeLong MR and Georgopoulos AP: Motor functions of the basal ganglia. In Brooks VB, editor: The nervous system, vol II; Motor control, part 2, Bethesda, Md, 1981, American Physiological Society.
5. DeLong MR: Motor functions of the basal ganglia: single-unit activity during movement. In Schmitt FO and Worden FG editors: The neurosciences, third study program, Cambridge, Mass, The MIT Press.
6. Evarts, EV: Relation of pyramidal tract activity to force exerted during voluntary movement, J Neurophysiol 31:14-27, 1968.
7. Grillner S. Control of locomotion in bipeds, tetrapods, and fish. In Brooks VB, ed: Handbook of physiology (section 1), The nervous system, vol 2; Motor control, part 2, Bethesda, Md, 1981, American Physiological Society.
8. Horak FB and Nashner LM: Central programming of postural movements: adaptation to altered support-surface configurations, J Neurophysiol 55:1369-1381, 1986.
9. Jackson H: The Croonian lectures on evolution and dissolution of the nervous system, Br Med J :591-593.
10. Kornhuber HH: Motor functions of cerebellum and basal ganglia: the cerebellocortical saccadic (ballistic) clock, the cerebellonuclear hold regulator, and the basal ganglia ramp (voluntary speed smooth movement) generator, Kybernetik 8:157-162, 1971.
11. Kuypers HGHM: Anatomy of the descending pathways. In Brooks VB, editor: The nervous system, vol II; Motor control, part 2, Bethesda, Md, 1981, American Physiological Society.
12. Lee DN and Arronson E: Visual proprioceptive control of standing in human infants, Perception and Psychophysics 15:527-532, 1974.
13. Marsden CD and others: The use of peripheral feedback in the control of movement. In Evarts EV and others, editor: The motor system in neurobiology, Amsterdam, 1985, Elsevier Biomedical Press.
14. Martin JP: The basal ganglia and posture, London, 1967, Pitman Publishing Ltd.
15. Mountcastle VB and others: Posterior parietal association cortex of the monkey: command functions for operations within extrapersonal space, J Neurophysiol 38:871-908, 1975.
16. Nashner LM and McCollum: The organization of human postural movements: a formal basis and experimental synthesis, Behav Brain Sci 8:135-172, 1985.

17. Newton R: Current perspectives on neural control. Proceedings of the Tenth International Congress of the World Confederation for Physical Therapy, Sydney, Australia, 1987, pp 394-398.

18. Roland PE and others: Supplementary motor area and other cortical areas in organization of voluntary movements in man, J Neurophysiol 43:118-136, 1980.

19. Rothwell JC and others: Manual motor performance in a deafferented man, Brain 105:515-542, 1982.

20. Schmidt RA: Motor control and learning: a behavioral emphasis, ed 2, Champaign, Ill, 1988, Human Kinetics Publishers Inc.

21. Taub E: Movements in nonhuman primates deprived of somatosensory feedback, Exercise Sport Sci Rev 4:335-374, 1976.

Chapter 4

LIMBIC SYSTEM
Influence over motor control and learning

Darcy Ann Umphred and Marlene B. Appley

As stated at the end of Chapter 2, the understanding of the nervous system is based on viewing it as a total entity. The puzzle may initially consist of 5 to 10 pieces that fit together, but when interlocked give the student a feeling of accomplishment and intellectual mastery. The process of unlocking and reassembling the puzzle while either subdividing each original puzzle piece or adding new pieces is the journey a student begins in school and can, if so chosen, continue throughout life.

The traditional way to analyze and study brain function is to first approach the hard-core science (i.e., anatomy and physiology). Then the learner studies normal function as it relates to anatomy and physiology. At this level, behavior patterns expressing the specific functions might be introduced. Finally, dysfunction is presented. The study of dysfunction often relates animal studies to potential function in humans. The validity of these correlations are always questionable.

The complexity of the anatomy, physiology, and neuro-chemistry of the limbic system baffles the minds of basic science doctoral students. Yet a therapist deals on a moment-to-moment functional level with the limbic system of clients throughout the day.

This chapter was initially written using a traditional educational and textbook presentation. When put together as a whole, the complexity of the limbic system became overwhelming. It became apparent that colleagues would drown in the basic science presentation before they reached the application. Thus, a nontraditional presentation has been used in this chapter. An overview of the limbic system is followed by a section on functional application, including limbic lesions and their influence on the therapeutic environment. The later sections introduce the anatomy and physiology at an in-depth level. The goal of this chapter is to persuade the student that limbic function drastically effects the clinical environment. Once acceptance of the primary objective is achieved, it is hoped that the reader will be enticed to study further the basic science sections to understand more fully the true function of the limbic system.

THE LIMBIC SYSTEM: ITS FUNCTIONAL RELATIONSHIP TO CLINICAL PERFORMANCE
Overview: the limbic system's role in motor control, memory, and learning

It is not easy to find a generally accepted definition of the "limbic system," its boundaries, and the components that should be included. Mesulam[25] likens this to a 5th century BC philosopher's quotation: "the nature of God is like a circle of which the center is everywhere and the circumference is nowhere." Brodal[7] suggests that functional

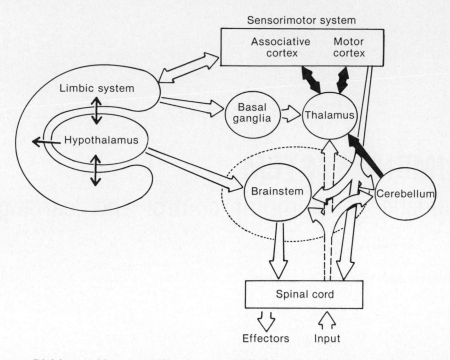

Fig. 4-1. Divisions and interconnections between the limbic and nonlimbic (sensorimotor) cortex.

separation of brain regions becomes less clear as we discover the interrelatedness through ongoing research. He sees the limbic system reaching out and encompassing the entire brain and all of its functional components and sees no purpose in defining such a subdivision.

Though the anatomical descriptions of the limbic system may vary from author to author, the functional significance of this system is widely acknowledged in defining human behavior and behavioral neurology.

Brooks[8] divides the brain into the limbic brain and the nonlimbic sensorimotor brain. The sensorimotor portion is involved in perception of nonlimbic sensations and motor performance. The limbic brain is primitive, essential for survival, sensing the "need" to act, and thereby initiating need-directed motor activity for survival. The limbic brain also has the capability for memory and can select what to learn from experience. Brooks also defines the two brain systems functionally and not anatomically, since their anatomical separation according to function is almost impossible and changes with the task (Fig. 4-1).

Kandel and Schwartz[18] state that behavior requires three major systems: the sensory, the motor, and the motivational or limbic. When analyzing a seemingly simple action, such as swinging a golf club, we recruit our sensory system for visual, tactile, and proprioceptive input to guide the motor systems for precise, coordinated muscle recruitment and postural control. The motivational (limbic) system does the following: (1) it provides intentional drive for the initiation, (2) it integrates the total input, and (3) it

draws on its "stored" memories of responses to come up with the appropriately scheduled and executed goal-directed behavior. The motivational system controls the two motor systems: the autonomic system, which is only involved in motor functions, and the somatic sensorimotor system. It thereby controls both the skeletal muscles through input to the motor cortex and the smooth muscles and glands through the hypothalamus, which lies at the "heart" of the limbic system (Fig. 4-2). Cotman[12] summarizes the function of the limbic system as "keeping a body on the beam."

Morgane[33] conceptualizes the limbic system as the cortical, midbrain, and brainstem output of the hypothalamus, which affects visceral and endocrine functions, and therefore, behavior. He stresses the importance of looking at "intersegmental effects" rather than on the effect of any one brain segment. He proposes that "functions" are not localized to a specific structure or region, pathway, or neurosecretion, but should be viewed as associated with "circuit interactions" (for further discussion see section on Long-term potentiation—LTP). In Morgane's view, structures of circuits themselves can influence the resulting effector activity. The loss of any link can affect the outcome activity of the whole circuit. Thus, damage to any area of the brain can potentially cause malfunctions in any or all other areas, and the entire circuit may need reorganization to restore function.

Morgane does not ascribe specific single functions to CNS formations, but sees each become a part of a system, participating to various degrees in the multitude of behav-

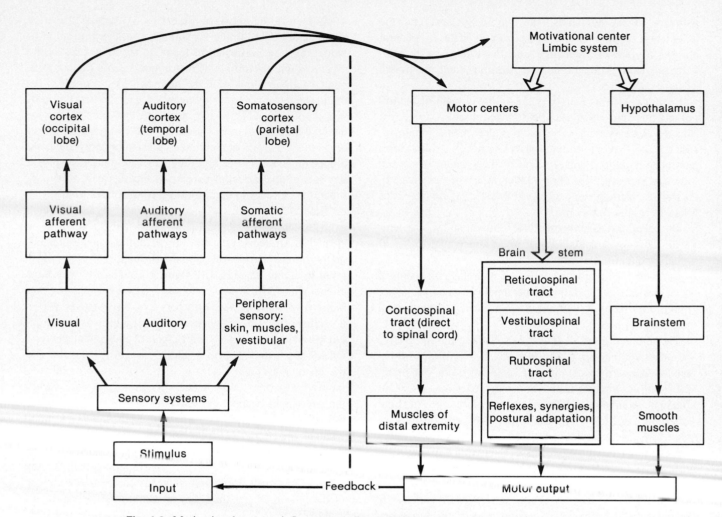

Fig. 4-2. Motivational systems influence over the sensorimotor and autonomic nervous systems. (Adapted from Kandel ER and Schwartz JH: Principles of neural science, ed 2, New York, 1985, Elsevier Science Publishing Co.)

ioral responses (see Chapters 2 and 3 for additional information). Therefore the loss of any part of higher centers or limbic system may not be clearly definable functionally, and the return of function is not always easy to predict. He suggests that there exists a "graded" localization of function that has a dynamic nature, assigning "specialized roles" in an integrated performance.

Recovery of function after injury may not involve a taking over by other brain areas, but may require a new "dynamic" system of interlinking areas of the brain. Morgane[33] calls it "behavioral reorganization during recovery." For complex behavior, such as in motor functioning requiring many steps, we should see for example the limbic system, cortex, hypothalamus, basal ganglia, and midbrain working as an integrated unit, with any damaged area causing the whole system to malfunction. A loss of function or a change in behavior cannot necessarily be localized as to the underlying cause. A lesion in one area may cause a malfunction of an area that is not actually damaged.

The complexity of the limbic system and its associative

influence over both the motor control system and cortical structures is enormous. A therapist dealing with a client with motor control or learning problems needs to understand how the limbic system affects behavioral responses. The knowledge base not only focuses on the client's deficits, but also on the integrative function of the therapist. This understanding should lead to a greater awareness of the clinical environment and which factors within the environment that cause change.

The limbic system's influence on behavior: its relevance to the therapeutic environment

Levels of behavioral hierarchies: where does the limbic system belong? Strub and Black[4] view behavior as occurring on distinct interrelated levels, which represent behavioral hierarchies. Starting at level one, a state of alertness to the internal and external environment must be maintained for motor or mental activity to occur. The brainstem reticular activating system brings about this state of general arousal by relating in an ascending pathway to the thalamus, the limbic system, and the association cortex. To proceed from a state of general arousal to one of "selective attention" requires the descending input from the cortex, thalamus, and the limbic system.

Level two of this hierarchy lies in the domain of the hypothalamus and its closely associated limbic structures. This level deals with subconscious drives and innate instincts. The survival-oriented drives of hunger, thirst, temperature regulation, and survival of the species (sex), and the steps necessary for drive reduction are processed here, as well as learning and memory. Most of these activities relate to limbic functioning.

On level three, only cerebral cortical areas are activated. This level deals with abstract conceptualization of verbal or quantitative entities.

Level four behavior is concerned with the expression of social aspects of behavior, personality, and life-style. Again, the limbic system and its relationship to the frontal lobe are vital here.

The interaction of all four levels leads to the integrative and adaptable behavior seen in humans. Our ability to become alert and protectively react is balanced by our previous learning, whether it be cognitive-perceptive, social, or affective. Adaptability to rapid changes in the physical environment, in life-styles, and in personal relationships results from the interrelationships or complex neurocircuitry of the human brain. When insult occurs at any one level within these behavioral hierarchies, all levels may be affected.

The limbic system MOVEs us. Moore[32] eloquently describes the limbic system as the area of the brain that moves us. The word *move* can be used as a mnemonic for the functions of the limbic system.

Limbic system function*

Memory/motivation: drive
1. Memory: attention and retrieval
2. Motivation: desire to learn, try, or benefit from the environment

Olfaction (especially in infants)
1. Only sensory system that does not go through the thalamus as its second-order synapse in the sensory pathway before it gets to the cerebral cortex

Visceral (drives: thirst, hunger, temperature regulation, endocrine functions)
1. Sympathetic and parasympathetic reactions
2. Peripheral autonomic nervous system (ANS) responses that reflect limbic function

Emotion: feelings and attitude
1. Self-concept and worth
2. Emotional body image
3. Tonal responses of motor system
4. Attitude, social skills, opinions

*Adapted from a lecture by Moore J, Fifteenth Annual Sensorimotor Integration Symposium, San Diego, July, 1987.

As seen in the above outline, the "M" depicts the drive component of the limbic system. Before learning, an individual must be motivated to learn, to try to succeed at the task, to solve the problem, or to benefit from the environment. Without motivation the brain will not orient itself to the problem and learn. However, once motivated the individual must be able to pay attention and process the sequential and simultaneous nature of the component parts to be learned, as well as the whole. The limbic amygdala and hippocampal structures and their intricate circuitries play a key role in this aspect of memory. Once learned, the information is stored and can be retrieved at a later time.

The "O" refers to the incoming sense of smell, which exerts a strong influence on alertness and drive. This is clearly illustrated by the billions of dollars spent annually on perfumes, deodorants, mouthwashes, and soap. This input tract can be used effectively by therapists who have clients with CNS lesions, such as internal capsule and thalamic involvement. The olfactory system synapses within the olfactory bulb and then with the limbic system structures before traveling to the thalamus and higher centers. Other senses may not be reaching the cortical levels, and the client may have a sensory-deprived environment. Olfactory sensations, which enter the limbic system before thalamic input connections, may be used to calm or arouse the client. The specific olfactory input may determine whether the person remains calm or emotionally aroused. Pleasant odors would be preferable to most people.

A comatose and seemingly nonresponsive client may respond to odor. The therapist needs to be *acutely* aware of the responses, for they may be autonomic instead of somatomotor.

The "V" represents visceral or autonomic drives. As noted earlier, the hypothalamus is nestled within the limbic system. Thus regulation of sympathetic and parasympathetic reactions, both of the internal organ systems and the periphery, reflect ongoing limbic activity. Obviously, drives such as thirst, hunger, temperature regulation, and sexuality are controlled by this system. Clients demonstrating total lack of inhibitory control over eating or drinking or manifesting very unstable body temperature regulation may be exhibiting signs of limbic involvement.

Less obvious autonomic responses that may reflect limbic imbalances often go unnoticed by therapists. When the stress of an activity is becoming overwhelming to a client, he or she may react with severe sweating of the palms or an increase in dysreflexic activity in the mouth area rather than heightened motor activity. A therapist must continually monitor this aspect of the client's response behaviors to ascertain that the behaviors observed reflect motor control and not limbic influences over that motor system.

If the input to the client is excessive, the limbic system will not function at the optimal level and learning will diminish. The client may withdraw physically or mentally, lose focus or attention, decrease his motivation, and get frustrated or even angry. All of these behaviors may be expressed within the hypothalamic/autonomic system as output. The evaluation of this system seems even more critical when a client's motor control system is locked, with no volitional movement present. Therapists often try to increase motor activity through sensory input, however, they must cautiously avoid indiscriminately bombarding the sensory systems. The limbic system may demonstrate overload while the spinal motor generators reflect inadequate activation. Although the two systems are different, they are intricately connected, and the concept of massively bombarding one while ignoring the other does not make sense in a learning framework.

"E" relates to emotions, the feelings and attitudes unique to that individual. This refers especially to the amygdaloid aspect of the limbic system. This is a primary emotional center, and it regulates not only our self-concept, but our attitudes and opinions toward our environment and the people within it.

Self-concept is the emotional aspect of body image. For example, assume that one morning I looked in the mirror and said, "The poor world, I will not subject it to me today." I then go back to bed and eat nothing for the rest of the day. The next day I get up and look in the same mirror and say, "What a change, I look trim and beautiful. Look out world, here I come!" In reality my physical body has not been altered drastically, if at all, but my attitude toward that body has changed. That is, the emotional component of my body image has perceptually changed.

A second self-concept deals with my attitude about my worth or value to society and the world and my role within it. Again this attitude can change with mood, but more often it seems to change with experience. This aspect of client/therapist interaction can be critical to the success of a therapeutic environment. Two examples will be given to illustrate this point, with the focus of bringing perceived roles into the therapeutic setting:

1. Your client is Mrs. S., a 72-year-old woman with a left cerebroventricular accident (CVA). She comes from a low socioeconomic background, and was a housekeeper for 40 years for a wealthy family of high social standing. When addressing you (the therapist) she always says "yes, ma'am" or "no, ma'am," and does just what was asked, no more and no less. It may be very hard to get this client to assume responsibility for self-direction in the therapeutic setting. Her perceived role in life may not be to take responsibility or authority within a setting that may have high social status, such as a medical facility. She also may feel that she does not have the power to assume such responsibilities. Success in the therapeutic setting may be based more on changing her attitudes than on motor control.
2. Your client is a 24-year-old lumberjack who suffered a closed head injury (CHI) during a fall at work. It is now 1 month since his accident, and he is

totally alert, verbal, angry, and has moderate to severe motor control problems. During your initial treatment you note that he responds very well to handling. He seems to flow with your movement, and with your assistance is able to practice much higher level motor control. At the end of therapy he sits back in his chair with much better function. Then he turns to you (the female therapist) and instead of saying "That was great," he says, "You witch, I hate you." The inconsistency between how his body responded to your handling and his attitude toward you as a person may seem baffling, until you realize that he has always perceived himself as a dominant male. Similarly, he perceives women as weak, to be protected, and in need of control. If his attitude toward you cannot be changed to see you in a generic professional role, he will most likely not benefit as much from your clinical skills.

Preconceived attitudes, social behaviors, and opinions have been learned by filtering the input through the limbic system. If new attitudes and behaviors need to be learned following a neurological insult, the intactness especially of the amygdaloid pathways seem crucial (see the section on anatomy). Damage to these limbic structures may prevent learning and thus socially maladaptive behavior may persist, making the individual less likely to adapt to his social environment.

As our feelings, attitudes, and values drive our behaviors both through attention and motor responses, the emotional aspect of the limbic system has great impact on our learning and motor control. Placing too little value on a motor output often leads to complacency and lack of learning. On the other hand, placing an extremely high value on a motor output or learning skills, such as in a cognitive test situation, can overload the system and decrease function.

Motivation and reward. Moore[32] considers motivation and memory as part of the MOVE system. Stellar and Stellar[45] link motivation with reward and help, illustrating how the limbic system learns through repetition and reward. They state that the concept of motivation includes drive and satiation, goal-directed behavior and incentive. They recognize that these behaviors maintain homeostasis and ensure the survival of the individual and the species. The hypothalamus and the other limbic components are involved in motivational behavior, which is a product of the balance of excitatory and inhibitory input from external and internal stimuli.[36]

Motivated behavior is geared to reinforcement and reward. Repeated experience of reinforcement and reward lead to learning, changed expectancy, changed behavior, and maintained performance.[33] Repetition with the feeling of success (reinforcement) is a critical element in the therapeutic setting, and consistently making the task more difficult just when the client feels ready to succeed will tend to decrease reinforcement/reward and thus lessen the client's motivation to try. With the pressure placed on therapists to produce changes quickly, repetition and thus long-term learning are often jeopardized and this may have a dramatic effect on the quality of the client's life and the long-term treatment effects once he or she leaves the medical facility.

Integration of the limbic system as part of a whole functioning brain. Motivation, alertness, and concentration are critical in motor learning because they determine how well we pay attention to the learning and execution of any motor task. These processes of learning and doing are inevitably intertwined: "we learn as we do, and we do only as well as we have learned."[8]

Both motivation or "feeling the need to act" and con-

centration are contributed by the limbic system. As discussed later in the neuroanatomy portion of this chapter, the amygdaloid complex with its multitude of afferent and efferent interlinkages is especially adapted for recognizing the significance of a stimulus and it assigns the emotional aspect of feeling the need to act. This leads to need-directed and therefore goal-directed motor activity. It also filters out the significant from the nonsignificant information by selective processing and storing the significant for memory, learning, and recall.

Goal-directed or need-directed motor actions are the result of the nervous system structures acting in an interactive hierarchy system, which is also a functional, dynamic

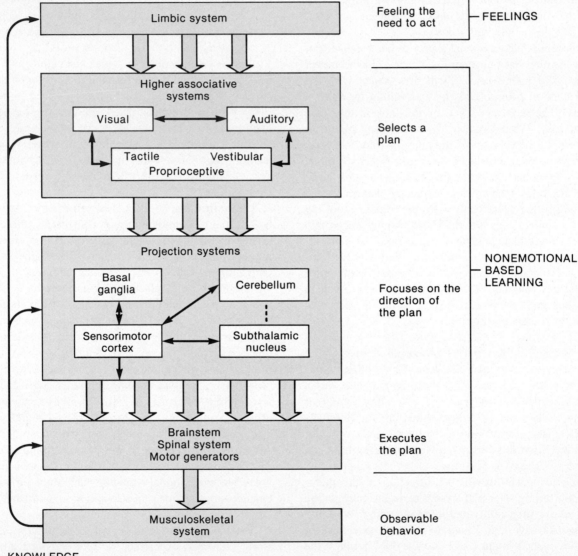

Fig. 4-3. Functional and dynamic hierarchy of systems based on both limbic and motor control interactions. (From Brooks VB: The neural basis of motor control, New York, 1986, Oxford University Press.)

hierarchy based on systems interacting together. In this system (Fig. 4-3), the highest level is represented by the limbic system and its cortical and subcortical components. In response to stimuli from the internal or external environment, the limbic system initiates motor activity out of the emotional aspect of feeling the need to act. This message is relayed to the association areas of the cerebral cortex, which could entail any one or all of association areas for visual, auditory, tactile, olfactory, gustatory, or proprioceptive input. These associative areas are located in the prefrontal, occipital, parietal, and temporal lobes, where they analyze and integrate sensory input into an overall strategy of action or a general plan that meets the requirements of the task. Therefore, the association cortex recognizes, selects, and prepares to act as a response to relevant sensory cues when a state of arousal is provided by reticular input. The thalamus, cerebellum, and basal ganglia contribute to the production of the specific motor plans. These messages of the general plan are relayed to the middle level or "projection system" represented by the sensorimotor cortex, cerebellum, basal ganglia, subthalamic nucleus, and the substantia nigra. The limbic system has even more influence over the sensorimotor cortex via the cingulate gyrus. The cingulate gyrus (limbic cortex) is linked to motor control structures not only via the association cortex, but also via the basal ganglia and pontine nuclei that project to the cerebellum and thalamus, which lead directly to the sensorimotor cortex.[18] These loops enable further control of limbic instructions over motor control. Here, in the middle level, the specifics are programmed and the tactics are given a strategy. In general, the "what" is turned into "how" and "when." The necessary parameters for coordinated movement are programmed here as to intensity, sequencing, and timing to carry out the motor task. These programs are then sent to the lower level, which involves the upper motor neurons, brainstem projection fibers, and the spinal system of the lower motor neuron, the final common pathway that sends orders for the specific motor tasks to the musculoskeletal system (see Chapter 3 for a more specific discussion of the motor control system). The actions of the lower level are constantly looped back to middle level structures for adjustments of intensity and duration, also the cerebral association cortex assesses feedback from sensory centers and from the middle and higher levels of the motor sequence described above. In summary, the highest level in this sequence is the limbic system, which generates need-directed motor activity that is sent to be analyzed and integrated by the association cortex, where the appropriate plan of action is selected that corresponds to the relevant sensory information received from the internal and external environment. This step is vital to client care, because we have to give clients the opportunity to correctly analyze both their internal environment (their current posture from which they start their exercise and their emotional state)

and their external environment (the world around them and the requirements of the task), so that they can produce an appropriate strategy for the task at hand. These instructions must be correct, so that the projection system (middle level) can instruct the lower level to carry out the motor activity through the musculoskeletal system.[47]

Verbants[47] stresses the significance of "knowledge of results feedback" as being the information from the environment that provides the individual with insights into task requirements. This insight helps the highest levels correctly select strategies that will successfully initiate and support the appropriate movements for accomplishing the task. This knowledge of results feedback is required for effective motor learning and to form the correct "motor engrams." Brooks[8] distinguishes between insightful learning, which is programmed and leads to skills when the performer has gained insight into the requirements, and discontinuous movements are replaced by continuous ones. This process is hastened when the clients understand and can demonstrate their understanding of what "they were expected to do." Improvement of motor skills is possible by using programmed movement in goal-directed behavior. Learning through insight into task requirements properly cues the interaction of the limbic system with the association cortex in the selection of the motor plan to be passed down the hierarchial or systems chain for producing movement.

Without the knowledge of results, feedback, and insight into the requirements for goal directed activity, the learning is performing by "rote," which merely utilizes repetition without analysis, and little meaningful learning or building of effective motor memory in the form of motor engrams will occur.

Verbants[46] suggests that to elicit this highest level of function within the motor hierarchy and to enable insightful learning, therapy programs should be developed around goal-directed activities. These activities direct the client to analyze the environmental requirements (both internal and external) by placing the client in a situation that forces development of "appropriate strategies." Goal-directed activities should be functional behavior and thus involve motivation, meaningfulness, and selective attention. All three components are limbic in nature. Verbants[47] further suggests that specific techniques such as proprioceptive neuromuscular facilitation (PNF), neurodevelopmental therapy (NDT), Rood, and Feldenkrais can be incorporated into goal-directed activities in the therapy programs. With insights into the learned skills, clients will be better able to adjust these to meet the specific requirements of different environments and needs, using knowledge of response feedback to guide them. The message then is to design exercise or programs that are meaningful and need directed, to motivate clients into insightful goal-directed learning. Thus, understanding the specific goals of the client is important. A therapist cannot assume that "someone wants to do something." The goal of running a bank may seem very different than that of bird-watching in the mountains, yet both may require ambulatory skills. If a client does not wish to return to work, then a friendly smile and stating, "Hi, I'm your therapist and I'm going to get you up and walking so you can get back to work," may lead to resistance and decreased motivation. In contrast, by knowing the goal of the client, a person highly motivated to ambulate may be present in the clinic every day to meet the goal of bird-watching in the mountains.

Clinical perspectives

The client's internal system influences observable behavior. At least once a year almost any local newspaper will carry a story that generally reads as follows:

Seventy-nine–year-old, 109-pound arthritic grandmother picks up car by bumper to free trapped 3-year-old grandson.

All of us read these articles and at first doubt their validity and then question the sensationalism used by the reporter. I (D.U.) would also question such news reporting if, at age 13, I had not seen three teenage boys pick up a 1956 Chevrolet and put it back in the garage in its correctly parked position. The boys had moved the car because they feared that if they did not put the car back into its original parked position, their parents would find out that they had driven the car without a license or permission. That elderly lady picked up the car out of fear of severe injury to her grandchild. Emotions can create tremendous high tonal responses, either static as in a temper tantrum or dynamic as in picking up the car.

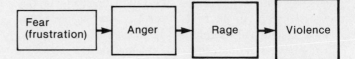

Fig. 4-4. Fear-anger-rage-violence: FARV continuum.

One sequence of behaviors used to describe the emotional circuitry of the amygdala is called the FARV (Fear, Anger, Rage, Violence) continuum[31] (Fig. 4-4). This continuum begins with fear, often exhibited as frustration by children. If the event inducing the fear continues to heighten, anger will often develop. From anger the person may go next into rage and finally violence. How quickly any individual will progress from fear to violence depends on many factors. First, the hard-wiring or genetic predisposition will influence their behavioral responses. Second, their soft-wired or conditioned responses resulting from environmental influences and reinforcement patterns will determine output. For example, it is commonly known that abusive parents were usually abused children; they learned that anger quickly lead to violence, and that the behavior was acceptable. Third, the stimulus and its intensity will determine the level of response.

Anger itself creates tone through the amygdaloid's influence over both the basal ganglia and associative cortex and their influence over the motor control cortex and output (Fig. 4-5). This is clearly exhibited in a child throwing a temper tantrum (Fig. 4-6) or an adult putting his fist through a wall.

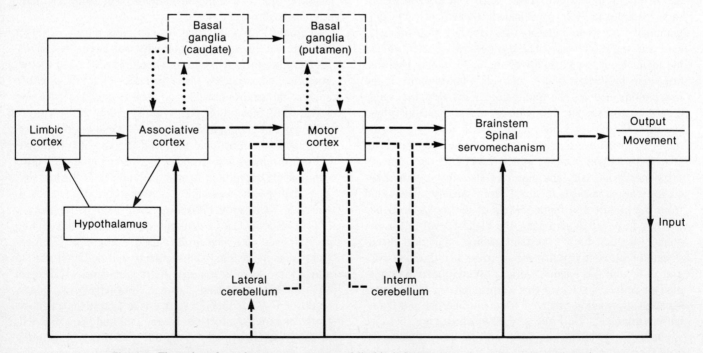

Fig. 4-5. Flow chart for voluntary movement and limbic influence over that movement. (Adapted from Brooks VB: The neural basis of motor control, New York, 1986, Oxford University Press.)

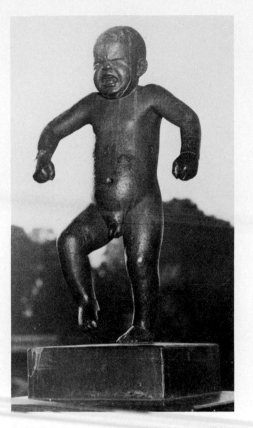

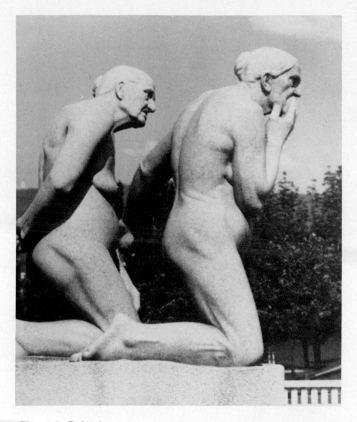

Fig. 4-6. Behavior responses caused by anger. ("Angry Boy," Vigelund Sculpture Grounds in the Frogner Park, Oslo, Norway. Adapted from photo by Normann.)

Fig. 4-7. Behavior responses elicited by concern, pain, grief. (Vigelund Sculpture Grounds in the Frogner Park, Norway. Adapted from photo by Normann.)

Emotions such as grief or depression can be exhibited within the motor system,[18] and one normally sees a decrease in motor output with these emotions. The behavioral responses are usually withdrawal, decreased postural adaption, and often a feeling of tiredness and exhaustion (Fig. 4-7). Sensory overload, especially in the elderly, can create the same pattern of response of flexion, internal rotation, and adduction. Again, it is hypothesized that these motor responses are the result of the limbic system's influence over motor control and not the motor control system itself.

Because of the potency of the limbic system's connections into the motor system, a therapist's sensitivity to the emotional state of a client would obviously be a key factor in understanding the motor responses observed during therapy. In Fig. 4-8 an entire spectrum of motor responses can be observed in the four statues. If a client is frustrated or angry and simultaneously has rigidity, spasticity, or general high tone, then a therapist might spend the entire session trying to decrease the motor response. If the client could be helped to deal with the anger or frustration during the therapy session, and thus release the emotion from the motor control system, then the specific motor control problems could be treated effectively. Differentiating the limbic system from the motor control system and establishing

treatment protocols for each may not be within the spectrum of a therapist's skills. Thus, working simultaneously with another professional such as a psychologist, social worker, or neuropsychologist may be an acceptable alternative approach. This cotreatment will allow all aspects of the client to be addressed simultaneously. Carryover of procedural learning (pure motor learning; see discussion of neurobiology of learning and memory for details) into adaptive motor responses need to be practiced with consistency.[18] The influence of the limbic system when the client is oscillating according to large mood swings may drastically dampen the procedural learning and limit the success of the therapeutic setting.

Limbic concepts influencing therapist/client interactions. How a clinician reacts at any given moment during a therapeutic session depends on both the client's and the clinician's declarative problem-solving skills and their procedural motor skills (see discussion of neurobiology of learning and memory). The limbic/declarative system drives our motor responses; therefore, the sensitivity of and the specific level of attention of the therapist toward the responses of the client depend on the clinician's limbic system.

When analyzing what differentiates a truly gifted or

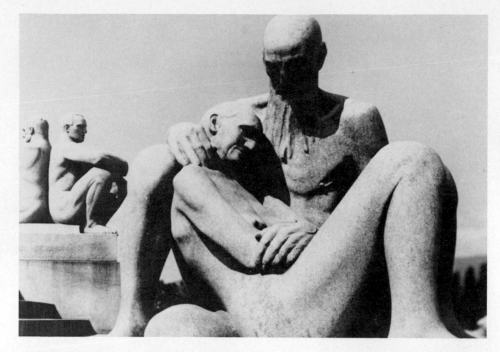

Fig. 4-8. Grief, depression and compassion responses are seen in the center figures, and rigid, stoic, distancing behaviors are observed in the left two male statues. (Vigelund Sculpture Grounds in the Frogner Park, Oslo, Norway. Adapted from photo by Normann.)

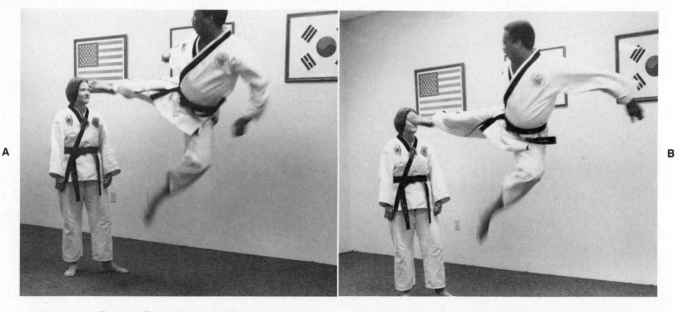

Fig. 4-9. Trust relaxes the limbic system's need to protect. **A,** The skill of the teacher is obvious. **B,** The student trusts that she is in no danger.

master clinician from a group of highly skilled and talented colleagues, the following philosophical concepts may be expressed:

1. That person has a rare gift.
2. That person seems to intuitively know what to do or what the client needs.
3. When that clinician treats a client, the two seem to flow together in their movements.
4. The client seems to totally trust that clinician; I have never seen that before.
5. I cannot believe that the client accurately did that with that clinician; before, the client was too afraid.

There are many factors in an interactive setting, such as therapy, that cannot be identified, but certain limbic/emotional factors that may play a role in that gifted clinician's skill can be mentioned.[21]

Trust/responsibility.[21] Trust is a critical component of a successful therapeutic session. The therapist gains the client's trust by his or her actions. Honesty and truth lead to trust.[21] Telling someone you will not hurt them and then continually ranging a joint beyond a pain-free range is neither honest nor truthful and will not lead to trust. That trust can be earned by stopping as soon as the client verbalizes pain or shows pain with a bodily response such as a grimace.

Once a client gives his or her trust, a clinician can freely move or move with a client and little resistance because of fear, reservations, or need to protect self will be felt or observed. Trust does not mean lack of awareness of potential danger; it means acceptance that although the danger is present, the potential of harm, pain, or disaster is very slight and the expected gain is worth the risk. In Fig. 4-9, *A* and *B*, the student's trust that the instructor will not hurt her can be seen by her lack of protective responses and by her calm, relaxed body posture. The student is aware of the potential of the kick, but trusts her life to the skills, control, and personal integrity of the teacher. Those same qualities are easily observed when watching a gifted clinician treat clients. The motor activities in a therapeutic setting are less complex that in Fig. 4-9, but in no way are they less stressful, less potentially harmful, or less frightening from the client's point of view.

Also, therapists must trust themselves enough to know that they can effect changes in their clients. Understanding their own motor system, how it responds, and how to use their hands, arms, or entire body to move someone else is based partly on procedural and partly on declarative learning (see Section IIB). Trusting that they have the skill to implement that motor response is limbic. If a therapist has self-doubts, it will change his or her motor performance, which will alter input to the client. This altered input can potentially alter the client's output and vary the desired responses.

Very close to the concept of trust is the idea of responsibility. Accepting responsibility for our own behavior seems obvious and is totally accepted as part of a professional role. Accepting and allowing the client the right to accept responsibility for his or her own environment is also a key element in creating a successful clinical environment and an independent person. Fig. 4-10 illustrates the concept through the following example:

The teacher (or therapist) asked the student (or client) to perform a motor act. In the figure, the act was to perform a kick to the teacher's head. The kick was to be very strong or forceful and completed. The student was told not to hold back or stop the kick in any way, yet the kick was to come within a few inches of the teacher's head. This placed tremendous responsibility on the

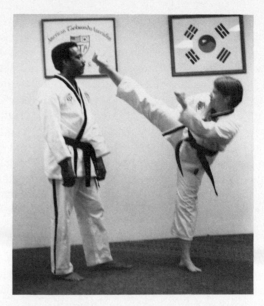

Fig. 4-10. The teacher relinquishes the task to the student and the student trusts the teacher is right even if self-doubt exists.

student. One inch too far might dangerously hurt the instructor, yet one inch too short was not acceptable. The teacher knew the student had the skill, power, and control to perform the task, and then passed the responsibility to the student. She was hesitant to assume the responsibility, for the consequence of failure could have been very traumatic, but the student trusted that the teacher would not ask for the behavior unless success was fairly guaranteed. That trust reduced anxiety and thus gave her more control over the act. Once the task was completed with success, the student gained confidence and could repeat the task with less fear or emotional influence while gaining refinement over motor control.

Although the motor activities are not as complex as in the example, the dynamics of the environment relate consistently with client/therapist roles and expectations. A gifted clinician knows that the client has the potential to succeed. When asked to perform, the client trusts the therapist and assumes the responsibility for the act. The therapist can facilitate the movement or postural pattern, thereby ensuring that the client succeeds. This feeling of success stimulates motivation for task repetition, which ultimately leads to learning. The incentive to repeat and learn becomes self-motivating and then becomes the limbic responsibility of the client. The task itself can be simple, such as a weight shift or a holding pattern, or as complex as climbing onto and off of a bus. No matter what the activity, the client needs to accept responsibility for his or her own behavior before independence in motor functioning can be achieved. Although the motor function itself is not limbic, many variables that lead to success, self-motivation, and feelings of independence are directly related to limbic circuitry.

Dedication to reality. Another component of a successful clinical environment deals with learning on the part of the therapist. A truly gifted therapist sees and feels what is happening within the motor control output system of the client. That therapist does not get stuck with what he or she has learned only because it was what was taught to them. Instead, learning is constantly related to past memories. Each client is a new map, only sketchy at the beginning and needs to be constantly revised as the client (terrain) changes. Similarly, the therapist will be able to transfer one motor activity into another spatial position. That is, the therapist can let go of an outdated map or treatment technique and create a new one as the environment and motor control system of the client changes. This transference or letting go of old maps or ideas is true for both the client and the therapist. If a position, pattern, or technique is not working, then the clinician needs to change the map or directions of treatment and let the client teach the therapist what will work. The ability to change and select new or alternative treatment techniques is based on the attitude of the therapist toward selecting alternative approaches. Willingness to be flexible is based on confidence in oneself, a truly emotional strategy or limbic behavior.

Vulnerability. To receive input from a client, a therapist has to be open to receive that information. If a clinician believes that he or she knows what each client needs and how to get those behaviors before meeting the client, then the client falls into a category of a recipe for treating the problem. Using the recipe does not mean the client cannot learn or gain better perceptual/cognitive, affective, or motor control, but it does mean that the individuality of the person may be lost. A more individualized approach would allow the clinician to identify through behavioral responses the best way for the client to learn, how to sequence the learning, when to make demands of the client, when to nurture, when to stop, when to continue, when to assist, when to have fun, when to laugh, or when to cry. An analogy might be that of going to a fast food restaurant versus a restaurant where each aspect of the meal is tailored to one's taste. It does not mean that both restaurants are not selling digestible foods. It does mean that at one eating place the food is mass produced with some choices, but individuality with respect to the consumer is not an aspect of the service.

To be open totally to processing the individual differences of the client, the clinician must be relaxed, nonthreatened, and feel no need to protect himself or herself from the external environment. It would seem that the clinician would be highly vulnerable, because of being open to new and as yet unanalyzed or unprocessed input. Being open must incorporate being sensitive to not only the variability of motor responses, but also the variability of emotional responses on the part of the client. This vulnerability leads to compassion, understanding, and acceptance of the client as a unique human being. All of these concepts are limbic, for they deal with the emotional component of declarative learning.

Limbic lesions and their influence on the therapeutic environment. There are many lesions or neurochemical imbalances within the limbic system that drastically effect the success or failure of physical, occupational, and other therapy programs. It is not within the scope of this chapter to discuss in detail specific problems and their treatment, but instead it is hoped that identification of the limbic involvement may help the reader develop a better understanding of specific neurological conditions.

Sensory overload. The autonomic responses to sensory overstimulation have been identified as following a specific course of behavioral changes and are referred to as the general adaptation syndrome (GAS).[35] The sequential stages of this syndrome directly relate to limbic imbalance and can play a dramatic role in determining client progress. Initial reaction to sensory overload creates a state of alarm or stress and triggers a strong sympathetic nervous system reaction. Heart rate, blood pressure, respiration, metabolism, and muscle tonus will increase. It is at this stage that the grandmother lifts the car off the child. If the overstimulation does not diminish, the body will protect itself from self-destruction and trigger a parasympathetic response. At this time, all the above symptoms reverse and the client exhibits a decrease in heart rate, blood pressure, and muscle tonus. The bronchi become constricted and the patient may hyperventilate and become dizzy, confused, and less alert. As the blood flow returns to the periphery, the face may flush and the skin becomes hot. The patient will have no energy to move, will withdraw, and again exhibit signs of flexion, adduction, internal rotation, and lack of postural tone.

There are 70 common symptoms identified in this overstimulation syndrome. If the acute symptoms are not eliminated, they will become chronic and the behavior patterns much more resistant to change.

GAS is often seen in the elderly, with various precipitating health crisis, and also in infants, head trauma victims, and other clients with neurological conditions. What causes the initial alarm can range from internal instability and minimal to mild external stress, to minimal internal instability and severe external sensory bombardment. Head traumas, inflammatory problems, and tumors often create hypersensitivity to external input such as noise, touch, or light. Normal clinical environments may create a sensory overload and trigger this general adaptation syndrome.

In the elderly, stresses such as change of environment, loss of loved ones, failing health, and fears of financial problems can each cause the client's system to react as if overloaded. Our elderly clients usually have two or more of these issues to deal with while trying to benefit from a therapeutic setting that demands their full attention for effective functioning. It is no wonder so many older clients shut down, withdraw from the therapeutic environment and eventually from the entire world, and become resistant and confused.

It is logical to assume that because of the autonomic responses that this syndrome evokes, strong interaction with the limbic system exists. Stress, no matter what the specific precipitating incident (confusion, fear, anxiety, grief, pain) has the potential of triggering the first steps in the sequence of this syndrome. The clinician's sensitivity to the client's limbic–emotional system will be the therapeutic technique that best controls and reverses the acute condition. Decreasing stimulation versus increasing facilitation may lead to attention, calmness, and receptiveness to therapy. When the client feels control over his or her life has been returned or at least the individual is consulted regarding decisions, often resistance to therapy or movement is released. Even semicomatose clients can participate to some extent. As a clinician begins to move a client, resistance may be encountered. If slight changes are made in rotation or trajectory of the movement pattern, the resistance is often lessened. If the clinician initially feels the resistance and overpowers it, total control has been taken from the client. Instead, if the clinician moves the patient in ways his or her body is willing to be moved, respect has been shown and overstimulation potentially avoided.

There is no one input that causes these reactions, nor is there one treatment to counteract its progression. Being aware of clinical signs is critical. Another important therapeutic skill is not prejudging withdrawn clients by assuming that they need more stimulation to regain function. The specific techniques appropriate for treating this syndrome are tools all therapists possess. How each clinician uses those tools is a critical link to success or failure in clinical interaction.

Alcoholism/drug abuse. Limbic epilepsy has been shown to be produced by systemic use of drugs such as cocaine and alcohol.[48] This type of seizure is often accompanied by sensory auras and alterations in behavior, with specific focus on mood shifts and cognitive dysfunction.[44] Obviously the precise association between behavior and emotions or temperolimbic and frontolimbic activity is not understood, yet the associations and thus their impact on a therapeutic setting cannot be ignored.

Whether they be street bought, medically administered, or ingested for private or social reasons, as in alcohol consumption, the effect of drugs and alcohol on the CNS can be dramatic. Korsakoff's syndrome, caused by chronic alcoholism and its related nutritional deficiency, is identified by the structural involvement of the diencephalon with specific focus on the mammillary bodies, and the dorsal medial and anterior nucleus of the thalamus[18] usually shows involvement (see the anatomy section and Fig. 4-11, *A*). This syndrome is not a dementia, but rather a discrete localized pathological state with specific clinical signs. The most dramatic sign observed in a client with Korsakoff's syndrome is the severe memory deficits. These deficits involve declarative memory and learning losses, but the most predominant problem is short-term

memory loss. As the disease progresses, the clients generally become totally unaware of their memory loss and are unconcerned. Initially, confabulation may be observed, but in time most clients with a chronic condition become apathetic, somewhat withdrawn, and are in a profound amnesic state. They are trapped in time, unable to learn from new experiences because they cannot retain memories for more than a few minutes and are unable to maintain their independence.[46]

Alzheimer's disease (see the anatomy section). In Alzheimer's disease, the hippocampus and nucleus basalis are the most severely involved structures, followed by neurofibrillar degeneration of anteriotemporal, parietal, and frontal lobes.[46]

Initially, the symptoms fall into several categories: emotional, social, and cognitive. Usually the symptoms have a gradual onset. Depression and anxiety often are seen during the early phases because of the neuronal degeneration within the frontal and limbic system.[39] During the second stage, the emotional, social, and intellectual changes become more marked. Clients have difficulty with demands, business affairs, and personal management. Their memory and cognitive processing continue to deteriorate while their awareness of the problem is often still insightful, causing additional anxiety and depression. The third phase manifests itself with moderate to severe aphasic, apractic, and agnostic problems. Object agnosia, the failure to recognize objects, is a typical sign of advancing Alzheimer's disease. Distractability and nonattentiveness are also common signs of this third stage. The final stage is marked by an individual who is noncommunicative, with little meaningful social interaction and who often takes on the features of the Klüver-Bucy syndrome. Thus, they exhibit emotional outbursts, inappropriate sexual behaviors, severe memory loss, constant mouth movements, and often a flexor type postural pattern. In this latter phase, the client is virtually decorticate and clinically indistinguishable from other dementias.[46]

The continual degeneration of the limbic system is a key distinguishing factor in Alzheimer's disease. Many clients are misdiagnosed as having other problems such as intracranial tumors, normal-pressure hydrocephalus, multi-infarct dementia, or alcoholic/chronic drug intoxication.[3] However, when correctly evaluated and diagnosed, it becomes obvious that the limbic-cortical area involved from phase one through the last phase is overlaying and constantly affecting the behavioral patterns of the patient.

Head injury

Traumatic injury

SHEARING[2,4]. One potentially severe limbic problem that can be present following traumatic closed head injury is diffuse axonal injury DAI.[26] The long associative bundles or fibers that transverse the cortex on a curved route can be sheared by an impact or a blow to the head. One of these long associative bundles is the uncinate fasciculus, which coordinates the amygdala and hippocampal projections to and from the prefrontal cortex. Many basic perceptual strategies, such as body schema, hearing, vision, and smell are linked into the emotional and learning centers of the limbic system through the cingulate fasciculus. Thus, declarative learning through sensory/cognitive processing can become impossible. If the hippocampal and amygdala tracts are sheared bilaterally, total and permanent global anterograde amnesia can be present.[46] If destruction of both tracts on one side occurs, but the contralateral is left intact, the individual can compensate, but learning will be slower or the rate of processing delayed.[31] If only one tract on one side is damaged, such as the hippocampal tract, the amygdaloid system on the same side will compensate, but be slower than without the lesion.[31] Thus, the specific degree of involvement will vary and depend on the extent of shearing. Those people with total shearing on both sides will usually be in a deep coma and will not survive the injury.[46] Those individuals with less severe insult will show signs ranging from total amnesia to minor delays in declarative learning.[4]

CONTUSIONS. Cerebral contusions (bruises) have long been a primary sign of traumatic head injury[37]. Regardless of impact, the contusions are generally found in the frontal and temporal regions. The regions most frequently involved are orbitofrontal, frontopolar, anterotemporal, and lateral temporal surfaces.[4] The limbic system's connection to these areas would suggest the potential for direct and indirect limbic involvement. The greater the contusions, the greater the likelihood that the limbic structures might simultaneously be involved. Impulsiveness, lack of inhibition, and hyperactivity are a few of the clinical signs associated with orbitofrontal–limbic involvement. The dorsolateral frontal region, involved in the Papez circuit (see the anatomy section) when damaged seems to induce a pseudodepressed state, including slowness and lack of initiation and perseveration. No matter what the symptoms are, the causes here reflect basolateral limbic system involvement, whereas in DAI the medial limbic system is the area most affected.

Nontraumatic head injuries: anoxic/hypoxic brain injury. Lack of oxygen to the brain, regardless of the cause, seems not only to have a dramatic effect throughout the cortex, but also selectively damages the hippocampal regions.[4] The loss of hippocampal declarative memory systems bilaterally would certainly provide one reason for the slowness in processing so commonly observed in head injury. A hypothesis could also be made regarding the limbic systems interrelation with other cortical and brainstem structures. In cases of hypoxia, many structures feeding into the limbic system are potentially affected, so information sent to the limbic system may be distorted. These distortions could cause tremendous imbalances within the limbic processing system, with not only attention and

learning problems but also hypothalamic irregularity often seen in head trauma.

Summary. The behavioral sequelae following any head injury reflects many signs of limbic involvement. In both pediatric and adult studies,[9,17,22,41] behaviors of impulsiveness, restlessness, overactivity, destructiveness, aggression, increased tantrums, and socially uninhibited behaviors (lack of social skills) are frequently reported. These behaviors all reflect a strong emotional or limbic component. After discussion of Moore's concept that the limbic system MOVEs us and the FARV continuum regarding emotional control over noxious or negative input, it is no wonder so many clients have difficulty with personal and emotional control over their reactions to the therapeutic world. If the imbalance is within the client, then the external environment would be one possible way to help center the client emotionally. This centering requires that the therapist be sensitive to the emotional level of the client. As the client begins to regain control, an increase in external environmental demands would challenge his limbic system. If the demand is excessive, the client's emotional reaction as expressed by motor behavior should alert the therapist to downgrade the activity level.

Head injuries affect so many areas of the CNS. A client with spasticity, rigidity, or ataxia may exhibit an increase in those motor responses when his or her limbic system becomes stressed. Learning to differentiate a motor control problem from a limbic problem influencing the motor control systems requires that the therapist be willing to address the cause of the problems and how to treat those causes. Each client is so different and each minute in time has the potential of affecting his or her limbic system with great variance. Thus, the therapist needs to give undivided attention to the client at all times and be willing to make moment-to-moment adjustments within the external environment to help the client maintain focus on the desired learning.

Cerebrovascular accidents. The most common insult results in middle cerebral artery occlusions.[18] When this occlusion is in the right hemisphere, studies have shown that clients are often confused and exhibit metabolic imbalance.[43] The primary problem of this confused state is inattention. After brain scans, it has been shown that focal lesions existed both within the reticulocortical and limbic cortical tracts, suggesting direct limbic involvement in many middle cerebral artery problems.[25]

Many clients with a CVA do not have direct limbic involvement, yet the stresses placed on the client, whether external or internal, are often reflected in the limbic system's influence over the motor control systems. Everyday existence, as well as performance of the motor task required during therapy, is usually valued highly in the client's life. This value or stress placed on the limbic system overflows into the motor system and never allows it to relax. This is observed by noting the increase of tonus in the nonaffected leg. The client is usually unaware of this buildup of tonus, but can release it once attention is drawn to it. If attention is never directed toward these tension buildups, a therapist trying to decrease tonus in the affected arm or leg will always be interacting with the associated patterns from the uninvolved extremities.

Tumor. Any brain tumor, whether directly affecting the limbic structures or not, will certainly arouse the limbic system because of the stress, anxiety, and emotional overlays of the diagnosis. The degree of emotional involvement will obviously affect the declarative learning of the client as well as the limbic system's influence over motor response.

Tumors specifically arising within limbic structures can cause dramatic changes in the client's emotional behavior and level of alertness. This is especially true in hypothalamic tumors. The behaviors reported include aggressiveness, hyperphagia, paranoia, sloppiness, manic symptoms, and eventual confusion.[24,40] Tumors within the hypothalamus cause not only behavioral abnormalities, but autonomic endocrine imbalances are also often present, including body temperature changes, menstrual abnormalities, and diabetes insipidus.[46]

When the tumor is located within the frontal and temporal lobes associated with limbic structures, psychiatric problems may manifest themselves, ranging from depression to schizoid psychosis.[46] Amnesia has been reported in tumor patients with dorsomedial thalamus, fornix, and midbrain lesions. This again reinforces the importance of the limbic system's role in storage and retrieval of intermediate memory.[46]

Ventricular swelling following spinal defects in utero, CNS trauma, and inflammation. Although the effects of ventricular swelling following trauma, inflammation, and in utero cerebrospinal malformations are not discussed in great detail in the literature with respect to limbic involvement, the proximity of the lateral and third ventricle to limbic structures cannot be ignored. It is common knowledge that most people, when exposed to hot, humid weather and thus begin to swell, become more irritable, less tolerant, moody, and may complain of headaches. Some people become aggressive, others lethargic. All these behaviors are linked to limbic function. Thus, ventricular swelling causing hydrocephalus, whether caused by trauma, inflammation, or obstruction, would potentially effect the limbic structures. Reported behavioral changes such as seizures, memory and learning problems, personality alterations, alertness, dementia, and amnesia can be tied to direct or indirect limbic activity.[18]

It is easy to identify limbic problems when the behaviors deviate drastically from normal responses. It is much more difficult to determine subtle behavior shifts in clients. The therapist should be sensitive to these minor mood shifts, for they may represent early signs of future problems. Similarly, noting that a particular client is always irritable and has difficulty learning on hot days should help direct the therapist toward establishing a treatment session that regulates humidity and temperature to optimize the learning environment.

BASIC ANATOMY AND PHYSIOLOGY OF THE LIMBIC SYSTEM
Anatomy and physiology

Basic structure and function. The limbic system can best be visualized as consisting of cortical and subcortical structures with the hypothalamus in the central position (Figs. 4-11, *A* and *B* and 4-12). The hypothalamus is surrounded by the circular alignment of the subcortical limbic structures vitally linked with each other and the hypothalamus. These structures are the amygdaloid complex, the hippocampal formation, the nucleus accumbens (belonging to the basal ganglia), the anterior nuclei of the thalamus, the septal nuclei, and the paraolfactory region (Fig. 4-11, *B*). These structures are again surrounded by a ring of cortical structures collectively called the "limbic lobe," which includes the orbitofrontal cortex, the subcallosal gyrus, the cingulate gyrus, the parahippocampal gyrus, and the uncus (Fig. 4-11, *B*). Other neuroanatomists also include the olfactory system and the basal forebrain area (Fig. 4-12). Vitally linked and often included in the limbic system as the "meso-limbic" part is the excitatory component of the reticular activating system and other brainstem nuclei of the midbrain. Shepard[42] considers the midbrain a very important region for emotional expression. He found that attack behavior aroused by hypothalamic stimulation is blocked when the midbrain is damaged, and that midbrain stimulation can be made to elicit "attack behavior" even when the hypothalamus has been surgically disconnected from other brain regions. This "septo-hypothalamic-mesencephalic" continuum, connected by the medial forebrain bundle, seems to be very vital to the integration and expression of emotional behavior. The linking of other brain structures to emotions comes from the work of Papez[38] when he proposed the so-called Papez circuit (Figure 4-13). His circuit starts at the mammillary bodies (nuclei of the hypothalamus) to the anterior nuclei of the thalamus (via the mammillothalamic tract) and then on to the cerebral cortex and cingulate gyrus, where they reach the level of "conscious, subjective emotional experiences." Further projections reach the hippocampus for integration to be relayed back to the hypothalamic mammillary bodies. Papez saw this as a way of combining the "subjective" cortical experiences with the emotional hypothalamic contribution. Earlier, Paul Broca[6] labeled the cingulate gyrus and hippocampus "circle" as "The Great Limbic Lobe." These concepts were combined by Paul Maclean[23] into the construct of the limbic system.

Other regions then were added, such as the amygdaloid complex located in the temporal lobe. In their studies on

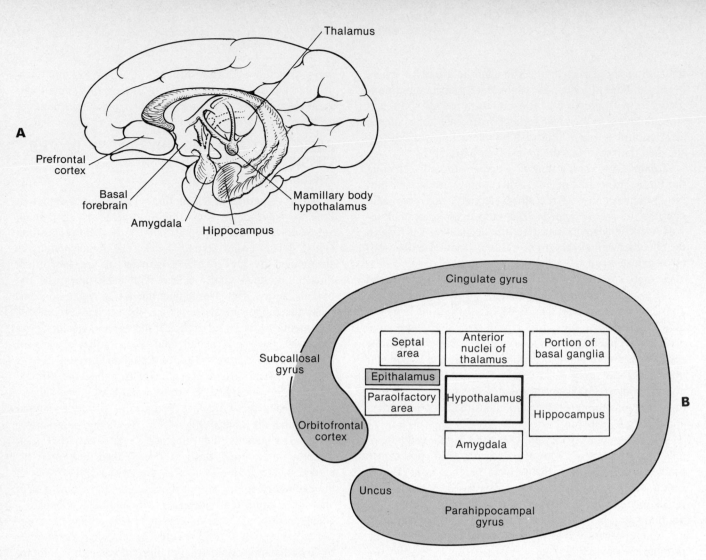

Fig. 4-11. Anatomy of the limbic system. **A,** Basic structures of the limbic system within a brain. **B,** Basic schematic diagram of the components of the limbic system.

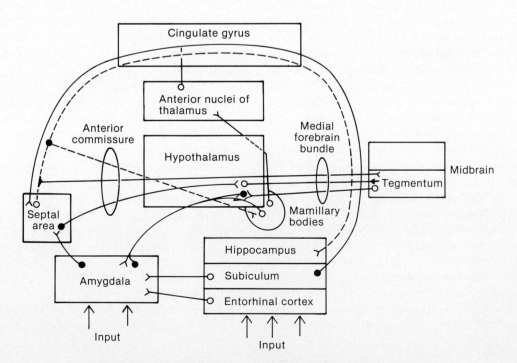

Fig. 4-12. Limbic system circuitry with medial forebrain bundle connections.

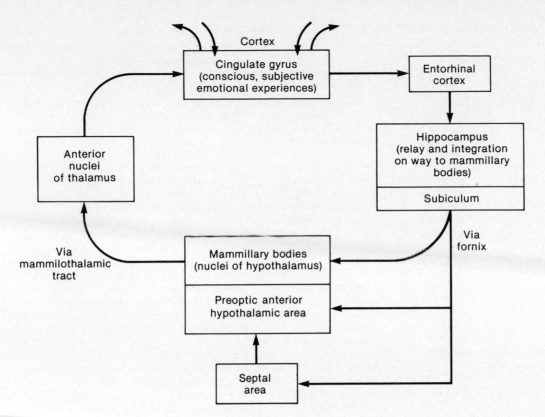

Fig. 4-10. Papez circuit. (Adapted from Kandel ER and Schwartz JH: Principles of neural science, ed 2, New York, 1985, Elsevier Science Publishing Co.)

monkeys, Klüver and Bucy[20] bilaterally removed the temporal lobes and reported the following changes in behavior which were subsequently specifically linked with loss of the amygdaloid complex input: (1) restless overresponsiveness, (2) hyperorality of examining objects by placing them in their mouths, (3) psychic blindness of seeing and not recognizing objects and the possible harm they may entail, (4) sexual hyperactivity, and (5) emotional changes, exhibiting loss of aggressiveness. These changes have been named the Klüver-Bucy syndrome. The amygdala has a myriad of connections linking it to the olfactory pathways, the frontal lobe and cingulate gyrus, the thalamus, the hypothalamus, the septum, and the midbrain structures of the substantia nigra, locus ceruleus, periaqueductal gray, and the reticular formation. The amygdala receives feedback from many of the above structures it projects to by reciprocal pathways. The amygdala is considered a part of the basal ganglia since it is fused with the tail of the caudate nucleus, the putamen, and the globus pallidus, thus forming "one large complex." Cotman[12] describes the amygdala as "listening" to the cerebral cortex and olfactory system and "talking" to many areas, with special communication with the hypothalamus. For further details see Table 4-1.

This neurological network between the amygdala and the basal ganglia may be the important connection that triggers the postural tone present in normal subjects when angry, upset, or when threatened. Similarly, if damage has occurred in either the limbic/amygdaloid structures or within the basal ganglia itself, a therapist might expect to see an increase in shoulder and hip contraction irrespective of spasticity, synergies, or volitional control. To differentiate whether the tonal rigidity was limbic or basal ganglia induced, the clinician would need to observe the emotional state and change within the client. If the abnormal state consistently alters with mood shifts, then limbic involvement causing motor control disturbances would be identified.

At the very heart of the limbic system is the hypothalamus, which oversees many functions. The specific nuclei relating to the limbic functions are the mammillary bodies and the lateral and ventromedial nuclei. The hypothalamus, in close reciprocal interaction with most centers of the cerebral cortex, the amygdala, hippocampus, pituitary gland, brainstem, and spinal cord, is a primary regulator of autonomic and endocrine functions and controls as well as balances homeostatic mechanisms. Autonomic and somatomotor responses controlled by the hypo-

Table 4-1. The components of the limbic system: their structure and functions

Structural definitions	Functions or effects	References
Amygdaloid complex		
Consists of 5 distinct nuclei	Involved in a variety of responses in the autonomic, endocrine, and somato-motor spheres related to motivation and emotions	7
Anatomically is grouped with basal ganglia, since it is fused with the tip of the caudate nucleus	Together with the hippocampus is necessary for storage of memory and subsequent recognition and recall	27
Gives rise to the stria terminales, which ends in the septal region	Some sensory input to the amygdala is from higher order association areas, which serve as storage areas for long-term memory. Therefore, the amygdala receives "highly processed information" of what is occurring now, but input also contains information of "how we reacted to similar stimuli in the past, i.e., memory component." Amygdala also matches input from transcortical pathways with that received from the hypothalamus regarding autonomic and motivational mechanisms. Efferent connections back to the hypothalamus allow amygdala to be a modulator of hypothalamus activity. Efferents also include those to the basal ganglia (amygdalostriatal projections), which provide direct input to the motor system, a feedback loop from the cortex to the basal ganglia, the thalamus, and returning to the motor and premotor cortices. Therefore, the amygdala communicates directly with both the sensorisomatomotor and the visceromotor parts of the nervous system.	16
Is tied to limbic system through the medial forebrain bundle	Sensory experiences acquire their emotional weight through the amygdala. When stimuli have emotional significance, positive associations will introduce the "reward" effect and select those stimuli for "selective attention," filtering out negative ones in a "gatekeeping" function. Therefore, emotions filter out what is perceived and learned and what subsequent actions result. "Gatekeeping" by the amygdala may also be enacted by control over the release of "opiates" in response to emotional levels originating in the hypothalamus.	29
Afferent connections bring amygdala in direct contact with all parts of the brain except the cerebellum	Within a given patient: repeated stimulation of the same site with the same or more intense parameters can evoke very different mental phenomena since the target sites "after discharges spread are themselves highly variable." The categories of mental phenomena evoked in a given patient are (at least in part) related to his or her personality, and the exact contents or quality of those phenomena are strongly influenced by the ongoing psychodynamic context. Stimulation of the amygdaloid complex often results in a general limbic activation which is "organized and integrated into a mental phenomenon according to the patient's habitual mechanisms for coping with emotional tension."	15
The amygdala of the right and left temporal lobes are functionally linked		
Hippocampus or hippocampal formation		
Situated on the floor of the temporal horn of the lateral ventricle, it forms an inwardly folded gyrus; innermost surface is the alveus, which gives rise to the fornix		7
The hippocampus proper is mapped into regions called CA_1, CA_2, and CA_3	Both the amygdala and the hippocampus are necessary for stimulus recognition and associative recall. Removal of both in temporal lobe removal results in the Klüver-Bucy syndrome in monkeys. The hippocampus is vital for memory of optical location of objects.	19, 29
The dentate gyrus is also part of the hippocampal formation; it follows the hippocampus, consisting of a thin area of cortex	The hippocampus is concerned with sensory and motor signals relating to the external environment, whereas the amygdala is concerned with those of the internal environment. The hippocampus is involved in procedural recall.	

Table 4-1. The components of the limbic system: their structure and functions—cont'd

	Structural definitions	Functions or effects	References
Subiculum	Medial to the hippocampal area lies a collection of nuclei called the subiculum	The subiculum is the major output of the hippocampus and has many reciprocal connections with other brain centers and supplies the fornix with fibers that carry messages to the hypothalamus (mammillary bodies) in a portion of the Papez circuit (see Fig. 4-13).	7
Entorhinal area	The subiculum adjoins the entorhinal area, which is the most important afferent input area to the hippocampus; the hippocampal connections to the hypothalamus travel through fornix from the subiculum	Input to the hippocampus is by way of entorhinal cortex and fornix. The entorhinal area receives input from the highest association cortex, where integration of this input facilitates learning by the addition of motivational and emotional factors. The entorhinal area, therefore, is the cortical limbic link.	8
Limbic lobe	Consists of a circular belt of cortex that borders the corpus callosum and the brainstem; parahippocampal gyrus (and the hippocampus dentate gyrus and the subiculum discussed above).	Collects sensory input of "all of the body's happenings," all converging here: integrates all of their input, stimulates and "maintains" responses, and "thereby provides for correctly scheduled goal-directed behavior. It keeps us on the beam."	12
	Cingulate gyrus	Affects aggressive behavior; ablation of this gyrus results in "increased tameness and social indifference."	7
	Subcallosal gyrus and the paraterminal gyrus together constitute the septal area (cortical portion; the subcortical part contain the septal nuclei)	The medial septal nucleus is continuous with the amygdaloid complex through the "diagonal band" (see Fig. 4-12). The septal nuclei also act as relay stations from the hippocampus via the fornix and are also reciprocally linked with the midbrain reticular function through the medial forebrain bundle (see Fig. 4-12).	10
	Orbitofrontal cortex	The orbitofrontal area of the limbic lobe is concerned with emotional responsiveness. Lesions here decrease normal aggressiveness and emotional responses. Electrical stimulation elicits sympathetic autonomic responses, imitates a state of general arousal.	18
Nucleus accumbens (part of basal ganglia)	Nucleus accumbens is developmentally related to the caudate nucleus and putamen	Nucleus accumbens is considered a part of the limbic system, tying it closely together with the basal ganglia. It projects directly to the globus pallidus and also the substantia nigra. Mesulam and Geschwind describe it as a part of the "limbic-inferior parietal lobe circuit concerned with attention evoking mechanisms."	10, 26

thalamus are closely aligned with the expression of emotions.

In the temporal lobe, anteromedially, are the amygdaloid complex of nuclei, with the hippocampal formation situated posterior to it. The hippocampal formation consists of the horn of Ammons, the subiculum, and the dentate gyrus (Table 4-1). Located close to the amygdala is a nucleus referred to as the "substantia innominata." This nucleus represents the center of the cholinergic system, which supplies acetylcholine to limbic and cortical structures involved in memory formation (see the neurochemistry section). Depletion of acetylcholine here in clients with Alzheimer's disease relates to their memory loss.

Interlinking the components of the system. The limbic system has many reciprocating interlinking circuits between its component structures, which provide for much functional interaction and also allow for ongoing adjustments with continuous feedback[13] (Fig. 4-14).

The largest pathway is the fornix. It has a C-shaped configuration that is almost circular. Its fibers arise from the hippocampus, for which it is the main efferent pathway extending to the hypothalamus and through its commissural portion to the contralateral hippocampus. The fornix fibers terminate in the mammillary bodies where they synapse with the neurons of the mammilothalamic tract heading for the anterior nuclei of the thalamus and eventually reach the cingulate gyrus of the limbic lobe. This circuit, called the Papez circuit (Figure 4-13), runs from the hippocampus along the fornix to the hypothalamus and on to the cingulate gyrus. The circle is completed by fibers to

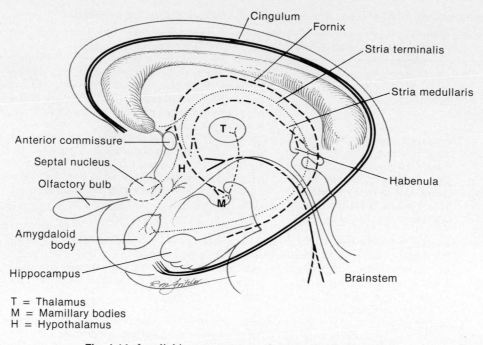

T = Thalamus
M = Mamillary bodies
H = Hypothalamus

Fig. 4-14. Interlinking neuron network within the limbic system.

the entorhinal cortex and back to the hippocampus.

Another limbic pathway is the stria terminalis, which originates in the amygdaloid complex and follows a course close to the fornix to end in the hypothalamus and septal regions. The amygdala and the septal region are also connected by a short direct pathway called the diagonal band of Broca. A third pathway, the uncinate fasciculus, runs between the amygdala and the orbitofrontal cortex.

The medial forebrain bundle (MFB) (Figure 4-12) is considered the most important connection of the limbic system. This pathway connects the septal region and the nucleus accumbans (basal ganglia) with the preoptic area and the amygdala. It courses through the lateral hypothalamus and terminates in the cingulate gyrus in its ascending limb and in the reticular formation of the midbrain in its descending part. These links enable the limbic system itself and the nonlimbic associated structures to act as one neural task system. It is important to realize that no portion of the brain, whether limbic or nonlimbic, has only one function.[12] Each area acts as an input-output station. At no time is it totally the center of a particular effect and each site depends on the cooperation and interaction with other regions.

Neurobiology of learning and memory
Functional applications for an intact system

"Ultimately, to be sure, memory is a series of molecular events. What we chart is the territory within which those events take place."[31, p. 687]

The brain stores sensory experiences as memory. In processing sensory information, most sensory pathways

from receptors to cortical areas send vital information to the components of the limbic system. For example, extensions can be found from the visual pathways into the inferior temporal lobe[29] (limbic system). Visual information is "processed sequentially" at each synapse along its entire pathway, in response to size, shape, color, and texture of objects. In the inferior temporal cortex, the total image of the item viewed is projected. In this way the sensory inputs are converted to become "perceptual experiences." This also applies to other sensory stimuli such as tactile, proprioceptive, and vestibular. The process of translating the integrated perceptions into memory occurs bilaterally in the limbic system structures of the amygdala and the hippocampus.

Before delving into the limbic system's impact on learning memory, a clear understanding of what is meant by these functions is needed.

Current theories support the view that a "dual memory system" using different pathways exists in the nervous system. Terms such as verbal and nonverbal,[13] procedural and declarative,[11] and habit versus recognition[28] have been given to these two memory systems. These systems are thought to operate autonomously, yet many therapeutic activities seem to combine these memory systems to achieve functional behavior.

For this discussion, two specific categories of learning, declarative and procedural, will be used. Declarative knowledge entails the capability to recall and verbally report experiences, whereas the procedural counterpart is the recall of "rules, skills, and procedures."

Procedural learning is vital to the development of pure

motor control. A child first receives sensory input from the various modalities via the thalamus, terminating at the appropriate sensory cortex. That information is processed and relayed to the motor cortex. From there, it is sent to both the basal ganglia and the cerebellum to establish plans for postural adaptations, refinement of motor programs, and coordination of direction, extent, timing, force, and tone necessary throughout the entire sequence of the motor act. Once back at the cortex (medial prefrontal cortex and posterior parietal association cortex), the established anticipatory tracts begin execution of the motor act. Storage and thus retrieval of memory of these semiautomatic motor plans is thought to occur throughout the motor control system (see Chapter 3, Motor control).

Procedural learning and memory do not necessitate limbic system involvement as long as no value is placed on the task; it deals with skills, habits, and stereotyped behaviors. This system is involved in developing procedural plans used in moving us from place to place or holding us in a position when we need to stop.

Declarative learning and thus memory (unlike procedural) requires the wiring of the limbic system. This type of thought deals with factual, material, semantic, and categorical aspects of higher cognitive and affective processing. There is a strong emotional and judgmental component linked with declarative thought. *Thus, as soon as a purely motor behavior has value placed upon the act, it becomes declarative as well as procedural and the limbic system may become a key element in the success or failure of that movement.* Most tasks or activities asked for in a clinical setting have value attached to them.

The two reverberating circuits within the limbic systems most intimately involved in declarative learning are: (1) the amygdaloid–dorsomedial thalamic–nucleus cortical pathways, and (2) the hippocampal–fornix–anterior thalamic nucleus–cortex.

The hippocampus may be more concerned with sensory and motor signals relating to the external environment, whereas the amygdala is concerned with those of the internal environment. They both contribute in relation to the significance of external or internal environmental influences.[19]

The amygdaloid tracts seem to deal with strongly emotional and judgmental thoughts, whereas the hippocampal tract is less emotional and more factual. These limbic circuits seem crucial in the initial processing of material that leads to learning and memory. Once the thought has been engrammed within the cortical structures, retrieval of that specific intermediate and long-term memory does not seem to require the limbic system, although new associations will need to be run through the system.

A third component in the memory pathway involves the medial diencephalon, a structure that contains both the thalamic and hypothalamic nuclei. When this region is destroyed by strokes, neoplasms, infections, or chronic alcoholism as in Korsakoff's syndrome, global amnesias are the consequence because of the destruction of the amygdala and hippocampus. The amygdala and hippocampus send fibers to specific target nuclei in the thalamus, and the destruction of these tracts also cause the same amnesic effect. It appears that the limbic system and the diencephalon cooperate in the memory circuits. The medial diencephalon seems to be another relay station along the pathway that leads from the specific sensory cortical region to the limbic structures in the temporal lobe to the medial diencephalic structures and ending in the ventromedial part of the prefrontal cortex (Fig. 4-15).

According to Figure 4-15, memories may be stored in the sensory cortex area where the original sensory input was interpreted into "sensory impressions." This may explain why damage to the limbic system structures does not destroy existing memory nor make it unavailable, since it is actually stored in some previous station of the pathway. The circular memory circuit reverts back to the original sensory area after activation of the limbic structures to cause the necessary neuronal changes that would inscribe the event into retrievable stored memory. This information can be recognized and retrieved by activation of storage sites anywhere along the pathway.

The last station or system to be added to the circuit is the "basal forebrain cholinergic system," which delivers the neurochemical acetylcholine to the cortical centers and to the limbic system with which it is richly linked. The loss of this neurotransmitter is linked to memory malfunctioning in Alzheimer's disease. Performance of visual recognition memory can be augmented or impaired by administration of drugs that enhance or block the action of acetylcholine.

It has also been shown that the amygdala and hippocampus are both interchangeably involved in recognition memory. The hippocampus is vital for memory of location of objects in space, whereas the amygdala is necessary for the association of memories derived through the various senses with a specific recognition recall. For example, a whiff of ether might bring to mind a painful surgical experience, or the sight of some food may cause a recall of its pleasant smell. Removal of the amygdala brings out the behavior shown in Klüver-Bucy syndrome. For clients with this neurologic problem, familiar objects do not bring forth the correct associations of memories experienced by sight, smell, taste, and touch and relate them to objects presented. Association of previously presented stimuli and their responses appear to be lost. Animals without amygdaloid input had different response patterns that ignored previous fears and aversions. Thus, the amygdala adds the "emotional weight" to sensory experiences.[30] Loss of the amygdala also loses the positive associations and reward, and thereby alters the shaping of perceptions that lead to memory storage.

When stimuli are endowed with emotional value or sig-

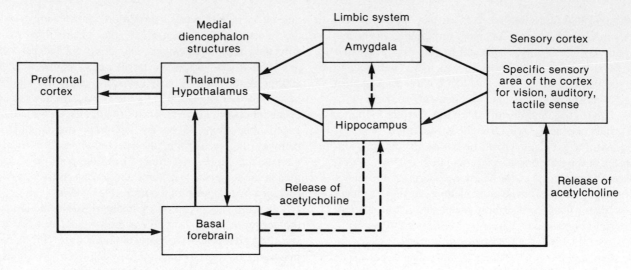

Fig. 4-15. The basal forebrain closes the circuit and causes changes in sensory area neurons, which could lead to correct perception and stored memory.

nificance, attention is drawn to those possessing emotional significance, selecting these for attention and learning. This would give the amygdala a "gatekeeping" function of selective filtering. The amygdala may enable emotions to influence what is perceived and learned by reciprocal connection with the cortex. Emotionally charged events will leave a more significant impression and subsequent recall. The amygdala alters perception of afferent sensory input and thereby affects subsequent actions.

Long-term potentiation: the key to limbic function. As discussed in the introduction, limbic functions may not be localized in specific structures or regions, but may be associated with "circuit interactions," and the structures themselves can influence the resulting effector activity. This can best be demonstrated by the concepts of reverberating circuits (Fig. 4-16) or oscillatory circuits. These circuits operate on positive feedback within the neuronal pool, which is arranged in a circular fashion. In this way the neuronal pool can feed back to re-excite itself in the circular circuit, and activity might be sustained for periods of time by repetitive discharges.[14] The mechanism of reverberating circuits may be used to "encode short-term memory" with brief excitation that can cause neural activity of long duration, producing memory traces or engrams.[18] These reverberating circuits could easily be demonstrated in the circular pathways of the limbic system, in pathways such as were suggested by the Papez circuit.

Slightly longer-term memory could be mediated by posttetanic potentiation. First, there must be a persistant train of high-frequency tetanic facilitary stimulation. This facilitation could last for hours, especially if this occurs in reverberating circuits. The chemical reaction to this continual volley of input creates a larger than normal influx of

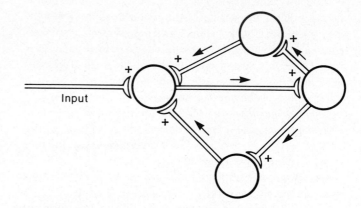

Fig. 4-16. Schema of a reverberating circuit, brief excitatory input could produce long-lasting neural activity.

calcium into the presynaptic terminal during the initial stimulation. This leads to increased release of transmitters from the terminals, causing larger than normal excitatory postsynaptic potentials (EPSP's). These potentials enhance synaptic transmission for an extended period of time.

This maintained excitation or processing is referred to as "the simplest kind of memory." The neuron remembers the increased train of impulses that increased the amount of calcium, and each action potential playing on this memory causes an increased amount of transmitter to be released, which will repeat the process in this posttetanic potentiation.[18]

In humans, memory functioning has been associated with the phenomenon of long-term potentiation (LTP) observed in hippocampal pathways. This potentiation of synaptic transmission, lasting for hours, days, and weeks, occurs after brief trains of high-frequency stimulation of hippocampal excitatory pathways.[5] Whether this phenomenon is caused by alteration at the presynaptic or postsynaptic terminals has not been established. The question remains as to whether there is an increased amount of neurotransmitter released presynaptically or is the expected amount producing a heightened postsynaptic response? Or are both sites involved?

Learning and memory evoke alterations in behavior that reflect neuroanatomical and neurophysiological changes.[1] These include the phenomenon of LTP as an example of such changes. The hippocampus demonstrates the importance of input of LTP in associative learning. In this type of learning, two or more stimuli are combined. Tetanizing of more than one pathway needs to occur simultaneously. When only one pathway is tetanized, the effect is decreased synaptic transmission. LTP, requiring the cooperative action of numbers of coactive fibers, is engendered and formed by the "associative" interaction of afferent inputs. LTP could, therefore, serve as a model for understanding the neural mechanism for associative learning.

Learning/memory problems following limbic involvement. For initial declarative learning and memory, the combination of hippocampus and amygdala of the limbic system are required.[30] For memory formation to occur, there must be a storing of the "neural representation" of the stimuli in the association and the processing areas of the cortex. This storage occurs when sensory stimuli activate a "cortico-limbo-thalamo-cortical" circuit.[30] This circuit serves as the "imprinting mechanism," reinforcing the pathway that activated it. On subsequent stimulation, a stimulus recognition or recall would be elicited. In associative recall, stored representations of any interconnected imprints could be evoked simultaneously.

A vital processing area for all sensory modalities is located in the region of the anterior temporal lobe. This area is directly linked with the amygdala and indirectly with the hippocampus. The hippocampus and amygdala are also linked both structurally and functionally to each other and to specific thalamic nuclei. Clients with temporal epileptic seizures and whose temporal lobes have been surgically removed developed global anterograde amnesia, that is, amnesia for all senses and no new memories could be formed. Experimental removal of only the hippocampus does not bring the above changes, although processing is slowed down. When both the hippocampus and the amygdala are removed bilaterally, the amnesia is both retrograde and global.[30] It is postulated that the amygdala is the area of the brain that adds a "positive association," the reward part to stimuli received and passed through processing. In this way, stimulus and reward are associated by the amygdala, and an emotional value is placed on it.

It appears that limbic involvement in the declarative memory process requires the participation of both the amygdala and the hippocampus for the cortical storage of "stimulus representation" necessary for subsequent recognition and recall of the information. As stated before, the amygdala adds the "affective value" to the recalled original stimulus, but apparently can do this without the contribution of the hippocampus if the latter is damaged. Without the amygdala, the stimulus might not be recognized for its proper emotional significance. With the loss of both the amygdala and the hippocampus, neither the stimulus recognition nor the associative recall is possible.[28,30]

When analyzing declarative and procedural learning from a clinical reference, a separation of functional mediation can be observed. Clients with brain lesions localized in the limbic system components of the amygdala and hippocampus have the ability to acquire and function with "rule-based" games and skills, but have lost the capacity to recall how, when, or where they gained this knowledge, or be able to give a description of the games and skills learned.[19] Relating this to clinical performance, clients may develop the skill in a functional activity but not the problem-solving strategies necessary to associate danger, or other potentially harmful aspects of a situation that may develop once out of the purely clinical setting.

Neurochemistry

Discussion of the limbic system's intricate regulation of many neurochemical substances is not within the scope of this chapter, yet therapists need to appreciate how potent this system can be with respect to neurochemical reactions.

The hypothalamus, the physiological center of the limbic system (see Figs. 4-1 and 4-3), is involved in neurochemical production and is geared for passage of information along specific neurochemical pathways. Guyton[15] considers it the major motor output pathway of the limbic system, which also communicates with every part of this system. Certain nuclei of the hypothalamus have been found to produce and release neuroactive peptides that have a long-acting effectiveness as neuromodulators. As such, they control the levels of neuronal excitation and effective functioning at the synapses. By their long-lasting effects, they regulate motivational levels, mood states, and learning. These peptide-producing neurons extend from the hypothalamic nuclei to the autonomic nervous system components and to the nuclei of the limbic system, where they modulate neuroendocrine and autonomic activities.[15]

Lesions in the medial hypothalamus affect hormone production and thus alter regulation of many hormonal control systems.[18] For example, clients with medial hypothalamic lesions may have huge weight gains because of the increase of insulin in the blood, which increases feeding and converts nutrients into fat. Similarly, this weight gain may be caused by hyperphagic responses resulting from the loss of satiety. General hyperactivity and signs of hostility after minimal provocation can also be observed. These problems are often encountered in patients with head trauma.

Lesions in the lateral hypothalamus lead to damage of dopamine-carrying fibers that begin in the substantia nigra and filter through the hypothalamus to the striatum. Lesions, either along this tract or within the lateral hypothalamus, lead to aphagia and hypoarousal. Decreased sensory awareness contributing to sensory neglect is also present in lateral hypothalamic lesions. The decreased awareness may be caused by a decrease of orientation to the stimuli versus awareness of the stimuli once they are brought to conscious attention.[19] These lesions cause the client to exhibit marked passivity with decreased functioning.[15]

As noted earlier, depression is a behavior clearly identified as a limbic function. A functional deficiency in monoamines, especially serotonin, is hypothesized to be a primary cause of depression.[19] The serotonin systems originate in the rostral and caudal raphe nuclei in the midbrain. Ascending serotonergic tracts start in the midbrain and ascend to the limbic forebrain and hypothalamus; they are concerned with mood and behavior regulation. Damage with direct or indirect limbic involvement results in the client exhibiting depression. Descending pathways to the substantia gelatinosa are involved in pain mechanisms and have also been linked through a complex sequence of biochemical steps to the increased sensitization of the presynaptic terminals of the cutaneous sensory neurons leading to a hyperactive withdrawal reflex or hypersensitivity to cutaneous input.[18] This would account for the behavior patterns seen in clients with head trauma, where the therapist sees a flexed posture with a withdrawn or depressed affect yet with an extremely sensitive tactile system.

It is hypothesized that the underlying pathophysiology of one form of schizophrenia involves an excessive transmission of dopamine within the mesolimbic tract system.[18] The dopaminergic cell bodies are located in the ventral tegmental area and the substantia nigra. Some of these neurons project to the limbic system. These projections go to the nucleus accumbens, the stria terminalis nuclei, parts of the amygdala, and to the frontal entorhinal and anterior cingulate cortex. It is the projection to the nucleus accumbens that seems critical, because of its influence over the hippocampus, frontal lobe, and hypothalamus. This nucleus may act as a filtering system with respect to affect and certain types of memory, and the dopaminergic projections may modulate the flow of neural activity.[18] The flat affect seen in clients with Parkinson's disease and the paranoid/schizophrenic behaviors observed in some clients with CNS damage may directly reflect back to these mesolimbic dopaminergic systems.

The specific roles of the noradrenaline pathway are numerous and affect almost all parts of the CNS. The center for the noradrenaline pathways is located within the caudal midbrain and upper pons. Its nucleus is referred to as locus ceruleus. This nucleus sends at least five tracts rostally to the diencephalon and telencephalon.[18] Of specific interest for this chapter are the projections to the hippocampus and amygdala. The axons of these neurons modulate an excitatory affect on the regions where they terminate.[35] Thus, the activation of this system will heighten the excitation of the two nuclei within the limbic system intricately involved in declarative learning and memory. Hyperactivation may cause overload or the lack of focus of attention. Decreased activity may prevent the desired responses. Attention to task may be dependent on on-going noradrenaline stimulation. It has been shown that these tracts from the midbrain rostrally play a key role in alertness. The correlation of alertness and attention to performance of motor tasks as well as to learning can be demonstrated.[18]

In conclusion, the neurochemistry of the limbic system is intricately linked to the neurochemistry of the brain. All systems within the limbic circuitry seem to be interdependent, with the summation of all the neurochemistry being the determinants of the specific processing of information. Similarly, the interdependence of the limbic system to almost all other areas of the brain and the activities of those areas at any time reflect the complexity of this system.

CONCLUSION

The complexity and interwoven neurological network of the limbic system may seem overwhelming. If the reader tries to grasp all parts on first study, he or she will feel lost and defeated, a true limbic emotion. Thus, this chapter was presented in two parts. The first part introduces the system and its potential clinical application. This section, in and of itself, has many interwoven components, for nothing in the limbic system functions in isolation. Yet the mysteries of this complex neurological network when solved may be the answers to many clinical questions regarding the art and gift of a master clinician. The second part introduces the basic anatomy and physiology of the limbic system. It is hoped that once the student/clinician has been drawn to the conclusion that this system may be a key to clinical success, he or she might be willing to delve into the science of the system. This path of exploration is challenging, difficult, and frustrating at times, but certainly worth the effort once understanding is achieved.

REFERENCES

1. Abraham WC and Goddard GV: Functions of different coactivity in long-term potentiation. pp. 459-465. In Lynch, McGaugh and Weinberger, editors: Neurobiology of learning and Memory, New York, 1984, The Guilford Press.
2. Adams JH and others: Diffuse axonal injury due to nonmissile head injury in humans: an analysis of 45 cases, Ann Newal 12:557-563, 1982.
3. Appel SH, editor: Current neurology, vol 6, Chicago, 1986, Year Book Publishing Company, Inc.
4. Auerbach, SH: Neuroanatomical correlates of attention and memory

disorders in traumatic brain injury: an application of neurobehavioral subtypes, J Head Trauma Rehab 1(3):1-12, 1986.

5. Bliss TVP and Dolphin AC: Where is the locus of long-term potentiation. In Lynch, McGaugh, and Weinberger, editors: Neurobiology of learning and memory, pp. 451-458, New York, 1984, The Guilford Press.

6. Broca P: Anatomie comparie des circonvoluntions cerebrales. Le grand lobe limbique et la scissure limblique dun la serie des mammiferes, Rhone Antropologie, I:385, 1878.

7. Brodal A: Neurological anatomy in relation to clinical medicine, ed 3, New York, 1981, Oxford University Press.

8. Brooks VB: The neural basis of motor control, New York, 1986, Oxford University Press.

9. Brown G and others: A prospective study of children with the head injuries. III. Psychiatric sequelae. Psych Med II:63, 1981.

10. Carpenter MB and Sutin J: Human neuroanatomy, ed 8, Baltimore, 1983, Williams and Williams.

11. Cohen NJ and Squire LR: Preserved learning and retentions of pattern-analyzing skill in amnesia: dissociations of knowing how and knowing that, Science 210, 1980.

12. Cotman CW and McGaugh JL: Behavioral neuroscience: an introduction, New York, 1980, Academic Press, Inc.

13. Gazzaniga MS and Le Doux JE: The integrated mind, New York, 1978, Plenum Press.

14. Guyton AC: Basic neuroscience anatomy and physiology, Philadelphia, 1987, WB Saunders Co.

15. Halgren E: The amygdala contribution to emotion and memory: current studies in humans. In Ben Ari Y: The amygdaloid complex, Amsterdam, North Holland, 1981, Bio Medical Press.

16. Heimer L: Hippocampus. In Ben-Ari Y: The amygdaloid complex, Amsterdam, North Holland, 1981, Bio Medical Press.

17. Hulsey PH: Serious disability from mild head injury. recognizing the silent epidemic, J Kansas Trial Lawyers 7(5):6, 1984.

18. Kandel ER and Schwartz JH: Principles of neural science, ed. 2, New York, 1985, Elsevier Science Publishing Co.

19. Kesner RP: The neurobiology of memory: implicit and explicit assumptions. In Lynch G, McGaugh JL, and Weinberger NM, editors: Neurobiology of learning and memory, New York, 1984, The Guilford Press.

20. Klüver H and Bucy PC: Preliminary analysis of functions of the temporal lobes in monkeys, Arch Neural Psychiatry 42:979, 1939.

21. Leonard G: The silent pulse, New York, 1981, Bantam Books, Inc.

22. Livingston MG, and others: Patient outcome in the year following severe head injury and relative's psychiatric and social functioning, J. Neural Neurosurg Psychiatry 48:876, 1985.

23. Maclean PD: Role of transhypothalamic pathways in social communication. In Morgane PJ and Panksapp J editors: Handbook of the hypothalamus, vol. 3, part B, New York, 1981, Marcel Dekker Inc.

24. Malamud N: Psychiatric disorders with intracranial tumors of the limbic system, Arch Neurol 17:113, 1967.

25. Mesulam M: Principles of behavioral neurology, Philadelphia, 1985, F.A. Davis.

26. Mesulam M and Geschwind: On the possible role of the neocortex and its limbic connections in the process of attention and schizophrenia: clinical cases of inattention in man, J Psych Res 14:249, 1978.

27. Mishkin MA: A memory system in the monkey, Philosophical Tranactions of the Royal Society of London, 1982, pp. 85-95.

28. Mishkin MA: memory in monkeys severely impaired by combined but not be separate removal of amygdala and hippocampus, Nature, 273:297, 1978.

29. Mishkin MA and Appenzeller T: The anatomy of memory, Sci Am 256:680, 1987.

30. Mishkin M and others: An animal model of global amnesia. In Cashin S editor: Alzheimer disease: a report of progress, New York, 1982, Raven Press.

31. Moore J: Neuroanatomical structures subserving learning and memory. In Fifteenth Annual Sensorimotor Integration Symposium, unpublished manual, San Diego, July 1987.

32. Moore J: Review of neurophysiology as it relates to treatment, Personal notes, San Francisco, 1980.

33. Morgane PJ and Panksapp J: Behavioral studies of the hypothalamus. In Morgane PJ and Panksapp J editors: Handbook of the hypothalamus, vol. I, New York, 1979, Marcel Dekker, Inc.

34. Murray RB and Huelskoetter MMW: Psychiatric mental health nursing-giving emotional care, Englewood Cliff, NJ, 1983, Prentice Hall.

35. Nicoll RA: Neurotransmitters can say more than just "yes" or "no," Trends Neurosci, 5:369-374, 1982.

36. Olds J and Milner P: Positive reinforcements produced by electrical stimulation of septal area and other lesions of the rat brain, J Comp Physiol Psychol 47:419, 1954.

37. Ommaya AIC and Gennarelli TA: Cerebral concussion and traumatic unconsciousness, Brain 24:1181, 1974.

38. Papez JW: A proposed mechanism of emotions, Arch Neurol Psych 38:725, 1937.

39. Reding M and others: Depression in patients referred to a dementia clinic, a three-year prospective study, Arch Neurol 42:894, 1985.

40. Reeves AG and Plum F: Hyperphagia, rage and dementia accompanying a ventromedial hypothalamic neoplasm, Arch Neurol 20:616, 1969.

41. Richardson F: Some effects of severe head injury: a follow-up study of children and adolescents after protracted coma, Dev Med Child Neurol 5:471, 1963.

42. Shepard GM: Neurobiology, New York, 1983, Oxford University Press.

43. Schmidley JW and Messing RO: Agitated confusional states in patients with right hemisphere infarctions, Stroke 15:883, 1984.

44. Spiers PA: Temporalimbic epilepsy and behavior. In Mesulum MM: Principles of behavioral neurology, Philadelphia, 1985, FA Davis.

45. Stellar JR and Stellar E: The neurobiology of motivation and rewards, New York, 1985, Springer Verlag.

46. Strub RL and Black FW: Neurobehavioral disorders: a clinical approach, Philadelphia, 1988, FA Davis.

47. Vrbantes: Personal communication, 1987.

48. Wasterlain, CG and others: Chemical kindling: a study of synaptic pharmacology. In Wade J, editor: Raven Press, 1981, New York.

Chapter 5

NORMAL SEQUENTIAL BEHAVIORAL AND PHYSIOLOGICAL CHANGES THROUGHOUT THE DEVELOPMENTAL ARC

C. Robert Almli

The study of the development of the relationships between the brain and behavior is interesting for people who want to know more about themselves. Such knowledge is also important as a background for understanding the anatomy and physiology of the nervous system and the behavior of human beings. Knowledge of neurological and behavioral ontogeny is also important for understanding the pathogenesis of developmental neurologic abnormalities, as well as for understanding the normal sequences of behavioral development.

The human developmental process is characterized by rather dramatic changes in both the physiology (e.g., nervous system) and the behavior (e.g., movement patterns) of the developing organism from conception through death at any age. In this sense the developmental process is lifelong. At present we have amassed considerable research and knowledge of the developmental process from conception through adulthood. However, study of the developmental process from adulthood through senescence and subsequent death is only beginning.

This chapter presents a survey of representative and critical characteristics of the human developmental process from conception through young adulthood, with the late prenatal through early childhood phases receiving the greatest attention. The late prenatal and early childhood phases are particularly important because of the extremely rapid changes that take place in both the physiology and the behavior of the human organism during that time and because of the organism's increased vulnerability to biological, environmental, and experiential influences. During these developmental phases, the normal sequential changes that occur in the CNS and the behavior of the developing human organism are stressed.

The first section of this chapter presents a general discussion of prenatal and postnatal physical development of the human organism. In the next section the development of the human nervous system is presented, and the development of the brain is emphasized. The final section is a representative look at general motor, sensory, language, and cognitive development of the human organism.

Human development data are presented when available; otherwise data for lower animals will be introduced. A basic knowledge of neuroanatomy is assumed of the reader.

PHYSICAL DEVELOPMENT OF THE HUMAN
Prenatal physical development

Prenatal development is often divided into three basic phases: the germinal phase, the embryonic phase, and the fetal phase (Table 5-1). The *germinal phase* begins at the moment of conception, or fertilization, and lasts through approximately the first 2 weeks of gestation. The germinal phase is the period of rapid cellular division and implantation of the embryo into the wall of the uterus. The next phase, the *embryonic phase,* begins at this time and continues through approximately 8 weeks of gestation. The embryonic phase is a period of rapid growth and differentiation of the major body systems and organs. The final prenatal phase, the *fetal phase,* begins at about 8 weeks of gestation and lasts through gestation term (birth) at approximately 38 weeks following fertilization. During the fetal phase, rapid growth and changes in the body form of the fetus are occurring.

During prenatal development, the human organism displays a physical developmental sequence that proceeds in a general rostral-to-caudal gradient, that is, development from the head region to lower body parts, and in a general proximal-to-distal gradient, that is, development from the central body parts and regions out to the peripheral body parts and regions. The averages and normative data presented in this chapter for the various growth measures are intended to communicate a general picture of growth and development of the human organism. The reader must keep in mind that these averages and norms vary consider-

ably, and "normal" in most cases can be only broadly defined.

Following fertilization, the fertilized ovum (zygote) begins division during the 3- to 4-day trip through the fallopian tube to the uterus. Upon arrival at the uterus, the future human is a fluid-filled sphere called a blastocyst. The cells around the edge of the blastocyst cluster to form the embryonic disk, from which the human organism will develop. The embryonic disk differentiates into two layers, the upper layer, or *ectoderm,* and the lower layer, or *endoderm.* A short time later a third layer, the *mesoderm,* or middle layer, will develop. These three germ layers give rise to all tissues and organs of the body (see Table 5-2).

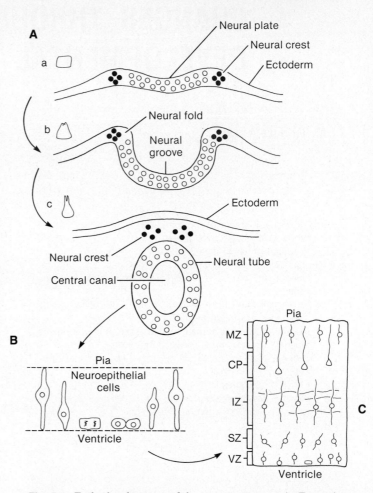

Fig. 5-1. Early development of the nervous system. **A,** Formation of the neural tube from the neural plate showing the relative positions of the ectoderm, neural crest, neural plate, neural folds, neural groove, neural tube, and central canal (ventricle). *a-c,* Relative changes in the shape of cells of the neural plate producing the neural folds and neural groove and ultimately, the neural tube. **B,** Cross section of the early neural tube showing the neuroepithelial or germinal cells at various stages of mitotic division. Postmitotic cells migrate out of this ventricular zone to form the intermediate or mantle zone. **C,** Cross section through the early forebrain showing the ventricular zone *(VZ),* subventricular zone *(SZ),* intermediate (mantle) zone *(IZ),* cortical plate *(CP),* and marginal zone *(MZ).*

Table 5-1. Phases of the human development process

Phase	Time
Prenatal (conception to birth)	
Germinal	Conception to 2 weeks
Embryonic	2 to 8 weeks
Fetal	8 to 38-40 weeks
Postnatal	
Newborn (neonatal)	Birth to 2 weeks
Infancy	2 weeks to 1 year
Childhood	1 to 12-13 years
Puberty	
Females	12 to 15 years
Males	13 to 16 years
Adolescence	15-16 years to 18-25 years
Adulthood	18-25 years to ?
Senescence	? to death

The ectoderm is the embryonic tissue from which the nervous system, sensory systems, and many other tissues develop (Fig. 5-1). The mesoderm differentiates into the muscles, skeleton, and other tissues, while the endoderm differentiates into the respiratory system and the digestive system, as well as other tissues.[76]

At 3 to 4 weeks of gestation the developing human is only a few millimeters long, yet morphogenesis is significantly advanced. The paraxial mesoderm of the embryo begins to divide into paired surface elevations, called somites, at about 20 days of gestation. Approximately 40 pairs of somites will shortly develop (occipital, cervical, thoracic, lumbar, sacral, and coccygeal), and these paired somites will eventually give rise to most of the skeleton, musculature, and dermis of the head, trunk, and limbs. By about 24 to 26 days of gestation, the primitive mouth begins to form as the mandibular and hyoid branchial arches become distinct. Also, the heart has developed to such an extent as to produce a bulge on the ventral surface of the embryo, and the primitive heart has begun to beat at approximately 65 beats per minute.[37] The upper limb buds and the otic pits (primordia of the inner ears) are recognizable by 26 days of gestation, followed by the lower limb buds and optic (lens) placodes at 28 days. Also during this period the primitive nervous system, kidney, liver, and digestive tract are continuing to differentiate (Table 5-2 and Fig. 5-2).

During the fifth week of gestation the upper limbs are paddle shaped and the hand plates have formed. The lower limbs and feet follow within a few days. The nasal pits become prominent during this week and the optic cups and vesicles are present. The embryo has grown to approximately 8 mm in length by the fifth week of gestation. Within the following week (sixth week of gestation) the upper limb buds have further differentiated and the elbow, wrist, and digital rays (fingers) are identifiable. The eyes become obvious at this age, because of the appearance of retinal pigments. By the seventh week of gestation the embryo has grown to approximately 16 to 18 mm in length and the eyelids are now forming. The trunk of the embryo is elongating and straightening, and notches are appearing between the finger rays.[76]

The embryo continues to grow until it is approximately 2.5 cm in length by 8 to 9 weeks of gestation. The face, mouth, eyes, ears, and nose are slowly becoming well defined, and the organism begins to resemble a very small baby. The arms, legs, hands, and feet have now become apparent and stubby fingers and toes can be distinguished by this age.[36] Development of the sex organs and muscle tissues have already begun at this time, and activation of muscles by neural input has achieved a functional, though primitive, level. Associated with the tremendous development of the brain that is occurring at this time, the head is quite large in comparison to the rest of the body. It makes up approximately one half of the total body length.

The development of the fetus extends from the end of the second month of gestation through gestation term. Development during the fetal period is characterized by growth and differentiation of the organs and tissues that evolved during the embryonic period. The rate of body growth is especially rapid between the ninth and twentieth weeks. During the early part of the fetal period, the fetus begins to respond to tactile (touch) stimulation with flexion of the trunk and extension of the head.[43,111] From this age onward, motor functions of the human organism become increasingly complex and differentiated. The earliest movements are of the generalized, whole-body type.

From 9 to 12 weeks of gestation the body length of the fetus doubles. The face is broad, the eyes are widely separated, and the ears are set low. The eyelids are now closed. By the end of 12 weeks the upper limbs have almost reached their final relative lengths, but the lower limbs are less well developed and are still relatively short. The neck region of the fetus is now well defined and the early fingernails are differentiating.[76]

At approximately 12 to 13 weeks of gestation the fetus has grown to about 7.5 cm in length and weighs over 40 gm. The muscles and the nervous system have greater connection and spontaneous generalized movements are made with the arms and legs. The head of the fetus now makes up approximately one third of its total body length and many organ systems are beginning to function. Further morphological differentiation of the fetus has occurred and

---

Table 5-2. Layers of the trilaminar embryonic disk and the tissues derived from the germinal layers

Germinal layers	Tissue and organ derivatives
Ectoderm	Central nervous system (brain and spinal cord); peripheral nervous system; sensory epithelia (eye, ear, nose); epidermis; hair; nails; mammary glands; pituitary gland; subcutaneous glands; tooth enamel; adrenal gland (medulla); pigment cells of the dermis; muscle, connective tissues, and bone of branchial arch origin; leptomeninges (pia-arachnoid)
Mesoderm	Bone, cartilage, and connective tissue; striated and smooth muscle; heart, blood, lymph vessels, and cells; kidneys, gonads (ovaries and testes), and genital ducts; serous membranes lining pericardial, pleural, and peritoneal body cavities; spleen; adrenal gland (cortex); microglial cells
Endoderm	Epithelial lining of the gastrointestinal, respiratory, urinary bladder, urethra, and auditory tracts and cavities; tonsils; thyroid, parathyroid, and thymus glands; liver; pancreas

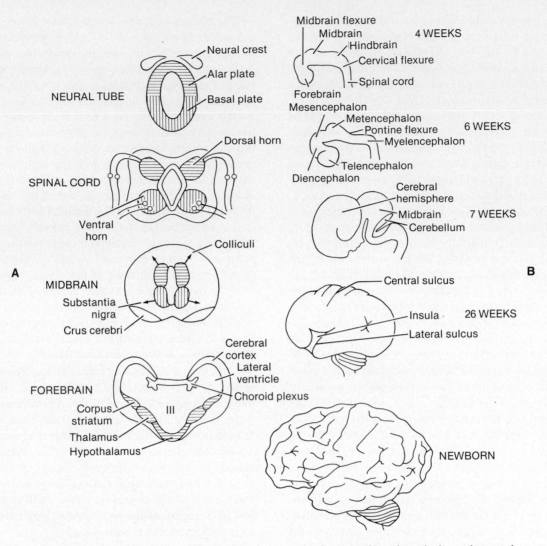

Fig. 5-2. Gross development of the nervous system. **A,** Cross sections through the early neural tube, spinal cord, midbrain, and forebrain. Horizontal cross-hatching indicates alar plate and vertical cross-hatching indicates basal plate. **B,** Lateral views of the developing nervous system from 1 month of gestation through gestation term (newborn). Noted are the brain flexures and the brain vesicles.

the lower limbs are increasing in relative length. The sex organs of the fetus can be identified by their external morphology, and the internal sex organs have primitive egg or sperm cells.

During weeks 12 to 16 of the fetal period, the nervous system continues to differentiate and grow at a rapid rate, and motor behavior daily becomes more complex. The fetus is now displaying movements resembling breathing and is swallowing amniotic fluid. In addition, the fetus at this age displays movement of the legs, feet, arms, thumbs, and head. The mouth opens and closes, and the fetus makes squinting movements in response to tactile stimulation of the eyelids. Touching the palm stimulates a closing of the hand into a fistlike shape, touching the lip region stimulates sucking movements, and stimulating the sole of the foot makes the toes fan out in response. Still present at

birth and for a period of time after birth, many of these reflexlike behaviors will drop out of the infant's repertoire during postnatal maturation. These are the primitive reflexes (Table 5-3).[120]

By 16 to 17 weeks of gestation, motor movement of the fetus has achieved a magnitude that allows the mother to actually feel the fetus moving around inside of her. The fetus at this age has grown to approximately 15 cm in length and weighs approximately 170 g. The reflexes and motor movements of the fetus become more brisk with age as the nervous and muscular systems continue to mature.

At 20 weeks of gestation, the fetus is approximately 19 cm in length and weighs about 400 g.[45] The mouth of the fetus shows all of the movements required for sucking, including opening, closing, and protrusion of the lips. The fetus also displays cyclic activity and quiet periods, which

Table 5-3. The primitive reflexes and ages at which they disappear

Reflex	Age (months) reflex disappears
Rooting	9
Moro	3-6
Grasping	2-3
Swimming	6
Tonic neck	2-7
Babinski	6-9
Walking	4-8
Placing	1

may signal the beginning of sleep-wake cycle development. During quiet periods, the fetus seems to display a "favorite" body position (or body lie) within the uterus. During active periods the fetus kicks, stretches, squirms, opens and closes the hands, and displays hiccup-like spasms. The fetal heartbeat can be clearly heard, yet the respiratory system remains quite immature. The fetus at this age shows coarse hair on the eyebrows and eyelids and fine hair on the head. A woolly type of hair, called lanugo, covers most of the body and will disappear shortly before or after birth.

When the fetus is at approximately 24 weeks of gestation, it has grown to about 23 cm in length and weighs about 800 g. Fat pads under the skin are developing, and the eyes are almost completely formed. The eyelids periodically open and close. Regular movements resembling breathing are seen, along with movements resembling crying. The grip of the hand has also increased in strength. A fetus born at this age might survive; however, the infant would probably have to overcome severe respiratory problems. The 6-month fetus truly resembles the human organism, complete with the appearance of taste buds on the tongue.[14]

At 28 weeks of gestation the fetus is approximately 27 cm in length and weighs about 1200 g. At this age the nervous, circulatory, and other body systems have sufficiently matured to allow the fetus a good chance of surviving birth; however, special care would be required. The fetus now displays well-developed motor movements, reflex patterns, and breathinglike inspirations and expirations. Crying, swallowing, and thumb sucking are part of the frequently observed behavior patterns. The fetus displays reactions to changes in temperature of its surroundings somewhat like those of the full-term infant, and when infants are born at this age they seem capable of differentiating the four basic tastes of sweet, sour, bitter, and salt.[16] These premature infants also display reactions to visual and auditory stimulation. Their responses to painful stimulation are attenuated when compared to responses of older infants.

At 8 months of gestation the fetus is about 30 cm in length and weighs about 2000 g. The movement of the fetus is somewhat decreased at this age, and this attenuated movement may be related to the cramped quarters within the uterus. The fetus continues to accumulate body fat layers that will help it to adjust more readily to temperature decreases in the environment.

In the final month of gestation the fetus displays a general slowdown in body growth, especially within the final week. The final weight of the fetus is approximately 3400 g with a final length of about 50 cm. Males tend to be a little longer and heavier than females at birth. The various organs of the body have now sufficiently developed to allow the newborn to survive extrauterine life; however, growth and differentiation do not stop here. The postnatal period is also one of tremendous growth, and the process continues.

Postnatal physical development

Postnatal development of the human is often considered to progress by stages (see Table 5-1). The *newborn* (or *neonatal*) *period* is the first 2 weeks after birth, and the *infancy period* is the first year after birth. During the infancy period the whole body grows very rapidly. The *childhood period* extends from the end of the first year through 12 to 13 years. This is a period of active ossification of the bones. Growth is rapid during the early part of this period and is slower toward the end. Just before puberty body growth accelerates during the prepubertal growth spurt. The *puberty periods* for females (12 to 15 years) and males (13 to 16 years) are signaled by the development of secondary sexual characteristics (e.g., pubic hair). *Adolescence* is the 3- to 4-year period following puberty, extending from the earliest signs of sexual maturity until adulthood. In our culture, these periods are not sharply defined. *Adulthood* is the period when growth and ossification are virtually complete; it begins at approximately 18 to 25 years of age. Growth of the human during the adulthood through senescence periods is considerably slowed.

Normal postnatal physical development follows a relatively strict course; however, the time at which individual infants reach specific milestones varies to a great extent. The first 3 years of postnatal life are years of tremendous body growth and change in body proportions. At birth males and females are approximately 19 to 20 inches in length (tall) and they weigh about 7 to 8 lb. By the end of the first year of postnatal life, infants have grown to approximately 30 in (75 cm) in length and weigh about 20 to 25 lb (9 to 10 kg). At 2 years of age they are about 35 in (85 cm) long and weigh about 27 lb (12 kg), while at 3 years of age they are approximately 38 in (95 cm) tall and weigh about 35 lb (15 kg).[122]

During the first few days following birth the neonate may lose up to 10% of its body weight, primarily because of a loss of fluids. By the fifth postnatal day body weight gains are seen, and birth weight is usually reachieved by about 10 to 14 days of age.[34]

The newborn infant is rather pale and pinkish in color because of thin skin, and the infant possesses varying amounts of lanugo. The head makes up about one quarter of the total body size. It may be elongated and misshapen because of the moulding that has occurred in utero and during the birth process. The skull bones have not yet fused and the separations between skull bones (fontanels) are overlaid with a thick membrane. The fusion of the skull bones occurs at approximately 18 months after birth.

The Apgar Scale[7] was developed to give a general assessment of the medical status of the newborn shortly after birth. The Apgar Scale continues to be widely used and is made up of five subtests. A score of 0, 1, or 2 is given to the newborn on the basis of its appearance (color), pulse (heart rate), grimace (reflex irritability), activity (muscle tone), and respiratory (breathing) evaluation. The maximum score on the Apgar Scale is 10 and scores are assigned at 1 and 5 minutes after delivery. For most normal deliveries (90%), an Apgar score of 7 or better is achieved. A score of 4 or less indicates that the infant requires immediate medical attention. Research has shown that low Apgar scores are fairly good predictors of later neurological problems.

Apgar scores at 1 minute after birth were found to be correlated with performance on the Bayley Scales of Infant Development at 8 months of age. Infants scoring 0 to 3 on the 1-minute Apgar test tend to score lower on the Bayley Scales of Infant Development administered at 8 months of age than infants who scored from 7 to 10 on the Apgar test.[105] Thus retrieval of the Apgar score from an infant's or child's record may provide information about the relationship between a child's difficulties and perinatal status.

Because of the required adaptation to the extrauterine environment, all newborns are closely monitored. At birth the respiratory status of the newborn is of great concern because of the effect of anoxia on the still-developing brain and because respiratory problems tend to be the major killer of newborns.[86,120] Many infants, especially those who are premature, develop a physiological jaundice, a yellowing of the eyeballs and skin, 3 to 4 days after birth. This jaundice is usually related to immaturity of the liver. The premature infant also has less fat than the full-term infant and thus has greater difficulty in regulating body temperature. Full-term infants can usually regulate body temperature around a slight decrease in environmental temperature by increasing their activity.[41] Premature infants also have a higher incidence of various pathological conditions, including periventricular and intraventricular hemorrhage.[120]

During the various stages of the postnatal period, there are changes in the portions of the body displaying the most rapid growth. For example, from conception to birth, the head grows faster than any other body part and is approximately 70% of adult size at birth. From birth through 1 year of age, the trunk is the fastest growing body segment. Trunk growth represents 60% of the total body growth in the first year. From 1 year of age through adolescence, the legs are the fastest growing body region, comprising 66% of the total body growth during this period. The trunk is again the fastest growing of body regions from adolescence through adulthood, comprising 60% of total body growth during this period.[118] Differential body growth during development has direct clinical implications. For example, because of these body growth spurts, orthotic devices may need to be reevaluated more frequently.

The pliable nature of the bones of infants is due to their lack of ossification. Different bone groups ossify at different times during development. The bones of the body are derived from cartilage tissue that becomes ossified or hardened by the deposition of minerals during development. The ossification process begins during the prenatal period and continues through adolescence. Some bones of the hand and wrist ossify by the end of the first year of life, and the six fontanels do not completely ossify until about 2 years after birth. Other bones ossify through late adolescence.[116]

Newborn infants essentially have their full complement of muscle fibers at birth; however, the muscle fibers are smaller than they should be even in relation to body size. There is a general rostral-to-caudal gradient in the development of muscle fibers, beginning in the head and neck region and extending to those of the lower limbs. Infant males already have a greater proportion of muscle tissue than females at birth, and this differential is maintained throughout life.[34]

Although males are generally larger than females, females develop faster. This sex difference begins during the prenatal period. As indicated above, the sexes also differ in body composition, with females having a greater proportion of fat and less muscle and water than males. At all ages females tend to be lighter and shorter than males except during the prepubertal growth spurt. Females are less variable than males in terms of physical growth characteristics, and physical growth of females is more stable over time than that of males. Skeletal development of a 2-year-old female is a better predictor of future skeletal development than that of a male at the same age.[1]

Physical growth increases rapidly during the preschool years, with no significant differences between males and females. During this time period, the muscular, nervous, and skeletal systems are rapidly maturing. As might be expected, factors such as nutrition and exercise can profoundly affect physical growth and development at these ages.[116]

During the middle childhood period, physical development is less rapid than earlier periods. Although males are typically taller and heavier than females at the start of this period, females attain the adolescent growth spurt earlier than males and thus tend to temporarily exceed the height of males. During the middle childhood period, the bodily and facial proportions of the child change a great deal, and it is now possible to predict future adult height relatively accurately for both males and females.

The adolescent period is a phase of rapid physical growth and maturation of reproductive functioning (primary and secondary sexual characteristics) associated with puberty. Both males and females show sharp growth in height, weight, muscular, and skeletal development—the adolescent growth spurt. The end of the adolescent period is diffuse rather than clearly demarcated, and it is often culturally specified. Growth during adulthood is complete and body weight changes are typically related to changes in body fat.

NORMAL HUMAN NERVOUS SYSTEM DEVELOPMENT
General principles of human nervous system development

During growth and development many impressive structural and functional changes take place within the human nervous system. These developmental changes are not homogeneous in rate throughout the nervous system and they do not occur in discrete stages. Rather, different neural regions develop at different rates, and they develop in a continuous fashion.[22,33] The development of the human nervous system can only accurately be characterized as a differential process over time, each alteration in structure and function representing at the same time the beginning, middle, and end of each preceding and each successive alteration. During human nervous system development there is a tendency for the more primitive neural regions to begin to form earlier than "higher" neural regions.[49] Those regions of the nervous system that appear first in phylogeny tend to appear first in ontogeny, whereas more recently evolved neural structures arise later in ontogeny. For example, neurons of the most recently evolved layers of the cerebral isocortex (outer layers) are the last cortical neurons to be generated during ontogeny.[64] However, the age at which a neural region attains functional maturity cannot be absolutely predicted by the age at which its neurons are derived during neurogenesis.[2] In addition, some neural regions (e.g., cerebellum) begin significant development relatively late in the prenatal period and, as a function of accelerated growth, achieve mature characteristics quite rapidly, whereas other neural regions (e.g., cerebral cortex) may have extremely elongated developmental periods. Thus the development of the human nervous system is not one of homogeneous accretion of substance but rather a process of differential rates and differential timing of growth changes within and between the various neural regions. Understanding these growth changes and the average age span in which they occur will help the clinician

dealing with clients of varying ages to identify areas most likely affected by neural trauma.

The major events that occur during the development of the human nervous system are presented in the following sections. These events appear to be common to the development of the nervous system in all mammals and represent the basic processes for building a brain.

Major events in human nervous system development. The major events in the development of the human brain and the peak times of their occurrence are (1) formation of the neural tube from the neural plate (called neurulation) at 3 to 4 weeks of gestation; (2) cellular proliferation at 2 to 4 months of gestation; (3) cellular migration at 3 to 6 months of gestation; (4) cellular organization at 6 months of gestation through many years after birth; and (5) myelination of neurons at birth through 10 or more years of age and continuing on into adulthood. Each of these major events is described more fully in later sections of this chapter.

The major events presented above may give the impression that brain development occurs in five stages or steps; however, this is not the case. First, there is considerable overlap of these events within and between neural areas. Second, neural regions are not homogenous for the onset and duration of these events. Third, different types of neurons within a given neural region display different time courses for these events. The considerable overlap of these events reinforces the notion that development of the human brain is a continuous process over time. The various events, stages, steps, and phases presented within this chapter are for organizational purposes only and do not accurately reflect the process of neural development as it occurs in nature. The burden on the reader is to keep in mind that these developmental processes are just that—continuous processes over time. However, an understanding of the general timetables for the various developmental events should help the reader gain insight into those neural areas affected when insult to the CNS occurs at different times during development (Fig. 5-3).

The processes of neurulation, cellular proliferation, cellular migration, cellular organization, and cellular myelination are part and parcel of the formation and development of the most complex and slow growing of human organs, the human brain and the remainder of the human nervous system. The vast complexity of the human brain is staggering when we merely consider one of its attributes, the number of neurons. The mature human brain contains on the order of 100 billion neurons (100,000,000,000 neurons)! If this number is not sufficiently impressive, consider further that each of these 100 billion neurons is capable of making literally thousands of functional contacts with other neurons. Because of the tremendous complexity of the mature human brain, many scientists have been studying the development of the brain, perhaps under the assumption that during development we would have a "simpler" system. Yet during the 9-month prenatal period, neurons are being generated at an average rate of approximately 250,000 neurons per minute!

While it may seem as though precise scientific study of the human brain is futile, this is really not the case. Major technological advances (e.g., microelectrode recording techniques, biochemical analyses, and autoradiography) used by creative scientists are continuously unlocking some of the secrets of the brain and its development. Thus, in spite of its complexity, our knowledge of human brain development is increasing at a rapid rate. The general characteristics of human brain development are detailed in the following sections.

Nervous system development during embryonic, fetal, and early postnatal periods

The development of the human nervous system during embryonic, fetal, and early postnatal periods is an awesome process; it is as intriguing as it is complex. From its embryonic beginnings, the human nervous system is dynamic and ever changing. During the embryonic and fetal periods, it grows from a strip of undifferentiated tissue to a recognizable brain that is distinctly human (Fig. 5-2). During the early postnatal period and continuing on for many years, the human nervous system displays further growth and development and is shaped in all of its detail into a mature organ capable of the highest human function. Basically, the embryonic and fetal periods show high rates of qualitative and quantitative growth, while the postnatal period is one of tremendous qualitative growth. Thus damage during any period of life, but especially the prenatal period, has the potential for producing drastic changes in CNS functioning.

The prenatal and postnatal development of the nervous system in humans can be characterized by nine major interactive and dependent processes.[22] Many of these processes, which are begun in the prenatal period, are continued through the postnatal period as well. The processes of building a human brain are (1) induction (formation) of the neural plate[100] followed by formation of the neural tube (neurulation);[51] (2) localized regional cellular proliferation of neurons and glia; (3) migration of neurons and glia to their final positions; (4) aggregation of cells into neural regions; (5) differentiation of immature neurons and glia; (6) formation of interneuronal connections as a function of dendritic and axonal growth and establishment of synapses; (7) selective neuronal death as result of "overproduction" of neurons;[21] (8) loss of some early interneuronal connections and stabilization of other interneuronal connections; and (9) myelination of axons. To varying extents, the fifth, sixth, seventh, eighth, and ninth process are active during postnatal life, and some of them are possibly active throughout the human life span (Fig. 5-3).

Formation of the neural plate and neural tube. At approximately 18 days after conception the human embryo is but 1.5 mm long, yet differentiation of two germ layers, the ectoderm and mesoderm, has begun.[54] Induced by an interaction between the ectoderm and the mesoderm, the ectoderm thickens along the embryonic midline as a function of migration of neuroepithelial cells (germinal cells) to form the neural plate. The neural plate is made up of approximately 125,000 neuroepithelial cells (see Fig. 5-1). In the formation of the nervous system, the neural plate is the smallest substrate that can give rise to the complete CNS.[49]

Neurulation is the process of forming the neural tube from the neural plate. During formation of the neural tube, the number of cells in the neural plate does not significantly change; instead, the neural tube results primarily from changes in the shape of cells of the neural plate.[39,51,100] The cells of the neural plate are initially cuboidal in shape. At the onset of neurulation, cells along the lateral edges (or margins) of the neural tube, as well as those of the midline, begin to elongate and constrict at one end (their dorsal surface). This change from cuboidal to flask shape results in a raising of the neural folds and a midline depression called the neural groove. As more and more cells of the neural plate change to the flasklike shape, the lateral edges of the neural folds curve over to meet at the midline. The changes in cell shape appear to be mediated by intracellular microtubules and microfilaments.[49] During closure to the neural tube, the lateral ectoderm is pulled dorsally and medially over the neural tube, which then sinks under and breaks away from the ectoderm. At the same time, cells at the margin of the neural folds and lateral ectoderm move to the dorsal aspect of the neural tube, where they form the neural crest.[49,78]

The initial fusion of the neural folds of the neural tube occurs at the presumptive "low medulla-cervical" level at approximately 22 days of gestation for the human. The fusion then spreads in both rostral and caudal directions until the tube has fully closed.[35] The rostral (brain end) fusion of the neural tube (anterior neuropore) is complete at approximately 24 days of gestation, and the posterior fusion of the tube (posterior neuropore) is complete to the first and second lumbar segments (presumptive or future segments) by approximately 26 days of gestation. The more caudal aspect of the neural tube, the presumptive lower spinal cord, is formed later. The lumen of the neural tube develops into the ventricular system of the brain and the central canal of the spinal cord.[54] Discussion of neural tube abnormality can be found in Chapter 14.

The neural plate and neural tube are the embryonic precursors of the brain and spinal cord—the CNS (see Table 5-2). This embryonic tissue is the source of neurons and macroglia (astroglia and oligodendroglia). Microglia are mesodermally derived and appear to enter the CNS via the vasculature.[66] The neural crest is the embryonic precursor of many cells intrinsic to the peripheral nervous system. Derived from the neural crest are cells such as the spinal

NEUROGENIC CYCLES

Neural induction: 3-6 wk G
Neuronal proliferation: 2-4 mo G
Glial proliferation: 2 mo G-yr P (?)
Neuronal migration: 3-5 mo G
Neuronal organization: 6 mo G-yr P (?)

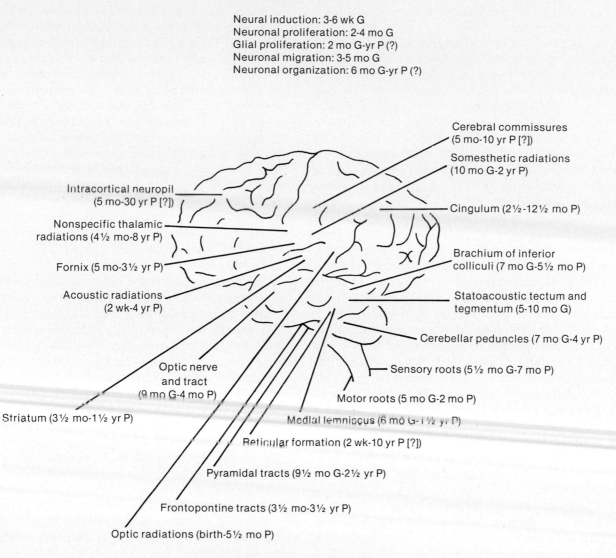

Cerebral commissures (5 mo-10 yr P [?])

Somesthetic radiations (10 mo G-2 yr P)

Intracortical neuropil (5 mo-30 yr P [?])

Cingulum (2½-12½ mo P)

Nonspecific thalamic radiations (4½ mo-8 yr P)

Brachium of inferior colliculi (7 mo G-5½ mo P)

Fornix (5 mo-3½ yr P)

Acoustic radiations (2 wk-4 yr P)

Statoacoustic tectum and tegmentum (5-10 mo G)

Cerebellar peduncles (7 mo G-4 yr P)

Optic nerve and tract (9 mo G-4 mo P)

Sensory roots (5½ mo G-7 mo P)

Motor roots (5 mo G-2 mo P)

Striatum (3½ mo-1½ yr P)

Medial lemniscus (6 mo G-1½ yr P)

Reticular formation (2 wk-10 yr P [?])

Pyramidal tracts (9½ mo G-2½ yr P)

Frontopontine tracts (3½ mo-3½ yr P)

Optic radiations (birth-5½ mo P)

MYELOGENIC CYCLES

G, Gestation
P, Postnatal

Fig. 5-3. Timetable of neurogenic and myelogenic cycles. Myelogenic cycles are detailed for selected neural areas showing the age at which myelination begins for that region and the age at which myelination is essentially complete for that neural area. Question marks *(?)* indicate that the maturation age is not determined. Gestation age *(G)* and postnatal age *(P)* are indicated.

dorsal root (sensory) ganglia, sensory ganglia of some cranial nerves, autonomic ganglia, Schwann cells, and cells of the pia-arachnoid (see Figs. 5-1 and 5-2). The dura mater is formed by an ectodermal-mesodermal interaction.[49]

The neural tube of the human embryo is formed at 3 to 4 weeks of gestation. At the time of closure of the neural tube, cellular proliferation becomes rapid: 250,000 neurons are generated per minute on the average during the prenatal period. As a result of rapid cellular proliferation, the cephalic (or brain end) of the neural tube becomes enlarged into the three primary brain vesicles by 4 to 5 weeks of gestation.[54,129] These vesicles are the prosencephalon (forebrain), which gives rise to the cerebral hemispheres and basal ganglia of the telencephalon, the thalamus and hypothalamus of the diencephalon, the mesencephalon or midbrain, and the rhombencephalon (hindbrain), which gives rise to the cerebellum and pons of the metencephalon and medulla of the myelencephalon (see Fig. 5-2). The caudal remainder of the neural tube develops into the spinal cord.

Cellular proliferation and migration. From the time of formation of the neural plate through formation of the neural tube at 3 to 4 weeks of gestation, the neural plate changes from a simple layer of neuroepithelial cells to a thick layer of cells whose nuclei lie at several levels (Fig. 5-1). Early in development, mitotic figures are confined to the layer of neuroepithelial or germinal cells lining the lumen of the neural tube.[49] The layer of germinal cells of the neural tube is called the *ventricular layer* (or zone). All of the cells of the ventricular zone are involved in cellular proliferation (mitotic activity), and the period of 2 to 4 months of gestation is the period of major proliferation of cells in the developing human brain.[24]

The germinal cells of the ventricular zone have cytoplasmic processes that extend from the lumen of the neural tube to its most superficial or peripheral extent. As neurogenesis proceeds, young neurons migrate out of the ventricular zone to form the *mantle* or *intermediate zone*.[103] The peripheral aspects of the cytoplasmic processes of germinal cells make up the outermost layer, the *marginal layer* or *zone*. Thus the early neural tube consists of the innermost ventricular zone, the intermediate or mantle zone, and the outermost marginal zone.[49]

The germinal cells of the ventricular zone are thought to give rise to both neurons and glial cells (Fig. 5-1). It has been suggested that a "common" germinal cell may give rise initially to young neurons and *later* to glioblasts (cells capable of further division). Glioblasts then give rise to all of the macroglia.[31]

The germinal cells are columnar in shape and extend from the inner to the outer surfaces of the neural tube (Fig. 5-1). The soma and nucleus are found within the ventricular zone. The nuclei of the germinal cells synthesize deoxyribonucleic acid (DNA), migrate toward the ventricular (luminal) surface, and divide (mitosis). The nuclei of the daughter cells then return to the outer surface of the ventricular zone and the cycle is repeated. This to-and-fro movement cycle is repeated for each occurrence of DNA synthesis and mitosis within the ventricular zone (Fig. 5-1). The number of proliferative cycles differs for cells destined to populate different neural regions and for different types of cells.[99] After a number of these proliferative cycles have been completed, cells destined to become neurons lose their capacity to synthesize DNA and migrate out of the ventricular zone or remain as ependymal cells.

Essentially all neurons and macroglia are generated from the ventricular and subventricular zones (a second germinal zone, to be discussed later) of the developing nervous system.[49] Using DNA as a chemical correlate of cell number, Dobbing and Sands[24] have identified two major phases of cellular proliferation in the developing human brain. The first phase, from 2 to 4 months of gestation, is the *phase of major neuronal proliferation*. The second phase, from 5 months of gestation to 1 year or more after birth is the *phase of major glial proliferation* (Fig. 5-3). There is some overlap in these two proliferative phases, especially in the cerebellum. It is also interesting to note that proliferation of the vasculature within the brain corresponds to the phase of neuronal proliferation. Development of arteries typically precedes that of veins.[54]

As early development proceeds, there is at first an increase in the number of germinal cells as the dividing cells continue to undergo mitosis repeatedly. Later, a steady state is reached for the number of germinal cells as one daughter cell of each pair migrates out of the germinal zone. Still later, as germinal cells cease dividing, the population of postmitotic cells increases and the population of germinal cells decreases. Ependymal cells lining the ventricles may represent the final differentiation of the neuroepithelial cells.

In developing mammals, including humans, large neurons are typically generated before small neurons, and neurons are produced before their associated glial cells.[49] It is possible that neural proliferation may actually stimulate glial proliferation.[67] Most glial proliferation occurs during the phase of neuron growth and differentiation. The proliferative cycle or cell cycle of glioblasts is typically much longer than that of neurons, and for some neural regions may be five times as long.[32] There also is a tendency for large neurons to be generated within the ventricular zone while most small neurons and essentially all macroglia are probably generated in a second germinal zone, the subventricular zone.[49] The subventricular zone develops between the ventricular and intermediate (or mantle) zones of the forebrain (Fig. 5-1). This zone retains mitotic figures during adulthood, presumably for glial cells only.[91] However, while most neuronal proliferation occurs during the prenatal period, there are examples of postnatal neuronal proliferation in the olfactory bulbs,[42] hippocampal formation,[3] brainstem nuclei,[115] and cerebellar cortex.[71]

During migration of a daughter cell out of the ventricular zone, the cell loses its basal or inner (ventricular) attachment, and it flows or is pulled *into* its external process as it migrates to the intermediate (mantle) layer. Differentiation of the cell proceeds within the intermediate layer. The remaining daughter cell prepares for another cycle of cell division.[99] In the telencephalon, the young neurons migrate to the intermediate (mantle) zone, which increases in size as a result of ingrowth of afferent axons and migration of cells. This zone forms the *cortical plate* (Fig. 5-1). As cells and fibers continue to invade this zone, the cortical plate of the telencephalon undergoes progressive differentiation to form the layers of the cerebral cortex.[49]

Most glioblasts, and the neuroblasts destined to become small neurons, migrate from the ventricular zone to a *second* germinal zone (located between the ventricular and intermediate zones) called the subventricular zone. One place the subventricular zone is found is in the forebrain.[90] The proliferating cells of the subventricular zone give rise to the *smaller neurons* of the cortex and deep structures of the cerebral hemispheres (such as the basal ganglia). Most of the glioblasts migrate to this subventricular zone, and following the period of major neuronal proliferation, the major period of glial proliferation begins. The macroglia retain their ability to proliferate throughout life.[3] Thus most glial cells are generated in the subventricular zone, and astroglia are typically generated before the oligodendroglia. The astroglia tend to be the primary glial cells found within the gray matter (e.g., cortex) and the oligodendroglia, because of their role in myelination, are the primary glial cells found within the white matter (e.g., fiber tracts).

Culminating with humans, there appears to be an evolutionary trend for an increase in the ratio of Golgi type II neurons to Golgi type I neurons. Golgi type I neurons are large neurons making up the major afferent and efferent pathways. Golgi type II neurons are smaller neurons usually functioning as interneurons or local circuit neurons. Many of these smaller neurons are generated postnatally, and thus they may be affected by the postnatal experience of the organism. The number of Golgi type I neurons in an organism's brain seems correlated with body mass, while the number of Golgi type II neurons is correlated with behavioral complexity.[48] In humans the ratio of granule cells (interneurons) to Purkinje cells (projection neurons) of the cerebellum is on the order of 1500:1.[12] There is also a phylogenetic trend for the glia to neuron ratio to increase up to humans.[30] These phylogenetic trends are primarily manifest in humans during the period of cellular proliferation.

Neuronal migration appears to be an actual ameboidlike movement of the cell out of the germinal zone to its final position within the nervous system. This migration process may take on different forms at different stages of neurogenesis.[49] Early in neurogenesis, when distances to be traveled are short, migrating cells may move while free of any attachment processes. Later in neurogenesis, when distances to be traveled are greater, migrating cells appear to have cytoplasmic attachment processes to both the inner (ventricular) and outer (pial) surfaces of the developing neural tube (Fig. 5-1). In this situation, the soma or nucleus is drawn or flows into the outer or leading process and the trailing process is withdrawn.[11] In still later stages of neurogenesis, when there are long distances and complex "terrain" with which to contend, cells appear to use specialized glial guides (radial glia cells) for migration.[89,108] The radial glial guides (Fig. 5-4) are found as early as 10 weeks of gestation in the human, and they persist throughout the period of neuronal migration.[6] The radial glia are probably associated with the subventricular germinal zone, and later they differentiate into astroglia.[104]

In the human brain the period of major neuronal migra-

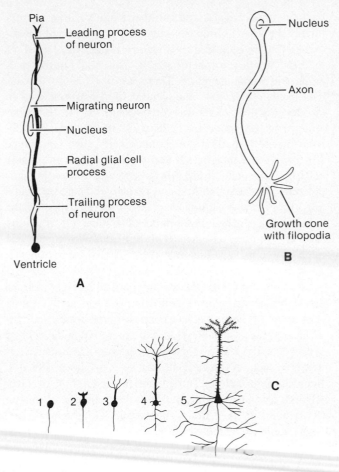

Fig. 5-4. Growth and migration of neurons. **A,** Schematic drawing of a neuron migrating along a radial glial guide. **B,** A growing axon with growth cone and filopodia. **C,** Sequence of development of the dendritic arbor of a pyramidal cell.

tion at 3 to 5 months of gestation overlaps and follows the period of major neuronal proliferation at 2 to 4 months of gestation. The two basic forms of migration are radial, as discussed above, and tangential. Tangential migration is found for both the cerebral and cerebellar cortex. Tangential migration is found for smaller neurons and glia of the superficial layers of the cerebral cortex, where cells of the subventricular zone migrate over the cortical surface, and then inward down through the cortical layer. Tangential migration is also found for granule cells of the cerebellum, where proliferative cells migrate from the ventricular layer in the alar plate of the medulla to the external granular layer. These germinal cells migrate over the surface of the cerebellum then inward to give rise to granule cells of the cerebellum.[114] As might be expected, migration of cells to their final positions takes longer as development proceeds, especially for the cerebral and cerebellar cortices, where distances to be traveled are long and tortuous.

The proliferation and migration of cells in the human CNS follow some general patterns that differ for different neural regions. For example, the cerebral cortex, optic tectum, hippocampus, and substantia nigra (laminar structures) show an inside to outside developmental gradient.[49,108] An opposite, outside to inside (or lateral to medial), gradient of neurogenesis is found for the thalamus and hypothalamus.[5] There are also rostral to caudal, caudal to rostral, and ventral to dorsal gradients in the development of the nervous system. In the cerebellar cortex the various cells develop in the following order from first to last. First are Purkinje cells, then Golgi type II neurons, and then basket and stellate cells, with granule cells being generated last. In the cerebral cortex, pyramidal cells are generated first and granule cells are generated last.[4] The largest neurons are also generated first in the spinal cord.[33] Thus the timing of trauma sustained by different regions of the CNS will differentially affect large and small neurons and also neuronal migration patterns.

In the motor cortex the thalamocortical afferent neurons arrive before and during cellular migration to the cortex (Fig. 5-5).[63] The first cells to appear in the cortex are cells of layer I, then Cajal-Retzius cells, then pyramidal cells of layers V and VI at 5 months of gestation, and then interneurons such as cortical basket cells of layer IV at 7 months of gestation. The pyramidal cells, first of layer III and second of layer II, reach their final positions at 7½ months of gestation. The various Golgi type II and small neurons complete migration during late prenatal periods.[63] Cells may be dormant within the cortex for many months before further differentiation and synaptogenesis take place. By 20 to 24 weeks of gestation, the cerebral cortex seems to have gained the majority of its neurons.

This section has presented the major characteristics of neuronal proliferation and migration, and these are summarized as follows.[22,24,90,91] First, the time at which a cell

ceases to synthesize DNA and ceases dividing (mitosis) appears to be rigidly (genetically?) determined (Fig. 5-1). Second, the cessation of mitosis seems to trigger migration of the cell to its final destination. Third, large cells with long processes (Golgi type I neurons) are generated and migrate before small cells with regionally confined or local processes (local circuit or Golgi type II neurons). Fourth, the sequence and timing of cellular proliferation and migration are characteristic for a given neural region. Fifth, some glial cells are generated with neurons, but most glial cells are generated at high rates after neuronal proliferation has essentially been completed. Sixth, the number of neurons for a given region is determined by the duration of the proliferation period for that region (ranging from days to several weeks for different regions), the duration of cell mitotic cycle (a few hours per cycle early in development to 4 to 5 days per cycle later in development), and the number of germinal or precursor cells. Seventh, more cells are generated for a given neural region than are found in the mature neural region. This cell loss results from cell death. Finally, most neuronal migration involves postmitotic cells, except those cells of special germinal zones such as the subventricular zone and the external granule layer of the cerebellar cortex.

Cellular differentiation and organization. While neurons are migrating, but to a greater extent when they have reached their final positions, neuronal differentiation and growth are the predominant events. In these later phases of neurogenesis, the developing telencephalon consists of the ventricular zone, the subventricular zone (which persists after birth and contains mitotic figures for glial cells throughout adulthood), the intermediate zone, which differentiates into the cortical plate (which further differentiates to form the layers of the cerebral cortex except layer I), and the marginal zone, which is sparsely

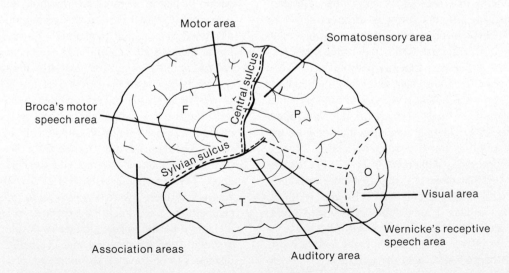

Fig. 5-5. Left cerebral hemisphere of the human brain with locations of sensory, motor, speech, and association areas. The occipital *(O)*, temporal *(T)*, frontal *(F)*, and parietal *(P)* lobes are indicated, as are the central and Sylvian sulci.

populated by neurons and forms layer I of the cerebral cortex (Fig. 5-1).[49]

The final position in the brain occupied by a migrating cell is primarily determined by its position in the germinal zone when the cell is generated.[44] Final neuronal aggregation and orientation within neural regions is most likely related to trophic factors and some characteristics of cell surface molecules.[22] Molecules on the cell surface (cell ligands) may function as receptor sites and serve to promote aggregation of cells. Different types of cells may have different ligands resulting in aggregation of like cells and exclusion of foreign cells.

The peak period of neuronal organization in the human brain occurs from 6 months of gestation through several years after birth (Fig. 5-3).[19] Development of the elaborate circuitry of the human brain is achieved through the following processes: the attainment of proper orientation and alignment of neurons such as seen in the cortical layers and columns, the elaboration of dendritic and axonal ramifications, the establishment of synaptic contacts, and the proliferation and differentiation of glia (Fig. 5-4). In addition, these organizational processes are influenced by developmental changes in a neuron's mode of transmission (e.g., to action potential from graded potential), in the formation of chemical synapses rather than electrical synapses (gap junctions), in the chemical transmitter finally utilized (e.g., norepinephrine or acetylcholine), and in the major ion of the action potential (e.g., calcium in the immature versus sodium in the mature).

Most newly differentiated neurons have many short processes and thus are multipolar neurons, the most frequent cell type of the mature brain.[68] Also, neurons typically generate their processes (axon and dendrites) after migrating to their final destination; however, exceptions are found. Recent studies suggest that the distinctive dendritic arbor of a neuron may be genetically determined, but that afferent input can influence this arbor to some extent (Fig. 5-4). Axons are usually well developed and complete with terminals before dendritic growth and expansion occur. The time elapsing between origin of a neuron and the time it is fully differentiated varies as a function of neuron type. Some neurons, such as Purkinje cells, originate early but have a long period of differentiation, while others such as cerebellar granule cells are generated relatively late and rapidly differentiate.[49]

Elongation of neuronal processes (axons and dendrites) is accomplished via the growth cones at the tips of growing processes.[49] Growth cones are enlarged areas of about 10 μm in diameter from which emerge fingerlike projections called filopodia, which are 0.15 to 0.30 μm in diameter and about 20 μm in length (Fig. 5-4). These filopodia wave, expand, and contract within periods of seconds. The filopodia are the sites of adhesion between the growing process and the substrate, and they may also function as tactile and/or chemosensory agents that test the environ-

ment within which they are growing.[49] The growth cone is also the site of incorporation or acquisition of new material that has been transported to the growth cone from the soma. The growth cone not only is the site of new growth of a process but also may be the site of process branching or bifurcation. Other processes may not have growth cones per se but may grow along gradients, glial channels, or "pioneer" axons. Throughout the nervous system, axonal process development tends to precede the development of dendritic processes.

The initial axon outgrowth appears to be genetically preprogrammed to aim in a particular direction. Later axonal growth and the reaching of its final destination(s) seems contingent on external forces, such as characteristics of the electrical, chemical, and physical substrate. Growth of the axon is at the tip and the materials for growth have been transported from the soma outward. Once an axon has grown to its general destination, axonal branching may or may not be random, and contacts with other neurons that do not become functional may eventually be eliminated.[49]

Dendritic differentiation starts later than axonal differentiation and proceeds long after axonal differentiation has been essentially completed. The dendritic tree of a neuron is characteristic of that neuron, yet the dendritic tree may be influenced by external factors.[40,49] Similar to the timetable for generation of neurons, dendritic development and elaboration seem to proceed first in large neurons and then in small neurons, and dendritic development occurs typically in a ventrodorsal or inside to outside sequence (Fig. 5-4). However, there are general exceptions to this trend. For example, Purkinje cells originate early and have a prolonged period of dendritic development, while cerebellar granule cells are generated late yet show rapid dendritic differentiation. Within the cerebral cortex, dendritic expansion is first radial (vertical) and then tangential (horizontal), for both pyramidal cells and local circuit neurons (Fig. 5-4).[77]

The dendritic tree of a "mature" neuron has 90% of its postsynaptic surface in the mature organism. However, early in neural development the dendrites are short, stout, varicose, and of an uneven diameter (Fig. 5-4). Fine hairlike protrusions are evenly distributed along the young dendrite. With further growth the proximal portions of the dendrites attain a more even diameter and the long hairlike protuberances remain. These hairs may be searching out growing axons. Further growth of the dendrites is associated with the formation of a substantial number of spines, some of which have dilated tips. As the dendritic tree reaches maturity, there is a gradual reduction of spine numbers and many of the early dendritic branches are lost or absorbed.

The building of a brain with all of its appropriate interneuronal connections is far from being understood. However, we are currently gaining some insights.[22,49,88] As indicated earlier, cells generated at the same time from the same region of the germinal matrix tend to stay together throughout migration and differentiation. Like cells tend to aggregate and thus are more likely to interconnect. Also, axons tend to grow with their neighbors. In addition, a number of trophic factors have been studied as possible guides for neuronal interconnections, such as nerve growth factor.[57] It has also been frequently observed that neurons tend to generate more processes and make more connections early in development than are found later in the fully mature neural region. Thus there seems to be a period of process retraction and connection elimination that contributes to neural organization during development. Finally, cell death seems to contribute to neural organization. More neurons are generated for a neural region than are found with maturation.[33] During the period of formation of neural connections, cell death may claim up to 85% of the neurons within a given region. The range of cell death varies from 15% to 85% of the neurons of regions studied to date. Cell death may be related to the size of the region innervated, the availability of functional contacts, or the amount of some trophic material.[22]

Synaptogenesis. Synaptogenesis within the human brain begins very early in prenatal development and continues to some extent throughout the life span of the human organism. It may occur, for example, with learning and with repair phenomena associated with brain damage (Fig. 5-3). Synaptogenesis is the establishment of a chemically mediated functional contact between neurons. The development of a synapse requires specialization of the presynaptic and postsynaptic membranes and neurotransmitter synthesis, release, storage, and inactivation. There are numerous known and putative neurotransmitters within the nervous system, for example acetylcholine and dopamine. Synaptogenesis is a prerequisite for communication and functional interaction between neurons.

While synaptogenesis in the human brain begins early in gestation, the highest rates of synaptogenesis occur during the early postnatal period.[49] However, it must be kept in mind that the rates of synaptogenesis differ for the various neuron types within and between neural regions. Chemical indices of synaptogenesis show a rapid increase in synapse formation from 2 months before birth to 2 years after birth. The increase in synapse formation from birth through 2 years of age is approximately threefold.

The process of developing a synapse (e.g., axodendritic synapse) requires the growth of an axon at the growth cone (filopodia) such that contact is made with a potential postsynaptic membrane, a dendrite for example. When a filopodia makes contact with a dendrite there is a period of about 30 minutes during which all filopodia activity ceases. The filopodia will then frequently resume its activity, either leaving the contact intact or breaking contact. If contact is preserved, a postsynaptic specialization begins to appear within a few hours, and this specialization elon-

gates with time. The synaptic cleft widens within about 2 days to achieve the normal adult distance of approximately 18 nm. Parallel with the postsynaptic specialization, a presynaptic dense projection develops. By approximately 1 day after initial contact, synaptic vesicles can be seen within the presynaptic terminals and the number of vesicles continues to increase with time. While synapse formation appears to be heavily dependent upon an interaction of presynaptic and postsynaptic membranes and intercellular contacts, the events associated with synapse formation seem not to be totally dependent upon functional activity per se.[78]

In the development of a synapse, the postsynaptic membrane may be sensitive to putative neurotransmitters before the synapse has fully developed. In fact, postsynaptic specializations may even develop before any interneuronal contacts are made.[93] Thus in most cases, the postsynaptic system interacts with the neurotransmitter showing a simultaneous development; however, this can occur even before development of neurotransmitter synthesis in the presynaptic terminals has reached adult levels. At the early or immature synapse, the receptors are few and sparse and there are low levels of synthesis and release of neurotransmitters. At this time there are very few recognizable synaptic structures or specializations. Later, rudimentary synaptic structures develop and there is a rapid increase in the number and density of postsynaptic receptors. Still later, biochemical maturation of presynaptic and postsynaptic components for synthesis, transport, and inactivation of neurotransmitters is achieved. Finally, all synaptic structures are present.[49]

The early appearance and maturation of neurotransmission in the absence of a morphologically and biochemically mature presynaptic apparatus seem a general development phenomenon for synaptogenesis. This may indicate that early synapses function under different and more primitive conditions than they do in the adult. A low release of neurotransmitter from an immature presynaptic terminal may be sufficient to trigger the process of neurotransmission and subsequent phases of synaptogenesis.

Synaptogenesis proceeds in an orderly sequence in various brain regions. However, the development of functional synapses appears to be different between neuron types and between neural regions. For example, synapses can be found in the human cerebral cortex as early as 8½ weeks of gestation.[75] These synapses are found above and below the cortical plate, never within the cortical plate. At 8½ weeks of gestation the density of synapses is low (five per square millimeter); then the number of synapses increases rapidly with age. The earliest synapses within the cortical plate are found at 23 weeks of gestation. The development of synapses in the cortical plate at this age may be associated with a second wave of axonal input to the cortex in conjunction with development of dendrites of neurons within the cortical plate. All of these cortical synapses are presumably the axodendritic variety. At these early ages, many of the presynaptic elements have vesicles, but presynaptic vesicles are fewer in number than in mature presynaptic terminals. This layering of synapses in the developing cortex, first above and below the cortical plate, then within the cortical plate, is an indication that development of synaptic strata may be a characteristic feature of immature cortex. This stratification may result from the fact that thalamocortical fibers reach the presumptive cortical layers before the migrating cortical neurons.[63]

Potential presynaptic and postsynaptic membranes do not appear different, morphologically, from other areas of the cell surface. However, spines of postsynaptic neurons tend to be associated with synapses, and this might indicate that areas of the spine surface membrane have a special capacity to initiate synaptic contacts. As dendritic spines are a prevalent site of synapse formation, the number of dendritic spines on a neuron may be used to estimate the number of synapses. Also, increases in dendritic length may be associated with increased numbers of spines and thus increased synapse formation.[49]

In the developing cerebrum there is a large prenatal and postnatal increase in total dendritic length, suggesting an increase in the number of synapses.[49,69] However, there is a general trend for the number of spines and synapses to increase during development, with a subsequent loss or regression of spines and synapses as nonfunctional synapses are eliminated. In the visual cortex of the human brain, the maximum rate of spine development occurs from 25 to 32 weeks of gestation.[88,119] In the hippocampus, the maximum rate of spine development occurs earlier, at 20 to 28 weeks of gestation, and the full complement of spines is achieved by approximately 6 months after birth.[80,81,87]

While change in the sensitivity of the presumptive postsynaptic membrane may be important for the development of a functional synapse, it may not be the only regulator of synaptic development. Synaptic development may also be regulated by some characteristic of afferent input.[49,93] For example, in the visual system, deafferentation results in a 50% decrease in the surface area of dendritic spines. It is also known that axons form contacts with large numbers of neurons in their projection field, but the final distribution of contacts is dependent in part upon competition with other axons for a limited number of synaptic sites on the receptor cell. Axons normally in the vicinity of a receptor cell will tend to form synapses preferentially with that cell. If those axons were destroyed, the receptor sites would be available to axons from other normally foreign neurons. Finally, the pharmacology of a synapse may be relatively flexible during development. For example, some neurons can become noradrenergic or cholinergic depending upon the types of postsynaptic membranes with which they come into contact.[49]

Myelination. The period of myelination within the human nervous system begins prenatally and extends well into adult life.[127,132] The period of most rapid myelination within the human brain is after gestation term (Fig. 5-3). It is thought that myelination of neurons improves coordinated behavior via an increase in neuronal conduction velocity. Myelinated fibers propagate impulses approximately six times faster than nonmyelinated fibers, and conduction velocity of myelinated fibers increases threefold from birth to adulthood in humans. While myelination is considered to be an important characteristic of neural development, it should be remembered that neurons are capable of carrying impulses before myelination. In other words, functional characteristics of neurons appear before myelin. However, myelination is often considered to be an index of total neuronal maturity.

Immediately preceding and overlapping the onset of myelination is a period of rapid proliferation of glial cells (presumably an increased proliferation of oligodendroglia that are associated with the processes of myelination) within the CNS (Fig. 5-4). This burst of cellular (glia) proliferation occurs at 20 to 30 weeks of gestation, a time that follows most of the neuronal proliferation.[24] From 30 weeks of gestation to gestation term there is a twofold increase in cells and a further twofold increase of cells from birth to 8 months of age. Smaller increases in cells continue through many years after birth.

Myelin formation is the major source of growth of the white matter in the CNS. Myelination begins close to the soma of a neuron and spreads distally. Myelin accumulates in two forms. Myelin increases in *thickness* as it circles an axon, and it increases as the axon *elongates* during development. It has been suggested that myelin formed early differs in some chemical characteristics from myelin formed later in development.[49,132] The accuracy and potential significance of this suggestion are unknown at this time. In the mature brain, myelin represents approximately 25% of total brain weight.[49]

Myelination of neurons occurs generally in the same order as neuronal generation and differentiation, and for a given level of the neuraxis, large neurons myelinate before small neurons.[132] The first myelination occurs in neurons of the peripheral nervous system when axons attain a diameter of approximately 1 to 2 μm. In general, axons generated earliest tend to be largest and those tend to myelinate earliest. The earliest myelinating axons are the ventral (motor) roots of the spinal cord, which begin myelination at approximately 4 months of gestation. Next to myelinate are the dorsal (sensory) roots of the spinal cord, which begin at 5 months of gestation and continue to develop over many months after birth (Fig. 5-3).

In the human nervous system, myelination tends to follow a general caudal to rostral gradient; however, different neurons *within* a neural region may myelinate at different rates. Homogeneous nerves and fiber bundles tend to myelinate as a group and display a relatively short cycle for myelin completion. More heterogeneous nerves and fiber bundles tend to take longer to complete myelination. The sequence of myelination within the nervous system parallels phylogenetic trends of regional neural development.[132]

Within the developing CNS there are gradients in the process of myelination. Myelination progresses from the lower lamina of the cortical plate to the outer lamina of the cortical plate and from the intracortical plexus of vertical fibers to the plexus of horizontal fibers. Myelination of fiber systems mediating sensory input to the thalamus and cortex generally precedes myelination of fiber systems mediating integration of sensory input into motor output (efferents). For example, myelination of the medial and lateral lemniscus, trapezoid body, brachium of the inferior colliculus, optic chiasm, optic tract, and optic radiations begins earlier than myelination of the pyramidal tract, corticospinal tract of the midbrain and pons, superior cerebellar peduncle, and frontopontine tract. Within the cerebral hemispheres, especially within the association areas, intracortical neuropil, and cerebral commissures, the process of myelination persists over decades of postnatal life (Fig. 5-3).[132]

One of the earliest myelinating systems in the brain is the vestibulocochlear system, which shows myelination in the tegmentum and tectal region by the end of the fifth month of gestation (Fig. 5-3). This is about 2 weeks earlier than myelination of the medial lemniscus (somatosensory function). The vestibulocochlear system at the brainstem level completes myelination before gestation term, while myelination of the medial lemniscus is not complete until approximately 1 year after birth. In the forebrain the first myelin appears at approximately 7 months of gestation and myelination becomes rapid in the thalamus, subthalamus, and pallidum during the last trimester of gestation.[132]

There is little myelin within the white matter of the cerebral hemispheres until about the last month of gestation. In the precentral gyrus (sensorimotor function), myelination begins at approximately 2 to 3 months after birth. It is interesting that, similar to the commissural and association fibers of the cerebral cortex, the fibers of the reticular formation show little myelin at gestation term and a very long postnatal period of myelin formation (Fig. 5-3).

Brainstem fibers of the vestibular and acoustic sensory systems (medial longitudinal bundle, lateral lemniscus) myelinate early, and myelination is well advanced by gestation term.[132] The brainstem fibers (medial lemniscus, inferior cerebellar peduncle, and brachium conjunctivum) of the proprioceptive and exteroceptive sensory systems begin myelination later than the brainstem fibers of the vestibular and acoustic sensory systems. Also, the duration of the period of myelin formation is elongated. In the forebrain the projections from the thalamus to the geniculocalcarine (optic), postcentral (somesthetic), and precentral (propriokinesthetic) cortices display rapid myelination during the first year after birth, while the thalamic projections to the geniculotemporal (auditory) cortices have a protracted period of myelination beyond the first year. With the exception of the latter, myelination of the thalamocortical projections precedes that of the corticofugal fiber systems of sensorimotor integration.

It is interesting to note that the prethalamic levels of the vestibuloacoustic system begin and complete myelin formation very early in comparison to the somatosensory, optic, and corticofugal fiber systems. However, at the cortical end, the optic system rapidly myelinates during the first year of postnatal life while the auditory system of the temporal lobe displays a protracted period of myelin formation beyond the first year of postnatal life. This sequencing of myelination suggests very early development of brainstem levels of vestibuloacoustic function as compared to other sensory systems.

Normal sequential human nervous system development

The development of the human nervous system begins with the formation of the neural groove and neural plate at about 18 days of gestation (see Figs. 5-1 to 5-5). This is followed, at 3 to 4 weeks of gestation, by formation of the neural tube, which is composed of the ventricular (innermost), mantle, and marginal (outermost) layers, and by formation of the neural crest. The neural tube differentiates into the CNS (brain and spinal cord), and the neural crest gives rise to most of the peripheral nervous system (cranial, spinal, and autonomic ganglia and nerves). The neural tube is the site of the four fundamental embryonic zones (ventricular, subventricular, intermediate, and marginal zones) involved in cellular proliferation and migration. The germinal zones involute or disappear with maturation. At this time the three primary vesicles of the brain are beginning to form: the prosencephalon or forebrain, the mesencephalon or midbrain, and the rhombencephalon or hindbrain. By the fifth and sixth weeks of gestation, the telencephalon, diencephalon, mesencephalon, metencephalon, and myelencephalon are beginning to differentiate and the cerebral hemispheres are bulging. The three primary flexures (cervical, pontine, and midbrain) of the brain are represented, nerves and ganglia are present, and sympathetic ganglia are forming segmental masses (Fig. 5-2).

The paired cerebral hemispheres, corpus striatum, thalamus, and hypothalamus are rapidly increasing in size at 7 weeks of gestation. Also, the pituitary gland is recognizable, and the choroid plexuses of the ventricle are appearing. At 8 weeks of gestation, the cerebral cortex begins to acquire its typical cells and the olfactory bulbs are visible. The dura mater and pia-arachnoid are distinct by this time. By 10 weeks of gestation the spinal cord has attained its internal structure (Fig. 5-2).

At 12 to 14 weeks of gestation, the hemispheres are readily recognized, the thalamus is enlarged, and the cerebellum has begun to develop. At this age the brain attains its general structural features, the spinal cord shows cervical and lumbar enlargements, and the cauda equina and filum terminale are appearing. The lateral ventricles of the brain are separated and connect the third ventricle via the interventricular foramen (of Monro), the cerebral hemispheres are not yet showing fissures, and neuroglia are beginning to differentiate (Fig. 5-2).

The cerebral hemispheres have bulged and lie over much of the brainstem at 16 weeks of gestation. The lateral (sylvian) fissure now separates the temporal lobe from the other neural lobes (frontal, parietal, and occipital), which are also recognizable at this time (Fig. 5-5). The cerebellum assumes some prominence at this age and the corpora quadrigemina (superior and inferior colliculi) are appearing. By 20 weeks of gestation the major brain commissures are in place and myelination of the spinal cord has begun. At twenty-five weeks of gestation the cerebral cortex begins to show its typical layering pattern, and at 28 to 30 weeks of gestation the fissures (central, calcarine, and parietooccipital sulci) and convolutions of the cerebral hemispheres are appearing rapidly (Figs. 5-2 and 5-5). By 8 months of gestation the pre- and postcentral gyri are prominent and the lateral sulcus remains wide, exposing the insula. Essentially all primary and secondary cortical sulci are represented at this age as are some tertiary cortical sulci. During the final month of gestation, myelination of the brain becomes rapid. The frontal, temporal, and occipital lobes are stubby or blunt, and the lateral sulcus is still wide. Most of the cerebral gyri are broad and plump and the fissures are shallow (Fig. 5-2).

At gestation term, the regions of the cerebral hemispheres posterior to the central sulcus are more developed than those regions anterior to the central sulcus (Fig. 5-5). The frontal and temporal poles are still short; however, the closure of the lateral sulcus almost covers the insula. The number of tertiary sulci on the cerebral cortex is still few. The subcortical white matter is not yet completely myelinated, and the brain has a soft gelatinous consistency. By 2 years of age the brain proportions are similar to those of the adult. Myelination of the brain is now quite advanced, the cerebral hemispheres show many tertiary sulci, and the brain is of a firmer consistency.[54,101,130,131]

The brain of the typical full-term newborn human infant weighs approximately 350 g and this represents approximately 10% of the newborn's total body weight. By 1 year of age the brain has increased in weight to about 1000 g.[24] At puberty the brain of a female weighs approximately 1250 g and the brain of a male weighs approximately 1375 g. The brain of a female generally grows more rapidly than that of a male up to the third year of age; thereafter the brain of a male grows faster than that of a female.

The human adult brain weighs approximately 1500 g and represents only 2% of the adult body weight. Thus it is clear that the major increase in absolute size and weight of the human brain occurs postnatally. The increase in brain size is twofold to threefold during just the first 12 months of postnatal life! This rapid brain growth period begins after the final neuronal number has been largely achieved (by midgestation) and is a function of glial multiplication, dendritic and axonal growth, establishment of synaptic connections, and myelination.[24]

In comparison to the remainder of the brain (forebrain and brainstem), the cerebellum shows a delay in reaching its peak period of cellular proliferation and weight increase. However, in spite of the delay, these measures reach adult values sooner in the cerebellum than in the forebrain or brainstem.[24]

Spinal cord and peripheral nervous system. In the portion of the neural tube that will become the spinal cord, two alar plates develop dorsolaterally and two basal plates develop ventrolaterally (Fig. 5-2). These plates (columns) are connected by roof and floor plates and separated by the sulcus limitans. The basal plate will contribute elements to motor units and it does not appear to extend beyond the mesencephalon in the rostral direction. The alar plate contributes elements to sensory units, extends to the forebrain, and contributes to development of the telencephalon and diencephalon, in addition to lower structures[54,101] (Fig. 5-2).

The basal plate gives rise to the ventral horn cells and cells of the intermediolateral cell column of the spinal cord. These cells will eventually make up the preganglionic sympathetic neurons, the intermediate motor neurons, the ventral motor neurons, and the motor neurons of certain cranial nerve nuclei. The alar plate gives rise to relay and internuncial (interneuron) neurons in the spinal cord. Peripheral sensory neurons are derived from the neural crest.[49] Fibers leaving the alar plate are found as early as the fifth week of gestation, and these are for intersegmental connections.

Up to 3 months of gestation, the spinal cord fills the entire vertebral column. With differential rates of growth between the spinal cord and the vertebral column, the end of the spinal cord is at the third lumbar vertebra at gestation term and at the first to second lumbar vertebra in the adult. This allows low lumbar punctures to be made without danger of spinal cord injury.

Cell bodies in the alar plates form the dorsal or posterior horns of the spinal cord gray matter. Likewise, cell bodies of the basal plates form the ventral (anterior) and lateral gray horns. Axons of the ventral horn cells grow out of the spinal cord to innervate somites, and the axons acquire myelin sheaths from Schwann cells (which are derivatives of neural crest cells). These axons form the ventral roots of the spinal nerves. The dorsal roots of spinal nerves are formed by unipolar neurons whose cell bodies reside in the dorsal root ganglia. These neurons are derived from neural crest cells, and some axons of these neurons enter the spinal cord and make synapses, while other axons ascend the spinal cord up toward the brain.[23]

The peripheral nervous system develops as follows (Table 5-2). Sensory ganglion (dorsal root) neurons are derived from the neural crest. Lower motor neurons are derived from the basal plate and their axons emerge through the ventral root to innervate muscles and glands. Neuroblasts of the neural crest and basal plate migrate peripherally to form the autonomic nervous system ganglia. The outgrowths of the neural crest and basal plate form early and invade the adjacent somites. As the somite differentiates and migrates to its final location in the body, the initial neuronal connections are maintained and carried away with the migrating somite. Since the number of nodes of Ranvier are fixed early in development, the carrying of the axon by the somite results in an elongation of the internodal segments of the axon.

A reciprocal relation exists between a peripheral nerve and peripheral tissue. For example, an uninnervated muscle cell is receptive to becoming innervated, but once it is innervated it will not usually accept any additional innervation. Because of this, muscle cells are spared potentially antagonistic axonal inputs. However, because of the branching capacity of nerve fibers, a single axon may branch repeatedly and thus innervate many muscle cells (a motor unit). This process of axonal branching increases the probability that all muscle cells will receive axonal input.

There is evidence to suggest that neural crest cells may be pluripotent, that is, they differentiate according to the sites in which they settle. The cells of the spinal sensory ganglia form compact cell aggregates under the influence of somites. Somites appear to be required for appropriate growth of spinal sensory neurons (Fig. 5-2).[49]

Cerebellum. The cerebellum develops from symmetrical thickenings of the dorsal parts of the alar plates, which eventually fold over the fourth ventricle (Fig. 5-2). At 9 to 10 weeks of gestation, the Purkinje cells move out of the ventricular zone to initiate the cerebellar cortex.[92] By 10 to 11 weeks of gestation, the external granule cells of the subventricular zone have migrated to the outer surface of the cerebellar cortex. At this time the cerebellar cortex already has many afferent inputs. From 16 to 25 weeks of gestation, the Purkinje cells enlarge and form apical dendritic trees.[133] Also at this time, the first granule cells appear in the cerebellar cortex followed by the appearance of basket cells. The normal maturation of the Purkinje cells is influenced by contacts with climbing fibers. All lobules of the cerebellar vermis can be identified as the major fissures develop at 15 weeks of gestation, and the fissures continue to develop up to 2 years of age.[61]

The two sources of neurons for the cerebellum are the ventricular-subventricular zones and the rhombic lip. The neurons migrate to form the cerebellum via radial and tangential migration (Fig. 5-1). Neuroblasts migrate to the mantle layer of the cerebellar plate and the mantle layer evolves into two strata. These strata are (1) the deep stratum, which differentiates to the deep cerebellar nuclei (fastigii, globose, emboliform, and dentate nuclei), and (2) the superficial stratum, which differentiates into the Purkinje and Golgi type II cells. Germinal cells of the rhombic lip migrate over the surface of the cerebellar cortical plate to form the external granular layer (another germinal zone). This layer gives rise to the granular cells of the granular layer and the stellate and basket cells of the molecular layer.[115]

While the Purkinje cells are forming their dendritic trees within the molecular layer, the granule cells are migrating down from the external granular layer through the molecular layer to the granular layer along the preexisting processes of Bergmann glial cells (a radial glial cell). The interaction between the migrating granule cells and the Purkinje cells results in the formation of the parallel fibers of the granule cells, the normal differentiation of the Purkinje cell dendritic tree, and the specific synaptic connections between these two neuron types. The timing of these developmental phenomena is remarkable. The final cerebellar development is complete within about 2 years after birth with the differentiation and growth of Golgi type II cells, stellate cells, basket cells, climbing fibers, and mossy fibers.[49]

Cerebral cortex. The neurons of the six-layer neocortex are derived from the ventricular and subventricular zones of the neural tube, and cells migrate to successively more peripheral layers. The first sign of neocortical development is a narrow plate of neuroblasts immediately beneath the marginal zone in the lateral wall of the presumptive hemisphere dorsolateral to the presumptive corpus striatum in the vicinity of the presumptive central sulcus. This cortical plate can be identified at approximately 8 weeks of gestation and progressively thickens by the addition of migrating cells (Fig. 5-1).[108]

Cells migrating to the cortex are simple: typically bipolar neurons with a 200 μm leading process. These neurons appear to attain their final positions via radially oriented glial guides. The presumptive cortex is already rich in afferent neurons from the thalamus as it gains in cells. The final positioning of cortical cells is a function of interactions of migrating cell processes with the processes of other cells.

In the motor cortex, thalamocortical afferent neurons arrive before and during cellular migration (Fig. 5-5). The first cortical cells to appear are the cells of layer I (an exception to the inside to outside gradient of neurogenesis), then the Cajal-Retzius cells, then the pyramidal cells of layers V and VI at approximately 5 months of gestation.

At approximately 7 months of gestation the cortical basket cells (interneurons) appear in layer IV, and by 7½ months of gestation the pyramidal cells have arrived in layers III and II. The various Golgi type II cells and other small neurons appear later during the prenatal and possibly the early postnatal periods.[63] The final appearing neurons in the cortex are intrinsic interneurons (stellate cells), neurons for lateral interactions (horizontal cells), interhemispheric callosal cells, and secondary extrinsic afferent neurons (association neurons).

During the development of individual pyramidal cells of the cortex, the apical dendrites appear first, then the basal dendrites (Fig. 5-4). The apical dendrites develop primarily during the late prenatal period while the basal dendrites develop primarily during the first year of postnatal life.[74] Axonal sprouts begin to leave the cortex after 8 weeks of gestation, and these are directed toward the diencephalon and lower centers. Many of the axons terminate within or dissect the corpus striatum, while others project through the internal capsule and on through the crus cerebri and pyramid to enter the spinal cord.

In the mature human cerebral cortex there are approximately 5 to 10 billion neurons. In addition to gaining neurons during development, the characteristics of the cortex change dramatically during the early growth periods. For example, in layer III of the midfrontal gyrus, there is a fivefold decrease in cell packing density from birth through 1 year of age. During the same 1-year period, there is a fourfold increase in cell body volume, a fivefold increase in dendritic branching, and a 16-fold increase in total dendritic length (Fig. 5-5). Between 1 year of age and adulthood, each of the above measures show a further change of approximately twofold (Fig. 5-4).

The cortex develops in a basic inside-to-outside gradient and in a basic caudal-to-rostral gradient. The laminar structure of the six-layer neocortex is partially a function to these neurogenesis gradients. The radial (vertical) pattern of neurogenesis is reflected in the cortical layers and also is apparent for the cortical columns. For at least the basal dendrites of the pyramidal cells of layers V, IV, III, and II, there is an inside to outside pattern of basal (lateral) dendritic formation of pyramidal cells within and across layers.[74] The tangential (horizontal) organization of cortical dendrites in humans persists through 2 years of age.[102] Tangential cortical development is also apparent for dendrites of Golgi type II cells and other small neurons with later-appearing dendrites.[77]

The synaptic input to the cortex also appears to develop in strata. A direct route of axons from the thalamus is through the presumptive corpus striatum in the outermost zone of the hemisphere wall. The thalamic projections separate into a deep and a superficial sheet around the cortical plate at approximately 8 weeks of gestation. A third stratum projects to the cortical plate forming synapses at approximately 23 weeks of gestation. Cortical cells typically form synapses at the time they reach their final positions. However, some cortical cells may be dormant for weeks or months before developing interconnections.

Changes in cortical thickness have been frequently studied and provide important data on human brain development.[88,129] In the presumptive hand area of the precentral gyrus (sensorimotor cortex), the increase in cortical thickness is rapid from 8 months of gestation through gestation term (Fig. 5-5). From birth to 6 years of age the increase in thickness of the cortex is slow, then is rapid again from 6 years through adulthood. In the presumptive motor area for speech (Broca's area), the thickness of the cortex increases rapidly from 8 months of gestation to about 1 month after birth; then further increase in cortical thickness is slow through 4 years (see Fig. 5-5). Little change in cortical thickness takes place after 4 years of age. In the presumptive orbital-frontal cortical area (higher cognitive function), the cortical thickness increases rapidly from 8 months of gestation through 2 years of age; from 2 years of age through adulthood, the increase in cortical thickness is slow and steady (see Fig. 5-5). While these developmental changes in cortical thickness tend to parallel behavioral development, the correspondence is not exact for these representative areas.[88]

The cerebral convolutions (sulci and gyri) appear in humans during the fifth month of gestation and they continue to develop postnatally (see Fig. 5-2). This time period corresponds to the period of maximal increase in volume of the cerebral cortex. The primary convolutions are the first to appear developmentally, and they are relatively constant in location, configuration, and relationship to cortical architectonic fields. The constancy of the primary and secondary cortical sulci may result from regional differences in growth of dendrites and thalamocortical projections to functionally distinct regions (see Fig. 5-5). The cortex on the gyrus tends to get strong thalamic projections while the cortex at the bottom of the sulcus gets weak thalamic projections. The major gyri also tend to receive heavy thalamic projections from distinct peripheral regions, which represents a functional mapping into the cortex.[125] The tertiary convolutions begin to develop during the third trimester of gestation and they mature postnatally. The tertiary convolutions appear random in their form and anatomical relationships, and they may be produced by intracortical forces, that is, mechanical forces generated by differential growth of the various cortical layers.[95]

None of the cortical convolutions make their appearance during neuronal proliferation; rather, convolutions begin to appear during the phases of glial production, growth of neuronal processes, and myelination. This is the period of the most rapid growth and increase in volume of the cortex. An earlier theory proposed that convolutions develop as a function of more rapid growth of the flexible cortex relative to the slower growth of the more rigid subcortical structures.[53] The more recent theory, presented in the preceding paragraph, is that convolutions are a result of relative growth differences within the cortex itself, that is, between layers and regions. The three outer cortical layers grow faster than the three inner layers of cortex, and different cortical regions grow at different rates as a function of growth of their thalamic projections.[95]

Postnatal development of the human brain

Brain growth spurts. Postnatal development of the human brain results primarily from growth of neurons and elaboration of their axonal and dendritic processes, glial proliferation, synaptogenesis, and formation of myelin. Among the principal features of growth of an individual neuron during the postnatal period are enlargement of the cell body, increase in the number of Nissl granules (ribonucleic acid, RNA), formation of neurofibrils, increase in numbers of mitochondria, branching of axons and increased axonal diameter, elaboration of the dendritic tree, increased numbers of axon terminals, and elaboration of myelin.[49] This neuronal growth produces developmental changes in characteristics of various neural regions. For example, because of the growth of neurons, cortical width increases with age, and concurrently, neuronal density decreases because of the relative expansion of the neuropil. At birth, cell bodies occupy approximately 14% of the volume of cerebral cortex and this decreases to approximately 6% cell bodies in the adult (Fig. 5-3). While each of the above are active processes during the prenatal period, they are all accelerated during the early postnatal period.

The late prenatal period extending through the early postnatal period is a time of rapid brain growth called the *brain growth spurt* by Dobbing and Sands.[27] The brain growth spurt was revealed by analysis of human brains ranging in age from 10 weeks of gestation through adulthood. The major variables measured were weight, DNA (cell number), cholesterol (myelin), and water content. The brain was analyzed as a whole and as parts (forebrain, brainstem, and cerebellum).

The brain growth spurt in the human is a transient period of rapid brain growth that begins when the final number of neurons has already been largely achieved.[24,128] The human brain growth spurt begins at approximately midgestation, and the onset of this spurt is correlated in time with the enormous multiplication of glial cells, not neurons. The later phase of the brain growth spurt is a function of elaboration and growth of axons and dendrites, increase in synaptogenesis, and myelination, as well as growth in neuron size. The deceleration of the brain growth spurt parallels the decrease in the rate of myelin formation. The brain growth spurt per se ends at approximately 2 to 4 years of age; however, subsequent brain growth continues at an attenuated rate (Fig. 5-4).[24]

These results reinforce the notion that significant human brain growth takes place during the postnatal period. This period of extremely high rates of growth begins during midgestation and is continued through the first 2 to 4 years. It is worth noting further that at least five-sixths of this brain growth spurt occurs postnatally. At the time of gestation term the human brain has achieved only 27% of the adult value for weight and cell number.[24] The human brain growth spurt may be a period of increased brain vulnerability to extraneous influences, for example, malnutrition, drugs, or trauma.

Epstein[26-28] has taken brain growth spurts a step further and uses indirect data to support the hypothesis that postnatal brain development occurs as a *series* of *growth spurts* and *plateaus* through at least the young adult years. He suggested that brain growth spurts occur for the human brain at 3 to 10 months, 2 to 4 years, 6 to 8 years, 10 to 12 or 13 years, and 14 to 16 or 17 years of age. During the intervening years the brain displays essentially no growth, that is, a plateau. The total increase in brain weight that occurs during these individual (five) brain growth spurts is approximately 35% of the total adult brain. Each of these brain growth spurts (e.g., increase in myelin or neuropil) would contribute to an increase in complexity and speed of interneuronal communication leading to more complex and more reliable neural networks.[26,27] The individual brain growth spurts appear to be correlated in time with developmental phenomena such as Piaget's stages of cognitive development,[84] the growth of mental age,[107] development of language,[55] sensory growth,[9,123] and electroencephalogram (EEG) changes.[50] These brain growth spurts appear to be related to total brain weight only, and there are no obvious brain regions that themselves show similar spurts. However, it is highly possible that telencephalic structures may be displaying growth corresponding to these postnatal brain growth spurts. This notion has interesting implications for education and therapy.

Development of hemispheric specialization. The existence of hemispheric specialization or lateralization has been known for many years. The left hemisphere of most right-handed individuals has a special role in language and the control of complex voluntary movement, while the right hemisphere has special functions associated with analysis of visuospatial dimensions of the world (see Fig. 5-5). Laterality of the hemispheres is relative, not absolute, and females appear to have less functional hemispheric asymmetry than males. Lenneberg[55] concluded from his research on brain-damaged developing humans that lateralization of function in the brain begins at the time of language acquisition and is complete by the age of puberty. Anatomical, electrophysiological, and pathological data indicate that hemispheric lateralization may be manifest as early as birth.

The evidence in favor of early hemispheric specialization and lateralization is quite strong across a variety of behavioral systems, including sensorimotor systems. In most individuals, the development of a right-hand preference is thought to indicate a left cerebral hemisphere specialization. However, if the frequency of reaching behavior is used to measure hand preference, infants at 4 to 5 months of age typically reach with their left hands. A switch to the right hand for reaching typically occurs at about 6 to 9 months of age, and this preference is strengthened through approximately 8 years of age. In contrast, grasp duration as an index of hand preference shows a right-hand preference as early as 1 month of age. Other observations supporting left hemisphere specialization for motor control by the age of 3 years or earlier include increased right-hand gesturing during speech, reduced speed of right-hand finger tapping when talking, a stronger right hand, a right-foot stepping, and preference for head positioned to the right.[112]

Hemispheric lateralization is also apparent in sensory function. Results of dichotic listening, evoked potential, and electroencephalographic research suggest hemispheric asymmetry in the auditory system of infants only a few weeks old. This research showed that by this age there was a lateralized preference for phonemes (left hemisphere) and notes or tones (right hemisphere). For the visual system, hemispheric asymmetry has been shown to develop between the ages of birth and 6 years depending on the measures used. For rhythmic visual stimuli, a right hemispheric specialization is found for newborn infants. Finally, head turning to the right predominates with perioral tactile stimulation. These results suggest that tests of hemispheric lateralization of sensory or motor function may be used in the evaluation of neurological development and pathology.

BEHAVIORAL AND PHYSIOLOGICAL CHARACTERISTICS OF DEVELOPMENT
Motor development

The acquisition of movement and motor skills occurs in a definite order during development, proceeding from the generalized and simple movements of the fetus to the highly specific and complex volitional movements of the mature human organism. With development there is displayed greater control and specificity of movement, from the trunk to the arms to the hands to the fingers. The earliest movements of the human are generalized whole body movements, which appear to develop into specific movements. A variety of these specific movements each become individually differentiated; then all of these differentiated movements are integrated into a complex behavior pattern. For example, individual leg, foot, and arm movements are ultimately integrated into the walking pattern. This represents a hierarchical integration or the integration of individual movements into more complex movements.[126]

Motor systems. The anatomical systems critical for the control of movement and tone begin their development during the early prenatal period, and the developmental process continues for many years postnatally (Fig. 5-5). Because the fetus has essentially its full complement of nerve and muscle cells before birth, the later development of the neuromuscular system is primarily a function of, for example, cellular growth, establishment of intercellular connections, and myelination. The establishment and development of neuromuscular circuits are required for regulating muscle contractions, and these circuits are basically established during the prenatal and early postnatal periods. Muscle contraction (spontaneous or stimulated) appears to be essential for normal muscular development to proceed during both the prenatal and the postnatal periods.

The major neural systems controlling motor movement via the lower motor neuron are (1) the primary motor efferent system comprising the corticospinal and corticobulbar tracts (pyramidal system), (2) basal ganglia, (3) cerebellum, (4) the rubrospinal, reticulospinal, vestibulospinal, tectospinal, and long spinal tracts, and (5) segmental reflexes. The corticospinal tract is concerned with movement of the axial and appendicular musculature (refined voluntary movements), while the corticobulbar tract is concerned with movements of muscles innervated by cranial nerves. The basal ganglia (caudate, putamen, globus pallidus, subthalamic nucleus, and substantia nigra) influence muscle power, tone, and movement primarily by their effects on cortical motor neurons. The cerebellum is concerned with coordination of motor activity, muscle tone, posture, and equilibrium. The other three tracts are concerned with muscle tone and flexor muscle groups (rubrospinal tract), muscle activity and tone (reticulospinal tract), and extensor muscle tone (vestibulospinal tract). The development of each of these systems appears to be associated with corresponding development of motor behavior. For example, the development of the rubrospinal tract may be related to the flexor posture (flexor tone) of the limbs of the term newborn, the reticulospinal system may mediate changes in tone of newborn infants during changes in level of alertness, and the vestibulospinal tract may mediate the reflex activity associated with vestibular input and extensor muscle activity, for example, tonic neck and Moro reflexes (Table 5-3).[120]

The development of muscle in the human organism goes through eight phases beginning in the first 5 weeks of gestation through gestation term. Axonal terminals contact the developing muscle cells as early as the eleventh week of gestation and motor endplates begin to appear by the fourteenth week of gestation. From 15 to 20 weeks of gestation, the nuclei of muscle cells migrate to the periphery of the myotube, and the period of 20 to 24 weeks of gestation is one of early histochemical differentiation. By 38 weeks of gestation the mature myocytic stage begins, which continues through approximately the age of puberty.[15]

During development it appears that the motor neuron plays a role in the determination of the muscle fiber type.[52] Thus not only do muscle fibers require motor innervation for normal growth, but the motor neuron influences the type of muscle fiber that eventually develops. In this fashion, type I fibers (slow, sustained activities) and type II fibers (rapid burst activities) are determined.

Because of the growth in diameter of an axon and the increasing thickness of myelin that occur during development, nerve conduction velocities are faster in adults than in newborns. The changes in motor competence that occur during development are thus a function of changes in muscle, changes in neural input to muscles, and changes in higher level inputs to lower motor neurons, as well as movement experience.

Prenatal motor development. The earliest movements of the human fetus in utero, as recorded by ultrasound, have been shown to occur at least as early as 6 to 7 weeks of gestation with smooth, wormlike movements of the body. At 8 weeks of gestation, rapid irregular wormlike movements of the body are measured, as well as quick flexion and extension movements of the trunk. Asymmetrical movements of the whole body and trunk flexion and extension are present at 9 weeks of gestation. The limbs and head begin to extend during the tenth week of gestation. At 11 weeks of gestation limb movements are wider and the fetus tends to jump and jerk, and at 12 to 13 weeks of gestation the head rotates and extends. Leg and arm movements are frequently in opposite directions, and the hands are often brought up to touch the face. Rotations of the head and trunk result in body position changes within the uterus.

At 13 to 14 weeks of gestation reciprocal and symmetrical limb movements become evident. Mouth and breathing movements begin at this age, and the lower limbs may extend and cross. At the fifteenth week of gestation, the fetus is "sucking" its fingers, turning its head, opening its mouth, and swallowing. At 16 weeks of gestation there is good coordination of the limbs, hands grasp, and the hands explore or feel the uterine walls. Full body extension from one side of the uterus to the other side of the uterus occurs at this age. During eighteenth to nineteenth weeks of gestation, the fetus displays simultaneous breathinglike and swallowing movements, and the fetus "explores" its own body with its hands. By 20 to 21 weeks of gestation, isolated movements of the fingers, feet, eyelids, and mouth are observed. Hiccuplike movements are displayed by the fetus at 22 weeks of gestation. At 24 to 25 weeks of gestation, mechanical stimulation provokes head rotation, and by 26 to 28 weeks of gestation, a sound will stimulate a startle reaction or trunk and head rotation.[46]

In addition to these developments an aborted fetus of 8 weeks of gestation displays unilateral body flexion in response to stimulation of the primitive mouth region. At 9½ weeks of gestation, similar stimulation produces bilateral body flexion. The fetus could also extend its trunk at 10 weeks, and the fingers would flex in response to a touch at 11 weeks of gestation. Some facial expression could be determined at 14 weeks of gestation, and the fetus could close and grip with its hands. A head turn at 20 weeks of gestation produces ipsilateral arm movements, and at 25 weeks of gestation, shallow rhythmic respiratory movements are measured.[38]

Using a pressure transducer placed on the uterus, a rolling movement of the fetus can be measured at 26 weeks of gestation. By 26 to 27 weeks of gestation, high-frequency, short, kick-type movements are displayed, as are respiratory movements. Simple short movements, which may be those of an extremity, are measured at 26 weeks of gestation.[117]

At 16 weeks of gestation the fetus kicks, squirms, rolls, stretches, breathes, and hiccups. Through the last trimester of pregnancy the fetus appears to be moving much of the time. There are fast and slow jerks and more sustained slow movements. The twisting and rolling of the fetus can produce a total change in body position within the uterus. A decrease in fetal movements and/or a change in pattern of fetal movements may signal fetal distress.[96]

Just as in later life, there are tremendous individual differences in the amount, type, and pattern of movements displayed by prenatal fetuses. Sontag[109] has classified these movements into three basic types. The first is the sharp kicking or punching movement of the extremities. These movements increase in frequency and amplitude from 6 months of gestation through birth. The second type of movement is the squirming or writhing slow movement, which is most observable at the sixth and seventh months of gestation. The third type of movement is the sharp convulsive movement, which resembles a hiccup or spasm of the diaphragm. It has also been suggested that fetal movement is a relatively good predictor of later activity, such that active fetuses tend to display advanced motor development at 6 months after birth.[94]

The results discussed in the preceding paragraphs demonstrate that the very young fetus is capable of a rich repertoire of movements that are occurring before and as soon as neuromuscular connections are made during development. These spontaneous and reflexive movements are occurring in a morphologically immature neural and muscular system.

Many of the reflexlike behaviors that are displayed by a fetus will also be seen for a period of months following birth. These reflexlike behaviors are often referred to as the *primitive reflexes* (Table 5-3). It is thought that these primitive reflexes are mediated by subcortical neuromuscular systems that are already quite mature even during the prenatal period. The disappearance of these primitive reflexes during the normal course of neuromuscular maturation is attributed to development of functional maturity of "higher" cortical mechanisms. Presence of these primitive reflexes beyond certain ages of development is considered a signal of possible neurological dysfunction.

The eight basic primitive reflexes elicited in the premature and full-term infant at birth are as follows (see Table 5-3). The *rooting reflex* is produced by stroking the cheek, which results in the infant turning the head toward the side of stimulation and opening the mouth. This primitive reflex disappears around 9 months of age. The *Moro reflex* is also a primitive reflex whereby infants first extend their arms, arch their backs, and extend their legs. These movements are then followed by a total flexor pattern. This reflex is elicited by a sudden intense stimulus of dropping of the head, usually into extension. This primitive reflex drops out at around 3 to 6 months of age. The primitive *darwinian* or *grasping reflex,* which consists of a strong fist and grip that allows the infant to carry its own weight, is a response to stroking the palm of the hand. The grasping reflex disappears at about 2 to 3 months of age. The *swimming reflex* is a release of well-coordinated swimming movements of the infant in response to placing the face in water. This primitive reflex disappears at approximately 6 months of age. The asymmetrical *tonic neck reflex* is the adoption of a "fencer" position while the infant lies on the back with the head turned to one side. The limbs on the side of the face are extended while the opposite limbs are flexed. This primitive reflex disappears at about 2 to 7 months of age. The *Babinski reflex* is a primitive reflex where the foot twists in and the toes fan out in response to a stroke of the sole of the foot. The Babinski reflex drops out at about 6 to 9 months of age. The primitive *walking reflex* is a series of steppinglike motions of the infant when held under the arms and with the feet in contact with a surface. This reflex disappears at approximately 4 to 8 weeks of age. In the primitive *placing reflex,* as the backs of the feet are drawn against the edge of a flat surface, the infant withdraws the foot. This reflex disappears at about 1 month of age.

It is thought that these reflexes are subcortically mediated and that they disappear with maturation of cortical inhibitory mechanisms. However, Bower[13] has suggested that many of these primitive reflexes are really repetitive processes that will come back into the infant's behavioral repertoire at some later stage of development. For example, the primitive *walking reflex* disappears at approximately 4 to 8 weeks of age, then comes back into the infant's behavioral repertoire at about 1 year of age when the child begins to walk independently. Also, it has been shown that if the primitive reflexes are exercised they may not disappear. For example, the walking reflex does not disappear if the infant is repeatedly exercised with it, and exercised infants walk unassisted earlier than nonexercised infants.[134] However, this may not apply for all primitive reflexes, especially those that have no function, such as the Babinski reflex.

Muscle tone in the premature or full-term infant is typically assessed by passive manipulation of the limbs with the head placed in the midline and careful observation of spontaneous posture.[36,38] Maturation of tone follows an approximate caudal-cephalic and distal-proximal progression, particularly for flexor tone. By 28 weeks of gestation the limbs show minimal resistance to passive manipulation in any direction. At 32 weeks of gestation the lower extremities display a distinct flexor tone. Flexor tone has become prominent in the lower extremities by 36 weeks of gestation, and flexor tone is palpable in the upper extremities at this age. The full-term infant displays a flexed posture of all limbs. These indices of tone are apparent in the quiet infant's posturing. However it must be noted that at all gestational ages, postures change very frequently.[120]

Related to muscle tone is the measure of muscle power. Neck flexor and extensor power are minimal in the infant born at 32 weeks of gestation as indicated by the complete head lag during the pull-to-sit test.[120] However, in an infant born at 36 weeks of gestation, neck extensor power can be observed. In the term infant neck extensor power has improved and neck flexor power is apparent. The full-term infant can usually hold its head upright for several seconds.[36,38]

It is apparent that considerable motor development has been achieved during the prenatal period, and subsequent motor development following birth appears to be an integration and refinement of the basic movement patterns already established in utero. As put forth by developmentalists, the embryonic organism is active before it reacts to stimulation, partial motor patterns differentiate from total patterns, and movement arises secondarily from local reflexes.[54] The existence of each of these orientations can be confirmed when human movement patterns during the prenatal period are analyzed.

Postnatal motor development. The initial spontaneous movements of the newborn are relatively generalized kicking of the legs and flailing of the arms and are under subcortical regulation. As more refined and specific movements emerge at around 4 months of age, the cortical regulation of movement may be responsible. From this age onward, voluntary directed movements become more frequent and precise, and balance and posture rapidly improve over subsequent months and years. Thus precision of movement and balance appear to be associated with vestibular, cerebellar, and cerebral maturation.

The general postnatal development of the human infant is an ever-expanding sequence of precision of individual and integrated movement patterns. Newborn through 1-month-old infants are typically capable of turning their heads from side to side while lying in a supine position and are also capable of lifting their heads to some extent while lying prone. The newborn demonstrates a variety of reflexes such as the grasp reflex.[20] In the second month after birth infants can lift and hold their heads up for a few seconds while prone. The 3- and 4-month-old infant can lift up the head and chest while prone and can kick the legs. At 4 months of age the infant is able to sit when supported.[106] The 5-month-old infant can hold the head erect and can roll over from a prone to supine position.[79] By 6 months of age infants can raise themselves on their wrists while prone and can sit in chairs. At 7 to 8 months of age the infant can sit without support and can stand when held.[106] The 7-month-old infant is also capable of a hook-grasp pattern (hand grasp without thumb opposition).[20] The 9- to 10-month-old infant can turn around on the floor and can creep and crawl.[79] The infant can also stand when holding furniture[106] and can walk when handheld.[79] The 9-month-old infant also displays a full hand grasp.[20] At 11 to 12 months, infants can pull themselves up to a standing position and can stand alone by 13 to 14 months of age.[106] The 15-month-old child can walk alone and can climb stairs when held. Walking while pushing toys is accomplished at about 16 months, and picking up toys from the floor while standing is displayed at 17 months of age. At 18 months the child can climb into a chair and sit, and the child can run. The 19-month-old child can climb up and down stairs and at 20 months the child can jump.[79] Children can walk up stairs alone at 22 months of age, seat themselves at the table at 23 months of age, and walk up and down stairs alone at 24 months of age. At 2 years of age the infant displays a nearly complete hand grasp with manipulation.[20]

The developmental sequencing of motor behaviors can also be seen during evaluation of spontaneous postures and spontaneous motility of the arms and legs. At birth the spontaneous posture of the arms and legs is predominately a flexion pattern and this pattern predominates for the first few weeks of life. Over the next few months the pattern evolves through semiflexion, extension, and finally, posture without a predominant pattern. This final pattern is achieved by approximately 6 to 7 months for the arms and 13 to 14 months for the legs. This developmental sequence parallels the development of goal-directed motility, and the progression through the sequence is most rapid for the arms. Likewise, the development of spontaneous motility of the arms and legs of infants progresses from a stereotyped alternating flexion-extension pattern characteristic of newborns through predominantly asymmetrical movements, predominantly symmetrical movements, symmetrical and voluntary movements, and finally, predominantly voluntary movements. The newborn pattern for the arms is displayed for about the first month. The arms show predominantly asymmetrical and symmetrical patterns at 2 to 4 months, the symmetrical voluntary pattern through approximately 7 to 11 months, and the voluntary motility pattern by 11 to 12 months. Infants tend to watch and play with their hands and grasp for objects at the same time that symmetrical motility patterns of the arms become manifest. This progression shows how movement patterns become incorporated into goal-directed activities during de-

velopment. The development of leg motility follows a similar sequence (asymmetrical pattern at 2 to 7 months, symmetrical pattern at 4 to 12 months, and voluntary pattern at 16 to 17 months); however, the developmental time course is elongated.[20]

The development of the grasp reflex of infants also shows a clear developmental sequencing. At 1 to 2 months of age, stimulation between the thumb and index finger produces adduction and flexion of these segments. This is the beginning of the development of the true grasp reflex. The true grasp develops by 3 to 4 months of age, when a stimulus to the medial palm produces sustained flexion and adduction of the fingers. The infant now begins to reach for things and utilizes a crude palmar grasp. At 4 to 5 months stimulation of the hand causes a supination or orienting response of the hand, and this is followed by groping after the retreating stimulus. By 8 to 10 months the hand gropes after the stimulus, adjusts, and grasps the object. This is the instinctive grasp reaction. It is now possible to fractionate the grasp reflex, that is, produce flexion in a single digit. When the grasp reflex can be entirely fractionated, a true pincer grasp with opposition of thumb and index finger characterizes the voluntary prehension of the infant.

The development of arm and leg posturing, motility, and hand grasp each show a sequencing pattern whereby each successive developmental component represents an integration and elaboration of each previous component. These behaviors progress from essentially stereotyped automatisms in the newborn through voluntary movements within the first year of life. Each of these behaviors also influence one another during development. Arm and leg posturing advances appear to directly influence the development of goal-directed or voluntary arm and leg movements, and voluntary arm movements appear to directly influence voluntary prehension patterns of the infant. This sequencing is continued during the development of eye-hand coordination, and so on through complete maturation of all sensorimotor function.

It is easy to see from the above developmental sequence that motor development in the human infant tends to proceed in a general proximal-to-distal (heads to hands) and rostral-to-caudal (head to legs) fashion. As postural and balance systems mature, the infant attains greater and greater control and locomotor skill. Prewalking locomotor behavior evolves through the crawling (wiggle or belly), hitching and scooting, bear walking, and creeping (on hands and knees) phases before bipedal locomotor skills are developed.

Compared to basic locomotor skills, precise hand manipulation tends to develop late and over a relatively long time course. According to Corbin,[20] eye-hand coordination develops in four sequential stages. The first stage, from birth through 16 weeks of age, is the period of static visual exploration where infants look at their hands. From 17 to

28 weeks of age, the period of active and repeated visual exploration, infants study objects with their eyes—a sort of ocular "grasping." The arms are flung toward the object in a crude attempt to grasp it. The period of initiation of grasp and/or manipulation lasts from 28 to 40 weeks of age, and infants correct their arm movements to enable the grasping of objects. In the final stage, the period of refinement and extension, the infant visually explores and grasps objects. This period begins at 40 weeks of age and continues for years with further development of precision of grasp and manipulation.

During the preschool years motor development improves vastly. Children show tremendous progress in large muscle, small muscle, and eye-hand coordination. These children are usually more advanced in gross motor skills relative to fine motor skills. The middle childhood period is one of improved motor development and coordination. By adolescence males tend to exceed females in physical achievement. This sex difference is most likely caused by social and physical interactions and does not always favor males, for example, in endurance and fine motor skills.

Sensory development

A considerable amount of research has been conducted on sensory function with prenatal humans, especially with the tactile and auditory systems (see the preceding section on motor development). Less is known about visual, vestibular, gustatory, and olfactory systems. However, at an anatomical level research suggests that most sensory receptors are morphologically mature before birth in humans. While morphologically mature receptors suggest sensory receptivity, such maturity may not be essential for early reflex responses for some sensory systems, such as the tactile system.[43] Nevertheless, the available data suggest that the tactile (1 to 6 months of gestation), taste (3 months of gestation), vestibular (4 to 6 months of gestation), auditory (6 months of gestation), and visual (mostly complete at birth) receptors mature morphologically while the human fetus is in utero. If these receptors are indeed functional, the developing human fetus must have the ability to monitor its surroundings while in utero.[73]

The sensory systems most likely stimulated within the prenatal environment are the gustatory, tactile, temperature, auditory, and vestibular systems. Fetal responses to stimulation of each of these modalities has been demonstrated in utero. While the fetus responds to these stimuli, such responses do not imply that the fetus can "perceive" such sensory stimuli. It is not until approximately 3 months after birth that the sensory receiving areas of the cerebral cortex begin their accelerated maturation (Fig. 5-5).[19]

Thus fetal receptors may mature in utero to prepare for function after birth, and the intrauterine environment may be ideal for sensory development based upon the level and quality of stimulation. Thus optimal stimulation of developing receptors may influence the subsequent formation of optimal neural connections in sensory pathways. This might suggest that normal sensory stimulation prenatally, like that postnatally, is essential for normal sensory development. It is also possible that prenatal sensory function allows the fetus to monitor its environment and thus adapt to that environment by making adjustments in behavior and position. For example, vestibular stimulation may be involved in the changes measured in fetal position in the uterus and gustatory stimulation may be a regulator of prenatal swallowing behavior. It is not known how these systems are affected by premature birth, although a considerable number of questions are now being generated.

Development of the visual system. Development of the visual system begins when the optic vesicle invaginates to the optic cup at 5 weeks of gestation. At 7 weeks of gestation the optic nerve fibers grow up the optic stalk from the retinal ganglia cells. These fibers reach the base of the brain at the optic chiasm. At 9 weeks of gestation the eyeball is about 1 mm in diameter, and the precursor muscle fibers are present. The optic tracts of the brain are being laid down at 10 weeks of gestation and the macula is distinguishable at 11 weeks of gestation. The rods and cones are differentiated by about 4 months of gestation. At birth the eye is fairly well developed, except for the photoreceptors in the foveal region. Myelin has reached the disk but there is little if any within the tracts (Fig. 5-4). During the first 4 months after birth the foveal cones are differentiating and the optic radiations are becoming myelinated. Differentiation of the occipital cortex is also nearly complete at this age (Fig. 5-5).

The newborn infant appears to have 20/150 vision and a fixed focus of about 20 cm and displays little accommodation. Accommodation is good by 4 months of age. Pupil light and blink reflexes are present by 29 to 31 weeks of gestation, and by 33 weeks of gestation there is a positive response to soft light. At 1 day after birth the newborn infant displays visual fixation and visual following.

Newborn humans blink to a bright light shown into the eyes and will shift their gaze to follow a moving light.[58] On the day of birth the infant will also follow a moving target,[97] and neonates seem to prefer curves and corners over straight contours, suggesting that the neonate's visual world is selective.[29] At 1 month of age infants can recognize their mothers based on visual information,[65] and they clearly display depth perception by 6 months of age.[121] There is also evidence suggesting that visual fixation ratings for newborns are better predictors of IQ at 3 to 4 years of age than are newborn neurological ratings.[72]

Color vision is demonstrable in infants of at least 2 months of age,[82] and preference for facial patterns develops between 10 and 15 weeks of age. A 1-month-old infant will actually imitate facial gestures.[70] The reader can refer to Chapter 25 for more in-depth review of visual-perceptual systems.

Development of the auditory system. The development of the auditory pontomedullary junction begins at the mid-hindbrain level at about 20 days of gestation with the initiation of the otic placodes. By 3 to 4 weeks of gestation the invaginations are closed, forming the otic vesicles (otocysts). The otic vesicle shows rapid development beginning at 4 weeks of gestation. By the fifth week of gestation the endolymphatic appendage, cochlear duct, utricle, and semicircular canals are all showing their beginnings. The development of the organ of Corti (auditory receptor) progresses rapidly and smoothly from 8 to 24 weeks of gestation. The internal and external hair cells (receptors) are differentiated by about 4 months of gestation, and all peripheral auditory structures appear present by 6 months of gestation. Central auditory structures mature postnatally (Figs. 5-4 and 5-5). Between 6 and 7 months of gestation, the fetus displays responses to external auditory stimulation.

As early as the thirteenth week of gestation, the human fetus has been shown to respond with convulsive movements to extreme auditory (vibratory) stimulation.[109] Newborns have been shown to produce heart rate acceleration in response to increasing sound intensity. Such responses have even been observed as early as 29 weeks of gestation with differential responses to different tones.[10,110] Newborns show a response threshold to sounds of 40 decibels in intensity.[113]

Using habituation design (decreased responding to repeated stimuli), newborn infants seem capable of sound localization and auditory-visual integration.[8,56] By 3 to 5 days of age infants are capable of auditory discrimination based upon intensity, pitch, and rhythm of sounds. These results suggest that cortical function is achieved very early in development based upon the temporal discrimination involved in rhythm of sounds. However, it must be remembered that auditory cortex myelinates quite late after birth (see Figs. 5-3 and 5-5). Intensity and pitch are thought to be at least partially mediated subcortically. Although total myelination occurs later, speech phonemic sounds are discriminated by infants as early as 1 month of age.[25] For additional background in speech and language development see Chapter 24.

Development of the vestibular system. The vestibular system is one of the most well-advanced sensory systems at birth, in terms of both morphology and function. At birth the vestibular apparatus has achieved the same configuration, size, and position as that of the adult. Early functional development of the vestibular apparatus is also indicated by vestibular responses to low threshold stimulation and vestibular responses, which are proportional to the intensity of the stimulus. These functional characteristics are already present at birth.

The vestibular system is embryologically and anatomically associated with the peripheral auditory system. The otic vesicle gives rise to the three vestibular end organs (the utricle, saccule, and semicircular canals and their specialized epithelial cells), which begin to differentiate during the fourth week of gestation. These end organs are innervated by the sensory endings of the vestibular portion of the eighth cranial nerve. The peripheral vestibular apparatus essentially completes morphogenesis by approximately 45 days of gestation; however, there is some continued development of the semicircular canals at later ages.[76] The late prenatal and early postnatal development of the vestibular system is primarily concerned with the elaboration of central connections. The vestibular system is made up of vast interconnections within the CNS, especially the spinal cord, cerebellum, and oculomotor nuclei. Many of the vestibular projections are the earliest fiber systems to myelinate within the brain, at approximately the fifth month of gestation (Fig. 5-3).[132]

One function of the vestibular system is the stabilization of body and eye positions for precise goal-directed movements.[101] This system is also involved in the control of muscular activity, balance or equilibrium, and position sense. Because of the advanced development of the vestibular system during the early prenatal period, this system may be quite functional in the fetus and may be related to the frequent changes in position of the fetus within the uterus.[73]

Indices of vestibular function are widely used in infant neurological examinations because vestibular function appears essential for maintenance of the body and head in space.[120] A majority of neonates produce active eye movements contrary to the direction of axial rotation while in supine suspension (doll's-eye phenomenon). This reaction is produced in infants as early as 30 weeks of gestation and it disappears or becomes latent with age. The Moro reaction (see the section on prenatal motor development and Table 5-3) is also thought to assess vestibular function. This reaction is present at birth and disappears by 3 to 6 months of age. Extension of the legs during the positive supporting reaction may also assess vestibular function. By 5 to 11 months of age most infants produce leg extension and bear their body weight on their legs for a few seconds.

A more direct measure of vestibular function is obtained by assessing postrotatory nystagmus. Developmental studies indicate that postnatal maturation of vestibular function does take place to some extent, in spite of precocious morphological maturation of this system.[120] A more intense postrotatory nystagmus is found in young children than in older children. The high amplitude responses of younger children may result from low-level reactions of central mechanisms to the vestibular sensory impulses, that is, immaturity of central systems that inhibit vestibular function.

Development of the somatosensory system. The somatosensory system includes the skin senses (touch, pressure, pain, temperature, itch, vibration, and tickle) and the body senses (joint position, muscle length and tension) (Fig. 5-5). This system has a wide variety of receptors and most of these receptors appear to mature during the prenatal period.[73] For example, Pacinian corpuscles, though immature, are found in the sole of the foot and thumb of the hand by approximately 20 weeks of gestation. Muscle spindles begin to differentiate at 12 to 20 weeks, and they become morphologically complex by 22 to 26 weeks of gestation. Mature receptors in the hand are found at 4 months (Merkel's) and 6 months (Meissner's and pacinian) of gestation. The functional development of the somatosensory system, as indicated by myelination (Figs. 5-3 and 5-5), proceeds from the dorsal roots (5 months of gestation), to the medial lemniscus (5 months of gestation through the first year after birth), to the cortical projections (1 or more years after birth).[132]

Somatosensory-evoked responses have been studied in premature infants. In infants as young as 29 weeks of gestation, somatosensory-evoked responses of the median nerve (wrist) show constant primary waveform components. The response pattern equivalent to that of the mature newborn is reached by infants at 37 to 38 weeks of gestation. These somatosensory responses appear a few weeks earlier than the comparable visual evoked potential. Both types of evoked potential (somatosensory and visual) display a linear decrease in response latency as a function of increasing gestational age.[120]

The development of receptive fields for tactile stimulation occurs initially in the perioral region and spreads down the trunk region. The earliest responses to tactile stimulation are generalized, and the responses appear to be avoiding or withdrawal responses. The earliest fetal (aborted) responses to tactile stimulation (touch) are from the perioral region at about 7½ weeks of gestation. The receptor fields for touch then spread to the nose and chin regions (8 to 9½ weeks), the eyelids and palms of the hand (10 weeks), the soles of the feet (11 weeks), the face, upper chest, thighs, and legs (11 to 12 weeks), the tongue and back (14 weeks), and finally the abdomen, buttocks, and inside thigh (32 weeks of gestation).

The premature infant of 28 weeks gestation appears to discriminate touch from pain.[120] Touch stimulation produces alerting and slight motor activity, while painful stimulation produces withdrawal and crying reactions. Thresholds for painful stimulation become lowered as the infant ages. The rooting reflex in response to tactile stimulation of the perioral region is well established by 32 weeks of gestation.[120]

Other details of somatosensory system development have been presented in the sections on motor, auditory, and vestibular system development.

Development of the olfactory and gustatory systems. The olfactory epithelium is differentiated before 2 months of gestation and then matures over the next prenatal months. In atricial species, such as humans and rats, a considerable amount of maturation of the olfactory system (bulb and projections) may occur postnatally.

Research with humans has shown early development of olfactory function. Infants as young as 32 weeks of gestation respond with sucking, arousal, or withdrawal to the odor of peppermint.[98] Newborn infants differentially respond to onionlike odors or anise oil,[59] as well as other substances. Infants can also discriminate the odor of a breast pad from their own mother from that of other mothers.[62]

The development of the gustatory system also begins early in the prenatal period. In the human fetus the presumptive taste buds (receptors) are present on the tongue as early as the first to second month of gestation, and these receptors are mature at about 3 months of gestation.[14] By 8 months of gestation the fetus responds to unpleasant stimuli within the amniotic fluid by decreasing its swallowing. The newborn infant is quite responsive to variations in taste of substances and can make relatively subtle gustatory discriminations. The newborn infant can discriminate between sweet, salty, and bland solutions.[60,124]

As olfactory and gustatory development coincide closely with primitive protective responses, they may play a protective, alertive role in neonatal development. Stimulation of these systems may be used as a treatment technique to arouse an infant whose response systems are delayed or nonresponsive.

Language and cognitive development

The development of language and cognitive (thinking, reasoning, memory, problem-solving, and planning) processes are obviously interrelated and interactive (Figs. 5-4 and 5-5). Language allows a form of communication of information (cognitive) that is uniquely human. During the second year of life, the infant already understands much of another's speech, and now the infant begins to speak the language. There is, however, little agreement between the various theories of language development.

The development of language and understanding of language have been studied for many years. Children learn to understand language before they can speak it. Shortly after birth neonates can determine the direction from which a sound comes and they can discriminate different sounds. By 2 weeks of age they can recognize the difference between voices and other sounds, and they can recognize the difference between different human voices at 2 months of age. By the end of the first year human infants can make fine discriminations between individual words.[55]

Before the acquisition of speech, infants display, in the order presented, the following expressions of sound. First is undifferentiated crying, which may be a reflexive form of communication, followed at 1 month of age by differentiated crying, which appears to communicate different need states. At about 6 weeks of age simple cooing sounds are made, and these sounds evolve into babbling at about 3 to 4 months of age. Lallation or imperfect imitation is displayed by infants during the second half of the first year, and children imitate many of their own sounds. During the ninth and tenth months the infant imitates the sounds of others (echolalia). By the end of the second year of life the child has developed a form of speech (a string of words) that is not yet completely communicative.

At approximately 1 year of age the child is capable of using one word sentences ("dada") and these expand into two word sentences ("me go") at about 2 years. These one- and two-word sentences are true language, since this telegraphic form of speech contains words that carry true meaning. By the age of 3 years the child has a vocabulary of approximately 900 words and the sentences become longer. By 4 to 5 years of age children are capable of using full, complex, adultlike sentences that demonstrate near mastery of the rules of grammar in their speech. By 6 years of age most children have amassed a vocabulary of about 8,000 to 14,000 words.

The preschooler's speech is of two main types: egocentric and socialized. Egocentric speech is used to guide the child's behavior, while socialized speech is intended to communicate with others. The younger the child, the more the use of egocentric speech. The environment of the preschool-age child can strongly influence the subsequent development of language.

The school-age child up to about 9 years of age displays an increased understanding of more complex syntax. Egocentrism is diminishing at this time and communication is increasing.

Two frequently studied theories of language development are the learning and the biological theories. The learning theories stress that language is acquired through reward and punishment or imitation. However, psycholinguists typically disagree with these theories. The biological theories propose that humans possess a built-in neural system that enables a child to process language[17,18] (Fig. 5-5). Piaget favors an interactionism theory, which acknowledges the mutual influences of heredity, maturation, and environmental stimulation.[83-85]

Although it seems intuitive that neonates and infants are capable of learning, the type and extent of learning in infants have been the subject of much controversy. However, there is research evidence that even very young infants are capable of several types of learning, including habituation, imitation, classical conditioning, and operant conditioning.

During the sensorimotor stage of cognitive development (defined by Piaget) the preverbal infant (birth to 2 years of age) exhibits intelligent (adaptive) behaviors.[83-85] The infant evolves from a primarily reflexive individual to one who is capable of rudimentary foresight, and the child develops the concept of object permanence.

The preoperational stage of cognitive development lasts from 2 to 7 years of age.[83-85] During this stage symbolic function develops; symbolic function allows children to represent and reflect upon their environments. Thought is gradually becoming more flexible, but the infant and child still cannot deal with adultlike abstractions. Symbolic function is manifest through language, deferred imitation, and symbolic play. The child is still egocentric and has difficulty with reversibility of events.

The age of 6 to 11 years is the stage of concrete operations.[83-85] The child now uses symbols (mental representations) to carry out operations and is becoming increasingly proficient at classifying and seriating objects and events, dealing with members, and perfecting the reality of conversation. The constraint of egocentrism on thought processes is diminishing at this time.

The adolescent years are the stage of formal operations during which the child develops the ability to think abstractly.[83-85] Thus the child can now solve problems, test hypotheses, and engage in hypothetical, deductive reasoning. The environment is of crucial importance during this stage, and thought progresses from extreme rigidity to flexibility.[47,83-85]

CONCLUSION

In this chapter basic characteristics of the development of the human organism have been covered from the time of conception through the age of adulthood. In each aspect of development covered, be it morphological, physiological, or behavioral (psychological), the pattern of development is clear: a series of interdependent and interactive processes over time (i.e., fine-tuning). This is seen in the development of the nervous system, motor movement systems, and sensory systems and is also seen in the development of cognitive and language processes.

Each phase of nervous system development is *dependent* upon each preceding phase, thereby allowing ever greater complexity of structure and function. Although many developmental changes reach a peak during the prenatal phase of development, most are active postnatally as well. There is considerable evidence for myelination of the nervous system to continue beyond the middle years of life in humans, and additional evidence exists for axonal, dendritic, and synaptic changes associated with postnatal experience. In this context we are only beginning to appreciate the true extent of postnatal development of the nervous system. The frequently used concept of "neural plasticity," as applied to the "mature" nervous system, may reflect nothing more than continuation of the developmental process. More research in this area is obviously needed in order to increase credibility for the use of postnatal neural developmental concepts as they are applied to learning and therapy.

Knowledge and awareness of neural and behavioral developmental processes are important for a complete understanding of normal ontogeny through the developmental arc, and such knowledge is important for an understanding of developmental neural-behavioral abnormalities. While development is generally characterized as a period of growth and building, periods of rapid development are also periods of increased vulnerability to biological, environmental, and experiential influences. These influences may or may not be pathogenic in nature. Pathological consequences of development are presented in other chapters of this volume.

The development of the human organism is a truly complex process that begins at conception and proceeds throughout essentially the total lifespan of humans. At each phase of development a unique biological substrate is achieved, and the ultimate behavioral capacity of the human is a function of the biological substrate at that time interacting with past and current environmental experiences. Each phase of human development is a function of, and dependent upon, each preceding phase. Thus development of the human organism cannot ever be considered to be static. The human is an adapting organism, forever developing.

REFERENCES

1. Acheson RM: Maturation of the skeleton. In Faulkner F., editor: Human development, Philadelphia, 1966, WB Saunders Co.
2. Almli CR: The ontogeny of feeding and drinking behaviors: effects of early brain damage, Neurosci Biobehav Rev 2:281, 1978.
3. Altman J: Autoradiographic and histological studies of postnatal neurogenesis. II. A longitudinal investigation of the kinetics, migration and transformation of cells incorporating tritiated thymidine in infant rats, with special reference to postnatal neurogenesis in some brain regions, J Comp Neurol 128:431, 1966.
4. Angevine JB Jr: Critical cellular events in the shaping of the neural centers. In Schmitt FO and Melnechuck T, editors: The neurosciences, New York, 1970, Rockefeller University Press.
5. Angevine JB Jr: Time of neuron origin in the diencephalon of the mouse, J Comp Neurol 139:129, 1970.
6. Antanitus DS and others: The demonstration of glial fibrillary acidic protein in the cerebrum of the human fetus by indirect immunofluorescence, Brain Res 103:613, 1976.
7. Apgar V: A proposal for a new method of evaluation of the newborn infant, Cur Res Anest Analg 32:260, 1953.
8. Aronson E and Rosenbloom S: Space perception in early infancy: perception within a common auditory-visual space, Science 172:1161, 1971.
9. Banks MS and others: Sensitive period for the development of human binocular vision, Science 190:675, 1975.
10. Bernard J and Sontag LW: Fetal reactivity to sound, J Genet Psychol 70:205, 1947.
11. Berry M and others: The pattern and mechanism of migration of the neuroblasts of the developing cerebral cortex, J Anat (London) 98:291, 1964.
12. Blinkov SM and Glezer I: The human brain in figures and tables, New York, 1968, Plenum Press.
13. Bower TGR: Repetitive processes in child development, Sci Am 235:38, 1976.
14. Bradley RM and Stein IB: The development of the human taste bud during the foetal period, J Anat 101:743, 1967.
15. Brooke MH and Engel WK: The histographic analysis of human muscle biopsies with regard to fiber types. 4. Children's biopsies, Neurology 19:591, 1969.
16. Carmichael L: The onset and early development of behavior. In Carmichael L, editor: Manual of child psychology, ed 2, New York, 1954, John Wiley & Sons, Inc.
17. Chomsky N: Syntactic structures, The Hague, 1957, Mouton Press.
18. Chomsky N: A review of verbal behavior by B.F. Skinner, Language 35:26, 1959.
19. Conel JL: The postnatal development of the human cerebral cortex, 6 vols, Cambridge, 1939-1960, Harvard University Press.
20. Corbin C: A textbook of motor development, Dubuque, Iowa, 1973, William C Brown, Inc.
21. Cowan WM: Neuronal death as a regulative mechanism in the control of cell number in the nervous system. In Rockstein M, editor: Development and aging in the nervous system, New York, 1973, Academic Press, Inc.
22. Cowan WM: The development of the brain. In The brain, a Scientific American Book, San Francisco, 1978, WH Freeman & Co, Publishers.
23. Detwiler SR: Observations upon migration of neural crest cells, and upon the development of the spinal ganglia and vertebral arches in amblystoma, Am J Anat 61:64, 1937.
24. Dobbing J and Sands J: Quantitative growth and development of human brain, Arch Dis Child 48:757, 1973.
25. Eimas PD and others: Speech perception in infants, Science 171:303, 1971.
26. Epstein HT: Phrenoblysis: special brain and mind growth periods. I. Human brain and skull development, Dev Psychobiol 7:207, 1974.
27. Epstein HT: Phrenoblysis: special brain and mind growth periods. II. Human mental development, Dev Psychobiol 7:217, 1974.
28. Epstein HT: Correlated brain and intelligence development in humans. In Hahn ME and others, editors: Development and evolution of brain size, New York, 1979, Academic Press, Inc.
29. Fantz R and Miranda S: Newborn infant attention to forms of contour, Child Dev 46:224, 1975.
30. Friede RL: The relationship of body size, nerve cell size, axon length and glial density in the cerebellum, Proc Natl Acad Sci USA 49:187, 1963.
31. Fujita S: An autoradiographic study on the origin and fate of the subpial glioblasts in the embryonic chick spinal cord, J Comp Neurol 124:51, 1965.
32. Fujita S: Application of light and electron microscopic autoradiography to the study of cytogenesis of the forebrain. In Hassler R and Stephan H, editors: Evolution of the forebrain, New York, 1966, Plenum Press.
33. Fujita H and Fujita S: Electron microscopic studies on neuroblast differentiation in the central nervous system of domestic fowl, Zeit Zellfor Mikroskop Anat 60:463, 1963.
34. Gain SM: Fat, body size and growth in the newborn, Hum Biol 30:265, 1958.
35. Geelen JAG and Langman J: Closure of the neural tube in the cephalic region of the mouse embryo, Anat Rec 189:625, 1977.
36. Gesell A: The embryology of behavior, New York, 1945, Harper & Row, Publishers, Inc.
37. Gesell A and Amatruda CS: Developmental diagnosis: normal and abnormal child development, New York, 1941, Harber.
38. Gesell A and Amatruda CS: In Knobloch H and Pasamanick B, editors: Developmental diagnosis, New York, 1974, Harper & Row, Publishers, Inc.
39. Gillette R: Cell number and cell size in the ectoderm during neurulation, J Exp Zool 96:201, 1944.
40. Greenough WT and Volkman FR: Pattern of dendritic branching in occipital cortex of rats reared in complex environments, Exp Neurol 40:491, 1973.
41. Hey EN: Thermal regulation in the newborn, Br J Hosp Med 8:51, 1972.

42. Hinds JW: Autoradiographic study of histogenesis in the mouse olfactory bulb. I. Time of origin of neurons and neuroglia, J Comp Neurol 134:287, 1968.

43. Humphrey T: The development of trigeminal nerve fibers to the oral mucosa, compared with their development to cutaneous surfaces, J Comp Neurol 126:91, 1966.

44. Hunt RK and Jacobson M: Neuronal specificity revisited. In Moscona A and Monroy A, editors: Current topics in developmental biology, vol 8, New York, 1974, Academic Press, Inc.

45. Hurlock EB: Child development, New York, 1950, McGraw-Hill Book Co.

46. Ianniruberto A and Tajani E: Ultrasonographic study of fetal movements, Semin. Perinatol. 5:175, 1981.

47. Inhelder B and Piaget J: The growth of logical thinking from childhood to adolescence, New York, 1958, Basic Books Inc, Publishers.

48. Jacobson M: Development and evolution of Type II neurons: conjectures a century after Golgi. In Santini M, editor: Golgi Centennial Symposium, New York, 1975, Raven Press.

49. Jacobson M: Developmental neurobiology, New York, 1978, Plenum Press.

50. John ER: Functional neuroscience, Hillsdale, NJ, 1977, Lawrence Erlbaum Associates, Inc.

51. Karfunkel P: The mechanisms of neural tube formation, Internat Rev Cytol 38:245, 1974.

52. Karpati G and Engel WK: "Type grouping" in skeletal muscles after experimental reinnervation, Neurology 18:447, 1968.

53. Le Gros Clark WE and Medavar PB, editors: Essays on growth and form, London, 1945, Oxford University Press.

54. Lemire RJ and others: Normal and abnormal development of the human nervous system, New York, 1975, Harper & Row, Publishers, Inc.

55. Lenneberg EH: Biological functions of language, New York, 1967, John Wiley & Sons, Inc.

56. Leventhal AS and Lipsitt LP: Adaptation, pitch discrimination and sound localization in the neonate, Child Dev 35:759, 1964.

57. Levi-Montalcini R and Angeletti PV: Nerve growth factor, Physiol Rev 48:534, 1968.

58. Lightwood R and others: Paterson's sick children, London, 1971, Baillière Tindall.

59. Lipsitt LP and others: Developmental changes in the olfactory threshold of the neonate, Child Dev 34:371, 1963.

60. Lipsitt LP and others: Effects of experience on the behavior of the young infant, Neuropadiat 8:107, 1977.

61. Loeser JD and others: The development of the folia in the human cerebellar vermis, Anat Rec 173:109, 1972.

62. MacFarlene A: Olfaction in the development of social preferences in the human neonate. In Parent-infant interaction, CIBA Foundation Symposium, New York, 1975, CIBA, Inc.

63. Marin-Padilla M: Prenatal and early postnatal ontogenesis of the human motor cortex: a Golgi study. I. The sequential development of the cortical layers, Brain Res 23:165, 1970.

64. Marin-Padilla M: Prenatal ontogenetic history of the principal neurons of the neocortex of the cat *(Felis domestica):* a Golgi study. II. Developmental differences and their significances, Z Anat Entwicklungsgesch 136:125, 1972.

65. Mauer D and Salapatek P: Developmental changes in the scanning of faces by young children, Child Dev 47:523, 1976.

66. Maxwell DS and Kruger L: Small blood vessels and the origin of phagocytes in the rat cerebral cortex following heavy particle irradiation, Exp Neurol 12:33, 1965.

67. McCarthy KD and Partlow LM: Neuronal stimulation of [^{3}H] thymidine incorporation by primary cultures of highly purified non-neuronal cells, Brain Res 114:415, 1976.

68. McMullen NT and Almli CR: Cell types within the medial forebrain bundle: a Golgi study of preoptic and hypothalamic neurons in the rat, Am J Anat 161:323, 1981.

69. Meller K and others: Synaptic organization of the molecular and outer granular layer in the motor cortex in the white mouse during postnatal development: a Golgi and electron-microscopical study, Z Zellforsch Mikrosk Anat Abt Histochem 92:217, 1968.

70. Meltzoff AN and Moore MK: Imitation of facial and manual gestures by human neonates, Science 198:75, 1977.

71. Miale IL and Sidman RL: An autoradiographic analysis of histogenesis in the mouse cerebellum, Exp Neurol 4:277, 1961.

72. Miranda S and others: Neonatal pattern vision: predictor of future mental performance? J Pediatr 91:642, 1977.

73. Mistretta CM and Bradley RM: Taste and swallowing in utero, Br Med Bull 31:80, 1975.

74. Molliver ME and Van der Loos H: The ontogenesis of cortical circuitry: the spatial distribution of synapses in somesthetic cortex of newborn dog, Ergeb Anat Ent Gesch 42:7, 1970.

75. Molliver ME and others: The development of synapses in the cerebral cortex of the human fetus, Brain Res 50:403, 1973.

76. Moore KL: The developing human, Philadelphia, 1977, WB Saunders Co.

77. Morest DK: The growth of dendrites in the mammalian brain, Z Anat Entwicklungsgesch 128:290, 1969.

78. Morest DK: A study of neurogenesis in the forebrain of opossum pouch young, Z Anat Entwicklungsgesch 130:265, 1970.

79. Nelson W and others: Textbook of pediatrics, ed 10, Philadelphia, 1975, WB Saunders Co.

80. Paldino AM and Purpura DP: Branching patterns of hippocampal neurons of human fetus during differentiation, Exp Neurol 64:620, 1979.

81. Paldino AM and Purpura DP: Quantitative analysis of the spatial distribution of axonal and dendritic terminals of hippocampal pyramidal neurons in immature human brain, Exp Neurol 64:604, 1979.

82. Peeples DR and Teller DY: Color vision and brightness discrimination in two-month-old human infants, Science 189:1102, 1975.

83. Piaget J: The origins of intelligence in children, New York, 1952, International Universities Press, Inc.

84. Piaget J: Psychology of intelligence, Totowa, NJ, 1969, Littlefield & Co.

85. Piaget J and Inhelder B: The psychology of the child, New York, 1969, Basic Books, Inc, Publishers.

86. Purpura DP: Stability and seizure susceptibility of immature brain. In Jasper HJ and others, editors: Basic mechanisms of the epilepsies, Boston, 1969, Little, Brown & Co.

87. Purpura DP: Dendritic differentiation in human cerebral cortex: normal and aberrant development patterns. In Kreutzberg GW, editor: Advances in neurology, New York, 1975, Raven Press.

88. Rabinowicz T: Some aspects of the maturation of the human cerebral cortex, Mod Probl Paediatr 13:44, 1974.

89. Rakic P: Mode of cell migration to the superficial layers of fetal monkey neocortex, J Comp Neurol 145:61, 1972.

90. Rakic P: Timing of major ontogenetic events in the visual cortex of the Rhesus monkey. In Buchwald NA and Brazier MAB, editors: Brain mechanisms in mental retardation, New York, 1975, Academic Press, Inc.

91. Rakic P and Sidman RL: Supravital DNA synthesis in the developing human and mouse brain, J Neuropathol Exp Neurol 27:246, 1968.

92. Rakic P and Sidman RL: Histogenesis of cortical layers in human cerebellum, particularly the lamina dissecans, J Comp Neurol 139:473, 1970.

93. Rees RP and others: Morphological changes in the neuritic growth cone and target neuron during synaptic junction development in culture, J Cell Biol 68:240, 1976.

94. Richards TW and Nelson VL: Studies in mental development: II. Analyses of abilities tested at six months by the Gesell schedule, J Genet Psychol 52:327, 1938.

95. Richman DP and others: Mechanical model of brain convolutional development, Science 189:18, 1975.

96. Roberts AB and others: Fetal activity in 100 normal third trimester pregnancies, Br J Obstet Gynaecol 87:480, 1980.

97. Rosenblith JE: The modified Graham behavior test for neonates, test-retest reliability, normative data and hypotheses for future work, Biol Neonate 3:174, 1961.

98. Sarnat HB: Olfactory reflexes in the newborn infant, J Pediatr 92:625, 1978.

99. Sauer FC: Mitosis in the neural tube, J Comp Neurol 62:377, 1935.

100. Saxen L and Toivonen S: Primary embryonic induction, London, 1962, Logos Press, Inc.

101. Schade JP and Ford DH. Basic neurology, Amsterdam, 1973, Elsevier Scientific Publishing Co, Inc.

102. Schade JP and others: Maturational aspects of the dendrites in the human cerebral cortex, Acta Morphol Neerl Scand 5:37, 1962.

103. Schaper A: The earliest differentiation in the central nervous system of vertebrates, Science 5:430, 1897.

104. Schmechle DE and Rakic P: Arrested proliferation of radial glial cells during midgestation in rhesus monkey, Nature 277:303, 1979.

105. Serunian S and Broman S: Relationship of Apgar scores and Bayley mental and motor scores, Child Dev 46:696, 1975.

106. Shirley MM: The first two years: a study of twenty-five babies, monograph, Institute of Child Welfare, Minneapolis, 1933, University of Minnesota Press.

107. Shuttleworth FK: The physical and mental growth of girls and boys, age six to nineteen in relation to age at maximum growth, Monogr Soc Res Child Dev 4:1, 1939.

108. Sidman RL and Rakic P: Neuronal migration, with special reference to developing human brain: a review, Brain Res 62:1, 1973.

109. Sontag LW: Implications of fetal behavior and environment for adult personality, Ann NY Acad Sci 134:782, 1966.

110. Sontag LW and Wallace RI: Changes in the heart rate of the human fetal heart in response to vibratory stimuli, Am J Dis Child 51:583, 1936.

111. Speidel CC: Studies of living nerves. VII. Growth adjustments of cutaneous terminal arborizations, J Comp Neurol 76:57, 1942.

112. Springer SP and Deutsch G: Left brain, right brain, San Francisco, 1981, WH Freeman & Co., Publishers.

113. Steinschmeider A: Developmental psychophysiology. In Brackbill Y, editor: Infancy and early childhood: a handbook and guide to human development, New York, 1968, The Free Press.

114. Taber-Pierce E: Histogenesis of deep cerebellar nuclei studied autoradiographically with thymidine-H^3 in the mouse, Anat Rec 157:301, 1967.

115. Taber-Pierce E: Time of origin of neurons in the brain stem of the mouse, Prog Brain Res 40:53, 1973.

116. Thompson H: Physical growth. In Carmichael L, editor: Manual of child psychology, New York, 1954, John Wiley & Sons, Inc.

117. Timor-Tritsch I and others: Classification of human fetal movement, Am J Obstet Gynecol 126:70, 1976.

118. Valadian I and Porter D: Physical growth and development, Boston, 1977, Little, Brown & Co.

119. Voeller K and others: Electron microscope study of development of cat superficial neocortex, Exp Neurol 7:107, 1963.

120. Volpe JJ: Neurology of the newborn, Philadelphia, 1981, WB Saunders Co.

121. Walk RD and Gibson EJ: A comparative and analytical study of visual depth perception, Psychol Monogr 75:170, 1961.

122. Watson EH and Lowrey GH. Growth and development of children, ed 5, Chicago, 1967, Year Book Medical Publishers, Inc.

123. Wedenberg E: Auditory training of severely hard-of-hearing preschool children, Acta Otolaryngol Suppl 110:7, 1954.

124. Weiffenback J and Thach B: Taste receptors in the tongue of the newborn human: behavioral evidence, Paper presented at the biennial meeting of the Society for Research in Child Development, Denver, 1975.

125. Welker WI and Campos GB: Physiological significance of sulci in somatic sensory cerebral cortex in mammals of the family Procyonidae, J Comp Neurol 120:19, 1963.

126. Werner H: Comparative psychology of mental development, Chicago, 1948, Follett Publishing Co.

127. Weston JA: The migration and differentiation of neural crest cells, Adv Morphogen 8:41, 1970.

128. Winick M: Cellular growth of cerebrum, cerebellum and brain stem in normal and marasmic children, Exp Neurol 26:393, 1970.

129. Yakovlev PI: Pathoarchitectonic studies of cerebral malformations. I. Arrhinencephalies (halotelencephalies), J Neuropathol Exp Neurol 18:22, 1959.

130. Yakovlev PI: Anatomy of human brain and the problem of mental retardation. In Bowman PW and Mautner HV, editors: Mental retardation, Proceedings of the First Conference on Mental Retardation, New York, 1960, Grune & Stratton, Inc.

131. Yakovlev PI: Morphological criteria of growth and maturation of the nervous system in man, Ment Retard 39:3, 1962.

132. Yakovlev PI and Lecours AR: The myelogenetic cycles of regional maturation of the brain. In Minkowski A, editor: Regional development of the brain in early life, Oxford, 1967, Blackwell Publisher, Ltd.

133. Zecevic N and Rakic P: Differentiation of Purkinje cells and their relationship to other components of developing cerebellar cortex in man, J Comp Neurol 167:27, 1976.

134. Zelazo NA and others: Walking in the newborn, Science 176:314, 1972.

ADDITIONAL READINGS

Almli CR and Finger S: Early brain damage; research orientations and clinical observations, vol 1, New York, 1984, Academic Press.

Amiel-Tison C: Neurological assessment during the first year of life, New York, 1986, Oxford University Press.

Battaglia FC and Meschia G: An introduction to fetal physiology, New York, 1986, Academic Press.

Finger S and Almli CR: Early brain damage: neurobiology and behavior, vol 2, New York, 1984, Academic Press.

Finger S and others: Brain injury and recovery: theoretical and controversial issues, New York, 1988, Plenum Press.

Guralnick MJ and Bennett FC: The effectiveness of early intervention. New York, 1986, Academic Press.

Krasnegor NA and others: Perinatal development, New York, 1986, Elsevier Publishing Company.

Obrzut JE and Hynd GW: Child neuropsychology, theory and research, vol 1, New York, 1986, Academic Press.

Purvis D and Lichtman JW: Principles of neural development. Sunderland, Mass, 1984, Sinauer Press.

Saint-Anne Dargassies S: The neuro-motor and pyscho-affective development of the infant. New York, 1987, Academic Press.

Smotherman WP and Robinson SR: Behavior of the fetus, Caldwell, NJ, 1988, Telford Press.

Chapter 6

CLASSIFICATION OF COMMON FACILITATORY AND INHIBITORY TREATMENT TECHNIQUES

Darcy Ann Umphred and Guy L. McCormack

A problem-oriented approach to treatment of any disability implies that flexibility is a key element. That flexibility, however, is not random, disjointed, or without parameters. It should be based on methods that provide the best combination of available treatment alternatives to meet individual needs and differences. This flexibility is not achieved by selecting one total approach, such as the Rood method, versus another total approach, such as neurodevelopmental therapy (NDT); either choice limits the clinician to a small number of clearly delineated methods. If, instead, flexibility means the therapist selects any component of any method that helps the client reach an objective, then the therapist is confronted with hundreds—if not thousands—of various treatment procedures. From a neurological standpoint, the nervous system has a limited capacity to process sensory input. The myriad of treatment procedures are transduced into chemical and electrical transmissions that must travel along a limited number of pathways. Thus, many treatment procedures must produce the same neurotransmission. The temporal and spatial sequencing or timing of the input will vary according to the technique and specific application. The clinician without a comprehensive understanding of the neurophysiology of the various techniques, let alone an entire approach, has an infinite number of options with little basis for decision making.

Appropriate selection of specific techniques can be overwhelming unless a classification schema is developed that categorizes these treatment techniques. The primary goal of this chapter is to help the reader develop such a classification system: a system based on the *primary* input modality used when introducing a stimulus. A discussion of the physiology of each sensory modality is presented. In-depth discussion of some basic treatment strategies, in addition to explanation of less familiar techniques, is also included. Those treatment strategies frequently practiced and whose physiology is commonly known are included only in the tables and lists. Although only the primary input system is identified, at no time do we suggest it is the only input system affected. For example, when a proprio-

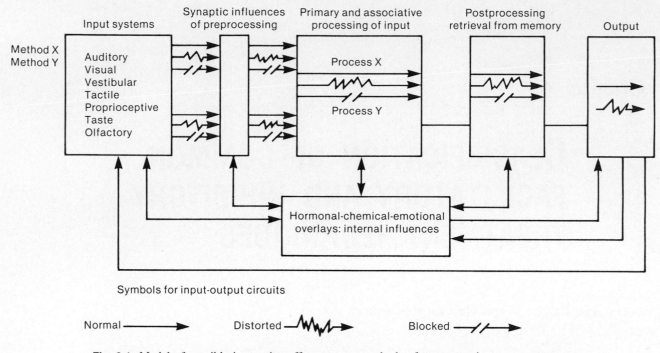

Fig. 6-1. Model of possible interactive effects among methods of treatment, input systems, processing and output systems, internal influences and feedback systems.

ceptor is facilitated, tactile input is simultaneously occurring. If there is a noise component (such as with vibration), then auditory input has been triggered. There is also evidence that a given sensory modality may "cross over" or fuse with a completely different modality, causing a synthesis of motor responses. These responses may occur in a modality that does not appear to be related. For example, olfaction may improve the tactile sensitivity of the hand. This concept is called *cross-modal stimulation* or *synesthesia*.[53,75] Yet a classification schema based on a primary modality promotes flexibility because the therapist can select from available treatment procedures that theoretically provide similar response patterns.

This type of classification system is based on identified input, observed responses, hypothesized neuromechanisms, and current research on the function of the central nervous system (CNS). An understanding of normal processing of input and its influence over response patterns helps the clinician evaluate and use the client's intact system as part of treatment. When response to certain stimuli does not elicit a desired output, then the classification schema provides the clinician with flexibility to select additional stimuli. This can be done by spatially summating input, such as using stretch, vibration, and resistance simultaneously, or temporally summating input, such as increasing the rate of the quick stretch. Many factors can influence desired output, such as method of instruction or the resting condition of the nervous system input of stimuli, synaptic connections, cerebellar or cortical processing, retrieval from past learning, motor output systems, or in-

ternal influences and balance. Fig. 6-1 illustrates this total system. Its clinical implications are clearer if the therapist retains a visual image of the client's total nervous system, including afferent input, processing, and efferent response. At any moment in time multiple stimuli are admitted into client's input system. Before that information reaches a level of primary processing, it will cross over at *least* one synaptic junction. At that time the information may be inhibited, it may be changed or distorted, or it may be allowed to continue without modification. If the information is inhibited, then no response will be observed. If it is changed, then the response will vary from the one that is anticipated. Furthermore, sensory processing can take place at many segments of the nervous system. At the spinal level the response may be phasic or reflexive. Brainstem mechanisms may evoke tonic or autonomic reactions. Subcortical and cortical feedback responses may be more adaptive and purposeful.[113]

The same three alternatives—inhibiting, distorting, or normal processing—can occur after the information reaches the primary processing areas or passes from primary processing to associative and postprocessing centers. Finally, motor output is elicited and thus response to the original input can be observed. If the response is normal, generally a clinician knows that the system is intact with regard to response to that stimuli. If the response is distorted or absent, little is known other than there is lack of the normal processing somewhere in the CNS. Internal influences also need to be considered since they affect each aspect of the system. Once normal processing is identified, understanding of deficit systems and potential problems can more easily be analyzed. This requires awareness of the totality of the individual, that is, the client's personal preference of stimuli and uniqueness of processing and internal influences. (Refer to Chapters 2, 3, and 4 for additional information.) Therefore stimuli that fall within one sensory categorization system may not be as effective as those within another and may create variability with respect to each client's response patterns.

It is the therapist's responsibility to select methods most efficient for each client's needs. This viewpoint, based on a variety of questions, leads to a problem-oriented approach to treatment. Since the output or response pattern is based on alpha motor neuron discharge and thus extrafusal muscle contraction, the first question is posed: what can be done to alter the excitatory state of the alpha motor neuron? Second, what input systems are available that will change this motor neuron's level of excitation? Third, which techniques use these various input systems as their primary modes of entry into the system? Fourth, what internal mechanisms need modification or facilitation to produce a desired behavior response from the client? Fifth, which input systems are available to alter the internal mechanism? Sixth, what combination of input stimuli will provide the best internal environment for the client to effect an optimal response pattern? For example, assume a hemiplegic client has a spastic lower extremity that produces the pattern of extension, adduction, internal rotation of the hip, extension of the knee, and plantar flexion inversion of the feet. The answers to the first two questions are based on the knowledge that the proprioceptive and exteroceptive systems can drastically affect alpha motor neuron excitation and that these systems are intact at a spinal level.

Appropriate selection of specific techniques—such as prolonged stretch using the tendon organ to inhibit the spastic pattern, quick stretch or light touch to the antagonistic muscle, or any other treatment modality within the classification schema—provides viable treatment alternatives. Awareness that the client's response pattern is an inherent synergistic pattern and that it is further facilitated by pressure to the ball of the foot leads to a better understanding of the clinical problem. Knowing that the client is unable to combine alternative patterns, such as hip flexion and knee extension, needed for the latter aspects of swing through and early aspects of heel strike in gait, the therapist can use the other inherent processes to elicit these and other patterns. Rolling, kneeling, half kneeling, and coming to stand can all be critical to breaking up the total extensor pattern. Lastly, techniques such as combining rolling with application of quick stretch, vibration, or rotation or having the client reach for a target or follow a visual stimulus provide a variety of combinations of therapeutic procedures to help the client learn or relearn normal response pattern. Further, this approach gives the clinician a choice of various procedures and promotes a learning environment that is flexible, changing, and interesting.

CLASSIFICATION ACCORDING TO SPECIFIC SENSORY MODALITIES

A variety of nerve fiber classification systems have been accepted by physiologists, neuroanatomists, and therapists. In order to avoid confusion about which nerve fiber is being discussed, the two primary methods of classification, along with a description of the functional component, have been included in Table 6-1 for easy referral.

Proprioceptive system

Muscle spindle. The muscle spindle consists anatomically of efferent and afferent, noncontractile tissue, and striated muscle. This entire feedback mechanism, which includes afferent and efferent fibers from the muscle structure to and from the spinal cord, is called the gamma loop or the fusimotor system[157] (Fig. 6-2). Varied in function, the system plays an important role in ongoing excitation of the alpha motor neurons innervating the extrafusal muscle within which it is lodged. It also facilitates polysynaptically agonistic synergies while inhibiting antagonistics and their synergies. Information is then sent via ascending pathways to the ipsilateral cerebellum and contralateral parietal lobe. Consequently, the spindle system seems to play an important role as an ongoing peripheral feedback mechanism to various centers within the CNS. These centers in turn regulate the continuous neuroexcitation at the spinal cord level and transmission of impulses along the reflex arc. Gamma innervation regulates the degree of internal stretch on the noncontractile portion of the spindle. Internal stretch, along with the external stretch of gravity, positioning, and therapeutic procedures, in turn regulates the afferent responses.

The afferent or sensory receptors are divided into Ia tonic and phasic, once referred to as annulospinal or primary endings; the II receptors are often called flower-spray or secondary endings. Ia tonic and II receptors are length receptors and respond to length changes placed on the noncontractile portion of the spindle. This length change can result from a mechanical external force, such as positioning or stretch to the muscle, or from an internal stretch caused by intrafusal muscle contraction. As long as the spindle has enough internal sensitivity, any therapeutic technique that creates a length change to the spindle has the potential of firing the Ia tonic receptors. If the intensity is great enough (such as increased range), the II receptors, which have a higher threshold, will also discharge. Their exact connections are not known. It was once hypothesized by Rood[155] that the II receptors are polysynaptic and may play a different role depending on the muscle type—tonic versus phasic—within which they were logged. This theory is now open for debate although the treatment procedures still seem effective.[179] The Ia phasic receptors re-

Table 6-1. Classifications of peripheral nerves according to size[85,92,136]

Gasser-Erlanger	Lloyd	Motor (functional component)	Sensory (functional component)
A fibers: large myelinated fibers with a high conduction rate			
Aα	Ia	Large, fast fibers of the alpha motor system (large cells of anterior horn to extrafusal motor fibers)	Muscle spindle: primary afferent endings, (primary stretch or low threshold stretch; Ia tonic responds to length, Ia phasic responds to rate)
	Ib		Golgi tendon organ for contraction: responds to tendon stretch or tension
Aβ	II		Muscle spindle: secondary afferent endings—tonic receptors responding to length
			Exteroceptive afferent endings from skin and joints: respond to light or low threshold stretch
Aγ 1 and 2	II	Gamma motor system (small cells of anterior horn to intrafusal motor fibers)	Bare nerve endings: joint receptors, mechanoreception of soft tissues—exteroceptors for pain, touch, and cold (low threshold)
AΔ	III		
B fibers: medium-sized myelinated fibers with a fairly rapid conduction rate			
Bβ		Preganglionic fibers of autonomic system (effective on glands and smooth muscle; motor branch of alpha): unknown function	
C fibers: small, poorly myelinated or unmyelinated fibers having the slowest conduction rate; augmentation and recruiting occurs within the nervous system after stimulation of these fibers has ceased			
	IV	Postganglionic fibers of sympathetic system	Exteroceptors: pain, temperature, touch

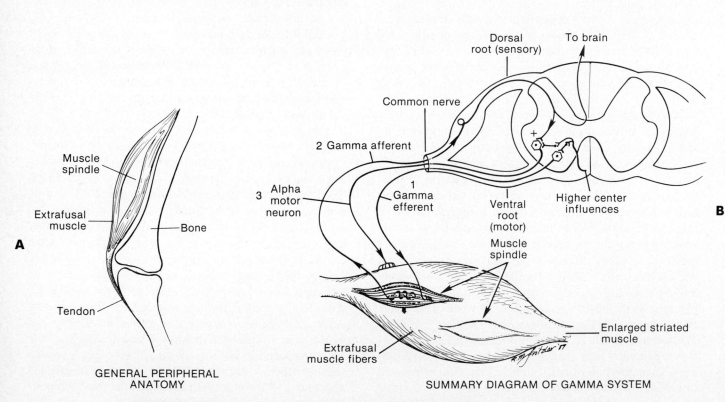

GENERAL PERIPHERAL ANATOMY

SUMMARY DIAGRAM OF GAMMA SYSTEM

Fig. 6-2. Summary diagram of gamma system. **A,** General peripheral anatomy of muscle spindle, joint, and bone. **B,** Enlarged striated muscle and spinal cord with gamma system neuroconnections: (1) γ efferent (motor); (2) γ afferent (sensory); (3) αMN (motor).

spond to rate versus length change. Techniques such as quick stretch, vibration, and tapping cause a rapid rate change within the spindle and thus potentially facilitate the Ia phasic receptors. Since from a neurological viewpoint regulation of the alpha motor neuron is the critical and final link to normal muscle contraction, techniques that raise and lower this excitatory state are certainly viable therapeutic techniques (Fig. 6-3).

Table 6-2 lists a variety of treatment procedures believed to use the proprioceptive muscle spindle system as a primary mode of sensory stimulation. The varying intensity, amount of tension, or rate of the stimuli, in addition to the original length of the muscle fiber before application of the stimulus, will determine which sensory receptor within the spindle is firing. When the Ia phasic or tonic receptors are excited, their response will be monosynaptic facilitation of the agonist. This important neurological connection at a behavioral level is referred to as "the monosynaptic stretch reflex." Simultaneously, polysynaptic circuitries are triggered that may (depending on the intensity and duration of the stimulus) lead to facilitation of

agonistic muscles and inhibition of the antagonist and antagonistic synergies (Fig. 6-4).

Resistance. Striated muscle has a unique ability to contract and thereby perform mechanical work. The physiology of muscle contraction includes a complex chain of neurological, histological, and chemical processes.

Resistance is often used to facilitate intrafusal and extrafusal muscle contraction. Resistance can be applied manually or mechanically. Although muscles can contract both in an isometric and isotonic fashion, most contractions are a mixture of the two. Certain muscle groups, such as the flexors, benefit from both isometric and isotonic exercise. Under normal circumstances, the flexors are employed for repetitive or rhythmic activities. The extensors, on the other hand, usually remain contracted in an effort to act against the forces of gravity. Therefore the extensor groups benefit best from isometric resistance.[50,94,184]

When resistance is applied to a voluntary muscle, spindle afferent fibers and tendon organs fire in proportion to the magnitude of the resistance. The motor response is also contingent on the amount of contraction needed to

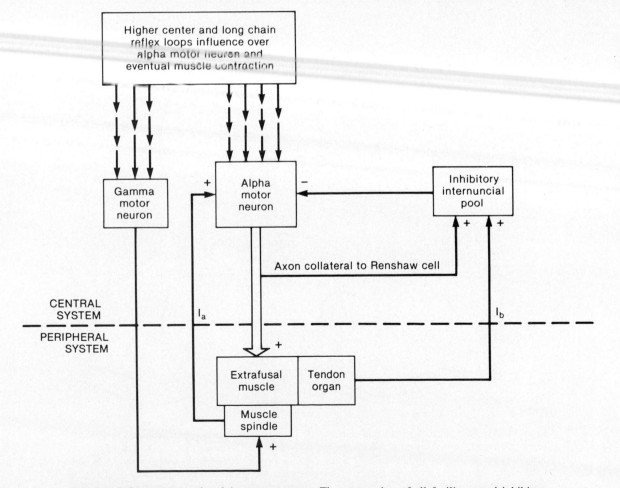

Fig. 6-3. Influences over the alpha motor neuron. The summation of all facilitory and inhibitory activity on the αMN will determine the response of the muscle.

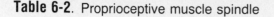

Table 6-2. Proprioceptive muscle spindle

Receptor	Stimulus	Nature of response
Ia tonic	Length	Monosynaptic and polysynaptic facilitation of agonist
Ia phasic	Rate of change in length	Polysynaptic inhibition of antagonist and antagonistic synergy
		Polysynaptic facilitation of agonistic synergy
		Input to cerebellum
		Input to opposite parietal lobe
		Specific responses open for question:
II	Length	Monosynaptic facilitation of agonist
		Polysynaptic facilitation of specific muscle groups, depending on muscle function of tissue where II originates
		Transmittal of information to higher centers

Possible treatment alternatives:
Resistance
Quick stretch to agonist
Tapping: tendon and muscle belly
Reverse tapping: gravity stretches; tapping agonist into shortened range
Positioning (range)
Electrical stimulation
Pressure or sustained stretch
Stretch pressure
Stretch release
Vibration within a facilitory frequency
Gravity as a prolonged stretched
Active motion

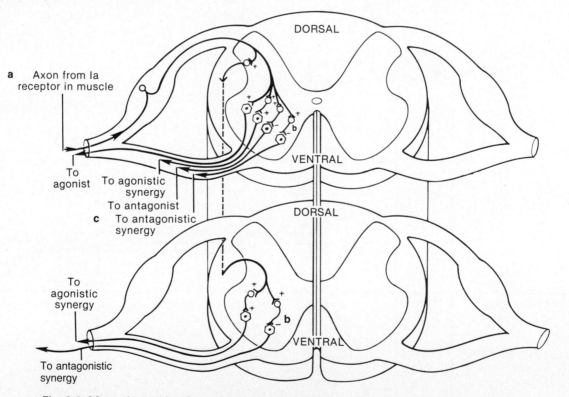

Fig. 6-4. Myo-tatic stretch reflex and relationship to muscle in synergy and agonists. *a,* Primary sensory afferent Ia (tonic and phasic) from muscle spindle. *b,* Interneurons: + = facilitory; − = inhibitory. *c,* Alpha (α) motor neurons going back to muscle tissue. If the interneuron at its synapse excites the alpha motor neuron, then the potential for firing has been heightened. If the interneuron inhibits the αMN, then potential for firing has been dampened. Note the Ia facilitates the αMN going back to the primary agonist via internuncials. The Ia has the potential of: (1) facilitating agonist synergies both at the level it enters the cord as well as other segments, and (2) inhibiting the antagonist at the level it enters and antagonistic synergies both at the entry level and other segments.

withstand the resistance force. Light resistance will activate a small number of motor units to develop a proportional amount of muscle tension. An increased load or resistance will generate more tension and require more motor units (recruitment) to respond with the appropriate amount of contraction.

Resistance to an isometrically contracted muscle is more facilitory than it is to an isotonic contraction.[7] As isometric resistance to isometric contraction continues, more motor units are recruited, thereby increasing the strength of extrafusal contraction.[157]

Isotonic contraction of muscles can be either concentric or eccentric. Concentric muscle contraction refers to shortening of muscle fibers while the joint is moving against gravity or resistance. Eccentric isotonic contraction refers to the lengthening of muscle fibers to resist force, as in lowering the arms while holding a heavy object. Eccentric contraction uses less metabolic output and promotes strength gains in less time.[157] However, all types of muscle contraction will promote increased strength. Isokinetics is a type of isotonic exercise that mechanically controls the rate of movement and resistance.

Theorists have used resistance in different fashions. Brunnstrom[30] uses resistance in conjunction with traction and joint compression to excite muscle synergies. Rood[155] used resistance and joint approximation greater than body weight to promote co-innervation. Kabot[100] used resistance and stretch to facilitate difficult volitional motor responses.

Tapping. Three types of tapping techniques are commonly used by therapists. Tapping of the tendon is a fairly nondiscriminatory stimulus. The tendon is tapped, which in turn causes the Ia phasic to discharge, causing a response similar to quick stretches of the entire muscle. This technique is used by physicians to determine degree of stretch sensitivity of a muscle. A normal response would be a brisk muscle contraction. Because of the magnitude of the stimulus, this technique is not highly effective in teaching a client to control or gradiate muscle contraction. Instead, tapping of the muscle belly, a lower-intensity stimulus, is more satisfactory. Reverse tapping, a less frequently described technique, is often used. The extremity is positioned so gravity promotes the stretch, instead of the therapist manually tapping or actively inducing muscle stretch. Once the muscle responds, the therapist taps or passively moves the muscle or a bony prominence to help the muscle obtain a shortened range. For example, assume the client is in a kneeling position and the therapist is kneeling behind the client. Instead of tapping the gluteus maximus to assist in hip extension, the therapist allows the client to momentarily drop out of full extension. This quick lengthening of the gluteus maximus is caused by gravity pulling the client toward the floor. As the muscle begins to contract, the therapist can apply a quick tap to the gluteus maximus to assist in obtaining a shortened

range. Another example would be reverse tapping the elbow when the client is bearing weight on extended elbows. Gravity quick stretches the triceps. Then the therapist taps the elbow into full extension. This tapping is usually performed at the elbow.

Positioning (range). The concept of submaximal and maximal range of muscles is highly significant to clinical application. Bessou and Laporte[15] monitored the neuronal firing of muscle spindles at different ranges of motion. Their finding contributed to the understanding that manual stretching of muscles causes the Ia endings to discharge at specific submaximal ranges; the secondary endings begin to fire near the maximum physiological length. It is important to note that upper motor neuron lesions can alter the sensitivity of the spindle afferent reflex arc fibers. As a result, the reflex arc becomes supersensitive to stretch. Therefore range of motion should be carefully assessed on an individual basis to determine what is maximal or submaximal range for an individual. For example, normal elbow range of motion extends up to 130 degrees. The submaximal range would be about 90 degrees of flexion or extension. The last 20 degrees of flexion or extension would place maximal range of stretch, and the secondary afferent fibers would begin to discharge. A client with upper-extremity spasticity resulting in a flexion contracture may be left with 30 degrees of motion. The submaximal range for this individual may be 10 degrees. Anything beyond 10 degrees of flexion or extension would place the extremity in maximal range, causing the secondary ending to fire. This would be counterproductive if the goal is to reduce tone in the biceps muscle. Additional stimulation of the secondary endings probably would cause further contraction of the biceps muscle, resulting in diminished range of motion. As an alternative, the therapist should position the joint and muscle in the submaximum range while stimulating the antagonist muscle(s).[101,106,179]

Electrical stimulation. For in-depth discussion of the use of electrical stimulation (ES) both as an evaluation and a treatment modality, see Chapter 26 on electrodiagnosis. Electrical stimulation is not generally identified as a muscle spindle facilitation technique. However, when any mixed nerve is stimulated, not only is the alpha motor neuron affected but both gamma efferent neurons and spindle afferent neurons are also stimulated. Afferent firing helps to increase the sensitivity of the alpha motor neuron for further firing. The gamma efferent system causes intrafusal contraction, afferent firing, and thus continued biasing of the alpha motor neuron. Thus electrical stimulation has the potential for being an excellent muscle spindle facilitory technique, especially if additional therapeutic tools, such as resistance, are used.

Stretch pressure. The muscle belly is the stimulus focus of stretch pressure. The thumb, fingertips, or palm of the hand is used. First, quick stretches are applied, followed by briefly maintained pressure. Both Ia phasic and tonic receptors have the potential of being stimulated. When the muscle is placed 30 to 50 degrees beyond midrange in a normal muscle, the II receptors should also fire. In a hypotonic spindle system, the length receptors may not fire because of a lack of internal tension. In that instance Ia phasic receptors are the focus of the technique until enough internal sensitivity has developed to fire the other length receptors. This approach would obviously not be used on a hypertonic muscle because it would increase the tone. But it could be used on the antagonist muscle in order to inhibit a hypertonic agonist.[53,67]

Stretch release. This technique is performed by placing the fingertips over the belly of larger muscles and spreading the fingers in an effort to stretch the skin and the underlying muscle. The stretch is done firmly enough to temporarily deform the soft tissue so the cutaneous receptors and Ia afferent fibers may produce facilitation of the target muscle.

Manual pressure. Manual pressure can be facilitory when applied as a brisk stretch or frictionlike massage over muscle bellies. The speed and duration at which the manual pressure is applied determine the extent of recruitment from receptors.

Vibration. Bishop[17,18] wrote an excellent series of articles on the neurophysiology and therapeutic application of vibration. High-frequency vibration (100 to 300 hertz [Hz] or cycles per second) to the muscle or tendon elicits a reflex response referred to as the tonic vibratory response (TVR). Each cycle of vibration elicits stretch to the muscle spindle and causes selective firing of the Ia afferent receptors. Tension within the muscle will increase slowly and progressively for 30 to 60 seconds and then plateau for the duration of the stimulus.[108] Certain researchers found that at cessation of the input, the contractibility of the muscle was enhanced for approximately 3 minutes.[108,181] Others found vibration to have a short duration period, lasting only as long as the stimulus was applied.[17,88,111]

By facilitation of the Ia afferent receptors through vibration, a variety of neurophysiological responses can be produced. Agonist facilitation and antagonistic inhibition, also called reciprocal innervation are physiological responses that have significant clinical application. To facilitate a hypotonic muscle the muscle belly is first put on stretch and then vibratory stimuli are applied.[80] To inhibit a hypertonic muscle the antagonistic muscle could be vibrated.[17,80] The use of vibration can be enhanced by combining it with additional modalities, such as resistance, position, and visually directed movement. Vibration also simulates cutaneous receptors, specifically the pacinian corpuscles and thus can be classified as an exteroceptive modality.[163] This is especially true with vibration of 60 cycles per second. Because of its ability to decrease hypersensitive tactile receptors, vibration is considered an inhibitory technique; it is also discussed in the section on exteroceptors—maintained stimulus (see Table 6-4).

Farber[53] summarized the use of vibration and clearly identified precautions that must be taken. Again, frequencies of 100 to 300 cycles per second can be used to effectively elicit the tonic vibratory response. However, we have observed that in a hypertonic muscle the resting threshold of the Ia afferent is lower (biased) and the normal inhibitory mechanisms are not present. As a result, 60 Hz is an adequate stimulus to cause contraction of superficial mobilizer muscles.[113] Frequencies over 200 Hz can be damaging to the skin. We have found frequencies over 150 Hz to cause discomfort and even pain. Thus it is recommended that vibrators registering 100 to 125 Hz be used. Most battery-operated hand vibrators function at 50 to 90 Hz.[57] Frequencies below 75 Hz are thought to have an inhibitory effect on normal muscle.[108] For that reason it is recommended that batteries be replaced when the frequency begins to drop. A common error is applying additional pressure to the muscle with the vibrator when the batteries begin to lose their charge. This additional pressure causes resistance and further decreases the frequency of the vibration. Cutaneous pressure is also known to cause inhibition, so if it is combined with vibration, it can only serve to cancel out the desired effects.

Amplitude or amount of displacement must also be considered when analyzing vibration as a modality. High-amplitude vibration has the potential of causing skin breakdown. An understanding of various responses and their neurophysiological explanation should be part of a clinician's background. Because of the potency of vibration as a treatment technique, its indiscriminate use should be highly discouraged. It has been reported that this technique causes adverse effects, especially in clients with cerebellar dysfunction[18]; thus keen clinical observation strategies should always be employed whatever the anticipated response.

The tendon organ. The tendon organ (TO) is a specialized receptor located in both the proximal and the distal musculotendinous insertions. In conjunction with the muscle spindle, the TO plays an important role in the mediation of subconscious proprioception.[121,90,188]

The principal role of the TO is to monitor muscle tension exerted by the contraction of the extrafusal muscles. Originally, it was believed that the TO had a high threshold to stretch and low threshold to contraction. The high-threshold organs are usually located in the insertions of the muscles. They are thought to be a protective mechanism designed to prevent structural damage when extreme tension is put on muscles and tendons. However, the TO is more than a protective device. Recent research has demonstrated that the tendon organ is highly sensitive to tension and acts conjointly with the muscle spindle to regulate tonicity and compliance of extrafusal muscles.[29,174]

TOs are innervated by Group Ib afferent fibers. Because the TO adapts slowly, it provides continuous information about extrafusal muscle contraction. Physiological studies have shown that, once activated, the TO discharges rapidly and then settles down to fire at a rate nearly proportional to the muscle tension. The TO (Ib) is signaling not only tension but rate of change of tension.[79]

Perhaps a better understanding of the TO can be achieved if it is compared and contrasted with the muscle spindle. A fundamental difference between the two proprioceptors is that the muscle spindle detects length whereas the tendon organ monitors tension. Motorically, the muscle spindle and the TO produce reflexes that are the exact opposite.[66,111,147] The muscle regulates reciprocal innervation whereas the TO modulates autogenic inhibition.

Again, the muscle spindle responds to an adequate stimulus with reciprocal inhibition. That is, the muscle receiving the stimulus is facilitated and the antagonist inhibited. In contrast, the TO responds to an adequate stimulus with autogenic inhibition. In other words, it inhibits the muscle receiving the stimulus if concurrent facilitory influences, such as resistance, are eliminated. In multiarthrodial muscles (superficial flexors and adductors), small-range repeated contractions will reduce hypertonicity in spastic muscles.[46,90] This is accomplished by synaptic connections to inhibitory interneurons in the spinal cord, which in turn produce a dampening effect on the alpha motor neurons from which the stimulus was derived. The TO was thought to be responsible for the pathological reflex described by Sherrington as the "clasped knife reflex," but this theory is now open to speculation.[101]

Clinically, this release phenomenon is seen in clients with upper motor neuron lesions. Usually the patient has some degree of hypertonicity. As the hypertonic extremity is passively moved through range of motion, resistance is felt and then suddenly "melts away," allowing more freedom of movement. This phenomenon is the result of autogenic inhibition. The hypertonicity and lengthening produce tension in the tendon, which stimulates the Ib endings, causing them to fire. The discharge synapses with an inhibitory interneuron, causing the homonymous muscle to be relaxed; the antagonist may be excited to further facilitate the unloading of tension.

According to Moore,[121] autogenic inhibition may not be a manifestation of the TO alone. There are a number of other joint receptors that have not been studied in great detail. It appears that other joint and cutaneous receptors could be sending signals to supraspinal centers as well.

There appears to be a delicate balance between the inhibitory loop of the TO and the excitatory loop of the fusimotor system. These systems provide feedback control mechanisms to inform the CNS about the length, speed of movement, and contraction of a given muscle. Therefore this balance of excitatory and inhibitory feedback mechanisms is basic to the precise integration of reflex activity and control of fine movements.[135,156] Table 6-3 lists a variety of known treatment approaches that use the TO as the primary mode for inhibition.

Inhibitory pressure. Pressure has been used therapeutically to inhibit or facilitate motor responses. Mechanical pressure, such as cones, pads, or the orthokinetic cuff developed by Blashy and Fuchs,[19] provides continuous pressure (force). Pressure on tendinous insertions activates deep receptors called *pacinian* corpuscles, which are rapidly adapting receptors. Vallbo[180] describes the pacinian corpuscle as the largest, most studied, and most highly structured end organ in cutaneous and tendon tissue. These receptors are usually found in the deep subcutaneous layers of skin in the palms of the hands, soles of the feet, mesentery, periosteum, tendon sheaths, and intramuscular connective tissue.[51,126] Tuttle and McClearly[176] studied the pacinian corpuscles in the mesentery of cats. They postulated that the pacinian corpuscle is a baroreceptor initiating vasomotor reflexes in the skin and muscles. Pertovaara,[144] studying the modification of pain thresholds in seven healthy adults, found that the pacinian corpuscles were activated by vibrotactile stimulation when the subjects were exposed to painful electrical stimuli. The pacinian corpuscles probably suppress other sensations in the receptor field.[181]

This inhibitory pressure technique also works when pressure is applied across the longitudinal axis of a tendon. The pressure is applied across the tendon with increasing pressure until the muscle relaxes. Constant pressure applied over the tendons of the wrist flexors will be inhibitory.

Pressure over bony prominences has facilitory and inhibitory effects. A common example is pressure on the medial aspect of the calcaneus, which inhibits calf muscles and allows contraction of the lateral dorsiflexors muscles, while pressure over the lateral side of the calcaneus also inhibits calf muscles to allow for contraction of the medial dorsiflexor muscles.[155] Localized finger pressure applied bilaterally to acupuncture points has been shown to relieve pain and reduce muscle tone.[115,116,160] This technique has also been found to be particularly effective when used in a low-stimuli environment and when combined with deep breathing.

The joint. A joint may be described as the articulating surfaces between two or more bones. Joints are usually classified according to the degree of movement they allow. On the basis of this interpretation, three types of joints are recognized: synarthrosis, amphiarthrosis, and diarthrosis.[153,187] Synarthrotic joints are relatively immovable and make up the sutures of the skull. Amphiarthrodial joints are partially movable because the adjacent bones are separated by a thick layer of cartilage—for example, the

Table 6-3. Proprioceptive tendon organs and joints

Receptor	Stimulus	Response
Tendon organ lb	Tension on extrafusal muscle	Polysynaptic inhibition of agonist, facilitation of antagonist

Possible treatment suggestions
1. Extreme stretch
2. Deep pressure to tendon
3. Passive positioning in extreme lengthened range
4. Extreme resistance: more effective in lengthen and shortened range
5. Deep pressure to muscle belly to put stretch on tendon
6. Small repeated contractions with gravity eliminated

Type of joint		Stimulus	Response
I	6-9 μ	Static and dynamic joint tension: muscle pull	?: Facilitates postural holding: joint awareness
II	9-12 μ	Dynamic: sudden change in joint tension	?: Facilitates agonist and awareness of joint motion: range
III	13-17 μ	Dynamic: linked to GTO traction; activates in extreme range	?: Inhibits agonist
IV	2-5 μ ≤ 2 μ	Pain	?: Inhibits agonist

Possible treatment alternatives
1. Manual traction (distraction) to joint surfaces to facilitate joint motion
2. Manual approximation (compression) to joint surfaces to facilitate cocontraction or postural holding
3. Positioning: gravity used to approximate or apply traction
4. Weight belts, shoulder harnesses, and helmets to increase approximation
5. Wrist and ankle cuffs to increase traction
6. Wall pulleys, weights, manual resistance
7. Manual therapy[109]

intervertebral joints and the pubic symphysis of the pelvic girdle. Diarthrosis means a joint in which there is a separation (cavity) between adjacent bones that allows them to be freely movable. The joint is encased in a ligamentous capsule. The inner layer of the capsule, except for the articular surfaces, is lined with the synovial membrane. This membrane generates synovial fluid, which serves to lubricate and nourish the joint. Diarthrodial joints are subdivided according to shape and the type of movement the joint performs.

From a neurophysiological standpoint, joint movement provides subcortical nuclei and the cortex with constant information about position and movement. It would appear that the diarthrodial joints contain the greatest number of receptors with the capacity to respond to the slightest change of angle between two bony articulations. In other words, joint receptors are arranged so that any change in the joint angle causes maximal discharge of designated receptors monitoring that degree of angle. Thus as a joint is moved through range of motion, each degree of movement activates a division of overlapping receptors sensitive to certain zones of movement. This arrangement of overlapping sensitivity zones is called *range fractionation*. What is most important is that the CNS receives continuous in-

formation about minute changes in joint positions.[102] However, receptors have been shown to have a certain amount of specificity. That is, some receptors are specifically sensitive to one form of energy. Receptor specificity is related to interaction of mechanical, chemical, electrical, and thermal energy tranduction. With the exception of some pain receptors, all joint receptors are mechanoreceptors. They signal mechanical distortion. They also give information about opposing ranges, such as abduction and adduction, based on the side of the joint on which they are found.

Numerous physiological studies have been conducted to determine the exact functions and threshold levels of joint receptors. To date many questions have been left unanswered, but from a clinical standpoint, the joint receptors are most amenable to facilitory and inhibitory techniques.*

The awareness of movement and position requires the integration of many receptors. Any detection of joint movement in the gravitational field causes the discharge of receptors in the somatic, visual, and vestibular afferent systems. Some joint receptors have absolute thresholds for specific ranges of motion, the sense of movement, and po-

*References 5, 15, 38, 48, 111, 155.

sition. In addition, a host of peripheral skin and muscle afferent fibers sense the movement.

Four major types of joint receptors are described in the literature. Anatomically, these receptors are localized in the joint capsules and ligaments. They include the Golgi-type endings, Golgi-Mazzoni corpuscles, Ruffini's corpuscle, and free nerve endings.[182,188] In general, the joint receptors are slowly adapting receptors. That is, they do not adapt completely but continue to send impulses to the CNS as long as the stimulus is present. With the exception of the free nerve endings, the joint receptors are subserved by well-myelinated type A alpha-neurons. Because they send ascending impulses via the lemniscal system to higher centers for precise interpretations, joint receptors provide discriminative information about movement and position. Last, joint receptors have different thresholds for the rate of movement and the degree of angulation.[5,171]

Type III, Golgi-type endings, are found primarily in the ligaments around the joints. These are the largest joint receptors and appear to be similar to the TOs in appearance. Their location in joint ligaments allows them to be stimulated very strongly by rate of joint movement and the force of gravity. Subsequently, the Golgi-type ending fires rapidly when the joint is first moved and then discharges at a steady lower rate. This slowly adapting joint receptor may also provide the brain with information about joint position.[111,188,192]

Type II, Golgi-Mazzoni corpuscles (paciniform corpuscles), resemble pacinian corpuscles in physical appearance. They are small, encapsulated receptors found sparsely in tendon surfaces and joint capsules. In comparison with the other joint receptors, Golgi-Mazzoni corpuscles are rapidly adapting. Higher concentrations have been found in the connective tissues of the hands. These corpuscles function principally as a detector of rapid joint movements. They have also been found to discharge under deep pressure and vibration stimulus.[171]

Type I, Ruffini's corpuscles, are exclusively joint receptors found in the fibrous joint capsules. These receptors have a lower threshold to stimulation than the Golgi-type ending. However, both receptors respond vigorously with a volley of impulses at the beginning of joint movement and taper off to a steady state of firing at different angular positions. Ruffini's corpuscles monitor both the rate and the direction of joint movement. These receptors also discharge when touch pressure is applied to joint surfaces.[76,192]

Free nerve endings are widely distributed throughout the body's soft tissues. Morphologically, they are more primitive than the encapsulated joint receptors. Moveover, the free nerve endings are contiguous with unmyelinated group IV or C fibers. The actual role the free nerve endings play in joint reception has not been identified. However, it has been speculated that they provide a crude awareness of initial joint movement and the signaling of joint pain.[58,111,180]

In summary, the final word on joint receptors does not seem to be in at this time. It would appear that joint receptors play a major role in the awareness of joint position and movement. However, studies have been conducted in which joint receptors have been selectively anesthetized in an effort to determine their exact function. The studies revealed that an unidentified set of muscle afferent fibers and cutaneous receptors also contribute to the sense of movement and position.[111] Hence it may be safe to say that the somatosensory system works cooperatively as a unit.[69]

Because joint receptors are stretched and compressed during joint movement, they are in a good position to transmit signals regarding joint position, direction, and velocity of movement, but not force. Force sensations seem to be mediated by the receptors of the muscles and TOs.

The joint receptors lend themselves well to facilitory and inhibitory techniques. As already stated, the joint receptors are both slow and fast adapting. They exert strong influences on musculature. Although the histological properties of the joint receptors are not entirely clear, certain techniques elicit predictable responses. Joint receptors are sensitive to movement, position, traction, compression, and palpation. Further studies to delineate the properties of individual receptors may not prove to be fruitful because the somatosensory system works as a whole. For clinical purposes there is a variety of potential treatment approaches that focus on the joint receptor (Table 6-3).

Combined proprioceptive techniques. Many techniques succeed because of the combined effects of multiple input. Some approaches that seem to combine two or more proprioceptive modalities are:

1. Jamming
2. Ballistic movements
3. Total positioning
4. Proprioceptive neuromuscular facilitation (PNF) patterns
5. Postexcitatory inhibition with stretch, range, rotation, and shaking
6. Heavy work patterns
7. Feldenkrais[55,56,96]

Jamming. Jamming is usually applied to the ankle and knee with the intent of inhibiting plantar flexion while facilitating postural cocontraction around the ankle. The client can be placed in side-lying position, can sit on a chair or mat, or can be positioned over a bolster with the hip and knee in some flexion. This flexion inhibits the total extension pattern, including the plantar flexor muscles. With release of plantar flexion these muscles are placed on extreme stretch to maintain the inhibition. At this time intermittent joint approximation of considerable force is applied between the heel and knee. If the client is sitting, this approximation can easily be applied by pounding the heel on the floor and controlling a counterforce at the knee. Once cocontraction is minimally palpated, the clinician should facilitate a movement pattern such as partial weight-bearing to further encourage the CNS to readapt to these two stimuli. This technique can also be used to inhibition dorsiflexion of wrist and fingers by focusing on appropriate upper-extremity patterns, releasing spasticity, and applying a large amount of joint approximation between the heel of the hand and the elbow.

Ballistic movement. Ballistic movements or pendular exercises are effective because of their combined proprioceptive interaction. The client is asked to begin a movement, such as shoulder flexion while prone over a table with the arm hanging over the side. As the muscle approaches the shortened range, the amount of ongoing gamma afferent activity decreases. Thus the agonist alpha motor neuron bias and the inhibition of Ia and II receptors of the antagonistic alpha motor neurons decrease. Simultaneously, the antagonistic muscle is being placed on more and more stretch. This stretch, as well as the lack of inhibition on the antagonistic alpha motor neurons, will encourage the antagonistic muscle to begin contraction and reverse the movement pattern. The TOs also play a key role in ongoing inhibition. As the muscle approaches the shortened range and tension on the tendon becomes intense the TO increases its firing, thus inhibiting the agonistic muscle in the shortened range while facilitating the antagonistic muscle. This technique is highly movement oriented, and the traction applied to the shoulder joint while swinging the arm further facilitates the movement.

Caution must be exercised by the clinician using this technique. Range of motion can easily be obtained through pendular movement. If limitation of motion is caused by superficial splinting of muscles whose function is to move (which now protects torn muscles), the technique will encourage the splinting muscles to relax; it will inhibit the postural patterns by traction and thus have the potential of tearing the muscle further by the pull and weight of the arm. Consequently, the clinician must always determine before therapy the reasons for specific clinical signs and whether the total problem will be corrected through an activity such as a ballistic movement. If only one component of the problem is alleviated, such as limitation of range, while lack of postural tone or joint stability possibly increases in severity, then additional techniques must be combined with this treatment modality. For example, assume the rotator cuff muscles were slightly torn and the movers of the shoulder are superficially splinting to prevent further tearing. Instructing the client to hold the humerus in the glenohumeral joint by active contraction of the rotator cuff muscles will facilitate postural holding and strengthen the torn muscles. Having the client simultaneously perform a ballistic movement with the arm will expedite shoulder movement, thus preventing unnecessary splinting and possible limitation of joint range.

Total positioning. In brief, positioning implies the use of *reflex-inhibiting postures* and gravity to release tonic reflex activity of the muscle spindle.[142] According to Bobath and Rood[21,155] normal muscle tone must be established before normal postures and movements can take place. With an understanding of the secondary spindle endings and the TOs, the therapist can position clients in total or partial reversals of the abnormal *postural set.* A vast number of sensorimotor systems are then brought into play: autogenic inhibition, reciprocal innervation, and labyrinthine and somatosensory influences.

Proprioceptive neuromuscular facilitation patterns. To analyze and learn the patterns and techniques that constitute proprioceptive neuromuscular facilitation, a total approach to treatment, refer to the texts by Kottke[101] and Sullivan.[169]

Postexcitatory inhibition with stretch, range, rotation, and shaking. The concept of postexcitatory inhibition (PEI) is based on the action potential or electrical response pattern of a neuron at the time of stimulation, as well as the entire phase response until the neuron returns to normal. At the time of stimulation the action potential will build and go through an excitatory phase. Following that phase the neuron enters an inhibitory phase or refractory period during which further stimulation is not possible. This is referred to as the postexcitatory inhibition phase or postsynaptic afferent depolarization (PAD).[53] Following the second stage an increase of excitation above resting level ensures, followed by return to normal of neuronal activity. These phase changes are extremely short and, in normal muscle, asynchronous with respect to multiple neuronal firing. In a spastic muscle more simultaneous firing occurs; with an increase of range, and thus tension, more fibers will be discharged. It is hypothesized that if the spastic muscle is placed at the end of its spastic range and a quick stretch is applied and held, then total facilitation followed by total inhibition will occur because of postexcitatory inhibition. As the inhibition phase is felt, the therapist can passively lengthen the spastic muscle until the facility phase sets in repolarization. At that time the clinician holds the lengthened position. Increased tone will ensue, followed by inhibition and continued lengthening. Holding the range (or not allowing concentric contraction during the excitatory phase) is critical. If shortening is permitted, the spindle will readapt to the new position and the therapist will find that the spastic muscle quickly becomes more spastic. In contrast, if the muscle is held as the tone increases, the resistance and stretch is then maximal and probably further facilitates the inhibitory phase.

At a certain point in the range, the spastic muscle will become inhibited and tone will disappear. It is thought that at this time the TO activity takes over and maintains inhibition, thus creating an inhibitory range where antagonistic muscles can be facilitated optimally. If this technique is performed in a pure plane of motion, the clinician will find it a time-consuming procedure. Range can be achieved quickly by integrating a few additional techniques—that is, incorporating rotatory patterns of movement. For example, if the spastic upper extremity is positioned in the pattern of shoulder adduction, internal rotation, elbow flexion, wrist pronation, and finger flexion, then a pattern in the exact opposite direction can be incorporated to include external rotation of the shoulder and supination of the wrist. Every time the clinician begins to lengthen the spastic extremity, those rotatory patterns should be used. This should be done both on initial stretch and hold and during the inhibitory phase. Rotation seems to lengthen the inhibitory phase and allows additional range. If the clinician adds a quick stretch to the antagonistic during the inhibitory phase of the agonistic muscle, then further facilitation of antagonist muscle will occur. Since the agonistic muscle is in an inhibitory phase, movement in and out of its spastic range should not affect it. Yet the quick stretch facilitation of the antagonistic muscle inhibits the spastic agonistic muscle and again lengthens the inhibitory phase. This entire procedure occurs quite quickly. An observer might say that the clinician shakes the spasticity out of the arm. The shaking action is thought to be the quick stretch. The degree of success depends on the therapist's sensitivity to the tonal shifts or phase changes occurring in the client. These tonal shifts are automatic and not under the client's conscious control. The technique does not teach the client anything and should be used to maintain range of motion and to create an optimal environment to facilitate normal antagonistic control.

Rood's heavy work patterns. See Stockmeyer's interpretation of the Rood approach.[168]

Feldenkrais. Moshe Feldenkrais's concepts[55,56] of sensory awareness through movement place emphasis on relaxation of muscle on stretch and distracting and compressing joints for sensory awareness. Both techniques reflect combined proprioceptive techniques. Taking muscles off stretch slows down general efferent firing and thus overload to the CNS. Compression and distraction of joints enhance specific input from a body part while simultaneously facilitating input of a lesser intensity from other body segments. This combined proprioceptive approach enhances body schema awareness in a relaxed environment.

Exteroceptors

The somatosensory system is usually subdivided into two distinct systems. One system is phylogenetically older and nonspecific in nature. The other system is phylogenetically newer and specific in function.

The concept of the dual quality of the somatosensory system was first suggested by Head.[84] The older sensory system was said to be *protopathic* in that it mediated primitive stimuli for protective responses. The newer sensory system was described as *epicritic* in that it mediated the discriminative aspects of somatic sensibility. The dual systems were further researched and elaborated on by Mountcastle and his associates.[126] Today the systems are described in more anatomical terms as the *spinothalamic* (protopathic) and the *lemniscal* (epicritic) systems.[7]

A fundamental understanding of the anatomy and physiology of the dual sensory systems is important before undertaking therapeutic intervention techniques. A brief explanation is presented here. The lemniscal system consists of pathways that are clearly distinguishable anatomically and neurophysiologically. Afferent signals are projected to two cortical regions of the parietal lobe from the spinal cord and the trigeminal nerve. From the spinal level, afferent impulses travel through the posterior columns, ascend through the medial lemniscus to the ventrobasal nuclei of the thalamus and on to specific regions of the cortex. The afferent impulses entering the CNS by way of the trigeminal nerve synapse with nuclei in the medulla and continue through the medial lemniscus, thalamus, and parietal region of the cortex. The fibers of the lemniscal system are large and well-myelinated. Therefore signals are transmitted rapidly, with a minimum of three synaptic relays. A striking characteristic of this system is its somatotopic organization. There is an orderly spatial topographic representation of the surface of the skin in the fiber bundles of the dorsal columns and the synaptic organization of the thalamus. This highly developed organization of sensory relays allows the lemniscal system to discriminate among specific tactile stimuli. This system transmits conscious and unconscious proprioceptive and kinesthetic information, such as touch, pressure, localization, contour, quality, and spatial details of mechanical stimuli. In general the receptors that feed into the lemniscal system are encapsulated, slowly adapting with type I and II (Aα) fibers. Many of these receptors are found in the joints, muscles, and glabrous (nonhairy) surfaces of the skin.[192,195]

The spinothalamic system is less well-defined anatomically than the lemniscal system. Different impulses are linked to this system by way of the anterior and lateral spinothalamic tracts or the reticulospinal tracts (anterolateral funiculus). Ascending impulses either terminate in or send collateral connections to the reticular formation. These fibers continue upward to synapse with the nonspecific thalamic nuclei (medial) and then diverge to make connections with practically all regions of the cerebral cortex. Other collaterals of this system project to the regulators of the autonomic nervous system, limbic system, and the so-called extrapyramidal nuclei.[147]

Since the spinothalamic system synapses with the reticular formation and the ANS, it serves more as an energizing or arousal mechanism to potentially harmful stimuli. Therefore this system is involved in perception of pain, light touch, pleasurable sexual sensations, and aversive stimuli and in the production of primitive orientations and protective responses.[147,154]

This subdivision into spinothalamic and lemniscal systems can mislead one into thinking that they can be activated separately. Most sensory stimuli will activate both systems simultaneously—for example, light touch. The lemniscal system can carry both exteroceptive and proprioceptive stimuli. However, it is possible to "load" one system more than the other by using selective stimuli in a fast or slow manner.[7]

Poggio and Mountcastle[147] suggest that the lemniscal system can have an inhibiting influence on the spinothalamic system. Ayers[8] has proposed that "tactile defensiveness" constitutes the predominance of the spinothalamic (protective) system over the lemniscal system. Many of the therapeutic techniques used in sensory integrative therapy are designed to activate the lemniscal system and establish a better balance between the two systems. In addition, the facial region receives its sensory innervation from the trigeminal nerve, which can be regarded as a third somatosensory system because it supplies a body surface that is outside of the dermatomal segments supplied by the spinal cord.[126] A soft, low-intensity stimulation to the facial region can elicit a relaxation response, because the soft tissues are also richly innervated by the parasympathetic nervous system.[76,97]

Cutaneous exteroceptive system. Exteroceptors are sensory end organs located in the superficial layers of the skin, the subcutaneous layers, and the external mucous membranes.[163] Some authors include the special sense organs, such as gustatory, olfactory, visual, and auditory, as part of the exteroceptive system. This section describes only the nonencapsulated and encapsulated end organs found in the skin and around hairs.

The skin is the organ of touch. Exteroceptors in the skin are activated by stimuli from outside the body. Therefore the exteroceptors inform the CNS about changes taking place in the external environment. These receptors tend to be especially sensitive to specific kinds of energy, such as pain, temperature, touch, and pressure. Before an exteroceptor will discharge, it must receive the appropriate amount of energy, which is called the adequate stimulus. Exteroceptors also have different thresholds. When the stimuli are adequate, the neuron reaches its action potential and discharges according to the intensity of the stimulus.[73,163] The duration of discharge depends on the receptor's ability to adapt. Some receptors adapt quickly while others adapt slowly. The exteroreceptors that adapt quickly are called *phasic* and the slowly adapting receptors are called *tonic*.

Exteroceptors transmit impulses along fibers of different diameters. Thick fibers are more myelinated and transmit impulses at a faster rate. Thin fibers have little or no myelin and transmit more slowly.[14,144] Exteroceptors innervate certain areas of the skin in an overlapping fashion. The area of skin innervation is called a receptor field. There is much variation in the number of receptors that innervate a given field of skin. Generally, the palmer surface of the hand contains a greater number of receptors with overlapping fields because the hands are used for prehension and touch. The shoulder region, on the contrary, has fewer receptors with less overlap and ability to discriminate stimuli. For example, the fingertips, lips, and tip of the tongue have a greater capacity for fine discrimination of touch stimuli. These areas contain more encapsulated receptors and more afferent neurons, and they transmit along the thicker fibers.[2,95,196]

Free nerve endings. Free or bare nerve endings are phylogenetically the oldest unencapsulated receptors. Free nerve endings transmit principally along thin fibers classified as Aδ (group III) or C fibers (group IV) (see Table 6-1). These fibers have little or no myelination. Free nerve endings are widely distributed throughout the dermis of the skin's connective tissue and in the viscera. Their greatest concentration is found along the midline axis of the body. For example, the area of the skin along either side of the vertebrae (the ramus posterior) has a 5:1 ratio of free nerve endings to other skin receptors.[73]

Free nerve endings transmit pain, temperature, and light touch sensations. Because these receptors are in greater concentration along the midline axis, pain sensitivity is 20 times greater in skin of the abdomen than in the skin of the fingertip. Pain awareness in the cornea has been estimated to be 30 times greater than in the abdomen. In addition, sensitivity to cold stimuli is 10 times greater along the midline than in the extremities. An exception to this midline rule can be found in the mucosal linings and the posterior surface of the tongue.[41,188]

Free nerve endings seem to serve as primitive protective receptors because they are centrally located and alert the organism to potential dangers to vital organs. Most of the impulses derived from free nerve endings travel to the CNS by way of the spinothalamic tracts. Touch stimuli are also transmitted via the dorsal columns.

Hair receptors. Hair follicles are quickly adapting receptors that discharge when displaced. Brushing against the natural direction of hairs sends impulses into the spinothalamic tract, which has many collaterals to the reticular-activating system. In general, this causes an excitatory response because the reticular-activating system links to the ANS. Stimulation to hair follicles or skin located on a dermatome at the same segmental level can facilitate the underlying muscle.[48] This stimulus activates a cutaneous fusimotor reflex. The reflex sends impulses carried along Aβ (group II) fibers to the fusimotor neurons and alpha motor neurons that terminate at the myoneural junction of the skeletal muscle.[48,81]

Merkel's disks. Merkel's disks can be found in the deepest layer of the epidermis, primarily in glaborous (non-hairy) skin. The greatest number are located in the volar surface of the fingers, lips, and external genitalia. Slowly adapting touch-pressure receptors, they are highly responsive to slow movements across the skin surface and to pressures. They transmit impulses along Aβ fibers (group II) and produce a prolonged discharge. These receptors have also been associated with the sense of tickly and pleasurable touch.[182,188]

Meissner's corpuscles. Meissner's corpuscles are highly developed, encapsulated receptors commonly found in the glaborous skin. The greatest numbers are found in the tip of the tongue, lips, fingertips, nipples of the breasts, and the pads of the feet. These receptors are highly discriminative, providing instantaneous sense of contact and flutter sensation. These receptors are used in two-point discrimination and stereognosis. Histological studies show that these receptors have a close relationship to the skin. In the fingertips they are uniformly arranged in line with the fingerprint patterns. During digital exploration, the neighboring sweat glands secrete and the liquid aids discriminative touch. Highly skilled braille readers are able to perceive 100 words/minute. There is some evidence that elderly individuals have a reduction of sensation resulting from a combination of skin inelasticity and loss of Meissner's corpuscles.[150,151]

Pacinian corpuscles. Pacinian corpuscles are the largest encapsulated and most studied cutaneous receptors. They are located very deep in the dermis of the skin; in viscera, mesenteries, and ligaments; and near blood vessels. Interestingly enough, they are most plentiful in the soles of the feet, where they seem to exert some influence on posture, position, and ambulation.[151] The pacinian corpuscles adapt very quickly, and they are activated by deep pressure and quick stretch of tissues.[48] In addition, they are responsive to vibration and show maximal discharge when vibrated at 250 to 300 Hz.[103] However, it has not been demonstrated that the pacinian corpuscles are implicated in the tonic vibration reflex.[153,188]

A list of treatment techniques using the tactile or exteroceptive system as their primary mode of entry can be found in Table 6-4.

Table 6-4. Exteroceptive input techniques

Receptors	Stimuli	Response
Free nerve endings: C + A fibers	Pain, temperature, touch	Seems to protect and alert, perception of temperatures, protective withdrawal
Hair follicles	Mechanical displacement of hair receptors	Increased tone of muscle below stimulus site
Merkel's disk	Touch, pressure receptors	Touch identification
Meissner's corpuscles	Discriminative touch	Postural tone; two-point discrimination
Pacinian corpuscles	Deep pressure and quick stretch to tissue, vibration	Position sense, postural tone and movement
Ruffini's corpuscles	Touch mechanoreceptor	Touch/spatial discrimination

Suggested treatment procedures using cutaneous stimuli
Quick phasic withdrawal
1. Stimuli
   a. Pain
   b. Cold: one sweep with ice cube—Rood's quick ice
   c. Light touch: brush (quick stroking), finger, feather
2. Response
   a. Stimulus applied to an extensor surface: elicites a flexor withdrawal
   b. Stimulus applied to flexor surface: may elicit flexor withdrawal or withdrawal from stimulus into extension
Repetitive icing or brushing (Rood's prolonged icing and brushing): not used because of rebound effect
Prolonged icing
1. Stimuli
   a. Ice cube
   b. Ice chips and wet towel
   c. Bucket of ice water
   d. Ice pack
   e. Immersion of body part or total body
2. Response: inhibition of muscles below skin areas iced
Neutral warmth
1. Stimulus
   a. Air bag splints
   b. Wrapping entire body or individual body part with towel
   c. Tight clothing such as tights, fitted turtle-neck jerseys
   d. Tepid water or shower
2. Response: inhibition of area under which neutral warmth was applied
Light touch/rapid stroking: to facilitate muscle below stimulus area
Maintained pressure or slow continuous stroking with pressure
● Response: adaptation of many cutaneous receptors to stimulus, thus decreasing exteroceptive input, decreasing reticular activity, and decreasing facilitation of muscles underlying stimulated skin

Treatment alternatives

For an overview of exteroceptive techniques, refer to Table 6-4.

Quick phasic withdrawal. The human organism reacts to painful or noxious stimuli at both the conscious and unconscious levels. If the stimulus is brief and of noxious quality, it will elicit a protective reaction of short duration, which is a spinal-level phasic withdrawal reflex (Fig. 6-5). Simultaneously, afferent impulses ascend to higher centers to evoke prolonged emotional-behavioral responses. Stimuli such as pain, extremes in temperature, rapid movement, light touch, and hair displacement are the most likely to cause this reaction by activating free nerve endings. It would seem that these stimuli are perceived as potentially dangerous, and most of the impulses are transmitted along C fibers and Aδ fibers. Although both sensory systems would be activated, the majority of the impulses would be channeled to the spinothalamic system. As already mentioned, this system communicates directly with the reticular-activating system and nonspecific thalamic nuclei. These structures have diffuse interconnections with all regions of the cerebral cortex, ANS, limbic system, cerebellum, and motor centers in the brainstem.

There are some real therapeutic limitations to using stimuli that "load" the spinothalamic system. A painful stimulus will be excitatory to the nervous system and produce a prolonged reaction after discharge. According to Wall's "gate-control" theory,[58,105,183] all sensory afferent neurons converge and synapse in the dorsal horn in an area called the substantia gelatinosa. Thick well-myelinated fibers—Aα, Bβ, and γ (group I and II)—synapse with cells in the substantia gelatinosa, causing an inhibition of the second-order tract (T) cells. Thus, according to the theory, the gate is closed and a limited number of impulses are permitted to ascend to higher centers. The thick fibers

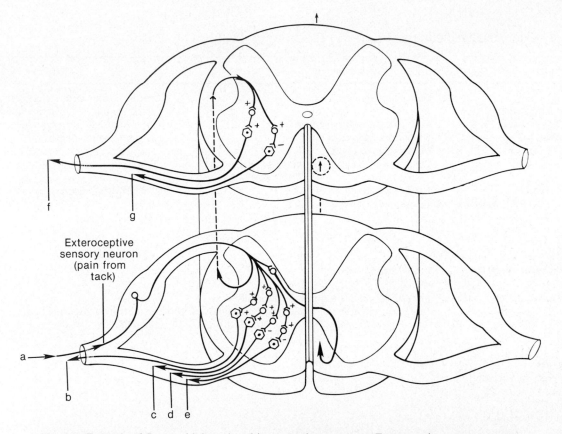

Fig. 6-5. Example of flexor withdrawal multisegmental response. *a,* Exteroceptive sensory neuron triggered by stimulus in skin—will elicit the entire quick phasic with manual/protective response. *b,* Primary flexor muscle to draw distal body part away from stimulus (facilitated). *c,* Flexor muscles in synergy with primary flexor and innervated at same segmental level (facilitated). *d,* Antagonist to primary flexor muscle (inhibited). *e,* Muscle in antagonistic synergy innervated at same segmental level (inhibited). *f,* Muscles in agonistic synergy at different segmental level (facilitated). *g,* Muscles in antagonistic synergy at different segmental level (inhibited). The quick phasic withdrawal visually elicits a flexor withdrawal pattern that facilitates a flexor synergy. This requires activation of flexor and extensor motor neurons at the cord level of the afferent stimulus as well as at other segments. Similarly, the antagonistic synergy is modified at multisegmental levels.

carry impulses from receptors in tendons, joint capsules, muscles, and deep-pressure receptors (pacinian corpuscles), whereas the fibers that conduct painful stimuli have less myelination, are thinner, and conduct more impulses than the thick fibers, but at a slower rate. These pain fibers have an inhibitory influence on the cells of the substantial gelatinosa, which in turn decreases the inhibition on the second-order T cells so that the gate is open and painful stimuli are allowed to ascend the spinothalamic tract. This phenomenon may have some positive implications for pain management because the "gate can swing both ways." Curiously, the large fibers outnumber the small fibers.[190] Therefore physical activity, frequent positioning, deep pressure, and proprioceptive and cutaneous stimulation should cause enough impulses to converge on the T cells of the substantia gelatinosa to close the gate and thus block transmission of pain messages to the brain. Recent studies have demonstrated that physical activity (types of physical stress) stimulates the production of endorphins, which in turn release opiate receptors and act as the body's own morphine.[24,109,117]

Stimuli, such as brushing or stroking the skin with a soft brush, would generate impulses along both spinothalamic and lemniscal pathways because they both transmit light touch and will elicit a withdrawal at the spinal level. What specific withdrawal pattern occurs depends on a variety of circumstances. If the stimulus is applied to an extensor surface, then a flexor withdrawal will be facilitated. If the stimulus is placed on a flexor surface, one of two responses occurs. First, the client might withdraw from the stimulus, thus going into an extensor pattern. Second, the stimulus may elicit a flexor withdrawal and cause the client to go into a flexor pattern. Which pattern occurs depends on biasing of tone as a result of positioning and the predisposition of the client's CNS. Both responses would be considered normal.

If resistance is immediately applied to the withdrawal pattern, the technique no longer is considered exteroceptive because spindle, joint, and tendon proprioception has been added. By adding such a procedure, the number of adverse effects, such as a rebound phenomenon caused by eliciting only a withdrawal reflex, can be drastically reduced. Quick phasic withdrawal responses are best elicited by applying the stimulus dermatomally to activate specific target muscles (myotomes). For example, a moving light-touch stimulus from midline to lateral along T10 can elicit a quick withdrawal response in the hip flexors.[52] A light-touch stimulus along dermatome C6 on the dorsum of the forearm can facilitate the extensor carpi radialis muscle and encourage extension of the wrist. The response occurs because the light touch causes rapid changes in muscle spindle sensitivity through a complex cutaneous fusimotor system reflex.[155,168] Stepping on a tack quickly elicits a strong total flexor withdrawal of the foot and leg (Fig. 6-5).

Repetitive icing and brushing. Cold is another stimulus that the nervous system perceives as potentially dangerous. The use of ice as a stimulus to elicit desired motor patterns is an early technique developed by Rood. An ice cube is rubbed with pressure for 3 to 5 seconds or used in a quick-sweep stimulus over the muscle bellies to be facilitated. Obviously, this method would activate both exterocepters and proprioceptors and cause a brief arousal of the cortex. This method can produce unpredictable results. At the spinal level it would elicit a phasic withdrawal pattern. Yet immediately after the reflex has taken place, the "rebound" phenomenon deactivates the muscle that has been stimulated and lowers the resting potential of the antagonistic muscle.[158] Therefore a second stimulus to the muscle originally stimulated may not elicit a reflex, but because of reciprocal innervation, the antagonistic muscle may effect a rebound movement in the opposite direction. Icing may also cause prolonged reaction after discharge in the connections to the reticular system, limbic, and ANS. Thus the ANS would be shifted toward the sympathetic end. Too much sympathetic tone causes a desynchronization of the cortex.[70] In addition, reflex activity requires a lot of energy to be expended in the skeletal muscles, causing oxygen debt. Too much muscle fatigue will reduce the effectiveness of treatment. Because of unpredictable response patterns to either Rood's repetitive icing or brushing, this technique is seldom used.

Ice should not be applied to the facial region above the level of the lips. Again, the spinothalamic system has two afferent pathways, the trigeminal and spinal. The trigeminal nerve innervates three divisions of the facial region the ophthalmic, maxillary, and mandibular. The trigeminal nerves have a powerful influence on the somatosensory system because they feed directly into the reticular formation. Thus icing around the forehead can set off unwanted behavioral and ANS responses. It is also ill advised to apply ice to the midline of the trunk because the greatest concentration of C fibers are in that region of the body.[41,153]

Ice should not be used behind the ear as it may produce a sudden lowering of blood pressure.[46] The therapist should also avoid using ice in the left shoulder region in patients with a history of heart disease. This is because referred pain secondary to angina pectoris manifests itself in the left shoulder area, indicating the cold stimulus might cause a reflexive constriction of the coronary arteries.[185]

In addition, the primary rami located along the midline of the dorsum of the trunk have sympathetic connections to internal organs. The cold stimulus may alter organ activity and perhaps produce vasoconstriction, causing increased blood pressure and less blood supply to the viscera.[64,137]

Ice can also have beneficial effects if the nervous system's inhibitory mechanisms are in place. For instance, in children with learning disabilities or sensory-motor delays, the application of ice to the palmar surface of the hands will cause arousal at the cortical level because of the increased activity of the reticular activating system. This arousal response presumably produces increased adrenal medullary secretions, resulting in various metabolic changes. Therefore icing should be used selectively. If the patient has an unstable ANS, it should be eliminated as a potential sensory modality.[65]

Prolonged icing. A variety of approaches incorporate prolonged icing techniques. The proprioceptive neuromuscular facilitation approach may be the most common.[100] Inhibition of hypertonicity or pain is the goal for use of any of these methods. With prolonged cold the neurotransmission of impulses, both afferent and efferent, is reduced. Simultaneously, the metabolic rate within the cooled tissue is reduced. (For further information on the use of cold see Chapter 27 on pain.) Caution must be exercised with regard to use of this modality. For effective treatment results, the client (1) should be receptive to the modality, (2) should be able to monitor the cold stimulus; thus sensory deficits should not be present, and (3) should have a stable autonomic system to prevent unnecessary adverse effects of hypothermia.

Neutral warmth. Like icing, this approach has been shown to cause inhibition. According to Farber,[52] the temperature range is between 35° and 37° C. The length of application depends on the client. A 3- to 4-minute tepid bath may create the same results as a 15-minute total body-wrapping procedure. As with any input procedure, the effects should be incorporated into the therapeutic session to maximize the effect and promote client learning.

Maintained stimulus or pressure. Because of the rapid adaptation of many cutaneous receptors, a maintained stimulus will effectively cause inhibition by preventing further stimuli from entering the system. This technique is applied to hypersensitive areas to normalize skin responses. Vibration, used alternately with maintained pressure, can be highly effective. It should be remembered that these combined inputs use different neurophysiological mechanisms. One of us (D.U.) has found that low-frequency maintained vibration is especially effective with learning-disabled children who have hypersensitive tactile systems that prevent them from comfortably exploring their environment. By having them hold and vibrate themselves on the extremities, their hypersensitive system seems to normalize and become receptive to exploring objects. If that exploration is accompanied by additional prolonged pressure, such as digging in a sandbox, the technique seems to be more effective.

Vestibular system

Sensory receptors and physiology. The vestibular apparatus is a proprioceptive organ.[74] Functionally, it is involved in the maintenance of head and body equilibrium. Because the vestibular system is intimately connected with the auditory, visual, proprioceptive, and motor systems, it works cooperatively with a number of other systems to modulate important functions. Research evidence suggests that the vestibular system relies on a variety sensory input to make adjustments in its sensitivity to position in space and movement.[141] The vestibular system has been credited with influencing muscle tone; maintaining visual gaze, spatial directionality, and head and body orientation; and influencing learning and emotional development.[194]

The vestibular apparatus is a membranous structure located in the temporal region of the skull. It is subdivided into the cochlea (which is primarily involved in hearing), the vestibule, and the three semicircular canals. Phylogenetically, the receptors of the vestibular system are similar to the receptors that transduce sound. In both cases the receptors are hair cells. However, the anatomical arrangement and the physiological properties allow the receptors to transduce different sensory modalities. Another commonality between the auditory and the vestibular system is that they share the same cranial nerve root. Yet the connections to brainstem nuclei and other neurological structures are explicitly different.

The vestibule (utricle and saccule) is located between the semicircular canals and the cochlea. It is often called the static labyrinth because it elicits tonic reflexes on postural muscles in response to changes in head and body positions and gravitational influences.[114] The vestibule contains two communicating chambers, the sacculus and the utriculus. The hair cells in the sacculus and utriculus are similar: each chamber contains a thickened patch of sensory hair cells called the macula. The hair cells are arranged in a fixed position so that their hair tufts project up through a gelatinous mass called the *otolithic membrane.* Embedded in this gelatinous substance are small calcium carbonate crystals called *otoliths* (otoconia). This anatomical arrangement allows the hair cells to be highly responsive to changes in head position. As the head is tilted to one side, the force of gravity displaces the otolithic membrane, which causes the cilia of the hair cell to bend. This bending or shearing action causes the hair cell to discharge and transmit afferent impulses to the CNS.

It should be emphasized that the hair cells are tonic receptors. Therefore even in the neutral position, the hair cells are constantly discharging. The bending of the cilia in a single hair cell in one direction will cause an increase in firing, and bending in the opposite direction will cause a slowing of the rate of discharge.[114,194] The mechanism that allows this to happen is inherent in the cilia of the hair cell. The cilia are arranged in a steplike gradation in length, getting progressively larger toward the end of the bundle of cilia. At the outer side of the bundle, a conspicuously large cilium called the *kinocilium* serves as a regulator. That is, if the cilia bend toward the kinocilium, the rate of firing increases; if the cilia bend away from the kinocilium, the rate of discharge is reduced.[113,141]

The sacculus lies between the utricle and cochlear duct. The majority of the cilia (hair cells) in the saccule are arranged in a side-lying fashion when the head is in the normal upright position. Therefore if the head moves in a vertical plane in linear acceleration and deceleration, the cilia will discharge. Any up and down motion, such as bouncing on a trampoline, is an adequate stimulus to the cilia in the saccule. In contrast, the majority of the cilia in the utricle are arranged vertically while the head is in the upright position. Thus, linear acceleration and deceleration in the horizontal plane is the adequate stimulus for the cilia in the utricle. One may think of a child in a prone position propelling down an incline on a scooter board. As the child hits the horizontal plane, the head is upright, causing the cilia to deflect and discharge. Quick deceleration, caused by running into a mat on the floor, causes the hair cells to whip forward, deflecting of cilia once again. In most instances, the cilia in both the sacculus and utriculus are sensitive to a variety of stimuli. For example, forward and backward movements will activate cilia in both chambers. In summary, the adequate stimuli for the cilia of the utricle and saccule (vestibule) are the static position of the head in space and linear acceleration and deceleration in horizontal and vertical planes. The greatest tonal changes occur in extensor groups of the postural muscles. In addition, the vestibule (saccule and utricle) contributes to the maintenance of righting reactions and equilibrium responses.

Rood[155] suggested that the side-lying position of the head is useful to diminish unwanted extensor tone caused by a poorly integrated tonic labyrinthine reflex. In this position the symmetrical input of the vestibule receptors on the vestibular nuclei is eliminated, modifying the outflow of the vestibulospinal tract and thus the tonic labyrinthine reflex.

The semicircular canals are referred to as the kinetic labyrinth, because they respond to movements of the head. The semicircular canals also exert influences on the limbs and the extraocular muscles of the eyes, as well as assist in equilibrium responses and orientation in space. The semicircular canals are arranged approximately at right angles to one another, one for each axis of rotation. The anterior and posterior canals are sensitive to movement in the sagittal plane. The horizontal canal reacts to rotation around the central body axis.[40]

The three membranous semicircular canals are contiguous with the vestibule. The canals are enlarged at the juncture where the canals terminate into the vestibule. This enlargement is called the *ampulla*; it contains neuroepithelial receptors similar to the vestibule. These receptors consist of mounds of cilia termed the *crista ampullaris*. The crista are composed of cilia attached firmly to the base of the

ampullae. The tufts of cilia project into a dome-shaped gelatinous substance called the *cupula*. The cupula differs from the otolithic membrane in that it does not contain otoliths. Instead it sits on top of the cilia like a hat and is stimulated by the movement of the endolymph in the canal. Therefore any angular (rotatory) acceleration or deceleration of the head will cause the endolymph to circulate through the canals, which in turn displaces the cupula and causes the cilia to fire.[141,194]

It should be emphasized that the cupula-endolymph mechanism has not evolved to be responsive to prolonged spinning at constant velocity. Numerous physiological studies[10,28,76] have demonstrated that during the beginning of rotation, the cupula is deflected from its resting position and the cilia discharge at a greater rate. If the rotation is continued, the cupula gradually reassumes its resting position in about 20 seconds and the ciliary firing is reduced. When rotation is stopped, the cupula is again deflected, but in the opposite direction because the endolymph continues to circulate through the canals. This bending of the cilia causes the firing to diminish until the endolymph comes to rest. After about 10 to 30 seconds, the endolymph stops circulating and the cupula returns to its resting position and resumes its tonic level of discharge. Based on this information, prolonged spinning is physiologically nonproductive. It should be remembered that the initial acceleration is the force that causes the cupula to be deflected and fire at a greater rate. Also, the semicircular canals are most responsive to short rotational movements as opposed to prolonged rotation. A good formula for semicircular canal stimulation is to spin the subject approximately 10 times in 20 seconds, stop abruptly, wait about 20 seconds, and spin again at the same rate in the opposite direction. It is also beneficial to consider the position of the head while spinning. For example, if the subject is side lying on a large spinning apparatus, the endolymph in both the anterior and posterior canals will circulate, causing a more powerful response.

Spinning is not to be used without proper precautions. In infants and disinhibited patients, it may induce seizures or depress respiration. It is best to allow patients to control the initial rate of spinning or vestibular stimulation so they can accommodate to the stimulus.

Because of its diffuse connections, the vestibular apparatus has a tremendous capacity to cause inhibitory and facilitory states in the nervous system. Generally, impulses are dispatched to key centers of the nervous system from the vestibular nuclei located at the pontomedullary junction. For instance, there are extensive interconnections to the 12 cranial nerve nuclei (III, IV, and VI in particular), the cerebellum (flocculomodular lobe), spinal motor centers, the ANS, extrapyramidal nuclei in the brainstem, postcentral gyrus of the cerebral cortex, and the reticular formation.[27,44]

To recapitulate, the receptors of the vestibule (macula) seem to be concerned with static orientation of the head in space and "directionality." In this context, directionality refers to the ability to move from a beginning point *A* to a designated point *B* without becoming disoriented or veering off in the wrong direction. For example, we rely on the macula for orientation when we are swimming under water. Because the feet are not in contact with the ground and gravitational forces are altered, the proprioceptors in joints and muscles provide little information about position in space. Thus the brain is not receiving its normal proprioceptive input from the legs and postural muscles. In addition, vision is of little assistance because to work properly, the cornea must have air in front of it. Water causes a refractive error, and vision becomes distorted.[74] Consequently, if the vestibular mechanism were not receiving gravitational feedback, the underwater swimmer would become disoriented and unable to determine the direction of the surface.

The semicircular canals detect movements of the head in all planes and are involved in the maintenance of the upright posture. The pathways of the semicircular canals are extremely important for visual gaze, ocular movements, and alignment of head and body. The connections of the semicircular canals and the otoliths work cooperatively with the joint receptors of the neck to accomplish head and neck-righting reaction.[6]

Treatment alternatives. Because the vestibular system is a unique sensory system, critical for multisensory functioning, it is a viable and powerful input modality for therapeutic intervention. Table 6-5 summarizes the receptor, stimulus, and response patterns of this system and also suggests treatment procedures. Since any static position, as well as any movement pattern, will facilitate the labyrinthine system, vestibular function and dysfunction play a

role in all therapeutic activities. To conceptualize vestibular stimulation as spinning or angular acceleration minimizes its therapeutic potential and also negates an entire developmental progression of vestibular treatment techniques.[52,85] Horizontal, vertical, and forward-backward movement occurs very early in development and should be considered one viable treatment modality. These movements seem to precede side-to-side and diagonal movements, followed by linear acceleration and ending with rotatory movements. All of these movements can be done with assistance or by the client independently in all developmental patterns. *It is important to remember that the rate of vestibular stimulation determines the facilitory or inhibitory effects. A constant, slow rocking tends to be inhibitory whereas a fast spin or linear movement tends to be facilitory.*

General inhibitory and facilitory techniques. As already indicated, slow, repetitive rocking patterns, irrespective of plane or direction, generally cause inhibition of the total body responses. Yet any stimulus has the potential of causing undesired responses, such as increased tone. When this occurs, the procedure should be stopped and reanalyzed to determine the reason for the observed or palpated response. For example, assume a client, whether a child with cerebral palsy, an adolescent with head trauma, or an adult with anoxia, exhibits signs of severe generalized extensor spasticity in supine position. To facilitate total body inhibition the therapist decides to use a slow, gentle rocking procedure in supine and discovers the spasticity has increased. Obviously the procedure did not elicit the desired response and alternative treatment is selected, but the reason for increased spasticity needs to be addressed.

It is possible that the static positioning of the vestibular system is causing the release of the original tone and that by increasing vestibular input the tone also increases. It

Table 6-5. Vestibular system

Receptor	Stimulus	Response
Static		
Vestibule (sacculus, utriculus)	Pressure on hair cells caused by position of head in space (linear movements)	Tonic reflexes in response to head position and gravity Tonic labyrinthine reflexes
Kinetic		
Semicircular canals	Pressure on hair follicles caused by change of direction of head in various planes (angular [rotatory] movements)	Tendency of slow movement to be inhibitory to muscle tone Tendency of rapid movement to be facilitory to muscle tone Linked to perception of space and directionality Linked to labyrinthine righting and equilibrium Linked to extraocular muscles to control visual gaze

may also be that the facilitory input did indeed cause inhibition but the movement itself caused fear and anxiety, thus increasing preexisting tone and overriding the inhibitory technique. Instead of selecting an entirely new treatment approach, a therapist could use the same procedure in a different spatial plane, such as side lying, prone, or sitting. Each position affects the static position of the vestibular system differently and may differentially affect the excessive extensor tone observed in the client. The vertical sitting position adds flexion to the system, which has the potential of further inhibiting extensor tone. This additional inhibition may be necessary to determine whether the slow rocking pattern will be effective with this client. It would seem obvious that if a vestibular inhibitory procedure were ineffective in modifying the preexisting extensor tone, then using a powerful facilitory procedure, such as spinning, is inappropriate. Selection of treatment techniques should be determined according to client needs and disability. Clients with either an acoustic tumor that perforates into the brainstem or with generalized inflammatory disorders may be hypersensitive to vestibular stimulation while other clients, such as a child with a learning disability, may be in need of massive input through this system. See Heiniger and Randolph[85] and Farber[52,53] for in-depth analysis of various specific vestibular treatment procedures commonly used in the clinic. A general discussion of the treatment suggestions is summarized in the box at right.

Total body inhibitory techniques. Any technique performed in a slow, continuous, even pattern will facilitate an inhibitory response.[92] During handling techniques, these procedures can be performed with the client in bed, on a mat while horizontal, sitting at bedside or in a chair, or standing. The movement can be done passively by the therapist or actively by the client. In a clinical or school setting, a client who is extremely anxious, hyperactive, and hypertonic may initiate slow rocking to decrease tone or feel less anxious or hyperactive. The reduction of clinical signs allows the client to sit with less effort and to be more attentive to the environment, thus promoting ability to learn and adapt.

It is not the technique that is critical but the type of movement employed. The concept of slow, continuous patterns is used in Brunnstrom's rocking patterns[30] in early sitting and in proprioceptive neuromuscular facilitation mat programs; the use of these patterns can be observed in every clinic. Although the therapist may be unaware of why Mr. Smith gets so relaxed when slowly rocked from side to side in sitting, this procedure elicits an appropriate response. The nurse taking Mr. Smith for a slow wheelchair ride around the hospital grounds may do the same thing. Once the relaxation or inhibition has occurred, the groundwork for a therapeutic environment has been created to promote further learning, such as activity of daily living (ADL) skills. The technique in and of itself will relax the individual but not create change. The change will

occur if the therapeutic sessions follow the inhibition because the relaxation response is a good neurophysiological state from which changes can be induced. For example, it allows time for the resting potentials to become established in membranes and synaptic junctures, thereby causing subsequent stimulation techniques to be more effective.[46,113]

Pelvic mobilization techniques in sitting often use relaxation from slow rocking to release the fixed pelvis. This release allows for joint mobility and thus creates the potential for pelvic movement performed passively by the therapist, with the assistance of the therapist, or actively by the client. This technique often combines vestibular with proprioceptive techniques, such as rotation and elongation of muscle groups, which physiologically modify existing static tonal response through spinal and joint responses. Simultaneously, slow, rhythmical rocking, especially on diagonals, is used to incorporate all planes of motion and thus all vestibular receptor sites to get maximal inhibitory responses. The same pelvic mobility can be achieve by

---

Treatment suggestions

Inhibitory techniques to total body

1. Slow rocking
2. Slow anterior-posterior: horizontal or vertical movement (chair, hassock, mesh net, swing, ball bolster, carriage)
3. Rocking bed or chair
4. Slow linear movements, such as in a carriage, stroller, wheelchair, or wagon

Facilitory techniques to postural extensors

1. Rapid anterior-posterior or angular acceleration
   a. Scooter board: pulled or projected down inclines
   b. Prone over ball: rapid acceleration forward
   c. Platform or mesh net: prone
   d. Slides
2. Rapid anterior-posterior motion in prone, weight-bearing patterns such as on elbows or extended elbows while rocking and crawling

Facilitory techniques influencing total body responses

1. Movement patterns in specific sequences
   a. Rolling patterns
   b. On elbows, extended elbows, and crawling: side by side, linear and angular motion
2. Spinning
   a. Mesh net
   b. Sit and spin toy
   c. Office chair on universal joint

Combined facilitory and inhibitory technique: inverted tonic labyrinthine

1. Semi-inverted in-sitting
2. Squatting to stand
3. Total inverted vertical position

placing the patient (child or adult) over a large ball. The ball must be large enough for the patient to be semiprone while arms are abducted and externally rotated and legs relaxed (either draped over the ball or in the therapist's arms). Again, this position allows for maintained or prolonged stretch to tight muscles both in the extremities and trunk while doing slow, rhythmical rocking over the ball. The pelvis often releases and the patient can be rolled off the large ball to standing on a relaxed pelvis, preliminary to gait activities.

Facilitory techniques for postural extensors. Any technique that uses rapid anterior-posterior or angular acceleration of the head and body while the client is prone will facilitate a postural extensor response. Scooter boards down inclines, rapid acceleration forward over a ball or bolster, going down slides prone, or using a platform or mesh net to propel someone will all facilitate a similar vestibular response of righting of the head with postural overflow down into shoulder girdle, trunk, hips, and lower extremities. Rapid movements while on elbows, on extended elbows, and in a crawling position can also facilitate a similar response. Depending on the intensity of the stimulus, the response will vary. In addition, the client's emotional level during introduction to various types of stimuli may cause differences in tonal patterns. Clinical experience has shown that facilitory vestibular stimulation promotes verbal responses and affects oral motor mechanisms. Children with speech delays will speak out spontaneously and respond verbally.

Because facilitatory vestibular stimulation biases the sympathetic branch of the ANS, drooling diminishes and a generalized arousal response occurs at the cortical level. Therefore the appropriate time to teach adaptive rehabilitative techniques is after vestibular stimulation.[113]

Facilitory techniques influencing total body responses. One primary reason movement facilitates motor responses is that vestibular influences over motor tracts regulate tone and behavioral mechanisms. Thus rolling patterns, a rocking pattern on elbows, and extended elbows and crawling—especially in fast side-to-side, linear, and angular motions—tend to elicit total-body responses. Tactile and proprioceptive inputs also assist in the regulation of the body's responses to movement.[7,53]

The vestibular system, when facilitated with fast, irregular, or angular-movement, such as spinning, not only induces tonal responses but also causes massive reticular activity and overflow into higher centers. Thus increased attention and alertness are often the outcome. It is necessary that the tracts going from the spinal cord, brainstem, and higher subcortical structure be sufficiently intact to permit the desired responses from this type of input. If a lesion in the brainstem blocks higher-center communication with the vestibular apparatus, then massive input may cause a large increase in abnormal tone. The therapist needs to closely monitor any distress or ANS anomalies.

Total body inhibition followed by selective postural facilitation. The use of the inverted position in therapy has become increasingly more popular in recent years. The tonic labyrinthine influences on posture were first studied by de Kleijn[45] and Magnus[107] in the 1920s. In a series of short papers Magnus described some studies performed with decerebrate cats, which entailed progressively positioning the cat until its head was in an inverted position. Magnus discovered that the inverted position activated the cilia of the vestibular system, which in turn promoted "extension maximum." Tokizane (cited by Payton, Hirt, and Newton[142]) replicated Magnus' and de Kleijn's work with human subjects. Tokizane used a tilt-table apparatus and electromyographic readings to gather data. Although there was a discrepancy in the angles used by the researchers, the net results were the same. Total inversion (angle of 0 degrees) produced maximal extensor tone, and the normal upright position elicited maximal flexor tonicity.[142] There seems to be much confusion in the literature about the clinical effects of inversion. Kottke[101] reports the static labyrinthine reflex is maximal when the head is tilted back in the semireclining position at an angle of 60 degrees above the horizontal. Conversely, minimal stimulation occurs when the head is prone and down 60 degrees below the horizontal position. Stejskal[167] studied the effects of the tonic labyrinthine position in spastic patients. This study failed to show labyrinthine reflexes in subjects with spastic hypertonia.

The explanation for this incongruity seems to be one of interpretation. Any time a subject is put on a tilt table or even a scooter board, the weight bearing of the body on the surface must cause firing of the underlying exteroceptors.[47] As the body shifts and presses onto the underlying surface, tonic stretch reflexes associated with posture must contribute some bias to muscle tone.[195] In addition, if the subject is flexing or extending the head, the proprioceptors of the neck (tonic neck reflex) could also alter the muscle tone of the limbs.[154]

Another factor that contributes to tonal changes in the extremities is the cervicoocular reflex.[9,10] Reflex eye movements to center the eyes as the body or neck rotates also exert influences on the muscles of the limbs. Since all the influences brought about by gravity and postural mechanisms in a clinical situation cannot be controlled, the inverted position does not elicit a purely tonic labyrinthine reflex (TLR). Instead, there appears to be an interplay of cutaneous receptors, proprioceptors, and tonal changes in the labyrinthine system.[141]

Several highly recognized therapists have reported using the inverted position as a therapeutic modality.[52,85,168] Generally, the inverted position produces three major changes: first, because of the gravitational forces on circulation, the carotid sinus sends messages to the medulla and cardiac centers that ultimately lower heart rate, respiration, and resting blood pressure through peripheral dilation.

This position may be contraindicated for certain patients with a history of cardiovascular disease, such as many with hemiplegia. Clients with unstable intercranial pressure, for example, those with traumatic head injuries, coma, tumor, or postinflammatory disorders, and many children with congenital spinal cord lesion would also be at high risk for further injury if the inverted position were used. However, this position has been used with some success for adult patients with hypertension. In any case, scrupulous recording of blood pressure and other ANS effects should be taken before, during, and after positioning.

Another benefit of the inverted position is generalized relaxation. Farber[52] recommends its use as an inhibitory technique. Because the carotid sinus stimulates the parasympathetic system, the trophotropic system is influenced and muscle tonicity is reduced. This has been found to be beneficial to patients with upper motor neuron lesions and also to children who exhibit hyperkinetic behavior.[165] Heininger and Randolph[85] report that severe spasticity in the upper extremities is noticeably reduced.

The third benefit of the inverted position is an increased tonicity of certain extensor muscles. This phenomenon is not purely a function of the labyrinth; it is also a result of activation of the exteroceptors being stimulated by the body's contact with the positioning apparatus.[141] Be that as it may, therapists have capitalized on this reaction to activate specific extensor muscles of the neck, trunk, and limb girdles.[101,154,167]

The inverted position can be achieved in a variety of ways. A child can be lowered over a ball or bolster into the inverted position. When the client is placed in a squat pattern, the head can effectively be lowered below the level of the heart. This position is more often used with children. Adults are usually seated and tilted forward until the head is in an inverted, semivertical position.[113]

Because the inverted position decreases hypertonicity and hyperactivity and facilitates normal postural extensor patterns, the responses to the technique should be incorporated into activities. For example, if the position of total inversion over a ball is used, then postural extension of the head, trunk, and shoulder girdles and hips should be facilitated next. Additional facilitation techniques, such as vibration or tapping, could help summate the response. Resistance to the pattern in a functional or play activity would be the ultimate goal. If the inverted position is used in a squat pattern, then squatting to standing against resistance would probably be a primary goal. This can be accomplished by the therapist positioning her or his body behind and over the child—not only to direct the child initially into the inverted position but also to resist the child coming to stand. If the inverted position is used in sitting, activities of the neck, trunk, and upper extremities would be the major focus following the initial responses.

As the inverted position elicits both labyrinthine and ANS responses, this technique needs to be cross-referenced within the classification schema. Because of its ANS influence, close monitoring is important for all clients placed in an inverted position. As with all labyrinthine treatment techniques, this approach, considered a normal, inherent human response, is used outside the therapeutic setting. For example, standing on one's head in a yoga exercise causes the same physiological state as that observed in the clinic. In many respects the yoga stance is done for the same reasons: decreasing hypertonicity (generally caused by tension), relaxation, and increasing postural tone and altered states of consciousness.

Autonomic nervous system

The ANS has become a focus of clinical interest over the last few years.[85] Traditionally, the ANS regulates, adjusts, and coordinates visceral activities. Many aspects of emotional behavior, and primative drives are controlled by the ANS.[65,135,137] Maintaining homeostasis within the body's internal environment is critical because it strongly influences the CNS response to the external world. The intricate interconnections between the ANS and CNS have led clinicians to discover viable treatment approaches that depend on both systems.[52,85] Input to the spinal cord, brainstem, cerebellum, thalamus, limbic system, and cerebrum has the potential of influencing both the somatic and visceral systems. Many tract systems, such as the reticulospinal tract, are common to both systems.[135] The importance of these interconnections seems obvious. If the external world is threatening the system, then both somatic and visceral systems need to modify responses in order to optimally protect the organism. For example, if your visual system identified an angry bear ready to attack you as you walk through the forest, both autonomic and somatic responses are needed. Your somatic system needs to ready your neuromuscular system for immediate action. Your autonomic system needs to ready your heart and respiration for increased rate to provide oxygen and nourishment to muscles for increased metabolism. Your emotional system needs arousal to attend to and deal efficiently with the crisis. All systems must react simultaneously and at appropriate intensities to protect the organism from imminent danger. If any system malfunctions and creates too little or too much output, imbalance and inefficiency results. This decreases your flexibility and ability to solve the problem and remove yourself from the dangerous environment.[185] Please refer to Chapter 4 for additional information.

The input and processing systems, as well as the ANS itself, are often impaired in clients with brain damage. This can create ANS responses not always appropriate to the situation. Understanding the intricate balance of sympathetic and parasympathetic responses of the ANS and how these behaviors affect functional output is important to conceptualizing the client's total needs. All systems of the person who perceives imminent danger, whether real or imaginary, will change; the clinician will observe these altered responses to the environment, for example, in a gait session or an ADL task. Anxiety level, emotional responses, increased blood pressure, heart rate, or respiration, hypertonicity, and hyperactivity are but a few of the signs a therapist might use to identify an ANS response. These signs should alert and orient the clinician to the causes of the change. Oftentimes slight alterations in the external environment are sufficient to produce homeostasis. For example, if a kneeling client feels about to fall forward, it is very important to check the patient's perception, even if the therapist believes it to be inaccurate. If the perception is wrong, then the clinician needs to help the client relearn perception of vertical. If the perception is correct, the client's response was appropriate and provided important internal feedback. Even more important than the first two reasons is the fact that the therapist has respected and responded to the opinion and judgment of the client. This helps begin and kindle trust and mutual respect, important clinical tools for modifying the client's ANS responses to new situations.[65]

The ability to differentiate tone created by emotional responses versus tone resulting from CNS damage is a critical aspect of the evaluation process. Emotional tone can be reduced when stress, anxiety, and fear of the unknown have been reduced. This is true for all individuals. The client with brain damage is no exception. Four treatment modalities that normally produce a parasympathetic response are:

1. Slow, continuous stroking for 3 to 5 minutes over the paravertebral area of the spine
2. Inversion, eliciting carotid sinus reflex and tonic labyrinthine response
3. Slow, smooth, passive and active assistive movement within pain-free range (Maitland's grade II movements)[109]
4. Maintained deep pressure on the abdomen, palms, soles of the feet, peroneal area, and skin rostral to the top lip

When pressure is applied to both the anterior and posterior surfaces of the body, measurable reductions can be recorded in pulse rate, metabolic activity, oxygen consumption, and muscle tone.[170,172]

These pressure techniques are identified as an intricate part of the many identifiable approaches such as therapeutic touch,[152,185] Feldenkrais,[55,56,96] Maitland,[109] rolfing, and myofacial release.[12,13,115,173,175] Although not verbally identified, other techniques (such as NDT,[23,34] Rood,[53,85,168] Brunnstrom,[30] and proprioceptive neuromuscular facilitation)[169] certainly place an important emphasis on the response of the patient to the therapist's touch.

Treatment alternatives

Slow stroking. Slow stroking over the paravertebral areas along the spine from the cervical through lumbar components will cause inhibition. The technique is performed while the client is in the prone position. The therapist begins by stroking the cervical paravertebral region in the direction of the thoracic area, using a slow, continuous motion with one hand. Usually a lubricant is applied to the skin and the index and middle fingers are used to stroke both sides of the spinal column simultaneously. Once the first hand is approaching the end of the lumbar section, the second hand should begin a downward stroking at the cervical region. This maintains at least one point of contact with the client's skin at all times during the procedure. The technique is applied for 3 to 5 minutes—and no longer—because of the potential for massive inhibition or rebound of the autonomic responses.[52,92] It is also recommended that at the end of the range of the last stroking pattern, the therapist maintain pressure for a few seconds to alert both the somatic and visceral systems that the procedure has concluded. Clients with large amounts of body hair or hair whorls are poor candidates for this procedure because of the irritating effect of stroking against the growth patterns and the sensitivity of hair follicles.

Inverted tonic labyrinthine therapy. See the section on vestibular procedures.

Slow, smooth, passive movement within pain-free range. Increasing range of motion in painful joints is a dilemma frequently encountered by therapists caring for clients with neurological damage. We have found that by having the client communicate the first perception of pain and then move the limb in a slow, smooth motion toward the pain range, a variety of behaviors occur. First, the client generally gestures or verbalizes that pain is present 10 to 15 degrees before it may, in reality, exist. We believe this occurs because on previous occasions, the therapist has responded to the client statement of pain by saying, "Let's just go a little farther." That additional range is usually 10 to 15 degrees. We have found that if we stop impinging on the stated pain range, go back into a pain-free area, and approach again—possibly with a slight variation in the rotatory direction—the client relinquishes the safety range and a true picture of pain range is obtained. The second finding is that if the motion toward the pain range is slow, smooth, and continuous, very frequently much of the range that was initially painful becomes pain free. The hypothesis is that slow, continuous motion is critical feedback for the ANS to handle imminent discomfort. The slow pattern provides the ANS time to release endorphins, (enkephalins) neuropeptides, thus relieving the perception of pain and allowing for increased motion. If the therapist stabilizes the painful joint and prevents the possibility of that joint going into the pain range, rapid, oscillating movements can often be obtained within the pain-free range. This maintains joint mobility and often, as an end result, increases the pain-free range. This technique is not unique to the treatment of clients with neurological problems; it is often used as a manual therapy procedure.[58,112,117]

Maintained pressure. Farber[52] discusses a variety of techniques that elicit a reduction of tone or hyperactivity.

Pressure to the palm of the hand or sole of the foot, to the tip of the upper lip, and to the abdomen all seem to produce this effect. The pressure need not be forceful, but it should be firm and maintained. It is hypothesized that some, if not all, of these responses are parasympathetic.[71]

Olfactory system: smell

The sense of smell is the least understood of all the senses. Because of the inaccessibility of the olfactory receptors, to date little research has been conducted. Unfortunately, there are more theories than facts about how we sense odors.[97]

Olfaction or the sense of smell is a chemical process. Receptors for smell are located in the olfactory epithelium in the roof of the nasal cavity between the median septum and the superior turbinate bone. The olfactory epithelium has a yellowish-brown color and contains three types of cells: the receptor cells, supporting cells, and basal cells. Interspersed among the epithelial cells are minute ducts from Bowman's gland, which secrete mucous substances onto the cells and aid in dissolving odorous materials.

The olfactory receptor cells are bipolar sensory neurons. Each cell has a single crownlike dendrite projecting to the surface of the epithelium. The distal end of this dendrite contains 10 to 20 cilia. These cilia are actually fine hairlike nerve endings. Aside from a thin layer of mucus, these nerve endings are virtually uncovered, making them the most exposed in the body.[97] Although the olfactory epithelium occupies an area only about the size of a dime, it is estimated to contain 100 million receptor cells.[3] These have an equal number of fibers but converge on principal neurons at a ratio of 1000:1.[124]

How the receptor cells transduce odors into meaningful perception of smell is not well understood. One theory, called the stereochemical theory, suggests that primary odors have specific molecular shapes. The molecular shapes of the odors are thought to correspond to molecular configurations of specific receptors. Thus certain receptors will accept a molecule the way a given lock accepts a particular shape of key.[41] There has been some support for this theory because action potential studies have shown that different odors do selectively activate some receptors and not others.[162] Other theories suggest that odorous molecules simply alter the sodium permeability of the receptor membrane and cause an inactivation of enzymes, thus changing its chemical reactions and electrical states.

Several attempts have been made to classify types of odors. In 1895, odors were grouped into nine classes, each of which contained two or more subdivisions.[197] Current findings indicate that humans can distinguish between 2000 and 4000 different odors. What is more confusing is that individual perception of the same odor will vary considerably; what is nauseating to one may be fragrant to another.[52,139]

Receptors for smell adapt rather quickly to a constant stimulus. Physiological studies indicate that olfactory receptors adapt as much as 50% in the first few seconds of stimulation.[33,148] The strength of the odor has to change by approximately 30% before the receptors are reactivated. There is also some evidence that part of the adaption takes place in the CNS.

The impulses arising in the olfactory mucosa pass along axons that pierce the cribriform plate of the ethmoid bone to enter the cranial cavity. In the cranial cavity the axons synapse on primary neurons (mitral and tufted cells) in the olfactory bulb. The axons of the olfactory bulb make up the olfactory tract (cranial nerve I) and cranial nerve V. This band of fibers courses posteriorly and fans out at the olfactory trigone. Some of the fibers terminate in the trigone while other fibers form three diverging striae; the lateral, medial, and intermediate. The lateral olfactory stria projects to the temporal lobe of the cortex (uncus, hippocampus). The fibers proceed rostrally to the prefrontal cortex. The medial stria projects to nuclei located in the septal area of the brain below the corpus callosum. The intermediate stria terminates in the anterior perforated substance. The medial and intermediate striae are not well developed in humans.[33,192]

There are also a number of secondary association fibers that course to important subcortical nuclei. For example, impulses are transmitted to the autonomic nuclei of the hypothalamus. Although this connection is not well understood, it has been demonstrated in mammals to be associated with reproduction.[124,125] It has also been demonstrated that olfaction is not mediated exclusively by the olfactory nerve. The nasal region also derives sensory innervation from branches of the trigeminal nerve. Experimental evidence shows that the trigeminal fibers respond to burn smells and also make a general contribution to the sense of smell. With some severe head injuries the cribriform plate and the olfactory epithelium are ruptured. Although the sense of smell is severely compromised, some odor sensation may be preserved via the fibers of the trigeminal nerve.[79]

One of the most remarkable characteristics of the olfactory system is that some impulses travel from the receptors to the temporal lobe without passing through the thalamus.[33] All other major sensory systems pass through a relay in the thalamus en route to the cortex.

The primary olfactory cortex (temporal lobe) projects efferent impulses to cortical and subcortical structures. Output to the thalamus, hypothalamus, and limbic system is believed to influence behavior and emotion. Pleasant odors, such as vanilla or perfume, can evoke strong moods. Unpleasant odors can facilitate primitive protective reflexes, such as sneezing and choking. Sharp-smelling substances like ammonia can elicit a reflex interruption of breathing.[122,124]

As a result of arousal, protective reflexes, and mood changes caused by odors, the use of smell as treatment modality has been implemented especially during feeding procedures. Odors such as vanilla and banana have been used to facilitate sucking and licking motions.[166] Ammonia and vinegar have been used clinically to elicit withdrawal patterns and increase arousal in semicomatose patients.[93] When using odors as a stimulant, the therapist must be aware of all behavior changes occurring within the client. Arousal, level of consciousness, tonal patterns, reflex behavior, and emotional levels—all can be affected by odor. Because of limited research in this area, caution must be exercised to avoid indiscriminate use of the olfactory system. Odors such as body odor, perfumes, hair spray, and urine can affect client's behavior even though the smell was not intended as a therapeutic procedure. Some clients, especially those with head traumas and inflammatory disorders of the CNS, often seem to be hypersensitive to smell. In these cases the therapist needs to be aware of the external olfactory environment surrounding the client and to make sure those odors that are present facilitate or at least do not hinder desired response patterns.[51]

Gustatory sense: taste

The sense of taste is a chemical sense, involving not only the receptors of the tongue but also olfaction and tactile receptors. Therefore the term *taste* encompasses not only gustatory sensations derived from food but the smell, temperature, and texture of the material to be ingested.[37]

Taste receptors are found in the tongue, soft palate, and the beginning of the throat. The receptors for taste are complicated end organs of the neuroepithelium commonly called taste buds. Most of the taste buds, which are located on the tongue, are distributed in definite patterns. Taste buds are surrounded by raised structures called papillae. These papillae are visible on the surface of the tongue and give it a roughened appearance. The papillae vary in shape and form, and each papilla is surrounded by a small depression or moat. Taste buds can be found on the crest of the papilla or more commonly in the depressions. The papillae are distributed in three different locations. On the base of the tongue are seven to twelve circumvallate papillae arranged in a V configuration. Scattered over the entire dorsal surface are small papillae called the fungiform. A third type, called *foliate papillae*, are closely packed along the sides of the tongue.[89] They are well developed in children but less numerous in adults.

Taste buds are embedded in the papillae in clusters of 20 to 25 cells in the shape of a goblet. Each goblet contains supporting cells, basal cells, and receptor cells. The receptor cells have hairlike projections (microvilli) passing into the pore opening. These microvilli increase the surface area and probably help to trap molecules flowing through the moat surrounding the papillae.[192]

The physiology of taste is rather complicated. Because it is a chemical sense, only substances that dissolve in water or saliva can be tasted. Once the water-soluble substances are bathed in fluid, they can diffuse through the taste pore and come in contact with microvilli of the receptor cells. Although the mechanism is not well understood, the contact appears to evoke generator potentials followed by action potentials in the nerve terminals.[53,138,145]

Four primary taste sensations have been identified: salty, sour, bitter, and sweet. These primary tastes are believed to blend together in various combinations to form additional tastes, similar to the way mixing the colors yellow and blue produces green. Histologically, the taste buds appear to be the same, yet they tend to be selective to specific stimuli. Action-potential studies have shown that any one taste bud will respond to all four primary tastes.[77] However, the quantitative responses differ considerably, allowing some buds to respond more vigorously to bitter and some to sour, sweet, or salty stimuli. It is also commonly known that regions of the human tongue vary in sensitivity to the four primary tastes. The base of the tongue best detects bitter, the sides sour, and the tip is sensitive to sweet substances. The ability of taste buds to discriminate changes in concentration of a substance is relatively crude; a 30% change in concentration is needed before a difference in taste intensity is detected.[138]

Taste receptors in the epithelium of the soft palate are more numerous in children. In the adult the number of taste buds range from 9000 to 10,000. Taste buds have a tremendous capacity to reproduce. The average life span of a taste bud is 7 to 10 days. Each cluster of taste buds (approximately 20) contains mature and young cells; the mature lie toward the center of the cluster.[69]

Afferent transmission of impulses from taste receptors may travel to the CNS by three cranial nerves. Taste sensations from the base of the tongue are served by the glossopharyngeal nerve (cranial nerve IX); the sides and the tip are served by the vagus nerve (cranial nerve X) and the facial nerve (cranial nerve VII). The pharyngeal surface of the tongue is innervated by the laryngeal branch of the vagal nerve (cranial nerve X). Taste buds begin to degenerate during the fifth decade of life, contributing to diminished taste sensation in the elderly.[41]

Taste sensation adapts rapidly. Action-potential studies have shown that when first stimulated, taste buds fire a burst of impulses and only partially adapt. As with the olfactory system, the additional adaption is suspected to come from the CNS.[124,125]

Afferent taste impulses transmitted from the tongue and pharyngeal region pass through branches of the appropriate cranial nerves (facial, glossopharyngeal, and vagal) to the tractus solitarius in the brainstem. The fibers of the first-order neurons terminate in portions of the nucleus solitarius. The second-order neurons send a number of collaterals to reticular nuclei before crossing to the opposite side of the brainstem and coursing to the ventral posteromedial nucleus of the thalamus. Before reaching the thalamus, other collaterals project to nuclei associated with reflex activity. The third-order neuron transmits signals to the somatesthetic region of the parietal lobe.[40]

Gustatory input is generally used as part of feeding and

prefeeding activities. As already mentioned, the oral region is sensitive not only to taste but also to pressure, texture, and temperature. For that reason feeding would be classified as a multisensory technique that uses gustatory input as one of its entry modalities. Specific input modalities are based on the combined taste, texture, temperature, and affective response pattern. That is, a banana and an apple both may be sweet, yet the textures vary greatly. When mashed, both fruits may have a puddinglike texture, yet the client's emotional response may differ. Disliking the taste of banana but enjoying apple may cause startling differences in the client's response to various sensations. Although feeding and other complex treatment procedures are discussed in more detail under the classification of combined sensory systems, the importance of the clinician's sensitivity to the client's response patterns within each sensory modality cannot be overemphasized.[53]

Auditory system

Next to vision, the auditory system is probably the second most important exteroceptive sense. Together with vision the auditory system enables us to perceive events in the external environment that take place at a distance from our bodies.

Originally, the eighth cranial nerve may have been involved purely in the maintenance of equilibrium and orientation in space.[40] As the human organism developed into a land vertebrate, the evolutionary change probably gave rise to a new division of the eighth cranial nerve; the auditory system. Phylogenetic studies indicate that the auditory and vestibular mechanisms developed as a unit.[120]

Audition is more than the act of hearing. The auditory process is fundamental to survival and also to human communication. The loss of hearing or exposure to "noise pollution" has been known to cause severe behavioral disturbance.[1]

The anatomy and physiology of the ear is described only briefly here—with greater emphasis placed on the characteristics of the auditory receptors.

The organ of hearing consists of three components: the external, middle, and internal ear. The ear receives sound waves that are radiated from some source in the external environment. Sound waves are directed by the external ear, travel through the auditory meatus, then strike the tympanic membrane (eardrum) and cause it to vibrate. These vibrations move a series of three small articulating bones (malleus, incus, and stapes) that extend from the tympanic membrane to the inner ear. The chain of three bones is attached to two muscles, the tensor tympani and stapedius. These minute muscles serve as a protective mechanism (tympanic reflex) during excessive stimulation. Strong sound waves elicit contraction of the tensor tympani muscle, causing increased tension on the tympanic membrane.[3,74]

The ossicles serve as a mechanical receptor that converts sound waves to fluid motion in the cochlea. The fluid motion causes pressure waves that stimulate receptor cells, and the stimulus is once again converted to an electrical-chemical impulse.[37]

The organ of hearing is located in the cochlea, which is a fluid-filled tube resembling a small shell that spirals around itself two and a half times. The space within the bony canal of the cochlea is divided into three compartments by the vestibular and basilar membranes. The upper compartment is called the scala vestibuli. The scala vestibuli ends at the oval window and receives pistonlike action from the stapes to produce pressure waves in the perilymph. The lower compartment, the scala tympani, ends at the round window. The round window serves as a dampening mechanism for the pressure waves. The scala vestibuli and scala tympani connect at the apex of the spiral, and both contain perilymph. The third compartment is the cochlear duct (scala media). It is bordered by the vestibular and basilar membranes. Lying on the basilar membrane of the cochlear duct is a complex structure consisting of numerous receptor cells. This is the organ of Corti, the sensory mechanism for hearing. The organ of Corti consists of cilia, groups of supporting cells, and fibers from bipolar neurons derived from the spiral ganglion. The receptor cells are cilia similar to the receptors of the vestibular system—with an estimated 23,000 cilia on the basilar membrane of each cochlea.[37,192]

The receptor cells of the organ of Corti have some specific characteristics. First of all, they do not have axons. Actually, they transmit directly to the dendrites of the bipolar cells in the spiral ganglion. The inner cilia may have only one dendrite attached while the outer cilia receive synaptic input from many bipolar ganglion cells.

The arrangement of the cilia and the tectorial membrane is such that a movement of the basilar membrane causes the cilia to bend against the tectorial membrane. Therefore when sound strikes the ear, vibrations are passed from the tympanic membrane to the ossicles and converted to hydrodynamic waves in the cochlea. The basilar membrane vibrates up and down in response to the frequency of the sounds. The mechanical bending or shearing of the cilia releases chemical transmitter substances at their basal pool. This constitutes the adequate stimulus, and action potentials in the bipolar cells cause neuronal transmission.

The auditory pathway to the CNS is very diffuse. Impulses pass from ciliary receptors along nerve fibers of the spiral ganglion to synapse on neurons in the posterior and anterior cochlear nuclei in the upper region of the medulla. The second-order neurons project mainly to the opposite side of the brainstem and terminate in the superior olivary nucleus. However, some of the second-order neurons do not cross and ascend to the superior olivary nucleus on the same side. Other collaterals pass directly to the reticular-activating system. There are also important connections to the cerebellum, particularly in the event of a sudden noise.

The majority of the impulses reaching the superior olivary nucleus ascend by way of the lateral lemniscus, which continues to the inferior colliculus. The next group of neurons continues to ascend and synapse in the medial geniculate nucleus, a sensory nucleus of the thalamus. From this juncture impulses fan out along the auditory radiation to reach the auditory cortex at the superior temporal gyrus, or area 41. At this very small area of the cortex, a sound is "heard," but more specific recognition requires connections with additional auditory associative centers.

Recently, efferent fibers have been discovered in all parts of the auditory pathway.[64,66] Their role is still speculative, but some physiologists believe that these fibers exert inhibitory influences, function as a feedback loop, and improve hearing acuity to specific stimuli.

Treatment alternatives. Because of the complexity of the auditory system, a potentially large number of input modalities exists. Although some of them might not be considered traditional therapeutic tools, they are nonetheless techniques that affect the CNS. Some treatment alternatives focus on:

Quality of voice (pitch and tone)
Quantity of voice (level and intensity)
Affect of voice (emotional overtones)
Extraneous noise (sound)
Auditory biofeedback
Language

Levels, volume, and affect of voice. The therapist's voice can be considered one of the most powerful therapeutic tools. Even, constant sound has the ability to cause adaptation of the auditory system and thus inhibition of auditory sensitivity.[31] Similarly, intermittent, changing, or random auditory input can cause an increase in auditory sensitivity.[66] Because of auditory system connections, an increase or decrease in initial input or auditory sensitivity has the potential of drastically affecting many other areas of the CNS. The connections to the cerebellum could affect the regulation of muscle tone. The collaterals projecting into the reticular formation could affect arousal, alertness, and attention, in addition to muscular tone. The importance of voice level has been acknowledged by colleagues for decades with respect to encouraging clients to achieve optimal output or maximal effort. The use of voice levels is a critical aspect of the entire PNF approach.[100] Yet the volume or intensity of a therapist's voice is only one aspect of this important clinical tool. Through clinical observation, we have observed that clients respond differently to various pitches. The response patterns and specific range of comfortable pitch seem to be client dependent. The concept that each individual may have a range within the musical scale or even a specific note that is optimal for his or her biorhythm function has been posed by one composer-musician.[26] This concept needs research verification but may prove to relate to one of those innate talents some therapists have that distinguish them as gifted therapists.

The emotional inflections used by the clinician certainly have the potential of altering client response. For example, assume the therapist asks Tim, a child with cerebral palsy, to walk. The specific response from the child may vary if the clinician's voice expresses anger, frustration, encouragement, disgust, understanding, or empathy. Knowing which emotional tone best coincides with a client's need at a particular moment may come with experience or sensitivity to others' unique needs.

Extraneous noise. The varying level of sound or extraneous noise in a clinical setting can at times be overwhelming. Dropping of foot pedals, messages over loud speakers, conversations, typewriters, telephones, moans, a jackhammer outside the clinic, water filling in a tank, a drip in a faucet, whirlpool agitators, a burn patient screaming, a child crying—all are encountered in the clinical environment, and all could be occurring simultaneously. A therapist, whose CNS is intact, usually can inhibit or screen out most of the irrelevant sound. A client with CNS damage may not have the ability to filter his or her sensitivity to all these intermittent noise sensations. The protective arousal responses these sounds might produce in a client could certainly elevate tone, block attention to the task, heighten irritability, and generally destroy client progress during a therapy session. Awareness of the noise environment and the client's response to it is important not only to treatment modalities; it is also critical to the problem-solving process.

Music as an adjunct to therapy has been suggested as a viable way to help clients develop timing and rhythm to a movement sequence (see Chapter 19 for a discussion of basal ganglia disorders). Consistent sound waves and tempos, such as soft music, allow the patient to develop a neuronal modal or an engram for the stimulus. The use of background music during therapy sessions enables the patient to make an association to the sounds, producing an autonomically induced-relaxation response to a particular musical composition.[42]

Auditory biofeedback. Biofeedback as a total therapeutic modality is discussed under the treatment section in Chapter 26, which deals with electrodiagnosis. Auditory biofeedback is generally thought of as a procedure in which sound is used to inform the client of specific muscle activity. The level or pitch may change in relation to strength of muscle contraction or specific muscle group activity. Yet auditory biofeedback also encompasses feedback as simple as a foot slap that communicates that a client's foot is on the floor or verbal praise following a successful therapeutic session. The importance of the auditory feedback system as a regulatory mechanism between internal and external homeostasis cannot be overlooked. However, the clinician should not assume that this system is intact and can automatically be used as a normal feedback mechanism for clients with CNS damage.[75]

Language. Although most therapists thoroughly appreciate the complexity of the language system as a whole, they have little if any in-depth background to help them understand the components or the sequences leading to the development of language. Thus many therapists are extremely frustrated when confronted with clients who show perceptual or cognitive deficits involving the auditory processing system. The reader is referred to Chapter 24 to better understand the development of the language system and alternative treatment methods appropriate for use with clients having difficulty within this area.

Visual system

Vision is considered the most important and relied-on sense. The eye is also the most complex of all the sense organs in our body. Its uniqueness is attributed to the biochemical or biophysical mechanism employed to transduce a light stimulus to a neurological action potential. Rather than review the anatomy of the eye in great detail, this discussion will focus on tracking a light stimulus through the eye and describing some of the salient processes that occur en route to visual perception.

The stimulus for vision is light. Light is electromagnetic energy that travels outward in waves at a rate of 186,000 miles per second.[41,66] Light entering the eye first passes through the cornea and then through a clear, viscous fluid called the aqueous humor. The next structure light passes through is an opening in the iris known as the pupil. The amount of light allowed through is regulated by the diameter of the pupil. Next, the light passes through the lens and vitreous humor (a gelatinous material) and reaches the retina, where light energy is transformed into neuronalelectrical impulses.[135,136]

The retina lines a major portion of the inside of the eye. It is composed of three distinct layers of cells: the photoreceptor layer, the bipolar cell layer, and the ganglion cells. Light must first travel through the ganglion and bipolar cells to reach the sensory photoreceptors. There are two types of photoreceptors: the rods and cones. The rods, which number about 120 million, are reactive to light intensity, that is, shades of gray. Unable to distinguish different colors, rods are said to provide "night vision." The cones (about 6 million) are responsible for color vision and require more light energy to become activated. The rods and cones are fairly evenly distributed throughout the retina. However, a central part of the retina, called the *fovea* (macula lutea), is in direct line with the lens and cornea. Therefore when we fixate on an object, the image of that object is projected upside down and backward on the fovea.[91]

The rods and cones are unique sensory receptors. As light enters the eye, it strikes the rod and cone cells and is absorbed by pigments (photopigments) contained in these cells. This stimulus produces a chemical reaction that results in a change in the movement of ions through the cell membranes of the bipolar cells. This ionic movement generates an action potential in the afferent axons of the bipo-

lar cells. Synaptic activity occurs between the bipolar and ganglion cells. The ganglion cell axons project posteriorly and leave the eye in an area called the optic disk. The ganglion axons combine to form the optic nerve.[77,156,159]

The rods and cones require a rich blood supply to maintain their metabolic functions. The major blood supply is derived from the choroid, a layer between the retina and the sclera. The choroid has a pigmented layer that absorbs light not transduced by the rods and cones. In addition, this structure is a storage site for vitamin A, a necessary element for reproduction of the visual pigments used by rods and cones for the absorption of light energy.

The visual pathway begins at the optic foramen. Each optic nerve consists of about 1 million nerve fibers. The combined 2 million nerve fibers of both optic nerves make up about 38% of all sensory and motor fibers entering and leaving the CNS.[192]

The optic nerve contains two types of fibers: large, fast-conducting fibers concerned with visual perception and small, slower-conducting fibers concerned with reflexive activity. The optic nerve fibers originate from nasal and temporal portions of the retina to form the retinogeniculate fibers. These fibers project directly to the optic chiasm just anterior to the pituitary gland. At this juncture a partial crossing of fibers takes place. Fibers originating in the nasal halves of each retina cross at the chiasm. Conversely, the fibers originating in the temporal portion of the retina pass through the chiasm without crossing. The fibers from the temporal side also carry the fibers from the fovea (macula), where visual acuity is sharpest.[91]

Once the optic nerve passes through the optic chiasm, it is referred to as the optic tract. The two optic tracts continue uninterrupted to the left and right lateral geniculate bodies of the thalamus and to midbrain centers (superior colliculus and pretectal region). Fibers terminating in the lateral geniculate bodies give rise to the geniculocalcarine tract (optic radiations). These fibers spread out as they go and turn posteriorly to the occipital lobe of the cortex. The principal location of the visual receptive cortex is the area surrounding the calcarine fissure, which encompasses Brodmann's areas 17, 18, and 19. Area 17 is the site where the optic radiations terminate. Functionally, area 17 is said to be associated with conscious but not with interpretive vision; areas 18 and 19 believed to be involved in associative aspects of visual perception.[91]

The visual system is extremely helpful to physicians and medical personnel for diagnosing disorders of the CNS. The eye provides a window through which a physician can examine the integrity of blood vessels and neurological tissue. Because the system extends through so much of the subcortical and cortical regions of the brain, many disorders manifest themselves in the visual system. Aside from the more obvious visual-field problems, nervous system disorders can interrupt visual reflexes and impede eye movements.

Eye movements are subserved at the cortical and subcortical levels. Areas 18 and 19 of the occipital lobe produce a reflexive visual pursuit in response to visual stimuli. Voluntary eye movements elicited on command derive from neurons in the frontal lobe of the cortex (area 8). Protective reflexes, such as blinking and quick localization of eyes, head, and neck toward a startling stimulus, are mediated by the retinotectal system (superior colliculus). Reflex eye movements activated by rotation of the head are mediated at the brainstem level by the vestibular system. The size of the pupil and lens is reflexly controlled by light stimulus. Pretectal areas, such as the Edinger-Westphal nucleus of cranial nerve III, act on the sphincter muscle of the iris and the ciliary muscle. Psychosocial research has demonstrated that pupils dilate and constrict in response to emotional feelings elicited by a visual stimulus.[41] Objects that are pleasing to the eye cause the pupil to dilate, whereas repugnant visual stimuli constrict the pupil. The higher-level cortical association pathways that enable this phenomenon to take place have not been fully mapped out.[146]

Child development studies suggest that the efficiency with which an infant uses its eyes is a strong indicator of verbal ability and performance on intelligence tests.[25] The therapist should reinforce eye pursuits by pointing out objects in the environment and by encouraging the hand to follow the eye toward the object. According to Stejskal,[167] as the eyes turn toward an object, the head has a natural tendency to turn, and when the neck rotates, a volley of neuromuscular events takes place (ATNR, TNR) that better enables the upper extremities to perform a task such as reaching. This is a very useful maneuver in the rehabilitation of patients with head injuries and cerebrovascular accidents.[113]

Because of the complexity of the visual system, treatment procedures can vary from simple to extremely complex. Simple treatment alternatives, such as hues or types of lighting, are often overlooked by therapists, yet they have the potential of altering patient response. Complex treatment procedures, such as those discussed in Chapter 25, are also often ignored by therapists because of lack of understanding of and frustration with the visual system. Although we are not suggesting that all therapists become experts in visual processing and training, clinicians should become more aware of this input system, its potency as a treatment modality, and, when damaged, its devastating effect on normal response patterns.

Treatment alternatives. To help the therapist obtain a better understanding of treatment alternatives, a variety of categories (each encompassing a spectrum of treatment considerations) follows.

1. Colors (such as room, clothes, objects)
   a. Hues: brightness usually alerts the CNS and increases tone, whereas dark colors decrease muscle tone[53]
   b. Colors and shades of color: for example, pinks versus blues
2. Types of lighting: fluorescent, incandescent, or sunlight
3. Degree of visual complexity within environment
   a. Isolated room, blank walls with one floor mat
   b. Busy clinic with a table mat in the center of the room
4. Cognitive-perceptual sequential treatment methods—for example, figure and ground, depth, visual object permanency, visual position in space, spatial relationships
5. Treatment approaches to compensate for deficits in other sensory systems

Because light is an adequate stimulus for vision, any light, no matter the degree of complexity, has the potential to affect a client's CNS. That input not only reaches the optic cortex for sight recognition and processing; it also descends to the spinal cord via the tectospinal tract, projects to the cerebellum via the tectocerebellar tract, and affects the reticular-activating and limbic systems via the interneuronal pathway.[57] Thus as long as light is entering a client's CNS, that stimuli has the potential of altering response patterns either directly—via the tectospinal system or the corticospinal system via occipitofrontal radiations—or indirectly through the influence of the ANS and limbic system on muscle tone resulting from emotional levels.

The five categories of visual-system treatment alternatives should not be considered fixed, all-inclusive, or without overlap. The first three categories (color, lighting, and visual complexity) are common everyday visual stimuli. Combined, they make up the visual world.

Colors. By varying the colors or by changing hues, tones, or the type of lighting and degree of complexity of the combined visual stimuli, the treatment modality changes. Because the visual system tends to adapt to sustained, repetitive, even patterns, any input falling under those parameters should elicit visual adaptation.[69,148] This response will lead to decreased firing of sensory afferent fibers and have an overall effect of decreasing CNS excitation. A clinician would expect to see or palpate a decrease in muscle tone, a calming of the client's affective mood, and a generalized inhibitory response. Cool colors, a darkened room, monotone color schemes—all tend to have an inhibitory effect.

In contrast, intermittent visual stimuli, bright colors, bright lights, and a random color scheme seem to alert the CNS and have a generalized facilitatory effect. Research in the area of criminology is producing evidence to suggest that specific shades of colors can produce either a sedating response (such as certain pinks) or general arousal (certain blues).[134] Although a tremendous amount of research is required to substantiate these results if the clinician is to apply them with confidence, there is reason to believe that specific shades of colors and hues may drastically affect a client's general response to the world and specific response to a therapy session. Within the next few years, many facts regarding the reaction of the CNS to specific visual stimuli may be uncovered, and the clinician will be responsible for integrating this new information into the present categorization scheme.

Lighting. Two types of lighting are found in a clinical environment. Fluorescent or luminescent lighting comes by definition from a nonthermal cold source. This type of lighting is generally emitted by a high-frequency pulse. Umphred[177] has found that many individuals within a normal population complain that this high-frequency flutter is irritating and causes distraction. For this reason, it is recommended that each clinician observe clients' responses to various types of lighting to determine whether fluorescent visual stimuli cause undesirable output. This is especially true with clients who already have an irritated CNS, such as with inflammatory disorders or head trauma. The clinician should also remember that clients frequently lie supine and look directly at overhead lighting, while the therapist looking at the client is unaware of that particular visual stimulus.

Incandescent lights by definition come from hot sources and emit a constant light without a frequency. The brightness of this type of lighting has the potential of altering CNS response. The visual system quickly responds to bright lights with pupil constriction. Following prolonged exposure to a bright environment, the visual system adapts and becomes progressively less sensitive to it,[69] Similarly, when exposed to darkness, the retina becomes more sensitive to small amounts of light. Because of the response of the visual system to incandescent lighting, it is recommended that a therapist monitor the brightness of the lighting, especially preceding any type of visual-perceptual training or visually directed movement.

Although the sun is a natural source of light, it is not generally the primary source in a clinical setting. The sun can effectively be used as indirect lighting, thus eliminating the problems produced by artificial lighting. Sunlight is also more acceptable psychologically.

Visual complexity. The visual system is the primary spatial sense for monitoring moving and stationary objects in space.[87] An infant continually refines the ability to discriminate objects in external space until capable of identifying specific objects amid a complex visual array.[148] When brain damage occurs, the ability to identify objects, localize them in space, pick them out from other things, and adapt to their presence may be drastically diminished.[8] Because of the distractibility of many clients, reducing the visual stimuli within their external space can help them cope with the stimuli to which they are trying to pay attention. Using rooms that have been stripped of such stimuli as furniture and pictures can reduce not only distractibility but also hyperactivity and emotional tone. If this method of reduction of stimuli is used, the clinician must remember that this procedure has a sequential component. The

client must build up ability to adapt to extraneous visual stimuli. Thus objects must be introduced into the controlled environment. The therapist can monitor the amount of input according to the response patterns of the client.

Cognitive-perceptual sequencing with the visual system. This large category is the focus of many professionals' entire career. In sighted individuals the visual system is important in integrating many areas of perceptual development, such as body schemes, body image, position in space, and spatial relationships.[8] Vision as a processing system is so highly developed and interrelated with other sensory systems that, when intact, it can be used to help integrate other systems.[86] Simultaneously, if the visual system is neurologically damaged, it can cause problems in processing of other systems. For example, assume a child is asked to walk a balance beam while fixating on a target. The child is observed falling off the beam. On initial assessment vestibular-proprioceptive involvement would be primarily suspected. On further testing the therapist might discover that the child, while looking at the target, switches the lead eye in conjunction with the ipsilateral leg. As the child switches from right to left eye, the target will seem to move. Knowing the wall is stationary, the child will assume the movement is caused by body sway, will counter the force, and will fall off the beam. The problem is a lack of bilateral integration of the visual system versus other sensory modalities. The visual system deficit is overriding normal proprioceptive-vestibular input in order to avoid CNS confusion. Unfortunately, the client is attending to a deficit system and negating intact ones.

This same problem of the visual system overriding other inputs is often seen when clients are trying to relearn the concept of verticality. Since the intact visual system can often be used to help reintegrate other sensory systems, the reverse should also occur. Teaching clients to attend to vestibular-proprioceptive cues while vision is occluded or visual stimuli tremendously reduced will help them orient to intact systems. Once the orientation is reestablished, visual input will often be perceived in a more normal fashion.

Familiarity with the visual-perceptual system and its interrelationships with all aspects of the therapeutic environment is crucial if the clinician is to have a thorough concept of the client's problem. (See Chapter 25 for specific information regarding visual deficits and treatment alternatives.)

Compensatory treatment alternatives. The visual system can be effectively used as a compensatory input system if the sensory component of the tactile, proprioceptive, or vestibular system has been lost or severely damaged. The procedure of using vision in a compensatory manner should not be attempted until the clinician is convinced the primary systems will not regain needed input for normal processing. Although vision can direct and control many aspects of a movement, it is not extremely efficient and seems to take a tremendous amount of cortical concentration and effort.[178] Vision was meant to lead and direct movement sequences.[87,167] If used to modify each aspect of a movement, it cannot warn or inform the CNS about what to expect when advancing to the next movement sequence. Thus using vision to compensate eliminates one problem but also takes the visual system away from its normal function. For example, assume a hemiplegic man is taught to use vision to tell him the placement of his cane and feet, thus decreasing his need to attend to proprioceptive cues. When advancing to ambulatory skills such as crossing the street, the client may be caught in a dilemma. As he is crossing the street, if he attends to the truck coming rapidly down the road, he will not know where his cane or foot are and thus become anxious and possibly fall. If, on the other hand, he attends to his foot and cane, he will not know if the truck is going to hit him. That may increase emotional tone and make it difficult to move. If normal sensory mechanisms could be reintegrated, this client would have freedom to respond flexibly to the situation. Thus caution should be exercised to avoid automatic use of this high-level system to compensate for what seem to be depressed or deficit systems.

CLASSIFICATION OF MULTISENSORY TREATMENT TECHNIQUES

Although all techniques have the potential of being multisensory, the specific mode of entry may focus on one sensory system, as already described, or it may target two or more input modalities. Table 6-6 categorizes a variety of treatment techniques that are clearly multisensory. Since new methods of treatment are discovered daily, this table is not all-inclusive, but it allows the clinician to identify familiar techniques and their multisensory input channels. The therapist, analyzing how the summated effect of the combined input influences client performance, gains direction in anticipating treatment outcomes in terms of the problem-solving process. Because the potential combinations of multisensory classification are enormous, only a few examples of combinations are included in the text to illustrate the process a clinician might use when classifying a new technique.

Combined approaches
Proprioceptive: tactile integration
Sweep tapping. Many isolated techniques, such as sweep tapping[53] or rolling,[30] would be considered primarily proprioceptive-tactile in sensory origin. During *sweep tapping* the clinician first uses a light-touch sweep pattern over the back of the fingers of one of his or her hands. This stimulus is applied quickly over the dermatome area, innervating the muscles the client is to contract. Second, the therapist applies some quick tapping over the muscle belly of the hypotonic muscle. The first technique is tactile and believed to stimulate the reflex mechanism within the cord to heighten neuroexcitation and increase the potential

for muscle contraction. The second aspect, tapping, is a proprioceptive stimulus used to facilitate afferent activity within the muscle spindle, thus further enhancing the client's potential for muscle contraction.

Rolling. Before Brunnstrom's rolling pattern is implemented, the client's upper extremity is placed above 90 degrees to elicit a Souques's sign, which decreases abnormal excessive tone in the arm, wrist, and hand.[30] This phenomenon may well be a proprioceptive reaction to stretch on hypersensitive muscles. The rolling technique consists of two alternating stimulus patterns. The wrist and fingers are placed on extensor stretch. The ulnar side of the volar component of the hand is the stimulus target. A light-touch sweeping pattern is applied to the hypothenar aspect, which has the potential of eliciting an automatic opening of the hand beginning with the fifth digit.[30] Immediately after the light touch, a quick stretch is applied to the wrist and finger extensors. These two techniques are applied quickly and repeatedly, thus giving the visual impression that the therapist is rolling his or her hand over the ulnar aspect of the dorsum of the client's hand. In reality, tactile and proprioceptive stimuli are being effectively combined to facilitate the extensor motor neurons leading to the wrist and fingers. Since the tone is felt in the client's extensors and thus induces relaxation of the spastic flexors, the therapist can easily open the client's hand. As the client obtains volitional control, some resistance can be added by the therapist to further facilitate wrist and finger extension. A hemiplegic client can also be taught to use this combined approach to open the affected hand and give it increased range.

Withdrawal with resistance. A therapist could combine the technique of eliciting a *withdrawal* with *resistance* to the withdrawal pattern. This can be an effective way to release spastic tone, especially in the lower extremities. The withdrawal can be elicited by a thumbnail, a sharp instrument, a piece of ice, or any adequate light-touch stimulus to the sole of the foot. As soon as the flexor withdrawal is initiated, the therapist must resist the entire pattern. Once the resistance is applied, the input neuron network changes and the flexor pattern is maintained through proprioceptive input. The one difficulty with this technique is the application of resistance. The withdrawal pattern directly affects alpha motor neurons innervating those muscles responding in the flexor pattern and simultaneously suppresses alpha motor neurons going to the antagonistic muscles. If the antagonistic muscles are spastic, then initially the spasticity is suppressed. Because of the pattern itself, as soon as the flexor response begins, a high-intensity quick stretch has been applied to the extensor muscles. If resistance is not applied to the flexors to maintain inhibition over the antagonistic muscles, the extensors will respond to the stretch. The client will very quickly return to the predisposed spastic pattern and may even exhibit an increase of abnormal tone. This extensor response is called a rebound phenomenon.

Table 6-6. Combined sensory systems: treatment modalities

Technique	Proprioceptive: joint, tendon, spindle	Exteroceptive	Vestibular	Gustatory	Olfactory	Auditory	Visual	ANS	Inherent response	
									Labeled	Not labeled
Sweep tapping[52]	X	X								
Brunnstrom's rolling (hand)[108]	X	X							Automatic extension of hand	
Raimiste's sign[108]	X	X								?
Stretch pressure[52]	X	X								
Digging in sand, etc.	X	X				?				
Gentle shaking[52]	X		X							
Prone activities over ball[32,52]	X	X	X				X		Automatic righting of head	
Sitting activities on ball[32]	X	?	X				X	X	OLR and equilibrium	
Mat activities	X	X	X			?	?			
Resistive exercises	X	X								
1. Resistive rolling	X	X	X			If verbal command	If visual leads			Rotatory integration
2. Resistive patterns: PNF[100]	X	X	Depends on pattern			X	X			
3. Resistive gait	X	?	Depends on pattern			If verbal command	X			
4. Isokinetics	X	Some					X			
5. Wall pulleys	X		X (if done in body rotation)				X (if guided toward target)			
6. Rowing	X	?	X			If verbal command	X			Body rotation
Feeding[32,52,127]										
1. Maintained pressure: walking to back of tongue	X	X		?	?					
2. Resistive sucking										
a. Straw	X	X		?	?					
b. Popsicle	X	X		X	X				X	
3. Use of textures	X	X		X	X				X	
a. Peanut butter										
b. Apple sauce										
4. Maintained pressure to top lip	X	X						X	Automatic closing of mouth	
Inverted TLR[52,85]	X		X			?	X	X		
Touch bombardment[52]	X	X	X					X	Decreased hypersensitive tactile system and thus withdrawal pattern: stereognosis	
1. Tactile discrimination in sand, etc.										
2. Pool therapy								X		

Continued.

Table 6-6. Combined sensory systems: treatment modalities—cont'd

Technique	Proprioceptive: joint, tendon, spindle	Exteroceptive	Vestibular	Gustatory	Olfactory	Auditory	Visual	ANS	Inherent response	
									Labeled	Not labeled
Joint compression more than body weight[109,168]	X	X								
Throwing and catching										
1. Balloon	?	X					X	?	? (withdrawal to light touch)	
2. Heavy ball	X	?					X	Result of light touch		
Variance in movement										
1. Quick action directed by vision	X		X				X			
2. Postural activities in front of mirror	X		?				X			
3. Therapist using voice command to assist client with movement	X		X			X				
High-level movement										
1. Walking balance beam	X		X			?	? If visually directed	X	Labyrinthine righting and equilibrium; possible OLR	
2. Trampoline activities	X		X				If visually directed	X	OLR and equilibrium	

Modification of a hypersensitive touch system. Another example of a proprioceptive-tactile treatment technique is modification of a hypersensitive touch system through a touch-bombardment approach. The goal of this approach is to bombard the tactile system with continuous input to elicit light-touch sensory adaptation or desensitization. Deep pressure is applied simultaneously to facilitate proprioceptive input and conscious awareness. Proprioceptive discrimination and tactile-pressure sensitivity are thought to be critical for high-level tactile discrimination and stereognosis. A hypersensitive light-touch system elicits a protective, altering, withdrawal pattern that prevents development of this discriminatory system and the integrated use of these systems in higher thought. This method of treatment can be implemented by having an individual dig in sand or rice. The continuous pressure desensitizes the touch system while the resistance and deep pressure facilitates the proprioceptive-discriminatory touch system.

Pool therapy can be used effectively for the same purpose with the added advantage of neutral warmth. Any client perceiving touch as noxious, dangerous, and even life threatening will not greatly benefit from any therapeutic-session in which touch is a component part. Touch includes such contacts as touching the floor with a foot, reaching out and touching the parallel bar railings, and touching the mat. The client may not respond with verbal clues such as "Don't touch me" or "When I touch the floor it hurts" but will often respond with increased tone, emotional or attitude changes, and avoidance responses. Nevertheless, this treatment approach has application in many areas of intervention with clients having neurological deficits. As an adjunct to this method, a clinician should cautiously apply light touch when in contact with the client. Deep pressure or a firm hold should elicit a more desirable response for the client even if the light-touch system is functional.[71,172]

The therapist may also consider systematic desensitization as strategy to integrate the touch system. By allowing patients to apply the stimuli to themselves, they can grade the amount that they can tolerate. For example, the therapist may place a box containing objects of different textures before the patient and encourage exploration and active participation to learn which textures are acceptable or offensive. A gradual exposure to the offensive stimuli will raise the threshold of the mechanoreceptors in the skin. There are also the benefits to the patient being in control of the stimulus and having awareness of the treatment objective. In addition vibratory stimuli through a folded towel provide proprioceptive input to desensitize the touch system.[8,71,181] Desensitizing the touch system from a need to protectively withdraw is an important process within the CNS if normal stereognosis is to develop.

Orthokinetic cuff. The use of an *orthokinetic cuff* is another example of a proprioceptive-tactile treatment approach. The concept of orthokinetics is credited to Julius Fuchs,[19] an orthopaedic surgeon who was dissatisfied with "common static devices" for the correction of fracture dislocations and scoliosis.[15] The term *orthokinetics* is derived from Greek; roughly translated it means "righting of motion." Having observed the problems of prolonged immobilization, Fuchs wanted to design a dynamic device that used tactile and proprioceptive stimulation.

Today, the orthokinetic cuff is made from rubber-reinforced elastic bandage material. Half of the bandlike cuff is designed to be elastic and to stretch; this is called the *active field*. The other half of the cuff is sewn in a crisscross fashion to reduce its stretch; this is referred to as the *inactive field*. The active field of the cuff is worn over the muscle belly to be facilitated, and the inactive field is placed over the antagonistic muscle. The client wears the cuff during therapeutic exercise or in some cases throughout activities of daily living.

Orthokinetic orthoses a have been reported to remediate both dyskinesia and pain.[9,128,131,132] Whelan [191] conducted a study on the use of orthokinetics on the upper extremity of the adult hemiplegic patient. She reported significant results in the reduction of spasticity and an increase in active range of motion. Blashy and Fuchs[19] reported successful results with 81 out of 100 clients over a 4-year period.

The neurophysiological rationale for the orthokinetic cuff has not been fully established. Nevertheless, some important variables have been identified. First, it appears that the best results are obtained when the cuff is worn on the extremities. It would appear that the postural muscles do not lend themselves to orthokinetics because of their more tonic function. Sensory receptors within extremity musculature tend to adapt, whereas receptors found in postural muscles do not readily adapt.[48] Second, the cuff should fit snugly—not enough to impede circulation but enough to apply circumferential pressure. Obviously, this cutaneous stimulation should activate the exteroceptors of the skin and Ia afferent neurons of the muscle spindle. Thus the active field of the cuff would provide touch pressure and a pinching stimulus. In theory, the active field elicits an action potential in the exteroceptors and also feeds into the muscle spindle, resulting in an increased tonicity. The inactive field would appear to provide sustained deep pressure via the TO, which produces an inhibitory response. The research to date confirms the need for combining active and inactive kinetic fields for the cuff to be effective. However, which field provides the strongest influence on the nervous system has not yet been verified.[34,71,131]

Another important component of orthokinetics is the use of therapeutic exercise. Incorporating active resistive exercises using the shoulder wheel, pulley apparatus, and the stationary bicycle should provide sustained resistance to promote Ia receptor input by way of the muscle spindle.[19,191]

The last and most obvious variable is the placement of the cuff. For patients with spasticity, the active (elastic) field should be placed over the weaker muscle in need of facilitation, whereas the inactive (inhibitory) portion should cover the spastic muscles.[133]

The concept of orthokinetics has given rise to dynamic splinting devices for upper-extremity spasticity. Several dynamic orthokinetic splints and slings have been developed in recent years, and they appear to be more successful than previous attempts at static splinting. Most of the devices are based on variations of the principles derived from orthokinetics. (For a more thorough discussion of the concepts of orthokinetics and the therapeutic application of orthotics, see Chapter 28.)

Proprioceptive, tactile, and gustatory input. The complexity of combined proprioceptive-tactile input becomes enhanced by adding another sensory input, such as taste. Implementations of one of a variety of feeding techniques clearly identifies the complexity of the total input system. When taste is used, smell cannot be eliminated as a potential input, nor can vision if the client visually addresses the food. The following explanation of feeding techniques is included to encourage the reader to analyze the sensory input, processing, and motor response patterns necessary to accomplish this ADL task.

Several feeding techniques have been developed by Knickerbocher,[99] Mueller,[127] Farber,[53] Rood,[155] and Huss.[92] These techniques are not easily mastered or understood through reading alone. Competency in feeding techniques is best achieved from empirical experience under the guidance of a skilled instructor. The following techniques are eclectic, and they have been adapted for basic understanding.

Oral motor facilitation. The facial and oral region plays an important role in survival. Facial stimulation can elicit the rooting reaction. Oral stimulation facilitates reflexive behaviors, such as sucking and swallowing. Deeper stimulation to the midline of the tongue causes a gag reflex. These reactions and reflexes are normal patterns for the neonate. When these reactions/reflexes are depressed or hyperactive, therapeutic intervention is a necessity. Oral facilitation is an important treatment modality for infants and children with CNS dysfunction. Therapeutic intervention during the early stages of myelination can be crucial to the development of more normalized feeding and speech patterns.

Similarly, adults suffering neurological impairment often have difficulty with oral motor integration. Problems with swallowing, tongue control, hypersensitive and desensitive areas within the oral cavity, and problems with mouth closure and chewing are frequently observed in adults with CNS damage.

Before describing basic feeding techniques, some significant neurology should be highlighted. The innervation of the facial and oral musculature is complex. Therefore only the salient information pertaining to feeding is described here.

Facial sensation is conveyed by the trigeminal cranial (V) nerve. The fibers of the trigeminal nerve are among the earliest to become myelinated. This nerve contains both sensory and motor components. The sensory root of the trigeminal nerve contains two types of fibers: exteroceptive and proprioceptive. The exteroceptive fibers originate from cutaneous receptors of the face and head and enter the trigeminal ganglion through three branches: ophthalmic, maxillary, and mandibular.[188] The ophthalmic and maxillary are purely sensory fibers; the mandibular division contains sensory and motor fibers. As the fibers from the three divisions come together in the trigeminal ganglion, they enter the brainstem at the level of the pons and terminate in one of two nuclei. Some fibers descend, becoming the spinal trigeminal tract, and send collaterals to the trigeminal nucleus. These descending fibers convey pain and temperature sensation and participate in reflex activity. Other fibers ascend and terminate in the principal sensory nucleus. These fibers subserve two-point discrimination, pressure and touch.[3] Cutaneous innervation of the occipital region of the scalp and the dorsum of the upper neck is supplied by spinal roots C2 and C3.[193]

Proprioceptive fibers rise from deep structures, such as the muscles of mastication, temporomandibular joint (TMJ), and ligaments and fasciae of facial expression. The proprioceptive fibers have their cell bodies in the mesencephalic nucleus of the trigeminal nerve in the caudal portion of the mesencephalon. This represents the only example of first-order neuron cell bodies located within the brain. The pathways from the mesencephalic nucleus are not well understood, but the nucleus is believed to have projections to the cerebellum, motor nuclei of the brainstem, reticular formation, and the thalamus.[50,79]

The motor branch of the trigeminal nerve controls the muscles of mastication. These muscles include the masseter, temporalis, and medial and lateral pterygoids. The integrity of the mastication muscles is evaluated by having the client move the mandible from side to side or bite down on a tongue depressor.[53]

The process of chewing is a complicated motion requiring movement in all four directions. This movement is permitted by the TMJ. The TMJ and its supporting ligaments provide proprioceptive feedback concerning jaw position and force of bite. The alignment of this joint is very critical. Slight malocclusion has been associated with chronic pain and headaches. Other branches of the motor root control the tensor tympani, tensor veli palatini, mylohyoid, and the anterior belly of the digastric muscle.[52]

The muscles of facial expression are innervated by the facial nerve. Sensory branches provide proprioception from muscles of facial expression, exteroception from the external ear, and taste sensation from the anterior two-thirds of the tongue. The facial nerve also has a motor component to the stylohyoid and digastric muscles, stapedius muscle of the ear, and various secretory glands of the eyes and mouth. Certain muscles of the soft palate and tongue are innervated by branches of the trigeminal, facial, hypoglossal, glossopharyngeal, vagal nerves.

The tongue is a versatile organ with tremendous mobility. It plays a role in taste sensation, mastication, swallowing, and speech articulation. The tongue is also a discrete tactile receptor. The most precise two-point discrimination in the body is found on the tip of the tongue. The tongue also contains muscle spindles. Tongue proprioception and movement are controlled by the hypoglossal nerve (cranial nerve XII).[78,192]

Feeding therapy is preceded by observation and assessment. With a pediatric client, the therapist should observe breathing patterns while the client is feeding to determine if the child can breathe through the nose while sucking on a nipple. In addition, the child's lips should form a tight seal around the nipple. Formal assessments should include reflex testing, developmental milestones, and behavioral manifestations. Medical charts and results from neurological examinations should be consulted for baseline data.

Postural mechanisms can influence feeding and speech patterns in clients with neurological dysfunction.[154,168] A client with a strong extensor pattern may have to be placed in the side-lying, flexed position to inhibit the forces of the TLR pattern. The ideal pattern for feeding is the flexed position, which has been found to promote sucking and oral activity. Basic reflexes such as rooting, sucking, swallowing, and bite and gag reactions should be elicited and graded in children and evaluated in adults.

As already indicated, the facial region and the mouth have an extraordinary arrangement of sensory innervation. Therefore oral facilitation techniques must be employed with utmost care. Anyone who has visited the dentist can attest to the feeling of invasiveness when foreign objects are placed in the mouth. With this in mind, the therapist should begin each treatment session by moving the autonomic continuum toward the parasympathetic end. Activation of the parasympathetic system should lower blood pressure, decrease heart rate, and, more important, increase the activity of the gastrointestinal system. Neutral warmth, the inverted position, and slow vestibular stimulation should help to promote parasympathetic "loading." Another inhibitory technique that is applicable to feeding techniques is the application of sustained and firm pressure to the upper lip. An effective inhibitory device is a pacifier with a plastic shield that applies firm pressure on the lips. Perhaps this is why a pacifier is a "pacifier." Adults can acquire resistive sucking patterns with a straw and plastic shield and achieve the same results.

Sometimes children or adults are not cooperative and will not open their mouths. Rather than pry the mouth open, the jaw is pushed closed and held firmly for a few seconds. On releasing the pressure, the jaw reflexively relaxes. The receptors in the TMJ and tooth sockets may be involved in the production of this response.

The facial and trigeminal nerves work in concert to augment reflexes in the muscles of mastication. A common problem seen in neurologically impaired infants and adults with head trauma is the "hyperactive tongue," which is often accompanied by a hyperactive gag reflex. To alleviate this problem, the receptors have to be systematically desensitized. The technique, called *tongue walking*, has met with clinical success.[52,85] It entails using an instrument such as a swizzle stick or tongue depressor to apply firm pressure to the midline of the tongue. The pressure is first applied near the tip of the tongue and progressively "walked back" in small steps. As the instrument reaches the back of the tongue, the stimulus sets off an automatic swallow response. The instrument is withdrawn the instant the swallow is triggered. This technique is repeated anywhere from 5 to 30 times a session, depending on individual responses.

Another technique, which might be called *deep stroking,* is used to either elicit or desensitize the gag reflex. Again, an instrument such as a swizzle stick is used to apply a light stroking stimulus to the posterior arc of the mouth. The instrument should lightly stretch the lateral walls of the palatoglossal arch of the uvula. Normally, the palatoglossus muscle elevates the tongue and narrows the fauces (opening between the mouth and the oral pharynx). Just behind the palatoglossal arch lies another called the palatopharyngeal arch. Normally, this structure elevates the pharynx, closes off the nasopharynx, and aids in swallowing. Touch pressure to either arc incites the gag reflex. This touch pressure should be carefully calibrated. A hyperactive gag reflex may be best diminished by prolonged

pressure to the arcs, whereas light, continuous stroking may be more facilitory in activating a hypoactive gag reflex. A child or adult who has been fed by tube for extended periods of time will often have both hypersensitive reactions in various parts of the oral cavity and hyposensitive areas in other locations. This needs to be assessed in order to formulate a complete picture of the client's difficulties.

The use of vibration over the muscles of mastication appears to be physiologically valid. Muscle spindles have been identified in the temporal and masseter muscles.[43] Thus it seems likely that the tonic vibration reflex can be elicited. Selected use of vibration on the muscles of mastication enhances jaw stability and retraction. To facilitate protraction the mandible is manually pushed in.[53,82]

The value of vibration alone over facial muscles is questionable because muscle spindles have not been located in histological preparations. However, a combination of moving vibration followed by stretch pressure does seem to have therapeutic value. The vibration is applied with a battery-operated vibrator at a frequency about 60 Hz. In this case vibration is used to desensitize hypersensitive skin. To facilitate sucking in a hypertonic infant, for example, the stimulus is applied to the orbicular (circular) muscle of the mouth. The vibrator is applied firmly and moved in a circumferential pattern around the mouth. Although the orbicular muscle does not have muscle spindles, the mouth has a host of cutaneous receptors. These receptors (Meissner's and pacinian corpuscles, Merkel's disks, and free nerve endings) will fire when exposed to a touch-pressure stimulus. Vibration, on analysis, is nothing more than a series of high-velocity touch pressures. There is some evidence that the pacinian corpuscles are sensitive to vibration and exert an inhibitory effect over other receptors. Once the skin is desensitized, the musculature below is released. The stretch pressure in the direction of fibers following the vibratory stimulus activates receptors in tendons and ligaments. Another factor often overlooked is that muscle tissue has a certain elastic recoil quality that causes it to pull back after it is stretched. Therefore in facilitating the orbicular muscle, the lips should be stretched laterally, the top lip stretched upward, and the lower lip stretched downward to promote recoil.

To promote swallowing, some therapists use manual finger vibration in downward strokes along the laryngopharyngeal muscles and follow up with stretch pressure. Ice has been found to be beneficial as a quick stimulus to the ventral portion of the neck or the sternal notch. In addition, chewing ice chips serves as a thermal stimulus to the oral cavity and a proprioceptive stimulus to the jaw and teeth; it also increases salivation for swallowing.

Certain foods can be used to stimulate salivation. The sight of a dill pickle has been known to stimulate salivation in certain individuals. Ingestion of milk tends to thicken saliva, while warm beef broth thins saliva. Sweet flavors are universally accepted, and secretion increases with taste concentrations that are watered down. Concentrations of the same flavor should be increased by 30% so that difference in taste intensity is detected.

The therapist can quickly realize that feeding as a proprioceptive, tactile, and gustatory input modality is extremely complex and often incorporates other sensory systems. Breaking down the specific approaches into finite techniques helps the clinician categorize each component and then reassemble them into a whole. The job of dividing and reassembling the parts becomes more and more difficult as the number of input systems enlarges.[185]

Proprioceptive and vestibular input. Proprioceptive and vestibular input is one of the most frequently combined techniques used by therapists. In fact, client success in almost all therapeutic tasks depends on the coordinated input of these two sensory modalities.

Head and body movements in space. If the head is moving in space and gravity has not been eliminated from the environment, vestibular and proprioceptive receptors will be firing. Depending on the direction of the head motion and the way gravity is affecting joints, tendons, and muscle, the specific bodily response will vary. Bed mobility, transfers, mat activities, and gait all incorporate these two modalities. For that reason alone a thorough assessment of the integrity of both systems and the effect of their combined input seems critical if any ADL activity is to be used as a treatment technique.

The use of a large ball or a gymnastic exercise ball can be classified under the category of proprioceptive-vestibular input. Many activites can be initiated over a ball. When a child or adult is prone on a ball, righting of the head can often be elicited by quickly projecting the child forward while the therapist exerts control through the feet, knees, or hips. As the head begins to come up, approximation of neck can be added. Vibration of the paravertebral muscles might also assist. Rocking forward or bouncing the client who is weight bearing on elbows or extended elbows would facilitate postural weight-bearing patterns via the two identified sensory input systems. Having a client sitting on a gymnastic ball doing almost any exercise will stimulate vestibular and proprioceptive responses. The combination seems to play a delicate role in maintenance of normal righting and equilibrium response so important in functional independence.

A trampoline, equilibrium board, or a similar apparatus has the potential of channeling a large amount of vestibular-proprioceptive input into the client's CNS. In fact, a trampoline is so powerful it can often overstimulate the client and cause excitation or arousal in the CNS.

The trampoline and equilibrium boards are generally used to increase equilibrium reactions, orient the client to position in space and to verticality, and increase postural tone. A client with poor equilibrium, poor postural tone,

or inadequate position in space and verticality perception may be justifiably fearful of these two apparatuses because of the rate and intensity of their stimuli. Because fear creates tone and that tone may be in conflict with the response the therapist hopes to elicit from the client, caution must be exercised with either modality.

Gentle shaking. A specific technique of gentle shaking can be listed under a combined vestibular, muscle spindle, and tendon category. This technique is performed while the client is in a supine position and the head ventroflexed in midline. The head is flexed 35 to 40 degrees to reduce the influence of the tonic labyrinthine reflex (TLR) and unnecessary extensor tone. This flexed position should be maintained throughout the procedure. The therapist places one hand under the client's occiput and the other on the forehead. Light compression is applied to the cervical vertebrae. This technique activates the deep-joint receptors (C1 to C3) and muscle spindles in neck, which have polysynaptic connections with the cerebellum and vestibular system. If the technique is performed slowly and continuously in a rhythmic motion, total body inhibition will occur. If the pattern is irregular and fast, facilitation of tone will be observed.

Any one of these techniques can be implemented as a viable treatment approach in considering vestibular-proprioceptive stimuli. The selection of an approach or a method will depend on client preference, client response, and the clinician's application skills.

Modalities: auditory, visual, vestibular, tactile, and proprioceptive

Most, if not all, therapeutic activities activate five sensory modalities: auditory, visual, vestibular, tactile, and proprioceptive. Auditory and visual input are used as the therapist talks to the client and demonstrates the various movement or response patterns to be accomplished during an activity. As the client moves, vestibular, tactile, and proprioceptive receptors are firing. Thus the complexity of any activity with respect to analysis of primary input systems is enormous. Even a sendentary activity like card playing requires a certain amount of proprioception for postural background movements, tactile input from supporting body parts and limbs, and visual input for perception and cognition.

The tactile and proprioceptive sensory information is usually filtered by the reticular formation so the cortex can be "sensitive" to the stimuli. At the same time, visual input is formulating higher-order perceptions of the images projected on the retina. The turning of the head, postural control, and quick ocular pursuits bring in the vestibular mechanism.

Thus when considering the categorization of techniques—such as a PNF slow reversal,[100] a Brunnstrom marking time,[30] marking time with music,[42] Feldenkrais' sensory awareness through movement,[55,56] neurodevelopmental therapies,[23,34] Rood's mobility on stability,[155,168] or any mat or ADL activity—the therapist must observe the sensory system being bombarded during the activity. At the same time, if the therapist has determined which sensory systems are intact, which are suppressed, and which seem to be registering faulty data, then altering duration and intensity of stimuli through any one system and the combined input through all modalities creates tremendous flexibility in the clinical learning environment. Highly gifted therapists seem to know instinctively which input systems to use. Simultaneously, they sense the quantity and duration of combined input that best meets the needs of the client. By analyzing and categorizing input as well as patients' responses, many therapists may develop skills that were initially considered out of reach.

INNATE CNS RESPONSES TO MULTI-INPUT

The responses of peripheral and central nervous systems (PNS and CNS) to various external stimuli determine the individuality of an organism and its survival potential in the environment. As organisms become more and more complex, the types of external stimuli as well as the internal mechanisms designed to deal with that input also increase in complexity. As the CNS develops structurally and functionally, inherent responses to certain common types of stimuli seem to be manifested. At the spinal level, ipsilateral and contralateral responses to cutaneous or exteroceptive stimuli occur respectively as the flexor withdrawal and cross extension.[59] At higher levels within the CNS, reflexes and reactions are also produced by specific stimuli. The specific explanation for how these stimulus-response patterns are neuroanatomically produced can be found in Chapter 2 and other references.[51,85,193] The discussion within this section deals not with the specific neuroanatomy or neurophysiology but rather the potential use of these innate response mechanisms as treatment procedures. The focus is on classification of alternative methods that activate these innate neuron networks to produce a desired response.

We do not recommend or discredit the use of any reflex or reaction as a treatment procedure; we are only acknowledging their presence and stressing the importance of knowing how these innate mechanisms affect client responses. Without this knowledge, therapists, working with either children or adults with CNS dysfunction, limit their understanding of the normal CNS and thus decrease their ability to analyze behavioral responses that vary from the norm. This limitation restricts clinicians' flexibility when using a problem-oriented approach to treatment and may increase frustrations when they deal with individual clients.

Levels of processing

Much of what we know about the levels of processing has been gleaned from animal preparations and clinical observations of human subjects with localized neurological lesions. Although aspects of postural control and movement patterns can be identified at segmental levels, the circuitry producing these responses is infinite. During its ontogenetic development, the nervous system unfolds in a sequential pattern, laying down the foundations for higher-level cognition. Reflexes and motor reactions are superimposed on one another to form the background for higher-level skills.

One way to conceptualize reflexes and motor reactions (see Chapter 3) is to picture development of the telephone system or any other simple-to-complex structure. Initially, the system consisted of a few circuits going from one building to a central receiving center and then to other buildings. A spinal reflex such as the withdrawal response may be equated with this simple telephone network. With this reflex there is a clearly identified stimulus, a spinal neuron network, and a stereotyped motor response. Although this neuron network is by no means simple, its complexity does not equal the task of hitting a softball with a bat. Similar to the development of the complex international telephone network, as the developing CNS adds more and more reflexes and reactions to the system, a highly complex organism evolves, which no longer responds on a one-to-one relationship. That is, even if a withdrawal reflex is elicited, other reflexes, such as the TLR, may combine, creating a net effect that does not resemble the anticipated response pattern of either reflex. Thus the clinician must remember that the more complex the action (e.g., dressing versus rolling), the greater the need for integration and coordination of all reflexes and reactions. Another way to express this concept would be that the more complex the action, the greater the potential for affective and cognitive gratification and also for failure.

Spinal level. The spinal cord regulates certain reflexes (Table 6-7). These reflexes are said to be *phasic* because

Table 6-7. Spinal level reflexes

Reflex	Input stimulus
Myotatic or stretch reflex	Proprioception: muscle spindle
Reverse myotatic reflex	Proprioception: TO
Flexor withdrawal	Any noxious exteroceptive stimuli
Extensor trust	Exteroceptive: light touch
Crossed extension	Exteroceptive
Reflex stepping	Exteroceptive and proprioceptive
Grasp reflex	Exteroceptive or proprioceptive
Automatic extension of wrist and fingers	Exteroceptive or proprioceptive
Galant or incurvation of the trunk	Exteroceptive
Automatic trunk extension	Proprioceptive: joints and spindle

they manifest a short burst of action and then seem to be extinguished. The spinal reflexes act on the "all or none" principle. Once a spinal reflex is elicited, the extremity rapidly accelerates into a pattern of total flexion or extension. The spinal reflexes are primitive protective responses. Therefore any quick high-intensity nociceptive stimulus will elicit the response. In addition, these reflexes mediate muscle tone and provide crude components for forward progression.

Spinal reflexes are elicited in infants and individuals with neurological involvement to assess the integrity of the nervous system. Some therapists elicit the spinal-level reflexes in patients with upper motor neuron lesions to promote movement patterns.[3,39] For instance, a quick stimulus to the pads of the feet causes flexion (withdrawal) of the lower extremity (Fig. 6-5). Continuous use of this reflex arc may activate dormant neurons and pathways to eventually redevelop volitional movement.

Another way the spinal reflexes can promote movement is by facilitation of reciprocal patterns. If the subject is supine with one leg flexed, a stimulus to the sole of the flexed leg causes a pushing off or extensor thrust pattern. Crossed extension is a reciprocal pattern where manual flexion of one leg will cause extension of the other leg (Fig. 6-6). This provides a neurological basis for walking or shifting body weight to the contralateral side for maintenance of posture.

The reverse myotatic reflex produces or results in autogenic inhibition. Severe lengthening of the tendon stimulates the tendon organs. Impulses are sent along Ib nerve fibers to the spinal cord. In the cord the impulses synapse on inhibitory neurons, which in turn inhibit alpha motor neurons supplying the muscle under tension. As a result the muscle appears to relax (lengthening reaction). At the same time, the antagonistic muscle is facilitated. This reflex, not easy to elicit in normal subjects, is seen in exaggeration as the "clasp knife" phenomenon in patients with spastic paralysis.

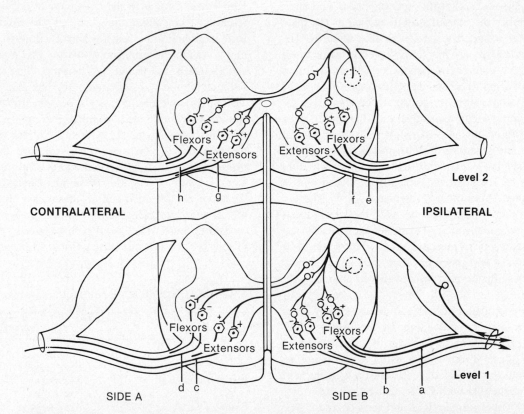

Fig. 6-6. Schematic representation of a neuronetwork of the cross-extension reflex. The stimulus enters at level one and elicits motor responses on both the ipsilateral and contralateral sides at the segmental level it entered and at other levels within the spinal cord. The specific response includes: *(a)* ipsilateral facilitation of flexor motor neurons at the same segmental level (level 1) going back to the leg; *(b)* ipsilateral inhibition of extensor motor neurons at the same segmental level going back to the stimulated extremity (level 1); *(c)* contralateral facilitation of extensor motor neurons at the same segmental level going to the other leg (level 1); *(d)* contralateral inhibition of flexor motor neurons at the same segmental level going to the other leg (level 1); *(e)* facilitation of ipsilateral flexor motor neurons located at other segmental levels but innervating the ipsilateral leg (level 2); *(f)* inhibition of ipsilateral extensor motor neurons located at other segmental levels (level 2); *(g)* facilitation of contralateral extensor motor neurons at other segmental levels (level 3); and *(h)* inhibition of contralateral flexor motor neurons at other segmental levels (level 2).

The reverse myotatic reflex is often employed to inhibit pathological patterns brought about by spasticity. A spastic child with cerebral palsy, for instance, shows extension and "scissoring" when the pads of the feet are stimulated. Sometimes the extension pattern is so strong that the child will arch backwards. Sustained positions that oppose pathological patterns are believed to elicit autogenic inhibition. Contraction-relaxation techniques also work on the autogenic inhibition principle.[100]

Just as spinal reflexes can be used to alter tone and elicit movement, they can also become obstacles when the therapist tries to coordinate complex movement patterns. A persistent grasp reflex is a common occurrence in children and adults with CNS insult. This dominant grasp is often triggered by the client's own fingers and frequently prevents functional use of the hand. If every time a client is touched, a withdrawal pattern is elicited, not only will the client be unable to explore the environment through the tactile-proprioceptive systems but will experience arousal by the influence of the cutaneous system over the reticular activating system. Severe agitation could likely be a behavioral outcome from such a persistent reflex.

As with any treatment procedure, a clinician should determine whether the technique will help the client obtain a higher level of function. As in the case of spinal reflexes that in and among themselves may be adequate for movement (see Chapters 2 and 9), lack of a controlling or regulatory system will prevent acquisition of functional skills. Thus, eliciting a withdrawal over and over again to get ankle eversion does not teach the client anything and will be effective only if it is incorporated into a higher-level activity. For example, initial use of withdrawal to elicit eversion followed immediately by resistance incorporates a spinal-level reflex with higher-order systems. As soon as the resistance is applied, the response pattern has changed and is no longer a pure spinal reflex.

The clinician must learn to recognize not only stimulus-response patterns but what combinations of responses to multi-stimuli would look like. If the reader overlayed Figs. 6-4, 6-5, and 6-6, a combined reaction to multiinput would be observed. The neuron network complexity of multiple input can be overwhelming, even at a spinal level. Thus, a therapist must always be observant of the specific behavioral response and the moment to moment changes in behavior during a treatment session, even if the specific neuron network is not understood.

Lower brainstem level. The lower brainstem includes the upper spinal cord, the medulla, the pons, and their substructures, especially (for our purposes) the facilitory portion of the reticular formation: the red nucleus and some vestibular nuclei.[101]

Reflexes mediated at this level are "tonically" activated: that is, the reticular formation activates motor neurons of the spinal cord (Table 6-8). These reflexes exert sustained influences and alter muscle tone throughout the body. The major motor influence at this level is directed toward the postural and antigravity muscles. The principal receptors are the joint and muscle proprioceptors of the neck (C1 to C3) and the otoliths and cristae of the labyrinth.

The tonic nature of these reflexes (if they are not controlled by other centers within the CNS) lends itself to prolonged static positioning of body parts. Clear descriptions of these reflexes and their effect on abnormal tone in clients with CNS dysfunction can be found in a variety of references,[20,59,60,72,143] which also identify the important role these reflexes play in development of the sensorimotor system. In a normally developing CNS the combined effort of these reflexes lays the foundation for integration of reaching, visual fixation, balance between flexors and extensors, turning of the head and body, bringing limbs to midline and across, and a myriad of other critical components leading to higher-level positioning and movement.[53]

Controversy exists as to whether these reflexes should be encouraged or discouraged as treatment procedures. Proponents of their use emphasize the importance of these reflex behaviors in the development of normal response patterns.[30] Opponents stress the difficulty clients encounter when obligated to assume the pattern once the stimulus is present.[20] Both groups are analyzing a similar system. It may be that both are viewing only half of the whole. Neither group wants a client dominated by a tonic pattern. Nor would either group teach the client to use the reflexes for functional movement since that option does not exist. Thus the first group teaches the client to use these reflexes to modify and control antagonistic function, which creates a more flexible dynamic interaction of muscle groups and encourages higher-level movement. The second group never teaches the clients to use the reflexes. These clinicians use the stimulus-response patterns only when they are effectively integrating these reflexes into inhibitory patterns exhibited by the client. These patterns modify the excessive abnormal tone and allow for facilitation of more integrated or functional patterns. Although the language sounds contradictory, clinical observation of both therapist behavior and client response would lead many observers to think clinicians in both groups were performing the same procedures.

Table 6-8. Reflexes of lower brainstem level

Reflexes	Stimulus
Tonic labyrinthine reflexes (TLR)	Static position of labyrinth
Tonic neck reflexes Symmetrical (STNR) Asymmetrical (ATNR)	Neck proprioceptors
Positive supporting reaction	Proprioceptors of hands and feet
Tonic lumbar reflex (? location in CNS)	Lumbar proprioceptors
Associated reactions	Proprioceptors and exteroceptors
Shifting reaction	Proprioceptors and labyrinth
Landau	Proprioceptors and labyrinth

Upper brainstem level. The upper brainstem includes pons, midbrain, and the diencephalon (thalamus and hypothalamus). It regulates postural adjustments and keeps the head aligned with the body. Animal preparations at this level are unable to initiate spontaneous movement but are able to assume and maintain the upright position. The principal reflexes (reactions) of the upper brainstem are termed *righting* or *displacement reactions.*[101]

A variety of reactions are thought to be processed at the pons, midbrain, and diencephalon level (Table 6-9).

Many available treatment alternatives incorporate the two general functions of righting reactions: rotation within the body axis to realign body parts and righting of the head to face vertical.

The first function, keeping the body in alignment, incorporates rotation with either flexion or extension. Rotation within the trunk axis or between the head and trunk elicits a variety of innate reactions: righting of neck, body on head, body on body, and body on body on head. Clinicians, no matter their orientation, have discovered that rotation within the client's body axis causes release of excessive tone in the trunk, shoulders, hips, and often into the extremities. The specific release of tone will depend on positioning of the client, direction of the rotatory pattern, and client's individuality. Brunnstrom's rowing technique in sitting position incorporates a large amount of trunk rotation.[30] This rowing maneuver releases trunk, shoulder, hip, and often upper-extremity excessive tone. Simultaneously, by actively moving the head in space, optic labyrinthine righting of the head (OLR) brings the head to face vertical. This tends to elicit a postural pattern in the neck, upper trunk, and shoulder girdle. PNF activities always incorporate rotation as a key element to facilitate normal patterns of movement.[100] Bobath and neurodevelopmental therapists using handling techniques to elicit righting reaction stress rotation as a critical element in eliciting normal coordinated movement.[22]

The importance of rotation as a treatment technique does not stop with movement within the trunk axis. Forearm rotation, usually into supination against spastic prona-

tors, will often elicit opening of the hand and release of elbow and wrist flexors. Often, shoulder flexion, internal rotation, and adduction are also reduced in tone.

When a client becomes spastic in shoulder or hip internal rotation, external rotation seems to be a key to releasing entire spastic patterns within the respective limb. Why the proprioceptive stimuli of rotation, which obviously stimulate spindle afferent fibers, joints, and tendons, has such a potent effect on abnormal excessive tone is not known. Yet clinical evidence through observation certainly reinforces rotation as a powerful therapeutic tool.

The second function of righting reactions is to orient the head to be upright and vertical—in prone OLR by extending the neck to orient the head to vertical and in supine OLR by facilitating flexors. With the client in a sitting position, the head should right to vertical no matter the plane or diagonal the body is tilted toward. In addition to the use of scooter boards, bolster platforms, and horizontal acceleration while the client is prone over a ball, techniques that automatically facilitate righting of the head to face vertical include (1) the second phase of the inverted tonic labyrinthine technique that elicits postural extension and righting of the head and (2) tipping off vertical while sitting.

These righting reactions often produce complex movement patterns. The specific stimulus, degree of rotation, or angle of the head off vertical determines the individual client's response. As the specific stimulus has a large degree of variance, so does the specific response. Therapists must be keen observers with respect to both the specific stimulus and the client's specific response to flexibly use righting reactions as a treatment modality.

Cerebellum. The cerebellum brings an added dimension to the upper brainstem functions. The cerebellum acts much like a computer in the integration of voluntary and involuntary motor activities. Generally, the cerebellum and its connections are the regulators of muscle tone. Within certain parameters the cerebellum monitors the range, rate, force, and direction of voluntary movement. It serves to correct errors in movement by informing the cortex about the current length and tension of skeletal muscles.

Cerebellar lesions affect the ipsilateral side of the body. Affected individuals may fatigue easily and exhibit ataxia, dysmetria, dysdiadochokinesia, asynergia, and intention tremor. The flucculonodular lobe of the cerebellum works intimately with the vestibular nuclei to orchestrate equilibrium and directional orientation.[40]

As the cerebellum modulates tone for posture and volitional movement, it relies on input from proprioceptive and vestibular mechanisms as well as higher-center regulatory mechanisms. Loss of higher-center feedback or peripheral input drastically affects the functional capacity of the cerebellum. (See Chapter 21) for specific treatment techniques that focus on cerebellar involvement.) Classifi-

Table 6-9. Reactions at the pons, midbrain, diencephalon level

Reaction	Stimulus
Neck righting	Rotation neck proprioceptors
Body on head righting	Rotation neck proprioceptors
Body on body righting	Rotation trunk proprioceptors
Body on body on head righting	Rotation trunk and neck proprioceptors
Labyrinthine righting	Gravity influence of labyrinth Vestibular and proprioceptors
Moro reflex	Neck proprioceptors
Emotional tone	ANS response to any arousal stimuli

cation of treatment modalities with respect to cerebellar integration can be divided into two areas. The first identifies the sensory input system while the second focuses on the rate, direction, and intensity of the stimuli. For example, assume resistance is the proprioceptive input. The intensity or amount of resistance would determine the rate of movement. By increasing the resistance and decreasing the rate, the cerebellum has more time to adjust and set appropriate base tone. Thus in a cerebellar categorization scheme, input needs to be cross-referenced with rate, intensity, and duration. In the example cited, optimal facilitation would correlate with a high degree of resistance. The gradient would sequence from maximal to minimal resistance in terms of the range of optimal to minimal facilitation.

Another proprioceptive input would be joint traction and approximation. Assume the two techniques are implemented with a weighted ankle cuff and a weighted waist belt respectively. Both techniques would increase the joint input and facilitate cerebellar function. Because of the added weight, both procedures would slow down the movement or rate component and thus give additional time for the cerebellum to regulate tone. Yet traction facilitates movement; approximation promotes joint cocontraction. Traction sends conflicting input to the cerebellum. The weight slows down and controls the movement, but the traction facilitates it. On the other hand, approximation summates input to obtain the desired response; it facilitates cocontraction to further control the movement. If the problem has already been identified as a rate deficit in which movement patterns occur too rapidly, then approximation rather than traction would be a preferred treatment. The specific technique for approximating—whether it be manual or with equipment such as a dental dam—would be the choice of the therapist. Please refer to Chapter 21 for additional information on the cerebellum's function in motor control.

Cortex and basal ganglia. The circuitry interconnecting the cortex, cerebellum, and basal ganglia has generated voluminous research (refer to Chapters 3 and 19 for more information on basal ganglia). The basal ganglia play an undisputed role in movement. This effect takes place through two systems. First, there appears to be a feedback circuit from the motor cortex to the basal ganglia. From the basal ganglia impulses travel to the thalamus, back to the cortex, and then to the spinal cord. The second system links the basal ganglia to descending pathways that synapse on motor centers in the brainstem. The basal ganglia have been credited with refining displacement reactions, mediating rhythmic automatic movement patterns and associated movements, and regulating postural tone in antigravity muscles.[3,39]

Lesions to the basal ganglia result in disturbances in muscle tone and involuntary movements. Clients exhibit resting tremors, hemiballismus, athetosis or choreo-type movements (hyperkinesia or hypokinesia).[104]

The cerebral cortex maintains an "advice and consent" relationship with the basal ganglia and cerebellum. The three structures interact cooperatively to complement voluntary skilled movement (refer to Chapter 3). The added dimension of the motor cortex enables the individual to isolate movement to one muscle or group of muscles during performance of a task. The cortex also permits rapid shifts of base of support when humans are displaced from their center of gravity. In order to accomplish this, the cortex has direct pathways to motor neurons in the spinal cord (corticospinal tracts). When fast and skillful movements are required, alpha motor neurons may predominate; when sustained postural movements are required, extrapyramidal and gamma motor neurons predominate.[16,164]

In terms of input and cortical-basal ganglia-controlled motor response, all sensory systems have the potential of altering output. The four categories of output that might be cross-referenced with the various sensory systems are praxis, optic righting, equilibrium reactions, and postural control.

The cortex is intimately involved in all learned skill. Thus all forms of praxis, no matter the sensory system(s) involved in the plan, would be considered a higher-level activity and linked to cortical function. (See the section on learning disabilities in Chapter 11 for a thorough discussion of praxis.)

Equilibrium reactions can be divided into two categories. The first includes the large, gross-movement responses called see-saw reactions, stepping, or hopping, and the second encompasses the small, postural-sway patterns over a base of support. Both types of responses either keep an individual's center of gravity over the base of support or replace the base of support back under the center of gravity. High-level movement requires equilibrium responses.[186] In order for the CNS to respond with the finite sensitivity needed for normal equilibrium, integration of spinal, brainstem, cerebellar, and basal ganglia areas are needed. If a client is dominated by abnormal tone or movement responses, then normal equilibrium reactions would not be expected. Thus before establishing the goal of normal equilibrium, a therapist needs to identify the client's CNS potential for integration. Similarly, before an attempt is made to elicit normal equilibrium reactions, normalization of tone should be established either innately by the client or through a therapist's help. Because of the complexity of equilibrium reactions, almost every combination of synergistic muscle action can be elicited. One of us (D.U.) has observed that once equilibrium responses can be facilitated, the client's freedom in all planes of space and thus control over functional activities are vastly improved. That improvement seems to simultaneously lead to client confidence and an ANS response that relaxes the individual and decreases the undesired emotional tone (refer to Chapters 4 and 13 for additional information).

Optic righting of the head (discussed with labyrinthine

righting) is placed at a cortical level of processing because of the level at which the optic nerve enters the CNS. Yet optic and labyrinthine righting are so intertwined that no one has clearly differentiated their levels for processing. From a clinical view, it is important that OLR become differentiated. The client needs to be able to look where he or she is falling—a visually guided activity—while maintaining the head in a near-vertical position to protect it from being hurt. It is believed that the labyrinths are responsible for the righting pattern and remain so throughout life.[6]

High-level cortical function with intact or adequately functioning lower levels is certainly the ultimate goal for all clients. The specific relationships and functional use of the various levels will depend on each client and on the therapist's ability to teach the client to reintegrate. The specific methods used will obviously vary from client to client and therapist to therapist. Flexibility and willingness to let the client teach the clinician which procedures best matches that individual's CNS are probably the most important therapeutic tools available. Unfortunately, this tool cannot be categorized within a specific scheme because it falls within all sensory systems and is critical at all levels within the CNS of both the client and the therapist.

Summary

The importance of understanding the various reflexes, reactions and synergistic responses inherent to the CNS is obvious. These interactions are one mechanism affecting the ultimate outcome of motor responses. It was once thought that the CNS was totally hierarchical and needed to be learned or retaught using a type of building-block design. Today, research has shown that there are a variety of systems affecting motor control (refer to Chapter 3). Each system can be approached as an inroad to the CNS. New theories and treatment approaches will be added to the clinical model as creative and visually astute colleagues challenge their clinical expertise and allow patients to show them alternative treatment techniques. Each therapist must be open to new advances while being analytical and cautious if those techniques are presented without any scientific or behavioral research or rationale.

HOLISTIC TREATMENT TECHNIQUES BASED ON MULTISENSORY INPUT

As already mentioned in this chapter and in Chapter 1, a variety of accepted treatment methodologies exist.* Each approach focuses on multisensory input introduced to the client in controlled and identified sequences. These sequences are based on the inherent nature of synergistic patterns[6,136] and the developmental patterns observed in humans[6,22,161] and lower-order animals[54] or a combination of

the two.[100,168] Each method focuses on the total client, the specific clinical problems, and alternative treatment approaches available within each established framework. Certain methods have traditionally emphasized specific neurological disabilities. Cerebral palsy in children[13,22,140,168] and hemiplegia in adults[21,30,35,118] are the two most frequently identified. In the last decade substantial clinical attention has been paid to children with learning difficulties.[7] Yet the concepts and treatment procedures specific to all the techniques have been applied to almost every neurological disability seen in the clinical setting. This expansion of the use of each method seems to be a natural evolution because of the structure and function of the CNS and commonalities in clinical signs manifested by brain insult.

Yet dogmatism still persists with respect to territorial boundaries identified by clinicians using specific methods. The question exists as to whether these boundaries are clearly delineated or superficially established. We believe there are many more commonalities than differences among approaches. For example, in the case of a hemiplegic client with a spastic upper-extremity pattern of shoulder adduction, internal rotation, elbow flexion, and forearm pronation with wrist and finger flexion, Brunnstrom would identify that pattern as the stronger of her two upper-extremity synergies.[30] Michels, although using an explanation similar to Brunnstrom's to describe the pattern, would elaborate and incorporate additional upper-extremity synergies.[118] Bobath would assert that the client was stuck in a mass-movement pattern resulting from abnormal postural reflex activity.[21] Although the conceptualization of the problem certainly determines treatment protocols, the pattern all three clinicians would work toward is shoulder abduction, external rotation, elbow extension, forearm supination, and wrist and finger extension. One clinician might describe the pattern as a reflex-inhibiting position. Another description might identify the weakest components of the various synergies, while still another might identify the extreme stretch and rotatory element that reciprocally inhibits the spastic pattern. How a clinician sequences treatment from the original spastic pattern to the goal pattern will again vary. Push-pull patterns in supine, side lying, and rolling; propping patterns in sitting; or a weight-bearing patterns in prone, over a ball or bolster, or in partially kneeling—all have the potential of eliciting the goal pattern and modifying the spastic pattern. It may be true that one method is better than others. That truth, however, stems not from the method itself but rather the preferential CNS biases of the client and the variability of application skills among clinicians themselves.

No matter the treatment methodology selected by a clinician, all techniques focus on the active learning process of the client. The client is never a passive participant, even if the level of consciousness is considered comatose. With a multiinput approach that requires a motor response,

*References 6, 13, 22, 30, 35, 36, 41, 61, 62, 68, 100, 118, 119, 152, 161, 168, 169.

whether that be an increase or a reduction of tone, movement, or postural holding, the client's CNS is being asked to process and respond to the external world. That response need not be at a cortical level, but it must be present.

Because of overlapping of treatment methodologies and the infiltration of therapeutic management into all avenues of neurological dysfunction, various multisensory models have developed over the last few years.[36,53,72,85,178] Although these models have attempted to integrate existing techniques, they may in reality have created a new set of holistic treatment approaches. The ultimate goal is to develop one all-encompassing methodology that allows the clinician the freedom to use any method that is appropriate for the needs and individual learning styles of the client as well as tapping the unique individual differences of the clinician. Although that approach does not yet exist, its development is the challenge to future therapists.

A CLINICAL EXAMPLE OF HOW TO USE A CLASSIFICATION SCHEME
Clinical problem: lack of head control

There is a potential for lack of head control following any severe injury to the CNS. For that reason it is a common clinical problem. Further, because of the importance of head and neck control, virtually all functional activities are affected by its absence.

Before discussing a classification schema, the clinical problem must be analyzed and identification made of those sensory and inherent systems to be facilitated. In considering the specific problem of lack of head control, let us assume that Barbara, a 16-year-old with a closed head injury, suffered a lesion within her CNS 3 months ago. She has the following signs regarding head control.

1. Mild extensor hypertonicity is present in supine, and Barbara is unable to flex and rotate her head off the mat.
2. In prone, extensor hypertonicity is gone, and hypotonicity prevails. The client is able to briefly bob her head off the mat in a hyperextension pattern. Mild tonal shifts occur to either side when the head is turned and when it is symmetrically flexed or extended.
3. Barbara is unable to roll or perform any functional activity in the horizontal plane.
4. When placed in long sitting, she is unable to hold the position or sit with flexed hips and extended knees. Her head remains in total flexion with her chin on her chest.
5. When sitting over a table mat, she is unable to hold her position. General hypotonicity prevails, although slightly more flexion is palpable. Her head remains flexed. When asked to pick up her head, she extends into a hyperextension pattern followed by a rebound into flexion. She is unable to hold the head in a vertical position.
6. Barbara does not mind being touched and responds well to handling techniques.

From the analysis of these clinical signs, the following clinical interpretations are presented.

1. In horizontal Barbara has persistence of a TLR. In this client this reflex is extensor dominant. While she is supine, extension prevails. While she is prone, extension is inhibited, although flexion tone is not dominant. Because of the persistence of this reflex, the ability to initiate rolling using a neck-righting pattern is prevented. Presence of mild ATNR to both sides and an STNR has been noted. In prone Barbara has the ability to move into a neck extension or OLR pattern but is unable to hold. Thus movement and range are present, but postural holding is missing.
2. As a result of ventroflexion of the head in sitting, the vestibular apparatus is placed in a similar position to that when prone. In a like manner, the total patterns remain fairly consistent. The increase in flexor tone may result from the positioning of hip and knee flexion and kyphosis of the back. The inability to flex the hips with knee extension suggests that total tonal patterns or synergies prevail. The client is unable to break out of those dominant patterns. Dominant OLR is not present.
3. Barbara, when asked, carries out the command to the best of her motor ability. This suggests the presence of some intact verbal processing, which is translated into appropriate motor acts. Similarly, when asked to pick up her head, she does just that, suggesting some perceptual integrity of body image, body schema, and position in space. Knowing where her head is in space and where to reposition it also suggest that some proprioceptive-vestibular input and processing are occurring.
4. Barbara's enjoyment of being moved in space with handling techniques again suggests proprioceptive-vestibular integrity. Similarly, her tactile systems seem to be functioning above the spinal level of withdrawal and arousal. Specific tactile perception would need a great deal of further testing.

Treatment sequence. Now that the clinical problem has been analyzed and the goal of development of head control set, a treatment sequence or protocol must be established. Barbara lacks head control in all planes and in all patterns of movement. Thus flexors and extensors must be facilitated to develop a dynamic cocontraction or postural holding pattern of the neck. The categorization scheme can now be of some assistance. The therapist can ask, "Are there any inherent mechanisms that facilitate flexors or extensors in a holding pattern?" OLR should elicit the desired response. Similarly, the clinician can ask, "Are there any inherent processes that would prevent righting of the head to face vertical OLR?" The TLR would block or inhibit the facilitation of OLR. Knowing the TLR is most dominant in horizontal and least dominant (if at all affected) in vertical is of clinical significance. It is also important to know that the OLR is most frequently tested in a vertical position and seems most active in that position. Awareness that the client is sensitive to total patterns (e.g., flexion facilitates flexion or extension facilitates extension) gives additional treatment clues.

After all this information is assimilated, the following treatment protocol could be established.

1. To facilitate neck flexors, the client will be placed in a totally flexed position in vertical with the head positioned in neutral. The client will be rocked backward toward supine, allowing gravity to quick stretch the flexors (Fig. 6-7, A). As soon as the neck flexors are stretched, the head should be tapped forward, back to vertical but not beyond. This avoids hyperextension, extreme stretch to the proprioceptors, and the horizontal supine position of the labyrinths—all of which inhibit the flexors and facilitate the extensors. The quick stretch and position should optimally facilitate OLR, which should activate the neck flexors. The total flexion of the body similarly facilitates the neck flexors. Once the neck flexors respond, Barbara can be rocked farther and farther backward while maintaining the head in vertical or ventroflexion (Fig. 6-7, B). Once Barbara can be rocked from vertical to horizontal and back to vertical while maintaining good flexor control, her CNS has demonstrated control and modification over the TLR in supine with respect to its influence over the

neck musculature. This rocking maneuver can be done on diagonals to facilitate flexion and rotation (Fig. 6-7, C), the key to eliciting a neck-righting, rolling pattern from supine to prone. The total flexed pattern can also be altered by adding more and more extension of the extremities. This decreases the external facilitation to the flexors and demands that Barbara's CNS take more and more control. Additional treatment procedures can be extracted from a variety of sensory categories. To add additional muscle-spindle proprioceptive input, any one of these listed techniques might be used. The rotation and speed of the rocking pattern will affect the vestibular mechanism.

a. Auditory and visual stimuli can be effectively used. If the therapist takes a position slightly below the client's horizontal eye level, the client (to look at the therapist) will need to look down and flex her head, thus facilitating the desired pattern. Any type of visual or auditory stimulus that directs the client into the desired pattern would be appropriate.

b. The therapist must remember that neck flexion was the goal. Rotation was added to incorporate and set the stage for facilitating additional desired inherent patterns. Since the extensor component still needs integration, total head control has not been attained.

2. To facilitate neck extension a procedure similar to the one for flexion can be established. A vertical position, thus eliminating the influence of the TLR, would again be the starting position of choice. With extension facilitating extension, the client should be placed in as much extension as possible without eliciting excessive extensor tone. Both an inverted tonic labyrinthine position or a kneeling position would be

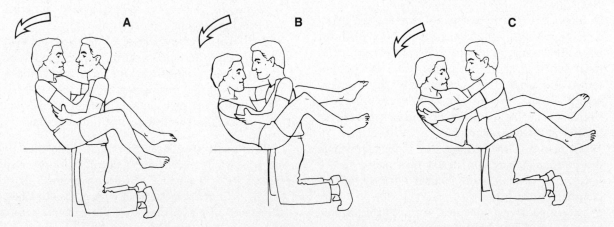

Fig. 6-7. Development of flexor aspect of head control. **A,** Vertical position: head midline and midrange (total body flexion) to optimally facilitate neck flexors. **B,** Facilitating symmetrical neck flexion, using position, gravity, and flexor positions. **C,** Facilitating flexion and rotation to develop pattern necessary for neck righting pattern.

viable spatial patterns to facilitate OLR of the head with focus on postural extensors. The vestibular system sensory category can be checked to identify the treatment procedure for use with an inverted TLR.

a. The kneeling position places the client in a vertical position with hip and trunk extension. Kneeling rather than standing is used because of the influence of the positive supporting reaction in standing and the massive facilitation of total extension. Kneeling avoids the total extension while maintaining a predominant extensor pattern. As a result of the gravitational pull of body weight through the joints, approximation to facilitate postural extension is constantly maintained. The upper extremities can be placed in shoulder abduction and external rotation, which tends to inhibit abnormal upper extremity flexor tone and facilitate postural tone into the shoulder. This extensor tone has the potential through associated spinal reactions to facilitate neck and trunk extension. The arms can be placed in this position over a bolster or ball or by the therapist handling the client from the rear (Fig. 6-8, *A*). The head should begin again in a neutral position. The client is rocked forward (Fig. 6-8, *B*) to facilitate OLR of the head and to elicit a quick stretch to the extensor. If the head begins to fall forward, the therapist can tap the client's forehead immediately following the quick stretch. This tapping action is the reverse tap procedure described under the muscle spindle proprioceptive category. The tapping is done to passively move the head back to vertical. A variety of additional procedures can easily be combined to summate facilitation to the extensors. Tapping, vibration, and approximation through the head to shoulders are only a few of the proprioceptive modalities. All

would be facilitory. A variety of auditory and visual stimuli could be used to orient the client to a position in space and thus righting of the head. Techniques listed under the exteroceptive and vestibular systems could also be part of the treatment protocol.

b. The therapist would want to sequence the client toward prone while the head remained in a vertical postural holding pattern. As the therapist rocks the client toward prone again, a rotatory component should be added (Fig. 6-8, *C*). The client will extend and rotate to counterbalance the movement, thus incorporating the neck-righting pattern of extension and rotation necessary when rolling from prone to supine. Resistance to neck extension with or without rotation is an important element in regaining normal spindle bias.

c. If the client is alert and has some functional use of the arms or legs, this rocking pattern in kneeling can be done as a functional activity. The therapist tells the client that she is going to reach toward an object with one upper extremity. The therapist can guide the client in the reaching pattern in a forward, sideward, or cross-midline direction. While reaching, the client can be rocked forward to elicit OLR. By incorporating an activity into the treatment of head control, the client not only is entertained but also attends to the task rather than to keeping her head up. In this way automatic head control is facilitated, and often postural patterns follow. In a partial kneeling pattern the client can be sequenced to on-elbow over a bolster or ball or on a chair. These activities should be sequenced from vertical to prone to ensure both total integration of the TLR prone and optimal integration of OLR.

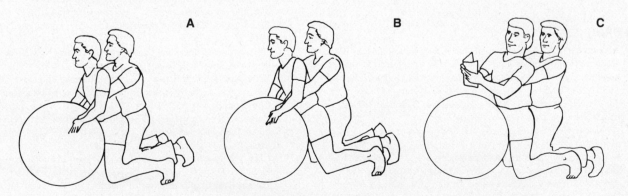

Fig. 6-8. Development of extensor aspect of head control. **A,** Vertical position: head midline with long extensor in midrange and postural extensors in shortened range; body in postural weight-bearing pattern, **B,** Facilitating symmetrical extension of head, trunk, and hips while inhibiting abnormal upper extremity tone. **C,** Facilitating head and trunk extension and rotation to encourage neck righting pattern; client reaches for an object, which is then placed on the opposite side.

Once the client can maintain good flexor, extensor, and rotational components of head control, the activity should, if possible, be practiced with eyes closed. If the client can still maintain head control, labyrinthine righting would be adequate for any functional activity. If the client loses head control, then additional labyrinthine facilitation would be indicated. If a client uses only vision to right the head, then any time vision is needed to lead or direct another activity, head control might be lost. Because symmetrical vestibular simulation plays a key role in facilitating the neck muscles to hold the head in vertical, it also is a key element leading to the perception of vertical and all the directional activities sequencing out of the concept of verticality.

• • •

Head control is a complex motor response. There are inherent mechanisms a therapist can facilitate to assist a client in regaining function. Simultaneously, there are multitudinous external input techniques classified under the various sensory modalities and combined modalities that can be used to give the client additional information. Awareness of one technique and the ability to categorize it appropriately allow easy identification and implementation of a large number of additional approaches.

SUMMARY

There are treatment techniques that are universally applied from the very young to the aged. The CNS is in a constant state of development throughout life. The brain is unique to each individual: it has idiosyncracies, but it also has an enormous number of predictable responses. Since these factors affect the success or failure of a client-clinician interaction, a classification scheme is only one of the many ways therapists can increase their repertoire while developing more clinical expertise. Both seem to be important factors in the growth and longevity of our professions. We hope this chapter will be useful for your practice.

REFERENCES

1. Abbott Laboratories: The internal ear, What's News 199:1-6, 1957.
2. Adrian ED and Zotterman Y: The impulses produced by sensory nerve endings. II. The response of a single end-organ, J Physiol 61:151-171, 1926.
3. Afifi A and Bergman R: Basic neuroscience, Baltimore, 1980, Urban & Schwarzenberg, Inc.
4. Alexander FM: The use of the self, Palo Alto, California, 1985, Centerline Press.
5. Andrew BL and Dodt E: The deployment of sensory nerve endings at the knee joint in a cat, Acta Physiol Scand 28:287-296, 1953.
6. Ayers AJ: Sensory integration and learning disabilities, Los Angeles, 1972, Western Psychological Services.
7. Ayers AJ: The development of sensory integrative theory and practice, Dubuque, Iowa, 1974, Kendall/Hunt Publishing Co.
8. Ayers AJ: Sensory integration and the child, Los Angeles, 1979, Western Psychological Services.
9. Barnes GR: Head-eye coordination in normals and in patients with vestibular disorders, Proceedings of the Barany Society, Uppsala, Sweden. In Adv Otorhinolaryngol (Basel) 25:15, 1978.
10. Barnes GR and Forbat LN: Cervical and vestibular afferent control of oculomotor response in man, Acta Otolaryngol (Stockh) 88:79-87, 1979.
11. Barnes JF: Benefits of myofascial release, craniosacral therapy explained, Physical Therapy Forum 1(2):1-5, 1984.
12. Barnes JF: The body is a self-correcting mechanism, Physical Therapy Forum 6:8-10, 1987.
13. Bertoti DB: Effect of therapeutic horseback riding on posture in children with cerebral palsy, Physical Therapy Forum 68(10):1505-1512, 1988.
14. Bessou P and others: Dynamic properties of mechanoreceptors with unmyelinated (C) fibers, J Neurophysiol 34:116-131, 1971.
15. Bessou P and LaPorte Y: Responses from primary and secondary endings of the same neuromuscular spindle of the tenesmus muscle of the cat. In Barker D, editor: Symposium of muscle receptors, Hong Kong, 1962, Hong Kong University Press.
16. Bickerstoff E: Neurology, ed 3, Kent, England, 1978, Hodder & Stoughton, Ltd.
17. Bishop B: Vibration stimulation. I. Neurophysiology of motor responses evoked by vibratory stimulation, Phys Ther 54:1273-1281, 1974.
18. Bishop B: Vibratory stimulation. II. Vibratory stimulation as an evaluation tool, Phys Ther 55:29-33, 1975.
19. Blashy MRM and Fuchs R: Orthokinetics: a new receptor facilitation method, Am J Therap 8:5, 1959.
20. Bobath B: Abnormal postural reflex activity caused by brain lesion, London, 1978, William Heineman Medical Books, Ltd.
21. Bobath B: Adult hemiplegia: evaluation and treatment, ed 2, London, 1978, William Heinemann Medical Books, Ltd.
22. Bobath K and Bobath B: Cerebral palsy. In Pearson PH and Williams CE, editors: Physical therapy services in developmental disabilities, Springfield, Ill, 1972, Charles C Thomas, Publisher.
23. Bobath B: Abnormal postural reflex activity caused by brain lesions, ed 3, Frederick, Md, 1985, Aspen Publications.
24. Booker J: Pain: it's all in your patient's head (or is it?), Nursing 82:47-51, 1982.
25. Borenstein M and Sigman M: Infant intelligence quotient predictable by gaze, Child Dev 57:251-274, 1987.
26. Brewer S: Personal correspondence with composer, pianist, and theoritician in use of sound in harmony with body rhythms, Aug 1983.
27. Brodal A and Pompliano V: Basic aspects of central vestibular mechanisms, Amsterdam, 1972, Elsevier/North Holland Biomedical Press.
28. Brookhart JM, Mori S, and Reynolds PJ: Postural reactions to two directions of displacement in dogs, Am J Physiol 218:719, 1970.
29. Brown D: Monograph on neuroscience review, unpublished outline, 1979.
30. Brunnstrom S: Movement therapy in hemiplegia, New York, 1970, Harper & Row Publishers, Inc.
31. Butler RA: The cumulative effects of differential stimulus repetition rates on the auditory evoked response in man, Electroencephalogr Clin Neurophysiol 35:337-345, 1973.
32. Buttram B and Brown G: Developmental physical management for the multi-disabled child, Tuscaloosa, 1977, University of Alabama Press.
33. Cain WS, editor: Odors, evaluation utilization and control, Ann NY Acad Sci 2371:439, 1974.
34. Campbell S: Clinics in physical therapy, vol 5, New York, 1984, Churchill-Livingstone, Inc.
35. Carr JH and Sheperd RB: A motor relearning for stroke, Frederick, Md, 1987, Aspen Publishers.
36. Carr JH and Sheperd RB: Movement science-foundations for physical therapy in rehabilitation, Frederick, Md, 1987, Aspen Publishers.

37. Case J: Sensory mechanisms: current concepts in biology, New York, 1966, MacMillan, Inc.

38. Cauna N: The effects of aging on the receptor organs of the human dermis. In Montagna W, editor: Advances in biology of skin, vol 6, Aging, New York, 1965, Pergamon Press, Inc.

39. Chusid JG: Correlative neuroanatomy and functional neurology, ed 18, Los Altos, Calif, 1982, Lange Medical Publications.

40. Clark R: Clinical neuroanatomy and neurophysiology, ed 5, Philadelphia, 1975, FA Davis Co.

41. Colavita F: Sensory changes in the elderly, Springfield, Ill, 1978, Charles C Thomas, Publisher.

42. Cook J: The therapeutic use of music: a literature review, Nurs Forum 20(3):252-256, 1981.

43. Cooper S: Muscle spindles in the intrinsic muscles of the human tongue, J Physiol 122:193, 1953.

44. Crosby EC, Humphrey F, and Laver EW: Correlative anatomy of the nervous system, New York, 1962, Macmillan, Inc.

45. deKleijn A and Magnus R: Korperstellung (body posture), Berlin, 1924, Julius Springer.

46. Downie RA: Cash's textbook of neurology for physiotherapists, Philadelphia, 1986, JB Lippincott Co.

47. Duensing F and Schaefer KP: The activity of various neurons of the reticular formation of the unfettered rabbit during head turning and vestibular stimulation, Arch Psychiat Nervenkr 201:97-122, 1960. (Ger)

48. Eldred E: Peripheral receptors: their excitation and relation to reflex patterns, Am J Phys Med 46(1):69-72, 1967.

49. Eldred E and Hagbarth KE: Facilitation and inhibition of gamma efferents by stimulation of certain skin areas, J Neurophysiol 17:59-65, 1954.

50. Ekelund LG: Exercise, including weightlessness, Ann Rev Physiol 31:85-116, 1969.

51. Eklund G and Hagbarth KE: Normal variability of tonic vibration reflexes in man, Exp Neurol 16:80-92, 1966.

52. Farber S: Sensorimotor evaluation and treatment procedures, ed 2, Indianapolis, 1974, Indiana University—Purdue University at Indianapolis Medical Center.

53. Farber S: A multisensory approach to neurorehabilitation. In Farber S, editor: Neurorehabilitation: a multisensory approach, Philadelphia, 1982, WB Saunders Co.

54. Fay T: The neurophysical aspects of therapy in cerebral palsy. In Payton OP, Hirt S, and Newton RA: Neurophysiologic approach to therapeutic exercise, Philadelphia, 1978, FA Davis Co.

55. Feldenkrais M: Awareness through movement, New York, 1977, Harper & Row, Inc, Publishers.

56. Feldenkrais M: The elusive obvious, Cupertino, Calif, 1981, Meta Publication.

57. Felton DL and Felton SY: A regional and systemic overview of functional neuroanatomy. In Farber SA, editor: Neurorehabilitation: a multisensory approach, Philadelphia, 1982, WB Saunders Co.

58. Fields HL: Pain, New York, 1987, McGraw-Hill Publishing Co.

59. Fiorentino MR: Normal and abnormal development: the influence of primitive reflexes on motor development, Springfield, Ill, 1972, Charles C Thomas, Publisher.

60. Fiorentino MR: A basis for sensorimotor development—normal and abnormal, Springfield, Ill, 1981, Charles C Thomas, Publisher.

61. Flynn J: "Snoezelen" Hartenberg, Ede, Holland, 1986, unpublished description of Institute de Hartenberg.

62. Freeman G: Hippotherapy/therapeutic horseback riding, Clin Man Phys Ther 4(3):20-25, 1984.

63. Gacek RR: Efferent components of the vestibular nerve. In Rasmussen G and Windle WF, editors: Neural mechanisms of the auditory and vestibular systems, Springfield, Ill, 1961, Charles C Thomas, Publisher.

64. Galambos R: Suppression of auditory nerve activity by stimulation of efferent fibers to cochlea, J Neurophysiol 19:424-437, 1956.

65. Gandhavadi B and others: Autonomic pain: features and methods of assessment, Pain 71(1):85-90, 1982.

66. Gardner E: Fundamentals of neurology, Philadelphia, 1975, WB Saunders Co.

67. Garliner D: Myofunctional therapy, Philadelphia, 1976, WB Saunders Co.

68. Gelb M: Body learning—an introduction to the Alexander technique, London, 1981, Auburn Press.

69. Geldard FA: The human senses, ed 2, New York, 1972, John Wiley & Sons, Inc.

70. Gelhorn E: Principles of autonomic-somatic integration: physiological basis and psychological and clinical implications, Minneapolis, 1967, University of Minnesota Press.

71. Gerhart KD and others: Inhibitory receptive fields of primitive spinothalamic tract cells, J Neurophysiol 46:1309-1325, 1981.

72. Gilfoyle EM, Grady AP, and Moore JC: Children adapt, Thorofare, NJ, 1981, Charles B Slack, Inc.

73. Granit R: Receptors and sensory perception, New Haven, Conn, 1962, Yale University Press.

74. Green JH: Basic clinical physiology, Oxford, 1973, Oxford University Press.

75. Greenberg JH and others: Metabolic mapping of functional activity in human subjects with the flourodeoxglucose technique, Science 212:678-680, 1981.

76. Groen JJ: Vestibular stimulation and its effects from the point of view of theoretical physics, Neurology 21:380, 1961.

77. Groër MW and Shekleton ME: Basic pathophysiology, ed 2, St Louis, 1983, The CV Mosby Co.

78. Grollman S: The human body—its structure and physiology, ed 2, New York, 1970, The Macmillan Co.

79. Guyton A: Structure and function of the nervous system, Philadelphia, 1972, WB Saunders Co.

80. Hagbarth KE and Eklund G: Tonic vibration reflexes in spasticity, Brain Res 2:201-203, 1966.

81. Hagbarth KE and Vallbo AB: Single unit recordings from muscle nerves in human subjects, Acta Physiol Scand 76:321-334, 1969.

82. Hagbarth KE and Wohlfart G: The number of muscle in cat in relation to the composition of the muscle nerves, Acta Anat 15:85, 1952.

83. Hannesson ME: Charting techniques and patterns of sensory stimulation, Preliminary draft of work manual for the Rood approach, Unpublished manuscript, 1963.

84. Head H: Studies in neurology, vol 2, Oxford, 1920, Oxford University Press.

85. Heiniger MC and Randolph SL: Neurophysiological concepts in human behavior, St Louis, 1981, The CV Mosby Co.

86. Heinsen A: Visual motor development, Palo Alto, Calif, 1973, Learning Opportunities: Stanford Professional Center.

87. Henderson A: Body schema and the visual guidance of movement. In Henderson A and Coryell J: The body senses and perceptual deficit, Boston, 1973, Boston University Press.

88. Hochreiter N and others: Effect of vibration on tactile sensitivity, Phys Ther 63:934-937, 1983.

89. Hodgson ES: Taste receptors, Sci Am 204(5):135, 1961.

90. Houk J and Hennemou E: Responses of Golgi tendon organs, J Neurophysiol 30:466-489, 1967.

91. Hubel D and Weisel T: Brain mechanisms of vision, Sci Am 241(3):130-162, 1979.

92. Huss J: Sensorimotor treatment approaches in occupational therapy, Philadelphia, 1971, JB Lippincott Co.

93. Huss J: Workshop, San Jose State University, Neurophysiological approaches to treatment, Unpublished class notes, 1980.

94. Huxley AF: Muscle, Ann Rev Physiol 26:131, 1964.

95. Iggo A: A single unit analysis of cutaneous receptor with C afferent fibers, CIBA foundation groups, Springfield, Ill, 1967, Charles C Thomas, Publisher.

96. Jackson O: Therapeutic considerations for the elderly, vol 14, Clinics in physical therapy, New York, 1987, Churchill-Livingstone.

97. Jacob S and Francone C: Structure and function in man, ed 3, Philadelphia, 1974, WB Saunders Co.

98. Kandel ER and Schwartz JH: Principles of neural science, ed 2, New York, 1985, Elsevier Medical Science Publishing Co, Inc.

99. Knickerbocker H: A holistic approach to the treatment of learning disorders, Thorofare, NJ, 1980, Charles B Slack, Inc.

100. Knott M and Voss DE: Proprioceptive neuromuscular facilitation, New York, 1968, Harper & Row, Publishers, Inc.

101. Kottke F: The neurophysiology of motor function. In Kottke F, Stillwell K, and Lehmann J, editors: Handbook of physical medicine and rehabilitation, ed 3, Philadelphia, 1982, WB Saunders Co.

102. Laidlaw RW and Hamilton MA: Quantitative measurement of apperception of passive movement, Bull Neurol Inst NY 6:145-153A, 1937.

103. LaMotte RH and Mountcastle VB: Capacities of humans and monkeys to discriminate vibratory stimuli of different frequency and amplitude: a correlation between neural events and psychological measurements, J Neurophysiol 38:539-559, 1975.

104. Levitt S: Treatment of cerebral palsy and motor delay, Oxford, 1977, Blackwell Scientific Publications, Ltd.

105. Lim RK: Pain, Annu Rev Physiol 32:269, 1970.

106. Loeb GE and Hoffer JA: Muscle spindle function. In Taylor A and Prochazka A, editors: Muscle receptors in movement control, 1981, MacMillan Publishing Co.

107. Magnus R: Cameron prize lectures on some results of studies in physiology and posture, Lancet 2:531-536, 1926.

108. Maisden DC, Meadows JC, and Hodgson HJ: Observations on the reflex response to muscle vibration in man and its voluntary control, Brain 42:829-846, 1969.

109. Maitland GD: Peripheral manipulation, Boston, 1977, Butterworth Publishers, Inc.

110. Marx J: Analgesia: how the body inhibits pain perception, Science 195:471-473, Feb 4, 1977.

111. McCloskey DI: Kinesthetic sensibility, Physiol Rev 58(4):763-813, 1978.

112. McCormack GL: Pain management: a role for occupational therapists, Am J Occup Ther 43:4, 1988.

113. McCormack GL: Neurophysiology of sensorimotor approaches to treatment. In Pedretti LW, editor: Occupational therapy practice skills for physical dysfunction, ed 2, St Louis, 1985, The CV Mosby Co.

114. Melwill-Jones G and Watts D: Muscular control of landing from unexpected falls in man, J Physiol (Lond) 219:729, 1971.

115. Melzack R: Myofascial trigger points: relations to acupuncture and mechanisms of pain, Arch Phys Med Rehabil 62:47-50, 1981.

116. Melzack R, Stillwell DM, and Fox EJ: Trigger points and acupuncture points for pain: correlations and implication, Pain 1:3-23, 1977.

117. Melzack R, Konrad KW, and Dubrobsky B: Prolonged changes in the nervous system activity produced by somatic and reticular stimulation, Exp Neurol 25:416-428, 1969.

118. Michels E: Motor behavior in hemiplegia, Phys Ther 45:759-767, 1965.

119. Mills M and Cohen BB: Developmental movement therapy, Amherst, Mass, 1979, The School for Body/Mind Centering.

120. Moore JC: Cranial nerves and their importance in current rehabilitation techniques. In Henderson A and Coryell J, editors: The body senses and perceptual deficit, Boston, 1973, Boston University Press.

121. Moore JC: The Golgi tendon organ and the muscle spindle, Am J Occup Ther 28(7):415-420, 1974.

122. Moore JC: The limbic system, Class notes from Bay Area Sensory Symposium, San Francisco, Calif, Feb 1980.

123. Moore JC: Recovery potentials following CNS lesions: a brief historical perspective in relation to modern research data on neuroplasticity, Am J Occup Ther 40(7):459-462, 1987.

124. Moulton DG and Beidler LM: Structure and function in the peripheral olfactory system, Physiol Rev 47:1, 1967.

125. Moulton DG, Turk A, and Johnston JW, editors: Methods in olfactory research, London, 1975, Academic Press, Inc.

126. Mountcastle VB: Sensory receptor and neural encoding: introduction to sensory processes. In Medical physiology, vol 2, ed 14, St Louis, 1979, The CV Mosby Co.

127. Mueller HA: Facilitating feeding and prespeech. In Pearson, PH and Williams CE, editors: Physical therapy services in the developmental disabilities, Springfield, Ill, 1972, Charles C Thomas, Publishers.

128. Neeman RL: Burn injury rehabilitation—hand dyskinesia and finger pain-treatment by orthokinetic orthoses, J Burn Care Rehabil 6:495-500, 1985.

129. Neeman RL: Post-polio sequelae—case report on orthokinetic treatment, Occupational Therapy Forum 2(8):17-20, 1986.

130. Neeman RL and Numan M: Clinical research-validation of orthokinetics, an established neuromuscular physiology-based treatment modality for dyskinesia. Paper presented at Ninth International Congress of Physical Medicine and Rehabilitation, Jerusalem, May 13-18, 1984 (abstract No 204).

131. Neeman RL and Numan M: Treatment of dyskinesia and pain by orthokineted orthoses in geriatric practice, Occupational Therapy Forum 2(15):19-21, 1986.

132. Neeman RL and Numan M: Treatment of pain by orthokinetic orthosis (cuffs), Occupational Therapy Forum 2(1):18-19, 1986, (northeast edition) and Occupational Therapy Forum 2(2):18-19, 1986.

133. Neeman RL, Numan HJ, and Numan M: A single-subject study of clinical utility and social validity of orthokinetics treatment for upper extremity dyskinesia in a subject with spastic quadriplegia, unpublished manuscript, 1986.

134. Ninth National Conference on Juvenile Justice: Open forum discussion, Atlanta, Ga, March 1982.

135. Noback CR: The human nervous system, New York, 1976, McGraw-Hill, Inc.

136. Noback CR and Demarest RJ: The human nervous system: basic principles of neurobiology, ed 2, New York, 1975, McGraw-Hill, Inc.

137. Normell LA: The cutaneous thermoregulatory vasomotor response in health subjects and paraplegic men, Scand J Clin Invest 4(33):133-138, 1974.

138. Oakley B and Benjamin RM: Neurological mechanisms of taste, Physiol Rev 46:173, 1966.

139. Ottoson D: Experiments and concepts in olfactory physiology, Progr Brain Res 23:83-138, 1967.

140. Page D: Neuromuscular reflex therapy as an approach to patient care, Am J Phys Med 46(1):816-837, 1967.

141. Parker DE: The vestibular apparatus, Sci Am 243(11):118-130, 1980.

142. Payton OD, Hirt S, and Newton RA: Scientific bases for neurophysiologic approaches to therapeutic exercise: an anthology, Philadelphia, 1978, FA Davis Co.

143. Peiper A: Cerebral function in infancy and childhood, New York, 1963, Consultants Bureau.

144. Pertovaara A: Modification of human pain threshold by specific tactile receptors, Acta Physiol Scand 107(4):339-341, 1979.

145. Pfaffman C: Taste, its sensory and motivating properties, Am Sci 52:187-206, 1964.

146. Phelps ME, Kuhl DE, and Mazziotta JC: Metabolic mapping of the brain's response to visual stimulation: studies in humans, Science 211:1445-1448, 1981.

147. Poggio GF and Mountcastle VB: A study of the functional contributions of the lemniscal and spinothalamic systems to somatic sensibility, Bull Johns Hopkins Hosp 106:266-316, 1960.

148. Pribram KH: Languages of the brain: experimental paradoxes and principles in neuropsychology, Englewood Cliffs, NJ, 1971, Prentice-Hall, Inc.

149. Quillian TA: Studies of the human hand and foot, Med Biol 15:140-142, 1965.

150. Quillian TA: Neuro-cutaneous relationships in fingerprint skin. In Kornhuber H, editor: The somatosensory system, Sachs, Germany, 1975, Thiene Publisher.

151. Quillian TA and Ridley A: The receptors community in the fingertip, J Physiol 216:15-17, 1971.

152. Quinn JF: Building a body of knowledge-research on therapeutic touch, 1974-1986, J Holistic Nurs 6(1):37-45, 1988.

153. Reith E and Breidenback B: Textbook of anatomy and physiology, ed 2, New York, 1978, McGraw-Hill, Inc.

154. Roberts TDM: Neurophysiology of postural mechanisms, New York, 1967, Plenum Publishing Corp.

155. Rood M: The use of sensory receptors to activate, facilitate and inhibit motor response, autonomic and somatic in developmental sequence. In Scattely C, editor: Approaches to treatment of patients with neuromuscular dysfunction, Third International Congress, World Federation of Occupational Therapists, Dubuque, Iowa, 1962, William Brown Group.

156. Schraidt R: Fundamentals of sensory physiology, Berlin, 1978, Springer-Verlag.

157. Scholz J and Campbell S: Muscle spindles and the regulation of movement, Phys Ther 60(11):1416-1424, 1981.

158. Selbach H: The principle of relaxation oscillation as a special instance of the law of initial value in cybernetic functions, Ann NY Acad Sci 98:1221-1228, 1962.

159. Selkurt E: Basic physiology for health sciences, Boston, 1975, Little, Brown & Co.

160. Serizawa K: TsuboL—vital points for oriental therapy, Tokyo, 1976, Japan Publishing, Inc.

161. Seufert-Jeffer U and Jeffer EK: An introduction to the VOJTA Method, Clin Man Phys Ther 2(4):26-29, 1982.

162. Shepard GM: Synaptic organization of the mammalian olfactory bulb, Physiol Rev 52:864-917, 1972.

163. Sinclair D: Cutaneous sensation, London, 1967, Oxford University Press.

164. Smith B: Differential diagnosis in neurology, New York, 1979, Arco Publishing, Inc.

165. Steinberg M and Rendle-Short M: Vestibular dysfunction in young children with minor neurological impairment, Dev Med Child Neurol 19:639-651, 1977.

166. Steiner JE: Innate discriminative human facial expressions to taste and smell stimulations, Ann NY Acad Sci 237:229-233, 1974.

167. Stejskal L: Postural reflexes in man, Am J Phys Med 58(1):1-24, 1979.

168. Stockmeyer SA: An interpretation of the approach of Rood to the treatment of neuromuscular dysfunction, Am J Phys Med 46:900-961, 1967.

169. Sullivan PE, Markos PD, and Minor MA: An integrated approach to therapeutic exercise, Reston, Va, 1982, The Reston Publishing Co.

170. Takagi K and Kobagasi S: Skin pressure reflex, Acta Med Biol 4:31-37, 1956.

171. Talbot WH and others: The sense of flutter-vibration: companion of the human capacity with response patterns of mechanoreceptive afferents, J Neurophysiol 31:301-334, 1968.

172. Tappan RM: Healing massage techniques: a study of eastern and western methods, Reston, Va, 1978, The Reston Publishing Co.

173. Taylor TC: Myofascial release techniques, Physical Therapy Forum 5(23):2-4, 1986.

174. Thompson E: The nervous system (monograph), Gainesville, 1978, University of Florida Medical School.

175. Travell J: Myofascial pain and dysfunction, Baltimore, 1983, Williams and Wilkins.

176. Tuttle R and McClearly J: Mesenteric baroreceptors, Am J Physiol 229(6):1514-1519, 1975.

177. Umphred DA: Clinical observations, 1967 to 1988.

178. Umphred DA: Integrated approach to treatment of the pediatric neurologic patient. In Campbell SK: Clinics in physical therapy: pediatric neurologic disorders, New York, 1984, Churchill Livingstone, Inc.

179. Urbscheit N: Reflexes evoked by group II afferent fibers from the muscle spindle, Phys Ther 59:1083-1087, 1979.

180. Vallbo AB and others: Somatosensory, proprioceptive, and sympathetic activity in human peripheral nerves, Physiol Rev 59(4):919 951, 1979.

181. Verrillo R: Change in vibrotactile thresholds as a function of age, Sens Processes 3:49-59, 1979.

182. Vierck C: Somesthesis (monograph), Gainesville, 1975, University of Florida Medical School.

183. Wall P: The gate control theory of pain mechanisms, Brain 101:1, March 1978.

184. Ward J and Fisk G: The difference in response of the quadriceps and the biceps brachii muscles to isometric and isotonic exercise, Arch Phys Med Rehabil 45:614-620, 1964.

185. Weiss SJ: Psychophysiologic effects of caregiver touch on incidence of cardiac dysrhythmia, Heart Lung 15(5):495-502, 1986.

186. Weisz S: Studies in equilibrium reaction. In Payton OD and others: Neurophysiologic approaches to therapeutic exercise, Philadelphia, 1978, FA Davis Co.

187. Wells K: Kinesiology, ed 4, Philadelphia, 1967, WB Saunders Co.

188. Werner J: Neuroscience: a clinical perspective, Philadelphia, 1980, WB Saunders Co.

189. Werntz DA: Breathing techniques selectively activate hemispheres, Hum Neurobiol 6:165-171, 1988.

190. West A: Understanding endorphins: our natural pain relief system, Nursing 2:50-53, 1981.

191. Whelan JK: Effect of orthokinetics on upper extremity function of the adult hemiplegic patient, Am J Occup Ther 18(4):141-143, 1964.

192. Williams P and Warwick R: Functional neuroanatomy of man, ed 35, Philadelphia, 1973, WB Saunders Co.

193. Willis WD and Grossman RG: Medical neurobiology, ed 3, St Louis, 1981, The CV Mosby Co.

194. Wilson V and Peterson B: The role of the vestibular system in posture and movement. In Mountcastle VB: Medical physiology, vol 2, ed 14, St Louis, 1980, The CV Mosby Co.

195. Young RR: The clinical significance of exteroceptive reflexes. In Desurdet JE, editor: New developments in electromyography and clinical neurophysiology, vol 3, Basel, 1973, Karger.

196. Zotterman Y: Sensory functions of the skin in primates, Oxford, 1976, Pergamon Press, Ltd.

197. Zwaardemaker H: Physiology of smell, London, 1895, Collier MacMillan Ltd.

Chapter 7

PSYCHOSOCIAL ASPECTS AND ADJUSTMENT DURING VARIOUS PHASES OF NEUROLOGICAL DISABILITY

Gordon Burton

OVERVIEW

Psychological adjustment appears to be elusive because it is a fluid process: all people are constantly changing. This is especially true for people who have recently become physically disabled. They do not reach a certain state of adjustment and stay there, but progress through a series of stages. Therapists commonly see clients in a crisis state[27] and therefore identify their adjustment pattern from this frame of reference. How well the client adjusts to crisis, however, does not necessarily indicate how well the individual will adjust to all aspects of the disability or the rate of progress from one stage to another. Disabilities are a massive insult to a person's self-perception.[80] A month, or even a year, after the injury may not be long enough to put the disability into perspective.

For most people progressing from the shock of injury to the acceptance of disability is a process fraught with psychological ups and downs. A number of authors have discussed the possible stages of adjustment and grieving.* The research of Kübler-Ross[59] into death and dying also has application to this topic of adjustment to disability. She discusses the concept of loss and grief in relation to life; loss of function may induce just as profound a reaction. Peretz[86] discusses the grieving process in relationship to loss of role function as well as loss of body function. These losses must be grieved for before the client can benefit from therapy or adjust to a changed life style and body. Therapists must be aware that the client can and must deal with the death of certain functional abilities.

The components of successful psychological adjustment to a physical disability are varied. To bring a client to a level of function that is of the highest quality possible for that individual, therapists must look holistically at the psychosocial aspects and at the adjustment processes involved, evaluate each component, and integrate the processes into the therapeutic milieu to promote growth in all areas. There is more to evaluation and treatment than just the physical component; the mind and body have interre-

*References 72, 80, 85, 89, 99, 100.

lated influences, and both must be understood, evaluated, and treated individually and as a whole.

The processes of adjustment and adaptation will be explored in this chapter as well as the influences of culture and societal values as they affect the physically disabled person. The importance of loss as a psychological component will be examined as it relates to the body, as well as to sexuality, the personality, and the family. Age will also be discussed as a factor in adjustment to disability. The importance of focusing on the strengths of the client, the family, and the support system, rather than on the weaknesses of the disability will also be explored.

This overview is designed to provoke therapists into thinking of the client as a whole person, not as a diagnosis to be handled in some prescribed way. As fellow human beings, therapist and client are in the rehabilitation process together.

Adjustment

Sequence process. Although each person has his/her own coping style and each should be allowed to be unique, Kerr's[52] research shows that there are five stages of adjustment:

1. Shock: "This really isn't happening to me."
2. Expectancy for recovery: "I will be well soon."
3. Mourning: "There is no hope."
4. Defense:
   a. "I will live with this obstacle and beat it." (healthy attitude)
   b. "I am adjusted, but you fail to see it." (neurotic attitude)
5. Adjustment: "It is part of me now, but it is not necessarily a 'bad' thing."

Shock. The client in shock does not recognize that anything is actually wrong. He or she may totally refuse to accept the diagnosis. The client may even laugh at the concern expressed by others. This stage is altered when the person has an opportunity to test reality and finds that the physical condition is actually limiting performance. If this stage continues, it may signify either a lack of mental health or an inability to cognitively realize the situation.

Expectancy for recovery. The client in this stage is aware that he/she is "ill" but also believes that recovery will be quick and complete. The person may look for a "miracle cure," and he or she may make future plans that require total return of function. Total recovery is the only goal, even if it takes a great deal of time and effort to achieve. Key signs of this stage are resentment of loss of function and the feeling that the whole body is necessary to do anything worthwhile. The staff can stimulate a change from this stage by giving clear statements to the client that the damage is permanent, by transferring the person home or to the rehabilitation unit, or by discontinu-

ing therapy. Any one of these occurrences can help make the client realize the permanence of the disability.

Mourning. It is during the stage of mourning that the individual feels all is lost; that he or she will never achieve anything in life. Suicide is often considered. The person may feel that characteristics of the personality (such as courage or fight) have also been lost and must be mourned as well. Thus motivation to continue therapy, to work on improving, may be absent. The prospect of total recovery can no longer be held, but, at the same time, there appears to be no other acceptable alternative. This feeling of despair may be expressed as hostility, and, as a result, therapists may view the individual as a "problem patient." It is possible for a client to remain at this stage with feelings of inadequacy, dependency, and hostility. However, it is also possible for therapeutic intervention to facilitate movement to the next stage by creating situations in which the client may feel that "normal" aspirations and goals can be achieved. In this circumstance, "normal" would not include such low-level activities as dressing or walking—activities that were taken for granted before the injury—but would include doing the work he/she was trained to do. These activities would also include playing with or caring for a child or family. This would be seen as self-actualization by Maslow.[70]

Defense. The defense stage has two components. The first represents a healthy attitude in which the client actually starts coping with the disability. The client can take pride in his or her accomplishments, work to improve independence, and become as normal as possible. The person is still very much aware that barriers to normal functioning exist and is bothered by this fact, but he or she also realizes that some of the barriers can be circumvented. This healthy defensive stage can be undermined and possibly destroyed by well-meaning family, friends, and therapists who encourage the individual to see only the positive aspects and who do not allow the client to examine his/her feelings about the restrictions and barriers of the handicapping condition. Conditions that lead to the final stage of adjustment may either be the client realizing that the whole body is not needed to actualize his or her life goals or that needs behind the goals can be actualized in other ways. A therapist should watch for opportunities to facilitate this transition.

The negative alternative during the defensive stage is the neurotic defensive reaction. This is typified by the client refusing to recognize that even a partial barrier exists to meeting normal goals. The client may try to convince everyone that he/she has adjusted.

Adjustment. In the final stage, adjustment, the person sees the disability as neither an asset nor a liability but as an aspect of the person, much like a large nose or big feet. The disability is not something to be overcome, apologized for, or defended against. Kerr[52] refers to two aspects or goals of this stage. The first goal is for the person to feel at peace with his god: the client does not feel that he or she is being punished or tested. The second goal is for the client to feel that he or she is an adequate person—not a second-class citizen. Kerr[53] believes that "It is essential that the paths to those more 'abstract goals' be structured if the person is to make a genuine adjustment." She also believes that it is the health professional's job to offer that structure.

Acceptance or adjustment is at least as hard to achieve and maintain in life for the disabled person as happiness and harmony are for the able-bodied person. Adjustment connotes putting the disability into perspective, seeing it as one of the many characteristics of that person. It does not mean negating the existence of or focusing on the condition. Successful adjustment may be defined as an ongoing process in which the person adapts to the environment in a satisfying and efficient manner. This is true for all human beings, able-bodied or disabled. There are always obstacles to overcome in attempting the goal of a happy and successful life.

People and circumstances change. Maintaining a balanced state of adjustment is not easy, especially for the disabled person. An individual known to this author as a woman who had achieved a stable state of acceptance of her quadraplegic condition called in a panic because, as she saw it, she "wasn't adjusted anymore." She had moved into a college dormitory and wanted to go out for a friendly game of football with her new friends, but suddenly saw how disabled she was. She had grown up in a hospital and had never had to face this situation. After discussing this, she was able to put things into perspective and was able to talk over her feelings of isolation with her friends, who, without hesitation, altered the game to include her. Keeping a balanced perspective is hard in a world that changes constantly.

White[112] states that without some performance, there can be no affecting the environment and thus, no sense of self-satisfaction. Skinner[78] points out that without satisfaction from affecting the environment, there is not sufficient reinforcement to carry on the behavior and the behavior will be extinguished. Thus satisfaction and performance must be linked. However, if the patient has not adjusted to his new body, little satisfaction can be gained from such everyday activities as walking, eating, or rolling over in bed.[78,89] To define adjustment on a purely performance basis is to run the risk of creating a "mechanical person" who might be physically rehabilitated, but, once discharged, may find that he lacks satisfaction, incentive, and purpose. The psychological state of adjustment is what makes self-satisfaction possible.

Adaptive process. The concept of the adaptive process can be used by the therapist to organize therapy sessions that promote the adjustment process as well as attain physical goals. In so doing, the therapist will be promoting and teaching performance and working toward the eventual achievement, client satisfaction.

The four characteristics of the adaptive process are described by King.[55] They can be worked on singly or simultaneously, and they can be thought of as the means to reach the goal of Kerr's[53] final stage of adjustment. These stages are active response, incorporation of the environment, response organized subcortically, and self-reinforcing adaptation.

Active response. In general, therapy encourages an active response by the client against the environment. The client is expected to produce action to improve. Interaction with environmental factors can be seen even if there is little functional ability, as in the case of a high-level quadraplegic client whose main avenue of interaction is verbal but whose influence can change the environment.

Incorporation of the environment. Another characteristic of the adaptive process is use of the environment to stimulate adaptive responses. An example of this would be setting up a graded walking program that takes the client from a smooth surface, to a rug, and eventually to grassy and rocky terrain. The adaptive process would be enhanced if at the time of discharge the client was not only able but also confident of his or her ability to walk over the lawn to reach the house from the surrounding perimeter.

Response organized subcortically. King[55] believes that a subcortically organized response most effectively achieved by directing the client's conscious attention to a task or an object while allowing the subconscious centers to integrate the response. The example in the previous paragraph can be used to illustrate this characteristic. The client's objective (conscious mind) may be set on getting across a lawn in order to get into her or his house, but the therapist's goal would be to stimulate automatic equilibrium reactions at a subconscious level. Subcortical adaptive responses generalize to other situations more easily than cognitively taught "splinter skill" reactions. As soon as the client cortically attends to equilibrium, the automatic postural changes are, by definition, lost.

Self-reinforcing adaptation. Each successful adaptation stimulates the next more complex step. It is essential for the client to succeed since this success stimulates progression to the next more complex "task." It should be remembered that the "task" is adjustment and that the activity only serves to facilitate adaptation or adjustment. Thus the therapist does not need to feel disheartened if the client learns to get into and out of his or her house but does not want to start mountain climbing: the goal of the adaptive process is adjustment in as near a normal pattern as possible for that client.

Combining knowledge of Kerr's stages of adjustment, as outlined previously, with the adaptive process gives the therapist a reality-based, evaluative treatment framework. The stage of adjustment can be assessed and the adaptive process characteristics can be drawn on in treatment to facilitate progression toward psychological acceptance of the disability as well as to promote physical improvement.

For example, if a person is in the mourning stage of adjustment, the therapist, knowing that the defense stage usually follows (p. 164), can encourage and support the client's entrance into this next stage by adapting a situation that meets the goal of the defense stage—beating the obstacles of disability. The adaptive process may also be used to structure the therapeutic activities that facilitate an active response to overcome the disability, using the environment to organize the response subcortically in such a way that it is self-reinforcing. For example, the client might to call his or her spouse and the therapist may be working cortically on increasing upper-extremity strength and wheelchair mobility. The client could be told that the only accessible phone is up a steep ramp and that the client must push him or herself up there to use the phone in privacy. The therapist might also add that it always seems that obstacles are in the way of the disabled and that the client must explore methods to deal with these problems. As the client accomplishes the task, not only will the objectives of strength and wheelchair mobility be realized, but the client may start thinking that he or she may be able to beat the effects of the disability, thus moving him from the mourning stage to the defense stage. No single experience will cause this to happen, but if therapy is designed to encourage adjustment and adaption, the client will tend to progress faster and with less trauma.

Awareness of psychological adjustment in the clinic

The problem for the therapist in treating a person with a disability is to see the disability in perspective: to see the whole person in the client's own world and in the context of society and a given time. After this difficult task is achieved, the therapist must develop a program that will appropriately stimulate the client and all significant others around the client to pursue the highest-quality life possible. The successful and skilled therapist evaluates the client's physical capabilities but does not stop there. At some level, assessment of the more subtle psychological aspects of the client's ability to function is needed. This includes the client's family network (support system) and its ability to adjust to the imminent change in life style.

The rest of this section will introduce the reader to some of the psychological change components that may be assessed. The last section will attempt to demonstrate possible ways that these components can be taken into account as an aspect of therapy.

Societal and cultural influences. From an early age, people in our society are exposed to misconceptions regarding the disabled person. Some of these misguided perceptions are that the physically disabled person is also retarded, not employable, dependent, helpless, asexual, unlovable, and miserable. If a first- or second-grade child is asked how a retarded person walks, the common response is the demonstration of a hemiplegic gait and posture with one arm going into a flexion synergy. This child has al-

ready learned not only the "role" of the physically disabled but will have also incorporated other misconceptions about how a disabled person acts. If these misconceptions were held before injury, then it is only reasonable for the newly disabled person to be inclined to fulfill these perceived role expectations. Thus the client may undergo a radical change in the perceived self (how the person sees him or herself) as a result of the "new" role expectations. Even worse, the family members may hold the same expectations of the disabled person and thus reinforce the helpless, dependent role.

If in the therapeutic environment, however, the client and family have their misconceptions challenged constantly, they may start reformulating their concept of the role of the disabled person. As this process progresses, therapists and other staff can help make the expectations of the disabled person more realistic. Therapists can schedule their clients at times when they will be exposed to people making realistic adjustments to their disabilities. Use of successfully rehabilitated individuals as staff members (role models) can help to dispel the misconception that disabled people are not employable.[68]

The cultural background of the individual also contributes to the perception of disability and to the acceptance of the disabled person. Trombley[107] states that perception and expression of pain, physical attractiveness, valuing of body parts, as well as acceptability of types of disabilities can be culturally influenced. One's ethnic background can also affect intensity of feelings toward specific handicaps,[92] trust of staff,[107] and acceptance of therapeutic modalities.[93]

The successful therapist will be sensitive to the cultural values of the client and will attempt to present therapy to the client in the most acceptable way. For example, in the Mexican culture it is not polite to just start to work with a client; rapport must first be established. Sharing of food may provide the vehicle to accomplish this. Thus the therapist might schedule the first visit with a Mexican client during a coffee break to allow time to establish rapport. The therapist must frequently remind herself that the dysfunctional client may be the one who can least be expected to adjust to the therapist and that the therapist may need to adjust to the client, especially in the early stages of therapy.

Gaining trust is one of the crucial links in any meaningful therapeutic situation.[58] Trust will create an environment that facilitates communication, productive learning, and exchange of information.[74] Trust is important in all cultures and will be fostered by the therapist who is sensitive to the needs of the client. This sensitivity is necessary with every client, but will be manifested in many different ways, depending on the background and needs of the individual in therapy. A client of one culture may feel that looking another person in the eyes is offensive, whereas in another culture refusal to look into someone's eyes is a sign of weakness or lack of honesty (shifty-eyed).[45] Thus, although it is impossible to be know every culture or subculture with which the therapist may come into contact, the therapist must attempt to be sensitive to the background of the client with whom he works. Even if the cultural norms are known by the therapist, not every person follows the cultural patterns, and thus every client needs to be treated as an individual in the therapeutic relationship. It should be the therapist's job to be sensitive to the subtle nonverbal and verbal cues that indicate the level of trust in the relationship.

Trust is often established in the therapeutic relationship through physical activities. The act of asking a client to transfer from the chair to the bed can either build trust or destroy the potential relationship. If the client trusts the therapist just enough to follow instructions to transfer but then falls in the process, it may take quite some time to reestablish the same level of trust, assuming that it can ever be reestablished. This trusting relationship is so complex and involves such a variety of levels that the therapist should be as aware of attending to the client's security in the relationship as to the physical safety of the client in the clinic.[58] If the client believes that the therapist is not trustworthy in the relationship, then it may follow that the therapist is not to be trusted when it comes to physical manipulation of a disabled body. If the client does not know how to use the damaged body and thus cannot trust the body, then lacking trust in the therapist will only serve to compound the stress of the situation[59] (refer to Chapter 4 for more information on some of the neurological components of this interaction).

The client's culture may be alien to the therapist, even though they may be from the same geographical region. A client's problems of poverty, unemployment, and a lack of educational opportunities[47] can all result in the therapist and client feeling that therapy will be unsuccessful, even before the first session has begun. Such preconceived concepts on both parts may not be warranted and must be examined.

Cultural and religious values may also result in the client feeling that he must pay for past sins by being disabled and that the disability will be overcome after atonement for these sins. If this is the case, such a client may not be inclined to participate in or enjoy therapy. The successful therapist does not assault the client's basic cultural or religious values, but may recognize them in the therapy sessions. If the therapist feels that the culturally defined problems are impeding the therapeutic process, he or she may offer the client opportunities to reexamine his or her cultural "truths" and may help the client redefine the way the disability and therapy is seen. Religious counseling could be recommended by the therapist, and follow-up support in the clinic may be given to the client to view therapy not as undoing what "God has done," but as a way of proving his religious strength. Note that reworking a person's cultural/religious (cognitive) structure is a very sensitive area, and it should be handled with care and respect and with the use of other professionals (social workers and religious and psychological counselors) if needed.

The hospital staff can be encouraged to establish groups in which commonly held values of clients can be examined and possibly challenged.[46] Such groups can lead the client to a better understanding of priorities and may help the person see the relevance of therapy and the need to continue the adjustment process. The therapist may be able to use information from such group sessions to adjust the way therapy sessions are presented and structured in order to make therapy more relevant to the client's values and needs. Value groups or exercises[46,94,101] can be another means used by the therapist for evaluation and understanding of the client.

Values, roles, and body parts may all be grieved for by the client. This is especially true during the mourning stage of adjustment. The following section will look at ways of grieving and will explore some possible losses the therapist may not be alert to.

Examination of loss. Reaction to loss has been examined by Peretz.[86] Nine types of bereavement states were described. They are as follows:

1. Normal grief
2. Anticipatory grief
3. Absent, delayed, and inhibited grief
4. Chronic grief
5. Depression
6. Hypochondriasis
7. Development of psychophysiological reactions
8. Acting out
9. Neurotic and psychotic states

The individual with normal grief alternates from shock and incomprehension to bewilderment and weeping, which may give way to guilt feelings, irrational anger, and even depressive symptoms. Progress can be judged by a gradual return to the client's level of functioning before the loss. The person with anticipatory grief is grieving for a loss that has not yet taken place. This may be grieving for loss of function or role even before the loss is documented. The client with absent, delayed, and inhibited grief may postpone grief until the crisis is past, or he or she may hide grief, not expressing it and not getting the necessary support. These individuals have been noted to experience "anniversary reactions" (reexperiencing loss at some later date such as the "anniversary" of the accident or diagnosis of the disability). With chronic grief the patient is in a state of persistent mourning, and no change in life style or environment will be tolerated. Sadness, tension, and gloom characterize the individual in the emotional state of depression. The client may feel sorry for him or herself and may be rendered nonfunctional. Psychotherapy or chemotherapy may be necessary. The patient with hypochondriasis may express anxiety regarding a physical concern (other than the disability) to avoid dealing with the disability. Usually there is no physical cause for the anxiety expressed, but the symptoms may exist. With development of psychophysiological reactions, depression or loss may be expressed through somatic symptom formation, such as a decreased immune defense system, colitis, hypertension, duodenal ulcers, and other illnesses. These illnesses may become so severe as to cause the person's death. Further research and documentation is needed in this area. Acting out is an attempt to avoid the pain of loss by turning attention to something else. This can be done through involvement in acceptable activities, such as work, or unacceptable activities, such as drug use (abuse). Neurotic and psychotic states may take numerous forms depending on the psychological predisposition of the person.

Knowledge of the types of bereavement as described by Peretz[86] can be used by the therapist to better understand the client's reactions to loss and will allow the therapist the possibility of adjusting the treatment approach to the client's type of bereavement.[59] This knowledge of the grief process can be applied to clients who have terminal illnesses in an attempt to increase the client's quality of life in his/her remaining time.[20,35]

Cognitive age and loss. The cognitive age of the person experiencing the loss is another aspect that therapists sometimes neglect to consider. Dunton[24] and Nagy[81] have pointed out that the age of the person dealing with death affects his reaction. It seems likely that this concept may be generalized to further understand loss of function.

The child under 5 years of age views loss as a temporary, reversible phenomenon. From age 5 to 9 years, the average child views death or loss as final but remote. The child thinks of the dead person as someone who went away on a long trip or as someone who will not be around anymore. It is not until the person is over the age of 9 that he perceives loss as permanent. Dunton cites the following case history:

A typical family with three children ages 11, 9, and 4½ years suffered the sudden loss of a beloved pet dog. When informed of the sad event the 11-year-old responded at first by saying nothing. Slowly the tears welled up in his eyes and he began to cry softly. When he regained his composure he said, "It's such a horrible thing—it's all over." The 9-year-old listened quietly to the news and said, "He has gone a long way. We'll have to get another one." The 4½-year-old looked puzzled and said repeatedly, "What happened? Why are you crying? Let's go get him!"*

As a result of brain damage or shock, cognitive levels in the adult may regress after injury, much as reflex development may regress. The client may be functioning at a low cognitive level and may not be capable of understand-

*Dunton HD: The child's concept of death. In Schoenberg B and others: Loss and grief: psychological management in medical practice, New York, 1970, Columbia University Press.

ing the permanence of the loss suffered. Disabled parents and spouses will have to deal with their children's reactions to the parent's loss in a manner appropriate to the cognitive level of each child.[32] Values clarification groups can be used to help the family deal with adjustment to loss.[46,94,101] The very act of being aware of cognitive levels of dealing with loss may help family members and therapists accept how the others are dealing (or not dealing) with the loss.

Preschool-age children often believe that the disability is a punishment and that they must have done something very wrong to deserve such a punishment. It is thus important to stress that a disability is not a punishment and that accidents and disabilities happen to good people as well as bad people. In this way the therapist dispels the next logical concept—that therapy is further punishment and that the client needs to be punished.

Loss and the family. In this chapter, the client's support system is referred to as the family. The family may be composed of spouses, parents, children, lovers (especially in gay and lesbian relationships), friends, employers, or interested others—church groups, civic organizations, or individuals. The people in the support system go through the same stages of reaction and adjustment to loss that the client does.

Family needs. The family will, at least temporarily, experience the loss of a loved member from the normal routine. During the acute stage the family may not have concrete answers to basic questions regarding the extent of injury, the length of time before the injured person will be back in the family unit, or possibly whether the person will live.

During this phase, the family network will be in a state of crisis. New roles will have to be assumed by the family members, and the "experts" will not even tell them for how long these roles must be endured. If children are involved, they will probably demand more attention to reassure themselves that they will remain loved. Depending on the child's age, the child will have differing capabilities in understanding the loss (see the section on examination of loss). Each member of the family may react differently to bereavement and each may be at a different stage of adjustment to the disability (see the section on adjustment). One member may be in shock and deny the disability while another member is in mourning and verbalizes a lack of hope. The family crisis that is caused by a severe injury cannot be overstated.

Role changes in the family may be dramatic. Members who have never driven may need to learn how; one who has never balanced a checkbook may now be responsible for managing the family budget; and those who have never been assertive may have to deal forcefully with insurance companies and the medical establishment.[108]

The family may feel resentment toward the injured member. This attitude may seem justified to them as they see the person lying in bed all day while the family members must take over new responsibilities in addition to their old ones. The medical staff may not always understand the stress that family members are under and may react to the resentment expressed either verbally or nonverbally with a protective stance toward the client. Siding with the "hurt" client may alienate the family from the medical staff and may also drive a permanent wedge between family members.

Parental bonding and the disabled child. The parent bonding process is complicated and is still being studied.[56,77] It has been found that this bonding process (attachment) may start well before the baby is even conceived.[56] The parents often think about having a child and plan and fantasize about future interactions with the child. After conception the planning and fantasizing about the child only increase. During the pregnancy the fetus is accepted as an individual by the mother[56] and the father, and after the birth of the child the attachment process is greatly intensified. The "sensitive period" is the first few minutes to hours after the birth. During this time the parents should have close physical contact with the child to strongly establish the attachment that will later grow deeper.[56] There is an almost symbiotic relationship between mother and child at this time; infant and mother behaviors complement each other (e.g., nursing stimulates uterine contraction). It is important at this point for the child to respond to the parents in some way so that there is an interaction. In the early stages of bonding, it is the seeing, touching, caring for, and interacting with the child that allows for the bonding process. When this process is disturbed for any reason, such as congenital malformations or hospital procedures for high-risk infants, problems have been found to occur later. The occurrence of battered child syndrome and failure to thrive has been noted to be higher than the norm when the child is born prematurely or when there is poor (or lack of) bonding at an early age.[56] Klaus and Kennell[56] have recommended elements that increase the chances of parental bonding, including (1) special needs during pregnancy and birth dealt with to support the parents, (2) parent preparation, education, and support, (3) need for a companion at labor and especially at birth, and (4) enhancing attachment—privacy and contact with the child and each other.

When the parents are told that their child is going to be malformed or disabled, it is a massive shock to the family. The parents must start a process of grieving. The dream of a "normal" child must be given up, and the parents must go through the loss or "death" of the child they expected before they can accept the new child. Parents often feel guilty. Poznanski[87] states that the parents feel the deformed child was their failure. Fathers have been found to be the most distressed about the child initially. The disabled child will always have a strong impact on the family, sometimes a catastrophic one.[75]

In the grieving process parents often appear to experience five stages—shock; disbelief (denial); sadness, anger, and anxiety; equilibrium; and reorganization. Klaus and Kennell have developed recommendations for dealing with the process.[56,89,90] Family education and support are the most beneficial aspects when raising a disabled infant. However, this has not always been accomplished in a refined manner.[22,89,90] As Davis has noted:

If the surgical treatment of the child's disability was planned as casually and haphazardly as are many parent education and treatment programs, these physicians would (or should) lose their licenses to practice.*

Parents must be encouraged to express their emotions and they must be taught how to deal with the issues at hand. Techniques for accomplishing this will be mentioned in later sections.

The child dealing with loss. In the event that a parent is injured, the young child may experience an overwhelming sense of loss. Child care may be a problem, especially if the primary caregiver is injured. The child will probably feel deserted by the injured parent and may demand the attention of the remaining parent. This will only increase the strain on all family members.

If the child is the client, his or her life will have undergone a radical change; every aspect of the child's world will have altered. Loved objects and people will help to restore the child's feeling of security. It is of major importance to explain to the child in very simple terms what is going on and to allow the child the opportunity to express his feelings both verbally and nonverbally (perhaps using play as the medium of communication).

The hospital setting is threatening to all people, but children are especially susceptible to loss of autonomy, feelings of isolation, and loss of independence. Bentovim[8] has stated that the severity of the disability is not as important a variable in the emotional development of the child as are the attitudes of the parents and family. The parents must attempt to be aware of the child's ability to understand the permanence (or transience) of the loss of function.[32] They will also need to help the child feel secure by bringing in familiar and cherished objects. A schedule should be established and kept to promote consistency. Play should be encouraged, especially that which allows the child to vent feelings and deal with the new environment. Any procedures or therapies should be presented in a relaxed way (fun, if possible), so that the child has time to think and to feel as comfortable as possible about the change.[26] The parents may often need to be reminded to pay attention to the nondisabled children in the family during this acute stage.

The adolescent dealing with loss. The adolescent is subject to all of the feelings and fears that other clients ex-

---

*Davis RE: Family of physically disabled children: family reactions and deductive reasoning, NY State J Med 75:1039, 1975.

press. Adolescents are in a struggle to obtain autonomy and independence, and they often feel ambivalent about these feelings. When an adolescent is suddenly injured and has to cope with being disabled, it can be a massive assault on the individual's development.

It has been noted[96] that the adolescent appears to react differently than other age groups to the knowledge of his own terminal illness. The adolescent often feels that he has gone through a very painful process (initiation) that will soon lead to the "joys and rights" of adulthood. Unlike persons in older age groups who might feel that they can look back and gain solace from the past,[109] the adolescent feels that he will have what Solnit and Green[105] term "death before fulfillment" and thus may react by feeling cheated by life. This same pattern may occur with the disabled adolescent. The therapist must be acutely aware of these feelings so that therapy may be presented in the most effective manner for the client to find challenge and fulfillment in life.

Family maturation. It should be noted that the family also has a maturational aspect. If the injured person is a child and if the family is young with dependent children at home, the adjustment may not be the problem that it would be for a family whose children are older. In the latter case, parents have begun to experience freedom and independence, and they may find adjusting to a return to a restricted life style, difficult, or even intolerable. They may have the feeling that they have already "put in their time" and should now be free. This is a very normal response but one that many parents feel guilty about and try to repress.

The reverse may also be true. The parents may be feeling that the children have left them ("empty nest syndrome"), and they may be too willing to welcome a "dependent" family member back into the home. This may lead to excessive dependence or anger toward the parents on the part of the client. All of these factors must be taken into consideration by the therapist when the therapy is presented to the client and family.

A greater understanding of the client and family members can be developed by the therapist if the therapist is aware of the normal human developmental patterns as discussed by Sheehy,[98] Lewis,[64] and Gould.[40] These patterns identify some of the major hurdles that must be overcome in the client's life.

Coping with transition. In the acute stage of a family member's injury, the family must be helped to deal with the crisis at hand. During this phase, the family must first be allowed to cope with the emotional impact of what is happening with a loved one. Second, the family should be helped to see the situation as a challenge that, if overcome, will facilitate growth. Third, adaptation within the family unit must occur to overcome the situation. Brammer and Abrego[12] have developed a list of basic coping skills that they have broken into five levels. In the first

level the person becomes aware of and mobilizes skills in perceiving and responding to transition and attempts to handle the situation. In the second level the person mobilizes the skills for assessing, developing, and using external support systems. In level three the person can possess, develop, and use internal support systems (develop positive self-regard and use the situation to grow). The person in level four must find ways to reduce emotional and physiological distress (relaxation, control stimulation, and verbal expression of feelings). In level five the person must plan and implement change (analyze discrepencies, plan new options, and successfully implement the plan). Using this model, the therapist and family can evaluate the coping skill-level of the family. The therapist and staff can then help promote movement toward the next level of coping with the transition. These levels are also broken into specific skills and subskills so that the therapist can gradate these them further.

One of the more damaging aspects of hospitalization to all involved is that the hospital staff focuses on the disability rather than on the individual's strengths. Centering upon the disability can lead to a situation where client, family, and staff see only the disability and not the potential ability of the client.

Decentering from the disability will be examined further in this chapter. If the family relationship was positive before the insult and if the client is cognitively intact, then the focus should be directed toward the relationship's strengths as well as toward the client's and family's individual strengths. In the initial acute stage of adjustment, crisis intervention may help the family use its strengths and at the same time deal with the situation at hand.

To adequately deal with the crisis, the family should:

1. Be helped to focus on the crisis caused by the disability
   a. Identify the situation in order to stimulate problem solving
   b. Identify and deal with doubts of adequacy, guilt, and self-blame
   c. Identify and deal with grief work
   d. Identify and deal with anticipatory worry
2. Be offered basic information and education regarding the crisis situation
3. Be helped to create a bridge to resources in the hospital and in the community for support as well as to see their own family resources
4. Be helped to remember how they have dealt successfully with crises in the past and to implement some of the same strategies in the present situation

An evaluation form has been developed by Holmes[50] to ascertain the state of crisis.

Working with the family as a unit during crisis will help strengthen the family and facilitate more positive attitudes toward the client, thus improving the client's attitudes or feelings toward the injury and hospitalization.[108] Encouraging family-unit functioning in this situation will decrease the amount of regression displayed by the client. If the family is encouraged to function without the client, however, more damage than good may be done.

Awareness of sexual issues

Sexuality is usually one of the last areas to be assessed, but it is one area recently mentioned as of great importance to family members and the client. Sexuality involves more than just the sex act; it incorporates characteristics such as sexual attraction, sexual identification, sexual confidence, and sexual validation.[7] It has been found to be a predictor of adjustment to disability,[111] of success in vocational training,[67] and of marital satisfaction when the woman is disabled.[97] Sexuality (sensuality) is representative of how the person is dealing with her or his world. If the person feels inadequate as a sexual, sensual, and lovable human being, there is little chance that he or she will also feel motivated to pursue other avenues of life.[63,73] Assessment of this area of function must be done with great sensitivity to the individual's feelings.[17]

The framework for assessing sexuality differs with the therapist. Some therapists see sexuality as an activity of daily living and incorporate it into this evaluation. Other therapists feel the client needs information about body mechanics to perform the sex act; thus positioning and reflex inhibiting patterns are assessed. Still others have found it a motivating force when range of motion and muscle control are worked on. For discussion of the anatomy and physiology of sex organs and their function refer to Chapter 29.

Development of sensuality (sexuality). Even before birth the sense of touch[33,74] and the ability to distinguish pleasurable and unpleasurable tactile sensations begin to develop. Pleasurable feelings are comforting, and attempts are made to prolong them; for example, a baby cries when nursing is stopped. If satisfaction is not derived from this interaction on a regular basis, a feeling of anxiety may develop and the child may withdraw from interaction with others and distrust may develop.[74] If pleasure in interaction with others is obtained in the first 3 years, the ability to maintain the warmth of being close and being nourished is translated into trust (that all needs will be satisfied by the caretaker) and lovability (bonding). It is here that a sense of intimacy is initiated.[4,33,74] Ego and sensuality are refined as the child develops the ability to stimulate and satisfy itself. By the age of 5, the ability to explore the world by using the hands and mouth, as well as other parts of the body, allows the person to develop communication, self-gratification, and a feeling of competence.[112]

This feeling of competence is derived from the effective use of the body to make itself feel good and to accomplish tasks. By the age of 8, body parts and body processes are usually named and the child perceives the body as good. At this time intimacy between the self and another person

is further refined, as are roles. During puberty body changes and sexual tension is heightened.[33,37,74] Self-acceptance is based on the person's perception of how effectively he or she has accomplished the previous tasks.

The preceding is an over-simplification of the first 20 years of life, but the role of sensuality and sensation cannot be overemphasized. This is especially true for those professionals who constantly interact with clients in a physical manner. The intervention the therapist provides when the client is, or feels he is, in a dependent state can have direct impact upon how the client may perceive himself in the future.

Pediatric sensuality. The child needs to learn to enjoy his body. The therapist should help the client to distinguish between therapeutic touch and "fun" sensual touch, such as tickling or cuddling. It is important for clients to distinguish between the two so that they do not "turn their bodies off" to touch. For example, a woman with cerebral palsy stated during an interview that therapy was either painful or so clinical that she disassociated herself from sensations in her body during therapy. Later in life this became a problem when she was married. She stated that it took 7 years of marriage before she could enjoy the sensations of being touched by her husband. She also stated that it was a revolutionary concept for her that a vibrator could be used to give pleasure!

The therapy session should also help the client develop a sense of personal ownership of the body.[58,69,74] This aspect is often neglected when working with children.[37,73,88] The therapist often does not ask permission to touch a client, thus suggesting that the client lacks the right to control being touched by others. The last thing the therapist would desire to communicate, especially to a child, is that any person has the right to handle and touch the client's body. Child molestation is just beginning to be recognized as a problem in this country, with possibly one third of the female and male population being victimized.[113] It is hard to think of a more likely victim than a person who has (unintentionally) been taught that he or she does not have the right to say NO to being touched, and who cannot physically resist unwanted advances and in some cases cannot even communicate that abuse has taken place.[113] The effects of this can be seen in adults. When one client was asked why tone increased in her lower extremities when she was touched, her response was "I was sexually abused by my father in the name of therapy, and therapy and sexual abuse are synonymous at this point." No wonder she had been resistant to reentering therapy!

One way of helping clients "own" their bodies (besides asking permission to touch) is by naming body parts and body processes using correct terminology (as opposed to baby talk), thus making it possible for the client to communicate and relate in an appropriate manner.[73,74] This can be accomplished as the need arises, or it can be encouraged through the use of anatomically correct puzzles or dolls during therapy sessions.

One goal of therapy may be to develop the concept that the body (in the case of persons with the congenital disabilities) or the "new body" (in the case of those with acquired disabilities) is acceptable and good,[37,58,69] thus giving the client a more positive attitude toward his or her body and toward therapy. This attitude can be encouraged by pointing out a particularly positive aspect of the client's body and mentioning this regularly.[113] The feature could be the hair, eyes, or a smile, but should be an aspect of the client that can be seen and commented on by others as well. Commenting on how well the body feels when it is relaxed or how good the sun feels on the body helps the client recognize that the body can be a positive source of pleasure.

Another message that can affect the client in later life is the concept that the disabled are asexual and will never have sexual needs or partners.[4,44,73] Although it is not be appropriate to deal directly with the concept in therapy with a child, the therapist might mention that he or she knows of a person with disabilities, such as the client's disability, who is married or who has children. In this way the therapist communicates that there is a possibility that the "normal" sex roles of the child may be fulfilled in the future. Without this possibility being presented, the child may think that there is no chance that all the movies, books, and television programs that deal with normal adult interactions apply to the disabled, a belief that leads to poor socialization and further alienation.[73]

Adult sexuality. Adaptive devices can be a detriment to one's perceived sexuality. It can be hard to see oneself as sexy with an indwelling catheter or braces, but by discussing this topic the client can get some ideas as how to handle difficult situations when they arise.[113] Discussing positioning to reduce pain and spasticity or to enable the client to more comfortably engage in sexual relations will help the client deal with problems before they reveal themselves.[58,69,74,113] Because sexual hygiene may be considered as an activity of daily living, it may fall within the domain of therapy.

The client may feel that his or her sexual identity is threatened by a newly acquired disability and may try to assert his or her sexuality through jokes, flirting, or even passes toward the therapist. In these cases it is important for the therapist to realize that what is often being looked for is the confirmation that the client is still a sexual and sensual human being, thus the therapist's response is very important.[44,57] If the therapist rejects or even ridicules the client, it may be a very long time before the client can even think of attempting such a confirmation of personal attractiveness. The client may feel that because the therapist rejects the client and the therapist is familiar with the disabled, then there is little chance anyone who is not familiar with the disabled could accept the client as lovable.[44] The therapist should not be surprised by such advances and should deal with the situation in a professional manner. The therapist should also realize that approximately 10% of the population is homosexual and be prepared for advances from clients of the same sex. The therapist may need to remember that therapy is not the time to attempt to change the client's sexual orientation nor is it time to be offended, but instead to be as professional in dealing with this client as with any other. All of the therapist's interactions should be directed toward creating an environment that will promote a stronger and more well-adjusted client.

Nowinski and Ayers[83] found that sexuality was of great concern to most people with physical disabilities. As Bogle and Shaul[10] stated, it is difficult to see oneself as lovable and huggable when surrounded by hard, cold, and usually unsightly braces. The therapist can assist the client in moving through the stages of self-awareness to the reinstatement of self-appreciation that precede positive feelings that he or she is still sensual, sexual, and huggable. This can be done through everyday interaction; this may entail encouraging the family to embrace the client and may even call for the therapist to role model these behaviors at times.[21] The therapist may provide reading materials to the client and family directly by reviewing and answering questions or indirectly by having such books as *Who Cares?*,[19] *Sexuality and Physical Disability*,[13] *Sexual Options for Paraplegics and Quadriplegics*,[76] or the Hite Report on female[48] and male sexuality[49] available. In this way, the individual and significant others are made aware of possible options for the expression of intimacy and of the fact that this part of life is not over.

Because the therapist is in a situation of one-to-one treatment involving touching, moving, and handling the client's body, he or she may frequently be a natural person from whom the individual may seek information. If this natural curiosity does not appear to be forthcoming, however, the therapist can give the client an opening. For example, during an evaluation of motor skills, the person may be asked if there are any problems in such areas as sexual positioning. The topic need not be pursued any further by the therapist, but when the client is ready to deal with the subject area, he or she will probably remember that the therapist brought it up and may be a person to approach when dealing with these issues.

Other ways of presenting sexual information are to have literature available on the client's ward so that those who are interested may pursue the topic in private, to have a group discussion (interested clients, clients and significant others, or whatever group the client and therapist might choose to assemble), or to have literature in the department waiting room.[3]

• • •

All of the clinical problem areas that need assessment and evaluation and that have been mentioned previously are examined in relation to treatment planning in the clinical setting in the following sections.

TREATMENT VARIABLES IN RELATION TO THERAPY

This section examines issues the therapist and staff should be alerted to in order to create a therapeutic environment that will facilitate psychological adjustment and independence of the disabled client. The physical and the attitudinal environment of the treatment facility plays a major role in the way the client views the services that are rendered.

Recall a time before you became a member of the medical community. Think about how awe-inspiring the people in white coats were, how strange the smells of the hospitals were, how busy it all seemed, and how puzzling the secret medical language was. It all seemed overwhelming then, and it still is to newcomers, especially newly admitted patients and their families. The hospital usually appears impersonal,[71] sterile, monotonous, and confusing, and all status accumulated outside the hospital means little inside.

The therapist needs to take the setting into account when dealing with the client. The environment can be altered in a variety of ways. Therapy staff could wear street clothes, decorate the department or hospital with posters and lively colors, and allow clients to bring some personal items into the hospital.

The nature of the therapy process can often lead the therapist to see only the disability and not the person. An example of this is when a client is referred to by his or her disability, rather than name. This stereotyping of disability can lead the therapist to concentrate on the lack of ability rather than on the strengths of the client. The real danger of this is that the client and family will also start to focus on the disability of the client and feel that their family relationship is now permanently altered. The accuracy of this perception may have to be evaluated as part of the adjustment process. The wife of a man with paraplegia said with a sudden burst of insight, "I didn't marry him for his legs—this doesn't change that much." Very often so much attention is directed toward the disability that tunnel vision develops. One way to try to get a better perspective is to look at the bigger picture. Ask some questions such as:

1. Who will marry this person and why?
2. What are his or her good points?
3. What will this person do for a living?
4. What will this person do for enjoyment?
5. How will this person bring others enjoyment?

After the therapist is aware of the strengths of the client, they may be capitalized on in therapy to help the client realize his/her strengths and build confidence. Clients often reported that they were not complimented in therapy and especially that they never received feedback that their bodies' were desirable[10] or that they were doing things correctly.[14] A logical thought by the client is "if the thera-

pist cannot see anything desirable about me, and the therapist deals with the disabled all the time, then there must not be anything good about me." Positive, sincere comments to client and family can add a motivational factor to treatment that may have been missing.[14]

The last, and possibly the most important aspect in creating an environment that will foster growth and adjustment in the client, is a staff that is well-adjusted and aware of their own personal needs. Just as coping skills are necessary for the client, the staff, too, must be capable of coping with the stresses of the emotional and physical pain of the client and the client's family. The therapist must also deal with his or her own personal reactions to the sometimes devastating situations others are in.[106] Exposure to such situations often elicits introspection on the part of the staff that can result in emotional turmoil for staff members and for their own personal relationships. This emotional energy needs to be directed in a productive way so that the energy does not turn into chaos within the staff and a destructive force on the client.

To decrease the possibly distractive nature of this emotional energy, the staff should be made aware of their own coping styles, and they should be allowed to vent their reactions to particularly distressing client loads in a positive, supportive group. Group meetings can be used to handle some of the inevitable tension, especially if there is a respected member who is skilled in group work. This is not a psychotherapy session but rather an opportunity to test reality and remove tension before it is incorrectly directed toward fellow staff members. These sessions can make use of the four elements of crisis intervention mentioned in the previous section, as well as information from Combs and others.[18] Other times that this stress reduction can be achieved is in supervision or during coffee breaks, as long as the sessions are productive.

The staff can use these sessions to better understand their reactions to stress and to explore their coping styles.[62,106] Ideally this knowledge of coping styles and stress reduction will decrease staff burnout as well as aid the staff to help clients and their families deal with stress more successfully. Industry has started using groups of this nature to increase productivity,[15] and these groups have been used in the mental health field to increase adjustment for the client and staff.[60]

The need to have a staff that is supportive is of paramount importance, because the attitude of rehabilitation personnel has emerged as one of the chief motivating factors in rehabilitation.[54] Rogers and Figone[90] developed several suggestions that the therapist could benefit from when trying to create a supportive environment:

1. It is helpful to use the same staff member to develop the relationship and to provide continuity of care.
2. Concerned silence is most appreciated, although pushing is sometimes necessary.

3. Staff members should anticipate the need to repeat information graciously.
4. Cumbersome and hard to repair adaptive equipment should not be used after discharge.
5. Give the client responsibility so that he feels he has some control over therapy.
   a. The client should be allowed to pick his or her own advocate from the team.
   b. The client should be given a choice of activities (e.g., which exercise comes first).
   c. Professionals should avoid placing the client in an inferior status. In time the client starts thinking this way (feeling like a second-class citizen).
6. Psychological support was attributed to noncounseling personnel—personal matters were better discussed with staff members with whom the client had developed a relationship.[79]
7. Willingness to allow the client to try and fail was more helpful than controlling the client.

CONCEPTUALIZATION OF ASSESSMENT AND TREATMENT
Assessment

The one component that weaves through all of Rogers and Figone's[90] seven points is the need for the therapist to be involved with the client in a therapeutic relationship, that is, to know where the client is "coming from." To know where the client is "coming from" is to be aware of and sensitive to the person's total psychosocial frame of reference.

The therapist who knows her own beliefs, reference points, and prejudices can evaluate whether an assessment result or treatment sequence reflects the client's needs and values or those of the therapist. In the first half of this chapter, several assessments were discussed that could be summarized into the following three major components:

1. Preinjury
   a. Values and prejudices (value systems, culture, and prejudgments) of the client and family members before the injury
   b. Developmental stage of the client and family members
   c. Cognitive level of the client and family members
   d. Ability of the client and family members to handle crisis
2. Components to be evaluated leading to adjustment
   a. Loss and grief process for the client and family members
   b. Adjustment process for the client and family members
   c. Transitional stages for the client and family members
   d. Role changes for the client and family members
   e. Age-cognitive level of client and family members
   f. Sexual adjustment for the client and spouse
3. Techniques used to elicit adjustment and independence
   a. Crisis intervention strategies
   b. Letting client and family take control
   c. Expression of emotion—both verbally and nonverbally
   d. Problem solving
   e. Role playing
   f. Praise
   g. Education
   h. Support groups

Once an assessment has been made of the client and family member's stages of psychological adjustment as well as of their preinjury attitudes and beliefs, a treatment protocol can be established. This protocol will need to incorporate steps toward stage change and possibly attitudinal change. Because these changes require learning on the part of the client and family, an environment that optimally facilitates these changes must be established.

Therapy can be seen as a form of education in which the client and the client's family are taught how the client should use his or her body. The education process is not limited to the physical aspects of therapy, however. The client is also taught how to look at and think about the body and the disability. If the staff is nonverbally telling the client and the family that the client is not capable of making decisions and of being independent, it follows that the client may indeed feel dependent and incapable of making decisions. Jellinek and others[56] stated that there was an inverse relationship between independence and distress. Distress causes further anxiety and decreases the learning potential of the client. There are ways, however, for the therapist to encourage independence on the part of the client and his family.

Treatment

Problem-solving process—independence. The family unit, including the client, should be encouraged to take active control over as much as possible of the client's care and decision making. This can be done in every phase of the rehabilitation process. A family conference with the rehabilitation staff should actively involve the client and family in all stages of planning and treatment up to and including discharge. The family (including the client) should be briefed ahead of time to prepare questions that they want answered or problems that need to be addressed. Rogers and Figone[90] report that conferences with family members that excluded the client engendered suspicion[6,103]; therefore, if the client is capable, the client may educate the family in regard to what is happening in the hospital and in rehabilitation. Conversely, family involvement has been found to facilitate and shorten the rehabilitation process.* Balcher and others[6] found that family rehabilitation planning resulted in 75% improvement, whereas lack of family involvement resulted in only 26% improvement. The family can also be educated regarding the side effects and interactions of medication with publications like the Physician's Desk Reference.[5] Later in the rehabilitation process the client and family can be encouraged to arrange transportation services, find and evaluate housing, and supervise attendent care. All of these activities allow the client and the family to be more in control of the environment and, thus, to feel independent.

In the context of one-to-one therapy, client responsibility and independence can be fostered by giving choices. Making decisions about the order of treatment activities (such as in which direction to roll first) can give the individual a sense of self-worth that can continue to grow. This should lead the client and family toward believing that they are strong, with rights that need to be met. Moving out of the role of the victim, the client begins to exercise responsibility and to take action, such as applying for extended health benefits or getting a second consultation when an important medical decision needs to be made. If the client and family start to realize that they do not have to be a casualty of the medical establishment and if they find ways to control the medical establishment,[110] they are better able to discard the role of victim.

In some centers, such as Ralph K. Davies in San Francisco, the client is even taught the art of self-defense to make sure that the client never has to fall into the victim (dependent) role. It should be noted, however, that this knowledge on the part of the client and family can be used in ways that the therapist may not always agree with. At such times it may help to adopt a philosophical attitude toward the situation and to view it as a positive direction for the client in terms of moving from victim to advocate in the rehabilitation process.

The steps of crisis intervention, which were mentioned in the previous section, can be used to help the family understand and analyze their needs in the crisis situation. Once the family has discovered that they are in crisis, they will then be able to create stategies that they can use to overcome present and future problems.

Problem solving is another element the therapist may use to help the client and family gain independence and control. Rather than having the client routinely learn how to accomplish a specific task, the client or family should be encouraged to think through the process, from the problem, to the solution, and to accomplishment of the task. To achieve this activity analysis, the client would have to know the basic principles behind the activity[90] and may then be responsible for educating the family. An example of this would be a transfer from the wheelchair to the toilet. If the therapist simply has the client memorize the

steps in the task, the client or family members will not necessarily be able to generalize this procedure to a transfer to the car. If the client learns the principles of proper body mechanics, work simplification, and movement, the client or family member may be able to generalize this information to almost any situation and to solve problems later when the therapist is unavailable. Rogers and Figone[90] have noted that even though the client and family may fail at times during these trials, the therapist should let them be as independent and responsible as possible: let them try it their way, even if they fail the first time.

Pictures or slides of a restaurant, movie theatre, or public building can be used to facilitate discussion and problem solving by the family unit when analyzing potential architectural barriers in the environment. Thus, in the future, when the family is presented with a problem or a barrier, they will have the resources to overcome it rather than be devastated by it. Chapter 30 has other examples of how social outings can be used to accomplish therapeutic goals.

Role playing can also be used to defuse potentially painful situations and operate independently. While still in the safe environment of the rehabilitation setting, simulations of incidents can be created for the family and client to practice problem solving with supervision. They can be asked what they would do when a stranger (possibly a child) approaches the client and asks why he is in a wheelchair or is disabled or what they would do when a waiter asks the family member to order for the disabled client. All of these situations are potentially devastating for all involved; however, if role playing is used in advance to help all members of the family (client included) to satisfactorily handle and feel in control of the situation, the family will not be as likely to be traumatized by a similar occurrence. The result is that the family will not be as inclined to be overwhelmed by social situations and will be able to socialize in a much freer, more gratifying way.[107]

Throughout the therapeutic process the client and the family need to be praised frequently, and credit needs to be given for the gains made by the client and family members. Granted, the therapist may have engineered the gains, but the family and client are the ones who need the reinforcement. Through gratifying experiences the family will unite to overcome the disability. They need to know that they can survive in the world without having the medical staff constantly there to solve the family's problems. In short, they need the strategies and resources that will allow them to be independent outside the medical model.

Yet another way to encourage independence can be applied to working with parents of disabled children.[28] The parents should be educated about normal and abnormal growth and development,[72] including physical, cognitive, and emotional growth,[41] so that the family can maintain some perspective and objectivity about their child's various levels. The parents can then better understand the needs of the disabled and nondisabled children in the family. Armed with this knowledge, the parents and children will not be frustrated with unreal expectations or unreal demands. Education of the parents could take place at local colleges, the hospital, or even in a parent's group.

Support systems. Groups are often used to increase motivation, provide support, increase social skills, instill hope, and help the client and family realize that they are not the only ones who have a disabled family member. This will help the client and family establish a more accurate set of perceptions about the disabled individual and allow for greater independence of the client and family. Problem solving can be encouraged and value systems can be clarified. Client and/or family support groups can be used to relieve pressure that might otherwise be vented in therapy. Goodell[39] found that in a chronic-care ward family involvement helped the client and the family improve their status. Smith[102] used support groups to teach women the use of transactional analysis (TA) to help them deal with husbands who had had strokes. She found that transactional analysis helped the family deal with situational change. Support groups can also be used to educate the client about the client's disability in order to increase independence. Smits[103] found that independent physical functioning and knowledge about one's condition were exceedingly important in moving through the phases of the rehabilitation process. A guide to facilitating support groups has been published by Boreing and Adler,[11] and it has been found to be useful, especially by lay people establishing such groups.

Establishment of self-worth and accurate body image. Self-worth is composed of many aspects, such as body image, sexuality, and the ability to help others and to affect the environment. The body image of a client is a composite of past and present experiences and of the individual's perception of those experiences. Because body image is based on experience, it is a constantly changing concept. An adult's body image is substantially different from that which he or she held as a child and will no doubt change again as the aging process continues. A newly disabled person is suddenly exposed to a radically new body, and it is that individual's job to assess the body's sensations and capabilities and develop a new body image. Because the therapist is at least partially responsible for creating the environmental experiences from which the client learns about this new body, he or she should be aware of the concept. In the case of an acute injury, the client has a new body from which to learn. The therapist can promote positive feelings as he or she instructs the client how to use this new body and to accept its changes.

Because in "normal" life we slowly observe changes in our bodies, such as finding one gray hair today and watching it take years for our hair to turn totally white, we have the luxury of slowly adapting to the "new me." This usu-

ally does not happen quite so slowly and "naturally" with a disability. This sudden loss of function creates a void that only new experiences and new role models can fill.

The loss of use of body parts can cause a person to perceive the body as an "enemy" that needs to be forced to work or to compensate for its disability. In all cases the body is the reason for the disability and the cause of all problems. The need for appliances can create a sense of alienation and lack of perceived "lovability" resulting from the "hardness of the hardware." People tend to avoid hugging someone who is in a wheelchair or who has braces around the body, because of the physical barrier and because of the person's perceived fragility;[74] the disabled person is certainly not perceived as soft and cuddly.[13,69,74] Both the perception that they are not lovable and their labored movements can sap the energy of the disabled for social interaction. To accept the appliances and the dysfunctional body in a way that also allows the disabled person to feel sexy and sensual is surely a major challenge.

In the case of a chronically disabled person, the therapist is attempting to teach the client how to change the previously accepted body image to one that would allow and encourage more normal function. In short, the therapist has two roles. One role is to take away the disabled body image of the chronically disabled person, such as the person with cerebral palsy or Parkinson's disease. The second is the opposite sequence, that is, to teach a disabled body image to a newly disabled person. The techniques may be the same, but in both cases the client will have to undergo a great amount of change. The chronically ill person has based his or her life on the concept that the reason for not accomplishing many things was the disability. If the therapist can change the client's ability level, the individual must now change self-expectations. The newly disabled person must now change expectations also; however, he or she has little concept of what is realistic to expect of this new body. At this point, role models can be used to help shape the client's expectations. If the client does not adjust to this new body and change his or her body image and self-expectations, life will be impoverished for that individual.[78] Pedretti[85] states that the client with low self-esteem often devalues his or her whole life in all respects, not just in the area of dysfunction.

One way the client can start exploring this new body is by exploring it for sensation and performance. The male client with a spinal cord injury may touch the whole body to see how it reacts.[98] For example, is there a way to get the legs to move using reflexes? What, if anything, stimulates an erection? Can positioning the legs in a certain way aid in rolling or make spasms decrease? Such exploration will start the client on the road to an informed evaluation of his abilities.

The therapist's role is to promote expansion of the client's realistic perceptions of body functioning. Exercises can be developed that encourage bodily exploration by the individual and, if appropriate, the significant other. Functioning and building an appropriate body image will be more difficult if intimate knowledge of the new body is not as complete as it was before injury.[25] Books on body massage or exercises, similar to those found in *Your Child's Sensory World*,[66] can be used to establish such programs. The successes the client experiences in the clinical setting coupled with the client's familiarity with his or her new body will result in a more accurate body image and will contribute to the client's feelings of self-worth.

As mentioned earlier in this chapter, sexuality and sensuality have an enormous impact on how the person feels about his or her adequacy and self-worth.[23] Societal members often evaluate each other on appearance and sensuality (or sexual attractiveness) and may avoid those who are perceived to have deficits.[10,104] Sensuality and sexuality are some of the major ways that humans express their intimate beings, and in Western society, the expression of the physical intimacy is closely associated with love. Thus if a client perceives himself incapable of expressing sensuality or sexuality, the individual may see himself as incapable of loving and being loved.[1] Because love and acceptance are primary driving forces in a human's life,[87] the inability to perceive the self as capable of loving would be devastating.

The last aspect of self-worth to be mentioned here is often overlooked in the health fields: it is the need that people have to help others.[36] People often discover that they are valuable through the act of giving. Self worth is increased by seeing others enjoy and benefit from the individual's presence or offering. Situations in which the client's worth can be appreciated by others may be needed. Unless the client can contribute to others, he is in a relatively dependent role, with everyone else giving to him without the opportunity of giving back. Achieving independence and then reaching out to others, with therapeutic assistance if necessary, facilitates the individual's more rapid reintegration into society. The therapist should take every opportunity to allow the client to express his self-worth to others through helping.

The adult client with brain damage. The adult client with brain damage and the needs of the family will be specifically, yet briefly, examined here since brain damage affects the cognitive and emotional system of the client. When a person receives brain injury and is hospitalized, emotional support for the family (client included) is the primary need to be met initially. Pearson[84] feels that it is not the function of the support but the emotional tone of the support that is most important. The therapist should attempt to convey warmth and a caring attitude, especially during the family's initial contacts. Typical complaints about the acute period involve impersonal hospital routines and lack of definite information about the patient's status.[71] Unfortunately, definite information is usually not available at the earliest stages.

Later, the family must deal with the physical changes in the client's body; what may be even more injurious to the family is the psychological, cognitive, and social changes in the client.[6,9,12,29,61] People with cerebral vascular accidents have been found to be more clinically depressed than orthopaedic patients.[29] The libido[9,30] and emotional systems[34] have also been shown to be affected.[30,31] It has further been shown that persons who survive a cerebrovascular accident and who have a full return of function do not return to normal life because of a lack of social and emotional skills.[61] Families of CVA victims have also reported that social reinterpretation is the most difficult phase of rehabilitation.[12,61] Lack of socially appropriate behaviors has been one of the most troublesome complaints of people who deal with the person with chronic brain injury.[6,12,31,61] Therapists may be able to help alter this syndrome by encouraging appropriate behavior and by structuring therapy situations to reteach the client interaction skills. A technique called structured learning therapy[22,38,42,43] has been used with schizophrenics, and although this approach has not been used by enough clinics to judge its effectiveness completely, it appears to be a promising approach.

Better follow-up care needs to be implemented when dealing with the adult with brain damage.[2] It may not be possible for the client and family to constantly come to the clinic for support and follow-up, but telephone conversations can be scheduled on a periodic basis, or the exchange of letters or audiotapes can also be used. With the increased availability of video recorders, the day may come when a follow-up may be done on videotapes sent by clients living in rural areas. Support groups, such as the family survival projects in northern California, are attempting to create an environment to facilitate growth for families who have a member who has chronic brain damage.

CONCLUSION
Clinical example: putting evaluations and techniques into practice

Joan, a married 30-year-old woman, has suffered a T2 spinal cord injury. She has worked as a computer programmer for the past 8 years, except for a short maternity leave when she gave birth to her daughter, who is now 6 years old. Joan was always very active physically and often stated that she felt sorry for her physically disabled neighbor because the neighbor could not hike, be active, or enjoy the outdoors. Joan's husband, age 33, is attempting to visit Joan regularly and care for their daughter, a role that is new for him.

The therapist has assessed several things regarding Joan's developmental stage, adjustment stage, social/cultural influences, and family adjustment reactions. The two adult family members are probably in Sheehy's[10] "catch-30" stage, in which the person reevaluates his or her life and relationships. Joan already "knows" that the physically disabled cannot enjoy a physically active life and is also feeling that everything she has worked for in her career is lost. She appears to be in the mourning stage of adjustment. Her daughter and husband are having to adjust to radical role changes. Cognitively, Joan's young daughter is not going to understand the permanence of the disability and may be inclined to act out as the result of the turmoil. The husband will have to be assessed to determine his stage of adjustment to her disability.

The therapist has determined that Joan's transfers need further work but would like to use the adaptive process to stimulate adjustment. The therapist has devised a treatment session to meet the goals of promoting the defense stage of adjustment, decreasing her prejudice against the disabled, encouraging problem solving, increasing her feelings of self-worth, proving to her that she can take care of her daughter through interacting with children, as well as having her decenter her focus from her disability to her ability. The therapist has contacted the recreational therapist (RT) (who is a paraplegic) to plan a collaborative session at the park across the street from the hospital. Because the RT works in the pediatrics ward, it is determined that the children with spina bifida should come and play tag transferring from log to log in the playground. The stage is now set. Joan will be asked to help supervise the children. The adaptive process will be used to teach Joan how to transfer using the environment. The transfer will be organized subcortically because she will be attending cortically to the children's needs and to the game itself. Joan will be actively affecting her personal environment, and if everything goes well, the act of helping the children will increase her self-worth and will also be self-reinforcing. Within this treatment session, the therapist has used the RT as a role model to change Joan's prejudice against the disabled being active in the outdoors as well as to show Joan that she can still be a parent even though she is disabled. The therapist may also increase Joan's knowledge of how to interact with children from a wheelchair by giving a few hints and then having Joan transfer up a set of stairs to reach one of the children. If we want to carry this fantasy further, the therapist could introduce Joan to a child who is interested in computers and who needs help with a programming problem (Joan's computer background will be used, which will increase Joan's feelings of self-worth and help her focus on her abilities rather than her disabilities). On the way back to the ward, the therapist and Joan may discuss how the family is dealing with the crisis they are in and help her realize how the family has made it through other crises in the past and how those previously successful strategies could be used in this situation. Support groups may be mentioned as resources. The session may end with Joan planning the next therapy session and thus starting to take control of her life.

REFERENCES

1. Anderson TP and Cole T: Sexual counseling of the physically disabled, Postgrad Med 58:117, 1975.
2. Anderson TP and others: Stroke rehabilitation: evaluation of its quality by assessing patient outcomes, Arch Phys Med Rehabil 59:170, 1978.
3. Annon J: The use of vicarious learning in the treatment of sexual concerns. In Lo Piccolo J and Lo Piccolo L, editors: Handbook of sex therapy, New York, 1978, Plenum Publishing Corp.
4. Askwith J: The role of social work in enhancing the sexuality of the physicaly handicapped, J Soc Work Hum Sex 1(3):83, 1983.
5. Baker EJ: Physicians desk reference, ed 36, Oradell NJ, 1982, Medical Economics Books.
6. Balcher SA and others: Independent living needs of postdischarge stroke persons: a pilot study, Arch Phys Med Rehabil 59:404, 1978.
7. Barnard MU and others: Human sexuality for health professionals, Philadelphia, 1978, WB Saunders Co.
8. Bentovim A: Emotional disturbances of handicapped pre-school children and their families—attitudes to the child, Br Med J 3:579, 1972.
9. Berrol S: Issues of sexuality in head injured adults in sexuality and physical disability. In Bullard DG and Knight DE, editors: Sexuality and physical disability, St Louis, 1981, The CV Mosby Co.
10. Bogle JE and Shaul SL: Body image and the woman with a disability. In Bullard DG and Knight DE, editors: Sexuality and physical disability, St Louis, 1981, The CV Mosby Co.
11. Boreing ML and Adler LM: Facilitating support groups: an instructional guide—Educational Monograph No 3, San Francisco, 1982, Dept of Psychiatry, Pacific Medical Center.
12. Brammer LM and Abrego PJ: Intervention strategies for coping with transitions, Counsel Psychol 9(2):19, 1981.
13. Bullard DG and Knight SE: Sexuality and physical disability, St Louis, 1981, The CV Mosby Co.
14. Capell B and Capell J: Being parents of children who are disabled. In Bullard DG and Knight SE: Sexuality and physical disability, St Louis, 1981, The CV Mosby Co.
15. Capra F: The turning point, New York, 1982, Simon & Schuster, Inc.
16. Carpenter JO: Changing roles and disagreement in families with disabled husbands, Arch Phys Med Rehabil 55:272, 1974.
17. Cole TM: Training for professionals in the sexuality of the physically disabled. In Pearsall FP and Rosenweig N, editors: Sex education for health professional, New York, 1983, Grune & Stratton, Inc.
18. Combs AW and others: Helping relationships, Boston, 1971, Allyn & Bacon, Inc.
19. Cornelius DA and others: Who cares?, Baltimore, 1982, University Park Press.
20. Craven J and Wald FS: Hospice care for dying patients, Am J Nurs 75:1816, 1975.
21. Daniels SM: Critical issues in sexuality and disability. In Bullard DG and Knight SE editors: Sexuality and physical disability, St. Louis, 1981, The CV Mosby Co.
22. Davis RE: Family of physically disabled children: family reactions and deductive reasoning, NY State J Med 75:1039, 1975.
23. Diamond M: Sexuality and the handicapped, Rehab Ret 35:34, 1974.
24. Dunton HD: The child's concept of death. In Schoenberg B and others: Loss and grief: psychological management in medical practice, New York, 1970, Columbia University Press.
25. Eisenberg MG and others: Sex and spinal cord injured: some questions and answers, Washington, DC, 1974, US Government Printing Office.
26. Fassler J: Helping children cope, New York, 1978, The Free Press.

27. Fink S: Crisis and motivation: a theoretical model, Arch Phys Med Rehabil 48:592, 1967.
28. Finnie NR: Handling the young cerebral palsied child at home, ed 2, New York, 1974, EP Dutton, Inc.
29. Folstein MF and others: Mood disorder as a specific complication of stroke, Neur Neurosurg Psychiatry 40:1018, 1977.
30. Ford A and Oriter A: Sexual behavior and chronically ill patient, Med Aspects Hum Sex 1:51, 1967.
31. Fowler RS: Stroke and cerebral trauma. In Stolov WC and Clowers MR, editors: Handbook of severe disability, Washington, DC, 1981, US Gov Printing Office.
32. Furman RA: The child's reaction to death in the family. In Schoenberg B and others: New York, 1970, Columbia University Press.
33. Gadpaille WJ: The cycles of sex, New York, 1975, Charles Scribner's Sons.
34. Gainotti G: Emotional behavior and hemispheric side of the lesion, Cortex 8:41, 1972.
35. Garner J: Palliative care: it's the quality of life remaining that matters, Can Med Assoc J 115:179, July 1976.
36. Geis HJ: The problem of personal worth in the physically disabled patient, Rehabil Lit 33(2):34, 1972.
37. Goldberg RT: Toward an understanding of the rehabilitation of the disabled adolescent, Rehabil Lit 42(3-4):66, 1981.
38. Goldstein AP and others: Skill training for the community living, New York, 1976, Pergamon Press Inc.
39. Goodell GE: Rehabilitation: family involved in patient's care, Hospitals 49:96, 1975.
40. Gould R: Transformations: growth and change in adult life, New York, 1978, Simon & Schuster Inc.
41. Greenfield PM and Tronick E: Infant curriculum, Santa Monica, 1980, Goodyear Publishing Co.
42. Gutride ME and others: The use of modeling and role playing to increase social interaction among schizophrenic patients, J Consult Clin Psych 40:408, 1973.
43. Gutride ME and others: The use of learning therapy with transfer training for chronic inpatients, J Clin Psych 30(3):277, 1974.
44. Hahn H: The social component of sexuality and disability: some problems and proposals, Sexuality and Disability 4(4):220, 1981.
45. Hall ET: The hidden dimension, Garden City, NJ, 1966, Doubleday Anchor Books.
46. Hamachek DE: Encounters with the self, New York, 1971, Holt, Rinehart & Winston.
47. Hammond DC: Cross-cultural rehabilitation. In Stublins J, editor: Social and psychological aspects of disability, Baltimore, 1977, University Park Press.
48. Hite S: The Hite report on female sexuality, New York, 1976, Dell Publishing Co, Inc.
49. Hite S: The Hite report on male sexuality, New York, 1981, Random House, Inc.
50. Holmes TH: Schedule of recent experience, Seattle, 1976, University of Washington School of Medicine.
51. Jellinek HM and others: Functional abilities and distress levels brain injured patients at long term follow up, Arch Phys Med Rehabil 63:160, 1982.
52. Kerr N: Understanding the process of adjustment to disability, J Rehabil 27(6):16, 1961.
53. Kerr N: Understanding the process of adjustment to disability. In Stubbins J, editor: Social and psychological aspects of disability, Baltimore, 1977, University Park Press.
54. Kerr N: Staff expectations for disabled persons. In Stubbins J, editor: Social and psychological aspects of disability, Baltimore, 1977, University Park Press.
55. King LJ: Toward a science of adaptive responses, Am J Occup Ther 32(7):429, 1978.
56. Klaus MH and Kennell JH: Maternal-infant bonding, ed 2 St Louis, 1982, The CV Mosby Co.
57. Kriegsman KH, and Celotta B: Sexuality in creative coping groups for women with physical disabilities, Sexuality and Disability 4(3):169, 1981.
58. Krueger DW: Rehabilitation psychology, Rockville, Md, 1984, Aspen Systems Corp.
59. Kübler-Ross E: On death and dying, New York, 1969, Macmillan Publishing Co.
60. Kutner G: Milue Therapy, J Rehabil 34(2):14, 1968.
61. Labi M and others: Psychosocial disability in physically restored long-term stroke survivors, Arch Phys Med Rehabil 61:561, 1980.
62. Lamb HR: Staff burnout in work with long-term patients, Hosp Community Psychiatry 30(6):396, 1979.
63. Lassiter RA: Work evaluation and work adjustment for severely handicapped people: a counseling approach, Int J Adv Couns 5(3):183, 1982.
64. Lewis SC: The mature years, Thorofare, NJ, 1979, Charles B Slack, Inc.
65. Lezak MD: Living with the characterologically, altered brain-injured patient, J Clin Psychiatry 39:592, 1978.
66. Liepmann L: Your child's sensory world, New York, 1973, Dial Press.
67. Lindner H: Perceptual sensitization to sexual phenomena in the chronic physically handicapped, J Clin Psychol 9:67, 1953.
68. Livneh H: A unified approach to existing models of adaption to disability, J Appl Rehabil Counsel 17(2):6, 1986.
69. Marinelli RP and Dell Orto AE: The psychological and social impact of physical disability, New York, 1984, Springer Publishing Co, Inc.
70. Maslow A: Motivation and personality, ed 2, New York, 1970, Harper & Row Publishers, Inc.
71. McCormick GP and Williams M: Stroke: the double crisis, Am J Nurs 78:1410, Aug. 1979.
72. McDaniel JS: Physical disability and human behavior, New York, 1969, Pergamon Press, Inc.
73. McKown JM and English BA: Disabled teenagers: sexual identification and sexuality counseling, Sexuality and Disability 7(12):17, 1984.
74. Mims FH and Swenson M: Sexuality: a nursing perspective, New York, 1980, McGraw-Hill Book Co.
75. Mitchell RG: Chronic handicap in childhood, its implications for family and community, Practitioner 211:763, 1973.
76. Mooney TO and others: Sexual options for paraplegics and quadriplegics, Boston, 1975, Little, Brown and Co.
77. Moore ML: Newborn family and nurse, ed 2, Philadelphia, 1981, WB Saunders Co.
78. Moos RH and Tsu VD: The crisis of physical illness. In Moos RH, editor: Coping with physical illness, New York, 1977, Plenum Medical Book Co.
79. Morgan ED and others: Psychological rehabilitation in UA spinal cord injury centers, Rehabil Psychol 21:3, 1974.
80. Mueller AD: Psychologic factors in rehabilitation of paraplegic patients, Arch Phys Med Rehabil 43(4):151, 1962.
81. Nagy M: The child's view of death. In Feifel H, editor: The meaning of death, New York, 1969, McGraw-Hill Book Co.
82. Nau L: Why not family rehabilitation? Rehabilitation 39(3):14, 1973.
83. Nowinski JK and Ayers T: Sexuality and major medical conditions: In Bullard DG and Knight SE, editors: Sexuality and physical disability, St Louis, 1981, The CV Mosby Co.
84. Pearson R: Support: exploration of a basic dimension of informal help and counseling, Personnel Guidance J 61(2):83, 1982.
85. Pedretti LW: Occupational therapy: practice skills for physical dysfunction, ed. 3 St Louis, 1989, The CV Mosby Co.

86. Peretz D: Reaction to loss. In Schoenberg B and others, editors: Loss and grief, New York, 1970, Columbia University Press.

87. Poznanski EO: Emotional issues in raising handicapped children, Rehabil Lit 34:322, 1973.

88. Rae WA: Body image of children and adolescents during physical illness and hospitalization, Psychiatr Ann 12(12):1065, 1982.

89. Rodrigue RR: Psychological crises of the ill and handicapped, Emotional First Aid 2(1):44, 1985.

90. Rogers JD and Figone JJ: Psychosocial parameters in treating the person with quadriplegia, Am J Occup Ther 33(7):432, 1979.

91. Rose MH: The concepts of coping and vulnerability as applied to children with chronic conditions, Issues in Comprehensive Pediatric Nursing 7(4-5):177, 1984.

92. Safilios-Rothschild C: The sociology and social psychology of disability and rehabilitation, New York, 1970, Random House, Inc.

93. Sanchez V: Relevance of cultural values: for occupational therapy programs, Am J Occup Ther 28(1):1, 1964.

94. Satir V: Peoplemaking, Palo Alto, 1972, Science & Behavior Books.

95. Schoenberg B and others: Loss and grief, New York, 1970, Columbia University Press.

96. Schowalter JE: The child's reaction to his own terminal illness. In Schoenberg B and others, editors: Loss and grief, New York 1970, Columbia University Press.

97. Schwab LO: Rehabilitation of physically disabled women in a family-oriented program, Rehabil Lit 36:34, 1975.

98. Sheehy G: Passages, New York, 1976, EP Dutton, Inc.

99. Shontz FC: Reactions of crisis, Volta Rev 67:364, 1965.

100. Simon JI: Emotional aspects of physical disability, Am J Occup Ther 25(8):408, 1971.

101. Simon SB and others; Values clarification, New York, 1972, Hart Publishing Co.

102. Smith CW: Releasing pressure caps: using TA with women whose husbands have strokes, Trans Analysis J 7:55, 1977.

103. Smits SJ: Variables related to success in a medical rehabilitation setting, Arch Phys Med Rehabil 55:449, 1974.

104. Snyder M and others: Avoidance of the handicapped: an attitude ambiguity analysis, J Personal Social Psych 37:2297, 1979.

105. Solnit AJ and Green M: The pediatric management of the dying child. In Solnit A and Provence S, editors: Modern perspectives in child development, New York, 1963, International Universities Press, Inc.

106. Stewart TD and Rossier AB: Psychological consideration in the adjustment to spinal cord injury, Rehabil Lit 39(3):75, 1978.

107. Trombly CA: Occupational therapy for physical dysfunction, ed 2, Baltimore, 1983, The Williams & Wilkins Co.

108. Verslys HP: Physical rehabilitation and family dynamics, Rehabil Lit 41(3-4):58, 1980.

109. Verwoerdt A and Elmore JL: Psychological reactions in fatal illness. I. The prospect of impending death, J Am Geriatr Soc 15:9, 1967.

110. Vickery DM and Fries JF: Take care of yourself: a consumers guide to medical care, 1976, Reading, Mass, Addison-Wesley Publishing Co, Inc.

111. Weiss AJ and Diamond MD: Sexual adjustment, identification, and attitudes of patients with myelopathy, Arch Phys Med Rehabil 47:245, 1966.

112. White W: The urge towards competence, Am J Occup Ther 26:(6)271, 1971.

113. Woods NF: Human sexuality in health and illness, ed 3 St Louis, 1984, The CV Mosby Co.

Part Two

MANAGEMENT OF CLINICAL PROBLEMS

Chapter 8

AT-RISK NEONATES AND INFANTS
NICU management and follow-up

Jane K. Sweeney and Marcia W. Swanson

Increasing numbers of regional neonatal intensive care units and high levels of technology in newborn medicine have contributed significantly to the decreased mortality and morbidity of preterm and other acutely ill neonates. Despite scientific and technological advances, 25% to 29% of infants requiring neonatal intensive care are estimated to be at *high risk* for neurological impairment or developmental delay.[123,186,188] Although the remaining 70% to 75% of infants discharged from intensive care nurseries are expected to be at low to medium developmental risk,

they still require careful developmental screening during medical follow-up in the outpatient phase. Pediatric therapists serve these increasing numbers of surviving neonates at developmental risk by: (1) offering valuable adjunctive diagnostic support in neurological and developmental assessment, (2) facilitating expedient interdisciplinary developmental case management for infants and parents, and (3) reinforcing the preventive aspects of health care by providing early intervention and long-term developmental monitoring.

This chapter focuses on at-risk infants and their parents during the clinical management phases of inpatient neonatal intensive care and outpatient monitoring. A theoretical framework for neonatal practice and an overview of neonatal neuropathology related to movement disorders are presented. In-depth discussion in the neonatal section includes indications for referral based on risk, neurological assessment instruments, high-risk profiles in the neonatal period, treatment planning, and therapy strategies in the neonatal intensive care unit (NICU). In the infant follow-up section discussion is focused on a service delivery model, neuromotor assessment, high-risk neuromotor markers in the first year of life, and selected intervention strategies.

THEORETICAL FRAMEWORK

Concepts of pathokinesiology, neonatal behavioral organization, and crisis intervention provide a theoretical framework for neonatal therapy practice. Synthesized from related literature and clinical problem solving, the theoretical models described below provide concepts to guide practitioners in the design and implementation of developmental intervention programs for at-risk infants and their parents.

Pathokinesiology model

Pathokinesiology, the science of abnormal human movement, has been described by Hislop[100] as the distinguishing clinical science of physical therapy. Applied to the neonatal population, a pathokinesiology model provides the practitioner with a framework for systematically analyzing the components of an infant's movement disorder from the cellular to the community level. Not limited to anatomical and physiological analyses, a pathokinesiological perspective also involves a hierarchy of biobehavioral components that outline the influence of neuromotor deficits on the person and the effect of a physically disabled child on the family and community.

A pathokinesiology hierarchy of spastic diplegia is illustrated in Fig. 8-1. The spastic diplegia hierarchy is adapted from Hislop's model and describes the category of cerebral palsy closely associated with a preterm birth. This paradigm presents a holistic biobehavioral framework for understanding the multiple components of a neonatal movement disorder.

Synactive model of infant behavior

The synactive model of infant behavioral organization is a major theoretical framework for establishing physio-logical stability as the foundation for the organization of motor, behavioral state, and attention/interactive behaviors in neonates. Als and others[3-5] described a "synactive" process of four subsystems interacting together as the neonate responds to the stresses of the extrauterine environment. They theorized that the basic subsystem of physiological organization must first be stabilized for the other subsystems to emerge and allow the infant to maintain behavioral state control and then interact positively with the environment (Fig. 8-2).

To evaluate infant behavior within the subsystems of function addressed in the synactive model, Als and others[5] developed the Assessment of Preterm Infant Behavior. With the development of this assessment instrument, a fifth subsystem of behavioral organization, self-regulation, was added to the synactive model. The self-regulation subsystem consists of physiological, motor, and behavioral state strategies used by the neonate to maintain balance within and between the subsystems.[124] For example, many preterm infants appear to regulate overstimulating environmental stimuli with a behavioral state strategy of withdrawing into a drowsy or light sleep state, thereby shutting out sensory input.

Fetters[78] placed the synactive model within a pathoki-

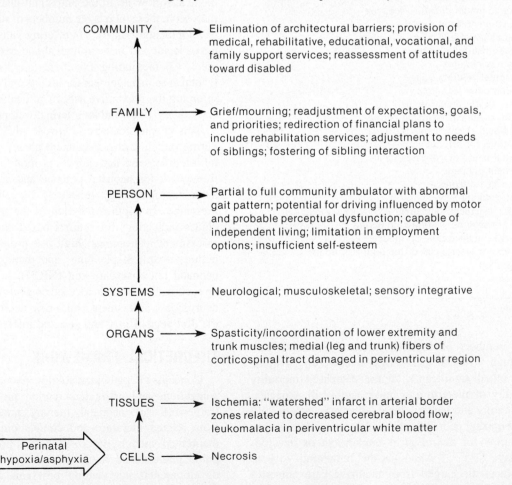

COMMUNITY → Elimination of architectural barriers; provision of medical, rehabilitative, educational, vocational, and family support services; reassessment of attitudes toward disabled

FAMILY → Grief/mourning; readjustment of expectations, goals, and priorities; redirection of financial plans to include rehabilitation services; adjustment to needs of siblings; fostering of sibling interaction

PERSON → Partial to full community ambulator with abnormal gait pattern; potential for driving influenced by motor and probable perceptual dysfunction; capable of independent living; limitation in employment options; insufficient self-esteem

SYSTEMS — Neurological; musculoskeletal; sensory integrative

ORGANS → Spasticity/incoordination of lower extremity and trunk muscles; medial (leg and trunk) fibers of corticospinal tract damaged in periventricular region

TISSUES → Ischemia: "watershed" infarct in arterial border zones related to decreased cerebral blood flow; leukomalacia in periventricular white matter

Perinatal hypoxia/asphyxia   CELLS → Necrosis

Fig. 8-1. Pathokinesiology hierarchy of spastic diplegia. (Adapted from Hislop HJ: The not-so-impossible dream, Phys Ther 55:1060, 1975.)

nesiology hierarchy to demonstrate the effect of a therapeutic intervention on an infant's multiple subsystems (Fig. 8-3). She explained that although a neonatal therapy intervention is offered to the infant at the level of the *person,* outcome is measured at the *systems* level where many subsystems may be affected. For example, the motor outcome from neonatal therapy procedures is frequently influenced by "synaction," or simultaneous effects, of an infant's physiological stability and behavioral state. Physiological state and behavioral state are therefore potential confounding variables during research on motor behavior in neonatal subjects. Neonatal therapists may find this combined pathokinesiology and synactive framework helpful in conceptualizing and assessing changes in infants' multiple subsystems from therapy procedures.

Hope-empowerment model

A major component of the intervention process in neonatal therapy is the interpersonal helping relationship with the family. A hope-empowerment framework (Fig. 8-4) may guide neonatal practitioners in building the therapeu-

tic partnership with parents, facilitating adaptive coping, and empowering them to participate in caregiving, problem solving, and advocacy. The birth or diagnosis of an at-risk or disabled infant may create both developmental and situational crises for the parents and the family system. The *developmental* crisis involves adaptation to changing roles in the transition to parenthood and in expansion of the family system. Although not occurring unexpectedly, this developmental transition for the parents brings life-style changes that may be stressful and cause conflict.[178]

A *situational* crisis occurs from unexpected external events presenting a sudden, overwhelming threat or loss for which previous coping strategies are either not applicable or are immobilized.[47,132] The unfamiliar, high-tech, often chaotic environment of the NICU creates many situational stresses that challenge parenting efforts and destabilize the family system. The language of the nursery is unfamiliar and intimidating. The sights of fragile, sick infants surrounded by medical equipment and the sounds of monitor alarms are frightening. The high frequency of seemingly uncomfortable but required medical procedures for the infant are of financial and humanistic concern to parents. No previous experiences in everyday life have prepared the parents for this unnatural, emergency-oriented environment.

The quality and orientation of the helping relationship in neonatal therapy affects the coping style of parents as they try to adapt to developmental and situational crises (Fig. 8-4). Although parents and neonatal therapists come into the partnership with established interactive styles and varying life and professional experiences, the initial contacts during assessment and program planning set the stage for either a positive or negative orientation to the relationship.

Despite many uncertainties about the clinical course, prognosis, and quality of social support, a positive orientation may be activated by validation or acknowledgment of parents' feelings and experiences. Validation then becomes a catalyst to a hope-empowerment process in which

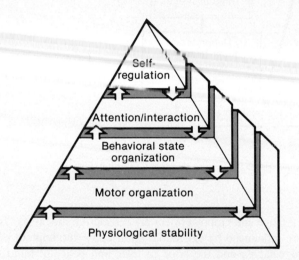

Fig. 8-2. Pyramid of synactive theory of infant behavioral organization with physiological stability at the foundation.

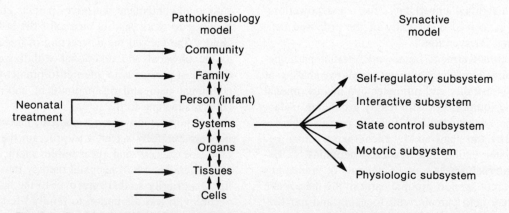

Fig. 8-3. Combined pathokinesiology and synactive models. (Adapted from Fetters L: Sensorimotor management of the high-risk neonate, Phys Occup Ther Pediatr 6(3/4):217, 1986.)

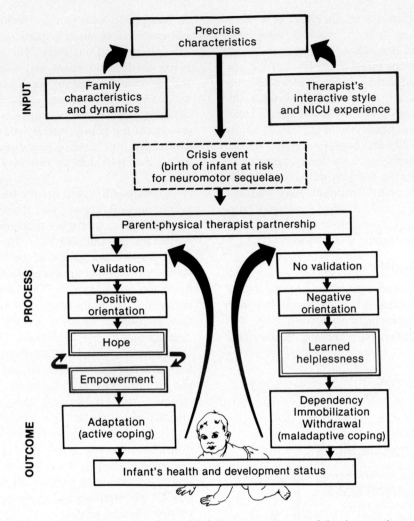

Fig. 8-4. Hope-empowerment versus learned helplessness processes of the therapeutic partnership between parents and neonatal therapist.

many crisis events, negative feelings, and insecurities are acknowledged in a positive, supportive, nonjudgemental context in which decision-making power is shared.[150] In contrast, a negative orientation may be facilitated by information overloading without exploration and validation of parents' feelings, experiences, and learning styles. This may lead to magnified uncertainty, fear, and powerlessness with the perceived complexity of the proposed neurodevelopmental intervention.

In a hope-empowerment framework, parent participation in neurodevelopmental intervention allows sharing of power and responsibility and promotes continuous, mutual setting and revision of goals with reality grounding. Adaptive power can be generated by helping parents stabilize and focus energy and plans and by encouraging active participation in intervention and advocacy activities.[150] Exploration of external power sources (Parents of Prematures or Parent-to-Parent support groups) early in the therapeutic relationship may help parents with focusing and mobilizing.[136]

Hope and empowerment are interactive processes. They are influenced by existential philosophy: the hope to adapt to what is, and the hope to later find peace-of-mind, regardless of the infant's outcome. In describing the effect of a prematurely born infant on the parenting process, Mercer[132] related that "hope seems to be a motivational, emotional component that gives parents energy to cope, to continue to work, and to strive for the best outcome for a child." She viewed the destruction of hope as contributing to the physical and emotional withdrawal observed frequently in parents who attempt to protect themselves from additional pain and disappointment and then have difficulty reattaching to the infant.

In a hope-empowerment context, parent teaching activities are carefully selected to program the parents and infants for success and pleasurable interaction. Integration and generalization of neonatal therapy into routine caregiving is a priority so that carryover to the home environment occurs with less disruption to family life-styles.

Conversely, if the parents' learning styles, goals, prior-

Table 8-1. Neuropathology of cerebral palsy

Category	Lesion	Event
Spastic diplegia	Periventricular leukomalacia involving medial fibers of the corticospinal tract	Ischemia
Spastic hemiplegia	Selective neuronal necrosis in cerebral cortex	Hypoxia
or	Parasaggital cerebral lesion	Ischemia
Spastic quadriplegia	Intraventricular hemorrhage	Increased perfusion
Ataxia	Selective neuronal necrosis in cerebellum	Hypoxia
Athetoid	Status marmoratus (hypermyelination) in basal ganglia	Brief, total asphyxia

ities, values, time constraints, energy levels, and emotional availability are not considered in the design of the developmental program, they are programmed for failure, destruction of self-esteem, powerlessness, immobilization, and dependency. Hopeless outlook, noncompliance, information overload, or negative interaction (power struggles) between infant and parent may be markers of an ineffective teaching style by the neonatal therapist, which can contribute to a learned helplessness outcome.[1]

New events in the infant's health or developmental status may create new crises and destabilize the coping processes.[55] In long term follow-up many opportunities occur within the partnership to validate new fears and chronic uncertainties within a hopeful, positively oriented helping relationship. The alleviation of hopelessness is a critical helping task in health care. This model provides a caring framework for sharing with parents the gifts of hope and power.

NEUROPATHOLOGY OF MOVEMENT DISORDERS

The pathogenesis of selected, major nonprogressive neurological deficits of spasticity, ataxia, and athetosis can be traced to hypoxic and/or ischemic insults. Four lesions have been associated with hypoxic-ischemic brain injury and are linked to the major categories of cerebral palsy.[53,99,219-221] The related neuropathology and neurological sequelae from these lesions are outlined in Table 8-1.

Selective neuronal necrosis

Selective neuronal necrosis is the random, widespread necrosis of neurons from a hypoxic-ischemic event in any of the following sites: the cerebellum (Purkinje cells, dentate nuclei), the deep layers of cerebral cortex including the hippocampus and brainstem (pons, medulla, oculomotor, troclear neurons), and the diencephalon (thalamus, hypothalamus, lateral geniculate body). Hypoxemia can result in an encephalopathy manifested by coma, hypotonia/proximal weakness of the upper extremities in full-term infants or of the lower extremities in preterm infants, seizures, and tremulous movement in a predictable pattern

during the first 72 hours following birth. The neurological sequelae associated with selective neuronal necrosis are related to the sites of necrosis and may include spastic hemiplegia, spastic quadriplegia, ataxia, deafness, seizures, or mental retardation. Only 20% to 30% of infants with both hypoxic-ischemic encephalopathy and seizures in the newborn period were neurologically intact at follow-up.[219] Computed tomography (CT) of the brain reveals moderate to marked cerebral atrophy.[102]

Status marmoratus

Status marmoratus refers to basal ganglia lesions in *full-term* infants resulting from acute, brief, total asphyxia. These lesions include neuronal loss and an overgrowth of myelin that causes a unique marbled appearance in the putamen, caudate, and thalamus. The primary neurological deficit associated with status marmoratus is choreoathetosis. This frequently appears in neonates as hypotonia until approximately 10 to 12 months of age, when athetoid cerebral palsy can be confirmed. Normal findings are usually present on the CT scan.[102]

Parasagittal cerebral injury

Parasagittal cerebral injury is the result of incompletely developed autoregulation of cerebral blood flow and the subsequent vulnerability of the brain of the newborn to fluctuations in blood pressure. Parasaggital injury is an ischemic insult in *full-term* infants resulting from generalized reduction in cerebral blood flow associated with intrauterine asphyxia and hypotension. Labeled the "watershed infarct," these lesions imitate a field irrigation system where the most distant section of the field may not get irrigated if the water force is suddenly reduced. The vulnerable "last field" in parasagittal injury is a result of a fall in pressure in the border zones between the "last fields" of the anterior, middle, or posterior cerebral arteries. This fall in blood pressure frequently occurs in a symmetrical distribution with cortical involvement of parietal, temporal, or occipital lobes. The neurological sequelae may include proximal weakness in the shoulder girdle more than in the pelvic girdle musculature during the neonatal period, perceptual dysfunction (particularly visual-motor), or mental retardation. Spastic hemiparesis or spastic quadriparesis may be present, depending on the topography of involvement of the motor cortex. CT scan data reveal cerebral atrophy from these lesions.[102]

Periventricular leukomalacia

Periventricular leukomalacia (PVL) refers to the "watershed infarct" in *premature* infants. This lesion results from a generalized reduction in cerebral blood flow in the periventricular white matter adjacent to the lateral ventricles. It is in this highly vulnerable periventricular region that the arterial "end-fields" of branches of the middle, posterior, and anterior cerebral arteries meet. Necrosis occurs if perfusion of blood flow is inadequate. The category of cerebral palsy closely associated with this ischemic lesion is spastic diplegia. Identified as the most common sensorimotor deficit in premature infants, spastic diplegia is clinically manifested by motor involvement of lower extremities more than upper extremities. Fig. 8-5 illustrates the neuroanatomical vulnerability of the medial (leg, trunk) corticospinal tract fibers from the motor cortex passing through the periventricular "end-field" to the legs.[158] CT analysis of this periventricular lesion may show an area of hemorrhage and dilated ventricles (Fig. 8-6). Bennett, and others[19] reported that premature infants who developed spastic diplegia had lower birth weights, smaller head circumferences, neurological depression with lower Apgar scores at 1 minute of age, and higher prevalence of intracranial hemorrhage and seizures than other preterm infants.

Areas of echodensity on cranial ultrasound are usually categorized according to their persistence, size, and location. A distinction is often made between transient echodensities, which resolve within 2 weeks, and "prolonged flare"—areas of echodensity that persist longer than 2 weeks but never evolve into cysts.[87] Periventricular leukomalacia generally refers to areas where cavitation or cysts have evolved, usually after 4 to 6 weeks.

The transient echodensities appear to be of no prognostic significance when the developmental outcome of affected infants is studied. In infants with prolonged flare, a low incidence (8%) of cerebral palsy has been reported and a relationship with later minor neuromotor abnormalities has been suggested.[87] The presence of cysts has been associated with cerebral palsy in 94% to 100% of the cases with the type and severity of cerebral palsy determined by the size and location of the lesions.[40,49,61,77] This strong relationship between cystic PVL and later cerebral palsy is an important finding relevant to high-risk infant follow-up and management. However, incidence of cystic PVL in the low-birth-weight population is reported to be only 2% to 4%.[40,86]

Intraventricular hemorrhage

In addition to the ischemic lesion of periventricular leukomalacia, the incidence of *intraventricular hemorrhage* (IVH) associated with preceeding perinatal asphyxia is

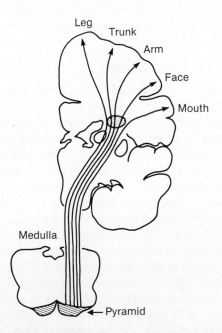

Fig. 8-5. Schematic diagram of corticospinal tract fibers that extend from the motor cortex through the periventricular region into the pyramid of the medulla.

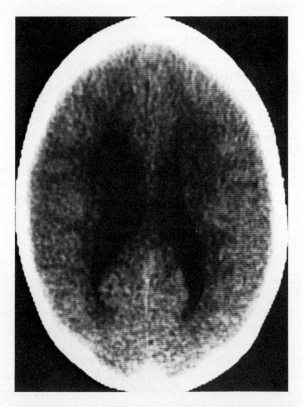

Fig. 8-6. CT findings of dilated ventricles from a child with spastic diplegia category of cerebral palsy.

high in the premature population. Papile and others[159] report that close to 50% of the infants with birth weights under 1500 g (3 lb 5 oz) showed intraventricular hemorrhages on CT scan. The thin-walled vasculature in the premature brain is fragile and poorly supported by the gelatinous subependymal germinal matrix in the periventricular region. This anatomic vulnerability and the impaired vascular autoregulation make the premature infant more susceptible to intraventricular hemorrhage if cerebral blood pressure is increased (as in resuscitation for asphyxia).[119,158,173,217,226]

The relationship between IVH and developmental outcome has been intensely investigated since the beginning of routine cranial ultrasound procedures for low-birth-weight infants. Attempts to compare the results of different studies have been complicated by the absence of a standard grading scale for these bleeds. The grading scale most commonly used is a four-level scale (Table 8-2).

When IVH in low-birth-weight infants is correlated with developmental outcome, the risk of major neurological handicap for infants with grades I and II bleeds is relatively low: often the degree of risk is not significantly different from that of infants with no IVH[137,160] (see Table 8-3). Infants with grade III have a significantly increased risk of major neurological impairment.

An infant with an identified grade IV intraventricular

hemorrhage can be considered at high risk for developing the neurological sequelae of hydrocephalus, mental retardation, deafness, seizure disorder, hemiplegia, or quadriplegia. Fig. 8-7 illustrates ventriculomegaly and hydrocephalus as a result of grade IV intraventricular hemorrhage.

The incidence of one or more major handicaps for infants with grade IV bleeds has been reported to be as high as 100%.[49,137] However, this has not been confirmed by a more recent investigation in which infants with periventricular leukomalacia were excluded from the study in an effort to evaluate the impact of the hemorrhage alone.[197]

CLINICAL MANAGEMENT: NEONATAL PERIOD

Pediatric therapists with precepted subspecialty training in neonatology and infant therapy can expand neonatal medicine efforts by creating clinical protocols designed to optimize the development and interaction of at-risk neonates and parents. The therapeutic partnership between parents and neonatal therapists during developmental intervention in the NICU sets the stage for competency in caregiving and compliance with follow-up in the outpatient period. General aims of NICU clinical management of infants at risk for neurological dysfunction, developmental delay, or orthopedic complications are to (1) promote normal movement experiences, (2) reduce active reinforcement of abnormal movement patterns and positions, (3)

Table 8-2. Grades of intraventricular hemorrhage (IVH)

Grade	Extent of hemorrhage
I	Hemorrhage confined to germinal matrix (no ventricular blood)
II	Intraventricular hemorrhage without ventricular distension
III	Intraventricular hemorrhage with ventricular dilation
IV	Intraventricular hemorrhage extending into brain parenchyma (hydrocephalus present)

Modified from Papile L and others: Relationship of cerebral intraventricular hemorrhage and early childhood neurologic handicaps, J Pediatr 103(2):273, 1983.

Table 8-3. Neurodevelopmental outcome of low-birth-weight (LBW) infants relative to intraventricular hemorrhage (IVH)[49,137,160,197]

Grade of hemorrhage	LBW infants with major handicap
No hemorrhage	7%–10%
Grade I	8%–25%
Grade II	10%–25%
Grade III	40%–67%
Grade IV	90%–100%

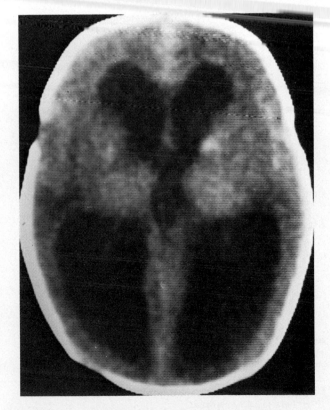

Fig. 8-7. CT findings of ventriculomegaly and hydrocephalus in an infant with a grade IV intraventricular hemorrhage.

decrease congenital musculoskeletal deformity and acquired joint-muscle contractures, (4) foster infant-parent attachment and interaction, (5) modify sensory stimulation in the infant's NICU environment to promote behavioral organization and physiological stability, (6) provide consultation or direct intervention for neonatal feeding dysfunction and oral-motor deficits, and (7) enhance parents' caregiving skills (feeding, dressing, bathing, positioning of infant for sleep, interaction/play, and transportation).

Educational requirements for therapists

Assessment and treatment of neonates are advanced-level, not entry-level, clinical competencies. Neonatology is a subspecialty within the specialty areas of pediatric physical therapy and pediatric occupational therapy. Campbell[45] advises that the development of a neonatal therapy program "requires specialized knowledge and skills in neonatal medicine, assessment of development in early infancy, early intervention, parent education, and interdisciplinary interaction in the specialized setting of the inten-

sive care nursery." She further describes the need for studying fetal development, neonatal physiology and pathophysiology, common neonatal medical conditions, nature and management of energy costs in preterm and at-risk full-term infants, parent-infant attachment and interaction and the ecology of the NICU.

No amount of literature review, self-study, or experience with other pediatric populations can substitute for clinical training with a preceptor in a NICU. The potential for causing harm to medically fragile infants during well-intentioned intervention is enormous.[163] The ongoing clinical decisions made by neonatal therapists in evaluating and managing physiological and musculoskeletal risk while handling small (2 or 3 lb), medically fragile infants in the NICU should not be a trial-and-error experience at the infants' expense. Therapists with adult-oriented training and even those with general pediatric training (excluding neonatal) are not qualified for neonatal practice without a supervised clinical practicum (usually 3 months duration). A position paper on advanced level competen-

Table 8-4. Prenatal, perinatal, and postnatal risk factors for neuromotor abnormalities

Study	Birth weight	Outcome age	Risk factors	
			High risk	Low risk
Pape (1978)	≤1000 g	2 years	Birth weight Acidemia ICH† Seizures	Asphyxia IRDS* Apnea Mechanical ventilation
Nelson and Ellenberg (1979)	All	7 years	Birth weight Microcephaly Low Apgar score: 5 and 10 minutes Seizures	Low Apgar score: 1 minute
Knobloch (1982)	≤1500 g	40 weeks	Birth weight Gestational age Low Apgar score: 5 minutes Seizures ICH† IRDS*	SGA‡ Head size
Bennett (1982)	≤2000 g	2 years	Birth weight Gestational age	IRDS*
Kraybill (1984)	≤1000 g	12-34 months	Mechanical ventilation	Birth weight Gestational age Low Apgar score SGA‡ Head size
Stanley (1986)	≤2000 g	6 years	Asphyxia score Low Apgar score: 1 minute	Birth weight Gestational age Low Apgar score: 5 minutes
Bull (1988)	≤1500 g	12-30 months	Mechanical ventilation BPD§ Meningitis	Birth weight Gestational age Low Apgar score

*IRDS; Idiopathic respiratory distress syndrome.
†ICH; Intracranial hemorrhage.
‡SGA; Small for gestational age.
§BPD; Bronchopulmonary dysplasia.

cies for the physical therapist in the NICU is available from the section on Pediatrics, American Physical Therapy Association.

Indications for referral

Research efforts in recent years have been directed toward determining which low-birth-weight infants will have a less-than-optimal outcome. One approach to this task has been the designation of risk factors: prenatal, perinatal, or neonatal conditions that are associated with infants considered to have a statistically higher chance of developing a neuromotor abnormality (Table 8-4). The studies in Table 8-4 represent different approaches to medical management at varying time periods and geographical sites. The risk criteria vary because of the absence of uniform definition and grading of conditions, differences in sample selection and follow-up procedures, and the absence of standard measures for neurodevelopmental outcome. Changes in obstetrical and neonatal procedures are occurring so rapidly that the findings from reported studies may not be completely relevant to developmental outcome from current practice.

Tjossem's categories[212] of biological, established, and social risk provide a logical framework for listing diagnoses and behavioral observations for neonatal therapy referral. A formal protocol for referral and clinical management validates the therapist as an integral part of the NICU team.[227] An overview of developmental risk categories and risk factors for neonatal therapy referral are listed in the box at right to assist clinicians in developing a referral mechanism for a clinical protocol based on risk categories.

Biological risk. Biological risk refers to developmental risk created by maturational or medically related complications in the prenatal, perinatal, or neonatal periods.[186,212] Biological risks may include fetoplacental abnormalities, labor/delivery complications, and teratogenic, iatrogenic, or physiological factors.

Birth weight has been found to be a strong predictor of outcome.[20,112,145] In general, the lower the birth weight, the greater the risk of a suboptimal neurodevelopmental outcome. This, however, is not a universal finding.[117,228] In some populations of very–low-birth-weight infants (1000-1500 g) or extremely low-birth-weight infants (less than 1000 g), the prevalence of cerebral palsy has been less than expected.[200] In one long-term follow-up study, birth weight was more predictive of the need for special education than for cerebral palsy.[218] Infants who were small for gestational age have been found to be at increased risk for cerebral palsy in some studies, whereas in others only the incidence of minor neurodevelopmental abnormalities is greater in these babies.[218]

Low Apgar scores, a measure of neonatal asphyxia, are a commonly used risk indicator.[25,83] Because Apgar scores also reflect the relative maturity and neurologic integrity of

the infant, low scores in preterm infants are not considered as reliable as those for full-term neonates.

Although the presence and severity of respiratory disease did not appear to be predictors of neurodevelopmental outcome in early studies,[20,157] recent comparisons of developmental status between ventilated and nonventilated infants showed that 80% of ventilated infants had developmental abnormalities.[117,177] In infants requiring ventilatory assistance, a relationship between duration of ventilatory assistance and outcome has been observed, with increased neurologic impairment associated with prolonged ventilatory assistance.[37]

Established risk. Established risk is the risk for neurodevelopmental deficits associated with a diagnosis easily established in the neonatal period. Included in this cate-

---

Developmental risk indicators for neonatal therapy referral

Biological risk

Birth weight of 1500 g or less
Gestational age of 32 weeks or less
Small for gestational age (less than 10th percentile for weight)
Ventilator requirement for 36 hours or more
Intracranial hemorrhage; grades III or IV
Muscle tone abnormalities (hypotonia, hypertonia, asymmetry of tone/movement)
Recurrent neonatal seizures (3 or more)
Feeding dysfunction
Symptomatic TORCH infections (toxoplasmosis, rubella, cytomegalovirus, herpes virus type II, syphilis)
Meningitis
Asphyxia with Apgar score less than 4 at 5 minutes

Established risk

Hydrocephalus
Microcephaly
Chromosomal abnormalities
Musculoskeletal abnormalities (congenitally dislocated hips, limb deficiencies, arthrogryposis, joint contractures, congenital torticollis)
Multiple births greater than twins
Brachial plexus injuries (Erb's palsy, Klumpke's paralysis)
Myelodysplasia
Congenital myopathies and myotonic dystrophy
Inborn errors of metabolism
HIV infection

Environmental/social risk

High–social risk (single parent, parental age less than 17 years, poor quality infant-parent attachment)
Maternal drug or alcohol abuse
Behavioral state abnormalities (lethargy, excessive irritability, behavioral state lability)

gory are congenital malformations, chromosomal abnormalities, CNS disorders, and metabolic diseases with known developmental sequelae.

Environmental/social risk. Environmental/social risk involves developmental risk related to competency in parenting roles and factors in family dynamics.[119,189] Such risk may be heightened by prolonged hospitalization of infants with suboptimal levels of stimulation and interaction (overstimulation or deprivation) in the intensive care nursery environment, inadequate infant-parent bonding, insufficient educational preparation of parents for caretaking roles, meager financial resources, and limited or absent family support to assist in taking care of and nurturing the infant in the home environment.

• • •

It is common for high-risk neonates to have a combination of risk factors from more than one major category. In-depth study of perinatal and neonatal medicine and related obstetrical, neonatal nursing, and neonatal therapy literature* are recommended before the development of a neonatal therapy protocol and participation as a member of the special care nursery team.

Neonatal neurological assessment

Multiple neonatal neurological, and neurobehavioral examinations have been developed to assess the integrity of the nervous system, to calculate gestational age, and to describe newborn behavior.[6,125,174,175,179] Five frequently employed instruments include the Clinical Assessment of Gestational Age,[70] the Neurological Examination of the Full-term Infant,[166] the Brazelton Neonatal Behavioral Assessment Scale,[33] the Neurological Assessment the Preterm and Full-term Newborn Infant,[5] and the Assessment of Preterm Infant Behavior.[5] These instruments were selected to familiarize clinicians with a range of neurological and behavioral assessments used in current practice for management of both preterm and full-term infants. Most of these assessment instruments offer *quality* data on motor performance and interactional behavior that are essential for the development of individualized treatment plans.

Clinical Assessment of Gestational Age in the Newborn Infant.[79] The Clinical Assessment of Gestational Age in the Newborn Infant[70] was developed by Dubowitz and others from a total of 167 preterm and full-term infants (28 to 42 weeks gestation) tested within 5 days of birth. It focuses on criteria for calculation of gestational age from a composite of 10 neurologic and 11 external features (see Appendix A).

This test rates criteria on a four-point scale; it is commonly administered by nurses or physicians in the new-

*References 11, 12, 18, 45, 46, 78, 80, 91, 97, 104, 110, 115, 125, 161, 198, 203.

born nursery. The accuracy (95% confidence limit) of the gestational age score is determined within a variation of ±2 weeks on any single assessment. This measurement error can be decreased to approximately ±1.4 weeks when two separate assessments are performed. From the analyses of multiple assessments on 70 of the 167 infants, the age score was equally reliable in the first 24 hours of age as during the next 4 days of life. The behavioral state(s) of the infant during the assessment is not considered a significant variable in the examination.

Calculation of gestational age is an important adjunct to all other neonatal assessment tools: it guides practitioners in interpretation of neurological and behavioral findings relative to the expected performance of infants at various gestational ages. Additional guidelines on gestational differences in neurological, physical, and neuromuscular maturation can be found in the work of Saint-Anne Dargassies,[179] Lubchenco,[125] Carter and Campbell,[43] and Amiel-Tison.[6,8,9]

Neurological Examination of the Full-term Infant.[166] The Neurological Examination of the Full-term Infant,[166] which is commonly administered by neonatal therapists, was designed by Prechtl to identify abnormal neurological signs in the newborn period. The examination was developed from an investigation of more than 1350 newborns and was standardized on infants born at the gestational age of 38 to 42 weeks. If used on premature infants who have reached an age of 38 to 42 weeks gestation, lower resistance to passive movements (lower tone) may be expected. Delay of testing until a minimum of 3 days of age is advised to maximize the stability of behavioral states and neuromotor responses for improved reliability and validity of results.

The pattern of examination includes an observation period and an examination period. A 10-minute screening examination is offered to determine if the full 30-minute assessment of posture, tone, reflexes, and spontaneous movement is required. Although specific requirements for examiner training are not addressed, Prechtl offers a flow diagram (Fig. 8-8) to assist clinicians with organizing the neurological examination process. Significant findings from the examination are summarized in the following categories: (1) the quality of posture, spontaneous movement, and muscle tone (consistency and resistance to passive movement), (2) presence of involuntary or pathological movements (clonus, tremor, athetoid postures or movements), (3) behavioral state changes and quality of cry, and (4) threshold/intensity of responses to stimulation.

From combinations of these findings, Prechtl identifies four clinical syndromes. The *hemisyndrome* identifies infants with three asymmetrical findings during assessment of movement, tone, posture, or reflexes. The *hyperexcitable syndrome* refers to a behavioral profile that may include instability of behavioral states, prolonged crying, presence of tremor and hypertonus, increased deep tendon

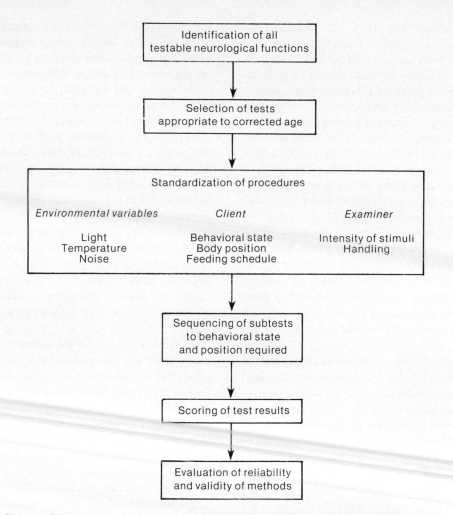

Fig. 8-8. Flow diagram illustrating decision steps in the neurological examination process.

reflexes, and hyperkinesis. The *apathetic syndrome,* a frequent precurser of the hemisyndrome, is manifested by hypotonia and a very high threshold for response to stimulation. The *comatose syndrome* is characterized by minimal or absent arousal to pain or other sensory stimuli and by the frequent presence of abnormal respiratory patterns. The presence of these syndromes in newborn infants strongly justifies the need for comprehensive interdisciplinary follow-up to manage potential developmental sequelae.

Neonatal Behavioral Assessment Scale (NBAS).[2,33,148,182,202] To document individual behavioral and motoric differences in full-term infants, Brazelton and others developed a neonatal behavior scale to assess neuromotor responses within a behavioral state context. The 30- to 45-minute examination consists of observing, eliciting, and scoring 28 biobehavioral items on a 9-point scale and 18 reflex items on a 4-point scale. The reflex items are derived from the neurological examination protocol of Prechtl and Beintema.[167]

The scale was designed to assess newborn behavior on healthy 3-day-old full-term (40-week gestation) white infants whose mothers had minimal sedative medication during an uncomplicated labor and delivery. Use of this examination with preterm infants requires modification of the examination procedure to the environmental constraints of an intensive care nursery and interpretation of findings relative to the gestational age and medical condition of the infant. For preterm infants approaching term (minimum of 37 weeks of gestation), nine supplementary behavioral items are offered. Many of these items were developed by Als and others[5] for use with preterm and physiologically stressed infants.

Although the mean scores are related to the expected behavior of 3-day-old full-term infants, the Neonatal Behavioral Assessment Scale is considered an appropriate assessment tool from 37 weeks of gestation until 44 weeks of gestation. Extended use of this scale for older infants was recently reported by Provost,[168,169] who described the methodology and results from administering the scale with Kansas Supplements (five additional items on a 9-point scale) to 11 normal, full-term infants during the first 4 months of life.

The Neonatal Behavioral Assessment Scale outlines 6

behavioral state categories: deep sleep, light sleep, drowsiness/semidozing, quiet alert, active alert, and crying. Behavioral state prerequisites are provided for each biobehavioral and reflex item to reduce the state-related variables in testing. During the assessment the examiner systematically maneuvers the infant from the sleep states to crying and back to the alert states to evaluate physiological, organizational, motoric, and interactive capabilities during stimulation. The scoring is based on the infant's *best* performance with flexibility allowed in the order of testing, repetition of items encouraged, and scheduling of the assessment midway between feedings to give the infant every advantage to demonstrate the best possible responses.

Four dimensions of newborn behavior are analyzed by the Brazelton Scale: interactive ability, motor behavior, behavioral state organization, and physiological organization. Interactive ability describes the infant's response to visual and auditory stimuli (Fig. 8-9), consolability from the crying state with intervention by the examiner, and ability to maintain alertness and respond to social/environmental stimuli.

Motor behavior refers to the ability to modulate muscle tone and motor control for the performance of integrated motor skills, such as the hand-to-mouth maneuver, pull-to-sit maneuver, and defensive reaction (i.e., removal of cloth from face). In the assessment of behavioral state or-

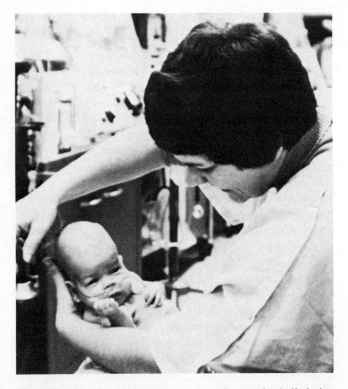

Fig. 8-9. Assessment of auditory orientation to the bell during neonatal assessment using the Brazelton Neonatal Behavioral Assessment Scale.

ganization, the infant's ability to organize behavioral states when stimulated and the ability to shut out irritating environmental stimuli when sleeping are analyzed. Physiological organization is analyzed by observing the infant's ability to manage physiological stress (changes of skin color, frequency of tremulous movement in the chin and extremities, number of startle reactions during the assessment).

Performance profiles of worrisome or deficient interactive-motoric and organizational behavior are described by Als and others[2] and Stengel[202] to identify clusters of behavior associated with potential developmental risk. The Brazelton Scale has proved to be more sensitive to the detection of mild neurological dysfunction in the newborn period than classical neurological examinations that omit the behavioral dimensions. In predicting neurological outcome at the age of 7 years in 53 high-risk neonates, the Brazelton Scale results provided a lower incidence of inaccuracy (a lower false-positive rate) in the prediction of neuropathology than a standard neurological examination.[213]

Definite strengths of the Neonatal Behavioral Assessment Scale are the well-defined indicators of autonomic stress, the analysis of the coping ability of high-risk infants to external stimuli and handling, and the quality of infant-examiner interaction. These features generate specific findings to assist therapists in grading the intensity of assessment and treatment within each infant's physiological and behavioral tolerance and in guiding the development of parent teaching strategies to address the individual behavioral styles of infants.

Participation of the parent in the newborn assessment may yield long-term, positive effects in infant-parent interaction and later cognitive and fine motor development. Widmayer and Field[225] reported significantly better face-to-face interaction and fine motor/adaptive skills at 4 months of age and higher mental development scores at 12 months of age when teenage mothers of preterm (mean gestational age at birth: 35.1 weeks) infants were given Brazelton Scale demonstrations. These demonstrations were scheduled when the premature infants had reached an age equivalence of 37 weeks gestation.

Nugent[149] developed parent teaching guidelines for using the Brazelton Scale as an intervention for infants and their families. Published by the March of Dimes, the guidelines offer strategies for interpreting each item according to its adaptive and developmental significance, descriptions of the expected developmental course of the behavior (item) over several months, and recommendations for caregiving according to the infant's response to the item.

Four films are available for examiner training.[35] In addition, the administration and scoring of the Neonatal Behavioral Assessment Scale on 15 to 25 infants is recommended to establish reliable testing and interpretation skills. Certification for use of the Brazelton Scales in research is offered in many university health science centers or university-affiliated child development centers.[34]

Neurological Assessment of the Preterm and Full-term Newborn Infant.[69] The Neurological Assessment of the Preterm and Full-term Newborn Infant[69] is a streamlined neurological and neurobehavioral assessment designed by Dubowitz and Dobowitz to provide a systematic, quickly administered (10 to 15 minute) examination applicable to *both* premature and full-term infants. A distinct advantage of this tool is the minimal training or experience required by the examiner.

The test includes multiple neurobehavioral components of the Brazelton Neonatal Behavioral Assessment Scale: the six behavioral state categories and nine neurobehavioral items are scored on a condensed five-point grading scale and sequenced according to the intensity of response. These neurobehavioral items, selected to reflect higher neurological functioning than the brainstem level reflex responses, consist of the following: (1) habituation to light and sound while sleeping, (2) auditory and visual orientation responses (Fig. 8-10), (3) quality and duration of alertness, (4) defensive reaction to a cloth over the face,

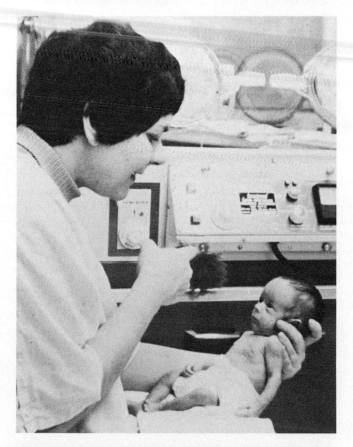

Fig. 8-10. Evaluation of visual orientation responses (i.e., visual fixation and horizontal tracking) during the Dubowitz Neurological Assessment.

(5) peak of excitement—the infant's overall responsiveness and variability of behavioral states during the examination, (6) irritability—the frequency of crying to aversive stimuli during reflex testing and handling throughout the examination, and (7) consolability—the ability after crying to reach a calm state independently or with intervention by the examiner. The appearance of the eyes (sunset sign, strabismus, nystagmus) and the quality of the cry are included in the neurobehavioral category since they also require the awake state for testing.

The 15 items that assess movement and tone and the six reflex items evolved from clinical trials on 50 full-term infants using the Clinical Assessment of Gestational Age by Dubowitz and others,[70] the Neurological Examination of the Newborn by Parmelee and others,[162] the Neurological Examination of the Full-term Newborn Infant by Prechtl,[166] and the abnormal inventory protocol described by Saint-Anne Dargassies.[179] The present format was then used during a 2-year period on over 500 infants of varying gestational ages. The authors did not present reliability data in the manual but described modification of the protocol during their clinical trial phase that promoted objectivity in scoring and a high interrater reliability among examiners, regardless of experience level.

The examination protocol is outlined and illustrated on a 2-page form with space allowed for comments. The illustrated form is constructed to accommodate both baseline and repeat assessments, and it can be effectively combined with an additional narrative impression and treatment goals/plan for neonatal therapy programs. Because a total or summary score is avoided in this examination and because emphasis is given instead to patterns of responses, selected parts of the protocol are appropriate for the assessment of premature or acutely ill infants on ventilators, in isolettes, or attached to monitoring or infusion equipment. It is recommended that the scheduling of examinations occur two-thirds of the way between feedings.

Dubowitz and Dubowitz[69,71] do not yet have long-term follow-up data beyond 1 year with this examination. Instead they present and discuss seven case histories, describe experiences using the tool in the evaluation of infants with intraventricular hemorrhage, and report outcome data at 12 months of age. The abnormal neonatal clinical signs that correlated with long-term neurological sequelae were persistent asymmetry, decreased lower extremity movement, and increased tone. Infants with intraventricular hemorrhage had significantly higher incidence of abnormally tight popliteal angles, reduced mobility, decreased visual fixing and following, and roving eye movements.

Dubowitz and others[72] reassessed 116 infants (27 to 34 weeks of gestation) at 1 year of age. Of 62 infants assessed as neurologically normal in the newborn period, 91% were also normal at 1 year of age. Of 39 infants assessed as neurologically abnormal in the newborn period, only 35% were found to be normal at 1 year of age.

Clinicians interested in using the Neurological Assessment for Preterm and Full-term Infants in clinical studies may assign numerical values to the range of descriptive criteria within the items under each major examination category. This technique was used by Morgan and others[138] in efforts to quantitate neonatal neurological status for data analysis.

Interpretations of evaluative findings from the Neurological Assessment for Preterm and Full-term Newborn Infants for neonatal therapy practice are well described in a case study format by Heriza[97] and Campbell.[46] In a recent publication, Dubowitz[68] discusses the clinical significance of neurological variations in infants and offers decision guidelines on when to worry, reassure, and intervene with developmental referrals.

Assessment of Preterm Infant Behavior. Als and others[3,5] designed the Assessment of Preterm Infant Behavior (APIB) to structure a comprehensive observation of a preterm infant's autonomic, adaptive, and interactive responses to graded handling and environmental stimuli. As described previously in the theoretical framework section, this assessment is derived from synactive theory and is focused on assessing the organization and balance of the infant's physiological, motor, behavioral state, attention/interaction, and self-regulation subsystems.

Administration and scoring of the Assessment of Preterm Infant Behavior may total 3 hours per infant. Although the APIB is an instrument of choice for the clinical researcher, it may not be practical (time efficient) for many neonatal clinicians with heavy caseloads.

Extensive training and reliability certification is required to safely administer and accurately score and interpret the test for clinical practice or research. The training is available in Boston and Tucson.[3]

Summary. It is essential that practitioners be aware of the normative and validation data and of the predictive characteristics of the test(s) administered to allow appropriate interpretation of test results. Specific clinical training with a precepter is advised to accurately administer, score, and interpret neonatal assessment instruments, to establish interrater reliability, and to plan treatment based on the evaluative findings.

Testing variables. Several variables that potentially affect neuromuscular status and interactional behavior in the newborn period can be identified. Increased reliability in examination results and in clinical impressions may occur when these variables are recognized.[11,53,83] *Medication* may produce side effects of low muscle tone, drowsiness, and lethargy. These medications include anticonvulsant medication, sedative medication for diagnostic procedures (CT scan, electroencephalography, electromyography), and medication for postsurgical pain management. *Intermittent subtle seizures* may produce changes in muscle tension and in the level of responsiveness. These may be mild, ongoing seizures that are manifested in the neonate by lip smacking or sucking, staring or horizontal gaze, apnea, bradycardia, or stiffening of the extremities more frequently than clonic movement. *Fatigue* from medical/nursing procedures can result in decreased tolerance to handling, decreased interaction, and magnified muscle tone abnormalities. Fatigue may also result when neurodevelopmental assessment is scheduled immediately after laboratory (hematologic) procedures, suctioning, ultrasonography, or respiratory (chest percussion) therapy. *Metabolic/physiological factors* such as tremulous movement in the extremities may be linked to conditions of metabolic imbalance (hypomagnesemia, hypocalcemia, hypoglycemia); low muscle tone may be associated with hyperbilirubinemia, hypoglycemia, hypoxemia, and hypothermia. *Racial factors* produce unique differences in infant temperament among racial groups. Freeman[82] describes the calm temperament of Chinese, Polynesian, and Navaho Indian newborns as clearly different from the comparatively more sensitive, irritable temperament of white or Japanese babies. Similarily in clinical practice, normal muscle tone variations among racial groups are commonly detected. These tone variations may involve decreased consistency to palpation in Oriental babies and increased muscular firmness in black infants as compared to white infants. The normal variations among racial groups in palpable muscle tension in the extremities have not yet been validated by quantitative measurement.

Treatment planning

Level of stimulation. The issue of safe and therapeutic levels of sensorimotor stimulation must be addressed in the design of developmental intervention programs for infants who have previously been unstable medically. The popular term, "infant stimulation," which was coined by early childhood educators to describe *general* developmental stimulation programs for infants, is highly inappropriate in an approach based on concepts of pathokinesiology and infant behavioral organization.

For intervention to be therapeutic in an intensive care nursery setting, the amount and type of stimulation must be individually graded to each infant's physiological tolerance, muscle tone category, movement patterns, unique temperament, and level of responsivity. Rather than needing more stimulation, many infants, especially those with hypertonus or those with tremulous, disorganized movement, have difficulty adapting to the routine levels of noise, light, position changes, and handling in the nursery environment. General stimulation can quickly magnify abnormal muscle tone and movement, increase behavioral state lability and irritability, and stress fragile physiological homeostasis when it is not individualized to the specific motor and interactive needs and responses of preterm or chronically ill infants. Implementation of careful physiological monitoring and graded handling techniques are essential to prevent compromise in patient safety and to facilitate development. Infant *modulation,* rather than stimulation, is the goal of intervention.

Physiological risk management. Many maturation-related anatomical and physiological factors predispose preterm infants to pulmonary dysfunction (Table 8-5). For this reason many at-risk neonates will require the use of a wide range of respiratory equipment and physiological monitors (Table 8-6). Pediatric therapists preparing to work in the NICU and those involved with designing risk management plans are referred to Crane's analysis[56-58] of neonatal cardiopulmonary management for therapists.

In this new area of pediatric practice, neonatal therapists are responsible for the prevention of physiological jeopardy in high-risk infants during developmental intervention in special care units. Before assessment, discussion with the supervising neonatologist is advised regarding specific precautions and the safe range of vital signs for each infant. Medical update and identification of new precautions by the nursing staff before each intervention session are recommended because new events in the last few hours may not be recorded or fully analyzed at the time therapy is scheduled. It is essential that the nurse be invited to maintain ongoing surveillance of the infant's medical stability during neonatal therapy activities in case physiological complications occur. If medical complications develop during or after therapy, immediate, comprehensive codocumentation of the incident with the supervising nurse and discussion with the neonatology staff are essential to analyze the events, outline related clinical teaching issues, and minimize legal jeopardy.

Areas of particular concern during neonatal therapy activities include the following: potential incidence of fracture or dislocation during the management of limited joint motion; skin breakdown or vascular compromise during splinting or taping to reduce deformity; apnea or bradycardia during movement therapy with potential deterioration to respiratory arrest; aspiration during feeding assessment or emesis with oral-motor therapy; hypothermia from prolonged handling of the infant away from the neutral thermal environment of the Isolette or overhead radiant warmer; propagation of infection from inadequate compliance with infection control procedures in the nursery. Signs of overstimulation may include labored breathing with chest retractions, grunting, nostril flaring, color changes (skin mottling to red or cyanotic appearance), frequent startles, irritability or drowsiness, trunk arching to withdraw from stimulation, sneezing, gaze aversion, bowel movement and hiccups.[3,124]

Even a baseline neurological assessment, usually presumed to be a benign clinical procedure, may be destabilizing to the newborn infant's cardiovascular and behavioral organization systems. The physiological and behavioral tolerance of low-risk preterm and full-term neonates to evaluative handling by a neonatal physical therapist was studied in 72 newborn subjects.[209,210] During and after administration of the Neurological Assessment of the Preterm and Full-term Newborn Infant, preterm subjects (30 to 35 weeks of gestation) had significantly higher heart rate, greater increase in blood pressure, decreased peripheral oxygenation inferred from mottled skin color, and higher frequencies of finger splay, arm salute, hiccups, and yawns than full-term subjects. Neonatal practitioners must examine the safety of even a neurological assessment and weigh the risks and anticipated benefit of the procedure given the expected physiological and behavioral changes in low-risk, medically stable neonates.

High-risk profiles. Three basic high-risk profiles can be established from a pathokinesiological perspective. These profiles identify major muscle tone abnormalities, related temperament/behavioral characteristics, and interactional styles associated with motor status.

The first high-risk profile involves the irritable *hyper-*

Table 8-5. Factors contributing to pulmonary dysfunction in preterm neonates*

Anatomical	Physiological
Capillary beds not well developed before 26 weeks gestation	Increased pulmonary vascular resistance leading to right-to-left shunting
Type II alveolar cells and surfactant production not mature until 35 weeks of gestation	
Elastic properties of lung not well developed	Decreased lung compliance
Lung "space" decreased by relative size of the heart and abdominal distention	
Type I, high-oxidative fibers compose only 10% to 20% of diaphragm muscle	Diaphragmatic fatigue; respiratory failure
Highly vascular subependymal germinal matrix not resorbed until 35 weeks of gestation, increasing the vulnerability of the infant to hemorrhage	Decreased or absent cough and gag reflexes; apnea
Lack of fatty insulation and high surface area to body-weight ratio	Hypothermia and increased oxygen consumption

*From Crane L: Physical therapy for the neonate with respiratory disease. In Irwin S and Tecklin JS: Cardiopulmonary physical therapy, St. Louis, 1985, The CV Mosby Co.

tonic infant. These infants classically have a low-tolerance level to handling and are frequently in a state of overstimulation from routine nursing care, laboratory procedures, and the presence of respiratory and infusion equipment. They express discomfort when provided with quick changes in position by the caregivers and when placed in any position for a prolonged time. Predominant extension patterns of posture and movement are associated with this category of infants. Quality of movement may appear tremulous or disorganized with poor midline orientation and limited antigravity movement into flexion as a result of the imbalance of increased proximal extensor tone. Vi-

Table 8-6. Equipment commonly encountered in the NICU

Equipment	Description
Radiant warmer	Unit composed of mattress on an adjustable table top covered by a radiant heat source controlled manually and by servocontrol mode. Unit has adjustable side panels. *Advantage:* provides open space for tubes and equipment and easier access to the infant. *Disadvantage:* open bed may lead to convective heat loss and insensible fluid loss.
Self-contained incubator (isolette)	Enclosed unit of transparent material providing a heated and humidified environment with a servo system of temperature monitoring. Access to infant through side portholes or opening side of unit. *Advantage:* less convective heat and insensible water loss. *Disadvantage:* infection control; more difficult to get to baby; not practical for a very acutely ill neonate.
Thermal shield	Plexiglass dome placed over the trunk and legs of an infant in an Isolette to reduce radiant heat loss.
Oxygen hood	Plexiglass hood that fits over the infant's head; provides environment for controlled oxygen and humidification delivery.
Mechanical ventilator: Pressure ventilator	Delivers positive-pressure ventilation; pressure-limited with volume delivered dependent on the stiffness of the lung.
Volume ventilator	Delivers positive-pressure ventilation; volume-limited delivering same tidal volume with each breath.
Negative-pressure ventilator	Ventilator that creates a relative negative pressure around the thorax and abdomen thereby assisting ventilation without endotracheal tube. NOTE: Difficult to use in infants weighing less than 1500 g.
Nasal and nasopharyngeal prongs	Simple system for providing continuous positive airway pressure (CPAP) consisting of nasal prongs of varying lengths and adaptor to pressure-source tubing.
Resuscitation bag	Usually a self-inflating bag with a reservoir (so high concentrations of oxygen may be delivered at a rapid rate) attached to an oxygen flowmeter and a pressure manometer.
ECG, heart rate, respiratory rate, and blood pressure monitor (cardiorespirograph)	Usually one unit will display one or more vital signs on oscilloscope and digital display. High and low limits may be set, and alarm sounds when limits exceeded.
Transcutaneous oxygen (Tc Po_2) monitor	Noninvasive method of monitoring partial pressure of oxygen from arterialized capillaries through the skin. The electrode is heated, placed on an area of thin epidermis (usually abdomen or thorax). The monitor has capability of providing both a digital display and a continuous recording of $TcPo_2$ values.
Intravenous infusion pump	Used to pump intravenous fluids, intralipids, and transpyloric feedings at a specified rate. Pump has alarm system and capacity to monitor volume delivered, obstruction of flow, and other parameters.
Neonatal vital signs monitor	Measures mean blood pressure and mean heart rate from plastic blood pressure cuff; values are digitally displayed on monitor.
Pulse oximeter	Measures peripheral oxygen saturation and pulse from a light sensor secured to the infant's skin; values are digitally displayed on the monitor; some models have continuous recording of values on strip charts.

*Modified from Crane L: Physical therapy for the neonate with respiratory disease. In Irwin S and Tecklin JS: Cardiopulmonary physical therapy. St Louis, 1985, The CV Mosby Co.

sual tracking and feeding may be difficult because of extension posturing or the presence of distracting, disorganized upper extremity movement. In addition, increased tone with related decreased mobility in oral musculature may complicate feeding behavior. Hypertonic infants frequently demonstrate poor self-quieting abilities and may require consistent intervention by caregivers. These temperament characteristics and the signs of neurological impairment discussed earlier place infants at considerable risk for child abuse or neglect as the stress and fatigue levels of parents rise and as coping strategies wear thin during the demanding care required by irritable, hypertonic babies.[108]

Conversely, the lethargic *hypotonic* infant excessively accommodates to the stimulation of the nursery environment and can be difficult to arouse to the awake states even for feeding. The crying state is reached infrequently, even with vigorous stimulation. The cry is characteristically weak, with low volume and short duration, related to hypotonic trunk, intercostal, and neck accessory musculature and decreased respiratory capacity. These infants are exceedingly comfortable in any position, and when held they easily mold themselves to the arms of the caregiver. Depression of normal neonatal movement and patterns is common. To compensate for low muscle tone, many preterm infants push into extension against the surface of the mattress in search of stability. Although successful in generating a temporary increase in neck and trunk tone, the extension posturing from stabilizing or "fixing" against a surface interferes with midline and antigravity movement of the extremities. Drowsy behavior limits these infants' spontaneous approach to the environment and decreases their accessibility to selected interaction by caregivers. Feeding behavior is commonly marked by fatigue, difficulty remaining awake, weak sucking, incoordination/inadequate rhythm in the suck-swallow process, and supplementation of caloric intake by gavage (oral or nasogastric tube) feeding. The risk for sensory deprivation and failure to thrive is high for hypotonic infants since they infrequently seek interaction, place few if any demands on caregivers, and remain somnolent.

The third high-risk profile is the disorganized infant with fluctuating tone and movement, who is easily overstimulated with routine handling but remains relatively passive when left alone. Disorganized infants usually respond well to swaddling or to containment when handled. When calm, these infants frequently demonstrate high quality social interaction and rhythmical feeding. When distracted and overstimulated, however, these infants appear hypertonic and irritable. Caregiving for intermittently hypertonic, disorganized, irritable infants can be frustrating for parents unskilled in reading the infant's cues and in implementing consolability and containment strategies.

While these profiles address the extremes in sensorimotor and interactional behavior, they suggest a need for different levels of stimulation and different approaches in managing neonates with abnormal tone and movement, even though long-term developmental goals may be similar. Few neonates will demonstrate all behaviors described in the high-risk profile, but outpatient surveillance of those neonates with worrisome or mildly abnormal motor and interactive behavior is advised to monitor the course of those behaviors and the developing styles of parenting.

Timing. The timing of developmental assessment and of treatment for infants with high-risk histories or diagnoses is based on the medical stability of the infant and, in some centers, gestational age. All therapy activities need to be synchronized with the intensive care nursery schedule so that nursing care and medical procedures are not interrupted.

Neonatal therapists should not interrupt infants in a quiet, deep sleep state, but instead wait about 15 minutes until the infant cycles into a light, active sleep or semiawake state. Higher transcutaneous oxygen saturation has been correlated with quiet rather than with active sleep in newborn infants. Preterm infants reportedly have a higher percentage of active sleep in contrast with the higher percentage of quiet sleep observed in full-term infants.[89] Allowing the preterm infant to maintain, rather than interrupting, a deep, quiet sleep is a therapeutic strategy for enhancing physiological stability.

Timing of parent teaching sessions is most effective when readiness to participate in the care of the infant is expressed. Some parents need time and support to work through the acute grief process related to the birth of an imperfect child before participation in developmental activities is accepted. Other parents find the neonatal therapy program to be a way of helping in the care of their child that assists them through the mourning process.

Treatment strategies

This section addresses components of treatment designed to normalize tone/movement, minimize contractures and deformity, facilitate normal patterns of movement, promote feeding behaviors appropriate to corrected age, develop social interaction behaviors, and foster attachment to primary caregivers. The areas of developmental intervention presented include management approaches to body positioning, extremity taping, graded sensorimotor intervention, neonatal hydrotherapy, oral-motor/feeding therapy, and parent teaching. In the management of an intensive care nursery caseload, the constant physiological monitoring, modification of techniques to adapt to the constraints of varying amounts of medical equipment, scheduling of intervention to coincide with visits of the parents and peak responsiveness of the infants, and ongoing coordination and reassessment of goals, plans, and follow-up recommendations with the nursery staff create many interesting challenges and demand a high degree of adaptability and creativity from the clinician. Willingness to change a

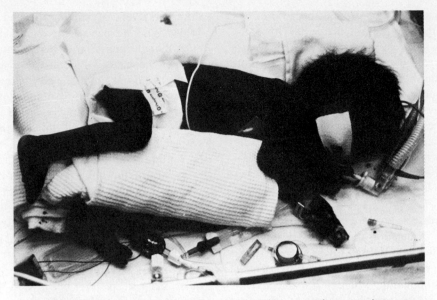

Fig. 8-11. Positioning with diaper rolls to reduce extension posturing.

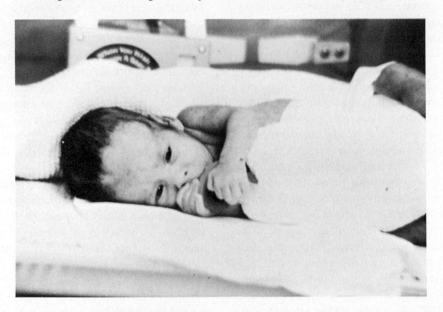

Fig. 8-12. Use of an anterior roll and a pacifier promotes stabilization in the flexed position.

preestablished assessment plan, treatment strategy, or therapy schedule to meet the immediate needs of the infant, parents, or nursery staff is paramount.

Positioning. A positioning program that is administered diligently can greatly assist infants on mechanical ventilators, under oxyhoods, or in isolettes to simulate the flexed, midline postures of the normal full-term newborn swaddled in a bassinet. Preterm infants characteristically demonstrate low postural tone with the amount of hypotonia varying with gestational age. Infants born prematurely do not have the neurological maturity or the prolonged positional advantage of the intrauterine environment to assist in the development of flexion. They are instead placed unexpectedly against gravity and presented with a dual chal-

lenge of compensating for maturation-related hypotonia and adapting to ventilatory and infusion equipment that frequently reinforces extension of the neck, trunk, and extremities.

The imbalance of excessive extension can occur quickly in preterm infants from repeated efforts to gain postural stability or containment in the nonfluid extrauterine environment by leaning into or "fixing" against a firm surface, usually the mattress. Fixing by the neonate is demonstrated initially as neck hyperextension in supine or sidelying positions and appears to block further development of mobility and cocontraction in the neck region. As described by Bly[25] and Quinton,[170] the neck hyperextension posturing may herald the development of a host of related

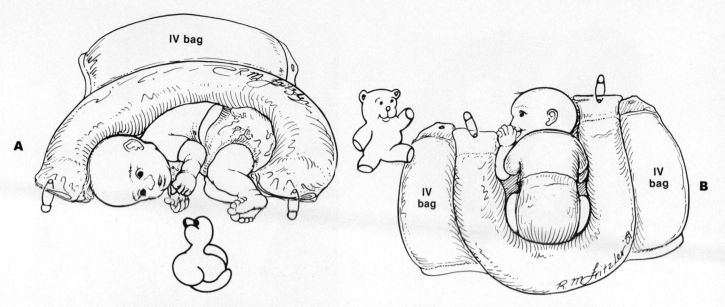

Fig. 8-13. Postural containment in flexion by body stabilization from a long blanket roll reinforced by a sand or intravenous fluid bag.

abnormal postural and mobility patterns to compensate for inadequate proximal stability. From neck hyperextension, abnormal postural fixing for stability can classically lead to sequential blocking in the shoulder, pelvis, and hip regions. In many preterm neonates, the active postural fixing to compensate for hypotonia contributes to a commonly observed postural profile associated with prematurity and the extension-producing forces of gravity. The components of this high-risk postural profile follow:

1. Hyperextended neck
2. Elevated shoulders with adducted scapulae
3. Decreased midline arm movement (hand-to-mouth)
4. Excessively extended trunk
5. Immobile pelvis (anterior tilt)
6. Infrequent antigravity movement of legs
7. Weight bearing on toes (supported standing)

The use of blanket or cloth diaper rolls or customized foam inserts in a neonatal positioning program can modify the increasing imbalance of extension in preterm or chronically ill infants and can promote movement and postural stability from positions of flexion. Postural principles to incorporate into a positioning program include elongation of neck extensor musculature for chin tucking, trunk flexion, shoulder protraction to encourage engagement of hands at midline, posterior pelvic tilt, and symmetrical flexion of the legs. After the infant is facilitated into a flexed position in the side-lying position, posterior rolls behind the head, trunk, and thighs provide a surface against which the infant can posturally stabilize while a flexed midline position is maintained (Fig. 8-11). An additional anterior roll between the extremities and the use of a pacifier may promote further midline stabilization in flex-

ion (Fig. 8-12).[9] Small neonates can be maintained in a flexed symmetrical position with a long blanket roll pinned to the mattress at each end. Larger neonates may need additional stabilization from a water bag, sand bag, or dextrose IV bag against the blanket roll (Fig. 8-13).

Endotracheal tube placement frequently contributes to the neck hyperextension posture in infants who require mechanical ventilation (Fig. 8-14). This iatrogenic compo-

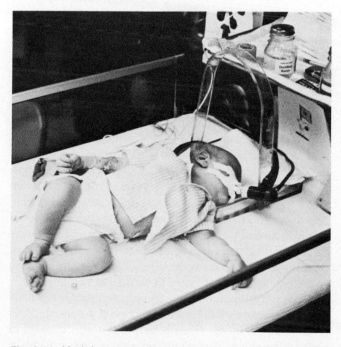

Fig. 8-14. Neck hyperextension posture magnified by the position of the endotracheal tube.

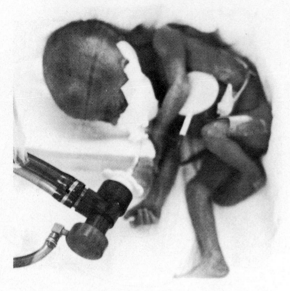

Fig. 8-15. Flexed posture maintained after repositioning of the endotracheal tube.

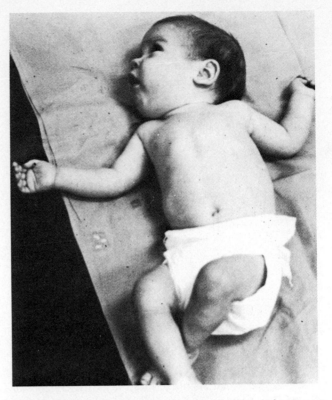

Fig. 8-16. Clinical presentation of contracture in neck extensor muscles related to hyperextension posture during prolonged mechanical ventilation.

nent can be avoided by repositioning the endotracheal tube to allow enough mobility for the tucked chin and flexed trunk postures (Fig. 8-15). For neurologically impaired infants with severe pulmonary disease necessitating prolonged ventilatory support, inattention to the alignment of the neck and shoulders can lead to the development of a contracture in the neck extensor muscles (Fig. 8-16) and occlusion of the airway.

Since flexion is enhanced in the prone position by the influence of the tonic labyrinthine reflex, the incorporation of prone positioning is strongly advocated even for infants on ventilators (Fig. 8-17). In fact, infants in the prone position have shown increased oxygenation[129,222] and less crying[31] than in those in the supine position. Placing infants on a sheepskin surface offers increased tactile input and has been correlated with increased weight gain in very–low-birth-weight infants compared with a matched group of infants on standard cotton sheets.[190]

Water mattresses are a highly effective adjunct to a nursery positioning program. They provide a soft, intermittently oscillating surface that is not conducive to postural fixing. Other recognized advantages of waterbeds include increased vestibular and proprioceptive stimulation, decreased apnea, reduced head flattening, and improved skin condition.[51,114,128] When moved from intensive care to intermediate care, transition from a waterbed to a standard mattress is recommended to allow time for adaption to the type of mattress likely to be used at home.

Extremity taping. The presence of perinatal elasticity encourages early management of congenital musculoskeletal deformities in the neonatal period (birth to 28 days of age). A temporary ligamentous laxity is presumed to be

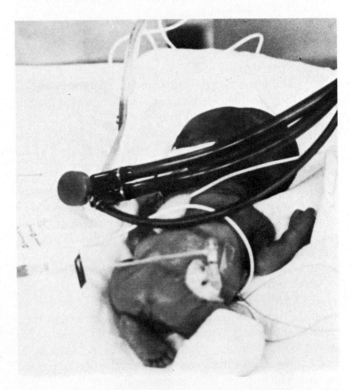

Fig. 8-17. Flexion posture enhanced in the prone position by the influence of the tonic labyrinthine reflex.

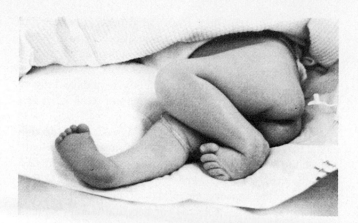

Fig. 8-18. Infant with lumbar meningomyelocoele demonstrating marked varus foot deformities before taping.

present in the neonate because of transplacental transfer of relaxin and estrogen from the mother. In addition to the influence of maternal hormones, the rapid growth of the neonate can foster correction of malalignment if the deforming forces are managed expediently. This peak period of hyperelasticity offers pediatric therapists with advanced orthopedic expertise many opportunities to manage congenital joint deformities.[96]

Intermittent taping of foot deformities (Fig. 8-18) has been more adaptable to the nursery setting than either casts or splints and is clearly more effective in gaining mobility than range of motion exercises. Access to the heel for drawing blood, inspection of skin and vascular status, and placement of intravenous lines can be accomplished with the tape in place or by temporary removal of the tape as needed. Therapists without a sound knowledge of arthroki-

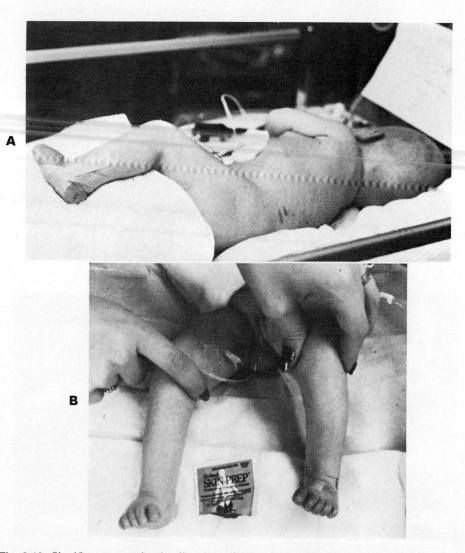

Fig. 8-19. Significant correction in alignment of varus foot deformities in neonate with a lumbar meningomyelocoele. **A,** Lateral stirrup with open heel taping procedure. **B,** Moderate correction.

nematic principles and techniques should not attempt the taping procedure, because it involves articulation of the joint(s) into a corrected position before taping. Other components of the taping process include application of an external skin protection solution under the tape, application of an adhesive removal solution when removing the tape, observance of skin condition and vascular tolerance, development of a taping schedule beginning with 1 hour and increasing by 1 hour intervals as tolerated, and clinical teaching with selected neonatal nurses for continuation of the taping if needed on night shifts and weekends. Infants with congenital foot deformities require shorter periods of casting in the outpatient period after taping of the extremity (Fig. 8-19) is implemented during the inpatient phase. In 6 years of experience by the author (JKS), using silk or knitted tape to reduce deformity in neonates, neither skin nor vascular complications have occurred, even in infants with absent lower extremity sensation resulting from meningomyelocele.

Infants with wrist drop from radial nerve compression related to intravenous line infiltration also benefit from the use of taping (Fig. 8-20). The wrist is supported in a functional position of slight extension. As muscle function returns, the taping is used intermittently to reduce fatigue and overstretching of the emerging but still weak wrist extensor musculature.

Sensorimotor intervention. The use of the sensory modalities of tactile, vestibular, proprioceptive, visual, and auditory stimuli to facilitate infant development has been reported* and reviewed[79,195] by many authors. Regardless of the sensory modalities or neurophysiological treatment approaches selected for neonatal therapy, attention to sensory overload and related physiological consequences should guide the type, intensity, duration, and frequency of intervention.

Primary aims of sensorimotor intervention are to assist

*References 52, 62, 113, 118, 142, 172, 183, 184, 185, 223, 224.

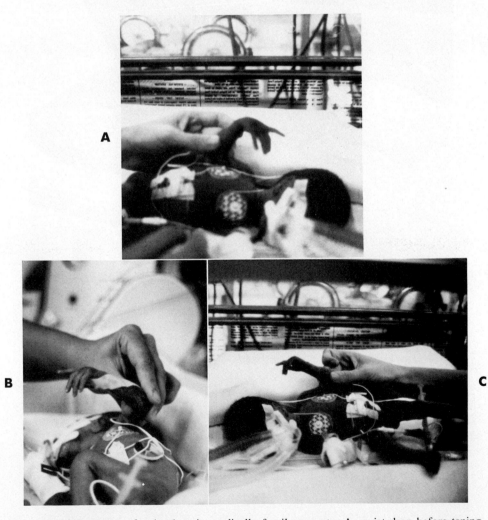

Fig. 8-20. Management of wrist drop in medically fragile neonate. **A,** wrist drop before taping. **B,** taping procedure. **C,** one week after taping.

the newborn to achieve maximum interaction with parents and caregivers and to facilitate the experience of normal postural and movement patterns. For lethargic, hypotonic infants, intervention may focus on arousal to the alert states and facilitation of cocontraction in the hypotonic proximal (neck, trunk) musculature. Conversely, movement therapy for irritable, hyperexcitable, hypertonic infants may be directed toward calming the infant to the quiet, alert state and inhibiting proximal hypertonus. Attainment of the quiet, alert behavioral state and temporary normalization of postural tone enhances opportunities for visual and auditory interaction and for normal movement experiences. These normal, early movement experiences include hand-to-mouth movement, shoulder protraction/retraction, anterior/posterior pelvic tilt, free movement of the extremities against gravity, and momentary holding of the head and midline.[44,46,60]

Preparation of the neonate for the development of righting reactions may include early-movement experiences in weight shifting and facilation of postural alignment in the side-lying position for trunk elongation on the weight-bearing side and lateral trunk flexion on the unweighted side.[25]

Behavioral state and movement abnormalities can be clinically influenced by swaddling and graded vestibular stimulation. Swaddling the infant in a blanket with flexed, midline extremity position appears to promote flexor tone, increase hand-to-mouth awareness, and inhibit jittery or disorganized movement. Slow, rhythmical vestibular stimulation (lateral or vertical rocking of the swaddled infant in the face-to-face position with caregiver) usually elicits a calming response in irritable infants. Slightly quicker,

more abrupt rocking movement without swaddling often generates an alerting response in drowsy infants. When employed by parents during visits to the nursery, these techniques help to elicit quiet, alert behavior and maximal infant-parent interaction. The techniques must be applied in a style consistent with the infant's responses: readiness for interaction or need for disengagement, a break in interaction because of sensory overload.

Incorporation of sensorimotor activities into routine nursing care in the neonatal intensive care unit greatly increases developmental opportunities for the neonate during prolonged hospitalization.[223] While feeding the infant in an isolette, the nurse may facilitate head lifting and momentary maintenance of the head in midline during the "burping process" in supported sitting (Fig. 8-21). Techniques for inhibition of trunk and lower extremity hypertonus may be added during diaper changes. Visual and auditory stimulation may be integrated into nearly all parts of child care (Fig. 8-22), or they may be specifically reinforced as appropriate (i.e., visual stimulation: human face, mobile, brightly colored toy, a picture with geometrical pattern; auditory stimulation: human voice, rattle, music box, radio). Easily overstimulated preterm infants may not tolerate multimodal sensory stimulation, but may instead respond to a single sensory stimulus.[23]

Implementation of a positioning program, oral-motor therapy, and reinforcement of developmental activities with parents can all be expertly managed by the neonatal nursing staff when ongoing clinical teaching and intermittent supervision by a pediatric therapist occurs.

A semi-inverted supine flexion position (Fig. 8-23) with preterm neonates should be used with caution to facilitate

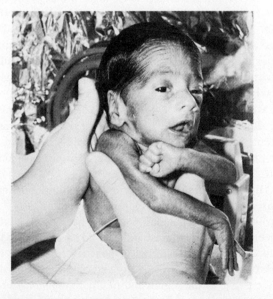

Fig. 8-21. Facilitation of head lifting by a neonatal nurse while "burping" the infant after feeding.

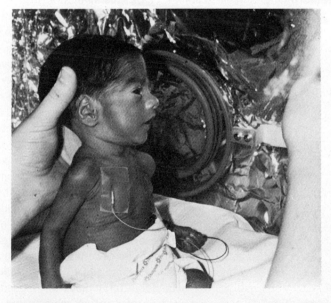

Fig. 8-22. Facilitation of visual following by a neonatal nurse during a change of the infant's position in the isolette.

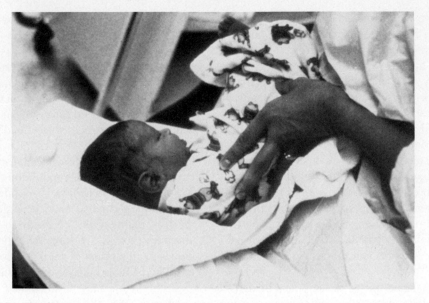

Fig. 8-23. Potential respiratory compromise to the infant from neck extensor muscle elongation in excessively flexed position while in supine position.

elongation of neck extensor muscles and decrease the neck hyperextension posture. This position may cause compromise of breathing from positional compression of the chest and from potential airway occlusion associated with maximal flexion of the neck. The use of a transcutaneous oxygen monitor or pulse oximeter during therapeutic handling activities is recommended for objective measurement of physiological tolerance. Although the peripheral oxygen saturation values from the monitors may be intermittently unreliable because of motion artifacts from either the infant's spontaneous movement or the therapist's handling of the infant, reliable readings of oxygen saturation may be taken approximately 1 minute after the infant's body is not moved.

Neonatal hydrotherapy. Modified for use in an intensive care nursery setting, the traditional physical therapy modality of hydrotherapy has been effectively implemented as an adjunct to individual developmental intervention for high-risk neonates. Neonatal hydrotherapy was conceptualized in 1980 at Madigan Army Medical Center in Tacoma, Washington.[208,211]

Indications for referral of medically stable infants to the hydrotherapy component of the developmental intervention program include the following: (1) muscle tone abnormalities (hypertonus or hypotonus) affecting the quality and quantity of spontaneous movement and contributing to the imbalance of extension in posture and movement (Fig. 8-24); (2) limitation of motion in the extremities related to muscular or connective tissue factors; and (3) behavioral state abnormalities of behavioral intolerance of graded "handling" to normalize muscle tone *or* excessive drowsiness during "handling" that prevents social interaction with

caregivers and contributes to depression of normal movement patterns and tone.

Infants are considered medically stable for aquatic intervention when ventilatory equipment and intravenous lines are discontinued and when resolution of temperature instability and apnea/bradycardia are demonstrated. A standard plastic bassinet is used with preparation of the water temperature at 99° to 101° F (37.2° to 38.3° C). Use of an overhead radiant heater decreases temperature loss in the undressed infant, thereby maximizing thermoregulation.

After receiving medical clearance and individualized criteria for the maximum acceptable limits of heart rate, blood pressure and color changes during hydrotherapy from the neonatal staff, the baseline heart rate and blood pressure values are recorded and pretreatment posture and behavioral states are observed. The undressed infant is then moved into a semiflexed, supine position, with the blood pressure cuff on one thigh, before being lifted into the water. After a short period for behavioral adaptation to the fluid environment, a second caregiver (i.e., nurse or parent) is recruited to stabilize the infant's head and shoulder girdle region while the pediatric therapist provides support at the pelvis.

The neuromuscular facilitation and inhibition techniques consistent with neurodevelopmental treatment[27-29,122,126] involve midline positioning of the head, proximal hand placement of the therapist and second caregiver, and slow, graded tone-normalizing movement (incorporating flexion and rotation) of the trunk, followed by progression distally to the pelvic girdle region and finally to the shoulder girdle and neck regions. After gentle elongation of cervical and trunk extensor musculature and facilitated dissociated

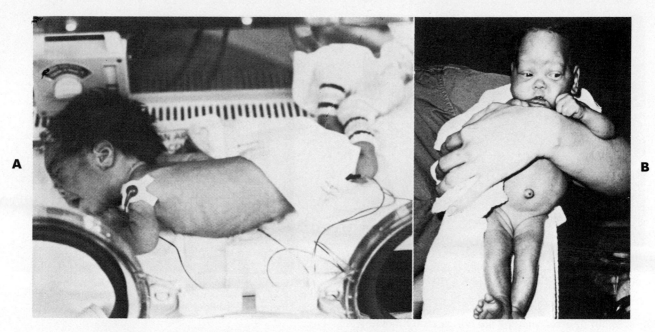

Fig. 8-24. Neonates demonstrating opisthotonic trunk posture, **A,** and marked lower extremity hypertonus, **B,** before hydrotherapy.

movement at shoulder or pelvic girdle, most infants will demonstrate active extremity movement in the water. The improved range and smoothness of spontaneous extremity movement is facilitated by the buoyancy and resistive properties of the water. Movement experiences in the supine, side-lying, and prone positions are offered as tolerated. If the movement therapy becomes too stressful, with resultant agitation or crying by the infant, the movement is immediately stopped, and the infant is either consoled or, if unconsolable, removed from the water and swaddled. Because the compromise of hemodynamic stability (increased heart rate, increased blood pressure, decreased respiratory rate) and a decrease in arterial oxygen tension during crying has been well documented in newborn infants recovering from respiratory distress syndrome,[63] careful monitoring of behavioral tolerance to hydrotherapy (with avoidance of crying) is considered critical for reducing physiological risk with hydrotherapy.

Multiple therapeutic benefits are obtained from selective use of 10- to 15-minute aquatic intervention sessions. Improvement of abnormal muscle tone and facilitation of semiflexed posture are obtained with less time and effort by the therapist and with higher behavioral tolerance by the infant than when a similar movement therapy approach is used without the medium of water (Fig. 8-25). Muscle tone changes are frequently maintained for 2 to 3 hours when aquatic intervention is followed by flexed, midline body positioning in the side-lying position on a water mattress. Enhancement of visual and auditory orientation responses (i.e., visual fixing and tracking, auditory alerting,

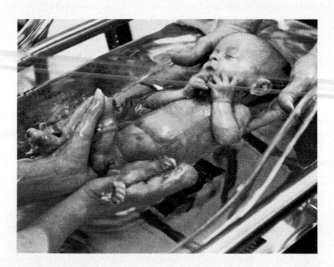

Fig. 8-25. Facilitation of flexed posture and hand-to-mouth movement with calm, behavioral response in infant previously irritable with handling.

and localization to human voices), prolonged high-quality alertness, and longer periods of social interaction with caregivers are demonstrated during and after hydrotherapy sessions. Significant improvement in feeding behavior can be effected when hydrotherapy is scheduled for 1 hour before feeding to prepare the infant for complete arousal and for flexed, midline postural changes conducive to optimal feeding. However, exhaustion of the infant and a deterioration in feeding abilities with a requirement for gavage feeding can occur if the side effects of fatigue and temper-

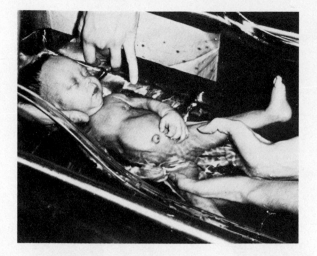

Fig. 8-26. Aquatic intervention for contracture control and inhibition of hypertonus.

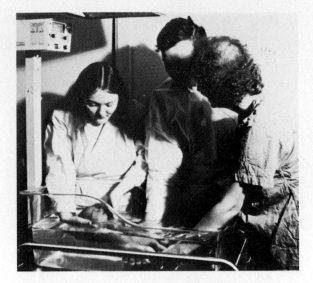

Fig. 8-27. Parents being trained in hydrotherapy techniques for later therapeutic bathing at home.

ature loss during hydrotherapy are not carefully monitored. Mild flexion contractures of knees and elbows and dynamic hip adduction contractures (Fig. 8-26) can be safely and quickly eliminated by gentle muscle/joint mobilization and elongation techniques in warm water as opposed to the traditional range-of-motion and stretching techniques frequently prescribed for adult orthopaedic clients.

Therapeutic bathing techniques are incorporated into the parent teaching program to foster early parent participation in child care and in specific developmental activities during the inpatient period to prepare for carryover into the home environment at hospital discharge. This early pleasurable involvement of parent and child in hydrotherapy and bathing can provide a strong base for future participation in aquatics as a family leisure sports activity and, if needed, as an adjunct to an outpatient developmental therapy program.

When oriented to treatment goals and trained in specific hydrotherapy techniques for individual infants, the nursing staff can effectively carry on the hydrotherapy program established by the pediatric therapist. This release of the pediatric therapist's role to the neonatal nurse allows additional use of hydrotherapy on evening and night shifts and continued teaching and supervision of parents during evening and weekend visits (Fig. 8-27).

An additional advantage of neonatal hydrotherapy is cost effectiveness. The use of equipment readily available in the newborn nursery and the short time period (10 to 15 minutes) required for therapeutic bathing in the nursing care plan and in the parent participation program in the nursery combine to make aquatic intervention cost effective for equipment, time management, and personnel resources.

Although many clinical benefits may be obtained by judicious use of hydrotherapy in the newborn nursery, pilot study data obtained on physiological changes in high-risk infants during hydrotherapy clearly indicate a physiological risk.[208] This physiological risk (increased blood pressure and heart rate) must be carefully evaluated relative to each infant's general medical stability and individual heart rate and blood pressure patterns before hydrotherapy can be included safely in an inpatient neonatal therapy program. In collaboration with the neonatology and nursing staff, preestablished criteria for general medical stability and the maximal limits during hydrotherapy for blood pressure, heart rate, and acceptable color changes are essential requirements for risk management. Physiological monitoring of mean blood pressure and heart rate by a neonatal vital signs monitor (i.e., DYNAMAPP Model 847 by Critikon, Inc., Tampa, Florida) during aquatic intervention is recommended. The blood pressure cuff is a pneumatically driven device that is not electronically connected to the infant and can be safely immersed in water. Since hypothermia is a recognized risk with hydrotherapy, routine measurement of body temperature using a thermometer with a digital display should occur before and after the hydrotherapy session. A risk-benefit analysis of the potential physiological risk to each infant and the expected therapeutic benefits is strongly advised before hydrotherapy techniques are incorporated into a neonatal therapy program.

Oral-motor therapy. Feeding difficulties are common among infants with neurological immaturity, abnormal muscle tone, depressed oral reflexes, or prolonged use of an endotracheal tube for mechanical ventilation. Because behavioral state affects the quality of feeding behavior, feeding performance may be improved significantly by specific arousal or calming procedures before feeding.

Other variables influencing feeding may include decreased tongue mobility, presence of tongue thrusting, decreased lip seal on nipple, nasal regurgitation, tactile hypersensitivity in the mouth, irregular respiratory patterns, insufficient proximal stability from hypotonic neck and trunk musculature, or hypertonic posturing of the neck and trunk in extension.[140,141]

Two instruments for assessing oral-motor and feeding behaviors in the nursery are the Neonatal Oral-Motor Assessment Scale (NOMAS)[32] and the Nursing Child Assessment Feeding (NCAF) Scale.[14] The NOMAS is used to evaluate the following oral-motor components during sucking: rate, rhythmicity, jaw excursion, tongue configuration, and tongue movement (timing, direction, and range). Tongue and jaw components are analyzed during nutritive and nonnutritive sucking activity. Cut-off scores were derived from a pilot study[32] with the instrument: a combined score of 43 to 47 indicated "some oral-motor disorganization"; a score of 42 or less indicated oral-motor dysfunction. Reliability and validity studies are not available on this new instrument.

The NCAF Scale is used to analyze parent-infant feeding interaction. It provides a method for evaluating the responsiveness of parents to infant cues, signs of distress, and social interaction opportunities during the feeding process. In concurrent validity studies, NCAF scores were positively correlated with the Home Observation for Measurement of the Environment Inventory at 8 months (r = .72) and at 12 months (r = .79).[14]

Management strategies during feeding may include semiflexed positioning with the chin slightly tucked and with elevated shoulder posture inhibited by elongation of the upper trapezius muscles through use of downward traction on the anterolateral shoulder region bilaterally (Fig. 8-28). Techniques of tactile facilitation of the facial muscles, tactile stimulation of specific intraoral structures, use of a pacifier during gavage feedings, manual stabilization of the jaw and thickening of formula are frequent components of oral-motor therapy programs.[91,139-141]

For some infants, oral intake by bottle may be improved by using a "premie nipple," which contains a larger hole and is more easily compressed than standard newborn nipples. The increasing popularity of breast-feeding has encouraged the development of breast-feeding aids (e.g., "Lact-Aid," Division of J.J. Avery, Inc., Denver). These devices allow supplementation of oral intake during breast-feeding through a small tube that goes to the mouth from a presterilized bag containing infant formula. The feeding performance of infants with severe cleft palate deformities is frequently improved by a dental obturator. This custom-fabricated prosthesis is inserted before feeding to cover the defect in the palate. The timing of movement therapy or neonatal hydrotherapy 1 hour before feeding may significantly improve performance by preparation of total body

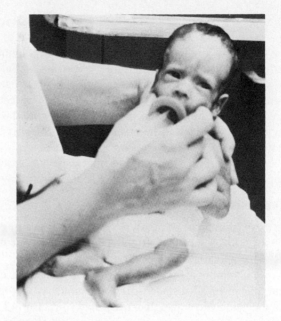

Fig. 8-28. Semiflexed feeding position with neck extensor and upper muscle elongation and occasional facilitation of buccinator muscles.

muscle tone, facilitation of oral musculature, and enhancement of alert responsivity.

Expected outcomes of oral-motor treatment supported by clinical research include: (1) increased number of nutritive sucks after perioral stimulation;[121] (2) increased volume of fluid ingested during nipple feedings;[214] (3) decreased number of gavage feedings, earlier bottle feeding[131] (4) accelerated weight gain[131] and (5) earlier hospital discharge.[131] Measel[131] found that use of a pacifier during tube feedings allowed a discharge 4 days earlier in experimental subjects (n = 29) compared with controls (n = 30). With the cost of NICU care at a minimum of $1000 per day, a discharge 4 days earlier for infants with alterations in feeding may represent a cost saving of at least $4000 per infant.

Monitoring the infant's physiological tolerance to oral-motor evaluation and intervention is crucial. Heart rate values may be monitored from the cardiorespirograph or the DYNAMAPP neonatal vital signs monitor. Tissue oxygen saturation may be followed from a pulse oximeter or transcutaneous oxygen monitor. Color changes and behavioral signs of stress should also be observed. Regurgitation with aspiration of milk or formula into the lungs may occur during oral-motor assessment or feeding therapy; complications of pneumonia, cardiopulmonary arrest, and associated asphyxia may also develop after aspiration. Significant physiological risk to the infant and medical-legal risk to the therapist are inherent in oral-motor treatment of medically fragile neonates.

Parent-infant interaction and perceived competency in

parenting may be negatively affected by feeding experiences in the NICU. Success during feeding activities has been identified as an important variable in developing a positive parent-infant relationship.[30] Parents of infants with feeding problems describe higher stress than parents of infants who "eat well."[178] Because alteration in feeding caused by oral-motor dysfunction has been reported as an early functional deficit in infants at high risk for later neuromotor sequelae,[189] early support to parents coping with a challenging feeding situation sets the stage for attitudes about and compliance with later developmental follow-up.

Parent teaching

Strong continuous support is essential to help parents through perhaps the most frightening crisis in their adult lives—the potential death or disability of their baby.[107,120] It is not uncommon for parents to initially establish emotional and physical distance from the infant as they cope with the knowledge that the baby may die. During this time of anticipatory grief, peer-group support by other parents of prematurely born children can be of immeasureable value. Actively listening to the parents' feelings and concerns is paramount. Although long-range plans include parent participation in all aspects of the developmental program, the timing and amount of initial teaching must be individualized to the levels of stress and acute grief present.

Components of the parent teaching process may include: (1) discussion of the program goals, purposes, and services in the NICU; (2) orientation to the follow-up plan after discharge; (3) guidelines for recognizing and understanding the baby's temperament and ability to interact with the environment; and (4) specific instructions on selected developmental activities and handling techniques. When used in conjunction with verbal instructions and demonstrations, a packet of written guidelines and pictures that are individualized to the infant's needs can improve parents' overall skills and understanding of the program. General handling guidelines for parents of preterm infants, written by pediatric therapists are available for purchase (Appendix B).

Occasionally when geographical distance prevents participation by parents in the inpatient phase of the developmental program, the developmental guidelines may be mailed and later reviewed during outpatient follow-up. During times of separation, telephone contact with parents is imperative to foster attachment to the baby, to explain the purpose and content of the home developmental intervention program, and to discuss the critical need for follow-up. Parents need this ongoing dialogue to make the baby seem real to them and to allow ventilation of their fears and concerns during the separation.

The teaching strategies are most effective when adapted to the learning style of the parents. This may involve more demonstrations and an increased opportunity for supervised practice for some parents, particularly those with reading difficulties that limit use of a written instructional packet.

In the inpatient period, the quality of infant-parent attachment and the comfort level and proficiency of participation in routine care and developmental therapy set the stage for later parenting styles. Helping parents find and appreciate some positive aspects of the newborn infant's neuromotor or other developmental behaviors gives them a spark of hope from which emotional energy can be generated to help them through the marathon of the NICU experience. Empowering parents early in their parenting experience with the infant is crucial. *In the life of the child, the effects of parent empowerment will last far longer than neonatal movement therapy and positioning.*

CLINICAL MANAGEMENT: OUTPATIENT FOLLOW-UP PERIOD
General purposes of follow-up period

Regular follow-up of the at-risk neonate after discharge from the NICU is a critical component of the total management of high-risk infants. The purpose of this follow-up is threefold:

1. To monitor and manage ongoing medical problems, such as respiratory complications and feeding difficulties
2. To provide support and instruction to parents in the care and nurturance of at-risk babies
3. To assess the neurodevelopmental progress of infants so that abnormalities may be identified and treated

Issues of assessment, intervention, and developmental profiles of the high-risk infant following discharge from the NICU are discussed in this section.

Medical management. The routine medical care of low-birth-weight infants following discharge may be provided by a pediatrician, family practitioner, or health clinic. The infant with medical or sensorimotor complications is often cared for later by a number of additional medical specialists, including neurologists, opthalmologists, cardiac or pulmonary specialists, nutritionists and gastrointestinal specialists, public health nurses, as well as physical and occupational therapists and infant educators. Communication among these specialists may be minimal, particularly when they are located at different sites. The parent or caregiver may be confronted with conflicting opinions, demands, and expectations of the family and their baby. The follow-up clinic can play a valuable role in this situation by designating one professional as case manager to assist the parents in coordinating services, to verify that all needs of the infant are being met, to set realistic and compatible goals, and to help set priorities

Table 8-7. Incidence of cerebral palsy relative to birth weight

Infant birth weight (g)	Rate of cerebral palsy (per 1000 live births)
All birth weights	2.0 to 2.5
>2500	3.3
1501 to 2500	13.9
<1501	90.4

Data from Ellenberg JH and Nelson KB: Birth weight and gestational age in children with cerebral palsy or seizure disorders, Am J Dis Child 133:1044, 1979 and Paneth N: Etiologic factors in cerebral palsy, Pediatric Annals 15(3):194, 1986.

Table 8-8. Incidence of major neurodevelopmental handicaps* in low-birth-weight infants[36,109,112,151]

Infant birth weight (g)	Neurodevelopmental handicap
1500 to 2500	10%
1000 to 1500	10% to 20%
<1000	15% to 40%

*Cerebral palsy, mental retardation, hydrocephalus, visual impairment, sensorineural hearing loss

among the multiple requirements placed on the family and infant.

Family support. The stress that a vulnerable, premature or at-risk infant brings to a family is well-documented. Anxiety, grief, anger, and depression are common reactions of parents of premature infants.[103,120] The primary caregivers of high-risk infants are required to become knowledgeable about complex medical terminology and equipment. At discharge they often become responsible for the administration of complicated feeding procedures requiring measurement and recording of intake and output, multiple medications of varying dosages and protocol, and cardiopulmonary procedures and equipment. Frequently, families must cope with a tremendous financial obligation and manage different billing agencies and funding sources.

The low-birth-weight infant is often irritable, hypersensitive to stimulation, less responsive to the affective interactions of his parents, and more irregular in sleeping and feeding schedules than the full-term infant.[7,60] The demands that such an infant places on the parents can have a long-term negative impact on the parent-infant relationship and the infant's social and affective development.[13,17,59] Regular follow-up by trained professionals who are knowledgeable about the developmental patterns and specific needs of the low-birth-weight infant is essential.

Assessment of neurodevelopmental status. Because low-birth-weight infants are at increased risk for neurodevelopmental disorders, close follow-up is necessary during the first 6 to 8 years of life. The prevalence of cerebral palsy is significantly greater in low-birth-weight babies than in full-term infants, and the frequency of handicap increases with decreasing birth-weight levels (Table 8-7).[74,156,199] Cerebral palsy is one of several major neurological conditions that are observed sequelae of prematurity; others include mental retardation, hydrocephalus, sensorineural hearing loss, visual impairment, and seizure disorder. When examined as a group, these major handicapping conditions occur with increased prevalence in low-birth-weight infants,

and again the frequency increases in the lower birth-weight groups[26,109,112,157,204] (Table 8-8).

The frequency of so-called minor neurodevelopmental and neurobehavioral abnormalities, observed in long-term follow-up of low-birth-weight infants, is also increased.* Problems in visual-motor skills, language comprehension, reading and math skills, static balance, coordination, as well as muscle tone abnormalities and behavior disorders, such as attention deficits and impulsivity, occur at greater frequency among children born prematurely. Outcome studies indicate that by school-age approximately one-half of low-birth-weight infants will have educational and learning deficits as compared with a reported rate of 24% in the general population.[39,73,146]

Overall, it is estimated that approximately 10% to 30% of low-birth-weight infants will have major neurological handicaps, and up to 40% will have "minor" neurological handicaps. A primary objective of developmental follow-up of at-risk infants is the early identification of neurodevelopmental abnormalities so that therapeutic intervention can be initiated. Low-birth-weight infants who participate in a follow-up clinic have demonstrated advanced performance on cognitive measures and receive more intervention services relative to nonmonitored infants.[196]

The benefits of early therapy have not been substantiated consistently by scientific research, although results of some studies indicate positive change.† However, early recognition of the presence of a developmental disorder is important for directing resources toward family support and/or school management. A developmentally delayed infant may evoke negative maternal responses of anxiety, frustration, and withdrawal even before a medical diagnosis is made.[135] Early recognition by professionals of a developmental problem enables them to assist the parents during this time of adjustment and to help maintain positive, affectionate interaction. A "minor" neurodevelopmental abnormality is not at all minor in the life of that child or his family.

*References 39, 67, 111, 146, 147, 191, 218.
†References 86, 98, 155, 164, 171, 194.

High-risk infant follow-up model

The neurodevelopmental progress of the at-risk infant requires careful monitoring with systematic evaluation at intervals in the first year of life. An organizational model of a high-risk infant follow-up clinic is shown in Figure 8-29. It is based on the format of the Neonatal Intensive Care Unit (NICU) Follow-up Clinic of the Child Development and Mental Retardation Center established at the University of Washington in Seattle, Washington.

Before discharge from the NICU, very-high-risk infants (infants with seizures, cystic PVL, grade IV bleeding, and obvious neurological abnormalities) are distinguished from infants at relatively low risk. The high-risk infant receives therapeutic intervention as described in the previous neonatal section. The infant who is not showing indications of abnormality is closely monitored, but usually without specific intervention. Instead, the role of the therapist with the low-risk infant is primarily to provide guidance to the nurses and parents regarding positioning and modulated developmental intervention.

At discharge, the high-risk or abnormal infant is referred to an ongoing therapy program in the community. It is recommended that the therapy services be provided in the home to minimize the stress to the infant and the family, although this objective cannot always be accommodated. The infants who do not require therapy are referred to the follow-up clinic for developmental follow-up and to their community pediatrician for medical management.

Age correction. Premature infants are scheduled for evaluation in the follow-up clinic according to their *corrected age* (age adjusted for weeks of prematurity). The issue of whether to adjust according to the gestational age of the infant when assessing psychomotor development is an ongoing question.[130,134,154,193] In several studies the authors have demonstrated that if uncorrected ages are used, the *normal* premature infant will have a lower developmental quotient and delayed acquisition of milestones relative to full-term peers.[134,154] If ages are adjusted for prematurity, the performance of the premature babies is comparable to that of full-term infants at 1 year. However, in assessment done before 1 year of age, adjustment for prematurity tends to result in overcorrection, particularly in infants less than 33 weeks gestation at birth. Consequently, abnormal infants have had developmental quotients in the normal range of standard tests when age was adjusted for prematurity.

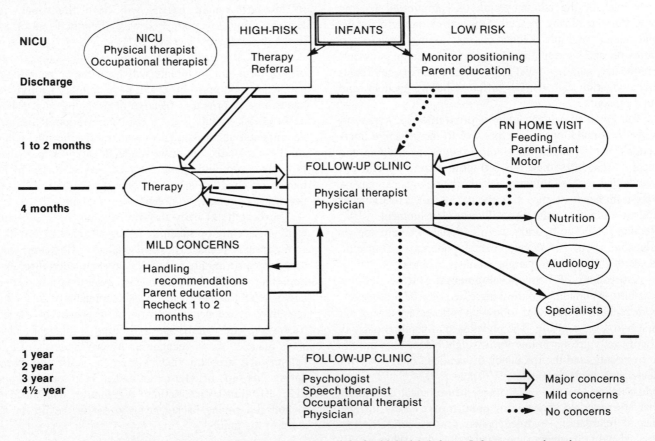

Fig. 8-29. Organizational model of a follow-up clinic for high-risk infants. Infants are evaluated through the interdisciplinary clinic from the time of discharge from the NICU. When problems are identified referral is made to appropriate specialist.

In a follow-up program, the decision of whether to correct for prematurity depends on the following factors: (1) testing instruments used, with attention to the competencies evaluated by the tool and the number of premature infants in the normative sample, and (2) the purpose of the assessment. If the objective is to detect infants who may be neurologically impaired, it is recommended that using uncorrected ages provides a more sensitive index of abnormality. If the purpose of the assessment is to document developmental progress of the at-risk infant relative to a normal population, using corrected age appears to be the more appropriate approach.

In the High-Risk Infant Clinic at the University of Washington, all premature infants are evaluated on the basis of their corrected age from infancy through school-age examinations to age 8 years. Developmental quotients in the normal range do not, however, preclude concerns or referral to intervention services when neuromotor or behavioral abnormality is observed.

Follow-up clinic evaluation schedule. The schedule of routine appointments for all infants in the follow-up clinic is shown in Table 8-9. Although the first *routine* appointment is at 4 months (corrected age), infants may be seen earlier at the recommendation of the hospital discharge team, physical therapist, community pediatrician, public health nurse or parent. The examinations typically performed by each specialist are listed in Table 8-9.

Home visit. At 4 to 6 weeks after discharge from the hospital, a pediatric nurse practitioner makes a home visit when geographically and logistically possible. In addition to providing support and assistance to the family in home management, she evaluates the baby's feeding and nutritional status, the parent-infant interaction, the infant's social and cognitive development, and the motor development of the baby. If there are concerns regarding neuromotor status, the infant is referred to the follow-up clinic for an early comprehensive assessment by the physical therapist.

Four-month evaluation. Four months of age has been determined to be an optimal time for the initial follow-up evaluation for the following reasons:

1. Examinations of older infants are better predictors than neonatal examinations. The neonatal period and the first 2 to 3 months of life are characterized by variability in infant behavior as well as instability of tone, reflex activity, and functional skills.[3] Predictive studies that have examined the results of sequential examinations have demonstrated that neonatal examinations are less accurate in their ability to predict neurodevelopmental outcome than examinations performed on older infants.[75,151,171]
2. Four months is a critical time in the developmental maturation of infants. In the normal infant, muscle

tone tends to be stable,[171] reflexes have minimal influence, balance reactions are emerging, and babies develop functional skills with an orientation to the midline (Fig. 8-30). At this time, when medical concerns about the high-risk infant are resolving, parents often begin to form questions about developmental expectations. Although for most infants it is not possible to make definitive statements about long-term prognosis at 4 months of age, a systematic evaluation at this age provides an important baseline

Table 8-9. High-risk infant clinic: scheduled evaluations

Corrected age of child	Examiners*	Standard tests administered
4 months	Physical therapist	Movement Assessment of Infants
		Bayley Scales of Infant Development (BSID)
	Pediatrician*	
1 year	Pediatrician	Denver Developmental Screening Test (DDST)
		Neurological examination
	Psychologist	BSID
	Audiologist	
	Physical therapist*	
2 years	Pediatrician	Neurological examination
		DDST
	Psychologist	BSID
	Physical therapist*	
3 years	Pediatrician	DDST
		Neurological examination
	Psychologist	Stanford-Binet
		Peabody Picture Vocabulary Test
	Physical therapist*	
	Speech/audiologist*	
4½ years	Pediatrician	DDST
		Neurological examination
	Psychologist	Wechsler Preschool and Primary Scale of Intelligence (WPPSI)
	Occupational therapist	Peabody Developmental Motor Scales
		Miller Assessment of Pre-School
	Physical therapist*	
	Speech/Audiologist*	
6 years	Pediatrician	DDST
		Neurological examination
8 years	Psychologist	Wechsler Intelligence Scale for Children—Revised (WISC-R) or WPPSI
		Peabody Individual Achievement Test (PIAT)
	Physical therapist*	
	Speech/Audiologist*	

*Consultant examiner.

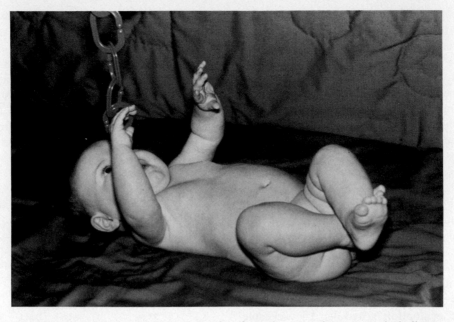

Fig. 8-30. A normal full-term infant at 4 months of age demonstrating symmetrical alignment of trunk and extremities, functional movement against gravity, and no influence of the tonic labyrinthine reflex.

for comparative assessment of developmental progress in subsequent evaluations.

3. When the initial follow-up evaluations occur at later ages, such as 6 or 9 months, the potential impact of the follow-up clinic in family support is diminished. Many adjustment crises and management problems occur before this time. Although neuromotor abnormality is usually more obvious and therefore more readily detected at later examinations,[206] equivocal findings are still common.[8,176] By delaying the time of assessment until the time when neuromotor abnormalities are conclusive, intervention for the baby and the family is also delayed.

• • •

At the 4-month evaluation the physical therapist assumes the role of case manager. Because infants at this age express their capabilities and consequently their neurological integrity through their movements, the therapist, as a specialist in movement, is the most highly skilled professional in observing and interpreting the motor activity of the infant. By using both the Movement Assessment of Infants (Appendix C) and the Bayley Scales of Infant Assessment, the therapist can examine the infant's neuromotor and developmental status. The developmental pediatrician provides medical consultation at the request of the therapist when health, neurological, or developmental concerns are noted during the examination. The infant is referred to a specialist for further investigation if problems are noted in nutrition, vision, hearing, or musculoskeletal alignment.

If the infant demonstrates normal neuromotor and developmental progress at the 4-month evaluation, the next scheduled evaluation is at 1 year (corrected age). The parents or caregivers are informed of their baby's level of function, given recommendations according to their child's performance, and advised regarding appropriate expectations for their baby in the next months. They are encouraged to call the therapist if questions arise in the interim period. If the therapist notes an area of minor concern, a telephone interview can be made with appropriate questions to the parents.

If the infant demonstrates definite abnormality, significant delay, or shows strong indications of neurological impairment, the child is referred to an appropriate intervention program. This could consist of physical therapy for the infant who demonstrates only motor impairment or a developmental program for the infant who is delayed in multiple areas.

At 4 months many infants demonstrate immaturity or mild neuromotor abnormality. The parents are given handling and positioning recommendations and are shown activities to facilitate developmental progress. The infant is scheduled for a reexamination at an appropriate interval relative to the level of concern, often 6 to 8 weeks. At that time, the infant is reassessed and may be referred for therapy if the concerns persist, reexamined in 2 months to confirm continuing improvement, or scheduled to return for the 1-year evaluation.

One-year evaluation. Beginning at 1 year, the follow-up evaluations become increasingly multidisciplinary as the infant becomes a more complex individual. The clinic schedule is designed to allow for maximum assessment of various areas of competency while not exhausting the infant and his family. Because the infant has been followed by the physical therapist throughout the first year of life, formal motor evaluation is not scheduled. Motor skills are assessed by the psychologist and the pediatrician using the Bayley Scales. The physical therapist is available to provide consultation when delay or deviance is noted. The protocol for the 2- and 3-year evaluations is similar in format to the 1-year evaluation.

Four-and-one-half year evaluation. A scheduled evaluation at 4½ years provides an opportunity to inform families of their child's developmental status as they are making decisions regarding school entry. In addition to assessment by the psychologist, speech pathologist, and pediatrician, the occupational therapist evaluates the child's motor development with particular attention to balance, coordination, and fine motor and perceptual motor dysfunction. The objective is to identify potential learning disorders before school placement and to minimize their effect on school performance.

Neuromotor assessment of the high-risk infant

Assessment tools. In addition to the tools designed to assess the neonate, a number of systematic assessments of the infant have been developed. Based on content and emphasis, these instruments can be viewed in two broad categories: developmental/behavioral and neurological. The Bayley Scales of Infant Development and the Denver Developmental Screening Test are well-known developmental tests, whereas Amiel-Tison's Neurological Assessment of the Infant is a neurological evaluation for the full-term and premature infant during the first year of life. The examination of Milani-Comparetti and the Movement Assessment of Infants are neuromotor examinations that include neurological components, such as the evaluation of reflexes, as well as assessment of some developmental functions.

The choice of instrument for a particular clinical situation will depend on the emphasis and focus of the clinic and the disciplines involved in its organization. Neurological findings tend to be more stable in the young infant and are less subject to the influence of the infant's affective state and the environment. However, individual neurological signs can be transient and may not be indicative of overall neurological competency, particularly in an infant who has been injured. Over time, neurological integrity is demonstrated best by the achievement of developmental skills. The results of a major collaborative follow-up study indicate that neurological abnormalities are predictive of later cerebral palsy only when they are associated with failure to perform one or more developmental milestones.[75]

A brief review of the infant assessments commonly used in follow-up clinics is presented below.

Neurologic Evaluation of the Newborn and Infant.[8] The Neurologic Evaluation of the Newborn and the Infant[8]
was developed by Amiel-Tison for the assessment of the neuromotor behavior of infants in the first 12 months of life. It was designed to be administered on a monthly basis, and its primary purpose is to detect neurological abnormalities or deviations.

The test includes examination of the skull, evaluation of muscle tone and primary reflexes, and observation of posture and movement. The assessment of passive muscle tone is based in part on methods described by Andre-Thomas.[10] Important factors include *extensibility,* in which the range of movement is expressed in terms of an angle or specific anatomical sign, and *passivity,* or flapping of the distal segments of the limbs. Active tone is assessed by observing the infant's motor responses to specific physical manipulation by the examiner. Control of the neck flexors and extensor musculature is emphasized as well as the traction response. Developmental milestones and functional skills are not assessed.

The infant's responses are recorded on a grid that provides a record of the infant's performance on successive tests throughout the year. Visual and written descriptions on the score sheet indicate how to score a particular response. Scores considered to be abnormal for a given item at a designated age are shaded on the record sheet. The individual scores do not yield a summary score. The examiner is given descriptive guidelines for formulating a clinical impression based on one examination and on the pattern of development on repeated evaluations.

The Neurologic Evaluation has a standardized procedure but normative data is not provided. Interrater reliability is available only for the passive tone items. Reported percentage of agreement ranges from 50% to 90%. Test-retest reliability is not given, and specific validity data have not been reported. The results of longitudinal studies of the outcome of infants evaluated with this instrument indicate that the abnormalities detected on early examinations frequently resolve. In a follow-up study of 168 low-birth-weight infants, 41% had abnormal examinations when examined at term age, with the principal findings including abnormalities of tone, hyperreflexia, and deviant eye movements. On follow-up examination at 12 months, only 13% of these infants had major neurodevelopmental disorders and another 20% infants had minor neurological abnormalities.[204]

Bayley Scales of Infant Development.[16] The Bayley Scales of Infant Development[16] is a standardized assessment of mental and motor abilities of infants and children between the ages of 2 months and 2½ years. The test is divided into two areas: the mental scale includes test items rating performance in the areas of problem solving, memory, visual-perception, learning and verbal communication; the motor scale evaluates gross and fine motor skills. For the infant younger than 12 months of age, successful performance on the mental scale requires competency in visual following and fine motor manipulation. The mental test becomes more heavily weighted towards language items at the older-age intervals. The motor scale is predominantly an assessment of gross motor milestones, with qualitative deviations and asymmetrical performance not recorded.

Administration procedures and grading criteria are clearly described in the manual. Items are scored on the basis of presence or absence of response. Basal and ceiling levels of performance are obtained on each scale. The raw scores are converted to standard scores, the Mental Developmental Index (MDI) and the Psychomotor Developmental Index (PDI), both of which reportedly have a mean of 100 and a standard deviation variation of ±16. These scores are based on standards set in 1969 from a sample of 1262 children in 14 age groups. Recent evidence suggests that this normative data is no longer valid and that the standard scores may overestimate an infant's performance relative to the normal population.[42]

Reliability of the Bayley Scales has been reported for both scales. For the motor scale the mean tester-observer percentage of agreement was 93 and mean test-retest percentage of agreement was 75. Concurrent validity with the Stanford-Binet is reported in the Bayley manual as .57.[16] No predictive validity is given. Numerous studies have evaluated the relationship between performance on the Bayley in infancy and later outcome. Although the Bayley Mental Scale appears to predict later cognitive development more accurately than the motor scale, the neurological status of a child at 7 years of age is predicted more efficiently by the motor scale.[21] The Bayley motor PDI reportedly identified cerebral palsy in 3-month-old infants with a sensitivity of 89%,[41] but this has not been confirmed by subsequent studies with 4-month-old infants.[94,151]

Milani-Comparetti Developmental Examination.[133] The Milani-Comparetti Developmental Examination[133] was an early attempt to evaluate neurological and developmental components of infant movement within one screening examination. The stated objective of this test is to selectively include items that reflect the "correlation between functional motor achievement and the underlying reflex structure."[133,p. 285] It assesses gross motor skills between birth and 24 months and the underlying postural reactions that support these skills: righting reactions, tilting reactions, and parachute reactions. Five primitive reflexes—the palmar and plantar grasp reflexes, asymmetrical and symmetrical tonic neck reflexes, and Moro—are included. Muscle tone is not assessed. The test reportedly can be administered in 3 to 10 minutes. This includes minimal time for observation of spontaneous movement, because the test primarily involves physical maneuvers applied to the infant.

In the original description of the examination, descriptive notes are provided for selected items with guidelines for administration and recognition of the desired reaction. Responses are graded only by presence or absence. Observations are recorded on a chart organized as a developmental grid extending from birth to 24 months, and items are arranged according to the time of "usual appearance" along the horizontal axis. Reflexes and reactions related to specific motor function are aligned along the vertical axis. The underlying assumption is that "a particular reaction must be present in order that a particular item of motor behavior can occur."[133, p. 295]

The Milani-Comparetti in its original form is not quantified and does not yield a numerical score. Subsequent modifications of the test have included numerical scoring systems with a total score achieved by summation.[76,196] Reliability was calculated for a revised version of the test. Interrater reliability was in the 90% to 93% range for mean percentage of agreement, whereas test-retest reliability was 93% for percent of agreement.[205] With a modified Milani-Comparetti scored on a 5-point scale, the test reportedly distinguished normal and abnormal infants at 6 months.[76] In subsequent studies the Milani-Comparetti administered at 3 months of age was not predictive of later neurodevelopmental outcome.[151,211] It was noted that the test did identify infants with severe cerebral palsy and that predictive validity was better at 6 months, although still not adequate for a screening tool. For additional information refer to Chapter 14, specifically Fig. 14-8.

Movement Assessment of Infants.[50] The Movement Assessment of Infants (MAI) was developed by Chandler, Andrews, and Swanson[50] specifically for use in a high-risk infant follow-up clinic. It is a systematic examination of muscle tone, primitive reflexes, automatic reactions of balance and equilibrium, and volitional gross and fine motor skills.

In the manual the authors recommend that the MAI be considered for the following purposes: (1) to identify motor dysfunction in infants up to 12 months of age, (2) to establish the basis for an early intervention program, (3) to monitor the effects of physical therapy on infants or children whose motor behavior is at or below 1 year of age, (4) to assist in data collection and clinical research on motor development through the use of a standard system of movement assessment, and (5) to teach skilled observation of movement and motor development through evaluation of normal and handicapped children.[50]

The 45-minute test period allows time for scoring, parent counseling, and rest/feeding breaks for the infant. A flexible order of testing is allowed, but grouping of items by infant position (supine, prone, sitting, vertical suspension, standing, prone suspension) is advised to minimize fatigue and stress.

The categories of primitive reflexes (14 items), automatic reactions (16 items), and volitional movement (25 items) are graded on a 4-point scale; muscle tone (10 items) is rated on a 6-point scale. Although the manual provides clear descriptions of the examination and scoring procedures, clinicians anticipating use of the Movement Assessment of Infants can improve reliability and overall understanding of the tool through postgraduate clinical training opportunities at the University of Washington, Seattle or during weekend seminars by the authors in selected cities.

The assessment provides a profile of motor behavior for 4- and 8-month-old infants, and a risk score indicating deviant or abnormal neuromotor function can be computed (see Appendixes C and D). Early data reported in the manual indicate that total-risk scores greater than 7 were suggestive of neuromotor delay or abnormality. The authors, however, recommended a higher cut-off point because of scoring revisions made before publication of the manual. This has been substantiated by more recent MAI data collected with full-term and premature infants.[90,187,207] Norms have not yet been established, although the performance of small samples of full-term and premature infants on the MAI at 4 and 8 months of age has been recorded. This preliminary information suggests that total risk scores *under 10* are within a normal range.

Early studies of interrater reliability based on percent of agreement reported a 90% level,[50] whereas a later study indicated a 72% interrater reliability and a 76% test-retest reliability.[92] Concurrent validity between the MAI and the Bayley Motor Scale has been reported as −.63.[93] The predictive validity has been examined in relation to later performance on the Bayley Scales as well as neurodevelopmental outcome. The correlation between the MAI at 4 and 8 months of age and the mental and motor scales of the Bayley at 1 and 2 years of age is highly significant.[93,206] The MAI at 4 months of age has been shown to be a more discriminating predictor of later outcome than several other tools, including the Milani-Comparetti and the Prechtl Neurological Examination.[151] The MAI was also more accurate in discriminating abnormality than the Bayley Motor Scale at 4 and 8 months of age.[206]

Chandler Movement Assessment of Infants Screening Test. The Chandler Movement Assessment of Infants Screening Test is a 15-minute screening tool for health professionals in primary care (pediatricians, family practice physicians, and nurse practitioners), designed to identify infants needing referral for definitive neurological and developmental assessment. The test retains the basic categories of the Movement Assessment of Infants, but it is limited to selected items considered predictive of movement disorders. Publication will occur after the collection of normative data has been completed.

• • •

Infant neuromotor assessment using an objective, standard instrument serves the following two major functions in a follow-up clinic:

1. It documents the infant's current neuromotor status relative to developmental norms and to the infant's previous examinations to determine progress, rate of change, and degree of delay, if any.

Table 8-10. Prediction accuracy of an infant test

Evaluation (at specified age)	Outcome (at specified age)	
	Normal	**Abnormal**
No-risk	Correct nonreferrals*	Under-referrals (false negatives)
Risk	Over-referrals (false positives)	Correct referrals†

Adapted from Stangler SR: Screening growth and development of preschool children, New York, 1980, McGraw-Hill Book Co.

$$*\text{Specificity} = \frac{\text{Correct nonreferrals}}{\text{Total normal}} \times 100 = \begin{array}{l}\text{Percentage of normal}\\\text{cases classified normal}\end{array}$$

$$†\text{Sensitivity} = \frac{\text{Correct referrals}}{\text{Total abnormal}} \times 100 = \begin{array}{l}\text{Percentage of}\\\text{abnormal}\\\text{cases identified}\end{array}$$

2. It identifies neuromotor abnormality indicative of a movement disorder, so that therapeutic intervention can be initiated. Early identification is not simply a task of recognizing signs of neuromotor deviation or central nervous system injury. The challenge is to distinguish among those infants with abnormal clinical signs the relatively few who will have an abnormal motor outcome. The goal of infant assessment is to predict the neurodevelopmental outcome of the child on the basis of a clinical examination of the infant.

Predictive Value of Infant Assessment Tools. The predictive accuracy of a test is stated in terms of sensitivity and specificity[201] (see Table 8-10). *Sensitivity* is the ability of the test to identify abnormal as abnormal. It is calculated as the percentage of abnormal children who were correctly identified as such when examined as infants. *Specificity* is the ability of the test to identify normal as normal. It is the percentage of normal children who were correctly identified as normal when examined as infants. Table 8-11 shows the sensitivity and specificity of several infant assessment tools.

When neonatal assessments are compared, it is evident that comprehensive instruments, such as the Prechtl,[166] have a good sensitivity. Low specificity indicates a high rate of "false positives": infants who were considered high risk on the basis of the infant examination, but were normal at the time of the outcome evaluation. Less comprehensive examinations, such as the Paine assessment,[153] had better specificity but lower sensitivity. This indicates a lesser ability to identify as abnormal infants who will later develop cerebral palsy.

The improved predictive ability of examination at 4 months compared with a neonatal examination is demonstrated by the higher sensitivity of the Paine evaluation at this age. The Movement Assessment of Infants, a comprehensive and detailed evaluation, demonstrated good sensitivity but low specificity when first examined.[93] More recent data with the MAI indicates better sensitivity and specificity at both 4 and 8 month evaluations.[206] In contrast, the sensitivity of the Bayley Motor Scale is low and the Bayley appears to offer little predictive value at 4 months.[93,206]

• • •

Prediction of neuromotor outcome is difficult in low-birth-weight infants because of several complicating factors.

Table 8-11. Predictive validity of infant assessment tools*

Assessment	Outcome age	Sensitivity (%)	Specificity (%)
Neonatal examinations			
Amiel-Tison (modified) (Stewart, 1988)[204]	1 year	80	67
Dubowitz (Dubowitz, 1984)[24]	1 year	83	67
Paine (Nelson and Ellenberg, 1979)[143]	7 years	57	88
Prechtl (Bierman-van Eendenburg, 1981, 1984)[22]	18 months	87	54
4-month examinations			
Bayley Motor Scale (Swanson, unpublished)	18 months	16	97
MAI (Harris, 1987)[94]	3 years	73	63
MAI (Swanson, unpublished)	18 months	83	78
Paine (Ellenberg and Nelson, 1981)[75]	7 years	64	89

*References 22, 24, 75, 94, 143, 204.

Impact of medical status on test performance. Low-birth-weight infants often exhibit delay and neurologic instability because of their medical status, not central nervous system dysfunction. This can occur at the following two levels:

1. Temporary depression or deviation in posture and movement because of weakness, shock, or medication. Abnormalities tend to diminish as the infant's condition stabilizes.
2. Prolonged retardation and neurological changes because of chronic disease, such as bronchopulmonary dysplasia. The babies with chronic lung disease typically exhibit low muscle tone, delayed gross motor function, and immature balance reactions (Fig. 8-31). Delay is evident as long as their pulmonary capacity is compromised, but developmental progress accelerates when the respiratory condition resolves.

Differences between premature and full-term infant neuromotor behavior. Premature infants demonstrate deviation from full-term infants in neuromotor function even when they have not experienced chronic illness and do not have neurological impairment. These variations may reflect predominant positioning during hospitalization, other extrauterine influences, or neurologic immaturity.

When compared with full-term infants, healthy premature infants demonstrate variations in their passive and active muscle tone. They initially show greater joint mobility, but may exhibit areas of increased tone, particularly in the hips and ankles, from 2 to 4 months of age.[76,181] Their movements reflect a tendency towards extension posturing, with shoulder retraction, and less antigravity movements in supine[83,215] (Fig. 8-32). Primitive reflexes, such as the asymmetrical tonic neck reflex, the Moro, and the positive support reflex, which are often less pronounced in the

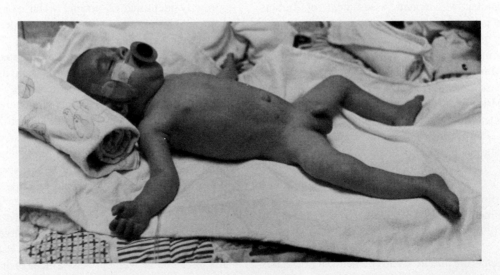

Fig. 8-31. A premature infant with chronic lung disease at 4 months of age with characteristic hypotonic posture and minimal movement against gravity.

young premature infant, tend to persist longer in low-birth-weight infants, even when assessed at corrected age.[127]

Balance reactions, including head righting, are immature in the healthy premature infant when compared with full-term infants of comparable age (Fig. 8-33, *A* and *B*). Gross and fine motor skills, especially activities requiring flexion control such as bringing hands to midline and feet to hands, are also less mature.

For most premature infants, these early variations in movement and posture eventually resolve. In the first months of life, however, they influence both the infant's performance on a neuromotor evaluation and the examiner's clinical impression.

Transient dystonia. Up to 60% of all low-birth-weight infants, as well as a number of full-term infants, exhibit abnormal neurologic signs that resolve without evidence of

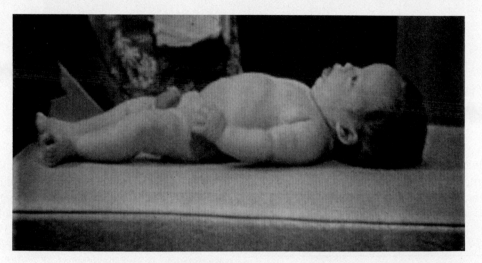

Fig. 8-32 A healthy premature infant at 4 months of age demonstrating shoulder retraction, neck hyperextension, and limited antigravity movement into flexion.

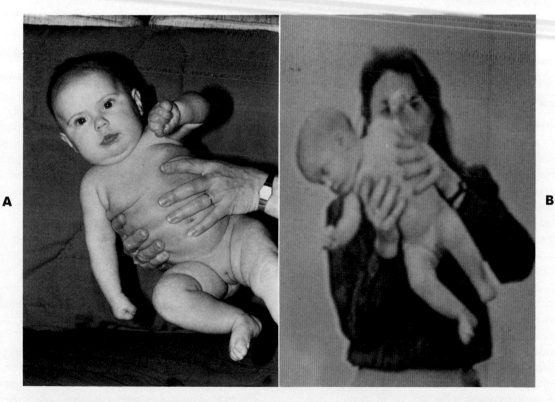

Fig. 8-33. A, A normal full-term infant at 4 months of age demonstrating lateral head righting. When tipped to the side she is able to maintain her head in midline. **B,** A healthy premature infant at 4 months of age demonstrating immature lateral head righting. When tipped to the side the head is not maintained in midline and falls to the side.

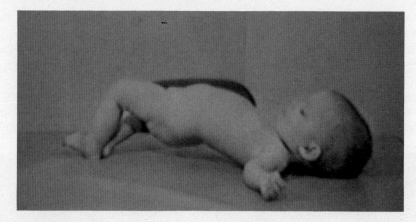

Fig. 8-34. A premature infant at 4 months of age demonstrating excessive arching and extension posturing in supine position, but developmental outcome was normal at 1 year.

Table 8-12. Clinical characteristics of dystonia and abnormality of movements in premature infants that often are transient and resolve spontaneously

Neonatal period	4 Months of age	6 to 8 Months of age
Neck extensor hypertonia	Hypertonicity: Extensor posturing Scissoring	Hypertonia of lower extremities
Hypotonia	Truncal hypotonia	Hypotonia
Irritability	Persistent reflexes: ATNR Positive support	Delayed postural reactions
Lethargy	Head lag	Delayed sitting

major neurologic sequelae.[65,88,179] This phenomenon is referred to as "transient dystonia." The abnormalities reportedly are observed in the first 4 months of life, they are most evident between 4 and 8 months, and they are resolved by 1 year of age (Fig. 8-34). The clinical characteristics of transient dystonia that have been most frequently described are given in Table 8-12.

Manifestation of these findings on examination presents a challenge to the examiner. Similar clinical signs have been reported to be indicative of developing cerebral palsy. It is usually not possible to distinguish the early signs of cerebral palsy from transient neurological signs on one examination. Moreover, long-term follow-up has revealed that even infants whose abnormalities are transient are at increased risk for minor neurodevelopmental abnormalities. Infants who demonstrate abnormal neurological findings in the first year, although developmentally normal at 1-year evaluations, have a higher rate of mental, motor, and behavioral deficits in preschool and schoolage assessments.[9,65]

It is evident that even transient abnormal neuromotor signs in the first year should not be considered as clinically insignificant. They may indicate a child who is at risk for neuromotor problems other than cerebral palsy that may not be functionally evident until school age. In addition, the abnormal behaviors of the infant, although transient, may interfere with the parent-infant bonding process. The infant who is arching instead of cuddling, the infant with poor head control and consequently diminished eye contact with his parents, or the infant who is irritable and less engaging threatens the quality of the affective and social environment. This may have a serious detrimental impact on the child's outcome with residual consequences long after the neurological signs have resolved.

High-risk clinical signs. Numerous attempts have been made to identify specific clinical signs that are early manifestations of cerebral palsy. Historically these were based on subjective qualitative impressions of experienced clinicians.[26,98,152] These observations were a major contribution to the effort to develop methods for early diagnosis of cerebral palsy. However, there were no standard criteria for the observed findings, no control for personal bias and interpretation, and, in general, there was no evidence that the observations were significantly related to outcome.

Recent data from follow-up studies based on objective measures has been examined to determine which individual clinical findings are most predictive of abnormal outcome. Conclusions are inconsistent, which may reflect the variability of infants as well as the lack of standard criteria for clinical variables and outcome measures. Results from these studies are summarized in Table 8-13.

Neonatal period. During the neonatal period, the clinical signs reported to be indicative of later cerebral palsy include jerky or abnormal movements and abnormal cry. The tone abnormality most frequently associated with later cerebral palsy is truncal hypotonia with head lag when pulled to sit.[179] However, this finding is not specific to ce-

Table 8-13. High-risk clinical signs indicative of neuromotor abnormality in infants

Neonatal period	4 Months of age	6 Months of age
Abnormal tone	Hypertonicity Lower extremities (hips/knees) Extensibility Neck extensor Hypotonia	Hypertonicity: Upper extremities (flexion) Lower extremities (ankles)
Tremulousness	Tremulousness	
Ankle clonus	Persistent reflexes: Asymmetrical tonic neck Tonic labyrinthine	Persistent asymmetrical tonic neck reflex
		Delayed postural reactions: Head righting Parachute
Abnormal or absent cry	Delayed motor skills: Head control	Delayed motor skills: Rolling
Jerky movements	Sit with support	Sitting
Abnormal eye movements	Support in prone Open hands Hands to midline Visual following	Reach Grasp

rebral palsy, because it is also a characteristic of many infants with normal outcome.[76] Although hypotonia and head lag are frequently observed in young premature infants, in *most* babies these conditions resolve as they mature.

Four months. By 3 to 4 months of age, the abnormal tone often associated with later cerebral palsy is hypertonicity, observed primarily in the lower extremities but usually not in the ankles at this age. Hypertonicity of the extremities in combination with truncal hypotonia is a particularly high-risk sign. The increased tone is detected by the "angles" method of passive assessment of tone used by the Amiel-Tison and Dubowitz examinations and the "extensibility" item of the MAI (Fig. 8-35). Neck extensor hypertonicity has been noted to be highly predictive of cerebral palsy.[7] However, although it was the single most predictive item in one study, the majority of infants (60%) who exhibited this clinical sign did not subsequently develop cerebral palsy.[75]

Persistent reflexes at 4 months have been equivocal. Reflexes and neurological signs such as the ATNR and tremulousness have been correlated with cerebral palsy in some studies[75,176,179] but not in others[41,95] (Fig. 8-36). Of the four sections of the MAI, "primitive reflexes" was found to be least predictive of later outcome.[93]

In contrast, the "volitional movement" section of the MAI was found to be most predictive at 4 months.[93] This finding is supported by other studies in which delayed de-

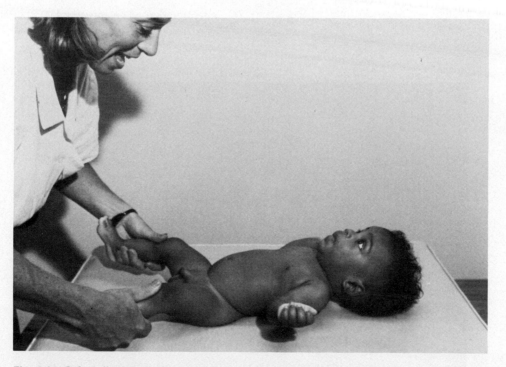

Fig. 8-35. Infant diagnosed with cerebral palsy at 5 months of age; limited hip abduction when passive mobility is examined.

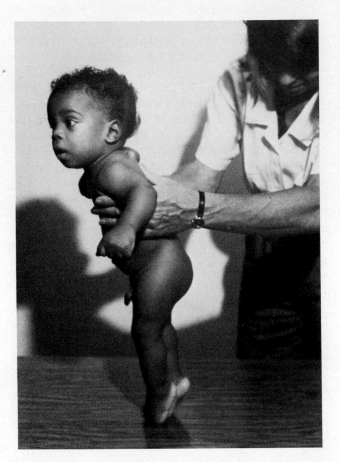

Fig. 8-36. Infant diagnosed with cerebral palsy at 5 months of age; persistence of the positive support reflex.

velopmental milestones were found to be significant predictors of later cerebral palsy[41,75] (Figs. 8-37 and 8-38). Asymmetry of tone and movement is often considered to be an early indication of neurological dysfunction, but this has not been documented.[75,95] It has been commonly observed in premature infants, but its presence does not correlate with later cerebral palsy. Fisting of the hands at this age is a significant finding.[95,179]

Six months. Because of the prevalence of transient neurological abnormalities in the low-birth-weight infant, 6 months is a less-than-optimal time for prediction of neurodevelopmental outcome on the basis of clinical observation.[9,176] Tone abnormalities most consistently associated with later cerebral palsy include hypertonicity of the upper and lower extremities. The increased tone in the lower extremities can be detected by examination of passive tone and in vertical suspension of the infant, which produces extension posturing of the legs. The upper extremity tone is commonly indicated by shoulder retraction and increased flexor tone.

Interpretation of infant assessment. A review of follow-up studies examining early identification of cerebral palsy indicates that the long-term predictive value of infant assessment, although limited, is of clinical importance. Although it is not possible to predict with certainty the outcome of a specific child, systematic, objective assessment does allow clinicians to make a reasonably accurate statement about a child's degree of risk. This information is important for appropriate medical and family management.

Interpretation of an infant assessment should reflect the following conclusions:

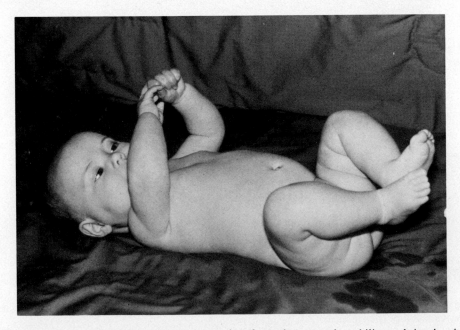

Fig. 8-37. A normal full-term infant at 4 months of age demonstrating ability to bring hands to midline and elevate legs with flexion and abduction of hips, dorsiflexion of ankles.

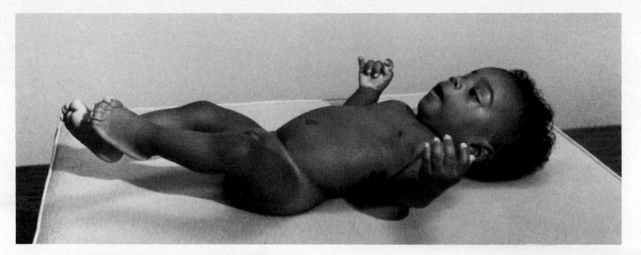

Fig. 8-38. Infant diagnosed with cerebral palsy at 5 months of age; inability to bring hands to midline because of shoulder retraction, extension and adduction of hips with limited movement into flexion, plantar flexion of ankles.

1. Risk is increased with specific abnormal neurological signs, but the majority of infants with any abnormal sign develop normally.
2. A normal neonatal or infant assessment is more predictive than an abnormal examination.
3. Multiple factors are more significantly related to outcome than single factors, indicating the need for a comprehensive evaluation.
4. Periodic examinations over time are the most useful method of determining the developmental outcome of an individual infant.

Intervention

Levels of intervention. Therapeutic intervention for the high-risk infant following discharge from the NICU occurs at multiple levels. Type and intensity of intervention depends on (1) the needs of the infant and his family, (2) the structure and organization of the follow-up clinic, and (3) the availability of therapy resources in a particular clinical and geographical setting.

Assessment as intervention. The clinical assessment of an infant by a therapist (or another professional such as a physician or pediatric nurse) is a unique opportunity for intervention on behalf of the infant and his family. For the full potential of this interaction to be realized, the parents or caregivers must be informed and involved participants, not passive observers. The focus of the intervention process during an assessment is parent support with two primary components: (1) parent education and (2) positive reinforcement for parenting skills.

Parent education involves demonstrating to the parents of an at-risk infant their child's unique capabilities, strengths, and ability to respond to and influence the environment. They learn about their infant's levels and types of responses to stimuli: what causes the child to pay attention and what elicits stress reactions. Parent education includes describing for parents typical temperamental and developmental patterns of the low-birth-weight or medically fragile infant that may differ from expectations based on observations and published descriptions of healthy full-term infants.

Parents of at-risk infants need to be informed about the appropriate level of function for their child and the sequence and pace of development so that they can be realistic in their expectations and interpretation of their infant's progress. This anticipatory guidance enables parents to prepare for and reinforce learning opportunities.

Opportunities to provide *positive reinforcement* to parents need to be emphasized. It is particularly important when working with an infant who may respond inconsistently to the caregiver's affective cues that the parents be given positive feedback for their investment of emotion and energy in their child. They should be reassured that they are providing beneficial parenting and that the infant's behavioral responses reflect neurobehavioral immaturity or instability rather than "personality" or negative affective feelings toward the caregiver.

Intervention as instruction in home management. A critical mode of intervention is the process of parent instruction in specific techniques for home management. This often occurs at the conclusion of a clinical assessment. The recommendations are based on knowledge of the individual infant's medical and neurological history, current health status, and assessment of neurodevelopmental progress. The objective may be to maximize a healthy child's growth potential or to promote developmental progress in an infant who demonstrates delay or neuromotor abnormality.

In either case it is crucial that the parent or caregiver has a clear understanding of the purpose of the activity, what it is intended to facilitate or counteract, the underlying neurodevelopmental process that this activity will support, and the desired response on the part of the infant. This enables the parent to participate more creatively in the process of intervention by adapting and modifying the recommendation according to the individual temperament of the infant (and parent).

Although handling recommendations are specific to the individual child, some intervention activities are appropriate for many preterm infants. These include the following:

1. Activities to counteract *shoulder retraction*. Fifty percent of low-birth-weight infants reportedly demonstrate shoulder retraction.[84] This predominant posture inhibits the infant's ability to move against gravity while supine and results in delayed upper extremity function and rolling. To overcome this retraction, play activities and carrying techniques that bring shoulders forward and hands to midline are demonstrated to parents of premature infants.

2. *Reaching*. Most premature infants are delayed in their reaching skills, decreasing their opportunity to interact with their environment. Although activities to counteract shoulder retraction will promote reaching, it is essential that the infants also be provided with opportunities for practice. Many infants are ready to develop this skill at 3 to 4 months of age, but have only a visually-stimulating mobile suspended *beyond their reach* in the crib. Parents are advised to hang toys within the child's reach in the crib, playpen, or other suitable place. Objects that are suspended, rather than handed to or placed in front of the baby, are ideal for the development of directed reach and grasp and shoulder stability (Fig. 8-39).

3. *Centering and symmetrical orientation*. Midline positioning of head with symmetrical alignment of trunk and extremities is encouraged to counteract the residual effects of asymmetrical positioning during

hospitalization. Midline orientation will also promote even development of tone and function in the right and left sides of the body. Asymmetry that is not caused by neurological dysfunction tends to resolve when positioning and environmental influences are modified.

4. *Prone positioning*. Active play time in the prone position is beneficial for the development of neck and back postural control and shoulder stability in weight-bearing, and to counteract the extension posturing of the supine position. However, parents of vulnerable premature infants are often hesitant to place their infants in the prone position. Low-birth-weight infants, particularly those babies who have relatively large heads and are very visually attentive, often demonstrate a low tolerance for prone positioning.

Parents are advised to gradually increase the baby's time in the prone position according to the infant's tolerance. When positioned on the floor in front of the baby, visually stimulating toys and objects, including mirrors and the faces of caregivers and siblings, increase acceptance of the prone position. A roll or wedge can facilitate positioning in prone, particularly for the infant with low muscle tone. The baby who is apprehensive or stressed when prone often accepts this position on the parent's chest, where reassuring eye contact can be maintained.

5. *Head balance*. Balance activities to develop head control are frequently recommended. Tilting responses are generally achieved most effectively with the infant in the parent's lap. During parent instruction, emphasis is placed on the importance of (a) adequate trunk support; (b) movement through small ranges; (c) slow, graded motion; (d) the desired head-righting response; and (e) indications of stress or fatigue.

6. Restricted use of infant jumper and walker. For infants with increased lower extremity tone or tendency toward toe-standing, the infant walkers and jumpers are not recommended because they tend to increase stiffness and extension posturing of the legs. However, these forms of infant equipment are often highly enjoyable for babies and may provide the parent of a very irritable infant with valuable moments of respite within a stressed household. Therefore, it is important to assist the parents in finding alternative methods of positioning and amusement for the infant while recommending that time in the walker or jumper be minimized. Caregivers are often reluctant to discard the walker, believing that it promotes early ambulation and is beneficial for infants. Informing them of the hazards of infant walkers and of studies showing that their use may delay the onset of independent ambulation encourages their cooperation.[105,106]

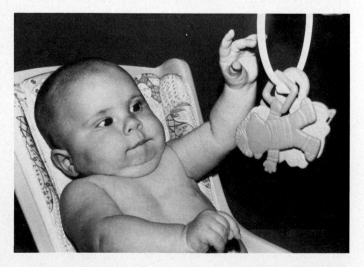

Fig. 8-39. Toys suspended directly in front of infant to encourage symmetrical reaching and midline orientation of head.

Intervention as ongoing therapy. Referral to a regular program of therapeutic intervention is usually made after at least two assessments and a trial period of interim home activities. Criteria for referral include the following:

1. Persistent or progressive indications of abnormal tone
2. Developmental delay in volitional skills or postural reactions
3. Increasing asymmetry or disparity between right and left sides of the body, especially if accompanied by tone differential
4. Loss of joint mobility
5. Feeding difficulties

A decision regarding therapy referral would be influenced by consideration of relevant factors including the following:

1. The infant's medical status
2. Parental concerns
3. Home environment
4. Availability of therapy services relative to geographical, financial, and personnel factors

Effectiveness of early therapy for infants. The effectiveness of therapy for high-risk or neurologically abnormal infants is an issue that is currently being investigated and discussed.[15,98,155,192,194] Numerous studies address this question with inconclusive and, at times, conflicting results. The clinical therapist involved in the treatment of infants needs to critically analyze these studies with respect to the validity of their research methodology and their clinical relevance. Specific questions to be addressed include the following:

1. The sample of infants receiving therapy: are they "at risk" or neurologically abnormal?
2. The frequency of therapy: is it an accurate representation of the standard of practice?
3. The duration and timing of therapy: is it appropriate to critical periods of development?
4. The therapy techniques used: are they specifically described?
5. The quality and amount of parent participation: is it realistic?
6. Assessment of results: are the outcome measures of the study appropriate relative to the goals of therapy?

A review of early intervention studies that demonstrated measurable positive change as a result of an infant intervention program suggests several characteristics critical to effective intervention[155,171,192]:

1. *High degree of parent involvement.* For the therapist this implies that the parent or caregiver must be a participant in the therapy session as well as the therapy program at home. This requires that the activities and techniques to be carried out by the parents are comprehensible and manageable by them.

2. *Comprehensive program of developmental intervention.* Motor skills cannot be addressed in isolation from other aspects of an infant's development. To improve quality of life, not just quality of movement, the therapist must explore a broad perspective of infant learning and incorporate a transdisciplinary approach.

3. *Well-defined curriculum of sequential activities.* Physical therapy for infants traditionally is accomplished through a flexible and variable selection of therapy activities rather than structured curriculum. However, a defined program of learning objectives and activities enables the therapist and parents (as well as daycare workers and others participating in the infant's care) to have a clear and consistent understanding of the current therapeutic activities, the goals of the program, and the steps involved in achieving those goals.

Design of an individualized therapy program. The therapy program for a specific infant should incorporate the above recommendations into a treatment plan that is individualized for the infant and his environment. Progress is monitored by systematic, quantified assessment performed at regular intervals. Effectiveness is determined relative to the rate of progress and the specified goals for each infant.

The long-range goals of an intervention program for a neurodevelopmentally impaired infant need to be realistic and stated in terms of clear, measurable objectives. When defining goals, it is important for therapists to make distinctions among (1) objectives that are generally accepted as achievable by therapists, (2) those believed but not yet conclusively demonstrated to be accomplishable by therapeutic intervention, and (3) changes that are not within the domain or capability of physical therapy. Examples of objectives in these categories are provided in Table 8-14.

For example, physical therapy cannot "cure" cerebral

Table 8-14. Efficacy and feasibility of physical therapy intervention for at-risk infants

Realistic goals of physical therapy	Potential goals of physical therapy not yet documented	Goals that are not in domain of physical therapy
Home management of disability (feeding, handling)	Change abnormal motor patterns	Cure cerebral palsy
Equipment design for position and function	Prevent physical deformities	Release contractures
Parent support and guidance	Predict outcome of at-risk infants	Diagnose abnormal neurological conditions
Document motor development in at-risk infants	Reduce impact of minor neurodevelopmental abnormalities by early therapy	

palsy (i.e., it cannot heal areas of infarcted brain tissue). Low-birth-weight infants who demonstrate neurological abnormalities, receive a course of physical therapy intervention, and subsequently exhibit no residual signs of abnormality demonstrate a clinical course typical of transient dystonia, in which the abnormalities resolve even without therapy. To imply that the therapy "cured" the cerebral palsy could be a misrepresentation and a disservice to families, funding agencies, and the profession. However, the value of the support and guidance provided by the therapist to the family during this critical time of intervention should not be underestimated.

Therapists are currently attempting to demonstrate and document their ability to change motor patterns and to improve motor function in neurologically impaired infants. While this effort is in progress, it is necessary to emphasize the unique professional skills and services that are indisputably provided, such as home management, equipment design, and functional training. Other aspects of intervention, such as the relationship between early therapy for "suspect" infants and later minor neurodevelopmental abnormalities, require further investigation.

CONCLUSION

This chapter on the NICU management and follow-up of at-risk neonates and infants presents three theoretical models for practice, reviews neonatal neuropathology related to movement disorders, and describes expanded professional services for at-risk neonates and infants in a relatively new subspecialty within pediatric practice. Pediatric therapists participating in intensive care nursery and follow-up teams in the care of high-risk neonates and their parents are involved in a new frontier of clinical practice that requires heightened responsibility for accountability and for precepted clinical training (beyond general pediatric specialization) in neonatology and infant therapy techniques.

Inherent in this new area of practice is the challenge to design comprehensive neonatal therapy protocols that include standardized evaluation instruments, comprehensive risk-management plans, long-term follow-up strategies, and systematic documentation of outcome. Ongoing analyses of the physiological risk–therapeutic benefit relationship of components of neuromotor and neurobehavioral treatment for chronically ill and prematurely born infants must guide the NICU intervention process.

Pediatric therapists working in nursery settings are encouraged to participate in follow-up clinics for NICU graduates to identify and analyze the development of movement dysfunction and behavioral sequelae that may, in the future, be minimized or prevented with creative neonatal treatment approaches. The important preventive aspect of neonatal treatment must be guided by careful analyses of neurodevelopmental and functional outcomes in the first year of life.

The low-birth-weight or medically fragile infant is at increased risk for major and minor neurodevelopmental problems that may be evident in infancy or not until later childhood. Prenatal and perinatal risk factors indicate infants who have a greater likelihood of neurological complications but the relationship between single factors and outcome is neither direct nor consistent. Abnormal neurological signs in the first year are also not reliably predictive of abnormal outcome. Attempts to identify factors that definitively indicate significant brain injury are complicated by changing NICU technology, management procedures, environmental variables, and the variability among and within individual infants.

In deciding whether and when an infant requires regular therapeutic intervention, consideration must be given to both the observed capacity for low-birth-weight infants to "normalize"[181] during the first year as well as the time span that may elapse before definitive evidence of cerebral palsy. The pediatric therapist's long-term clinical management of the at-risk infant is guided by the developmental course of the individual infant over time, including behavioral and cognitive growth as well as neuromotor progress, considered within the context of the priorities and values of the family. For additional information regarding treatment of those neonates who develop the motor impairments of the clinical problem of cerebral palsy, please refer to Chapter 9.

REFERENCES

1. Abramson and others: Learned helplessness in humans: critique and reformulation, J Abnorm Psychol 87:49, 1978.
2. Als H and others: The Brazelton neonatal behavioral assessment scale, J Abnorm Psychol 5:215, 1977.
3. Als H: A synactive model of neonatal behavioral organization: framework for the assessment of neurobehavioral development in the premature infant and for support of infants and parents in the neonatal intensive care environment, Phys Occup Ther Pediatr 6 (3/4), 3, 1986.
4. Als H and others: Dynamics of the behavioral organization of the premature infant: a theoretical perspective. In Field TM, editor: Infants born at risk, 173-192, New York, 1979, Spectrum Publications.
5. Als H and others: Toward a research instrument for the assessment of preterm infants' behavior (APIB). In Fitzgerald HE and others, editors: Theory and research in behavioral pediatrics, New York, 1982, Plenum Press.
6. Amiel-Tison C: Neurological evaluation of the maturity of newborn infants, Arch Dis Child 43:89, 1968.
7. Amiel-Tison C and others: Neck extensor hypertonia: a clinical sign of insult to the central nervous system of the newborn, Early Hum Dev 1(2):181, 1977.
8. Amiel-Tison C and Grenier A: Neurologic evaluation of the newborn and the infant, New York, 1980, Masson Publishing USA, Inc.
9. Amiel-Tison C and Grenier A: Neurological assessment during the first year of life, New York, 1986, Oxford University Press.
10. Andre-Thomas and others: The neurological examination of the infant, London, 1964, William Heinemann Medical Books Ltd.
11. Avery GB, editor: Neonataology, ed 2, Philadelphia, 1981, JB Lippincott Co.

12. Babson SG and others: Management of high risk pregnancy and intensive care of the neonate, ed 3, St. Louis, 1975, The CV Mosby Co.

13. Barnard KE and others: Developmental changes in maternal interactions with term and preterm infants, Infant Behav Dev 0:101, 1984.

14. Barnard KE and Eyres SJ: Feeding scale. In Child Health Assessment (DHEW Publication No HRA 79-25), Hyattsville, Md: U.S. Department of Health, Education, and Welfare, Health Resources Administration, Bureau of Health Manpower, Division of Nursing.

15. Barrera ME and others: Early home intervention with low-birth-weight infants and their parents, Child Dev 57:20, 1986.

16. Bayley N: Manual for the Bayley scales of infant development, New York, 1969, The Psychological Corp.

17. Beckwith L and others: Caregiver-infant interaction and early cognitive development in preterm infants, Child Dev 47:579, 1976.

18. Behrman RE: Neonatal-perinatal medicine: diseases of the fetus and newborn, ed 2, St. Louis, 1977, The CV Mosby Co.

19. Bennett FC and others: Spastic diplegia in premature infants, Am J Dis Child 135:732, 1981.

20. Bennett FC and others: Hyaline membrane disease, birth weight, and gestational age, Am J Dis Child 136:888, 1982.

21. Berk RA: The discriminative efficiency of the Bayley scales of infant development, J Abnorm Child Psych 0:113, 1979.

22. Bierman-van Eendenburg MEC and others: Predictive value of neonatal neurological examination: a follow-up study at 18 months, Develop Med Child Neurol 23:296, 1981.

23. Blackburn ST: Fostering behavioral development of high-risk infants, JOGN Nurs 12:76, 1983.

24. Blackburn ST: Assessment of risk: perinatal, family, and environmental perspectives, Phys Occup Ther Pediatr 6(3/4):105-120, 1986.

25. Bly L: The components of normal movement during the first year of life. In Slayton DS, editor: Development of movement in infancy, Chapel Hill, 1981, University of North Carolina Press.

26. Bobath K and Bobath B: The diagnosis of cerebral palsy in infancy, Arch Dis Child 31:408, 1956.

27. Bobath B and Bobath K: The neurodevelopmental treatment of cerebral palsy, Phys Ther 47:1039, 1967.

28. Bobath B and Bobath K: The motor development in the different types of cerebral palsy, London, 1975, William Heinemann Medical Books Ltd.

29. Bobath K and Bobath B: Cerebral palsy. In Pearson PH, and Fieber N, editors: Physical therapy services in the developmental disabilities, Springfield, Ill, 1972, Charles C Thomas.

30. Bowlby J: The child's tie to his mother: attachment behavior. In Attachment and loss, vol 1: Attachment, 1969, New York, Basic Books.

31. Brackbill Y and others: Psychophysiologic effects in the neonate of prone versus supine placement, J Pediatr 82:82, 1973.

32. Braun MA and Palmer MM: A pilot study of oral-motor dysfunction in "at-risk" infants, Phys Occup Ther Pediatr 5:13, 1985.

33. Brazelton TB: Neonatal behavioral assessment scale, ed 2, Clinics in Developmental Medicine, No 88, Philadelphia, 1984, JB Lippincott Co.

34. Brazelton neonatal behavioral assessment scale certification program: Child Development Unit, Children's Hospital Medical Center, 300 Longwood Avenue, Boston, Mass.

35. Brazelton neonatal behavioral assessment scale training films: Educational Development Corporation, 8 Mifflin Place, Cambridge, Mass.

36. Brothwood M and others: Mortality, morbidity, growth and development of babies weighing 501-1000 grams and 1001-1500 grams at birth, Acta Paediatr Scand 77:10, 1988.

37. Bull MJ, Bryson CQ, and Schreiner RL: Perinatal status and neonatal treatment as predictors of the neurologic integrity and development of very low birth weight infants, J Perinatol 5:16, 1988.

38. Burns WJ and others: Developmental assessment of premature infants, J Dev Behav Pediatr 3:12, 1982.

39. Calame A and others: Neurodevelopmental outcome and school performance of very–low-birth-weight infants at 8 years of age, Eur J Pediatr 145:461, 1986.

40. Calvert SA and others: Periventricular leukomalacia: ultrasonic diagnosis and neurological outcome, Acta Paediatr Scand 75:489, 1986.

41. Campbell SK and Wilhelm IJ: Development from birth to 3 years of age of 15 children at high risk for central nervous system dysfunction, Phys Ther 65:463, 1985.

42. Campbell SK and others: Evidence for the need to renorm the Bayley scales of infant development based on the performance of a population-based sample of 12-month-old infants, Top Early Child Spec Ed 6:2, 1986.

43. Campbell SK: The developing infant: neuromuscular maturation. In Wilson J, editor: Infants at risk: medical and therapeutic management, ed 2, Chapel Hill, 1982, University of North Carolina Press.

44. Campbell SK: Seminar on development and neuropathology of high-risk infants, Wauwatosa, Wisconsin, 1982.

45. Campbell SK: Organizational and educational considerations in creating an environment to promote optimal development of high-risk neonates, Phys Occup Ther Pediatr 6(3/4):191, 1986.

46. Campbell SK: Clinical decision making: management of the neonate with movement dysfunction. In Wolf SL, editor: Clinical decision making in physical therapy, Philadelphia, 1985, FA Davis Co.

47. Caplan G: Patterns of parental response to the crises of premature birth, Psychiatry 23:365, 1970.

48. Carter RE and Campbell SK: Early neuromuscular development of the premature infant, Phys Ther 55:1332, 1975.

49. Catto-Smith AG and others: Effect of neonatal periventricular haemorrhage on neurodevelopmental outcome, Arch Dis Child 60.8, 1985

50. Chandler LS and others: Movement assessment of infants: a manual, Rolling Bay, Wash, 1980, published by the authors.

51. Clark JE: Waterbeds: therapeutic devices for handicapped children, Phys Ther 61:1175, 1981.

52. Clarr DL and others: Vestibular stimulation influence on motor development in infants, Science 196:1228, 1977.

53. Coleman M: Congenital brain syndromes. In Coleman M, editor: Neonatal neurology, Baltimore, 1981, University Park Press.

54. Coolman RB and others: Neuromotor development of graduates of the neonatal intensive care unit: patterns encountered in the first two years of life, J Dev Behav Pediatr 6:327, 1985.

55. Cowan D: Personal communication, School of Nursing, University of Washington, August, 1987.

56. Crane L: Physical therapy for the neonate with respiratory disease. In Irwin S and Tecklin JS, editors: Cardiopulmonary physical therapy, St. Louis, 1985, The CV Mosby Co.

57. Crane L: Cardiorespiratory management of the high-risk neonate: implications for developmental therapists, Physical Occup Ther Ped 6(3/4):255, 1986.

58. Crane L: The neonate and child. In Frownfelter DL, editor: Chest physical therapy and pulmonary rehabilitation: an interdisciplinary approach, ed 2, Chicago, 1987, Year Book Medical Publishers.

59. Crnic KA and others: Social interaction and developmental competence of preterm and full-term infants during the first year of life, Child Dev 54:1199, 1983.

60. Davis DH and Thoman EB: Behavioral states of premature infants: implications for neural and behavioral development, Dev Psychobiol 20:25, 1987.

61. DeVries LS and others: Neurological, electrophysiological and MRI abnormalities in infants with extensive cystic leukomalacia, Neuropediatrics 18:61, 1987.

62. Dickson JM: A model for the physical therapist in the intensive care nursery, Phys Ther 61:45, 1981.

63. Dinwiddle R and others: Cardiopulmonary changes in the crying neonate, Pediatr Res 13:900, 1979.

64. Drillien CM: Aetiology and outcome in low-birthweight infants, Dev Med Child Neurol 14:563, 1972.

65. Drillien CM: Abnormal neurologic signs in the first year of life in low-birthweight infants: possible prognostic significance, Dev Med Child Neurol 14:575, 1972.

66. Drillien CM and Drummond MB, editors: Neurodevelopmental problems in early childhood, Oxford, England, 1977, Blackwell Medical Publishers.

67. Drillien CM and others: Low-birthweight children at early school-age: a longitudinal study, Dev Med Child Neurol 22:26, 1980.

68. Dubowitz L: Neurologic assessment. In Ballard R, editor: Pediatric care of the ICN graduate, Philadelphia, 1988, WB Saunders Co.

69. Dubowitz L and Dubowitz V: The neurological assessment of the preterm and full-term newborn infant, Clinics in Developmental Medicine, No 79, Philadelphia, 1981, JB Lippincott Co.

70. Dubowitz L and others: Clinical assessment of gestational age in the newborn infant, J Pediatr 77:1, 1970.

71. Dubowitz L and others: Neurologic signs in neonatal intraventricular hemorrhage: a correlation with real-time ultrasound, J Pediatr 99:127, 1981.

72. Dubowitz L and others: Correlation of neurologic assessment in the preterm newborn infant with outcome at 1 year, J Pediatr 105:452, 1984.

73. Eilers BL and others: Classroom performance and social factors of children with birth weights of 1,250 grams or less: follow-up at 5 to 8 years of age, Pediatrics 77:203, 1986.

74. Ellenberg JH and Nelson KB: Birth weight and gestational age in children with cerebral palsy or seizure disorders, Am J Dis Child 33:1044, 1979.

75. Ellenberg JH and Nelson KB: Early recognition of infants at high risk for cerebral palsy: examination at age four months, Dev Med Child Neurol 23:705, 1981.

76. Ellison PH and others: Development of a scoring system for the Milani-Comparetti and Gidoni method of assessing neurologic abnormality in infancy, Phys Ther 63:1414, 1983.

77. Fawer CL, Dievold P, and Calame A: Periventricular leucomalacia and neurodevelopmental outcome in preterm infants, Arch Dis Child 62:30, 1987.

78. Fetters L: Sensorimotor management of the high-risk neonate, Phys Occup Ther Pediatr 6(3/4):217, 1986.

79. Field T: Supplemental stimulation of preterm neonates, Early Hum Dev 4:301, 1980.

80. Fitterman C: Physical therapy in the NICU. In Connolly BH and Montgomery PC, editors: Therapeutic exercise in developmental disabilities, Chattanooga, 1987, Chattanooga Corp.

81. Forslund M and Bjerre I: Growth and development in preterm infants during the first 18 months, Early Hum Dev 10:201, 1985.

82. Freedman DG: Ethnic differences in babies, Hum Nature, p. 36, Jan. 1979.

83. Freeman JM and Nelson KB: Intrapartum asphyxia and cerebral palsy, Pediatrics 82:2, 1988.

84. Georgieff MK and Bernbaum JC: Abnormal shoulder girdle muscle tone in premature infants during their first 18 months of life, Pediatrics 77:664, 1986.

85. Georgieff MK and others: Abnormal truncal muscle tone as a useful early marker for developmental delay in low birth weight infants, Pediatrics 77:659, 1986.

86. Goodman M and others: Effect of early neurodevelopmental therapy in normal and at-risk survivors of neonatal intensive care, Lancet 1327, 1985.

87. Graham M and others: Prediction of cerebral palsy in very low birthweight infants: prospective ultrasound study, Lancet 593, 1987.

88. Hack M and others: The very low birth weight infant: the broader spectrum of morbidity during infancy and early childhood, J Dev Behav Pediatr 4:243, 1983.

89. Hansen N and Okken A: Transcutaneous oxygen tension of newborn infants in different behavioral states, Pediatr Res 14:911, 1980.

90. Hardy S: Personal communication, Toronto, Ontario, January, 1988.

91. Harris M: Oral-motor management of the high-risk neonate, Phys Occup Ther Pediatr 6(3/4):231, 1986.

92. Harris SR and others: Reliability of observational measures of the Movement Assessment of Infants, Phys Ther 64:471, 1984.

93. Harris SR and others: Predictive validity of the Movement Assessment of Infants, J Dev Behav Pediatr 5:335, 1984.

94. Harris SR: Early detection of cerebral palsy: sensitivity and specificity of two motor assessment tools, J Perinatol 7:11, 1987.

95. Harris SR: Early neuromotor predictors of cerebral palsy in low-birthweight infants, Dev Med Child Neurol 29:587, 1987.

96. Hensinger RN and Jones ET: Neonatal orthopedics, New York, 1981, Grune & Stratton Inc.

97. Heriza C: The neonate with cerebral palsy. In Scully R and Barnes ML, editors: Physical therapy, in press, Philadelphia, JB Lippincott Co.

98. Herndon WA and others: Effects of neurodevelopmental treatment of movement patterns of children with cerebral palsy, J Pediatr Orthop 7:395, 1987.

99. Hill A and Volpe JJ: Seizures, hypoxic-ischemic brain injury, and intraventricular hemorrhage in the newborn, Ann Neurol 10:109, 1981.

100. Hislop HJ: The not-so-impossible dream, Phys Ther 55:1060, 1975.

101. Illingworth RS: The diagnosis of cerebral palsy in the first year of life, Dev Med Child Neurol 8:178, 1966.

102. Ito M: Computed tomography of cerebral palsy: evaluation of brain damage by Volume index of CSF space, Brain Dev 4:293, 1979.

103. Jeffcoate JA and others: Disturbance in parent-child relationship following preterm delivery, Dev Med Child Neurol 21:344, 1979.

104. Kaback MM, editor: Prenatal diagnosis, Pediatr Ann 10:13, 1981.

105. Kauffman IB and Ridenour M: Influence of an infant walker on onset and quality of walking pattern of locomotion: an electromyographic investigation, Percept Mot Skills 45:1323, 1977.

106. Kavanagh CA and Banco L: The infant walker: a previously unrecognized health hazard, Am J Dis Child 136:205, 1982.

107. Kennell JH and Klaus MH: Caring for parents of a premature or sick infant. In Klaus MH and Kennell JH, editors: Maternal-infant bonding, 1976, St Louis, The CV Mosby Co.

108. Kennell J and others: Parent-infant bonding. In Helfer RE and Kempe CH, editors: Child abuse and neglect, Cambridge, Mass, 1976, Ballinger Publishing Co.

109. Kitchen WH and others: Collaborative study of very-low-birth-weight infants, Am J Dis Child. 137:555, 1983.

110. Klaus MH and Fanaroff AA: Care of the high-risk neonate, Philadelphia, 1973, WB Saunders Co.

111. Klein N and others: Preschool performance of children with normal intelligence who were very low-birth-weight infants, Pediatrics 75:531, 1985.

112. Knobloch H and others: Considerations in evaluating changes in outcome for infants weighing less than 1,501 grams, Pediatrics 69:285, 1982.

113. Korner AF and Thoman EB: The relative efficacy of contact and vestibular-proprioceptive stimulation in soothing neonates, Child Dev 43:443, 1972.

114. Korner AF and others: Effects of waterbed flotation on premature infants: a pilot study, Pediatrics 56:361, 1975.

115. Korones SB: High risk newborn infants, ed 3, St Louis, 1981, The CV Mosby Co.

116. Krabill E: Who is the infant at risk for CNS deficit? In Wilson J, editor: Infants at risk: medical and therapeutic management, ed 2, Chapel Hill, 1982, University of North Carolina Press.

117. Kraybill EN: Infants with birth weights less than 1,001 g, Am J Dis Child 138:837, 1984.

118. Kukla A, Fry C, and Goldstein FJ: Kinesthetic needs in infancy, Am J Orthopsychiatry 30:452, 1960.

119. Lacey DJ and Terplan K: Intraventricular hemorrhage in full-term neonates, Dev Med Child Neurol 24:332, 1982.

120. Leander D and Pettett G: Parental response to the birth of a high-risk neonate: dynamics and management, Phys Occup Ther Pediatr 6(3/4):205, 1986.

121. Leonard E and others: Nutritive sucking in high risk neonates after perioral stimulation, Phys Ther 60:299, 1980.

122. Levine MS and Kliebhan L: Communication between physician and physical and occupational therapists: a neurodevelopmental based prescription, Pediatrics 68:208, 1981.

123. Lindahl E and others: Neonatal risk factors and later neurodevelopmental disturbances, Dev Med Child Neurol 30:571, 1988.

124. Linton PT: Behavioral development of the premature infant, Pediatrics 29:175, 1986.

125. Lubchenco LO: The high risk infant, Philadelphia, 1976, WB Saunders Co.

126. Manning J: Facilitation of movement—the Bobath approach, Physiotherapy 58:403, 1972.

127. Marquis PJ and others: Retention of primitive reflexes and delayed motor development in very low birth weight infants, J Dev Behav Pediatr 5:124, 1984.

128. Marsden DJ: Reduction of head flattening in preterm infants, Dev Med Child Neurol 22:507, 1980.

129. Martin RJ and others: Effect of supine and prone positions on arterial oxygen tension in the preterm infant, Pediatrics 63:528, 1979.

130. Matthauen D: The value of correction for age in the assessment of prematurely born children, Early Hum Dev 13:257, 1987.

131. Measel CP: Non-nutritive sucking during tube feedings: effect on clinical course in premature infants, Obstet Gynecol Neonat Nurs 8:265, 1979.

132. Mercer RT: Nursing care for parents at risk, Thorofare, New Jersey, 1977, Slack Inc.

133. Milani-Comparetti A and Gidoni EA: Routine developmental examination in normal and retarded children, Dev Med Child Neurol 9:631, 1967.

134. Miller G and others: Follow-up of preterm infants: is correction of the developmental quotient for prematurity helpful? Early Hum Dev 9:137, 1984.

135. Minde K, and others: Impact of delayed development in premature infants on mother-infant interaction: a prospective investigation, J Pediatr 112:136, 1988.

136. Mitchell JS: Taking on the world: empowering strategies for parents of children with disabilities, New York, 1982, Harcourt Brace Jovanovich.

137. Morales WJ: Effect of intraventricular hemorrhage on the one-year mental and neurologic handicaps of the very low birth weight infant, Obstet Gynecol 70:111, 1987.

138. Morgan AM and others: Neonatal neurobehavioral examination, Phys Ther 68:1352, 1988.

139. Morris SE: Assessment and treatment of children with oral-motor dysfunction. In Wilson JM, editor: Oral-motor function and dysfunction in children, Chapel Hill, 1974, University of North Carolina Press.

140. Morris SE: The normal acquisition of oral feeding skills: implications for assessment and treatment, New York, 1982, Therapeutic Media Inc.

141. Mueller HA: Facilitating feeding and prespeech. In Pearson PH and Fieber N, editors: Physical therapy services in the developmental disabilities, Springfield, Ill, 1972, Charles C Thomas.

142. Neal MV: Vestibular stimulation and developmental behavior of the small premature infant, Nurs Res Rep 3:2, 1968.

143. Nelson KB and Ellenberg JH: Neonatal signs as predictors of cerebral palsy, Pediatrics 64:225, 1979.

144. Nelson KB and Ellenberg JH: Children who "outgrew" cerebral palsy, Pediatrics 69:529, 1982.

145. Nelson KB and Ellenberg JH: Antecedents of cerebral palsy, N Engl J Med 315:81, 1986.

146. Nickel RE, Bennett FC, and Lamson FN: School performance of children with birth weights of 1,000 g or less, Am J Dis Child 136:105, 1982.

147. Noble-Jamieson CM and others: Low birth weight children at school age: neurological, psychological, and pulmonary function, Semin Perinatol 6:266, 1982.

148. Nugent JK: The Brazelton neonatal behavioral assessment scale: implications for intervention, Pediatr Nurs 42:18, 1981.

149. Nugent JK: Using the NBAS with infants and their families: guidelines for intervention, White Plains, New York, 1985, March of Dimes Birth Defects Foundation.

150. O'Neil S: Personal communication, School of Nursing, University of Washington, Seattle, Wash, May, 1986.

151. Paban M and Piper MC: Early predictors of one year neurodevelopmental outcome for "at risk" infants, Physical Occup Ther Pediatr 7:17, 1987.

152. Paine RS: Early recognition of neuromotor disability in infants of low birthweight, Develop Med Child Neurol 11:455, 1969.

153. Paine RS: Neurologic exam of infants and children, Ped Clin North Am 0:471, 1960.

154. Palisano RJ and others: Chronological vs. adjusted age in assessing motor development of healthy twelve-month-old premature and full-term infants, Phys Occup Ther Ped 5:1, 1985.

155. Palmer FB and others: The effects of physical therapy on cerebral palsy, N Engl J Med 318:803, 1988.

156. Paneth N: Etiologic factors in cerebral palsy, Ped Ann 15:193, 1986.

157. Pape KE and others: The status at two years of low-birth-weight infants born in 1974 with birth weights of less than 1,001 gm, J Pediatr 92:253, 1978.

158. Pape KE and Wigglesworth JS: Hemorrhage, ischemia and the perinatal brain, Clinics in Developmental Medicine, Nos 69 and 70, Philadelphia, 1979, JB Lippincott Co.

159. Papile L and others: Incidence and evolution of subependymal and intraventricular hemorrhage: a study of infants with birth weights less than 1,500 gm, J Pediatr 92:529, 1978.

160. Papile L and others: Relationship of cerebral intraventricular hemorrhage and early childhood neurologic handicaps, J Pediatr 103:273, 1983.

161. Parer JT: Evaluation of the fetus during labor, Curr Probl Pediatr 12:1, 1982.

162. Parmelee AH and Michaelis MD: Neurological examination of the newborn. In Hellmuth J, editor: Exceptional infant, vol 2, New York, 1971, Brunner/Mazel Inc.

163. Peabody JL and Lewis K: Consequences of newborn intensive care. In Gottfried AW and Goither JL, editors: Infant stress under intensive care, Baltimore, 1985, University Park Press.

164. Piper MC and others: Early physical therapy effects on the high-risk infant: a randomized controlled trial, Pediatrics 78:216, 1986.

165. Piper MC and others: Resolution of neurological symptoms in high-risk infants during the first two years of life, Dev Med Child Neurol 30:26, 1988.

166. Prechtl H: The neurological examination of the full-term newborn infant, ed 2, Clinics in Developmental Medicine, No 63, Philadelphia, 1977, JB Lippincott Co.

167. Prechtl H and Beintema D: The neurological examination of the newborn infant, Clinics in Developmental Medicine, No 12, London, 1964, Heinemann Educational Books Inc.

168. Provost B: Normal development from birth to 4 months: extended use of the NBAS-K, Part I, Phys Occup Ther Pediatr 2:39, 1980.

169. Provost B: Normal development from birth to 4 months: extended use of the NBAS-K, Part II, Phys Occup Ther Pediatr 1:19, 1981.

170. Quinton M: Personel communication, Neurodevelopmental treatment baby course, Puyallup, Washington, July 1982.

171. Resnick MB and others: Developmental intervention for low birth weight infants: improved early developmental outcome, Pediatrics 80:68, 1987.

172. Rice RD: Neurophysiological development in premature infants following stimulation, Dev Psychol 13:69, 1977.

173. Robinson RO: Pathogenesis of intraventricular hemorrhage in the low-birthweight infant, Dev Med Child Neurol 21:815, 1979.

174. Rosenblith JF: Relations between neonatal behaviors and those at eight months, Dev Psychol 10:779, 1974.

175. Rosenblith JF and Anderson-Huntington R: Behavioral examination of the neonate. In Wilson J, editor: Infants at risk: medical and therapeutic management, ed 2, Chapel Hill, 1982, University of North Carolina Press.

176. Ross G and others: Perinatal and neurobehavioral predictors of one-year outcome in infants < 1500 grams, Semin Perinat 6:317, 1982.

177. Rothberg AD: Infants weighing 1,000 grams or less at birth: developmental outcome for ventilated and nonventilated infants, Pediatrics 71:599, 1983.

178. Russell C: Transition to parenthood: problems and gratifications, J Marriage Fam 36:294, 1974.

179. Saint-Anne Dargassies S: Neurodevelopmental symptoms during the first year of life, Dev Med Child Neurol 14:235, 1972.

180. Saint-Anne Dargassies S: Long-term neurological follow-up study of 286 truly premature infants 1: neurological sequelae, Dev Med Child Neurol 19:462, 1977.

181. Saint-Anne Dargassies S: Normality and normalization as seen in a long-term neurological follow-up of 286 premature infants, Neuropadiatrie 10:226, 1979.

182. Sameroff AJ, editor: Organization and stability of newborn behavior: a commentary on the Brazelton neonatal behavioral assessment scale, Monogr Soc Res Child Dev No. 5–6, 1978.

183. Scarr-Salapatek S and Williams ML: a stimulation program for low birth weight infants, Am J Public Health 62:662, 1972.

184. Scarr-Salapatek S and Williams ML: The effects of early stimulation on low–birth-weight infants, Child Dev 44:99, 1973.

185. Scafidi FA and others: Effects of tactile/kinesthetic stimulation on the clinical course and sleep/wake behavior of preterm neonates, Infant Behav Dev 9:91, 1986.

186. Scheiner AP and Abroms IF: The practical management of the developmentally disabled child, St Louis, 1980, The CV Mosby Co.

187. Schneider JW, Lee W, Chasnoff IJ: Field testing of the Movement Assessment of Infants, Phys Ther 68:321, 1988.

188. Scherzer AL: The changing face of cerebral palsy, Dev Med Child Neurol 29:550, 1987.

189. Schertzer AL and Tscharnuter I: Early diagnosis and therapy in cerebral palsy, New York, 1982, Marcel Decker.

190. Scott S and others: Weight gain and movement patterns of very low birthweight babies nursed on lambswool, Lancet, October 29, 1983, p. 1014.

191. Sell EJ and others: Early identification of learning problems in neonatal intensive care graduates, Am J Dis Child 139:460, 1985.

192. Shonkoff JP and Hauser-Cram P: Early intervention for disabled infants and their families: a quantitative analysis, Pediatrics 80:650, 1987.

193. Siegel LS: Reproductive, perinatal, and environmental variables as predictors of development of preterm (< 1501 grams) and fullterm children at 5 years, Semin Perinatol 6:274, 1982.

194. Simeonsson RJ, Cooper DH, and Scheiner AP: A review and analysis of the effectiveness of early intervention programs, Pediatrics 69:635, 1982.

195. Simeonsson RJ, Cooper DH, and Scheiner AP: A review and analysis of the effectiveness of early intervention programs, Pediatrics 69:635, 1982.

196. Slater MA and others: Neurodevelopment of monitored versus non-monitored very low birth weight infants: the importance of family influences, Dev Behav Pediatr 8:278, 1987.

197. Sostek AM and others: Developmental outcome of preterm infants with intraventricular hemorrhage at one and two years of age, Child Dev 58:779, 1987.

198. Spellacy WN, editor: Management of the high-risk pregnancy, Baltimore, 1975, University Park Press.

199. Stanley FJ: The changing face of cerebral palsy, Dev Med Child Neurol 29:263, 1987.

200. Stanley FJ and English DR: Prevalence of and risk factors for cerebral palsy in a total population cohort of low-birthweight (< 2000 g) in infants, Dev Med Child Neurol 28:559, 1986.

201. Stangler SR and others: Screening growth and development of preschool children, New York, 1980, McGraw-Hill Book Co.

202. Stengel TJ: The neonatal behavioral assessment scale: description, clinical uses, and research implications, Phys Occup Ther Pediatr 1:39, 1980.

203. Stevenson RE: The fetus and newly born infant—influences of the prenatal environment, St Louis, 1973, The CV Mosby Co.

204. Stewart A and others: Prediction in very preterm infants of satisfactory neurodevelopmental progress at 12 months, Dev Med Child Neurol 30:53, 1988.

205. Stuberg W and others: The Milani-Comparetti motor development screening test: test manual, Omaha, Nebraska, 1987, Meyer Children's Rehabilitation Institute.

206. Swanson MW and others: Identification of neuromotor abnormality at 4 and 8 months by the Movement Assessment of Infants, Abstract, Dev Med Child Neurol 30:23, 1988.

207. Swanson MW: Unpublished data, 1988.

208. Sweeney JK: Neonatal hydrotherapy: an adjunct to developmental intervention in an intensive care nursery setting, Phys Occup Ther Pediatr 3:20, 1983.

209. Sweeney JK: Physiological and behavioral effects of neurological assessment in preterm and full-term neonates. Unpublished thesis (PhD), University of Washington, Seattle, 1987.

210. Sweeney JK: Physiological adaptation of neonates to neurological assessment, Phys Occup Ther Pediatr 6:155, 1986.

211. Sweeney JK: Neonatal hydrotherapy: a risk-benefit analysis. In Wilhelm WJ, editor: Advances in neonatal special care, Chapel Hill, 1986, Division of Physical Therapy.

212. Tjossem TD: Early intervention: issues and approaches. In Tjossem TD, editor: Intervention strategies for high risk infants and young children, Baltimore, 1976, University Park Press.

213. Tronik E and Brazelton TB: Clinical uses of the Brazelton neonatal behavioral assessment scale. In Friedlander BZ, Sterritt GM, and Kirk GE, editors: Exceptional infant, vol 3, New York, 1975, Brunner/Mazel, Inc.

214. Trykowski L and others: Enhancement of nutritive sucking in premature infants, Phys Occup Ther Pediatr 1:27, 1982.

215. Valvano J and DeGangi GA: Atypical posture and movement findings in high risk pre-term infants, Phys Occup Ther Pediatr 6:71, 1986.

216. vanderLinden D: Ability of the Milani-Comparetti developmental examination to predict motor outcome, Phys Occup Ther Pediatr 5:27, 1985.

217. Vaucher YE: Understanding intraventricular hemorrhage and white-matter injury in premature infants, Inf Young Children 1:31, 1988.

218. Vohr BR and Garcia Coll CT: Neurodevelopmental and school per-

formance of very low-birth-weight infants: a seven year longitudinal study, Pediatrics 76:345, 1985.

219. Volpe JJ: Perinatal hypoxic-ischemic brain injury, Pediatr Clin North Am 23:383, 1976.

220. Volpe JJ: Neurology of the newborn, ed 2, Philadelphia, 1987, WB Saunders Co.

221. Volpe JJ and Koenigsberger R: Neurologic disorders. In Avery GB, editor: Neonatology, ed 2, Philadelphia, 1981, JB Lippincott Co.

222. Wagaman MJ and others: Improved oxygenation and lung compliance with prone positioning of neonates, J Pediatr 94:787, 1979.

223. Webb ZW: Developmental care in the neonatal intensive care unit, Dimens Crit Care Nurs 1:221, 1983.

224. White JL, and Labarba RC: The effects of tactile and kinesthetic stimulation on neonatal development in the premature infant, Dev Psychobiol 9:569, 1976.

225. Widmayer SM and Field TM: Effects of Brazelton demonstrations for mothers on the development of preterm infants, Pediatrics 67:711, 1981.

226. Wigglesworth JS and Pape KE: An integrated model for haemorrhagic and ischaemic lesions in the newborn brain, Early Hum Dev 2:197, 1978.

227. Wilhelm IJ: The neurologically suspect neonate. In Campbell SK, editor: Pediatric neurologic physical therapy, New York, 1985, Churchill Livingstone.

228. Williamson WD and others: Survival of low–birth-weight infants with neonatal intraventricular hemorrhage, Am J Dis Child 137:1181, 1983.

APPENDIX A

App. A. Evaluation Form of Clinical Assessment of Gestational Age in the Newborn Infant. (From Dubowitz LMS and others: J. Pediatr. 77:1, 1970.)

Scoring system for external criteria					
External sign	**Score***				
	0	**1**	**2**	**3**	**4**
Edema	Obvious edema of hands and feet; pitting over tibia	No obvious edema of hands and feet; pitting over tibia	No edema		
Skin texture	Very thin, gelatinous	Thin and smooth	Smooth; medium thickness; rash or superficial peeling	Slight thickening; superficial cracking and peeling especially of hands and feet	Thick and parchment-like; superficial or deep cracking
Skin color	Dark red	Uniformly pink	Pale pink, variable over body	Pale; only pink over ears, lips, palms, or soles	
Skin opacity (trunk)	Numerous veins and venules clearly seen, especially over abdomen	Veins and tributaries seen	A few large vessels clearly seen over abdomen	A few large vessels seen indistinctly over abdomen	No blood vessels seen
Lanugo (over back)	No lanugo	Abundant; long and thick over whole back	Hair thinning especially over lower back	Small amount of lanugo and bald areas	At least half of back devoid of lanugo
Plantar creases	No skin creases	Faint red marks over anterior half of sole	Definite red marks over > anterior half; indentations over < anterior third	Indentations over > anterior third	Definite deep indentations over > anterior third
Nipple formation	Nipple barely visible; no areola	Nipple well defined; areola smooth and flat, diameter <0.75 cm	Areola stippled, edge not raised, diameter <0.75 cm	Areola stippled, edge raised, diameter >0.75 cm	
Breast size	No breast tissue palpable	Breast tissue on one or both sides, <0.5 cm diameter	Breast tissue both sides; one or both 0.5-1.0 cm	Breast tissue both sides; one or both >1 cm	
Ear form	Pinna flat and shapeless, little or no incurving of edge	Incurving of part of edge of pinna	Partial incurving whole of upper pinna	Well-defined incurving whole of upper pinna	
Ear firmness	Pinna soft, easily folded, no recoil	Pinna soft, easily folded, slow recoil	Cartilage to edge of pinna, but soft in places, ready recoil	Pinna firm, cartilage to edge; instant recoil	
Genitals Male	Neither testis in scrotum	At least one testis high in scrotum	At least one testis right down		
Female (with hips half abducted)	Labia majora widely separated, labia minora protruding	Labia majora almost cover labia minora	Labia majora completely cover labia minora		

From Dubowitz, L.M.S., Dubowitz, V., and Goldberg, C.: Clinical assessment of gestational age in the newborn infant, J. Pediatr. **77:**1, 1970.
*If score differs on two sides, take the mean.

APPENDIX B

Parent education materials

LITERATURE BY PEDIATRIC THERAPISTS

Parents' guide: developmental support of low-birth-weight infants
Susan Dockendorf Thurber, PT
Lynda Brookshire Armstrong, OTR
Source: Office of Educational Resources
Texas Children's Hospital
P.O. Box 20269
Houston, TX

Handling your young premature baby at home
Joanne Valvano, PT
Rochelle Givens, MS
Source: R.R. Givens
P.O. Box 2922
Alexandria, VA 22301

Guiding your child through pre-term development
Tim Healy MS, PT
Source: Tim Healey MS, RPT, Inc.
Infant and Child Development Specialist
221 S. Glassell St
Orange, CA 92666

Understanding my signals: help for parents of premature infants (*complimentary user's guide for professional staff enclosed)
Brenda Hussy MS, OTR
Source: VORT Corporation
P.O. Box 60132
Palo Alto, CA 94306

LITERATURE BY PARENTS

Harrison H and Kasitsky A: The premature baby book: a parent's guide to coping and caring in the first years, New York, 1983, St. Martin's Press.
Nance S: Premature babies: a handbook for parents by parents, New York, 1984, Berkley Publishing Corp.

National agency:
Parents of Premature and High Risk Infants International, Inc.
33 W. 22nd Street, Suite 1227
New York, NY 10036

APPENDIX C

Movement Assessment of Infants with 4-Month Profile

Name _____   Date of examination _____

Case number _____   Birth date _____

Examiner _____   Chronological age _____

Gestational age _____

Total risk score [   ]   Corrected age _____

Muscle tone

Items 1 to 6, 9, and 10 should be coded by the scale below.
Code items 7 and 8 as explained in the instructions for these items in the manual.

0 — Item omitted
1 — Hypotonic
2 — Greater than hypotonic but less than normal
3 — Normal
4 — Greater than normal but less then hypertonic
5 — Hypertonic
6 — Fluctuating, variable

								Distribution variations		Asymmetries		
								Upper	Lower	Left	Right	
1	2		4	5	6	____	1.	Consistency	____	____	____ ____	1
1	2		4	5	6	____	2.	Extensibility	____	____	____ ____	2
1	2		4	5	6	____	3.	Passivity	____	____	____ ____	3
1	2		4	5	6	____	4.	Posture in supine	____	____	____ ____	4
1	2		4	5	6	____	5.	Posture in prone	____	____	____ ____	5
1	2		4	5	6	____	6.	Posture in prone suspended	____	____	____ ____	6
		3	4			____	7.	Asymmetry				
		3	4			____	8.	Distribution variation				
1	2		4	5	6	____	9.	Summary of tone extremities			____ ____	9
1	2		4	5	6	____	10.	Summary of tone truck			____ ____	10

[   ]

Primitive reflexes

Items 1 to 12 should be coded by the scale below.
Code items 13 and 14 as explained in the instructions for these items in the manual.

0 — Item omitted
1 — Integrated or not elicited
2 — Incomplete response
3 — Complete response
4 — Dominant

							Asymmetries		
							Left	Right	
2	3	4	____	1.	Tonic labyrinthine reflex in supine		____	____	1
2	3	4	____	2.	Tonic labyrinthine reflex in prone		____	____	2
	3	4	____	3.	Asymmetrical tonic neck reflex (evoked)		____	____	3
	3	4	____	4.	Asymmetrical tonic neck reflex (spontaneous)		____	____	4
	3	4	____	5.	Moro		____	____	5
	3	4	____	6.	Tremulousness		____	____	6
	3	4	____	7.	Palmar grasp		____	____	7
		4	____	8.	Plantar grasp		____	____	8
	3	4	____	9.	Ankle clonus		____	____	9
	3	4	____	10.	Neonatal positive support		____	____	10
	3	4	____	11.	Walking reflex		____	____	11
	3	4	____	12.	Trunk incurvation (galant)		____	____	12
	3	4	____	13.	Asymmetry				
	3	4	____	14.	Summary of primitive reflexes				

[   ]

App. C. Scoring sheet for Movement Assessment of Infants with 4-month profile. (From Chandler LS and others: Movement assessment of infants: a manual, Rolling Bay, Washington, 1980. Copyright © 1980 by Lynette S. Chandler, Mary Skillen Andrews, Marcia W. Swanson.)

Automatic reactions

Items 1 to 14 should be coded by the scale below.
Code items 15 and 16 as explained in the instructions for these items in the manual.

0 — Item omitted
1 — Complete and consistent response
2 — Incomplete or incorrect response
3 — Partial response
4 — No response

			Item		Asymmetries		
					Left	*Right*	
	3	4	_____	1. Head righting (lateral)	_____	_____	1
2	3	4	_____	2. Head righting (extension)	_____	_____	2
	3	4	_____	3. Head righting (flexion)	_____	_____	3
		4	_____	4. Landau	_____	_____	4
		4	_____	5. Rotation in trunk	_____	_____	5
		4	_____	6. Equilibrium reactions in prone	_____	_____	6
			_____	7. Equilibrium reactions in sitting	_____	_____	7
			_____	8. Equilibrium reactions in vertical suspension	_____	_____	8
			_____	9. Downward parachute	_____	_____	9
			_____	10. Protective extension (forward)	_____	_____	10
			_____	11. Protective extension (side)	_____	_____	11
			_____	12. Protective extension (backward)	_____	_____	12
	3	4	_____	13. Placing of feet	_____	_____	13
	3	4	_____	14. Placing of hands	_____	_____	14
	3	4	_____	15. Asymmetry	_____	_____	15
	3	4	_____	16. Summary of automatic reactions	_____	_____	16

Volitional movement

Items 1 to 23 should be coded by the scale below.
Code items 24 and 25 as explained in the instructions for these items in the manual.

0 — Item omitted
1 — Complete and consistent response
2 — Incomplete or incorrect response
3 — Partial response
4 — No response

			Item		Asymmetries		
					Left	*Right*	
		4	_____	1. Hearing	_____	_____	1
	3	4	_____	2. Visual following	_____	_____	2
	3	4	_____	3. Peripheral vision	_____	_____	3
		4	_____	4. Vocalization	_____	_____	4
2	3	4	_____	5. Head centering	_____	_____	5
	3	4	_____	6. Head position (anterior/posterior)	_____	_____	6
	3	4	_____	7. Head balance	_____	_____	7
	3	4	_____	8. Active weight bearing through shoulders	_____	_____	8
	3	4	_____	9. Open hands	_____	_____	9
	3	4	_____	10. Hands to midline	_____	_____	10
			_____	11. Large grasp	_____	_____	11
			_____	12. Small grasp	_____	_____	12
			_____	13. Reaches out	_____	_____	13
			_____	14. Combines	_____	_____	14
			_____	15. Transfers	_____	_____	15
		4	_____	16. Back straight in sitting	_____	_____	16
		4	_____	17. Active use of hips	_____	_____	17
			_____	18. Rolling	_____	_____	18
			_____	19. Prone progression	_____	_____	19
			_____	20. Sits when placed	_____	_____	20
			_____	21. Coming to sit	_____	_____	21
			_____	22. Coming to stand	_____	_____	22
			_____	23. Walking	_____	_____	23
	3	4	_____	24. Asymmetry	_____	_____	24
	3	4	_____	25. Summary of volitional movement	_____	_____	25

App. C, cont'd. Scoring sheet for Movement Assessment of infants with 4-month profile.

APPENDIX D

Movement Assessment of Infants with 8-Month Profile

Name _____   Date of examination _____

Case number _____   Birth date _____

Examiner _____   Chronological age _____

Total risk score [ ]   Gestational age _____

Corrected age _____

Muscle tone

Items 1 to 6, 9, and 10 should be coded by the scale below.
Code items 7 and 8 as explained in the instructions for these items in the manual.

0 — Item omitted
1 — Hypotonic
2 — Greater than hypotonic but less than normal
3 — Normal
4 — Greater than normal but less then hypertonic
5 — Hypertonic
6 — Fluctuating, variable

			Distribution variations		Asymmetries	
			Upper	Lower	Left	Right
1 2 4 5 6 ___	1.	Consistency	___	___	___	___ 1
1 2 4 5 6 ___	2.	Extensibility	___	___	___	___ 2
1 2 4 5 6 ___	3.	Passivity	___	___	___	___ 3
1 2 4 5 6 ___	4.	Posture in supine	___	___	___	___ 4
1 2 4 5 6 ___	5.	Posture in prone	___	___	___	___ 5
1 2 4 5 6 ___	6.	Posture in prone suspended	___	___	___	___ 6
3 4 ___	7.	Asymmetry				
3 4 ___	8.	Distribution variation				
1 2 4 5 6 ___	9.	Summary of tone (extremities)				___ 9
1 2 4 5 6 ___	10.	Summary of tone (trunk)	___	___	___	___ 10

[ ]

Primitive reflexes

Items 1 to 12 should be coded by the scale below.
Code items 13 and 14 as explained in the instructions for these items in the manual.

0 — Item omitted
1 — Integrated or not elicited
2 — Incomplete response
3 — Complete response
4 — Dominant

			Asymmetries	
			Left	Right
2 3 4 ___	1.	Tonic labyrinthine reflex in supine	___	___ 1
2 3 4 ___	2.	Tonic labyrinthine reflex in prone	___	___ 2
2 3 4 ___	3.	Asymmetrical tonic neck reflex (evoked)	___	___ 3
2 3 4 ___	4.	Asymmetrical tonic neck reflex (spontaneous)	___	___ 4
2 3 4 ___	5.	Moro	___	___ 5
2 3 4 ___	6.	Tremulousness	___	___ 6
2 3 4 ___	7.	Palmar grasp	___	___ 7
4 ___	8.	Plantar grasp	___	___ 8
2 3 4 ___	9.	Ankle clonus	___	___ 9
2 3 4 ___	10.	Neonatal positive support	___	___ 10
2 3 4 ___	11.	Walking reflex	___	___ 11
2 3 4 ___	12.	Trunk incurvation (galant)	___	___ 12
3 4 ___	13.	Asymmetry		
2 3 4 ___	14.	Summary of primitive reflexes		

[ ]

App. D. Scoring sheet for Movement Assessment of Infants with 8-month profile. (From Movement assessment of infants, PO Box 4631, Rolling Bay, Washington, 98361. Copyright © 1980 by Lynette S. Chandler, Mary Skillen Andrews, Marcia W. Swanson.)

Automatic reactions

Items 1 to 14 should be coded by the scale below.
Code items 15 and 16 as explained in the instructions for these items in the manual.

0 — Item omitted
1 — Complete and consistent response
2 — Incomplete or incorrect response
3 — Partial response
4 — No response

	Asymmetries	
	Left	*Right*

Code	Item		Left	Right	#
2 3 4	_____ 1.	Head righting (lateral)	_____	_____	1
2 3 4	_____ 2.	Head righting (extension)	_____	_____	2
3 4	_____ 3.	Head righting (flexion)	_____	_____	3
3 4	_____ 4.	Landau	_____	_____	4
2 3 4	_____ 5.	Rotation in trunk	_____	_____	5
2 3 4	_____ 6.	Equilibrium reactions in prone	_____	_____	6
3 4	_____ 7.	Equilibrium reactions in sitting	_____	_____	7
3 4	_____ 8.	Equilibrium reactions in vertical suspension	_____	_____	8
3 4	_____ 9.	Downward parachute	_____	_____	9
2 3 4	_____ 10.	Protective extension (forward)	_____	_____	10
2 3 4	_____ 11.	Protective extension (side)	_____	_____	11
	_____ 12.	Protective extension (backward)	_____	_____	12
2 3 4	_____ 13.	Placing of feet	_____	_____	13
2 3 4	_____ 14.	Placing of hands	_____	_____	14
3 4	_____ 15.	Asymmetry	_____	_____	15
2 3 4	_____ 16.	Summary of automatic reactions	_____	_____	16

Volitional movement

Items 1 to 23 should be coded by the scale below.
Code items 24 and 25 as explained in the instructions for these items in the manual.

0 — Item omitted
1 — Complete and consistent response
2 — Incomplete or incorrect response
3 — Partial response
4 — No response

	Asymmetries	
	Left	*Right*

Code	Item		Left	Right	#
2 3 4	_____ 1.	Hearing	_____	_____	1
2 3 4	_____ 2.	Visual following	_____	_____	2
2 3 4	_____ 3.	Peripheral vision	_____	_____	3
3 4	_____ 4.	Vocalization	_____	_____	4
2 3 4	_____ 5.	Head centering	_____	_____	5
2 3 4	_____ 6.	Head position (anterior/posterior)	_____	_____	6
2 3 4	_____ 7.	Head balance	_____	_____	7
2 3 4	_____ 8.	Active weight bearing through shoulders	_____	_____	8
2 3 4	_____ 9.	Open hands	_____	_____	9
2 3 4	_____ 10.	Hands to midline	_____	_____	10
2 3 4	_____ 11.	Large grasp	_____	_____	11
4	_____ 12.	Small grasp	_____	_____	12
2 3 4	_____ 13.	Reaches out	_____	_____	13
	_____ 14.	Combines	_____	_____	14
2 3 4	_____ 15.	Transfers	_____	_____	15
3 4	_____ 16.	Back straight in sitting	_____	_____	16
3 4	_____ 17.	Active use of hips	_____	_____	17
2 3 4	_____ 18.	Rolling	_____	_____	18
2 3 4	_____ 19.	Prone progression	_____	_____	19
2 3 4	_____ 20.	Sits when placed	_____	_____	20
4	_____ 21.	Coming to sit	_____	_____	21
	_____ 22.	Coming to stand	_____	_____	22
	_____ 23.	Walking	_____	_____	23
3 4	_____ 24.	Asymmetry	_____	_____	24
2 3 4	_____ 25.	Summary of volitional movement	_____	_____	25

App. D, cont'd. Scoring sheet for Movement Assessment of Infants with 8-month profile.

Chapter 9

CEREBRAL PALSY

Christine A. Nelson

OVERVIEW
Definitions, parameters, anticipated changes

Cerebral palsy presents a conglomerate of complexities.[2] The diagnosis has historically referred to a lack of oxygen or some related insult to the brain shortly before or during the birth process. The repercussions of that insult to the brain fall into patterns that are not always neatly organized. Earlier categorizations of the types of cerebral palsy have proved inconsistent because a single child may move from one diagnostic category to another during the maturation process. There may be associated perceptual and learning problems, as well as developmental deprivation of movement experience. Record keeping is inaccurate because of the various definitions applied. In one center a child is identified as having cerebral palsy, whereas in an-other the same child is labeled as having "psychomotor dysfunction" or developmental delay. At times the diagnosis is applied rather carelessly to infants who have sustained gross damage to the entire brain or who have conditions such as primary microcephaly. As we are confronted by new concepts of brain functioning,[16] we may have to completely revise our hypotheses of causation.

The Little Club, named for the physician who first defined the condition of cerebral palsy, described it as "a persistent disorder of movement and posture appearing early in life and due to a developmental nonprogressive disorder of the brain."[37] Dr. Bobath elaborates that "the lesion affects the immature brain and interferes with the maturation of the central nervous system, which has specific consequences in terms of the type of cerebral palsy which develops, its diagnosis, assessment, and treatment."[9]

Another controversy has been the span of time over which the diagnosis may be applied. Vining and others[52] report that their center uses a limit of 3 years of age for applying the diagnosis, whereas the American Association for Cerebral Palsy (AACP) recognizes damage occurring to the CNS before 5 years. The age limit set is somewhat arbitrary, but it intends to recognize the early plasticity of the immature brain.[27] This also creates some confusion in specific diagnosis, since there is immediately an overlap with traumatic head injuries, brain infections, near-drownings, and episodes that directly affect brain function. However, the alert therapist will find more similarities than differences in the treatment for the clinical consequences of these events. More complete coverage of these conditions may be found in Chapters 13 and 16.

Milani-Comparetti has recently presented for consideration a new classification of cerebral palsy based on characteristic fetal movement patterns.[38] Ultrasound now permits professionals to appreciate the wide variability of movements in utero, as well as the movement responses to specific changes in the external environment. Researchers have also identified changes in the rate and type of movement that precedes death of the fetus.

Clinically, therapists have to deal with the observable signs. These observable changes can be evaluated early in a child's development.[11] Therapists are attempting to evaluate the interference of pathological signs and symptoms in comparison to normal or nearly normal responses made by the child. The lack of or distortion of righting reactions against gravity is a strong clue to the presence of a neuromotor disorder.[6] As these righting reactions normally occur early in development, they provide one means of early identification of the infant who is in trouble.[7] Informed individualized home handling can change the outlook for this population. Older children also change significantly with intensive physical treatment that takes into account the tactile, proprioceptive, and vestibular aspects of the condition. It is essential for therapists to realize that they are dealing with a developing human being with emotional needs—an emerging personality within a personal environment. Physical limitations as well as perceptual distortions are to be assessed. Nothing less than a holistic view of the problem will serve to change the life pattern of the client who requests assistance to change.[32]

The pathological signs observed in cerebral palsy can be related to postural adjustments against gravity. The interference with function is therefore greater as normal developmental tasks demand control of the body in an upright alignment. To the naive observer, the increased difficulty may give the erroneous impression that the basic condition is worsening. There is no evidence to suggest that the condition itself worsens, but the will of children directs them to use whatever movement potential they possess to explore their environment and to become acquainted with their own bodies. Vining and others state unequivocally that cerebral palsy "is not a specific disease state with an accepted cause, pathogenesis, pathological picture, clinical presentation, treatment, or prognosis."[52] Bobath[8] has documented the course of development in the presence of various forms of cerebral palsy, but also stresses the uniqueness of each child and that child's particular constellation of pathological and normal responses. It is true that active use of the abnormal patterns of movement tends to reinforce the pathology and consequently block the expression of the more differentiated normal developmental progression[7] (Fig. 9-1).

The osteopathic profession calls our attention to their correlation of constellations of physical characteristics with cranial findings that offer the possibility of relieving specific pressures that impede proper craniosacral rhythms as well as venous and cerebrospinal fluid circulation.[51] Documentation of cranial abnormalities in the newborn has been in the literature for the last 40 years.[1] The infant or young child treated in this way by the cranial osteopathic

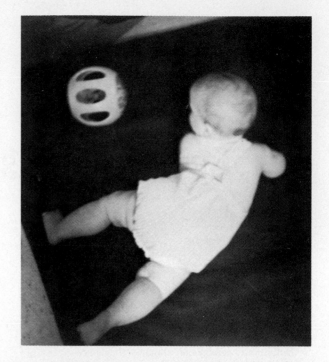

Fig. 9-1. Normal babies accumulate a multitude of experiences as they move smoothly in their environments.

physician tends to move the head more appropriately and postural tone is modified. General alertness is often affected in a positive way. The intervention is accomplished in a limited number of sessions, and the child generally is better able to retain the changes obtained by the therapist in direct therapeutic handling.

Because early development is so heavily dependent on motor responses, all areas of development are potentially affected.[47] There can also be primary physiological limitations. The most common of these is the limited movement of the eyes when head control fails to develop. Malnourishment, often compounding the intrauterine conditions, can develop because of poor sucking patterns and inadequate processing of ingested food. In fact, low-birth-weight for age is a significant feature of infants who become identified as having cerebral palsy.[25] Poor circulation relates directly to inadequate respiratory patterns and lack of movement. The sensory system is deprived from the beginning and consequently fails to mature appropriately. There is no question that cerebral palsy must be considered a sensorimotor dysfunction (Fig. 9-2).

The parents' concern and their feelings of inadequacy in dealing with this atypical infant further compound the developmental frustrations and thus affect personality development. Early therapeutic and educational programming can play a strong role in fostering emotional health for the child and the family. It is essential to support positive developmental responses and to avoid overidentification of inabilities. Parents are caught in the therapist's profes-

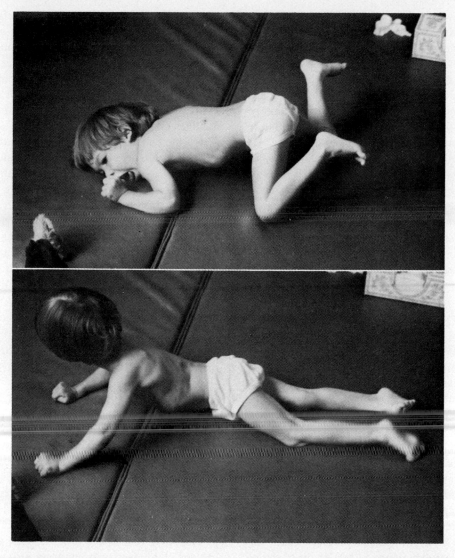

Fig. 9-2. The intelligent child will attempt movement even when the effort results in abnormal patterns.

sional dilemma of symptomatic diagnosis. The very characteristics that constitute the base for the labeling process are those features that change with the application of treatment strategies. This makes documentation of change vital for the continued learning of family and professional alike. Slides, film, or videotape sequences can provide a sample of a child's function on a particular date. The therapist gains much from the review of such visual aids and has a base from which change may be evaluated more objectively.

The overwhelmingly positive aspect of cerebral palsy is that its outcome can be positively influenced by informed and specific therapeutic intervention. Changes in population statistics have been clearly documented.[33] Individual cases can also be used as their own control, because the presence of pathology makes certain outcomes predictable with no intervention. Intelligence and motivation also have

their role in anticipating potential direction of change, particularly as the child grows older and initiates activity.

Family reactions

No one ever expects to give birth to a disabled child. Parents are looking for normal, healthy responses from their infant and, consequently, allow a wide latitude in their labeling of "normal."[2] In spite of this, most parents identify a problem long before it is acknowledged by professionals. Well-intentioned pediatricians are more fully prepared to cope with the medical needs of the normal child and tend to believe that this child will follow the majority of high-risk infants and "outgrow" the problematic delay. At our present level of knowledge, only the more severely damaged child can be identified at birth.

As the early months pass, suspicions accumulate to the point that they can no longer be ignored. Even when a "problem" is acknowledged, a formal diagnosis may not be applied. Humanistically, this is an advantage to the infant who joins the ranks of the "normal" after a relatively brief period of intensive treatment. A series of visits to specialists may be the next experience of the family. It must not be assumed that the parents do not make clear observations of developmental difficulties during this period, but in general they do not have the background to relate one finding to another nor the cause to the effect. Because there tends to be a reluctance on the part of professionals to begin intervention without a diagnosis, this period of searching by the family may require extended expenditure of time, energy, and financial investment. This investment without immediate return results in varying levels of frustration. Siblings may be somewhat neglected during this critical search for help. It is no wonder that parents appear suspicious and less than totally cooperative when they first arrive in the therapeutic environment.

Diagnosis and the time of intervention

In some instances there is an early diagnosis, which offers the possibility for better parental understanding. However, an early diagnosis may be accompanied by dire predictions as to the limited future of the child. Because these forecasts are presented to the parents in a moment of extreme emotional stress, they tend to make a strong impression. This colors the interaction between parent and infant and severely restricts the expectations of the parents. The therapist needs to be aware of these early experiences and the parents' view of their child when discussing treatment goals. Even early communicative attempts on the part of the child may be rejected as "not possible" and thus not reinforced. Inexperienced therapists should learn from this situation and avoid giving a specific prognosis until they have sufficient clinical experience to be certain of the observations made. It is important to encourage the parents to be alert to responses of the infant and young child and to offer consistent psychosocial stimulation. If the infant has merely spent developmental time resting in bed, the therapist may find deprivation compounding the physical and sensory limitations (Fig. 9-3). In actual practice, parents more often need help in seeing the positive responses and specific changes of their child. They need to acknowledge the child as a unique human being.

Although there is reason to supplement the young child's learning environment when definite limitations exist, clinicians must also maintain a strong sense of respect for the child's capacity to compensate. There are numerous examples of persons developing better than normal intelligence in spite of their inability to move or even speak.[45] Therapists do not have all the answers for how this is accomplished. By keeping a balanced perspective, therapists can offer meaningful help at a moment when the parents are ready to receive it. The child never exists in a vacuum, nor is treatment the only activity in the life of the family.

The most important contribution of therapists may be their ability to provide practical information based on clinical experience with similar children.[14] It is vital that the guidance offered be appropriate to the family's view of the situation. Once the parents begin to see results from the new positioning and home handling (Fig. 9-4), they find their tension sufficiently reduced and begin to ask questions and regain some of their lost assurance. A problem that is unknown is always more threatening and "impossible" than one that is understood.

Parents sometimes need specific reminders to avoid focusing all their energy on the disabled child.[55] Siblings often feel as helpless and guilty as the adults in this situation. Their life experience has been altered dramatically. Older children may profit from talking with the therapist

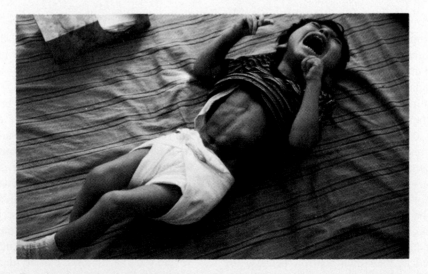

Fig. 9-3. Emotional reactions are also translated into further spasticity (see Chapter 4 on the limbic system).

directly to understand the movement problems of their sister or brother. It is important to enlist their cooperation in avoiding overstimulation that strengthens abnormal reactions. Some children born into the family after the disabled child may accept the situation without question. However, others may have vague fears that something like that could happen to them. At times, children may find it appealing to have the attention received by the disabled child. Normal siblings may even "wish" to have cerebral palsy themselves.

Cultural and familial value systems bear directly on the interaction of the family with the professional help they seek and receive. Socioeconomic factors and the existence of insurance may determine what assistance the family is able to offer the child. It is always helpful to determine how the family is currently viewing the problem and what they consider to be the major difficulty of the moment. The more therapists take these psychosocial factors into account, the more effective their influence will be to help the child. (See Chapter 7 on psychosocial adjustment.)

Diagnostic categorization of the characteristics of cerebral palsy

In general, diagnosis of cerebral palsy suggests that the individual in question has some central disorder of posture and movement. In addition, the labeling process often identifies the parts of the body that are primarily involved. Diplegia, hemiplegia, and quadriplegia indicate respectively that the lower extremities, one side of the body, or all four extremities are affected.

The clinician must be aware that the categorization of cerebral palsy is based on descriptions of observable characteristics: it is a symptomatic description. Both Dr. Little, who first identified the condition, and Dr. Winthrop Phelps, who differentiated the characteristic types of cerebral palsy, were describing the spontaneous movement attempts away from the resting posture. These characteristic movement patterns were identified as spasticity, athetosis, hypotonicity, and ataxia (Fig. 9-5).

The hypertonus of spasticity prevents a smooth exchange between mobility and stability of the body. Incrementation of postural tone occurs with an increase in the speed of even passive movement. Although diagnostic terms reflect the distribution of excessive postural tone, the entire body must be considered to be involved. Spasticity by nature involves less movement, which makes its distribution easier to identify.

The term athetosis refers to a lack of posture. The excessive peripheral movement occurs without central stability. Athetosis may occur with greater involvement in particular extremities, although it most often interferes with postural stability as a whole. Athetoid distribution of postural tone is changeable, particularly during attempted movement.

Hypotonicity is another category of cerebral palsy, but may also mask undiagnosed degenerative conditions (see Chapter 8). The hypotonic picture in a young infant may also be a precursor of athetosis. Often the athetoid move-

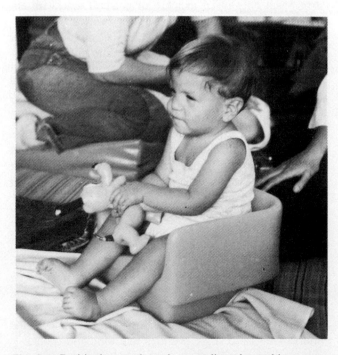

Fig. 9-4. Positioning need not be complicated to achieve a new play opportunity while primitive abduction is inhibited.

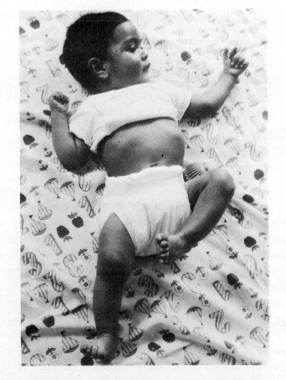

Fig. 9-5. Asymmetry in this immobile 8-month-old infant is a clue to right hemiparesis caused by porencephaly.

ments are not noticed until the infant is attempting anti-gravity postures, although there may be some disorganization apparent to the careful observer. Tone changes with attempted movement may be present even without the peripheral signs of athetosis.

Ataxia is a cerebellar disorder that is seen more frequently as a sequela of tumor removal (see Chapter 20) than as a problem occurring from birth. Probably because of changes in delivery practices, it seems to occur with less frequency now than it did when Dr. Phelps categorized the types of cerebral palsy. Ataxic reactions are often noted in the gait of an athetoid individual. However, more specific analysis may reveal compensatory responses to the athetoid tone changes while the body is in motion through space. (See Chapter 3 on motor control.)

There are also individuals who demonstrate athetoid tone changes within a range of spasticity or spastic distributions of postural tone superimposed on athetotic disorganization. The developing child may also move from one predominant postural tone to another. Treatment intervention may reveal finer nuances of difference in the distribution of postural tone as total patterns are inhibited[49] and reflexive reactions are integrated.

These classifications, when accurately applied, give the therapist a general idea of the treatment problem. Supplementation of this information will occur with a specific analysis of posture and movement, an interview for home-care information, and assessment of treatment responses. The therapist is then ready to establish treatment priorities for the individual child.

Many of the characteristics described in the preceding paragraphs also apply to children who have suffered closed head traumas or brain infections. Further information can be obtained in Chapters 13 and 16. Some of the treatment suggestions that follow may also be applied in such cases. As with cerebral palsy, early positioning and handling may deter many problems later.

EVALUATIVE ANALYSIS OF THE INDIVIDUAL CHILD
Initial observations

Assessment of the individual child begins with careful observation of the interaction between parents and the child, including parental handling of the child that occurs spontaneously (Fig. 9-6). While observing the child, the experienced therapist may extend this initial interaction by eliciting from the parents their view of the problem. By listening carefully, the therapist will also be able to discern the emotional impressions that have surrounded previous experiences with professionals.

The next general step is to observe, in as much detail as possible, the spontaneous movement of the child. Is the child very passive? Are there abnormal patterns of movement to reach a toy (Fig. 9-7)? Are clearly normal responses occurring with specific interference by reflexive

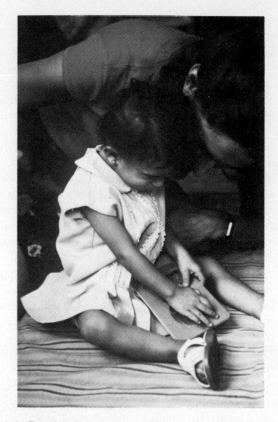

Fig. 9-6. Emotional nurturing by the parent is vital for the child's optimal development.

synergies or total patterns of movement? Does the child rely heavily on visual communication? Does an effort to move result only in an increase of postural tone with abnormal distribution?

These observations are valuable, because movement patterns directly reflect the state of the central nervous system and can generally be obtained while the parent is still handling the child. Once the child is on the mat, one can more easily remove outer clothing to observe movement patterns. Movement responses of the child can gradually be influenced directly by the therapist. Many disabled children associate immediate undressing in a new environment with a doctor's office, and the chance to establish rapport is lost. In some instances it is preferable to have the parent gently remove the child's clothing.

Assessment of the child's status is more likely to be adequate if the therapist follows the child's lead where possible. Notes can later be organized to conform to a specific format. It is often possible to jot down essential information while observing the child moving spontaneously or while the parent is still holding the child. After the session one can dictate the salient information into a tape recorder. Attention should be given to the normal movements of the child as well as to those postures that the child spontaneously attempts to control. In noting abnormal reactions and compensatory movement patterns, one must also indicate

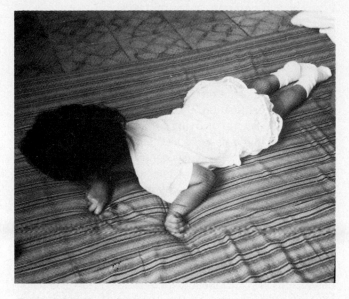

Fig. 9-7. Play experience or exploration for this child is limited to abnormal patterns of movement.

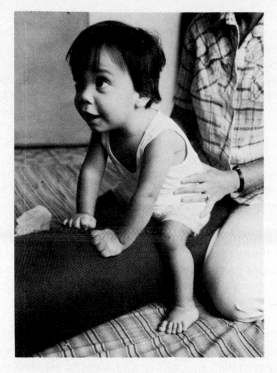

Fig. 9-8. Simple positioning can facilitate head lift and visual contact with the environment.

the position of the body with respect to gravity. One tends to compile more pertinent data by following the lead of the child. Children are vibrant beings. Choices of position tell us something about their habits and how comfortable they are in this situation. To be the slave of a preformulated sequence destroys the decision-making initiative appropriate to the situation at hand. This is true for the therapist as well as the child.

Each child will differ in ability to separate from his or her parents. Spontaneity of movement, general activity level, and communication skills will also vary from child to child. Responding to the specific needs of the child enables the therapist to set priorities more effectively. If fatigue is likely to be a factor, it is important to evaluate first those reactions that present themselves spontaneously. Those for which there is a major interference by spasticity or reflexive responses may better be checked at the termination of the assessment.

Reactions to placement in a position

If the child totally avoids certain postures during the spontaneous activity, these are likely to be the more important positions for the therapist to evaluate. Placement of the child in the avoided position will permit the therapist to feel the resistance that prevents successful control by the child. The parent should play an active role in the assessment whenever possible. Continued dialogue with the parent reveals such factors as the frequency of a poor sitting alignment at home or a habitual aversion to the prone position. These contributions by the parent establish the importance of good observation and the need for parent and therapist to work cooperatively.

Following the guide of normal development,[24,36] in-

fants should be able to maintain a posture in which they are placed before they acquire the ability to move into that position alone.[34] The problems presented by cerebral palsy occur primarily as a reaction to the field of gravity in which the child moves.[7] It is therefore helpful to attempt placement of the infant or child into developmentally appropriate postures that are not assumed spontaneously (Fig. 9-8). Resistance to placement indicates an increase in postural tone, the presence of spasticity, or a structural problem. It is important to keep in mind that a movement that resists control by the therapist will be even less possible for the child. What appears to be a passive posture may in some children hide rapid increases in postural tone when movement is initiated. Such a child has learned to avoid excitation of the unwanted reactions. Another child may enjoy the sensory experience of accelerated postural tone changes and deliberately set them off.

Abnormal interferences

Abnormal responses that interfere with postural adjustments by the infant or child with cerebral palsy may have been normal at some point in development. Reflexive reactions that are retained beyond the point at which they should have been integrated block the normal differentiation of movement. Postural transitions or movement sequences become distorted and poorly timed. In normal development the integration of reflexive reactions follows a sequence that correlates with the acquisition of motor skills.[6] Fiorentino[21] and others [10,24] view these early reflexive reactions as the establishment of patterns of movement that are used even in adult life. They may also be viewed as systematic, organized cues that guide the motor responses. Hellebrandt and others[28] predictably elicited the asymmetrical tonic neck reflex (ATNR) in normal college students by placing them in a prone position across a hammock type support. With the subjects blindfolded and the arms unsupported, voluntary turning of the head to the side was resisted by the examiner. The response obtained in the arm position was the typical ATNR. Children with cerebral palsy will also vary greatly as to the amount of stress required to activate a reflexive synergy. The most severely involved almost never move out of the reflex patterns, whereas the mildly involved child who runs or reacts emotionally to a situation becomes transiently bound by reflexes. The level at which the reflexive responses interfere with function is most significant. The therapist must also be aware of the reflexive synergies most active in each position of the body (Fig. 9-9, *A* and *B*).

These abnormal patterns of movement may also be used by the child to accomplish functional skills of daily living. In such cases reflexive reactions and abnormal distribution of postural tone are reinforced by constant use. Differentiated levels of motor control are prevented, and the child seems to plateau in motor development. At this point parents may seek help to elaborate the necessary sensorimotor base for more sophisticated function. It is more effective to avoid the child's early use of abnormal patterns than to attempt to change established habits superimposed on the use of abnormal synergies.

Primary and compensatory patterns

Compensatory patterns must also be taken into account when assessing function. They commonly are mistaken for primary postural reactions, possibly resulting from the distribution of spasticity. One of the most common misunderstandings occurs with the presence of the "toe-walking" response. The distribution of postural tone usually is stronger in flexor patterns, serving to pull the individual down into gravity. In the standing alignment, as the body weight is displaced forward, it is accentuated by hip flexion and the forward position of the center of gravity. With undifferentiated responses of the legs and lack of lateral weight shift, the spastic child counteracts the pull of flexion with a total pattern of extension. The plantar flexion of the foot is only one small component of the total postural picture.

Careful analysis of the postural adjustments and movement patterns of the cerebral palsied child is crucial to initiating effective therapeutic intervention. The interaction of many factors creates the final picture (Fig. 9-10). Normal reactions to abnormal distribution of tone may distort gait as easily as a lack of adequate trunk extension or marked pelvic immobility. In addition to the physical factors, the sensory aspects of the condition often interfere with the quality of movement. Tactile sensitivity may interfere with foot placement or prevent sustained grasp of a toy or an eating utensil. This tendency to "drop" objects can be misleading to the examiner, who may mistake it for lack of interest. It also prevents the learning experiences associated with firm pressure input to the hands and feet and the consequent normal evolution of the sensory sys-

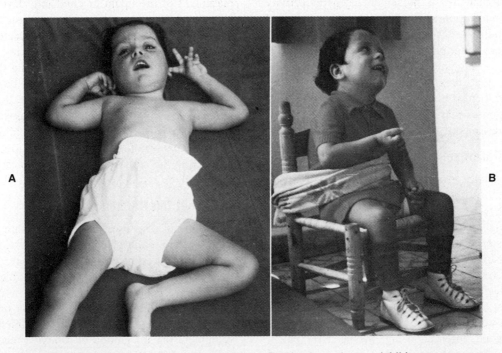

Fig. 9-9. A, Strong asymmetry and abnormal tone. **B,** Simple seating can inhibit strong asymmetry and make function a possibility.

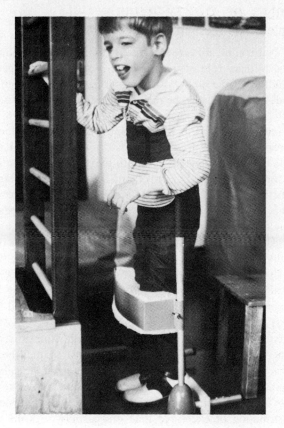

Fig. 0 10. The upright position can help to integrate abnormal postural patterns.

tem. The therapist may want to simulate normal weight-bearing by the application of firm pressure against the palms of the hands and the soles of the feet. Slight movement of the extremity will facilitate the adaptation. This experience of firm pressure tends to inhibit the withdrawal.

Consideration of foot support is crucial to influence a more normal distribution of postural tone and a better alignment. Heavy controls and limitation of ankle mobility are to be avoided. Detailed attention to the dynamic balance of the foot itself, a stability that permits mobility in gait, brings greater successful adaptation.

The independence finally achieved by the older child reflects his or her intelligence and motivation, as well as the family attitude toward the child and the disability. The most debilitating "handicap" of cerebral palsy may be social or psychological in nature, when the child is not accepted by the family and therefore cannot accept himself or herself.[55] Early treatment not only prevents physical limitations but also assists the parents in understanding their child and the disability.

DIRECT TREATMENT OR CASE MANAGEMENT

Simple documentation of observed changes in a child over a series of regular clinic visits is still too common for many children with cerebral palsy. Regular appointments,

with periodic assignment of a new piece of apparatus, does not constitute active treatment. Although physical intervention in the form of direct handling of the child is considered a "conservative treatment" by most physicians,[46] there are relatively few children who receive sufficient physical treatment at an early age.[29]

The prognosis for change in cerebral palsy is too often based on records of case management rather than on the effect of direct treatment. Bobath[8] documented more accurately the developmental sequence expected in the presence of spasticity or athetosis. This volume[8] consolidates some observations of older clients that help professionals understand the uninterrupted effects of the cerebral palsy condition. In any institution one can observe the tightly adducted and internally rotated legs, the shoulder retraction with flexion of the arms, and the chronic shortening of the neck so common as the long-term effects of spasticity. The athetoid component provides movement to avoid contractures while creating a need to experience reliable postures for stability.

Responsible surgeons now recognize the improved outcome of their intervention if physical treatment, or a "conservative approach," is applied before and after the surgical procedure.[39] Tendon lengthenings for older children with average intelligence may be preceded by "muscle energy" work, in which the therapist assists the child in activating the desired muscle group. The therapist may then follow the controlled release with isometric activity inside the cast. Early standing in casts is to be highly recommended, as are specific footplates, to reduce potential sensory deprivation and to promote more rapid healing with improved circulation.[4,50,53]

There is clear documentation[28,33] of epidemiological or population changes as a result of early intervention while the CNS is in a period of rapid growth and change. It is also important to offer the flexibility that permits short periods of intensive treatment for an individual child. Informed evaluation by developmentally knowledgeable physicians permits optimal use of effective treatment. We have long had evidence that neurological change occurs in small mammals as a result of physical handling and specific environmental experiences.[26] Now evidence for change in the human CNS as a result of therapeutic intervention is accumulating rapidly.[40]

Dr. Josephine Moore[3] has highlighted some important points for therapists in her concept of "forcing" the system and her observations of the significance of the neck structures in developmental sequences. The righting reactions used by both Rood and Bobath are completely dependent on neck functions. Spastic children are often observed to have a lack of developmental elongation of the neck, whereas athetoid children lack neck stability as well as postural stability. Moore suggests that our concept of "cephalo-caudal development" should be amended to consider development beginning at the neck and moving in both a "cephalo" and "caudal" direction. This is useful to the therapist who realizes that tone change most often originates with changes in the delicate interrelationship between head and body.

In applying Dr. Moore's notion of "forcing" the system, professionals must first gain an understanding of the function of various subsystems as well as the integrative action of the CNS as a whole. Appreciation of the abundance of polysynaptic neurons and polysensory receptors[3] will provide a much more optimistic view of the therapist's role as a "facilitator" of the system. At the same time, therapists have a responsibility to interpret and apply the feedback that they receive from the entire organism. Any stimulus that is of sufficient strength to make a positive change is also capable, under the right circumstances, of making a negative change to influence the quality of "output" in that moment. For example, excessive treatment to obtain extensor responses in the prone position can result in failure of the neck to elongate and inadequate balance of flexor tone to permit normal standing. Treatment intervention is far from innocuous when responsibly applied. A truly "eclectic" treatment approach comes only after years of experience and a comprehensive understanding of various approaches. The effective therapist will gradually formulate a personal philosophy of treatment, with space for new ideas that arise from treatment feedback or from new knowledge about the CNS. One can never learn "too much" about the intricacies of normal development and its implications.

ROLES OF THE THERAPIST
Role of the therapist in direct intervention

Nature of direct treatment for specific problems. The primary role of the therapist is in direct treatment or handling of the child with cerebral palsy. This should precede and accompany the making of recommendations to parents, teachers, and others handling the child. As with the initial assessment, there are many interventions that will cause a reaction unique to the particular youngster.[18,43] It is the role of the therapist to ascertain the response of the child before recommending to others activity, positioning, or handling (Fig. 9-11). It will then be possible for other persons to manage play activities and supervise independent functioning that reinforces treatment goals.[48]

The child who is bound within the limitations of spasticity suffers first of all from a paucity of movement. As early attempts to move have resulted in the expression of total reflexive postural patterns, the child generally loses incentive to attempt movement. The easily observed tightness in the limbs is not the major problem of these children. Looking past the obvious, one sometimes discovers that the stability that should be present in the shoulder structure to support good arm movement or in the pelvis to free the leg is replaced by mobility and low tone. The limb has then taken on the role of "stabilizer" with the abnormal distribution of excessive tone or spasticity. As the trunk tone is normalized, the abnormally high tone in the limbs will be reduced.

Postures that are associated with an abnormal distribu-

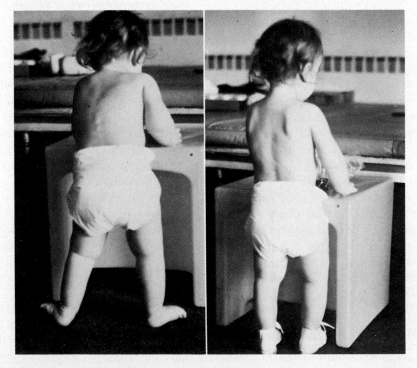

Fig. 9-11. Supportive shoes for the low-tone child unquestionably facilitate more normal trunk reactions and permit use of the hands for play.

tion of postural tone or that express abnormal patterns of movement should be avoided initially. Later in the treatment process the therapist will want to return to these positions to reduce tone in the active posture and gradually to turn over control to the child. One might think here of the child who lies in the supine position with extreme pushing back against the surface. The therapist would initially eliminate the supine position entirely but would incorporate into the treatment plan the activation of normal flexor tone in sitting with variations of pelvic tilt. Only gradually would the child be reintroduced to the independently controlled supine position.

A primary consideration for the spastic child is sufficient mobility of the chest wall and abdominal area to allow for near-normal respiration. Because rotation within the longitudinal axis of the body is frequently of poor quality or completely absent, respiratory patterns remain immature and spontaneous; differentiated or segmental rolling does not occur. A lack of sitting or antigravity postural control will limit even the physiological shaping of the rib cage itself, because the ribs do not have an opportunity to change their angle at the spine. Initial treatment sessions with an older child must take into account the physiological stress induced by respiratory adaptation. The therapist is literally "forcing" an adaptation in the breathing pattern, which will then serve to reinforce postural tone changes in the trunk itself. Normal adaptable respiration will help to maintain normal trunk tone.

When working to change spasticity, the therapist may find it useful to inhibit unwanted posturing, such as extension, by placing the body in an opposite alignment, such as flexion. While controlling the flexed position, one can deliberately stimulate extension by changing the body position in space or by weight-bearing over the extensor surface. From a flexed body posture maintained by the therapist, the child might protectively extend an arm for support. Once the hand makes contact, the therapist can move the body weight over the limb to further normalize the postural tone while preventing the expression of total extensor patterns. In this way the threshold is gradually altered so that the child begins to tolerate some stimulation without immediately responding with the unwanted posturing—in this case, extension. When there are distinct differences between the two sides of the body, the same control of position might be used in company with lateral weight shifts in standing. For example, the supporting leg may be maintained in extension while the body weight is guided over that side. Frequently, changes near midline are some of the more difficult stimuli for the disorganized system to accept. Thus it may be necessary for the therapist to offer more specific cues for the change and even repeat the experience with a marked pause to allow integration of the new alignment at the sensory-proprioceptive level and time for the CNS to process the information.

While working with CNS disorders, the therapist often uses an intensity of stimulation somewhat beyond the range that is generally considered "normal." However, therapists must take into account that they are addressing a system that is deficient in its ability to perceive and to use the available input. If the microcosm of experience given the child during a treatment session is no more intense than an equal amount of time in his or her everyday living environment, the therapist has failed to utilize this unique opportunity to deliver a meaningful message that developmentally integrates the system.

Reassessment of direct treatment. The therapist actually functions as an extension of the child's CNS, organizing input as to intensity, frequency, and distribution to anticipate a desired response. The child may react positively, negatively, or inadequately to the sensory experience. The therapist immediately is confronted with the need to evaluate the quality of the motor response, much as an intact system monitors its own output and seeks further experience. Has the needed relaxation been achieved? Is the body tolerating symmetry in a resting position? Is the movement of a limb graded and without unwanted associated reactions in other parts of the body? Is the child now ready to take over more independent control?

The therapist acts on the judgment made regarding the nature of the response obtained. The next "feedback" provided for processing by the child's CNS needs to challenge the system while assuring success and moving towards more normal control. In various ways, depending on the technique found to be most effective, the therapist is interrupting the child's customary abnormal feedback. At times the input of the therapist may only be a slight modification of the child's own response, such as an elongation of a limb as it is being moved. At other times the therapist may introduce a substitute for missed experiences. For example, with firm pressure on the sole of the foot, approximation of the lower extremity gives the system an impression similar to the pushing of a foot against the surface during normal movement within the home environment. This can be considered a component of the sensory experience of normal development (Fig. 9-12).

Too often professionals consider sensory input to be on a simple graded continuum. The picture is not so elementary.[17] It must be considered as at least a three-dimensional and possibly a four-dimensional phenomenon. Multiple sensory systems are simultaneously activated by most therapeutic input, while a variety of sights and sounds may be available in the immediate environment. Memory, previous learnings, and cognition are often activated by the therapist-child interaction. The therapist must be accustomed to continuous reassessment of the child's experiential needs as compared with the current input provided. The entire CNS is activated by the treatment experience.

To philosophically explore the developmental meaning attached to the sensory experience of normal movement,

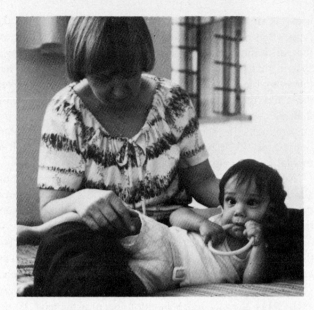

Fig. 9-12. Treatment sessions can consider a child's need for a teething experience while facilitating good postural patterns and tone distribution.

therapists must take into account the ability to process contrasting stimuli. While several parts of the body are stable, another is moving. Stability of the proximal body permits a limb to extend forcefully or to be maintained in space. Each new level of differentiation or disassociation of movement increases the complexity of processing by the CNS (Fig. 9-13). Stimuli from within the body and from the environment impinge simultaneously on the CNS. This is easily illustrated with a review of self-feeding. Initially the process of guiding a full spoon into the mouth engages the child's full attention. In time this aspect of the task becomes automatic as the child participates in social exchanges with the family at the same time.

A solid understanding of normal developmental sequences is essential for the clinician. These insights confirm that earlier, simpler responses of the normal infant are constantly being integrated more completely by the acquisition of new developmental competence. (Elaboration of balance in sitting only occurs with the ability to pull to standing.) How is this knowledge to be applied by the therapist? The implication is that the therapist, functioning to screen input for the child's nervous system, can offer the child the experience of postural activities at a higher level than his or her present function permits. To sit well, the child must experience standing (Fig. 9-14). To walk well, the child may need to run with control by the therapist. At the same time, some of the treatment session is spent filling in gaps that represent missed experiences, such as squatting to play or coming to stand from kneeling. Preparation of the entire body with the most normal alignment and postural tone is vital to maximize the sensory experience of postural control. Specific techniques can be reviewed thoroughly in Chapter 6.

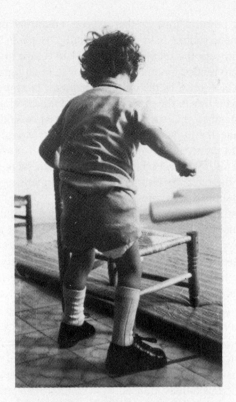

Fig. 9-13. This hemiplegic boy tries to move a chair by orienting only his more active side to the task and bearing weight only briefly on the more affected side.

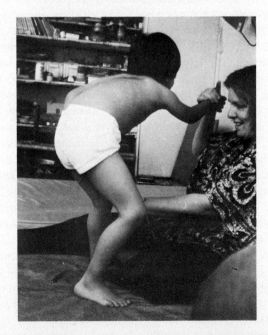

Fig. 9-14. The experience of coming to standing over the more affected side activates diagonal patterns of postural adjustment.

With the athetoid child, the therapist's role relates primarily to organization and grading of seemingly erratic movement. Initially, therapists provide the postural control never achieved by the child. Through their handling of the child they give stability from which movement can emerge. At a more sophisticated level the therapist grades the movement of limbs by structuring the postural control of the proximal body. In some instances a limb may be maintained in position by the therapist to elicit active proximal adjustments that are the basis of true postural control. The astute therapist will find that careful analysis of tone changes reveals, in many cases, a predictable pattern. One particular movement will initiate the interfering spasm or series of spasms that interrupt stability. This may be part of a reflexive pattern, or it may be an isolated reaction. In the ambulatory athetoid child it is often the spontaneous depression or elevation of a scapula or the protraction of a shoulder that initiates tone change throughout the body. If this particular initiating action can be effectively inhibited, while righting reactions of the head and trunk are stimulated, the body begins to build a repertoire of responses that does not include the customary interference. With functional use of the upper extremity for support, reach, and grasp, the client shares with the therapist inhibition of the abnormal response. Gradually, the more normal use of the whole upper trunk integrates the interfering response, resulting in improved control for a variety of independently controlled postures. The therapist continues to introduce graded stress during treatment sessions to normalize even further the threshold for the unwanted reaction. Environmental stimuli such as sights, sounds, and social interaction should be considered as stimuli along with positional stress. This concept of graded stress is considered more thoroughly in Chapter 6.

Direct intervention for the hemiplegic child takes into account the obvious difference in postural tone between one side of the body and the other. However, treatment that addresses itself only to the more affected side of the body has seldom proved effective. The critical therapeutic experience seems to be that of integration of the two sides of the body. Normally, this begins early, with the lateral weight shifts of the infant in a variety of developmental patterns and the same postural organization that permits later reaching for a toy. The hemiplegic child needs assistance to experience those developmental patterns that include rotation within the longitudinal body axis and lateral flexion of the trunk. The therapist will find it profitable to spend time achieving active lateral flexion responses in the trunk. This may be controlled initially in side lying and coming to sitting before active responses are expected in sitting and in prone. As with other instances of spasticity, one may find that true flexion of the more affected side of the body is fully as difficult for some children as the initial elongation of that side. These children also seem to have difficulty in sustaining a posture against the influence of gravity. This is a characteristic that may contribute to the development of seemingly "hyperactive" behavior. The therapist must also be cognizant of the possibility that hyperkinetic responses in one side of the body may compensate for the inactivity in the opposite side. One goal of treatment is to approximate these divergent response levels.

The limbs of the hemiplegic child will change in postural tone as the trunk reactions are brought under control. Specific attention must also be given to sensory normalization. The two hands need to sustain the body weight simultaneously, as do the two feet. In effect, the discrepancy between the experiences of the two sides seems to lead the system to reject one of the messages. This can lead to distortions in verticality and is a major interference in bilateral integration. As body weight is shifted to the more normal side, flexor withdrawal patterns of the limbs increase in frequency and strength. One important therapy goal is the achievement of true weight shift in the pelvis during ambulation. Treatment preparation must incorporate a wide variety of more basic developmental alignments in which pelvic weight shift is a factor. The choice of prone, half-kneeling, or a simple weight shift, for example, will depend on the constellation of factors observed by the therapist at the time. Dynamic foot supports will facilitate this lateral weight shift when the child is not in treatment. Careful attention must be given to pelvic alignment and mobility, because the more affected side of the pelvis is often rotated back, which causes hip flexion and may easily mislead the therapist during analysis of leg position. Although the more affected hand may not have sensation adequate for skilled activity, it needs to acquire sufficient shoulder mobility to move across the body midline and to assume a relaxed alignment during ambulation. This goal is best reached through a wide variety of weight-bearing postures, from the obvious developmental alignments to horizontal protective responses against a wall from the standing position (Fig. 9-15).

The low-tone child is perhaps the greatest challenge for therapist and parent alike. Adequate developmental stimulation is difficult unless positioning can be varied. Placing the child in a more upright alignment, even though it is achieved with complete support initially, seems to aid the incrementation of postural tone. Strong proprioceptive input, while ensuring accurate postural alignment, is an important part of the treatment session. Direct "tapping," as described by the Bobaths,[9] also assists in maintaining antigravity positions. At all times the therapist must be cautious of high-tone responses only belatedly evident. This spasticity, which can be distributed in the deeper musculature, contributes to fixation rather than differentiated postural control. Similarly, even though the child's motor output may remain low, the sensory and emotional systems may be on overload; thus keen observation by the therapist is critical.

Developing a personal philosophy of treatment. The practicing therapist can never learn too much about the nuances of normal human development.[16] The dynamic interaction of developmental components rises to a new level of significance as the clinician gains awareness of this phenomenon as a reflection of CNS maturation. Increasing knowledge of the functional nature of sensory systems and CNS processing will influence the choice of treatment

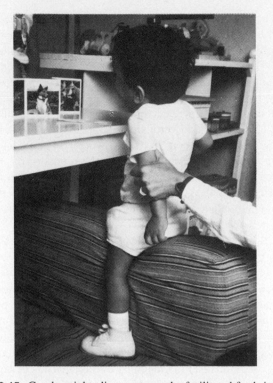

Fig. 9-15. Good upright alignment may be facilitated for brief periods of time to utilize the proprioceptive experience and to inhibit interfering tone changes.

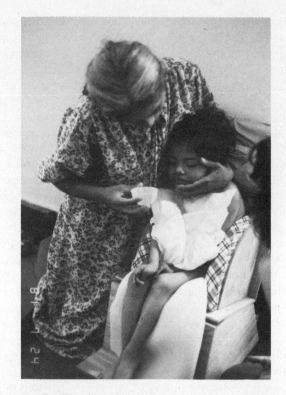

Fig. 9-16. Feeding the child with severe cerebral palsy requires patience and is made easier by an understanding of abnormal reactions and how to avoid them.

techniques (Fig. 9-16). This knowledge will offer more depth and specificity to concepts of posture and movement, as well as a better understanding of the disorders of posture and movement in cerebral palsy. Based on individual experience, each therapist must develop a personal philosophy of treatment to incorporate emerging ideas and new perceptions of the problem of CNS dysfunction. Without this base, it is easy to become "victimized" by each promising treatment idea that presents itself. The therapist, without an internalized treatment goal toward which independent "techniques" are applied, remains ineffective and unconvincing. The therapist in a direct treatment situation must be secure in a concise, personalized visualization of what is to be achieved in the particular session with the individual child.

Intentionally, little has been said of training the cerebral-palsied child in specific skills. Intelligent children will often develop personal "shortcuts," and the therapist only has to limit the use of abnormal reactions. All of treatment, like all of development, is potentially a preparation for functional skills. Adaptations and equipment may be useful in initiating independent activity. Nancy Finnie[20] has given many practical suggestions along these lines. With some help in providing structure to the situation and adaptations where necessary, parents can experience success when eliciting play responses from their disabled child. The acquisition of self-help skills must respect the

individual child's rate of development, emotional separation of self, and physical readiness. Brereton and others[12] have done an excellent job of grading perceptual-motor tasks and suggest alternate presentations that may better suit the individual child. Furth and Wachs[23] have also presented precognitive skill development according to the thinking strategy employed by the child in a useful reference that is organized for the busy therapist.

Active involvement of the family. Active treatment entails active home follow-up in the form of both physical and psychological handling of the child. Parents must be helped to understand the importance of their participation. This is not always easy, because parents may have suffered in their own self-image when they learned of their child's disability. Although they should not be expected to become therapists per se, close observation of treatment sessions offers insight as to the child's current strengths and weaknesses. Parents can consequently adapt their expectations in keeping with the child's ongoing change. Parenting a child with cerebral palsy is no easy task, and the therapist will do well to develop respect for this demanding role. No one provides more for the cerebral-palsied child than the nurturing parent who guides the child to self-acceptance without destroying initiative.

The therapist must give serious thought to priorities in home recommendations. To be considered are the size of the family, outside employment of mother and father, physical capacity of the child, general health status of the child, and psychological acceptance of the problem within the family. The emotional needs of some parents demand a period of less, rather than more, direct involvement with the child. Other parents must be cautioned that repetition of an activity more times than recommended will not result in faster improvement. Both parent and therapist must ap-preciate the need for the CNS to have some time to inte-grate new experiences and to perfect emerging control of postural adjustments. Health needs for good nutrition and adequate rest must also be considered.

Equipment recommendations must take into account the physical space in the home and the amount of direct treat-ment available to the child (Fig. 9-17). Young children, in particular, can often use normal seating with slight adapta-tions. This is not only more socially acceptable, but also permits changes as required by developmental progress. Portability of supportive seats or standers encourages the family to take the apparatus along for weekend outings. Chair designs should also place children at an age-appro-priate level in their environments. This permits a better quality of visual exploration and facilitates social exchange with siblings and visiting peers.

Criteria for equipment recommendations. When planning the amount of physical support needed by the child, the therapist will do well to consider varying the structural control in relation to activity (Fig. 9-18). The child who is merely watching the play of others or a tele-vision presentation may successfully control trunk and head balance. However, concentration on hand skills or self-feeding may necessitate trunk control by a chair insert to avoid the use of abnormal reactions. As the postural re-actions become more integrated and hence more auto-matic, support should be diminished.

Particularly for the more severely disabled child, equip-ment should be easily and completely washable. Mothers, using one free hand, should be able to place special seat-ing inserts into wheelchairs or travel chairs. Pleasing color, good quality upholstery, and professional finishing are important not only for the child but also for the family

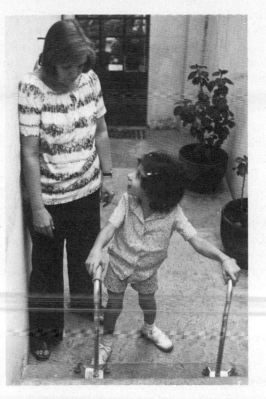

Fig. 9-17. True ability to "walk" must include problem solving for architectural barriers in the child's own environment.

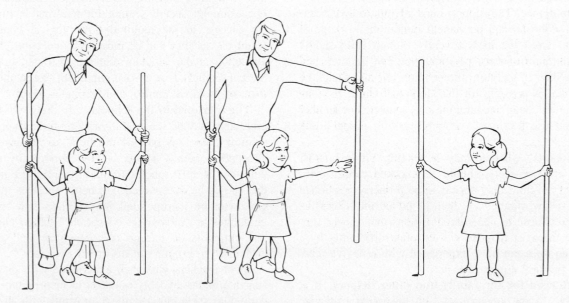

Fig. 9-18. The use of poles was introduced by the Bobaths as a transitional support for increas-ingly complex postural adjustments in standing.

who is accepting the equipment as part of a personal living environment.

As prices rise, cost effectiveness must be considered more carefully by the therapist. Parents are often desperate to do everything possible for their child and tend to be very susceptible to high-powered advertising and reassuring sales personnel. The therapist, by providing a list of essential equipment features, will aid the parents in becoming informed consumers. Perusal of several catalogs permits some comparison of quality and prices. Investment in expensive equipment also has the hidden effect of influencing both parent and therapist to continue its use when its effectiveness as a dynamic supplement to treatment has passed. For this reason more than any other, large investments must be thoroughly researched as to their long-term applicability.

Role of the therapist in indirect intervention

For many children with cerebral palsy, active treatment is not available. Geographic isolation, socioeconomic factors, and lack of qualified therapists may interfere with the delivery of direct service. The therapist must then assume the role of teacher, counselor, or consultant. More often the new role emerges as one in which the therapist tries to meet a combination of needs and is frequently frustrated by lack of time, energy, and community resources. The therapist may be a member of a community team that includes a psychologist, a social worker, and a public health nurse. This sometimes creates more of a behavioral than a traditional medical orientation. Therapists can also be primarily responsible to the public school systems, introducing therapeutic positioning to classroom teachers.

Physical positioning for the child who lacks direct treatment. When the therapist is seeing children who have no access to direct treatment, positioning is of paramount importance. The support must attempt to avoid contractures, scoliosis, and permanent limitations in range of movement. Even the most severely limited child should have a minimum of three positions that can be alternated during the day. In addition, the position selected should be as functional as possible for the individual child. In some cases this may mean encouraging eye contact. For another child, hand use becomes a possibility with proper trunk support.

All supports, whether they be chairs, prone boards, standers, or floor seats, should be checked carefully for their effect. A child may appear to be properly positioned for the first few minutes and then be pulled into excessive flexion or collapse to one side. Positions that appear simple to the therapist may be viewed quite differently by a person who does not have experience with reflexive reactions and postural alignments.

Consultation for the family and other helpers. If at all possible, some opportunity for in-service exchange should be provided when persons with a variety of professional backgrounds are brought together to accomplish a task. The therapist, along with other specialists, must forfeit some professional jargon in the interest of true communication to benefit the child. One may practice with familiar persons who lack training in therapy. The therapist can try talking this volunteer through the task of positioning a child or feeding the child according to written directions. The therapist should then note the areas of miscommunication and adapt the instructions accordingly.

Therapists should encourage parents, teachers, and others to understand why certain positions are being used. This will make them more conscious of both positive and negative changes that may call for further adaptations. It is safer to overexplain than to leave persons with a partial understanding or outright confusion as to why the positioning may have an effect on the child's development. When feasible, it is helpful to let persons caring for the child assume some of the abnormal postures to personally experience the difficulties that the child experiences.

For the infant, avoidance of abnormal patterns may be sufficient to facilitate normal developmental responses that integrate the more primitive reactions. Some children will need additional help to experience success in the movement required for reach, grasp, or visual following once therapeutic positioning is introduced. The older child has learned to use abnormal patterns of movement to function.

Communication systems for the more severely disabled child should be evaluated by the therapist to determine which normal patterns may be utilized. Repeated activation of total patterns of flexion or extension will eventually interfere with trunk control in sitting and may cause a child to regress physically. Use of a simple, normal response will help toward the goal of better function. All activities that are repeated on a daily basis should be examined in light of possible interference by abnormal patterns. For example, secure seating for toileting is fundamental for success in the required physiological control. Self-feeding assistance can be most effectively introduced with abduction at the shoulder and the overhand grasp of the normal toddler. This normal alignment fosters the development of proximal control and facilitates grasp.

The therapist in the schools. Children with mild cerebral palsy may be successfully incorporated in physical education classes as part of the trend to "mainstreaming." Teachers generally appreciate the opportunity to discuss with the therapist specific limitations and those movements that should be encouraged. For better success, the disabled child can be incorporated into a class that follows the guidelines of "movement education," which places much less emphasis on intragroup competition and encourages each child to progress at his or her own rate.

Most teachers who lack experience with disabled persons are understandably reluctant to incorporate a disabled child into their classroom. A meeting with the therapist might be used to help the child demonstrate his or her strengths and physical independence. The child may also be a part of the problem solving necessary for a successful classroom experience. Children may have their own ways of managing the water fountain, the locker door, or personal care needs. This reinforces strengths rather than limitations and arms the child with some positive responses for curious peers.

New directions in the community

As programs that hire therapists move into prevention and early intervention, the therapist is dealing directly with a population that is not familiar with therapy per se nor aware of the need for this intervention. The therapist may discover a need to reorient previously accepted concepts of rehabilitation. Clarification in one's own mind is essential to effective communication with others. In some instances active intervention will precede the labeling process. Philosophically, therapy may become an enhancement of normal development rather than a remedial process.

The movement toward a health orientation as opposed to crisis intervention for illness will also affect services for children and adults with cerebral palsy. This population does not have an illness or active disease process. Many adults with neuromotor disabilities express their preference to participate in the decisions that are made for them regarding their ultimate life-style. Certainly, optimal health for the person with residuals of cerebral palsy has yet to be described.

PSYCHOSOCIAL FACTORS IN CEREBRAL PALSY

We have defined cerebral palsy as a condition existing from the time of birth or infancy. The developing child has no memory of life in a different body. Movement limitations circumscribe the horizon of the child's world unless the family is able to provide compensatory experiences. The development of both intelligence and personality relies heavily on developmental experiences and self-expression.

The spastic child may be hesitant in making decisions or reaching out for a new opportunity because the world may seem overwhelming and somewhat threatening. The child may find it easier to withdraw toward social isolation. Parents and professionals can help to avoid these reactions by encouraging independence in thought and in physical tasks. Early choices can be made by the child regarding which clothes to wear or which task to do first. Understanding of the child's limitations helps build successes rather than failures. To function in spite of the constraints of spasticity demands considerable effort.

Athetoid children, in contrast, have adapted to failures as a transient part of life. However disorganized their movements, they repeatedly attempt tasks and eventually succeed. Their social interactions reflect this life experience. Most people will sooner or later succumb to the pos-

itive smiling approach without assessing the underlying communication offered by the child. These children are difficult for parents to discipline and structure during their early years. Early treatment with concomitant guidance for young parents does ameliorate some of the problems by making more appropriate the developmental expectations for the child.

Intelligent children with low tone demand that the world be brought to them. Mentally limited children may fail to receive sufficient stimulation for optimal development. Whatever the learning potential of the child with cerebral palsy, it is not always evident early. Parents find it difficult to know how to guide a child when they are not certain that an assigned task is understood.

Parental guidance of the disabled child is also influenced by the adults' adaptation to their offspring's problem. They need to have resolved in their own way the emotional impact of the child's disability. Most parents feel inadequate, ignorant, and relatively helpless at being unable to remedy the situation for their child. They need help in feeling good about themselves before they can effectively guide the child toward acceptance of himself or herself as an adequate human being.

The therapist plays an important role in the psychosocial development of children who receive regular treatment. The child may perceive the therapist as a confidant, disciplinarian, counselor, or friend at various stages of development. Some children accept the therapist as a member of their extended family. This is natural considering the extent to which therapists influence clients' own self-awareness through changes in their physical bodies. However, it also places a personal responsibility on the therapist to be cognizant of the ongoing interaction and its effect on the maturational process.

Any evaluation of personality characteristics in a disabled child must take into account the unnatural life-style that is superimposed by the need for therapy, medical appointments, and hospitalization, for example. The child is expected to separate from parents earlier than the average child and usually confronts many more novel situations. There is little time or physical opportunity for free play. Continuous demands are placed on children to prove their intellectual potential in evaluations of various types. Their social interaction is most often monitored by adults, while they assume a dependent role. Nonetheless, these children's social acceptance frequently rests on their skill in interacting with persons in their environments. It is not easy to evaluate the evolution of personality without consideration of these experiential factors.

MEDICAL INFLUENCES ON TREATMENT

Because the problems of cerebral palsy are so varied, the condition lends itself to diverse interventions, some of which have a longer life than others. The cerebellar implant so popular in the late 1970s offered the possibility of regulating tone by supplementing cerebellar inhibition.[15,16,54] As time goes on the procedure is used less often and patients have difficulty getting repairs or replacement parts for the implant. The procedure that largely replaced the cerebellar implant was the placement of four electrodes in the cervical area to offer more control over postural tone.[30] These had the advantage of being adjustable so that the individual or a family member could make daily choices as to the optimal tone distribution. In some cases early success gave way to disappointment as the system adapted to the inputs.[30] Therapy was always recommended after the procedure, although the nature of the program was left to the family to decide.

In 1908 a rhizotomy procedure was developed by Dr. Otfrid Foerster and some success was reported.[35] It remained for Dr. Peacock to apply the procedure more selectively and functionally and to bring it to the United States from South Africa.[41] Based on his experience, he insisted on daily Neurodevelopmental (Bobath) Treatment for at least 1 year after the surgical intervention. Because it is necessary to use an electrophysiological system to determine which nerves are creating the spasticity in the lower extremities and the child needs to cooperate later in treatment, the procedure works best with intelligent children. There is a need to have some trunk function and fairly normal underlying tone.[13,30] The child must also adapt psychologically to the temporary loss of physical control, since the previous ability to walk or move about may be impaired for some months as new patterns of movement are learned. The long-term gains can be impressive,[19] although experienced therapists state the need for 1 to 3 years of treatment after surgery because of the child's completely new tone distribution. The foundation for success is accurate selection of the child, an experienced surgeon, and accurate analysis of therapy goals.

RECORD KEEPING AND CLINICAL RESEARCH

Data collection is an important task in the treatment of cerebral palsy. Change occurs at variable rates, but it is important to document the cause and effect of change whenever possible. Slides, super 8 film, or videotapes are useful in recording functional comparisons over time. Film lends itself to a formal frame-by-frame analysis. A motor drive unit or "automatic advance" on a 35 mm single lens reflex (SLR) camera also records a sample of movement five or more times per second. By placing the subject against a spaced grid in the same alignment to perform the same movement task, efficiency of movement can be measured. These ideas may be applied to documentation of treatment effectiveness or elaborated for a statement regarding similar movement problems.

Matching of groups is an approach doomed to failure or at least to considerable inaccuracy in cerebral palsy because of a wide range of individuality. It is analogous to making a statement regarding the mean in a widely vari-

able population. This does not mean that methods of intervention or treatment are not measurable nor that research is inapplicable to the problems of cerebral palsy. Once a specific question has been formulated, systematic recordings of appropriate data can be gathered over a period of time to accumulate the number needed for a viable study.

The way in which therapists are taught to view a problem determines, to a large extent, the potential range of solutions available to them. Cerebral palsy is a complex of inabilities that cluster about the inadequacy of CNS control. For the purpose of productive study, therapists may look critically at qualities of movement, postural adjustments, timing of movements, or changes in range of functional movement. Therapists are improving a disorder of posture and movement through their treatment. Analysis of the postural components and movement characteristics will help them toward meaningful research more quickly than reliance on the traditional definitions of the condition.

REFERENCES

1. Arbuckle BE: The selected writings of Beryl E Arbuckle, Newark, Ohio, 1947, American Academy of Osteopathy.
2. Arnold GG: Problems of the cerebral palsy child and his family, Va Med Monthly 103:225-227, March 1976.
3. Bach-y-Rita P, editor: Recovery of function: theoretical considerations for brain injury rehabilitation, Berne, Switzerland, 1980, Hans Huber, Publishers.
4. Bertoti DB: Effect of short leg casting on ambulation in children with cerebral palsy, Phys Ther 66(10):1522-1529, 1986.
5. Bleck E: Orthopedic management in cerebral palsy, Philadelphia, 1987, JB Lippincott Co.
6. Bobath B: The very early treatment of cerebral palsy, Dev Med Child Neurol 9(4):373-390, 1967.
7. Bobath B: Abnormal postural reflex activity caused by brain lesions, London, 1975, William Heinemann Medical Books, Ltd.
8. Bobath B: Motor development in the different types of cerebral palsy, New York, 1975, William Heinemann.
9. Bobath K: A neurophysiological basis for the treatment of cerebral palsy, ed 2 of CDM 23, Clinics in Developmental Medicine, no 75, London, 1980, William Heinemann Medical Books, Ltd.
10. Brazelton TB: Infants and mothers: differences in development, New York, 1969, Dell Publishing Co, Inc.
11. Brazelton TB: Neonatal behavioral assessment scale. In Clinics in Developmental Medicine, no 50, London, 1973, William Heinemann Medical Books, Ltd.
12. Brereton B and others: Cerebral palsy: basic abilities, Mosman, NSW, Australia, 1975, The Spastic Centre of New South Wales.
13. Cahan LD and others: Electrophysiologic studies in selective dorsal rhizotomy for spasticity in children with cerebral palsy, Appl Neurophysiol 50(1-6):459-462, 1987.
14. Conner F and others: Program guide for infants and toddlers with neuromotor and other developmental disabilities, New York, 1978, Teacher's College Press.
15. Cooper IS and others: Correlation of clinical and physiological effects of cerebellar stimulation, Acta Neurochir (suppl)(Wien), 30:339-344, 1980.
16. Davis R and others: Cerebellar stimulation for spastic cerebral palsy: double-blind quantitative study, Appl Neurophysiol 50(1-6):451-452, 1987.
17. Davis R and others: Cerebellar stimulation for cerebral palsy, J Fla Med Assoc 63:910-912, Nov 1976.
18. Denhoff E and others: Treatment of spastic cerebral palsied children

with sodium dantrolene, Dev Med Child Neurol 17(6):736-742, Dec 1975.

19. Fasano VA and others: Long-term results of posterior functional rhizotomy, Acta Neurochir (suppl)(Wien), 30:435-439, 1980.
20. Finnie NR: Handling the young cerebral-palsied child at home, New York, 1975, EP Dutton, Inc.
21. Fiorentino MR: A basis for sensorimotor development: normal and abnormal, Springfield, Ill, 1981, Charles C Thomas, Publisher.
22. Frymann V: Relation of disturbances of craniosacral mechanisms to symptomatology of the newborn: study of 1,250 infants, J Amer Osteo Assoc 65:1059-1075, June 1966.
23. Furth H and Wachs H: Learning goes to school, New York, 1974, Oxford University Press, Inc.
24. Gilfoyle EM and others: Children adapt, Thorofare, NJ, 1981, Slack, Inc.
25. Haberfellner H and Müller G: Sequelae of head and neck positions on auditory performance, Neuropädiatrie 7(4):373-378, 1976.
26. Hagberg BA: Epidemiology of cerebral palsy: aspects on perinatal prevention in Sweden, Neonatal Neurological Assessment and Outcome Report of the 77th Ross Conference on Pediatric Research, 1980.
27. Held R: Plasticity in sensory-motor systems, Sci Am pp 71-80, Nov 1965.
28. Hellebrandt FA and others: Methods of evoking the tonic neck reflexes in normal human subjects, Am J Phys Med 41(90):263-269, 1962.
29. Hochleitner M: Control study of children with cerebral palsy with and without early neurophysiological treatment, Austrian Med J 32(18):1091-1097, 1977.
30. Hugenholtz H and others: Cervical spinal cord stimulation for spasticity in cerebral palsy, Neurosurgery 22(4):707-714, Apr 1988.
31. Illingworth RS: The development of the infant and young childi ab normal and normal, ed 7, Edinburgh, 1980, Churchill Livingstone.
32. Keshner EA: Re-evaluating the theoretical model underlying the neurodevelopmental theory, Phys Ther 61(7):1033-1040, July 1981.
33. Knoblock H and Pasamanick B, editors: Developmental diagnosis, Hagerstown, Md, 1974, Harper & Row, Publishers, Inc.
34. Köng E: Very early treatment of cerebral palsy, Dev Med Child Neurol 8:68-75, 1966.
35. Laitinen LV and others: Selective posterior rhizotomy for treatment of spasticity, J Neurosurg 58:895-899, June 1983.
36. Leach P: Babyhood, New York, 1977, Alfred A Knopf, Inc.
37. MacKeith RC and others: The Little Club memorandum on terminology and classification of cerebral palsy, Cerebral Palsy Bulletin 1(27):34-37, 1959.
38. Milani-Comparetti A: Neurophysiologic and clinical implications of studies on fetal motor behavior, Semin Perinatol 5(2):183-189, April 1981.
39. Niswander KR: The obstetrician, fetal asphyxia, and cerebral palsy, Am J Obstet and Gynecol 133(4):358-361, Feb 1979.
40. Palmer FB and others: The effects of physical therapy on cerebral palsy: a controlled trial in infants with spastic diplegia, N Engl J Med 318(13):803-808, 1988.
41. Peacock WJ and Arens LJ: Selective posterior rhizotomy for the relief of spasticity in cerebral palsy, S Afr Med J 62:119-125, July 1982.
42. Pearlstone A and Benjamin R: Ocular defects in cerebral palsy, Eye, Ear, Nose, Throat Monthly 48:87-89, July 1969.
43. Pettitt B: Surgery of the lower extremity in cerebral palsy: considerations and approaches, Arch Phys Med Rehabil 57:443-447, Sept 1976.
44. Prechtl H: The neurological examination of the full-term newborn infant, Philadelphia, 1977, JB Lippincott Co.
45. Restak RM: The brain: the last frontier, New York, 1979, Doubleday & Co, Inc.
46. Rosenthal R and others: Levodopa therapy in athetoid cerebral palsy, Neurology 22(1):21-24, Jan 1972.
47. Rosenzweig M and others: Brain changes in response to experience, Sci Am, Feb 1972.
48. Soboloff HR: Trends in cerebral palsy treatment, Tex Med 66(12)82-91, Dec 1970.
49. Sussman M and Cusick B: Preliminary report: the role of short-leg tone-reducing casts as an adjunct to physical therapy of patients with cerebral palsy, Johns Hopkins Med J 145(3):112-114, Sept 1979.
50. Tardieu G and Tardieu C: Cerebral palsy: mechanical evaluation and conservative correction of limb joint contractures, Clin Orthop 219:63-69, 1987.
51. Upledger JE and Vredevoogd JD: Craniosacral therapy, Seattle, 1983, Eastland Press.
52. Vining E and others: Cerebral palsy: a pediatric developmentalist's overview, Am J Dis Child, 130:643-649, 1976.
53. Watt J and others: A prospective study of inhibitive casting as an adjunct to physiotherapy for cerebral-palsied children, Dev Med Child Neurol 28(4):480-488, 1986.
54. Whittaker CK: Cerebellar stimulation for cerebral palsy, J Neurosurg 52(5):648-653, May 1980.
55. Wright BA: Physical disability—a psychological approach, New York, 1960, Harper & Row, Publishers, Inc.

ADDITIONAL READINGS

Ames LB and others: The Gesell Institute's child from one to six: evaluating the behavior of the preschool child, New York, 1979, Harper & Row, Publishers, Inc.

Aptekar R and others: Light patterns as means of assessing and recording gait. II. Results in children with cerebral palsy, Dev Med Child Neurol 18(1):37-40, Feb 1976.

Bach-y-Rita P: Brain mechanisms in sensory substitution, New York, 1972, Academic Press, Inc.

Beintema DJ: A neurological study of newborn infants. In Clinics in Developmental Medicine, no 28, London, 1968 William Heinemann Medical Books, Ltd.

Black R: Visual disorders associated with cerebral palsy, Br J Opthalmol 66(1):46-52, 1982.

Boehme R: Improving upper body control: an approach to assessment and treatment of tonal dysfunction, Tucson, Arizona, 1988, Therapy Skill Builders.

Bower TGR: The visual world of infants, Sci Am 251(6):349-357, 1966.

Bower TGR: A primer of infant development, San Francisco, 1977, WH Freeman & Co, Publishers.

Briggs DC: Your child's self-esteem, ed 2, Garden City, NJ, 1975, Dolphin Books.

Buscaglia L: The disabled and their parents: a counseling challenge, Thorofare, NJ, 1975, Slack, Inc.

Eccles JC: The understanding of the brain, ed 2, New York, 1977, McGraw-Hill Book Co.

Featherstone H: A difference in the family: life with a disabled child, New York, 1980, Basic Books, Inc, Publishers.

Feldenkrais M: Awareness through movement, New York, 1977, Harper & Row, Inc, Publishers.

Ford E and Englund S: For the love of children, Garden City, NY, 1977, Anchor Press.

Gahm NH and others: Chronic cerebellar stimulation for cerebral palsy: a double-blind study, Neurology (NY) 31(1):87-90, 1981.

Goffman E: Stigma: notes on the management of spoiled identity, Englewood Cliffs, NJ, 1963, Prentice-Hall, Inc.

Graham M and others: Prediction of cerebral palsy in very low birthweight infants: prospective ultrasound study, Lancet 2(8559):593-595, 1987.

Haeusserman E: Developmental potential of preschool children, New York, 1958, Grune & Stratton, Inc.

Hannon C: Parents and mentally handicapped children, London, 1975, Penguin Books, Ltd.

Harrell R and others: Can nutritional supplements help mentally retarded children? An exploratory study, Proc Natl Acad Sci USA, 78(1):574-578, 1981.

Holt KS: Developmental paediatrics, postgraduate paediatrics series, London, 1978, Butterworth & Co.

Hulme JB and others: Effects of adaptive seating devices on the eating and drinking of children with multiple handicaps, Am J Occup Ther 41(2):81-89, 1987.

Jones FP: Body awareness in action: the Alexander technique, New York, 1976, Schocken Books, Inc.

Kane P: Food makes the difference: a parent's guide to raising a healthy child, New York, 1985, Simon and Schuster.

Katayama M and Tamas LB: Saccadic eye-movements of children with cerebral palsy, Dev Med Child Neurol 29(1):36-39, 1987.

Katz K and others: Seat insert for cerebral-palsied children with total body involvement, Dev Med and Child Neurol 30(2):222-226, 1988.

Kock J: Total baby development, New York, 1976, Wyden Books.

Leboyer F: Loving hands: the traditional Indian art of baby massage, New York, 1976, Alfred A Knopf, Inc.

Menken C and others: Evaluating the visual-perceptual skills of children with cerebral palsy, Am J Occup Ther 41(10):646-651, 1987.

Montagu A: Touching, the human significance of the skin, ed 2, New York, 1978, Harper & Row, Publishers, Inc.

Nelson KB and others: Children who "outgrew" cerebral palsy, Pediatrics 69(5):529-536, 1982.

Nwaobi OM: Seating orientations and upper extremity function in children with cerebral palsy, Phys Ther 67(8):1209-1212, 1987.

Ornstein R and Sobel D: The healing brain, New York, 1987, Simon and Schuster.

Pearson P and Ethun-Williams C: Physical therapy services in the developmental disabilities, Springfield, Ill, 1972, Charles C Thomas, Publisher.

Penn RD: Chronic cerebellar stimulation—a review, Neurosurgery 10(1):116-121, 1982.

Prechtl Heinz FR: Continuity of neural functions from prenatal to postnatal life, Philadelphia, 1984, JB Lippincott Co.

Restak R: The brain, New York, 1984, Bantam Books.

Rolf IP: Rolfing: the integration of human structures, New York, 1978, Harper & Row, Publishers, Inc.

Rose S: The conscious brain, updated edition, New York, 1976, Vintage Books.

Samples B: Open mind whole mind: parenting and teaching tomorrow's children today, Rolling Hills Estates, California, 1987, Jalmar Press.

Scherzer A and Tscharnuter I: Early diagnosis and therapy in cerebral palsy, New York, 1982, Marcel Dekker, Inc.

Scherzer AL and others: Physical therapy as a determinant of change in the cerebral palsied infant, Pediatrics 58:47-52, 1976.

Stockmeyer SA: An interpretation of the approach of Rood to the treatment of neuromuscular dysfunction, Am J Phys Med 46, 1977.

Stone LJ and others: The competent infant, research and commentary, New York, 1973, Basic Books, Inc, Publishers.

Sweeney JK: The high-risk neonate: developmental therapy perspectives, New York, 1986, The Haworth Press.

Szasz S: The body language of children, New York, 1978, WW Norton & Co, Inc.

Tjossen TD, editor: Intervention strategies for high-risk infants and children, Baltimore, 1976, University Park Press.

Touwen B: Neurological development in infancy. In Clinics in Developmental Medicine, no 58, London, 1976, William Heinemann Medical Books, Ltd.

Verny T and Kelly J: Secret life of the unborn child, New York, 1981, Delta Books.

Willemson E: Understanding infancy, San Francisco, 1979, WH Freeman & Co, Publishers.

Witkin K: To move, to learn, New York, 1977, Schocken Books, Inc.

Chapter 10

GENETIC DISORDERS

Susan R. Harris and Wendy L. Tada

Genetic disorders in children frequently include severe neurological impairment as part of the symptom complex. This chapter discusses various types of disorders of known genetic origin that may be represented in a developmental therapist's case load. Minor, isolated anomalies of known genetic origin will be addressed only briefly. In the section on identification of the problem, the definition and discussion of the categories of genetic disorders are presented, followed by specific examples of each type. Examples have been chosen that are most representative of those disorders or syndromes that are found among patients in a developmental therapy setting. Included in the discussion of each of these examples is a description of the typical clinical characteristics and symptoms, the incidence or prevalence of each, and the underlying neuropathology. A summary of typical clinical signs for genetic disorders in general concludes the section.

The section on chromosomal abnormalities addresses the developmental therapist's role in the clinical manage-ment of children with genetic disorders. Evaluation procedures, areas of concern in the habilitation of deficits, and treatment strategies are discussed. The medical management and psychosocial aspect of genetic disorders, including genetic counseling, are also presented.

AN OVERVIEW: TYPES OF GENETIC DISORDERS WITH REPRESENTATIVE CLINICAL EXAMPLES

Genetic disorders may be divided into two major categories: chromosomal abnormalities and specific gene defects. Chromosomal abnormalities can be further subdivided into autosomal trisomies, sex chromosome abnormalities, and partial deletion syndromes.[87] Specific gene defects may be transmitted through three different modes of inheritance: autosomal dominant, autosomal recessive, and sex-linked. Fig. 10-1 shows the categories and subcategories of genetic disorders with clinical examples of each.

Chromosomal abnormalities

According to Smith,[87] the defect that produces a chromosomal abnormality is usually one of quantity rather than quality of genetic material. Most chromosomal abnormalities appear as an extra chromosome or as a missing chromosome, the latter being even more lethal than the former. The incidence of chromosomal abnormalities among spontaneously aborted fetuses may be as high as 50% to 60%.[11] Of the chromosomally abnormal fetuses that survive to term, about half represent sex chromosomal abnormalities and the other half represent autosomal trisomies.[87]

The autosomal trisomies (trisomies 13, 18, and 21) are discussed first because these chromosomal abnormalities are more apt to include serious neuromotor problems than

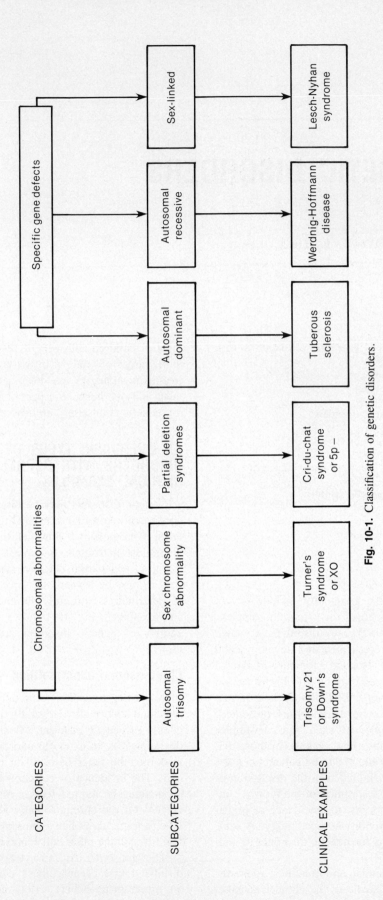

Fig. 10-1. Classification of genetic disorders.

are the sex chromosome abnormalities. Finally, two deletion syndromes (4p− and 5p−) will be briefly described.

Autosomal trisomies

Trisomy 21. Down's syndrome represents the most common chromosomal cause of moderate to severe mental retardation.[81] The presence of an extra twenty-first chromosome (trisomy 21) accounts for 91% of all cases of Down's syndrome. The exact cause of the presence of the additional chromosome is unknown.[20] Remaining cases include mosaic and translocation forms of Down's syndrome (Fig. 10-2).

First described clinically as "mongolism" in 1866 by Dr. Langdon Down, the cause of Down's syndrome as the presence of an extra chromosome in the G group was discovered by Lejeune in 1959. Down's syndrome occurs in one out of every 660 live births overall with the incidence increasing with advanced maternal age.[81] A list of 10 features characterizing newborns with Down's syndrome was published by Hall in 1966.[37] These features include hypotonicity, poor Moro reflex, joint hyperextensibility, excess skin on the back of the neck, flat facial profile, slanted palpebral fissures, anomalous auricles, dysplasia of the pelvis, dysplasia of the midphalanx of the fifth finger, and simian creases. In his study of 48 newborns with Down's syndrome, Hall found the frequency of these characteristics to vary from 45% to 90%.[37]

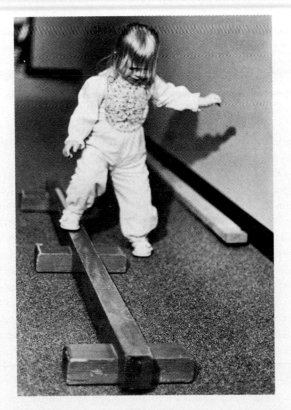

Fig. 10-2. Three-year-old child with Down's syndrome attempting to walk on balance beam.

Skeletal anomalies prevalent in Down's syndrome include short metacarpals and phalanges in the hands, pelvic hypoplasia with outward flaring of iliac crests,[88] and a tendency toward atlantoaxial dislocation.[96] It is particularly important that developmental therapists who work with Down's syndrome infants and children are aware of this propensity for atlantoaxial dislocation, which has been shown through radiogram in up to 20% of a sample studied.[96] Although dislocation is relatively rare, cases have been reported where quadriplegia has occurred.[96]

Other clinical features that have been described include brachycephaly, small stature, epicanthal folds, speckled iris (Brushfield's spots), convergent strabismus, and nystagmus.[35] Frequently associated impairments include hearing loss[14] and congenital cardiac anomalies, which are present in 40% of individuals with Down's syndrome.[30] Down's syndrome is equally distributed between the sexes.[94]

The neuropathology associated with Down's syndrome has been explored by a number of researchers in addition to Crome, Cowie, and Slater.[28] The relatively small size of the cerebellum and brainstem has been widely reported.[5,27,62,78,83] Whereas the overall brain weight of Down's syndrome individuals averages 76% of the brain weight of normal individuals, the combined brainstem and cerebellum weight averages only 66% of normal.[26]

The reduction in size of the cerebral hemispheres is especially apparent at the frontal poles, causing Cowie[24] to speculate that this particular aspect of the neuropathology may have some bearing on the clinical persistence of the palmar grasp reflex since a lesion in the frontal lobe of an adult may result in a forced grasp.

Other gross neuropathological findings include the more rounded shape of Down's syndrome brains, which may be secondary to the brachycephaly associated with this syndrome.[78] The brains of Down's syndrome infants show smaller convolutions than those of normal infants of comparable age, indicating their relative neurological immaturity.[5]

In addition to these gross neurological differences, there are a number of cytological distinctions that characterize the brains of Down's syndrome individuals. Marin-Padilla[64] studied the neuronal organization of the motor cortex of a 19-month-old Down's syndrome child and found various structural abnormalities in the dendritic spines of the pyramidal neurons of the motor cortex. He suggested that these structural differences may underlie the motor incoordination and mental retardation characteristic of Down's syndrome. Loesch-Mdzewska,[62] in his neuropathological study of 123 Down's syndrome individuals aged 3 to 62, also frequently found neurological abnormalities of the pyramidal system in addition to the reduced brain weight noted by other researchers cited previously.

Benda[5] noted a lack of myelinization of the nerve fibers in the precentral areas, frontal lobes, and cerebellum of

Down's syndrome infants, indicating a lack of CNS maturity. As McGraw[67] has pointed out, the amount of myelin in the brain reflects the stage of developmental maturation. The delayed myelinization characteristic of Down's syndrome newborns and infants is thought to be a contributing factor to the generalized hypotonicity apparent during this time,[5] as well as to the persistence of primitive reflexes characteristic of this group.[23]

In her longitudinal study of 79 Down's syndrome infants from birth to 10 months of age, Cowie[24] administered comprehensive neurological examinations during the neonatal period at 6 weeks, at 6 months, and at 10 months of age. In addition to the universal finding of marked hypotonicity (which appeared to gradually diminish with age), Cowie also noted a persistence of several primitive reflexes past the time when they should normally disappear. These reflexes included the palmar and plantar grasp reflexes, the stepping reflex, and the Moro reflex. The third major neurological finding was a delay in the development of normal postural tone as indicated by the severe head lag evident during elicitation of the traction response and the lack of full antigravity extension noted when the Landau response was tested. Cowie speculates that the possible neurological causes for these clinical findings are delayed cerebellar maturation, the relatively small size of the cerebellum and brainstem, and the maturational delay of cortical pathways from the motor cortex.[28]

Trisomy 18. Trisomy 18 is the second most common of the trisomic syndromes to occur in term deliveries, although far less prevalent than Down's syndrome. The incidence has been reported as 1:4500 live births.[22] Known also as Edwards' syndrome, trisomy 18 generally produces far more serious organic malformations than does Down's syndrome.[94] Included among the typical malformations observed in individuals with trisomy 18 are cardiovascular, gastrointestinal, urogenital, and skeletal malformations. At birth, these infants are characterized by low birth-weight and small stature, long narrow skull, low-set ears, flexion deformities of the fingers, hypotonicity, and rocker-bottom feet[94] (Fig. 10-3).

Advanced maternal age is also positively correlated with trisomy 18 as it is with Down's syndrome. The mean maternal age for women giving birth to infants with trisomy 18 is 32.[35] Only 10% of infants born with trisomy 18 survive past the first year of life with the survival rate of females averaging 7 months compared with that of males with a mean survival of 2 months. Initially characterized by limpness or hypotonicity, these infants soon progress to hypertonicity.[94] Based on our experience in providing developmental therapy to two sisters with trisomy 18, the period of hypertonicity in the early years once again gave way to low tone and joint hyperextensibility by preschool and school age. Common skeletal malformations, which may warrant management by the developmental therapist, include scoliosis,[34] limited hip abduc-

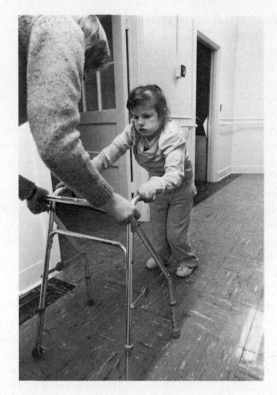

Fig. 10-3. Fourteen-year-old girl with trisomy 18 during assisted ambulation.

tion, flexion contractures of the fingers, rocker-bottom feet, and talipes equinovarus.[94] Profound mental retardation is another clinical factor that affects the delivery of therapy services for the child with trisomy 18.

Grossly abnormal neuropathological findings include microcephaly, abnormal gyri, cerebellar anomalies, myelomeningoceles, hydrocephaly, and corpus callosum defects.[94] Cytological abnormalities such as heterotopic ganglion cells and abnormal stratification of the cerebellum have also been noted.[94]

Trisomy 13. Described in 1960 by Patau,[76] trisomy 13 is the least common of the three major autosomal trisomies with an incidence of 1:14,500 live births.[21] Characterized by microcephaly, anopthalmia or micropthalmia, cleft lip and palate, and polydactyly of the hands and feet,[94] infants born with trisomy 13 are obviously severely impaired. Less than 5% of individuals with this syndrome survive past the third year of life.[35] As in trisomy 18, infants with trisomy 13 frequently have serious cardiovascular and urogenital malformations.[94] Reported CNS malformations include arrhinencephalies, cerebellar anomalies, defects of the corpus callosum, and hydrocephaly.[93] As in the other trisomic syndromes, advanced maternal age is correlated with an increasing incidence of trisomy 13.[21]

Skeletal deformities and anomalies include flexion contractures of the fingers, as in trisomy 18, and polydactyly of hands and feet.[94] Rocker-bottom feet have also been reported, although less frequently than in trisomy 18. The severe to profound mental retardation that characterizes individuals with this syndrome also has implications for choosing the appropriate developmental therapy approach.

Sex chromosome abnormalities

Turner's syndrome. The two most prevalent sex chromosome anomalies are Turner's syndrome and Klinefelter's syndrome. Known also as gonadal dysgenesis or XO syndrome, Turner's syndrome has been shown to be the most common chromosomal anomaly present among spontaneous abortions.[18] First described in 1938 by Turner,[92] who noted three primary characteristics of sexual infantilism, congenital webbed neck, and cubitus valgus, Turner's syndrome has an incidence of 1:2500 female births.[69] Other clinical characteristics noted at birth include dorsal edema of hands and feet, hypertelorism, epicanthal folds, ptosis of the upper eyelids, and elongated ears.[94] Growth retardation is particularly noticeable after the age of 5 or 6, and sexual infantilism, characterized by primary amenorrhea, lack of breast development, and scanty pubic and axillary hair, is apparent during the pubertal years.[94] Ovarian development is severely deficient as is estrogen production.[94]

Congenital heart disease is present in 25% to 40% of individuals with Turner's syndrome.[80] Two-thirds of Turner individuals have kidney malformations.[94] There are numerous incidences of skeletal anomalies, some of which may be significant enough to require the attention of a pediatric therapist. Included among these latter deformities are hip dislocation, pes planus and pes equinovarus,[91] deformity of medial tibial condyles,[35] and osteoporosis.[46] Idiopathic scoliosis is common.[34,60]

Sensory impairments include moderate hearing losses, decrease in gustatory and olfactory sensitivity,[94] and deficits in spatial perception and orientation.[70] Although the average intellect of individuals with Turner's syndrome is within normal limits, the incidence of mental retardation is more frequent than in the general population.[94] Unlike the autosomal trisomy syndromes, there is no correlation between an increase in births of Turner infants with advanced maternal age.

Klinefelter syndrome. Eighty percent of males with Klinefelter's syndrome possess a karyotype of XXY, 10% are mosaic, and the remaining 10% include karyotypes of XXXY, XXYY, and XXXXY.[35] Described in 1942 by Klinefelter and others,[53] the most common type of Klinefelter's syndrome, XXY, is usually not clinically apparent until puberty, when the testes fail to enlarge and gynecomastia occurs.[35] The incidence of XXY is 1.3:1000; the incidence of all types of Klinefelter's syndrome is about 2:1000.[35]

Most XXY individuals have normal intelligence with a somewhat passive personality. Libido is reduced and nearly all nonmosaic individuals are sterile. Advanced maternal age is positively correlated with an increase in births

of XXY males.[35] Klinefelter XXY has been found to occur in combination with Down's syndrome.[33]

The most severe karyotypes (XXXY and XXXXY) tend to display a more severe clinical picture. Individuals with XXXY usually have severe mental retardation and multiple congenital anomalies, including cases of microcephaly, hypertelorism, strabismus, and cleft palate.[94] Skeletal anomalies include radioulnar synostosis, genu valgum, malformed cervical vertebrae, and pes planus.[35] Parental age does not appear to be a factor in the incidence of the more severe types of Klinefelter's syndrome.[35]

Partial deletion syndromes. Two types of partial deletion syndromes that result in severe handicaps are the Wolf-Hirschhorn (4p−) syndrome and the cri-du-chat (5p−) syndrome. The 4p− syndrome is less common than the 5p− syndrome and will be discussed first.

Wolf-Hirschhorn syndrome (4p−). Described separately by Wolf and others[97] and Hirschhorn and others[45] in 1965, this syndrome appears karyotypically as a partial deletion of the short arm of chromosome 4.[35] As of 1976, 45 cases of 4p− had been described.[51]

Characterized clinically by severe psychomotor and growth retardation, hypotonicity, seizures, and microcephaly, one-third of these infants die within the first 2 years of life.[35] Other congenital anomalies include ocular hypertelorism, cleft lip or palate, and heart malformations. Skeletal deformities such as dislocated hips, club feet, and proximal radioulnar synostosis may also be present.[35]

Cri-du-chat syndrome (5p−). As of 1977, approximately 150 cases of cri-du-chat or cat-cry syndrome had been identified.[35] First described in 1963 by Lejeune and others,[58] cri-du-chat syndrome results from a partial deletion of the short arm of chromosome 5. This syndrome accounts for about 1% of the institutionalized population with IQs of less than 35.[35] Primary identifying characteristics at birth include the definitive high-pitched catlike cry, microcephaly, and evidence of intrauterine growth retardation.[94] Other signs include hypertelorism, strabismus, "moon face," and low-set ears.[94] Severe mental retardation and muscular hypotonicity are associated with this syndrome, although cases with hypertonicity have also been noted.[84] Associated musculoskeletal deformities include scoliosis, hip dislocations, clubfeet, and hyperextensibility of fingers and toes.[84]

The appearance of this disorder is not correlated with advanced parental age. Although approximately 70% of those cri-du-chat cases identified at birth are female, there is an unexplained higher prevalence of older cri-du-chat individuals who are male.[13]

Specific gene defects

Other genetic disorders commonly encountered among the developmentally disabled population include those that occur as a result of specific gene defects. Over 300 congenital malformations arising from specific gene defects have been identified.[66] There are three types of specific gene defects: autosomal dominant, autosomal recessive, and sex-linked. Each of these types of inheritance are discussed separately. Several examples of syndromes or disorders associated with each type are presented. Examples selected include those that most commonly appear among the developmentally disabled population and those that are of specific neurological importance to pediatric therapists.

Autosomal dominant disorders. McCusick has identified more than 150 disorders of autosomal dominant inheritance. Many of these are specific, isolated anomalies that may occur in otherwise normal individuals,[94] such as extra digits, short fingers, and lobster claw deformity. Other autosomal dominant disorders include syndromes that are characterized by profound neurological handicaps. Autosomal dominant disorders arise when one parent is affected with the disorder, although spontaneous cases with no family history have also been reported.[94] Each child of a parent with an autosomal dominant trait faces a 50:50 risk of inheriting that trait.

Three examples of autosomal dominant disorders are presented: osteogenesis imperfecta, tuberous sclerosis, and neurofibromatosis. Individuals with these disorders may require intervention from a developmental therapist because of musculoskeletal deformities commonly associated with each.

Osteogenesis imperfecta. The complete syndrome of osteogenesis imperfecta includes brittle bones, blue sclerae, and deafness,[94] although a number of individuals may possess only one or two symptoms of the triad. Characterized by an extreme tendency for fractures, osteogenesis imperfecta may lead to severe physical disability with shortening and deformity of the extremities and deformity of the rib cage, which predisposes these individuals to life-threatening respiratory infections.[94] In severe cases infants may sustain multiple fractures in utero.

Frequency of appearance of this disorder is 1:25,000.[22] Autosomal dominant inheritance has been demonstrated in two-thirds of the cases of osteogenesis imperfecta, but the remaining cases show no family history of the disorder.[44] There is wide individual variability in the number and severity of symptoms.[88] Commonly appearing skeletal deformities include pectus carinatum or excavatum, bowed tibiae, small facial bones, and kyphoscoliosis.[88] Hypotonicity,[2] poor muscle development, and joint hyperextensibility[88] also occur (Fig. 10-4). Severely involved individuals have extremely small stature and short limbs[88] and are usually wheelchair dependent. The long bones of the lower extremities are most susceptible to fractures, particularly between the ages of 2 to 3 years and 10 to 15 years.[88] Deafness, secondary to otosclerosis, does not appear until adulthood, with 35% of individuals showing hearing loss by the third decade of life.[88] Those individuals who survive childhood have a good life expectancy.[82]

Intramedullary rods inserted in the tibia or femur may

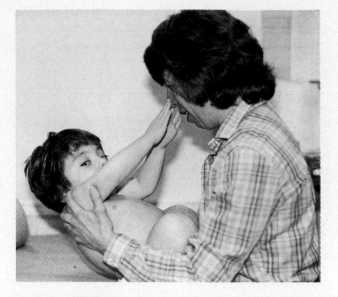

Fig. 10-4. Child with osteogenesis imperfecta during physical therapy session.

minimize recurrent fractures.[82] Prevention of fractures through careful handling and positioning is the most important goal in working with individuals with osteogenesis imperfecta.[94] We have found the use of pool therapy to be a valuable treatment strategy for a child with osteogenesis imperfecta.

Tuberous sclerosis. Characterized by a triad of symptoms of seizures, mental retardation, and sebaceous adenomas,[82] the most severe form of tuberous sclerosis accounts for 0.5% of the institutionalized retarded population.[88] Although inherited through autosomal dominance, 86% of cases occur as spontaneous mutations with older paternal age a contributing factor. The sexes are affected equally.[94] Infants are frequently normal in appearance at birth, but 70% of those who go on to show the complete triad of symptoms display seizures during the first year of life.[94] Ultimately, 93% of severely affected individuals develop seizures, usually of myoclonic type in early life and later progressing to grand mal.[88] Delayed development is noted during infancy,[25] particularly in the achievement of motor and speech milestones.

The first appearance of sebaceous adenomas occurs between the ages of 4 to 5 years with early individual brown, yellow, or red lesions of firm consistency in the areas of the nose and upper lips.[94] These isolated lesions may later coalesce to form a characteristic butterfly pattern on the cheeks.[94] Known also as hamartomas or tumorlike nodules of superfluous tissue, the skin lesions are present in 83% of cases of tuberous sclerosis.[88] There is wide variability in expression of the symptoms, with some individuals displaying skin lesions only.[88]

Seizure development is secondary to nodular lesions in the cerebral cortex and white matter.[88] Tumors are also

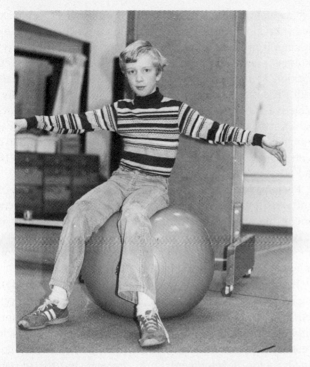

Fig. 10-5. Child with neurofibromatosis during therapy session.

found in the walls of the ventricles.[94] Neurocytological examination reveals a decreased number of neurons and an increased number of glial cells as well as enlarged nerve cells with abnormally shaped cell bodies.[94] Cyst formation in the long bones and in the bones of the fingers and toes contributes to osteoporosis.[94] Other associated anomalies include retinal tumors and hemorrhages, glaucoma, and corneal opacities.[82] Catatonic schizophrenia has also been found in individuals with tuberous sclerosis.[82]

With frequency of 1:30,000 births, tuberous sclerosis is a relatively rare developmental disability, but because of the retardation in motor development as well as associated rigidity or hemiplegia seen in some cases,[94] children with this disorder may require intervention from a pediatric therapist. Mental retardation occurs as well in 62% of cases.[88] Surgical excision of seizure-producing tumors has been successful in some cases.[82]

Neurofibromatosis. First described by von Recklinghausen in 1882, neurofibromatosis is characterized by flat, light brown skin patches known as café au lait spots as well as by neurofibromas or connective tissue tumors of the nerve fiber fasciculus.[94] Neurofibromas may be found in either the peripheral or central nervous system[89] and may lead to secondary disabilities such as optic and acoustic nerve damage,[94] paraplegia, quadriplegia,[82] or hemiparesis.[49] Neurofibromas may also develop in the kidneys, stomach, or heart[88] (Fig. 10-5).

Infants usually appear normal at birth, with the initial symptoms of café au lait spots first appearing in early

childhood.[88] Ultimately, 47% develop some type of neurological impairment.[88] A slowly progressive disease, the course of neurofibromatosis is characterized by an increase in number of tumors with increasing age.[94] Family history is apparent in 50% of cases, with fresh mutations apparently responsible for the remaining 50%.[88] The incidence of this disorder is relatively common, appearing in one out of every 2500 to 3200 births.[29] Ten percent of affected individuals are mentally retarded and 12% have seizure disorders.[88]

Skeletal lesions or impairments occur in up to 50% of individuals with neurofibromatosis,[50] with scoliosis representing the most common skeletal deformity.[94] Severe kyphoscoliotic deformities may lead to spinal cord compression or impaired cardiopulmonary function.[94] Other skeletal deformities include pseudoarthrosis of tibia and fibula,[94] tibial bowing, rib fusion, and dislocation of radius and ulna.[94] Differences in leg length have also been noted and may contribute to scoliosis.[94]

Autosomal recessive disorders. McCusick[66] has identified more than 150 congenital malformations that can be acquired through autosomal recessive inheritance. Certain types of limb defects, familial microcephaly, and a variety of syndromes such as Laurence-Moon-Biedl and Hurler's syndromes are passed on through autosomal recessive genes. When parents are unaffected carriers of the trait, they are heterozygous for the abnormal gene, and each of their offspring faces a 25% chance of demonstrating the defect.[94] When two homozygous, affected parents mate, there is a great risk that all children will be similarly affected with the disorder.[94] Consanguinity or marriage between close relatives increases the chance of passing on autosomal recessive traits.

Three examples of autosomal recessive disorders that may be of interest to developmental therapists are presented in this section: Hurler's syndrome, phenylketonuria, and Werdnig-Hoffmann disease.

Hurler's syndrome (gargoylism, mucopolysaccharidosis I). Hurler's syndrome was the first of the mucopolysaccharidoses to be identified.[82] An inborn error of metabolism, Hurler's syndrome involves abnormal storage of mucopolysaccharides in many different tissues of the body.[2] Infants born with Hurler's syndrome are usually normal in appearance at birth[82] and may be larger in birth weight than their normal siblings.[94] Symptoms of this progressively deteriorating disease usually appear during the latter half of the first year of life[87] with the full disease picture apparent by 2 to 3 years.[94] A preponderance of male cases of this disorder has been noted.[2]

Characteristic physical features include a large skull with frontal bossing, heavy eyebrows, edematous eyelids, corneal clouding, small upturned nose with flat nasal bridge, thick lips, low-set ears, hirsutism, and gargoyle-like facial features.[2] Progressive mental and physical deterioration lead to early death, usually before adulthood.[2]

Death is usually secondary to deposits of mucopolysaccharides in the cardiac valves, myocardium, or coronary arteries.[2] Growth retardation results in characteristic dwarfism.[2] Other frequently associated anomalies include deafness, hydrocephaly,[2] enlarged tongue,[88] hepatosplenomegaly, and delayed dentition with small, pointed teeth.[82]

Because of many associated neuromotor and orthopaedic problems, infants and children with Hurler's syndrome may benefit from developmental therapy services. Delayed motor milestones have been noted in later infancy and early childhood.[94] Spastic paraparesis or paraplegia[2] and ataxia[94] have also been observed. Orthopaedic deformities include flexion contractures of the extremities, thoracolumbar kyphosis, genu valgum, pes cavus,[2] hip dislocation, and claw hands secondary to joint deformity.[88]

Gross neuropathological findings include reduced brain size and weight.[94] Cytological findings reported are distended pyramidal cells, peripherally displaced nuclei, and a decrease in number of Nissl bodies.[94] Mucopolysaccharide deposits in neurons have also been noted.[2] Although most cases of Hurler's syndrome are acquired through autosomal recessive inheritance, there are also some cases of males with Hurler's syndrome who have acquired the disorder through sex-linked inheritance modes; these cases are usually less severe.[94] Some individuals with the physical characteristics of Hurler's syndrome are of normal intelligence, but the vast majority are mentally retarded.[94]

We have had experience in providing developmental therapy to a 10-year-old boy with Hurler's syndrome who was profoundly retarded and had accompanying spastic paraplegia and severe plantar flexion deformities of the ankles. Because of the ankle deformities, this child was basically a "knee-walker" but occasionally ambulated short distances with weight borne on the dorsum of his feet.

Phenylketonuria. Phenylketonuria (PKU) represents one of the more common inborn errors of metabolism.[85] Absence of phenylalanine hydroxylase prevents the conversion of phenlalanine to tyrosine, which results in an abnormally excessive accumulation of phenylalanine in the blood and other body fluids.[85] If untreated, this metabolic error leads to the pathological characteristics associated with this disorder, which include mental and growth retardation, seizures, and pigment deficiency of hair and skin.[85] Children born with PKU are usually normal in appearance, with delayed development becoming apparent toward the end of the first year.[85] Parents usually become concerned with their child's slow development when the child reaches preschool age.[85]

A simple blood plasma analysis, which is mandatory for newborns in many states in the United States, can detect the presence of elevated phenylalanine levels. This test is ideally performed when the infant is at least 72 hours old.[85] If elevated phenylalanine levels are found, the test is repeated along with further diagnostic procedures. Placing the infant on a low phenylalanine diet can prevent the mental retardation and other neurological sequelae characteristic of this disorder.[85] Follow-up management by an interdisciplinary team consisting of a nutritionist, a psychologist, and appropriate medical personnel is advised in addition to the specialized diet. If untreated, individuals with PKU may go on to develop hypertonicity (75%), hyperactive reflexes (66%), hyperkinesis (50%), or tremors (30%),[55] in addition to mental retardation. In rare cases, untreated PKU individuals with normal intelligence have been reported, but in general the IQ level is between 10 and 50.[85]

Phenylketonuria is most prevalent among individuals of northern European ancestry and is practically nonexistent among blacks. The frequency among the former group is 1:10,000 to 15,000 births compared with 1:1,000,000 among blacks.[87] It is estimated that one out of every 50 individuals are heterozygous for PKU.

Werdnig-Hoffmann disease (spinal muscular atrophy). A progressive, degenerative disorder of the anterior horn cells, Werdnig-Hoffmann disease is characterized clinically by hypotonicity, generalized symmetrical muscle weakness, absent deep-tendon reflexes, and markedly delayed motor development.[43] A prenatal history of decreased fetal movements during the third trimester frequently accompanies the other neurological signs present during early infancy.[43] Neuropathological examination reveals abnormal and decreased numbers of neurons in the spinal cord and medulla as well as demyelinization of anterior roots and peripheral nerves.[48] Other definitive clinical signs are fasciculation and atrophy of the tongue secondary to hypoglossal nucleus involvement.[43]

Diagnosis may be accomplished through electromyogram (EMG) and muscle biopsy, which reveal neurogenic atrophy.[43] Poor head control, froglike positioning of lower extremities,[48] and better use of distal than proximal musculature[43] are other clinical symptoms. Intellect, sensation, and sphincter functioning are normal.[43] Smiling and recognition are developmentally appropriate.[43] Intercostal muscle weakness leads to a diaphragmatic breathing pattern and contributes to the greatly increased susceptibility to pulmonary infection,[43] which usually results in death before the age of 2.[48] A few individuals with Werdnig-Hoffmann disease have survived to adolescence but are unable to stand without support.[48]

We recently participated in the interdisciplinary evaluation of a 13-month-old girl with Werdnig-Hoffmann disease. Pronounced trunk and proximal muscle weakness were noted, and the infant was unable to sit, crawl, or creep. On the Mental Scale of the Bayley Scales of Infant Development,[4] the child was found to be functioning in the mildly delayed range, but it must be noted that the completion of certain fine motor items was compromised by the proximal upper-extremity weakness. Examination by the neurologist on the team revealed tongue fasciculations and many of the other neurological signs noted above. Referral was made to a pediatric physical therapist to provide the parents with positioning techniques and breathing exercises for the infant.

Sex-linked inherited disorders. The third mechanism for transmission of specific gene defects is through sex-linked inheritance. Two well-known sex-linked inherited diseases are Duchenne's muscular dystrophy and hemophilia. In sex-linked inherited disorders, the abnormal gene is carried on the X chromosome. Females carrying one abnormal gene will not show the trait because of the dominant normal gene on the other X chromosome. However, each son born to a carrier mother has a 50:50 chance of inheriting the abnormal gene and thus demonstrating the disorder. Each daughter has a 50:50 chance of becoming a carrier of the trait. McCusick[66] has identified more than 30 congenital malformations or syndromes that are passed on through sex-linked inheritance. Two of these syndromes, which include profound neurological handicaps, are discussed in this section: Lowe's syndrome and Lesch-Nyhan syndrome.

Lowe's syndrome (oculocerebrorenal syndrome). First described by Lowe and others in 1952,[63] Lowe's syndrome is characterized by progressive mental deterioration, renal tubular dysfunction, and cortical cataracts with or without glaucoma.[88] In the 70 cases of Lowe's syndrome studied by Abassi and others in 1968,[1] it was noted that although the characteristic eye changes were usually present at birth, there was no evidence of metabolic disturbance at this time; by 6 months of age, however, metabolic acidosis occurred.[2] Other clinical symptoms that become apparent during infancy include hypotonicity, joint hyperextensibility, growth retardation and failure to thrive,[86] frontal bossing,[94] and a shrill, piercing cry.[2] Other physical characteristics such as scaphocephaly (long, narrow skull), large low-set ears, pale skin, and blond hair are also characteristic of Lowe's syndrome[2] (Fig. 10-6).

Because of the sex-linked inheritance, all Lowe's syndrome individuals are boys. Additional neuromuscular findings include diminished or absent deep-tendon reflexes and muscle hypoplasia with fatty infiltration.[88] Moderate to severe mental retardation, hyperactivity, and abnormal electroencephalogram (EEG) findings are also present.[88] Blindness, secondary to the cataracts and glaucoma, adds an additional handicap later on.[94] Osteoporosis is nearly always present as well.[88] Neuropathological findings of demyelination and gliosis in the CNS have been noted.[2] Death usually results from renal failure.[2]

Lesch-Nyhan syndrome. Another of the sex-linked disorders that leads to profound neurological deterioration is Lesch-Nyhan syndrome or hereditary choreoathetosis. First described in 1964 by Lesch and Nyhan,[59] over 150 cases have been identified.[47] Although normal in appearance at birth, infants with this disorder begin to self-mutilate at 1 to 2 years by biting their lips and later progress to

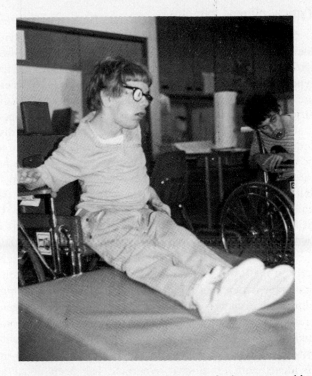

Fig. 10-6. Boy with Lowe's syndrome transferring to mat table.

more severe forms of self-mutilation in which they have been known to bite off their finger tips.[47] The primary metabolic symptom that characterizes this disorder is a marked overproduction of uric acid (hyperuricemia),[17] which results in a deficiency of hypoxanthine guanine phosphoribosyltransferase (HGPRT) in the brain, liver,[52] and amniotic cells.[12] This disorder is detectable through amniocentesis, and genetic counseling is advisable for parents who have already given birth to an affected son.[12]

Although motor development is often normal during the first 6 to 8 months, progressive spastic paresis and athetosis become evident during the latter half of the first year of life.[47] Other neuromotor symptoms include chorea, ballimus, tremor, hyperactive deep-tendon reflexes, severe dysarthria, and dysphagia.[47] Growth retardation is also apparent as well as moderate to severe mental retardation.[47] Bilateral dislocation of hips may occur secondary to the spasticity.[47] In spite of the extreme self-mutilation that characterizes this disorder, pain perception appears to be normal among individuals with Lesch-Nyhan syndrome.

Although blood levels of uric acid have been successfully decreased through the administration of allopurinol, there has been no effective treatment developed for alleviating the neurological symptoms of this syndrome.[65] Death usually occurs before adolescence and is often secondary to uremia from gouty neuropathy or to generalized debilitation.[47]

Typical clinical symptoms

Specific examples of genetic disorders in children, with their accompanying symptomatology, have been presented in the foregoing section. In the present section some of the typical clinical signs common to many of these disorders are discussed, particularly those that are relevant for pediatric therapists. Table 10-1 summarizes this information.

Disorders of tone are characteristic in many genetic disorders. Marked to extreme hypotonicity has been shown to be universally present in a sample of Down's syndrome infants, although it tends to improve with increasing age.[23] Initial hypotonicity has also been reported in trisomy 18 children, but has been shown to progress to hypertonicity in later childhood.[94] Our clinical experience in treating two sisters with trisomy 18 has shown a reversal of this picture, with initial hypertonicity during infancy, particularly in the lower extremities, progressing to hypotonicity and joint hyperextensibility in later childhood. Werdnig-Hoffmann disease is also universally characterized by generalized hypotonicity,[43] as is Lowe's syndrome.[88] Hypotonicity has also been noted in infants and children with partial deletion syndromes, although increased tone in individuals with cri-du-chat syndrome has been noted as well.[35]

Hypertonicity, in the form of hemiparesis, is occasionally found in tuberous sclerosis[94] and neurofibromatosis.[49] Spastic paresis may accompany Hurler's syndrome[2] and is usually present in Lesch-Nyhan syndrome during later infancy and early childhood.[47]

A number of skeletal deformities and anomalies are found among children with genetic disorders. In the examples cited earlier, the most profound skeletal deformities are associated with osteogenesis imperfecta, in which numerous bony irregularities are present.[88] Scoliosis, kyphosis, or kyphoscoliosis are commonly associated deformities in the following syndromes: osteogenesis imperfecta,[88] cri-du-chat syndrome,[84] neurofibromatosis,[94] Hurler's syndrome,[88] and Turner's syndrome.[60] Hip dislocation has been noted in Turner's syndrome,[94] Wolf-Hirschhorn syndrome,[35] cri-du-chat syndrome,[84] Hurler's syndrome,[88] and Lesch-Nyhan syndrome.[47] Individuals with Klinefelter's and Hurler's syndromes are predisposed to demonstrating genu valgum.[2,35]

Many types of ankle and foot deformities have been reported among children with genetic disorders. Rocker-bottom feet characterize trisomy 18 and, more commonly, trisomy 13.[94] Talipes equinovarus has been noted in individuals with trisomy 18,[94] Wolf-Hirschhorn syndrome,[35] and cri-du-chat syndrome.[84] Foot deformities that have been noted in Turner's syndrome are pes planus and pes equinovarus;[94] pes planus may also be associated with Klinefelter's syndrome.[94] Hurler's syndrome individuals may demonstrate pes cavus.[2] Tibial bowing is frequently noted in cases of osteogenesis imperfecta[88] and may also occur in individuals with neurofibromatosis.[88]

Upper-extremity deformities may also occur. Flexion contractures in the upper extremities are common in Hurler's syndrome,[2] and flexion contractures of the fingers are frequently observed in trisomies 13 and 18[94] (Fig. 10-7). Radioulnar synostosis has been noted in Klinefelter's and Wolf-Hirschhorn syndromes (Fig. 10-7).[35] Several skeletal deformities that occur primarily in a specific syndrome include the tendency toward atlantoaxial dislocation in Down's syndrome,[96] pseudoarthrosis of the tibia and fibula

Table 10-1. Typical clinical symptoms

Genetic disorder	Hypotonicity	Hypertonicity	Hip dislocation	Spinal deformities	Upper extremity deformities	Other spinal deformities	Motor delays	Cognitive delays	Cerebellar dysfunction
Trisomy 21	X					X	X	X	X
Trisomy 18	X	X			X	X	X	X	
Trisomy 13					X	X	X	X	
Turner's syndrome			X	X		X			
Klinefelter's syndrome					X	X			
Wold-Hirschhorn syndrome (4p−)	X				X	X	X	X	
Cri-du-chat syndrome (5p−)	X	X	X	X		X	X	X	
Osteogenesis imperfecta				X		X	X		
Tuberous sclerosis		X					X	X	
Neurofibromatosis		X		X		X			
Hurler's syndrome		X	X	X	X	X	X	X	X
Untreated PKU							X	X	X
Werdnig-Hoffmann syndrome	X						X		
Lowe's syndrome	X						X	X	
Lesch-Nyhan syndrome		X	X				X	X	X

in neurofibromatosis,[94] and pectus excavatum or pectus carinatum in osteogenesis imperfecta.[88]

Typical of most genetic syndromes cited in the foregoing examples is delayed motor development. Delay in the achievement of developmental motor milestones has been noted in children with Down's syndrome,[19] trisomies 13 and 18,[94] cri-du-chat syndrome,[84] Wolf-Hirschhorn syndrome,[35] osteogenesis imperfecta,[94] tuberous sclerosis,[25] Hurler's syndrome,[94] untreated phenylketonuria,[85] Werdnig-Hoffmann disease,[43] Lowe's syndrome, and Lesch-Nyhan syndrome.[47]

Mental retardation is also a frequent finding in genetic disorders. Moderate to severe mental retardation is characteristic of the following syndromes: Down's,[81] trisomy 13 and trisomy 18,[94] cri-du-chat,[84] Wolf-Hirschhorn,[35] tuberous sclerosis,[82] Hurler's,[2] untreated phenylketonuria,[85] Lowe's,[88] and Lesch-Nyhan.[47] In Turner's syndrome[94] and neurofibromatosis,[88] there is a greater incidence of mental retardation than among the normal population, but most individuals with these disorders function within normal IQ ranges. Intellectual functioning is generally within normal limits for children with Werdnig-Hoffmann disease [43] and osteogenesis imperfecta.[8] Children with phenylketonuria who have been diagnosed at birth and treated with a low phenylalanine diet also have a good prognosis for normal intellectual functioning.[82]

Symptoms of cerebellar dysfunction may be found in a number of genetic disorders. The balance and coordination

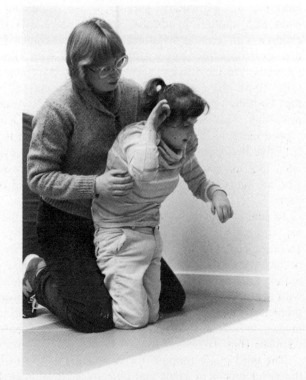

Fig. 10-7. Teenager with trisomy 18 who exhibits kyphoscoliosis and flexion contractures of distal joints of fifth digits.

deficits typical of Down's syndrome children may be caused, in part, by delays in cerebellar maturation and a disproportionately small cerebellum.[28] Ataxia has also been noted in Hurler's syndrome.[94] Tremors occur in 30% of individuals with untreated phenylketonuria[55] and are also displayed by individuals with Lesch-Nyhan syndrome.[47] For additional information on cerebellar dysfunction and treatment, refer to Chapter 21.

In summary, many of the more severe genetic disorders are characterized by accompanying neuromotor, cognitive, and orthopaedic problems of which the pediatric therapist should be cognizant. Although only 15 clinical examples of genetic disorders have been presented in this chapter, these were chosen because they were felt to be most representative of the types of disorders that might appear in children who would require the services of a developmental therapist. The following part of this chapter focuses on the clinical management of genetic disorders in children.

CLINICAL MANAGEMENT OF GENETIC DISORDERS

Genetic disorders in children frequently result in multiple handicapping conditions to which the developmental therapist must be alerted. In most genetic disorders, clinical symptomatology is present at birth or becomes apparent during early infancy. Because of the congenital nature of these disorders, the pediatric therapist is usually concerned with habilitation rather than rehabilitation. Habilitation of the child with a congenital syndrome or disease must be directed at three major domains of learning: sensorimotor, emotional-affective, and cognitive-perceptual. In dealing with the infant or young child, a transdisciplinary approach may be espoused,[39] and the developmental therapist, in functioning as the transdisciplinary specialist, must be concerned with all three areas of habilitation. The first step toward habilitating a child with a genetic disorder is a careful evaluation of the child's strengths and deficits.

Evaluation procedures

A child's diagnostic label will be valuable initially to aid in the selection of appropriate assessment tools and to alert the therapist to any medical problems or contraindications associated with the specific syndrome that could affect the evaluation procedures. However, it is vitally important that such labels do not bias the therapist or other developmental specialists into developing preconceived opinions about the child's capabilities based on how other children with similar diagnostic labels have performed. It is important to remember that there are wide behavioral and performance variabilities within each genetic disorder. For example, children with Down's syndrome may vary in intellectual functioning from mild to profound mental retardation. Wide variability in the achievement of developmental motor milestones has also been reported among children with Down's syndrome.[61,68]

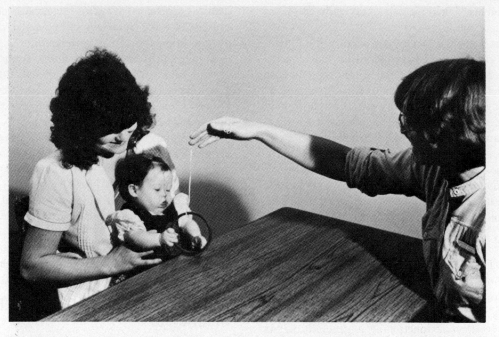

Fig. 10-8. Four-month-old infant with Down's syndrome being assessed on the Bayley Scales of Infant Development

It is far more pertinent to concentrate on the strengths and deficits that appear clinically than to focus directly on the child's diagnostic label. Through comprehensive evaluation procedures, the therapist not only can determine the child's functional or developmental level but also can ascertain what problems may be interfering with the achievement of age-appropriate developmental milestones.

The problem-oriented approach to evaluation has been described in detail by Campbell in the assessment of self-care skills.[16] This approach has applicability for assessment in all domains of learning. The steps involved in the problem-oriented approach are as follows:

1. Observe the child's general behavior in the specific skill area.
2. Identify the specific problem or problems interfering with the acquisition of the skill.
3. Hypothesize and test possible reasons for the problems (pathological neuromotor problems or noncompliant behavior).
4. Devise alternative strategies to minimize the effect of the interfering behavior.
5. Formulate programming objectives:
   a. Specify the skill to be acquired.
   b. Specify the problem to be remediated.

There are three primary purposes for conducting a developmental therapy evaluation for a child with a genetic disorder: (1) to establish the child's developmental level so that developmental gains may be monitored, (2) to provide verification of developmental delay so that the child may qualify for special programs or special funding, and (3) to develop long-term programming goals and short-term therapy objectives.

Unfortunately, there are few published assessment tools that are particularly appropriate for evaluating the child with multiple handicaps, as is the case with most children with genetic syndromes. Three assessment tools that have been used repeatedly for infants with Down's syndrome are the Bayley Scales of Infant Development[4] (Fig. 10-8), the Gesell Developmental Schedules,[54] and the Griffiths Mental Development Scales.[36] Another promising assessment tool for young or severely handicapped children that is currently being field tested is the Adaptive Performance Instrument, a comprehensive evaluation tool for assessing severely handicapped individuals who are functioning below the developmental level of 2 years.[3]

In addition to assessing developmental levels in the areas of cognitive, motor and adaptive/self-help skills, assessment of the child's neuromuscular functioning should be included. Primitive reflexes, automatic reactions, and muscle tone will be important areas to assess in children with neuromotor problems. For children with orthopaedic problems, standard range of motion measurements and manual muscle testing will be important assessments to complete (Fig. 10-9).

The third major purpose for conducting an evaluation, the development of goals and objectives, is addressed in the next section.

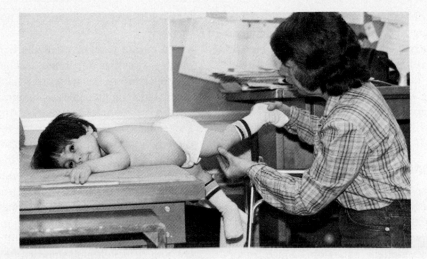

Fig. 10-9. Evaluating range of hip extension in a child with osteogenesis imperfecta.

Establishment of goals and objectives

With the enactment of Public Law 94-142 in 1975,[79] physical and occupational therapists working in public school settings were required to establish long-term, annual goals and short-term therapy objectives.[75] Similar requirements are now in effect for infants with handicapping conditions as a result of the enactment of Public Law 99-457 in 1986. An Individualized Family Service Plan (IFSP) must be written after a multidisciplinary assessment is completed.[32] The IFSP must contain: (1) a statement of the child's present levels of development (cognitive, speech/language, psychosocial, motor, and self-help); (2) a statement of the family's strengths and needs related to enhancing the child's development; (3) a statement of major outcomes expected to be achieved for the child and family; (4) the criteria, procedures, and timelines for determining progress; (5) the specific early-intervention services necessary to meet the unique needs of the child and family including the method, frequency, and intensity of service; (6) the projected dates for the initiation of services and expected duration; (7) the name of the case manager; and (8) procedures for transition from early intervention to the preschool program.[32] The establishment of goals and objectives for the infant or child with a genetic disorder is vitally important to the overall intervention plan.

Public Law 94-142 requires that annual goals and short-term objectives be established within the framework of each child's Individual Education Program (IEP). The components of an IEP are as follows[75]:

1. A statement of the child's present levels of educational performance
2. A statement of annual goals, including short-term instructional objectives
3. A statement of the specific special education and related services to be provided to the child

4. The projected dates for initiation of services and the anticipated duration of the service
5. Appropriate objective criteria and evaluation procedures and schedules for determining, on at least an annual basis, whether short-term instructional objectives are being achieved

The development of behaviorally written, measurable therapy objectives is crucial in monitoring the effects of intervention in a child with a genetic disorder. Many of the clinical symptoms listed in the descriptions of genetic disorders described earlier in the chapter may be monitored through systematic, periodic, data-keeping procedures. One example would be the monitoring of range of motion measurements of the flexion contractures frequently associated with trisomy 13, trisomy 18, and Lesch-Nyhan syndromes. A behavioral program for decreasing the self-mutilating behaviors characteristic of individuals with Lesch-Nyhan syndrome might also be part of the overall therapy intervention plan. Periodic vital capacity measures for a child with osteogenesis imperfecta or Werdnig-Hoffmann disease could reflect progress toward a goal of maintaining respiratory function. Following are some examples of behaviorally written, developmental therapy objectives for infants with Down's syndrome:

1. N. will stand independently for 15 seconds, 2 out of 3 trials by 6/89.
2. J. will maintain prone-on-elbows position with head at a 45 degree angle for 15 seconds, 1 out of 2 trials by 6/89.
3. In 30 seconds, S. will progress forward on abdomen 12 feet by 6/89.

Through systematic and periodic data-keeping procedures, therapists can graph and monitor trends toward the achievement of short-term therapy objectives. Objectives that appear to be too difficult to obtain as a result of analyzing the graphed data may be modified. As other individual objectives are achieved, new objectives can be written by following a developmentally appropriate hierarchy. It is vitally important that pediatric therapists become accountable for effecting change in their clients.[41] Failure to systematically document the effects of intervention is unfair to the child, his or her family, and other professionals working with the child.

General treatment principles

Once the evaluation has been completed, with goals and objectives established, a treatment program may be initiated. The goal of therapy is to maximize the child's potential through alleviation of any interfering neuromotor deficits or noncompliant behaviors. Since abnormalities in muscle tone and developmental delay are two of the most common problems observed in children with genetic disorders, a treatment approach that emphasizes normal sensorimotor development and focuses on the total needs of the child is critical.[9] Harris[39] has advocated such an approach for use with infants with Down's syndrome that stresses normalization of muscle tone and facilitation of normal postural and movement patterns (Fig. 10-10). Other treatment approaches have been described in the physical and occupational therapy literature that also emphasize normal sensorimotor development as the foundation for its treatment methods.[9,42] These approaches generally include techniques to improve muscle tone and foster development of normal patterns of movement.

To ensure carry-over of the beneficial effects of treatment, instruction of parents, teachers, and other caregivers in proper lifting, carrying, and handling techniques should be included in the therapy program.[38] The therapist can become a more effective role model for demonstrating proper handling and positioning techniques by integrating therapy into the classroom or infant program setting. Sternat and others[90] advocate an integrated therapy model where the therapist provides intervention within the child's everyday setting. In this model the therapist assesses the child within the classroom or home environment and determines which motor activities are most functionally or educationally appropriate for that child. The teacher and parent join in developing appropriate therapy goals and specific short-term objectives. In such a setting, small group activities to facilitate normal movement patterns can be encouraged, with less physically handicapped classmates serving as peer models. The therapist can benefit by learning from teachers and parents about appropriate strategies for reinforcing positive behaviors and decreasing negative or inappropriate behaviors. Additionally, the child will benefit by not being withdrawn from important classroom activities. Although not all aspects of therapy can best be carried out in an integrated setting, a creative therapist who is concerned with the well-being of the "whole child" can usually develop strategies for integrating many types of intervention modes into the child's natural environment.[90]

This important consideration for the emotional as well as the physical well-being of the child should be remembered when making recommendations for home therapy programs. As much as possible, recommended activities should be incorporated into the daily routine of the child in activities such as dressing, bathing, and playtimes.[38] Sensitivity to the time constraints and capabilities of family members is important to ensure that the therapy needs of the child do not overshadow the needs of the family for normal parent-child relationships.

In planning a treatment program, general knowledge of the specific genetic disorder is important to alert the therapist to any precautions or contraindications that might affect the treatment program. The treatment program will need to be modified, for example, for the child with osteogenesis imperfecta because of the high risk of fractures. Likewise, respiratory problems in a child with Werdnig-Hoffmann disease may limit the amount of time the child is able to tolerate one particular position.

Therapists should also be alert for behavior problems, such as noncompliance, self-stimulation, or self-abuse, that will interfere with the therapy program and significantly affect the acquisition of new skills. Knowledge of basic behavior management techniques will be important for pediatric therapists, who should work with parents,

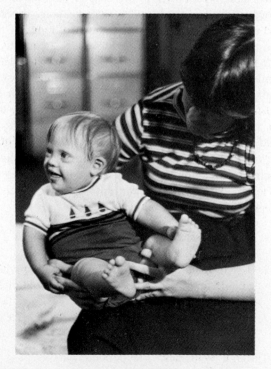

Fig. 10-10. Facilitating truncal equilibrium reactions in a 10-month-old child with Down's syndrome.

teachers, and other staff members to develop a consistent management program for problem behaviors.

In the following section, common problems observed in children with genetic disorders that are of particular concern to therapists will be presented. Basic treatment procedures and management strategies will also be discussed, but are intended to serve only as guidelines to assist in the planning of the treatment program. The often unique variety of problems presented by children with genetic disorders will provide a challenge to therapists, who will need to continually adapt the treatment program to meet the needs of the individual child. As noted earlier, developmentally based treatment objectives will assist the therapist in this process by providing a systematic method of measuring and monitoring the effectiveness of therapy.

Common problems and general treatment strategies

Hypertonicity. Differences and similarities observed in children with hypertonicity and hypotonicity are listed in Table 10-2. In these children it is important to facilitate more normal muscle tone to allow normal postural reactions, such as head righting and equilibrium reactions, to develop. For children with hypertonicity, as in Lesch-Nyhan and Hurler's syndromes, techniques to reduce hypertonicity, such as rotation of the trunk between shoulder girdle and pelvis[10] and the use of positions that reduce abnormal tone, may be helpful. Inhibitive casting is another relatively new technique used to reduce hypertonicity throughout the body.[31,91]

The motor development of children with hypertonicity is often further interfered with by the retention of primitive reflexes. Retention of reflexes such as the asymmetrical tonic neck reflex (ATNR) and the symmetrical tonic neck reflex interfere with normal movement patterns because the position of the extremities is determined by the position of the head. These reflexes must therefore be discouraged by proper positioning and handling.[10,38] For example, midline orientation should be encouraged for the child

Table 10-2. Hypotonicity and hypertonicity: differences and similarities

	Hypotonicity	Hypertonicity
1. Characteristics	Low tone, floppy, "rag doll"	High tone, spastic or rigid
2. Distribution	Generalized; symmetrical	Generalized; often asymmetrical
3. Range of motion	Excessive; joint hyperextensibility	Limited to midranges
4. Risk for contractures and deformities	Risk for dislocation (jaw, hip, atlantoaxial joint)	Risks for contractures (flexor), dislocations (hip), and deformities (scoliosis, kyphosis)
5. Deep tendon reflexes	Hypoactive	Hyperactive
6. Integration of primitive reflexes	Hyporeflexive; sometimes delayed integration	Often delayed
7. Achievement of motor milestones	Delayed (amount of delay correlates with severity of tone abnormality)	Delayed (amount of delay correlates with severity of tone abnormality)
8. Influence of body position	Tone remains same	Tone fluctuates with changes in body position
9. Consistency of muscles	Soft, doughy	Hard, rocklike
10. Passivity	Wide-ranging, continuous excursions	Stiff, limited range of excursions
11. Respiratory problems	Shallow breathing; choking secondary to decreased pharyngeal tone	Decreased thoracic mobility; limited inspiration and expiration
12. Speech problems	Secondary to respiratory problems—little sustained phonation	Dysarthria secondary to hypertonicity in oral muscles
13. Feeding problems	Hypoactive gag reflex, open mouth and protruding tongue, incoordination in swallowing	Hyperactive gag reflex, tongue thrust, bite reflex, rooting reflex
14. Change with increasing age	Tone improves; becomes more normal	Hypertonicity often increases because of use of abnormal reflexes and abnormal movement patterns
15. Therapy techniques (to normalize tone)	Joint compression through spine and extremities Bouncing and tapping	Relaxation in prone position over therapy ball or lap Use of reflex-inhibiting postures and positions
16. Neuropathology	Disturbance in cerebellar function	Release of reflex activity from cortical control (inhibition)

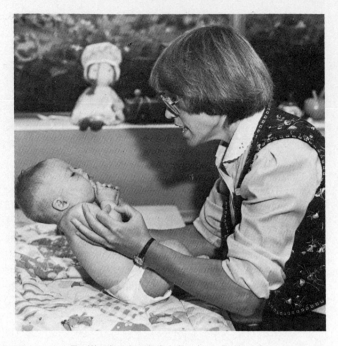

Fig. 10-11. Facilitating head righting into flexion for a 4-month-old infant with Down's syndrome.

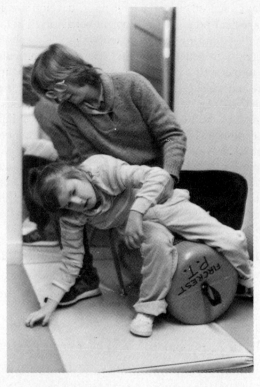

Fig. 10-12. Facilitating sideways protective extension for a girl with trisomy 18.

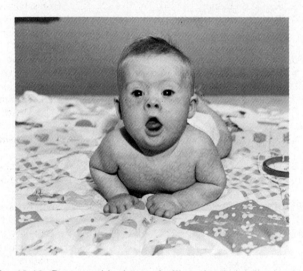

Fig. 10-13. Prone positioning to facilitate head righting into extension for a 4-month-old infant with Down's syndrome.

with a retained asymmetrical tonic neck reflex. Because the ATNR is often stronger in the supine position, alternate positions, such as side-lying, should be encouraged.[10,38]

The tightening and splinting of spastic muscles often limits movements of the hypertonic child to the midranges. Movements tend to be in total flexion and extension patterns, with selective movements of individual joints, such as flexing the wrist with the elbow extended, being very difficult. To reduce the spasticity and allow the development of more selective movement, these total patterns of movement must be discouraged.[10] For example, the total extension pattern of hip adduction, extension, and internal rotation with knee extension and plantar flexion is often effectively inhibited by keeping the hips abducted. This can be done while lifting and carrying the child and can be incorporated into positioning programs. An abduction wedge can be used, for instance, in adapted seating devices, prone boards, wheelchairs, and sidelying positioners.

Hypotonicity. For the child displaying hypotonicity, as in Down's syndrome, trisomy 18, and Lowe's syndrome, techniques such as joint compression, tapping, and resistance may be used to improve muscle tone.[40,86] The use of these techniques should be carefully monitored because initial hypotonicity may develop into hypertonicity, as has been reported in children with trisomy 18.

Although retention of primitive reflexes is less likely to interfere with the development of normal movement patterns, delay in the development of head righting, equilibrium reactions, and protective extension reactions is a ma-

jor concern. Development of these reactions can be promoted through direct handling (Figs. 10-11 and 10-12) as well as through positioning programs.[38] The development of extension against gravity, for example, can be facilitated by positioning the child in the prone position (Fig. 10-13). Head and trunk extension will be encouraged as well as weight bearing on upper extremities to improve stability of the shoulder girdle.

For the child who lacks adequate head and trunk control to maintain the prone position for extended periods of time, adaptations may be necessary. For example, the child can be placed prone on a wedge cushion with head and arms extending over the wide end of the cushion and arms reaching the surface. If a child has difficulty keeping elbows forward to prop on, a small roll or bolster can be placed behind the elbows. For the more advanced child who is able to easily prop on extended arms but is not yet able to maintain a quadruped position, a bolster can be placed under the abdomen for additional support.

Although movements of the hypertonic child are generally limited to the midranges, children with hypotonicity typically display movements in the extremes of the range. Low muscle tone and delays in the development of automatic reactions force these children to assume positions of excessive flexion or extension. The head, for example, is often held in excessive extension, resting on the shoulders to maintain an upright position, and this should not be mistaken for normal head control. Additional problems that may arise from persistent positioning in excessive extension are discussed in the next section.

Hyperextensible joints. Hyperextensible joints are commonly observed in children with hypotonicity and are noted in many children with genetic disorders. The therapy program may need to be modified to avoid undue stress to these joints and the surrounding ligaments. Positions that encourage knee and elbow joints to lock into extension, for example, should be avoided. Activities to encourage weight bearing on upper extremities may need to be encouraged on flexed, instead of extended, arms if elbows persistently lock into hyperextension. Likewise, standing activities may need to be limited if knees are continually held in hyperextension. Control in upright positions may then need to be facilitated in a kneel-stand or half-kneel position.[38] If hyperextensible feet and ankle joints cause excessive foot pronation in standing, additional support may be desirable in the form of shoe modifications or other orthoses.

Protection of hyperextensible joints also needs to be considered in activities such as pulling a child to sit from supine. In a hypotonic child lacking adequate head control and muscle tone, holding the child by the hands and pulling to sitting is likely to be stressful to shoulder and neck muscles. Instead, the activity can be modified by holding the child more proximally at the upper arms to provide additional support until head and shoulder stability improve (Fig. 10-11). As noted earlier, therapists should be particularly aware of the importance of avoiding such stress to children with Down's syndrome because of the propensity for atlantoaxial dislocation and the added risk for spinal cord injury in these children. Activities such as gymnastics, tumbling, and diving should be avoided in these children at risk for subluxation or dislocation.[34]

Contractures and deformities. Skeletal deformities and anomalies are associated with many genetic disorders. The pediatric therapist may work with orthopaedists, prosthetists, and orthotists to prevent existing problems from progressing. The therapist should be aware of factors that can contribute to the development of deformities in order to prevent or minimize such problems. For example, the child with hypertonicity is at high risk for developing joint contractures because of the abnormal reflex patterns and abnormal patterns of movement that limit movement to small ranges. Although joint contractures are less likely to occur in a child with hypotonicity, there is an added risk for other deformities, such as hip dislocation, from the typical positioning of lower extremities in hip abduction and flexion. Spinal deformities, such as lumbar lordosis and kyphosis, are also common problems in children with abnormal muscle tone (Fig. 10-7). An asymmetrical distribution of muscle tone or muscle strength or other problems that encourage asymmetrical postures and use of one side of the body increase the risk of scoliosis.

To help prevent or minimize these deformities, proper positioning is important. Wheelchairs, special seating devices, and other adaptive equipment should be adjusted and modified to allow the best possible alignment of the spine and extremities. Specific exercise programs and handling techniques that facilitate movement through the full range of motion should also be included in the therapy program. For some children, standard range of motion exercises and the use of positioning or other orthoses may be appropriate.

Although maintenance of normal joint range is generally desirable, there may be occasions where joint contractures may improve functional capabilities. An elbow flexion contracture, for example, may be more functional for the child with osteogenesis imperfecta to assist in feeding and other self-care activities.

Respiratory problems. Respiratory problems are often observed in children with hypotonicity as well as in children whose respiratory functioning is compromised by chest and skeletal deformities. Deep breathing and chest expansion exercises as well as postural drainage may be required for these children. In addition, frequent changes of positions and adapted positioning devices may be required for those children whose respiratory status makes it difficult to tolerate one position for extended periods of time.

Our experience in treating a child with Werdnig-Hoffmann disease necessitated the modification of a prone board as an alternate positioning device. The child was unable to tolerate a completely prone position because of respiratory problems and became easily fatigued when sitting for extended periods, often needing her hands to support her head in an upright position. A standard prone board with desk was modified to include an anterior head rest. This allowed her to rest her neck muscles and free her hands for other activities, and it did not compromise her respiratory status.

Adaptive equipment needs. As noted previously, an important adjunct to direct therapy services is the use of adaptive equipment and proper positioning techniques in the classroom or home setting.[17] The use of wedges, prone boards, corner chairs, and side-lying positioners is as important for many children with genetic disorders as it is for children with cerebral palsy, and it is the therapist's responsibility to instruct parents, teachers, and other professionals in the use of this equipment.

Because the problems of children with genetic disorders are often unique, special modifications to meet the needs of the individual child are often necessary. For the child with normal cognitive functioning, as in Werdnig-Hoffmann disease and osteogenesis imperfecta, the challenge increases to provide every opportunity for independent functioning (Fig. 10-14). Adaptive equipment needs may vary from dressing, feeding, and other self-care equipment to writing aids and alternative seating devices to enhance the child's learning and participation in classroom activities. Mobility aids, including electric wheelchairs for those children with normal intelligence who do not have the potential for independent ambulation, should also be considered at an early age.[15]

Cognitive delays. Mental retardation is associated with many of the genetic disorders discussed in this chapter. The degree of retardation will obviously affect the therapy program and must be considered when establishing appropriate goals and objectives.

Techniques that encourage automatic movements rather than requests for conscious volitional effort will be necessary for the child with severe mental and physical impair-

ments. For these children, emphasis should be placed on proper positioning and handling techniques to assist parents, teachers, and staff in caring for the child (Fig. 10-15).

For the retarded child with only minor physical limitations, emphasis should be placed on achieving the necessary motor, perceptual, and social skills for independent living. Therapists may offer consultation to classroom teachers and parents in the areas of independent feeding, dressing, and toileting skills. Adaptive self-help aids as well as clothing modifications should be considered to assure the highest level of independent functioning possible. For the older child, social skill and survival skill training will be vitally important.

Medical management

It is important for the physical or occupational therapist to be aware of some aspects of medical management of the child with genetic disorders in addition to being cognizant of particular developmental therapy strategies that may be employed. Unfortunately, few known medical therapies have been successful in the treatment of genetic disorders in children, although a number of strategies for ameliorating isolated symptoms have been reported. In the genetic disorders discussed in this chapter, the only one for which dramatic results have been achieved through early medical management is phenylketonuria. With early diagnosis and immediate implementation of a low phenylalanine diet, the infant with PKU can be spared the severe mental retardation and other progressive neurological impairments that result in untreated individuals.[85]

Medical treatment for the other disorders described in

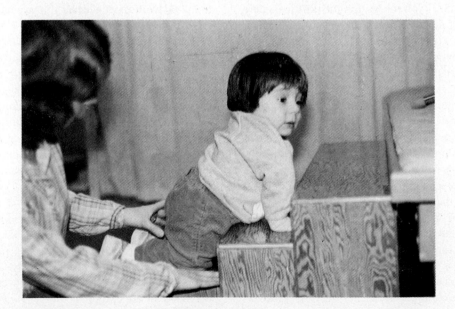

Fig. 10-14. Encouraging developmentally appropriate, functional activities for a child with osteogenesis imperfecta.

this chapter is not curative but rather either palliative or directed at specific associated anomalies. The congenital heart defects present in an estimated 40% of individuals with Down's syndrome[30] may, in some instances, be corrected by cardiac surgery. Orthopaedic surgery in the form of insertion of intramedullary rods in the tibia or femur may minimize the recurrence of repeated fractures associated with osteogenesis imperfecta.[82] Surgical correction of scoliosis may be warranted in individuals with neurofibromatosis or Werdnig-Hoffmann disease,[56] if the deformity is severe and bracing[72] is not successful. Surgical removal of obstructive or malignant tumors is advisable in certain cases of neurofibromatosis,[47] as is removal of cerebral

nodular growths in individuals with tuberous sclerosis for the control of seizures.[82]

Respiratory therapy is an important adjunctive treatment strategy in individuals with Werdnig-Hoffmann disease[56] and may be implemented as part of the overall developmental therapy program. Specific medical therapies include estrogen therapy to promote feminization in individuals with Turner's syndrome and testosterone therapy to enhance masculinity in Klinefelter males.[71] The use of anticonvulsants is an important part of seizure management in individuals with tuberous sclerosis.[6] To assist in the management of metabolic acidosis and rickets, which are often present in Lowe's syndrome, alkali supplements and

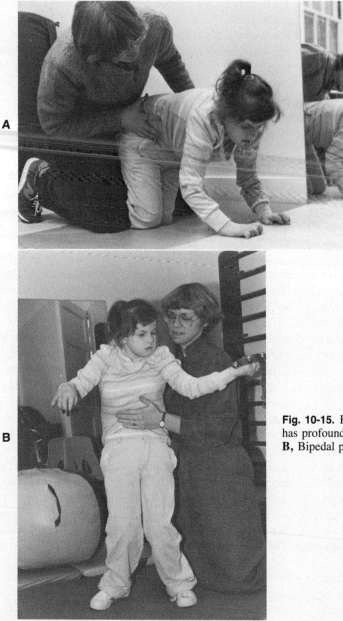

Fig. 10-15. Facilitating positions for a girl with trisomy 18 who has profound mental retardation. **A,** Quadrupedal position. **B,** Bipedal position.

vitamin D therapy have been used.[47] Allopurinol has been used for individuals with Lesch-Nyhan syndrome to prevent urologic complications, although it has no effect on the progressive neurological symptomatology.[47]

In light of the limited medical treatment strategies available for children with genetic disorders, the developmental therapist must be concerned with maximizing the child's developmental or functional potential within the limitations imposed by the lack of possible cures and the prospect of the shortened life span that characterizes many of these disorders. Therapy must be directed at maintenance of current functioning levels or at minimization of expected decline.

Psychosocial aspects of genetic disorders

Though the adjustment to the birth of any handicapped child is always difficult for parents, the birth of a child with a genetic disorder can be even more traumatic because of the implications for similar disorders occurring in future offspring, particularly in the case of specific gene defects in which the risk for future offspring being similarly affected may be as high as 50%. Solnit and Stark [89] discuss the mourning experienced by parents at the "loss" of the expected normal child when a handicapped child is born: "The mourning process makes it possible to progress from the initial phase of numbness and disbelief; to the dawning awareness of the disappointment and feeling of loss with the accompanying affective and physical symptoms; to the last phase of the grief reaction in which intense re-experiencing of the memories and expectations gradually reduce the hypercathexis of the wish of the idealized child" (p. 116). The authors point out that it is vitally important for professionals who are dealing with parents of a recently identified handicapped child to be cognizant of the mourning process. By realizing that the acceptance level for coping with this unexpected loss of the wished-for normal child may vary, depending on which stage of the grieving process the parents are in, professionals can gauge their discussion of the diagnosis and prognosis for the child to the most appropriate time.

Even when, and if, acceptance of the child's condition is achieved, a host of practical problems still face the parents. These have been elaborated by Robinson and Robinson[81] and include medical costs, transportation, finding day-care and baby-sitting services, and selecting an appropriate school or intervention program. The amount of attention required from parents to be directed toward a special child may reduce their ability to spend time with the child's siblings and may result in feelings of jealousy and anger toward the handicapped child. It is important for pediatric therapists who work with children with genetic disorders to be aware of the psychosocial aspects of the family's adjustment to the child, because these may impact greatly on the child's responses to therapy. Therapists who work intensively with children with genetic disorders may find themselves filling the role of counselor, particularly since they may be the medical professionals who work most closely with the child and the family.

Because of the intensive contact that therapists frequently have with children with genetic disorders and their families, they may occasionally assume the role of advocate in facilitating the placement of the child in the least restrictive educational environment.[79] Particularly in the case of the child with severe physical handicaps who has normal intelligence, such as a child with osteogenesis imperfecta or Werdnig-Hoffmann disease, the pediatric therapist may be the primary advocate for assuring that the child is placed in a regular classroom or preschool setting with peers of comparable age and IQ.

Genetic counseling

Of crucial importance in dealing with the child with a genetic disorder is a knowledge of genetic counseling. Developmental therapists must have an understanding of the modes of inheritance of the various genetic disorders as well as information about the services that can be offered through genetic counseling. Although the physician has primary responsibility for informing the parents of a child with a genetic disorder about the availability of genetic counseling, therapists also must be informed about the risks of recurrence of specific disorders, because they may have a closer professional and personal relationship with the parents. As recently as 1979, a Down's syndrome infant was born to a 37-year-old mother who had received no counseling or information from her physician about the increased risks of giving birth to a chromosomally abnormal child at her advanced maternal age.

Although we are certainly not advocating that the therapist serve in the role of genetic counselor, it *is* important that therapists be aware of the availability and location of such services so that they may be assured that parents of a child with a genetic disorder are informed of their availability. Most major university-affiliated medical centers provide genetic counseling. Six steps or procedures in genetic counseling have been discussed by Novitski.[73] The first is to make an accurate medical diagnosis of the child's disorder. In the case of a suspected chromosome abnormality, this usually involves conducting a karyotype of the affected child as well as karyotypes of parents and siblings. Other diagnostic procedures may include a medical examination, muscle biopsy, other laboratory tests, and radiographic examinations. If it is determined that the disorder is of genetic origin, further procedures should follow.

The next step in genetic counseling is to construct a pedigree or family tree of all known relatives and ancestors of both parents.[73] Pedigree information should include the age and cause of death of ancestors, a history of stillbirths and spontaneous abortions, and a history of appearance of any other genetic defects or unknown causes of mental retardation. The country of origin of ancestors is also important, because certain genetic defects, such as phenylketonuria, are far more prevalent in families of a particular ethnic origin.[73] Once the defect has been identified and a pedigree constructed, Novitski[73] advises that further information be obtained from one of the comprehensive resource texts on genetic disorders.

The third procedure in genetic counseling is to estimate the risk of recurrence of the disorder.[73] In specific gene defects, the probability of recurrence is fairly straightforward, with a risk of 25% for autosomal recessive disorders and a 50% risk for each male child in sex-linked disorders. These figures do not hold true in cases of spontaneous mutations, however. In cases of chromosomal abnormalities, such as Down's syndrome, karyotyping is mandated to determine if the child has the translocation type of Down's syndrome, in which the risk of recurrence is much greater than with a history of standard trisomy 21 Down's syndrome.

Educating the parents in the probability of recurrence is the next procedure discussed by Novitski.[73] He points out the common misunderstanding that if a risk is 1:4 for an affected child to be born, as in an autosomal recessive disorder, many parents may assume that if they have just given birth to a child with the disorder, the next three children should be normal. It is important to explain that each subsequent child faces a 1:4 risk of inheriting the disorder regardless of how many handicapped or uninvolved siblings have already been born.

The fifth step in genetic counseling is for the parents to decide on the course of action they will take for future pregnancies once all available facts have been presented to them by the counselor.[73] Some parents may choose not to have any further children; others may elect to undergo prenatal diagnostic procedures for subsequent pregnancies. These decisions rest entirely with the parents and may be influenced by their individual religious or ethical preferences.

Follow-up counseling and review of the most recent advances in medical genetics represent the final step in the genetic counseling procedure.[73] The effect of the handicapped child on the family may modify the parents' earlier decision to have or not to have subsequent children. Recent medical advances may allow a more certain prenatal diagnosis of specific genetic disorders.

The most common prenatal diagnostic procedure is amniocentesis, a method for detecting early genetic disorders in the fetus at 14 to 16 weeks gestation by inserting a long, slender needle through the mother's abdominal wall and into the placenta to extract a small amount of amniotic fluid.[95] Laboratory tests of amniotic fluid will reveal all types of chromosome abnormalities as well as a number of specific gene defects, including Tay-Sach disease and Lesch-Nyhan syndrome, and some disorders of polygenic multifactorial inheritance, such as neural tube defects. Although certain sex-linked disorders are not as yet detectable through laboratory analysis of amniotic cells, it is possible to determine the sex of the fetus and thus elect to abort male offspring who have a 50:50 chance of inheriting the disorder. Recently, chorionic villi sampling has gained increased acceptance as a prenatal diagnostic procedure because it allows for detection of some genetic disorders as early as 10 to 12 weeks gestation.[77]

SUMMARY

Because genetic disorders make up about 20% of all birth defects,[7] it is important for pediatric physical and occupational therapists to be knowledgeable about the etiology, clinical characteristics, management, and psychosocial aspects of many of these disorders. Two of the more common pediatric disorders of genetic origin, which are of particular interest to developmental therapists, are Duchenne's muscular dystrophy and myelomeningocele. Congenital spinal injuries are discussed in Chapter 14 of this volume. The present chapter has addressed a number of chromosomal abnormalities and specific gene defects, which are also apt to appear in children in a typical developmental therapy caseload. Because over 300 specific gene defects have been identified, it was not possible to provide descriptions of all the genetic disorders that might be represented in a pediatric setting. Readers are encouraged to consult the reference list at the end of this chapter for further information about genetic disorders not described herein. The references by Aita,[2] Holmes and others,[47] McCusick,[66] Rubin,[82] and Smith[88] may be particularly helpful. A recent text by Goldberg,[38] which provides an orthopaedic perspective on many childhood genetic disorders, is especially appropriate for physical therapists.

REFERENCES

1. Abassi V and others: Oculo-cerebro-renal syndrome: a review, Am J Dis Child 115:145, 1968.
2. Aita JA: Congenital facial anomalies with neurologic defects, Springfield, Ill, 1969, Charles C Thomas, Publisher.
3. American Association for the Education of the Severely and Profoundly Handicapped, Consortium on Adaptive Performance Evaluation (CAPE), Committee on Infant Assessment (CIA): Adaptive assessment for evaluating the progress of severely/profoundly handicapped children functioning between birth and two years. The annual report of a field-initiated research project funded by the Bureau of Education for the Handicapped, grant no G007702139, 1978.
4. Bayley N: Bayley scales of infant development, New York, 1969, Psychological Corporation.
5. Benda CE: The child with mongolism (congenital acromicria), New York, 1960, Grune & Stratton, Inc.
6. Berg BO: Convulsive disorders. In Bleck EE and Nagel DA, editors: Physically handicapped children: a medical atlas for teachers, New York, 1975, Grune & Stratton, Inc.
7. Birth defects: the tragedy and the hope, White Plains, NY, 1975, The National Foundation/March of Dimes.
8. Bleck EE: Osteogenesis imperfecta. In Bleck EE and Nagel DA, editors: Physically handicapped children: a medical atlas for teachers, New York, 1975, Grune & Stratton, Inc.
9. Bobath K and Bobath B: The facilitation of normal postural reactions and movements in cerebral palsy, Physiotherapy 50:246, 1964.

10. Bobath K and Bobath B: Cerebral palsy. In Pearson PH and Williams CE, editors: Physical therapy services in the developmental disabilities, Springfield, Ill, 1976, Charles C Thomas, Publisher.

11. Boué JG: Chromosomal studies in more than 900 spontaneous abortuses, Teratology Society meeting, 1974.

12. Boyle JA and others: Lesch-Nyhan syndrome: preventive control by prenatal diagnosis, Science 169:688, 1970.

13. Breg WR and others: The cri du chat syndrome in adolescents and adults: clinical findings in 13 older patients with partial deletion of the short arms of chromosome no 5 (5p−), J Pediatr 77:782, 1970.

14. Brooks DN and others: Hearing loss and middle ear disorders in patients with Down's syndrome (mongolism), J Ment Defic Res 16:21, 1972.

15. Butler C and others: Powered mobility for young disabled children, Dev Med Child Neurol 25:472, 1983.

16. Campbell PH: Daily living skills. In Haring NG, editor: Developing effective individualized education programs for severely handicapped children and youth, Washington, 1977, Bureau of Education for the Handicapped.

17. Campbell PH and others: Approximating the norm through environmental and child-centered prosthetics and adaptive equipment. In Sontag E: Educational programming for the severely and profoundly handicapped, Reston, Va, 1977, Council for Exceptional Children.

18. Carr DH: Chromosome anomalies as a cause of spontaneous abortion, Am J Obstet Gynec 97:283, 1967.

19. Carr J: Mental and motor development in young mongol children, J Ment Defic Res 14:205, 1970.

20. Coleman M: Down's syndrome, Pediatr Ann 7:90, 1978.

21. Conen PE and Erkman B: Frequency and occurrence of chromosomal syndromes. I. D-trisomy, Am J Hum Genet 18:374, 1966.

22. Conen PE and Erkman B: Frequency and occurrence of chromosomal syndromes. II. E-trisomy, Am J Human Genet 18:387, 1966.

23. Cowie VA: Neurological aspects of the early development of mongols, Clin Proc Child Hosp DC 23:64, 1967.

24. Cowie VA: A study of the early development of mongols, Oxford, 1970, Pergamon Press, Ltd.

25. Critchley M and Earl CJC: Tuberose sclerosis and allied conditions, Brain 55:311, 1932.

26. Crome L: Pathology of Down's disease. In Hilliard LT and Kirman BH, editors: Mental deficiency, ed 2, Boston, 1965, Little, Brown & Co.

27. Crome L and Stern J: Pathology of mental retardation, ed 2, Edinburgh, 1972, Churchill Livingstone.

28. Crome L and others: A statistical note on cerebellar and brainstem weight in mongolism, J Ment Defic Res 10:69, 1966.

29. Crowe FW and others: A clinical, pathological, and genetic study of multiple neurofibromatosis, Springfield, Ill, 1956, Charles C Thomas, Publisher.

30. Cullum L and Liebman J: The association of congenital heart disease with Down's syndrome (mongolism), Am J Cardiol 24:354, 1969.

31. Cusick B and Sussman M: Short leg casts: their role in the management of cerebral palsy, Phys Occup Ther Ped 2:93, 1982.

32. Department of Governmental Relations, The Council for Exceptional Children: New federal early intervention program under PL 99-457, Reston, Va, 1986.

33. Ford CE and others: The chromosomes in a patient showing both mongolism and Klinefelter syndrome, Lancet 1:709, 1959.

34. Goldberg MJ: The dysmorphic child: an orthopedic perspective, New York, 1987, Raven Press.

35. Gorlin RJ: Classical chromosome disorders. In Yunis J, editor: New chromosomal syndromes, New York, 1977, Academic Press, Inc.

36. Griffiths R: The abilities of young children: a comprehensive system for mental measurement for the first eight years of life, London, 1970, Child Development Research Centre.

37. Hall D: Mongolism in newborn infants, Clin Pediatr 5:90, 1978.

38. Hanson MJ and Harris SR: Teaching the young child with motor delay: a guide for parents and professionals, Austin, Tex, 1986, PRO-ED.

39. Harris SR: Transdisciplinary therapy model for the infant with Down's syndrome, Phys Ther 60:420, 1980.

40. Harris SR: Effects of neurodevelopmental therapy on motor performance of infants with Down's syndrome, Dev Med Child Neur 23:477, 1981.

41. Harris SR: Early intervention: does developmental therapy make a difference? Top Early Child Spec Ed 7(4):20, 1988.

42. Harris SR and Tada WL: Providing developmental therapy services. In Garwood SG and Fewell RR, editors: Educating handicapped infants, Rockville, Md, 1983, Aspen Systems Corp.

43. Haslam RHA: Neurological disorders. In Smith DW, editor: Introduction to clinical pediatrics, ed 2, Philadelphia, 1977, WB Saunders Co.

44. Herndon CN: Osteogenesis imperfecta: some clinical and genetic considerations, Clin Orthop 8:132, 1956.

45. Hirschhorn K and others: Deletion of short arms of chromosome 4-5 in a child with defects of midline fusion, Humangenitik 1:479, 1965.

46. Hoffenberg R and Jackson WPU: Gonadal dysgenesis: modern concepts, Br Med J 2:1457, 1957.

47. Holmes LB and others: Mental retardation: an atlas of diseases with associated physical abnormalities, New York, 1972, Macmillan Publishing Co, Inc.

48. Holvey DN, editor: The Merck manual of diagnosis and therapy, Rahway, NJ, 1972, Merck & Co, Inc.

49. Hudson LH and Cox TR: Brown-Séquard syndrome with bilateral elephantiasis in neurofibromatosis, JAMA 161:326, 1956.

50. Hunt JC and Pugh DG: Skeletal lesions in neurofibromatosis, Radiology 76:1, 1961.

51. Johnson VP and others: The Wolf-Hirschhorn (4p−) syndrome, Clin Genet 10:104, 1976.

52. Kelley WN: Hypoxanthine-guanine phosphoribosyltransferase deficiency in the Lesch-Nyhan syndrome and gout, Fed Proc 27:1047, 1968.

53. Klinefelter HF Jr and others: Gynecomastia, aspermatogenesis without aLeydigism, and increased excretion of follicle-stimulating hormone, J Clin Endocrinol 2:615, 1946.

54. Knobloch H and Pasamanick B, editors: Gesell and Amatruda's developmental diagnosis: the evaluation and management of normal and abnormal neuropsychologic development in infancy and early childhood, ed 3, New York, 1974, Harper & Row, Publishers, Inc.

55. Know WE: Phenylketonuria. In Stanbury JB and others, editors: The metabolic basis of inherited disease, ed 3, New York, 1972, McGraw-Hill Book Co.

56. Koehler J: Spinal muscular atrophy of childhood. In Bleck EE and Nagel DA, editors: Physically handicapped children: a medical atlas for teachers, New York, 1975, Grune & Stratton, Inc.

57. Lejeune J: Le Mongolisme. Premier exemple d'aberration autosomique humane, Ann Genet 1:41, 1959.

58. Lejeune J and others: Trois cas de délétion partielle du bras court d'un chromosome 5, Compt rend Acad Sc (Paris) 257:3098, 1963.

59. Lesch M and Nyhan WL: A familial disorder of uric acid metabolism and central nervous system function, Am J Med 36:561, 1964.

60. Levin B: Gonadal dysgenesis: clinical and roentgenologic manifestations, Am J Roentgenol 87:1116, 1962.

61. Levinson A and others: Variability of mongolism, Pediatrics 16:43, 1955.

62. Loesch-Mdzewska D: Some aspects of neurology of Down's syndrome, J Ment Defic Res 12:237, 1968.

63. Lowe CU and others: Organic aciduria, decreased renal ammonia production, hydropthalmos, and mental retardation, Am J Dis Child 83:164, 1952.

64. Marin-Padilla M: Pyramidal cell abnormalities in the motor cortex of

a child with Down's syndrome: a Golgi study, J Comp Neurol 167:63, 1976.

65. Marks JF and others: Lesch-Nyhan syndrome treated from the early neonatal period, Pediatrics 42:357, 1968.

66. McCusick VA: Mendelian inheritance in man: catalogs of autosomal dominants, autosomal recessives, and X-linked phenotypes, Baltimore, 1966, Johns Hopkins University Press.

67. McGraw MB: The neuromuscular maturation of the human infant, New York, 1966, Hafer.

68. Melyn MA and White DT: Mental and developmental milestones of noninstitutionalized Down's syndrome children, Pediatrics 52:542, 1973.

69. Mikamo K: Sex chromosomal anomalies in newborn infants, Obstet Gynecol 32:688, 1968.

70. Money J and Alexander D: Turner's syndrome: further demonstration of the presence of specific perceptual deficits, J Med Genet 3:47, 1966.

71. Myhre SA and others: The effects of testosterone treatment in Klinefelter's syndrome, J Pediatr 76:267, 1970.

72. Nagel DA: Temporary orthopedic disabilities in children. In Bleck EE and Nagel DA, editors: Physically handicapped children: a medical atlas for teachers, New York, 1975, Grune & Stratton, Inc.

73. Novitski E: Human genetics, New York, 1977, Macmillan Publishing Co, Inc.

74. Nyhan WL: Clinical features of Lesch-Nyhan syndrome. Introduction—clinical and genetic features, Fed Proc 27:1027, 1968.

75. O'Neill DL and Harris SR: Developing goals and objectives for handicapped children, Phys Ther 62:295, 1982.

76. Patau K and others: Multiple congenital anomaly caused by an extra chromosome, Lancet 1:790, 1960.

77. Pescia G and The HN, editors: Chorionic villi sampling (CVS), Contrib Gynecol Obstet 15:1, 1986.

78. Penrose LS and Smith GF: Down's anomaly, London, 1966, Churchill.

79. Public Law 94-142. Education for all handicapped children act of 1975 (S.6), 94th Congress, 1st Session, 1975.

80. Rainier-Pope CR and others: Cardiovascular malformations in Turner's syndrome, Pediatrics 33:919, 1964.

81. Robinson NM and Robinson HB, editors: The mentally retarded child: a psychological approach, New York, 1976, McGraw-Hill Book Co.

82. Rubin A: Handbook of congenital malformations, Philadelphia, 1967, WB Saunders Co.

83. Rubinstein TH: Cranial abnormalities. In Carter CH, editor: Medical aspects of mental retardation, ed 2, Springfield, Ill, 1978, Charles C Thomas, Publisher.

84. Schneegans E and others: Un cas de maladie du cri du chat. D'aael'aaetion partielle du bras court du chromosome 5, Pédiatrie 21:823, 1966.

85. Scott CR: Inborn enzymatic errors. In Smith DW, editor: Introduction to clinical pediatrics, ed 2, Philadelphia, 1977, WB Saunders Co.

86. Semans S: The Bobath concept in treatment of neurologic disorders, Am J Phys Med 46:732, 1967.

87. Smith DW: Clinical diagnosis and nature of chromosomal abnormalities. In Yunis, J, editor: New chromosomal syndromes, New York, 1977, Academic Press, Inc.

88. Smith DW: Recognizable patterns of human malformation, ed 3, Philadelphia, 1982, WB Saunders Co.

89. Solnit A and Stark M: Mourning and the birth of a defective child. In Menolascino FJ, editor: Psychiatric aspects of the diagnosis and treatment of mental retardation, Seattle, 1971, Special Child Publications.

90. Sternat J and others: Occupational and physical therapy services for severely handicapped students: toward a naturalized public school service delivery model. In Sontag E: Educational programming for the severely and profoundly handicapped, Reston, Va, 1977, Council for Exceptional Children.

91. Sussman MD and Cusick B: Preliminary report: the role of short-leg, tone-reducing casts as an adjunct to physical therapy of patients with cerebral palsy, Johns Hopkins Med J 154:112, 1979.

92. Turner HH: A syndrome of infantilism, congenital webbed neck, and cubitus valgus, Endocrinology 23:566, 1938.

93. Warkany J and others: Congenital malformations in autosomal trisomy syndromes, Am J Dis Child 112:502, 1966.

94. Warkany J: Congenital malformations, Chicago, 1971, Year Book Medical Publishers, Inc.

95. Werch A: Amniocentesis: indications, techniques, and complications, South Med J 69:894, 1976.

96. Whaley WJ and Gray WD: Atlanto-axial dislocation and Down's syndrome, Can Med Assoc J 123:35, 1980.

97. Wolf U and others: Deficiency an den kurzen Armen eines Chromosomes Nr 4, Humangenitik 1:397, 1965.

Chapter 11

LEARNING DISABILITIES

Sharon A. Cermak and Anne Henderson

AN OVERVIEW OF LEARNING DISABILITIES
Characteristics

Difficulties in learning may manifest themselves in various combinations of impairment in perception, conceptualization, language, memory, and control of attention, impulses, or motor functions.[70,111] The symptomatology of a child with learning disabilities is diverse and varied. All of the symptoms are not present in all children, and the symptoms that are present vary in degree of severity from child to child.

The most commonly recognized deficits in learning are those that pertain to academic success. In most instances, attention has been given to deficits in verbal learning, including deficits in the learning of arithmetic, in the acquisition of spoken and written language, and in reading. However, there are deficits in nonverbal learning that are equally important, such as disturbances in directional con-

cepts (e.g., right and left, up and down) and body orientation, in the meanings of facial expressions and the behaviors of others, and in music and rhythm.[153,246]

In addition to disorders in the perceptual, conceptual, language, or academic areas, children with learning disabilities often have correlated behavioral disorders that include hyperactivity, lack of attention, and general maladaptive behavior.[4,172] The 10 characteristics most often reported by clinicians of the child with learning disabilities are: hyperactivity, perceptual-motor impairment, emotional lability, general coordination deficits, disorders of attention (short attention span, distractibility, perseveration), impulsiveness, disorders of memory and thinking (concept formation and problem solving), specific learning disabilities (reading, arithmetic, or spelling), disorders of speech and hearing, and soft neurological signs.[211]

Definition. Many disciplines have focused on the child with learning disabilities, and each has described the problem according to its own frame of reference. Because numerous names and labels have been given to children who experience difficulties in learning,[4,45,46,111,189] there is a great deal of confusion about terminology in the literature.[242] In general, the terms fall into two broad categories: etiological and behavioral.[4,172] Medical professionals tend to label the disability in terms of cause, and they generally relate it to a deficit in the brain, particularly to cerebral dysfunction. Terms such as *brain-injured*,[283] *minimal brain dysfunction*,[70] and *psychoneurological disorder*[219] imply a neurological cause as an explanation for the deviation in development.

Educators tend to describe the child's disability in behavioral terms that address the disordered function rather than identify the cause, even though some of the terms may imply a CNS deficit. These terms include *perceptual handicap, perceptual-motor deficit, clumsy child syndrome, conceptual disability, reading disability* or *dyslexia, hyperkinetic disorder,* and *learning disability.* Regardless of the terminology, adequate motor ability, average to high intelligence, adequate hearing and vision, and adequate emotional adjustment together with a deficiency in learning are the salient features that constitute the basis for homogeneity.[153]

The term that is used in this chapter as a general name for this type of dysfunction is *learning disabilities.* This includes children with minimal brain dysfunction, although not all learning-disabled (LD) children have been identified as having minimal brain dysfunction. The definition of learning disabilities that is accepted by the United States Office of Education and the National Advisory Committee on Handicapped Children and that is also accepted for the purposes of this chapter states that:

Children with specific learning disabilities exhibit a disorder in one or more of the basic psychological processes involved in understanding or using spoken or written language. These may be manifested in disorders of listening, thinking, talking, reading, writing, spelling or arithmetic. They include conditions which have been referred to as perceptual handicaps, brain injury, minimal brain dysfunction, dyslexia, developmental aphasia, etc. They do not include learning problems which are primarily due to visual, hearing, or motor handicaps, to mental retardation, emotional disturbance or to environmental disadvantage (p. 322).[51]

This definition of learning disabilities has been controversial, and new definitions have been proposed by various organizations.[4] For example, the National Joint Committee for Learning Disabilities (NJCLD), which consists of seven major organizations concerned with learning problems, felt that the definition adopted by the United States Congress was confusing, ambiguous, and too restrictive and proposed the following definition:

Learning disabilities is a generic term that refers to a heterogeneous group of disorders manifested by significant difficulties in the acquisition and use of listening, speaking, reading, writing, reasoning or mathematical abilities. These disorders are intrinsic to the individual and presumed to be due to central nervous system dysfunction. Even though a learning disability may occur concomitantly with other handicapping conditions (e.g., sensory impairment, mental retardation, social and emotional disturbance) or environmental influences, it is not the direct result of those conditions or influences (p. 336).[135]

The NJCLD proposed definition was adopted by six of its seven member organizations. However, the Association for Children and Adults with Learning Disabilities (ACLD) refused to accept the NJCLD definition, and in 1984 proposed the following definition:

Specific learning disabilities is a chronic condition of presumed neurological origin which selectively interferes with the development, integration, and/or demonstration of verbal and/or nonverbal abilities.

Specific learning disabilities exists as a distinct handicapping condition in the presence of average to superior intelligence, adequate sensory and motor systems, and adequate learning opportunities. The condition varies in its manifestations and in degree of severity.

Throughout life, the condition can affect self-esteem, education, vocation, socialization, and/or daily living activities.[181]

What is interesting is that both the NJCLD and the ACLD definitions suggest, as did most early leaders in the field, that learning disabilities result from CNS dysfunction—minor neurological problems that interfere with effective processing. The legal definition, however, does not refer to proposed etiology, and thus is not restricted to those with such problems. The legal definition and the ACLD definition exclude individuals with visual, hearing, or motor handicaps, emotional disturbance, environmental deprivation, or mental retardation from being considered to have a learning disability, but the NJCLD states that although a learning disability is not the direct result of these conditions or influences, it may occur concomitantly with them. Finally, a unique feature of the ACLD definitions is its emphasis that the condition persists into and throughout adulthood and that it may influence not only school achievement but also areas such as self-esteem, daily living skills, family and community living, and vocation.

Incidence. The incidence of children with learning disabilities is estimated at from 1% to 30% of the school population, depending on the criteria used to determine the disability.[4,183,254,310] A more conservative estimate has been made by the National Advisory Committee on Handicapped Children, which estimated that the incidence of children with significant learning disabilities constituted approximately 1% to 3% of the school population.[172] Whichever estimate is used, it is clear that a tremendous number of children are involved.

Students diagnosed as learning disabled are currently the largest percentage of enrollments in special education programs.[4] Most observers agree that learning problems are far more common in boys than in girls. In general, learning disabilities occur at least five times more frequently in males than in females, although some writers have extended the ratio to as high as 10:1.[153]

Subtypes. The search for the single description of learning disabilities has not been successful. Rourke[247] has stated that "the confusion that abounds in the literature dealing with the group of clinical problems known as learning disabilities is, in many ways, a direct reflection of the failure of many scientists and practitioners in this field to acknowledge and address the heterogeneity and diversity extant among the learning disabled population." It is now recognized that subgroups of children with learning disabilities exist who manifest differing clusters of deficiencies in higher cortical functions.[193] There is growing evidence that children with learning disabilities show different patterns of disorders.* However, the categorization of learning disabilities appears to vary largely with the orientation of the researcher, the types of observations made, and the age and nature of the sample.[247]

Based on neurological examinations of 190 children with learning disabilities, Denckla[92] indicated that certain clusters or symptom complexes emerged from the more frequent signs of minimal brain dysfunction. She found that about 30% of the children could be divided into three subgroups based on easily recognizable clusters of signs; 70% showed an unclassifiable mixture. Of the 30%, the first subgroup was classified as children having specific language disability. These children, who were failing in reading and spelling, showed a pattern of inadequacy on repetition, sequencing, memory, language, motor, and other tasks, all of which required rote functioning. The second group had what was termed a *specific visuospatial disability*: they were children with at least average performance in reading and spelling who were poor in arithmetic, who were seriously inadequate in writing and copying, and who were all socially and/or emotionally maladjusted. The third group manifested a dyscontrol syndrome and included children who had poor motor and impulse control, who were behaviorally immature, and who were normal in language and perceptual functioning.

Mattis and others[193] identified three groups among children with reading retardation: a language disordered (anomic) group, a group exhibiting articulatory and graphomotor dyscoordination, and a group showing a visuospatial-perceptual disorder. On the basis of the analysis of the type of spelling error, Boder[48] identified three types of dyslexia: children with dysphonic dyslexia have a basic deficiency in letter-sound integration and in learning phonetically; children with dysdeitic dyslexia have a basic difficulty in perceiving words as gestalts; and children with dysphonetic-dysdeitic dyslexia manifest difficulty both in phonetic analysis and whole-word learning.

In a series of factor analysis studies and clinical observations, Ayres[12-14,17,21,29] identified a number of different types of sensory integration dysfunction that characterize some children with learning disabilities. One type of disorder is tactile defensiveness, which is characterized by an aversive response to certain types of tactile stimuli. Another type of disorder is developmental dyspraxia, a motor planning deficit that is usually associated with dysfunction in tactile perception. A number of different types of vestibular dysfunction have also been reported, including shortened duration of postrotary nystagmus, gravitational insecurity, and postural and ocular dysfunction. In addition, a disorder characterized by shortened duration of postrotary nystagmus and bilateral integration problems has been identified.

Through subtype analysis, Strang and Rourke[282] have

identified a type of learning-disabled child who has many of the same characteristics as children seen for occupational and physical therapy services. Academically, this child is characterized primarily by problems in mechanical arithmetic (as compared with spelling, reading, and 'automatic' [overlearned] language skills all of which are in the average range). Neuropsychological assessment indicated difficulty in complex tactile perceptual abilities and in psychomotor performance. Left-hand performance was particularly impaired as were visual-perceptual organizational skills and handwriting. Social skills were also inadequate. Strang and Rourke[282] referred to this as the "nonverbal perceptual-organizational-output disability" (NPOOD). These children exhibit many of the same characteristics as do the dyspraxic children described by Ayres.

Some researchers, in attempting to identify types of learning disabilities, have drawn on research with adult patients with brain damage that used the Wechsler Adult Intelligence Scale (WAIS). This scale yields both a "verbal IQ" (based primarily on language tasks) and a "performance IQ" (based primarily on visual-perceptual tasks and perceptual-motor tasks). Research with adults with brain damage found that patients with left hemisphere damage tended to show a low-verbal–high-performance WAIS profile and language deficits. Those patients with right hemisphere dysfunction showed predominantly visuoconstructive deficits and a WAIS profile of high-verbal–low-performance. Subgroups of learning disabled children ages 9 to 14 have also been identified on the bases of the pattern of their Wechsler Intelligence Scale for Children (WISC) scores.[159,246,248,249] The performance of the high-verbal–low-performance group was superior to that of the high-performance–low-verbal group on those tasks involving verbal, language, and auditory-perceptual skills. In contrast, the performance of the high-performance–low-verbal group was superior to that of the high-verbal–low-performance group on tasks that primarily involved visual-perceptual skills. The investigators suggested that the WISC verbal/performance discrepancy reflected the differential integrity of the two cerebral hemispheres in older children with learning disabilities. However, these same patterns were not identified in the younger children with learning disabilities. Some researchers believe that it is particularly difficult to draw inferences about brain function based on behavioral responses in children and that pattern analysis (e.g., WISC verbal/performance discrepancies) is very difficult in children since the relationship between performance on tests and subtests often does not correspond to specific types of CNS dysfunction in the same fashion as is exhibited by adults.

In a recent text on subtype analysis of learning disabilities, attempts are made to identify subgroups of learning disabilities within different academic areas such as reading,[96] spelling,[284] and arithmetic.[282] In addition, personal-

---

*References 12, 13, 14, 17, 18, 21, 44, 50, 70, 77, 92, 247, 256.

ity and socioemotional dimensions of learning disabilities are examined through subtype analysis.[231,236,282]

Clinical observations by educators, therapists, and researchers suggest that learning disability is not a unitary syndrome but that it is heterogeneous in nature.[16,92,101,193] This has resulted in numerous categorization systems. The relationship between these various systems has been only minimally explored; there is no one, agreed-on classification, although for some time it has been recognized that children with learning disabilities need to be classified into subgroups in order to best plan appropriate treatment interventions.*

Summary. A great deal of attention has been focused on the definition of *learning disabilities,* and many attempts have been made to identify different "types" of learning disabilities. Recent research has attempted to relate brain mechanisms to the different types of learning disabilities. According to Rourke,[246,247] an important problem is whether and to what extent dysfunction at the level of the cerebral hemispheres causes learning disabilities. Etiological considerations of learning disabilities contribute to the understanding of the nature of developmental cerebral dysfunction and they have very practical applications.[246] A number of theories about learning disabilities have been proposed. These are discussed in the following sections, with greatest emphasis given to those theories that consider the role of brain function.

Brain dysfunction theories

Numerous hypotheses have been proposed about the causes of learning disabilities, including those related to psychosocial/emotional causes and those related to neurological causes. For example, Peck and Stackhouse[234] hypothesized that children with reading disabilities were experiencing difficulties as a result of familial conflict. Bannatyne[31] stated that there is a type of dyslexia, termed *primary emotional communicative dyslexia,* that results from a poor communicative (language) relationship between the mother and infant.

Other researchers hypothesize that learning disabilities result from an interaction of organic and nonorganic factors.[200] Keough[162] suggested that hyperactive children may have different conceptual styles than nonhyperactive children. Other investigators suggested that situational influences play an important role in eliciting maladaptive behavior in children with brain damage, and they have suggested that the behavior is not maladaptive because of the brain damage, but rather that such children are likely to find themselves in situations in which they are continuously frustrated in achieving their hopes and aspirations.[197]

Although some researchers have emphasized emotional and social causes of learning disabilities, the majority of

*References 12, 13, 24, 29, 141, 247.

recent research has focused on the role of neurological factors in learning disability. In general, however, the cause of learning disabilities is presently unknown. It is likely to be multifactorial and heterogeneous with no single cause sufficient to explain the varied symptomatology. In addition, cause may well be multiple even in any one child assessed. Diverse causes have received varying degrees of empirical support but none has been demonstrated to exist for all learning disabled/minimal brain dysfunction children.[144,302] Frequently studied etiological factors include: (1) brain damage or dysfunction from such causes as birth injury, perinatal anoxia, head injury, fetal malnutrition, encephalitis, and lead poisoning; (2) allergies; (3) biochemical abnormalities or metabolic disorders; (4) genetics; (5) maturational lag; and (6) environmental factors, such as neglect and abuse, a disorganized home, and inadequate stimulation.[101,291]

Because learning disabilities are frequently associated with neuropsychological symptoms, such as disorders of speech, lateral dominance, spatial orientation, perception, coordination, and activity level, and because neuropsychological deficits tend to occur concomitantly, various researchers have attempted to identify aspects of the brain that may be dysfunctional. A number of these theories will be discussed, but it must be recognized that theories of brain dysfunction are, to some extent, speculative.[179] Many of these theories of the cause of learning disabilities have been based on experimental studies of animals, studies of adults who have received gunshot wounds or other forms of cerebral trauma, research on epileptics who have undergone brain surgery and, more recently, research that has been implemented through the use of specific techniques, such as CT scans and magnetic resonance imaging (MRI).

Left-hemisphere maturational lag or damage. Some researchers have suggested that reading problems are a result of a lag in the lateralization of the cerebral hemispheres, particularly the left hemisphere.[256,274,275] Patterns of behavioral deficits in children with dyslexic learning disabilities (including right-left confusion, finger agnosia, calculation difficulty, writing difficulty, visuoconstructive impairment, depressed verbal intelligence, and reading problems) are quite similar to those of adults who have sustained damage to the left cerebral hemisphere.[116] In addition, dyslexic children, as well as patients with lesions restricted to the left inferior parietal cortex, show impaired performance in cross-modal tasks, particularly auditory-visual ones.

In support of the hypothesis that retarded readers demonstrate a lack of specialization of the language-dominant (left) hemisphere, researchers found that poor readers did not show the normal pattern of right visual field (left-hemisphere) superiority for word recognition.[127,190,223] Some dichotic listening studies have also shown that children with reading problems have diminished lateralization of language and linguistic auditory function in the left hemisphere.[22,63,310]

Although there exists a similar pattern of behavioral deficits in dyslexic children and adults with a brain injury to the left hemisphere,[256] several researchers have postulated that in dyslexic children there is a delay in the lateral development of the functions of the left hemisphere, rather than damage to the left hemisphere.[256,274,275] These authors have suggested that there is a maturational lag in the differentiation of motor, somatosensory, and language functions subserved by the dominant left hemisphere, and they further suggest that the pattern of deficits observed in dyslexic children resembles the behavioral patterns of chronologically younger normal children rather than representing a unique syndrome of disturbance. Geschwind and Galaburda[117] have proposed an elaborate model in which underdevelopment of the left hemisphere is attributed to the effects of testosterone, which selectively inhibits maturation of the left hemisphere. Recently, an abnormal cellular organization in a portion of the left hemisphere was identified at autopsy in the brain of a person with dyslexia.[112,113]

Lack of hemispheric specialization. Specialization of function of the cerebral hemispheres is generally considered an optimal neural basis for learning.[18] Whether a possible cause for learning disorders is the failure of one hemisphere to establish "dominance" for language and skilled hand usage and of the other hemisphere for visuospatial skill has long been a controversial issue. Ayres[14] suggested that in some children with learning disabilities, the two hemispheres do not specialize in their functions and thus develop similar functions, with neither hemisphere being as effective. Levy and others[187] reviewed a number of studies that support the hypothesis that development of language function in both hemispheres is achieved at the expense of the development of visual-spatial-perceptual-skills.

While many researchers have hypothesized that learning-disabled children have left-hemisphere dysfunction as a result of developmental lag or focal damage, Witelson[304] has hypothesized that these children have bilateral representation for spatial function rather than representation of spatial function in the right hemisphere as seen in normal children. Specifically, she suggested that the left hemisphere does not exhibit the "normal" focal organization but rather exhibits the right hemisphere type of diffuse organization as described by Semmes.[260] As a result, children with learning disabilities tend to use predominantly spatial, parallel, holistic modes of processing. This leads to poor performance on such linguistic tasks as reading, which demands sequential analysis.

Inadequate interhemispheric communication. The importance of adequate communication between the two sides of the brain, particularly between the cerebral hemispheres, has been emphasized frequently in theories that propose that reading is a process that requires the active participation of both hemispheres and the transfer of information between them.* Gazzaniga[115] suggests that some aspects of minimal brain dysfunction may reflect problems in the "shuttling of information between various specialized processing centers in the brain." Myklebust[220] states that the primary deficit of some learning-disabled children is an impairment of the ability of one hemisphere to communicate with the other; this is reflected cognitively by the child's inability to convert verbal learning (left hemisphere) into nonverbal meanings (right hemisphere) and to convert nonverbal learning into verbal meanings. Frostig[110] also reports that disturbances caused by a deficit in integrative functions (between the hemispheres), particularly lack of integration of verbal and nonverbal functions, are frequent among children with learning disabilities. Hardy and others[137] have shown that auditory-to-visual processing is critical to academic achievement.

Support for the hypothesis of impaired interhemispheric communication comes from computer analysis of brain wave patterns of dyslexic children that show a consistent abnormality in interrelations between the two hemispheres and within the dominant hemisphere.[273] Further support comes from a tachistoscopic study in which right visual half-field scores were at about the same level of accuracy for both poor and good readers while the poor readers showed considerable deficit in their left visual half-field scores.[308] In the latter study, because the material presented was linguistic in nature and because the response mode was verbal, these authors suggested that the poor readers might suffer from some form of processing deficit in the right hemisphere or that the transmission from the right to the left hemisphere was degraded. Gross and others[127] found that students with reading disabilities showed a greater difference between thresholds for left and right hemifield stimuli than normal readers. They suggested that this perceptual asymmetry may reflect inefficient interhemispheric transfer of visual information.

Adequacy of interhemispheric communication has also been assessed using motor tasks. Badian and Wolff[30] examined motor sequencing abilities in boys 8 to 15 years old with reading disabilities, using both single-hand tapping and alternating-hand tapping. The authors found that in the single-hand trials, boys with reading disabilities tapped as well as boys without reading disabilities. However, the boys with the disability showed marked deterioration of performance when tapping with two hands in alternation, resulting primarily from the left hand's performance. The authors suggest that the motor sequencing deficit was the result of inadequate interhemispheric cooperation necessary to coordinate control over the motor actions in the left hand (right hemisphere) and hemispheric specialization for temporal sequencing (left hemisphere).

*References 62, 115, 235, 296-298, 308.

Inadequate intersensory integration. Because reading is a task that requires translation from an auditory to a visual code and vice versa,[107] Birch and Belmont[42] suggested that reading impairment is a failure of cross-modal (visual-auditory or auditory-visual) integration. They compared intersensory and intrasensory functions in normal groups and in groups with brain damage. Although the two groups did not differ from one another in their intrasensory abilities, a significant impairment in intersensory integration existed in the group with brain damage. Other researchers compared intersensory integration between normal and disabled readers and also found the reading disabled to be significantly impaired.[42,43,72,215,252] Vellutino and others[297] believe that poor readers did not have visual-perceptual deficits as proposed by Orton,[224] Kephart,[163] and others, but rather find it difficult to integrate and/or retrieve the verbal equivalent of input in the form of visual representation.

Although data support the hypothesis of intermodal difficulty, Bryant[55] pointed out that because intrasensory controls had not always been run, there was no evidence regarding the adequacy of intramodal functions. Indeed, recent studies of audiovisual pattern-matching have indicated that retarded readers were impaired intramodally as well as between modalities.*

Sensory integration dysfunction. Ayres[16,18,20,25,29] views learning disorders as a reflection of deviation in neural function and hypothesizes that certain types of learning disorders are a result of dysfunction in the ability to organize and interpret sensory information. This dysfunction has been termed *sensory integration dysfunction.* Ayres[25] has suggested that higher-level perception, language, and cognition are dependent on the ability of the brainstem/midbrain to organize and integrate sensory processes. Normal development is considered dependent on intersensory integration, particularly from the somatosensory and vestibular senses. This processing is considered significant because of the phylogenetically and ontogenetically early development of these systems and because of the many interconnections of the vestibular and tactile system throughout the brain. The functioning of these systems is considered to affect the functioning of the brain as a whole. Impairment in this processing can result in immature postural reactions, poor eye/motor control, and motor planning problems, and it can also result in language and learning disabilities. Elaboration of this theory is presented in the treatment section. This theory is especially useful to therapists because it provides an organizing framework for treatment.

Summary. Various researchers have attempted to explain the underlying nature of learning disabilities, and various theories of learning disabilities have been proposed, including psychological and/or social explanations

*References 56, 196, 215, 252, 278, 295, 311.

as possible causative factors. However, the majority of theorists have suggested that learning disabilities are the result of some type of brain dysfunction, with an emphasis placed on anomalous hemispheric specialization. After a review of the findings, however, Hiscock and Kinsbourne[144] concluded that "there is very little reason to believe that behavioral skill is in any way correlated with hemispheric specialization." These authors emphasized that "the heterogeneity of learning disabilities militates against a single etiology" and suggested that "the neural basis of learning disorders appears to be brain pathology rather than anomalous brain organization per se." In contrast, Geschwind and Galaburda[117] feel that it may be the anomalous dominance that causes both dyslexia as well as neonatal and birth problems.

A multidisciplinary approach to learning disabilities

Evaluation and treatment of the learning-disabled child are essentially interdisciplinary procedures since the complex cause of learning disabilities results in differing constellations of problems and since remediation is beyond the competency of any individual professional group. Most learning disabled children are seen by a group of professionals, the make-up of which depends on the purpose, the location, the philosophical orientation, or the available resources of a particular program. The box on p. 289 lists the different professionals and specialists within professions who might participate in assessment or remediation of learning disabilities. The types of professionals are grouped into the four categories of education, medicine, psychology, and special services, and they have been listed only once although some professions could be categorized more than one way. Indeed, the number of potential professional disciplines is enormous.

The label of learning disability is given to a child if he/she has a primary problem in academic learning. Furthermore, the management of learning disabilities takes place most commonly in a school setting. Therefore the center of a child's program is education, and a number of educational specialists have emerged to meet programming needs. Categories of educators include those teaching children directly and those evaluating and/or supervising teaching.

In some educational settings, children with learning disabilities are given full-time instruction in a special classroom with a small group of other learning-disabled children. A special education teacher or a learning disability teacher is in charge of the classroom. More commonly, the child is placed in a regular classroom and leaves his/her class for special instruction for some part of the day. He/she may go to a resource room, where a special education teacher provides regularly scheduled remedial education for children with a variety of educational handicaps, or he/she may receive tutoring from a reading specialist or a private tutor. In any of these patterns the educational program

---

Types of specialists working with learning disabled children

Education

Classroom teacher
Special educator
Learning disability
   specialist
Psychoeducational
   diagnostician
Reading specialist
Early childhood
   education teacher
Physical educator
Adaptive physical
   educator

Medicine and nursing

Family physician
Pediatrician
Pediatric neurologist
Psychiatrist
School nurse
Biochemist
Geneticist
Endocrinologist
Electroencephalogist
Nutritionist
Ophthamologist
Otologist

Psychology

Clinical psychologist
Neuropsychologist
School psychologist
Child psychologist
Counseling psychologist
Guidance counselor

Special services

Occupational therapist
Physical therapist
Speech and language
   pathologist
Psycholinguist
Audiologist
Optometrist
Social worker
Recreational therapist
Motor therapist
Perceptual-motor trainer
Vocational education
   specialist

---

done by clinical psychologists, school psychologists, or clinical neuropsychologists who specialize in diagnosis of learning disorders with an organic base. The second role of psychologists is to provide mental health service. Children with learning disabilities often have problems with self-esteem and peer relationships, resulting from either primary behavior problems or from reactions to failure.

A learning-disabled child with a primary behavior problem, such as impulsiveness, disinhibited behavior, or hyperkinetic activity, may receive special treatment for the behavior disorder. A behavior modification specialist may be working with parents and teachers to help the child control his/her behavior. The child may receive psychotherapy from a psychologist or psychiatrist, or family therapy may be provided by a social worker, psychologist, or psychiatrist. These latter interventions are usually provided by public or private mental health clinics. Learning-disabled children with general adjustment problems in peer relationships are often treated within the school setting. School adjustment or guidance counselors offer support and advice on specific academic difficulties, social conflicts, and affective issues. The school psychologist, in addition to the diagnostic role, may offer psychological counseling to students and may help plan strategies for classroom management. Alternatively, the child may be seen outside of the school program by a psychiatrist or psychologist.

Among the professionals listed in the box at left as providing special services, a number are concerned with motor and perceptual-motor education. The physical therapist is primarily concerned with, although not limited to, the purely motor and postural functions and efficient use of the body. The occupational therapist has similar concerns for the postural basis of movement but stresses fine motor abilities, sensory integration, visual, spatial, and perceptual functions, and activities of daily living. Within the educational system, in addition to physical educators, are a group of perceptual-motor specialists, often special educators, who have received training in the techniques devised by Kephart and other perceptual-motor theorists. Finally optometrists, whose special concern is visual functions, such as visual acuity, visual perception, visual memory, and visual motor learning, may provide perceptual-motor training programs.

In other areas of function, speech and/or language therapists serve children who have problems with stuttering, vocabulary, word finding, articulation, sound sequencing, auditory attention, as well as the comprehension and processing of complex language. Audiologists are concerned with hearing, auditory perception, and auditory training. A related area of language study is psycholinguistics, which combines psychology and linguistics in the study of how language is acquired. This has also been applied to the educational setting.

The liaison between the child's family and the various service organizations may be a social worker. Social work-

might be supervised by a psychoeducational specialist or a learning disabilities specialist in consultative positions. These professionals are specialists in educational measurement and are involved in psychoeducational diagnosis as a basis for planning remedial education. Within the school system are the physical educators, both those generally trained and the adaptive physical educator who works with the child with handicaps.

Since therapists are familiar with the roles of the various medical specialists and of primary care physicians, these specialists will not be described here. School nursing is mentioned, however, because it is a specialty within nursing. The school nurse is usually the key health professional in a school system and is responsible for maintaining information about the child's health history, current health status, medication, home environment, family cooperation, and family problems. The school nurse is the primary liaison between the child and the doctor or health clinic and relays information from the school to medical professionals.

Psychologists have two distinct and often separate roles in the management of learning disorders. The first role is in psychodiagnosis. Psychological testing is essential in the identification of specific learning problems and may be ers may also provide family therapy or serve as program coordinators. Finally, recreational therapists or vocational education specialists may be available to provide their special services.

While a single child is rarely seen by all of these professionals, a child with multiple problems may see many specialists. As an example, we describe the program of Paul, a learning-disabled child.

CASE STUDY: PAUL

Paul, an 8-year-old boy, came to the Sargent College Occupational Therapy Clinic at Boston University because of the severe motor coordination problems that accompanied his learning disability. In addition to Paul's weekly treatment sessions, suggestions were made to his mother for a home program to be done two to three times a week for 15 to 30 minutes each time. Meanwhile, Paul also received other services. Although he was mainstreamed into a regular classroom in accordance with the special education law, he was seen by the resource room teacher on a daily basis and by the adaptive physical education teacher twice weekly in order to meet his specialized needs. Paul's regular teacher told Paul's mother that it was imperative for Paul to read at least one book a night because he needed additional reading practice. A reading tutor came to Paul's house Saturday morning. Paul also had oculomotor problems so he was evaluated by an optometrist who recommended weekly visits plus ocular exercises for one-half hour a day. Paul developed secondary emotional problems, partly because he was very bright yet aware of his learning disability and frustrated by it. Thus Paul saw a psychotherapist on a weekly basis. The psychotherapist recommended participation in weekly group sessions, in addition to Paul's individual sessions, to help improve peer relationships. Thus, in all, Paul's "therapists" had developed a 12-hour-a-day program for him and his family. It is no wonder that Paul had difficulty in developing peer relationships—he never had time. Paul's schedule also affected interaction in his own family. His mother felt that her being a "therapist" interfered with her being a mother. She felt unable to carry out the home programs and felt guilty for not doing it.

What became apparent with Paul is that although a number of professionals were involved with him and although each contributed to the evaluation and treatment, the massive input, to some extent, had a detrimental effect on Paul and his family. The potential problems with multiple interventions and the need for coordinated services are discussed in the next section.

Coordinating multiple interventions. Learning disabilities are complex, multifaceted problems. The varied symptoms have brought the child with learning disabilities to the attention of many disciplines. Over the years, the number of therapeutic disciplines involved in the assessment and therapeutic management of learning disabilities has steadily increased. However, the involvement of so many specialists is both a problem and a benefit. The skill and interest of these disciplines constitutes the benefit. However, the view that the more service the better may result in a service delivery overkill, as was the case with Paul. According to Kenny and Burka,[161] our society, because it values highly trained specialists, is in jeopardy of expanding itself to the "point of logistic chaos."

Cruickshank[78] indicated that one of the major problems confronting the child with learning disabilities was the lack of a true interdisciplinary approach. Each discipline has traditionally been concerned with its own viewpoint of the learning disability field, with the result that research and subsequent remediation of learning problems has been limited in scope. According to Weiner,[301] efforts to educate the child with minimal brain dysfunction have been reminiscent of the fable of the blind man and the elephant. Depending on which part of the elephant was being touched, the elephant was described as "a huge leaf waving in the breeze," "a broad table top," "a short, dangling rope," "a twisting snake," "a wide wall," "a tree trunk," or "a spear." Weiner suggested that similar failures to perceive the whole and to appreciate the behavioral uniqueness of the individual are in part a result of the skewedness and skimpiness of special professional preparation. He emphasized that "the task of educating the child with minimal brain dysfunction requires a repertoire of information, insights, and competencies that draw across arbitrary lines of profession proprietorship" (p. 283).[301]

Kenny and Burka[161] have identified factors that impact on the process of achieving effective coordination of intervention services. One problem area is that treatment approaches fall in the skills and domain of a number of disciplines, and the territories often overlap. There is a strong need for each discipline to prove its expertise with the result being the development of territoriality. According to Gaddes,[111] the "proponent of each of these methods (treatment approaches) frequently recommends his or her system with an emotional fervor that reflects a stronger relationship with professional prejudices than with the objective behavior of the child" (p. 376).[111] It is for reasons of this nature that diagnosis of the same child may be different depending on differing professional responsibilities and goals.[39] Kenny and Burka[161] emphasize the need for each discipline to accept fully the skills and competence of other disciplines. Gaddes[111] emphasizes that territoriality is not necessary since none of the procedures by themselves is complete and adequate for dealing with all learning-disabled children or with all the disabilities of one child, and the superiority of any one method over another has generally not been demonstrated for all learning-disabled children. Johnson[152] supports this belief, stating that there is no simple response or treatment program for the learning-disabled population because of the variability and complexity of the problems.

Another problem that has been identified in achieving effective coordination of intervention services is that no single discipline has trained its students to handle that role.[161] Rather, it seems to be an assumption that all professionals acquire the ability to coordinate services by virtue of learning their own special skills. Kenny and Burka[161] stress the need for a person to act as coordinator for the management and integration of the multiple interventions received by the learning-disabled child. They suggest that leadership be delegated on a functional rather than on a hierarchical basis. By this, they suggest that the coordinator be the team member who could best service the needs of the child.

THE LEARNING-DISABLED CHILD WITH MOTOR DEFICITS
Concept of the clinical problems

Rationale for emphasizing this aspect. Motor deficits are only one aspect of the problems facing the learning-disabled child. This aspect, however, has been selected for the focus of this chapter since physical and occupational therapists working with learning disabled children generally deal with the motor problems. Denckla[91] reported that, across the entire spectrum of developmental disabilities, the most frequent signs leading to medical referral are those related to motor output. However, selection of this aspect is not meant to imply that the motor deficits are the paramount problems of the learning-disabled child or that motor deficits should receive priority over other symptoms. It is critical for the therapist who works with the learning-disabled child to be aware of the overall strengths and deficits of the child and of the characteristics of the child's educational program in order to plan optimal intervention strategies.

Terminology. A frequently cited characteristic of the child with learning disabilities is a problem in motor coordination. Developmental clumsiness has been documented since at least the early 1900s, when Collier used the term *congenital maladroitness*.[104] Orton [224] recognized that disorders of praxis and gnosis resulted in clumsiness in physical performance that was different from that rising from pyramidal, extrapyramidal, or cerebellar dysfunction. He described developmental apraxia as similar to the right-handed person trying to use his left hand, and said that the child seemed to have two left feet. The learning-disabled child with motor incoordination has been variously described as being "clumsy,"[128-131,142,151,299] "congenitally maladroit,"[104] or as having developmental apraxia,[12,18,25,299] psychomotor syndrome,[104] choreiform syndrome,[238] "developmental clumsiness,"[240] or sensory integration dysfunction.[16] Whereas some of these terms, such as *clumsiness,* are general terms that encompass a variety of motor coordination problems, other terms, such as *developmental apraxia,* are more specific.

In this chapter the terms *motor dysfunction, deficit, disorder,* or *disturbance* are used as general terms that encompass all disorders that have a motor component. We identify two classes of motor function, which we term *motor coordination* and *visual-motor function*. Motor coordination refers to functions that are more clearly and traditionally defined as motoric and includes gross motor, fine motor, and motor planning (praxic) functions. *Gross motor coordination* is defined as motor behaviors concerned with posture and locomotion, ranging from early develop-

ing behaviors to finely tuned balance.[145] *Fine motor coordination* includes such motor behavior as manipulation, discrete finger movements, and eye-hand coordination. *Praxis* and *motor planning* are used only in the specific sense to denote the ability to plan and execute skilled, nonhabitual tasks.[16]

Although visual-motor function is in fact an aspect of motor coordination as we have defined it, it is predominantly used in the literature as a synonym for visuoconstructional abilities and refers to the ability to copy or draw forms or other visual stimuli. Visual-motor functions as thus defined are generally the concern of the special educator or the occupational therapist and are described and discussed in another chapter of this book. Therefore the emphasis in the discussions of evaluation and treatment is on motor coordination deficits.

Both sensory integration and perceptual-motor function encompass motor coordination, visual-motor function, and sensory/perceptual functions. *Sensory integration* is defined in detail in the following pages. *Perceptual-motor function* is defined variously by different authors and is used only in the discussion of the theorists who made the term popular.

Incidence. Various researchers have attempted to identify the incidence of motor problems in learning-disabled children. In a recent National Collaborative Perinatal Project, of the more than 2300 children who had positive total "neurologically soft signs" ratings, the most common symptom, poor coordination, was present in nearly three-quarters of the children. Other frequently noted signs were abnormal reflexes, abnormal gait, mirror movements, and impaired position sense.[91] Tarnopol[285] reports that about 90% of children with learning disabilities have motor coordination or visual-motor defects. Clements[70] reports that 98% of children with minimal brain dysfunction (MBD) showed poor, slow, labored handwriting. In a study of 9- to 12-year-old hyperactive children, Prechtl[237] found that the majority of these children were clumsy and that almost all had poor fine motor control. Other estimates of motor deficits were more conservative and ranged from 50% to 60%.[173] Bender[40] notes that a high percentage of problem learners had some degree of residual symmetrical tonic neck reflex. Thus a significant percentage of children with learning disabilities evidence some type of motor coordination deficit.

Descriptions of motor deficits in the learning-disabled child. Although many children with minimal brain dysfunction or learning disabilities have disorders of motor control, there is no consistent correlation between motor dysfunction and minimal brain dysfunction.[188] Because motor functions are the result of complex neurophysiological mechanisms and since the concept of learning disability or minimal brain dysfunction is controversial and not well defined, it is difficult to draw a clear, valid generalization from the study of the relationship between a complex function and a not well-defined concept.[188]

The motor deficits of the learning-disabled child are quite variable, and there does not appear to be any single characteristic pattern.[64] Patterns of movement in children are influenced by age, individual variability, and the environment.[188] For example, research has indicated that younger learning-disabled children show perceptual-motor signs more frequently and in a greater degree of severity than older learning-disabled children.[83,173]

Because there is not a single pattern of motor deficits, two approaches are being used to describe the characteristic motor deficits. This serves to enhance the therapist's awareness of the varied symptomatology and may familiarize the therapist with the focus and type of description that various disciplines provide. The first approach is a descriptive and observational approach and includes the general characteristics of the motor problems. These characteristics are frequently those reported by parents and teachers. The second approach, called the neurological approach, focuses primarily on the soft neurological signs. These signs include both motor and nonmotor signs. When evaluating the learning-disabled child, the pediatric neurologist generally looks for soft neurological signs as part of the examination.

Descriptive/observational. Although many developmentally dyspraxic children are not referred for evaluation until they reach school age, many parents report longstanding clumsiness and associated difficulties.[64] Children are described as falling excessively, continuously knocking into things and dropping things, and having more than the usual number of bruises. Although motor milestones such as rolling, sitting, standing, and walking may be within normal or slow to normal limits, there is often a history of relative slowness in self-care skills. The child often appears excessively awkward in daily activities, and there is a history of slowness in dressing, such as buttoning a coat or sweater or tying shoes. Feeding, including handling a spoon, fork, and knife, is often delayed. Play skills, such as learning to ride a tricycle and bicycle, skipping rope, and catching a ball, are often achieved at a later age and seem to take extra effort for the child to perform.

Fine motor coordination problems are also evident. They may be manifested in reluctance to engage in, or incompetence in, small motor tasks such as block building, or constructive manipulatory play such as tinker toys, tracing, and cutting with scissors. Inefficiencies of fine motor performance may manifest themselves educationally in the impairment of the ability to write or draw. Impaired drawing ability is characterized both by poor motor control and spatial disorientation. Handwriting is often labored and spacing problems are evident. Letters are irregular in shape and poorly organized on the page. To compensate for inadequate pencil manipulation, the child may develop a maladaptive grasp that further contributes to making writing prolonged and laborious. Associated articulatory deficits are often present, probably because of the fine motor nature of the demands of articulation.[16,25,65,185]

Although poor motor coordination may be present as difficulty with total-body balance, ineptness may be most apparent when complex motor activities are attempted. Physical education class often presents major problems. A 9-year-old boy described his motor problems as follows: "When the gym teacher tells us to do something, I understand exactly what he means. I even know how to do it, I think. But my body never seems to do the job."[186]

Children with motor coordination problems cannot keep up with other children in sports. They often prefer to play more sedentary games, to play alone, or to play with younger children. They are often described as children with whom other children will not play because they are "no fun." These children often get into fights.

There are a number of characteristics that are associated with the motor coordination problems. Problems often cited include overactivity or underactivity, a short attention span, spatial disorientation, constructional apraxia, finger agnosia, right-left discrimination problems, low self-esteem, poor peer relationships, and assorted behavior problems.[25,93,262]

CASE STUDY: PAUL

The following is a mother's description of her child, Paul, who had motor coordination problems and was learning disabled:

"I think when Paul was first born I tried to ignore the problem. Paul is a child who never climbed or ran or drew pictures the way other kids did. But until he went to nursery school, I didn't pay much attention to it. Maybe I didn't want to pay attention to it. Maybe I knew it was there and I didn't want to know about it. I'm not sure. But Paul was always a very verbal child and a very creative and imaginative child. He and I had something special because I used to enjoy that kind of creative imaginative play. We used to have our own world of various fantasies, heroes, and places."

"Paul sat up at about 7 months, he crawled and crept on time. He didn't learn to walk until he was about 15 months old. He walked very cautiously holding on and wouldn't let go of anything. He walked late but he talked early. He said his first clear word, 'cat', at 6 months. He knew what a cat was and could relate to it. My husband and I were so enthusiastic about his sounds. In those days they said that if you stimulated your child and talked to him and got him ready to talk, that this was the important thing, and he could read early. I was very concerned that Paul would be able to talk and have a marvelous vocabulary and read because I had a reading disability and a spelling disability."

"When Paul was 4 years old and in nursery school, at my first conference, the teacher said, 'Look out the window, Mrs. B. See Paul sitting at the bottom. All the other kids are climbing on top of the jungle gym.' And then she showed me some art work. Paul couldn't cut, he couldn't paste, he couldn't do any of it. We could definitely, at the age of 3½ or 4, see his problems. He was very bright but he couldn't cut, paste, or draw, he couldn't climb, he really didn't know how to run. That was where his handicaps were first being noticed, more by other teachers and professionals than by my husband and myself."

"When we had to make the decision as to whether to put Paul into kindergarten or hold him back, we were very frustrated by it because Paul was very very bright and very alert. He has always known everything that was going on in the world."

"Now, the kids Paul knows and the kids who know Paul, know that he can't do motor tasks and they'll come over and play rocket ships with him. But there will come a time, as the kids are getting older, that they won't want to do this."

Paul's mother, who was also learning disabled, described her own disability as follows:

The hardest course for me was gym. I was unfortunate enough to have the same gym teacher throughout high school. The teacher always used to think I was a lazy kid, that I just never wanted to try to do the exercises. Although I tried, I couldn't do the stunts and tumbling for anything. The other girls would do a somersault and I would still do it like a 4-year-old. I'd just about get over.

I took dance a couple of times. I never could figure out as a kid why I couldn't point my toes. The teacher would say "Point your toes" and it never made any sense to me. I always curled my toes up. Only when somebody sat down with me and actually showed me, did I know that that was how you were supposed to point your toes. With other kids, they just did what the teacher did. Nobody had to stop and tell them. I was the clutsy kid. I never could do the nice leaps across the floor. But I would try. After two or three sessions my mother stopped giving me lessons. She was probably embarrassed.

As a girl, it wasn't as traumatic not being athletic. As I got older, the need for a woman to be athletic tended to decrease, whereas for a boy, the need to be athletic and competitive tends to increase. I forsee this as one of the major problems for Paul.

Most of my life my friendships with people have always relied upon other people. I met most of my friends through other friends because I've gone along to things. I think it goes back to being teased as a child, about the things I couldn't do or the way I looked. If you looked at me, I probably looked like a lot of the learning-disabled kids that you see . . . clothes were not put together properly, shoelaces were untied, my hair was never quite combed properly.

It was very difficult for me learning how to put on make-up, to use a hairblower. It would take many hours of trying to learn. For a long time, my finger nails were cut very short because I didn't know how to file them. It is still very hard for me to put on eye make-up . . . to look in the mirror and try to figure it out. I still don't feel as though I am completely put together. And I put a lot of effort and energy into looking good.

Neurological approach/soft neurological signs. Although children with learning disabilities have many symptoms that appear similar to those exhibited by the adult with brain damage, for the most part, they do not demonstrate problems identified by classical neurological examination.[125] Rather, they demonstrate "soft neurological signs."[241,262,289,290] These signs suggest minor abnormalities in function of the central nervous system.

Several studies have shown that a high percentage of learning-disabled children display certain soft neurological signs. These signs may include psychological, linguistic, motor, sensory, and neurological responses. The following are examples of soft neurological signs:

Motor awkwardness
Fine motor incoordination
Mild dysphasias
Choreiform movements
Finger agnosia
Exaggerated associated movements
Borderline hyperreflexia and reflex asymmetries
Tremor
Ocular apraxia
Endpoint nystagmus
Dysdiadochokinesia
Whirling
Graphesthesia
Mixed laterality and disturbances of right-left discrimination
Pupillary inequalities
Extinction to double-tactile stimulation
Avoidance response to outstretched hands
Awkward gait
Unilateral winking defect
Strabismus

Although a higher proportion of children with learning disabilities manifest soft neurological signs than does a normal control group, neurological involvement is not a necessary concomitant of learning disabilities.[4,305]

Most of the neurological evaluations of learning-disabled children do not attempt to identify a specific site of neurological deficit or to evaluate sensory functions or frank reflexes. Rather, they emphasize the consideration of how the signs may affect a child's functional performance in tasks involving motor skills, spatial understanding, perceptual tasks, and the integration of various modalities for adaptation to demands in the environment. Kinsbourne[169,170] stressed the need to view soft signs from a developmental perspective and stated that "soft signs differed from hard signs in that the child's age is the factor that determines whether the sign represents an abnormality." Accordingly, in a younger child the same sign, would be considered normal. Denckla[90] divided soft signs into two groups—developmental and neurological. Developmental signs imply a state of immature neurological function that would be considered normal in a younger normal child. These include awkwardness of motor skills, functional articulatory substitution or distortion, motor overflow and impersistence, persistence in late childhood of extinction to double-tactile stimulation, right-left confusion, and mild oculomotor difficulties. Neurological soft signs, such as reflex asymmetries, are subtle abnormalities that do not occur at any time during normal development and are sufficient but not necessary evidence for brain damage. See Touwen and Prechtl[288, 289] and Levine and others[186] for evaluation of soft neurological signs.

Social and emotional consequences of motor deficits. Poor motor coordination often results in significant social and emotional consequences. Play, which in the early years is in large part motoric, is essential to psychosocial aspects of development, including self-concept and ego development.[11] As early as 1912, Montessori[208] believed that movement is the basis for personality. In addition, the stimulation that comes from socialization and play is essential to the development of motor behavior.[11] Thus the child with poor play and manipulative skills loses both ways.

Development of gross motor skills and the child's ability to master his/her body movements serve to enhance feelings of self-esteem and confidence. To the extent that the child's perceptual or motor difficulties impede success, his/her self-concept suffers.[161,244] Children who are clumsy may be ostracized by their peers. Learning-disabled boys with poor motor coordination were found to have lower ratings on measures of self-esteem and lower same-sex social relationships and happiness than a matched group of learning-disabled boys with good motor coordination.[263] Shaw, Levine, and Belfer[263] called this phenomenon 'double developmental jeopardy', which refers to the double risk factors for poor self-esteem possessed by learning-disabled with motoric impairments. Being unable to compete with peers or feeling self-conscious because of their lack of coordination, learning disabled children often shy away from participation in games. Failure at play and the inability to succeed at school serve to compound the child's feelings of worthlessness, increasing his/her inappropriate responses to the demands of society.[11] Antisocial behavior may occur. Motor performance affects social behavior as exemplified in this statement by a learning disabled child with motor deficits:

They always pick me last. This morning they were all fighting over which team had to have me. One guy was shouting about it. He said it wasn't fair because his team had me twice last week. Another kid said they would only take me if his team could be spotted four runs. Later, on the bus, they were all making fun of me, calling me a 'fag' and a 'spaz.' There are a few good kids, I mean kids who aren't mean, but they don't want to play with me. I guess it could hurt their reputation (p. 83).[186]

Statements like these highlight the close relationship between motor output, effectiveness, self-image, and social interaction.

Evaluation of motor deficits in the learning-disabled child

Disciplines involved in the evaluation of the learning disabled child. The disciplines of physical education, special education, occupational therapy, physical therapy, and optometry all are involved in the evaluation and training of motor dysfunction in learning-disabled children. Techniques of evaluation have been borrowed as needed between disciplines, and there may be considerable overlap in areas that are assessed both informally and in the tests and test batteries. It should be noted that, even though one motor evaluation may resemble another superficially, there are differences between professions in their orientation and rationale for evaluating dysfunction. The unique training of the particular profession influences both the selection of tests and the qualitative aspects of evaluation that come from observation of a child's performance.

Some of the differences in professional orientation and emphases in evaluation and treatment are as follows. Physical educators and physical therapists have a common concern for purely motor activities and physical fitness. Physical therapists are more concerned with early motor developmental functions, such as reflex integration, postural efficiency, and sensorimotor functions. Physical educators usually include evaluation of sports-related activities such as ball play and broad jump. Perceptual-motor therapists and optometrists evaluate gross motor skills as a part of a developmental evaluation leading to visual perception and eye-hand coordination in pencil and paper activities. The special attention of an optometrist is on eye movement functions as they relate to visual-motor and visual-perceptual skills. Occupational therapists evaluate sensory integrative functions as well as motor functions and perceptual and spatial abilities and are particularly concerned with the impact of motor deficits on functional abilities.

The areas assessed and the particular tests chosen by a therapist depend on the make-up of the professional team serving children in a particular setting. Careful planning is required in designing an evaluation protocol. Unnecessary duplication of assessment must be avoided: both the child's and the therapist's time are too valuable. Free exchange of information between professionals evaluating motor function is absolutely essential, both of the tests that are used and of the rationale underlying evaluation. The therapist must be aware of information on motor function that is available from other professionals and of information that should be shared with those professionals.

Assessing motor deficits: areas to examine. The learning-disabled child with motor dysfunction performs motor tasks with a level of strength, flexibility, speed, and coordination that is virtually normal by the standards of evaluation used by neurologists as well as by occupational therapists and physical therapists with more severely physically handicapped children. The child's difficulty with skilled, purposeful manipulative tasks or with finely tuned balance activities may not be readily apparent in the classroom. This appearance of normality, which leads to expectations of age-level motor performance, can create problems and misunderstandings for these children. Therefore identification of subtle motor handicaps is very important.

Areas of testing commonly used in physical therapy, such as muscle strength, range-of-motion, and ambulation, those used in occupational therapy, such as eye-hand coordination and fine motor function, and those used in both professions, such as evaluation of reflex integration and postural control, are appropriate. However, evaluation techniques have, for the most part, been developed for children with moderate to severe neurological impairments. To evaluate learning-disabled children, levels of expected performance in these areas must encompass borderline dysfunction. For example, a child might have a normal gait but lack steadiness standing on one leg or be unable to tandem walk with his/her eyes closed.

While the specific system of evaluation reflects the philosophy and objectives of a center or therapist, evaluation of the following areas should be included for the assessment of motor abilities in learning-disabled children: (1) postural control and gross motor performance, including muscle tone, reflex integration, vestibular function and equilibrium, posture, and gross motor skills; (2) fine motor performance, including fine motor movements, eye-hand coordination, and fine motor skills; (3) motor planning; (4) sensory integration and perceptual functions; and (5) physical fitness, including muscular strength and endurance, flexibility, and cardiorespiratory endurance. Each of these interrelated functions is described here as an area of clinical assessment. However, because the motor dysfunction of learning-disabled children is subtle, a greater reliance on tests with normative data may be necessary, especially for the new therapist or one without experience with neurological disorders. Information on age-appropriate performance is not always available, but sources for provisional information are included when possible. Formal tests and test batteries described in Appendix A provide sources of normative data that can be used as guides for clinical assessment.

Postural control and gross motor performance

Muscle tone. Low muscle tone and poor cocontraction have been identified as characteristic of some learning-disabled children.[2,16] Increased tone is not common in children with learning disabilities and may be indicative of minimal cerebral palsy. Judgments of inadequate muscle tone and cocontraction are primarily clinical observations, for example, muscle groups may be poorly defined, muscles may feel "mushy," and joints may appear hyperextensible. A common method of evaluating muscle tone in learning-disabled children involves putting all the flexors on stretch and examining the degree of extension (hyperextension) at the elbow, knee, and hip.[16] The therapist also palpates muscles for tone and checks for right/left differences. The child's ability to stabilize his or her neck musculature is evaluated by asking the child to "freeze" while the therapist attempts to move the head slightly back and forth. Cocontraction of the arms and shoulders is similarly tested. Evaluation of both muscle tone and cocontraction is subjective and depends on the clinical experiences of the therapist and on a knowledge of normal performance.

Integration of primitive postural reflexes. Although stereotyped obligatory reflexes occur only in pathology and

although preferences for reflex postures are not seen in the normal child past infancy, integration of postural reactions is not fully established until 8 or 9 years of age[271] or even later.[136,253] This lack of full integration in school-age children cannot usually be demonstrated in the test positions designed for testing infants and cerebral-palsied children,[47,59,60,102] but it may be elicited in other positions, such as on the hands and knees.[136,232,233,253] Using this technique, it has been shown that some learning-disabled children show abnormally persistent asymmetrical tonic neck reflex (ATNR), symmetrical tonic neck reflex (STNR), and righting reflexes.[16,213,232,253,271]

An early test of reflex integration in school-age children is Schilder's Arm Extension Test.[268] In this test the child stands with his or her arms extended with forward flexion of the arms and with his or her eyes closed. Righting reactions, which are expressed as "swinging the arms and body to the side when the head is turned," and ATNR reactions, which are expressed in asymmetry in arm flexion, are normal in 6- and 7-year-old children. Older children, however, should be able to maintain arm position with only slight deviations. Arm extension tests are also used in neurological examination for observing involuntary and associated movements.[289]

The most widely reported method of testing the ATNR response in learning-disabled children is with the child in the quadruped position. The child assumes the quadruped position, the head is passively or actively rotated, and the degree of flexion of the skull arm is measured with a goniometer or a scaling device. Rating scales and age expectation can be found in research studies.[97,232,233,266] Ayres[16] has designed reflex-inhibiting postures in the quadruped positions that increase stress and that can be used when disorders are subtle. Sieg and Shuster[266] compared several methods of testing the ATNR and concluded that the reflex-inhibiting position was the most sensitive but that the quadruped position identified all but the most subtle disorders.

DeQuiros and Schrager[95] described the use of a sitting posture for eliciting the ATNR: they call this position the "ATNR Sunshine Position." The child sits on the examination table, leaning backward on extended arms with the head turned passively to one side. If the ATNR response of flexion at the elbow on the skull side is elicited, inadequate integration is assumed. Age-related expectations are not discussed. DeQuiros and Schrager also observed signs of the ATNR in their tests of vestibular function.[95] When a child walks on a balance beam or stands on one foot, the ATNR generates extension and abduction of the arm ipsilateral to the weight-bearing leg. In learning-disabled children this normal response is exaggerated. Asymmetric responses are also noted.

The Purdue Reflex Test[40] was designed to detect abnormal persistence of the STNR. The child creeps forward and backward on his or her hands and knees against manual resistance. Scoring is based on specific postures or behaviors shown during performance of the test. The STNR can also be tested in the static quadruped position and in dynamic balance tests.[16,20]

Vestibular function and equilibrium. The tests of vestibular function discussed here are those that could be conducted by a therapist in the clinic and include tests of nystagmus and of prone extension as well as tests of equilibrium.

In the Southern California Postrotary Nystagmus Test,[19,28] a child sits cross-legged on a board with his/her head tilted forward. The board is rotated by the examiner 10 times in 20 seconds and then stopped abruptly; the child's eye movements are then observed. The test is done with rotation first to the left and then to the right, and the score is the duration of nystagmus following cessation of rotation. Normative scores for children 5 to 9 years of age have been obtained.[19,28,168,239] Using the Southern California Postrotary Nystagmus Test, various researchers have found that many children with learning disabilities have a shortened duration of postrotary nystagmus.[24,213] Steinberg and Rendle-Short[277] described a similar test using a padded scooter board and a pair of special glasses (Frenzel glasses) that prevented fixation. A method of testing nystagmus in infants has been described by Kantner and others.[156]

Difficulty in assuming and holding the prone extension posture has been considered by several researchers as a manifestation of vestibular dysfunction.[20,57,80] This has been supported by its relationship to hyporeactive postrotary nystagmus in learning-disabled children.* Ayres[20] suggested that an inability to maintain the prone extension position reflects inadequate facilitation of the extensor muscles via the vestibulospinal pathways. Provisional data on age-related performance of prone extension have been obtained by Dunn[97] in 5-year-olds, by Harris[138] in 4-, 6-, and 8-year-olds, and by Roach and Kephart[243] using the Kraus Weber Test.

A series of tests of vestibular function was reported by DeQuiros and Schrager.[95] Traditional tests of vestibular function include: (1) the Romberg position—standing with feet together and eyes closed; (2) Mann's position—standing with feet in tandem position (heel to toe) and eyes closed; and (3) standing on one leg with eyes open and eyes closed. These tests are not timed. Observation is made of a tendency to fall to one side, swaying, abduction of the arms more to one side than to the other, and associated movements of the mouth and hands.

Another method of testing vestibular function is the use of the changing consistency board. A changing consistency board is a wide walking beam in which irregular lengths of polyurethane foam are alternated with wood

*References 20, 24, 80, 225, 229, 230.

to provide a change in consistency of the walking surface. The board is covered to look solid. DeQuiros and Schrager[95] believe that this test demonstrates vestibular proprioceptive disassociation. The reader is referred to their work for a full description of reflex and vestibular tests.

DeHaven and others[82] have stated that "Balance is of little diagnostic value in differentiating children with the diagnosis of minimal cerebral dysfunction from normal children when visual cues are present, but takes on greater importance when visual cues are absent" (p. 156). However, since some learning-disabled children perform as well or better without vision than with vision,[294] balance should be assessed with eyes both open and closed. Fregly[106] has reported the development and use of the Floor Ataxia Test with persons with vestibular dysfunction. The test consists of several balance tasks, including walking a line with the eyes closed and with the eyes open. Cunningham and Goetzinger[79] reported provisional norms for children ages 8 to 18 on the Floor Ataxia Test. Many of the standardized tests described in the Appendix also have tests of balancing on one foot and of walking on a balance beam, measures that assess aspects of equilibrium. The new Sensory Integration and Praxis Tests[28] include a 16-item test of standing and walking balance.

Posture. The posture of some learning-disabled children is poor.[11,16] Lordosis may be seen well beyond the age at which it normally disappears, and recurvation of the knees is common. Posture in the sitting position may also be poor during fine motor tasks. It is important to observe the effects of fatigue since both sitting and standing posture may deteriorate over the course of a day. The relationship between posture and muscle tone must be considered.

Gross motor skills. Learning-disabled children with perceptual-motor or sensory-integrative dysfunction may attain reasonably high degrees of motor skills in specific activities; however, these motor accomplishments remain highly specific to particular movements or to a series of movements and do not generalize to other activities, regardless of their similarities. Whenever variation is required in the motor response, the response breaks down and the motor behavior becomes inaccurate and disorganized.[64,164] Thus, although the learning-disabled child sits, stands, and walks with apparent ease, he or she may be awkward in rolling, coming to standing, running, and hopping. The child may be unable to balance on his or her knees or to alternate his/her feet when climbing stairs.

Therefore evaluation of motor skills should include developmentally earlier skills as well as age-appropriate skills. Quality of performance must be considered. Gilfoyle and others[119,120] have illustrated qualitative differences in gross motor skills by describing and photographing twins, one of whom was normal while demonstrated motor dysfunction. Hughes and Riley[147] have described several gross motor tasks useful in evaluating minor motor dysfunction. Tests of balance, such as those described in the section on vestibular function and in the standardized tests, are important in monitoring achievement as well as in observing exaggerated postural responses. The Test of Motor Proficiency by Bruininks[52] and the Peabody Developmental Motor Scales[103] are examples of standardized assessment of motor skills (see Appendix).

Trampolines have been used to evaluate both basic motor functions and movement skills. Arnheim and Sinclair[11] have translated a checklist for Movement Evaluation on the Trampoline, which was developed in Europe. Evaluation is in the four categories of general movement control, presence of involuntary movements, differences between left and right sides, and hypertonicity of the extremities. The checklist is designed for use with children from 4 to 12 years of age, but norms have not been established.

Fine motor performance

Fine motor movements. The soft neurological signs assessed by neurologists include tests of fine motor movements that can be incorporated into screening and evaluation. Descriptions of the neurological assessment of children with minimal cerebral dysfunction include methods for the evaluation of many of the abilities, such as diadochokinesis, thumb and finger touching, and synkinesis. There are a number of excellent sources on assessing soft neurological signs, many of which provide provisional information on age-appropriate performance.*

A second source of methods of evaluation of fine motor movements are research studies, some of which provide provisional normative data as well as describe an evaluation technique. For example, Denckla[88] tested 5- to 7-year-old right-handed children on the speed of repetitive and successive finger movements. Grant and others[126] tested finger movements and diadochokinesis under stressed and nonstressed conditions in 4- to 8-year-old children and developed a scoring system based on quality of performance. Kendrick and Hanten[160] tested extremity coordination and found it to differentiate between learning-disabled children and normal children their age. A number of other investigators have also examined and described the performance of learning-disabled children on neuromotor tasks.[121,182,262,264,309]

Eye-hand coordination and fine motor skills. The evaluation of eye-hand coordination and fine motor skills is best achieved by using tests or portions of the standardized tests described in the Appendix, specifically Gubbay's Test of Motor Proficiency,[128,130] the Motor Accuracy Test of the Southern California Sensory Integration Test,[26] the Bruininks-Oseretsky Test of Motor Proficiency,[52] the Peabody Developmental Motor Scales,[103] and the Purdue Pegboard Test.[287] The formal tests should be supplemented by

*References 89, 128, 186, 217, 289, 290, 305.

an evaluation of activities of daily living requiring dextrous hand use (e.g., buttoning buttons, lacing and tying shoes, cutting with a knife and fork, and turning a key in a lock). The grasp and manipulation of pencils and other tools should also be a part of the assessment.

Motor planning. Motor planning, as defined here, is the performance of new and different motor acts. Clumsiness as well as difficulty adapting motor responses to changes in external conditions, which have been described in Kephart,[164] are often a reflection of a child's inability to plan his or her movements. Motor planning can be evaluated informally through observation of the child's coordination in a variety of motor tasks. Standardized assessments of praxis include the tests of Postural Praxis, Sequencing Praxis, Praxis on Verbal Command, Oral Praxis, Constructional Praxis, and Design Copying of the new Sensory Integration and Praxis Tests.[28] (See the Appendix for a description of these tests.)

Sensory integration and perceptual functions. Although this chapter focuses on the motor deficits of learning-disabled children, it must be remembered that the children may also have deficits in sensory and perceptual processing. It is the deficits in these areas that may be responsible for the poor performance noted in motor functions. Kinesthetic perception has a particularly close association with motor performance. Laszlo and Bairstow[180] have developed a Kinaesthetic Sensitivity Test that measures acuity, perception, and memory. These authors also report on the initial development of a perceptual-motor abilities test in which the emphasis is on the assessment of the perception and use of kinesthetic information.

Hulme and Lord[149] emphasize that when they refer to motor skills, they are really referring to perceptual-motor skills because almost all movements require the coordination of motor information with perceptual information. Whereas Ayres' research has repeatedly linked poor tactile and kinesthetic perception with problems in motor planning, other researchers have emphasized the visual and kinesthetic contributions to movement.[142,148,150,180,221]

Other methods of evaluation of sensory integration, perceptual-motor, and visual-motor functions are included in the section on standardized testing.

Physical fitness. The child with motor dysfunction often performs poorly in games and athletic activities and consequently is reluctant to participate. As a result, the level of physical fitness, strength, muscular endurance, flexibility, and cardiorespiratory endurance deteriorates. One task of the physical therapist is to differentiate between poor physical fitness secondary to low motor activity and problems of low muscle tone, joint limitations, low strength and endurance that reflect a developmental lag or deviation in motor function. The collaboration of the physical educator and the physical therapist is of special importance in these areas. The reader is referred to Arnheim and

Sinclair[11] for further discussion of physical fitness and a developmental program for learning-disabled children.

Standardized screening and diagnostic tools for assessment of motor deficits. A number of standardized or partially standardized tests of motor function have been used for the evaluation of children with learning disabilities. The use of a standardized test battery can help both to examine the overall developmental status of a child and identify patterns of disability that provide clues to underlying disabilities.[180] A selection of standardized tests is described in the Appendix to provide an overview of the kinds of tests available for the assessment of motor dysfunction in learning-disabled children and to indicate the uses and limitations of the individual tests and test batteries. These tests, as a whole or in part, should be used only by individuals who have knowledge and understanding of the rules of the use and interpretation of standardized tests in general. Furthermore, the use of an individual test requires specific training and/or practice with that test. An examiner should always be thoroughly familiar with all aspects of the administration and scoring procedures of a test and should comply with the requirements for training described in the test manual. Administration and interpretation of some tests (for example, the Sensory Integration Tests) requires special certification.

In the test descriptions included in the Appendix, comment is generally made on test construction and reliability but not on validity. Criteria for a satisfactory standardized test should include validation against external criteria. However, it is difficult to say what external criteria should be selected to validate a motor test because of the fragmentary state of knowledge about patterns of motor deficit and their functional implications. Few of the tests for learning-disabled children reach a desirable level of external validity.[124] In any case, the judicious use of the tests described here must rest on the content validity of the test items. This means that the clinical judgment of the examiner is all-important in the selection of tests for an evaluation protocol. The tests must be logical for testing attributes of concern to the user, and the interpretation must be made within the overall frame of reference for the evaluation and treatment of children with minimal motor dysfunction.

Setting goals. The treatment process begins with a statement of the child's specific difficulties and with corresponding statements of the type and quality of behavior desired as a result of therapy.[32] In other words, the therapist must set treatment goals.

It is not simple to interpret test data, integrate findings, identify problem areas, and formulate goals. It may be necessary at times to form initial clinical impressions, which will result in the need for further evaluation in order to formulate refined goals. This additional assessment may involve formal testing or observation during initial ther-

apy. All therapy is, in a sense, evaluation, and the therapist refines the goals and the methods of achieving these goals.

Setting goals for the learning-disabled child with motor problems, as with any child, should be based on a number of factors. These include:

1. Referral information
2. Medical, developmental, and sensory processing history
3. Parents/teachers' perception of child's strengths and deficit areas
4. Educational information
   a. Major difficulties experienced in school
   b. How motor problems are interfering with the child's school performance
   c. Current services being received
5. Child's peer relationships
6. The therapists' observation/evaluation of the child through informal and formal assessment, both standardized and nonstandardized

In addition, the age of the child and current external (school and home) demands and expectations must be considered.

Goals for the learning-disabled child can be stated in terms of long-term and/or short-term objectives. According to Arnheim and Sinclair,[11] the major long-term objectives in remediation of motor deficits of the clumsy child should be:

effective total body management in a wide variety of activities requiring dynamic balance and agility, object management including manipulation, propulsion and reception, emotional control, ability to socialize effectively, a positive self-concept and a sense of enjoyment in movement.*

A therapist would also add the prevention of maladaptive motor patterns. In general, whether a goal is long term or short term depends, in part, on the performance level of the child. The following sample of objectives may be appropriate for the learning-disabled child with motor deficits.

1. To develop a stable and efficient base from which to perform more skilled activities
2. To enhance integration of primitive postural reflexes
3. To enhance maturation of postural responses and related proprioceptive mechanisms
4. To develop the basic motor repertoire: basic gross motor patterns of flexion in supine and extension in prone, portions of the basic flexion and extension synergies, gross diagonal patterns

*Reference 11, p 156.

5. To facilitate righting and equilibrium reactions and static and dynamic balance
6. To promote trunk rotation
7. To enhance neural integration, especially of the tactile and vestibular systems
8. To reduce tactile defensiveness
9. To reduce fear of movement (gravitational insecurity)
10. To enhance body awareness, body image, and body scheme
11. To develop the capacity to motor plan
12. To encourage interaction of the two sides of the body and space
13. To increase speed, accuracy, and strength of manipulative skills
14. To assist the child in the acquisition of tool use (e.g., pencil skills, cutting skills, crayon skills)
15. To improve eye-hand coordination
16. To assist the child in the development of basic and higher-level activities of daily living skills (e.g., dressing skills, such as zipping, buttoning, and tying show laces, feeding skills, such as opening milk containers, and hygiene skills, such as nose blowing)
17. To promote physical fitness including strength, muscular and cardiorespiratory endurance, flexibility, speed, and agility
18. To promote good posture
19. To provide structuring of the environment (e.g., adaptive equipment, positioning) to facilitate the child's optimum performance
20. To improve play skills, especially with peers
21. To increase self-esteem through mastery of physical activity
22. To provide an opportunity for physical activity in situations where children are not made to feel embarrassed by their awkwardness so that they may learn to derive pleasure from physical activities
23. To assist the child (and family and teachers) in understanding the nature of the problem

In recent years there has been a trend in education to state both long-term and short-term objectives in behavioral terms. This serves to enable the educator/therapist to identify measurable changes in behavior and provides for an ongoing evaluation process. Moreover, the professional is accountable for the educational/therapeutic program. In school systems an Individualized Education Program (IEP) must be developed for each student covered by PL 94-142 the right to education law. The student's IEP must include a statement of annual goals as well as short-term objectives.[178] Many references are available to assist the therapist in writing behavior objectives generally, as well as for motor problems specifically.[11,174]

Treatment of the learning-disabled child with motor deficits

What is remediation? In treating the deficits of the learning-disabled child, an important question is, do you try to improve brain function or do you drill the child in the specific perceptual and cognitive and motor skills? Direct therapy is teaching the child what you want him/her to learn, and indirect therapy is "training the brain."[111]

Indirect therapy is based on the assumption that learning disabilities result from dysfunction of the central nervous system and that the CNS dysfunction affects one (or more) basic perceptual motor or language ability. Treatment is directed toward the improvement of the underlying abilities. Pioneers in the treatment of learning-disabled children followed this orientation and developed techniques directed toward the improvement of underlying perceptual, perceptual-motor and psycholinguistic abilities.[4] Direct therapy follows a behaviorist orientation. The presence of CNS dysfunction is not denied, but training in underlying abilities is not considered to be of use. Treatment approaches emphasize behavior modification, programmed and criterion-referenced instruction, and direct teaching of skills.[4]

The direct approach, teaching the child specific cognitive and academic skills, has been expounded by Sapir,[255] who believes that one should teach to the child's strengths, but at the same time develop methods to help the child deal with interfering deficits. The child should be encouraged to become an active collaborator in diminishing his or her own weaknesses by developing an awareness of the problem and by using his or her conceptual ability to consciously approach his or her perceptual problems and develop compensatory mechanisms. Sapir feels that mobilization of the child's strengths is more effective than training the perceptual skills and hoping for transfer.

Sensory integration procedures is an example of the indirect approach. According to Gaddes,[111] this is one of the most articulate and best-developed programs of sensorimotor training for learning-disabled children. The objective of sensory integration procedures is modification of the neurological dysfunction interfering with learning rather than dealing with the specific behavior associated with the dysfunction.[16] This approach emphasizes the role of subcortical functions and structures, including the brainstem, thalamus, and vestibular mechanisms, because they are considered functionally important. The goal of therapy is to improve sensory integration at all levels of the CNS. According to Ayres,[16] "If the brain develops the capacity to perceive, remember and motor plan, the ability can then be applied toward mastery of all academic and other tasks, regardless of the specific content." A sensory integration approach to treating learning disorders differs from many other procedures in that it does not teach specific skills, such as matching visual stimuli, learning to remember the sequence of sounds or movements, or differentiating one sound from another. Rather, the objective is to enhance the brain's ability to learn how to do these things. Ayres emphasizes, however, that sensory integration procedures must be coupled with an educational program to enable optimal integration of sensory and motor functions that subserve language and higher cortical functions.

These descriptions of the approaches of Sapir[255] and Ayres[16] illustrate direct and indirect therapy used primarily in the remediation of perceptual and cognitive deficits. The same differentiation occurs in the remediation of motor deficits. The issue then becomes whether one should try to build the underlying foundation abilities or try to develop specific skills. Often the objective of influencing brain function is inherent to the theoretical framework of building foundations. For example, sensory integration theory holds that by increasing integration at all levels of the nervous system, particularly at subcortical levels, the brain also develops better performance. In sensorimotor therapy, as well as in neurodevelopmental therapy (NDT) and proprioceptive neuromuscular facilitation (PNF), techniques are directed toward influencing the CNS through sensory input. These are all indirect approaches in which increased integration of sensation or of basic reflex responses is expected to result in improved specific skills. Kephart[163,165] and other perceptual-motor theorists also emphasize underlying foundations, although they do not really mention the brain. Kephart's concept that motor patterns that are generalizable should precede the development of specific skills is similar to that of sensorimotor therapy and sensory integration procedures.

One of the concerns of proponents of indirect therapy is that teaching a child the specific motor skills that he/she needs in everyday life will result in the development of "splinter skills," a term used to describe skills that have been learned by the child but that are inefficient because the child did not have the prerequisite sensory integration, postural functions, or movement patterns. For example, in the case of a child with poor balance affecting his/her ability to sit in a chair, having the child attend to his/her balance develops a splinter skill. Research has indicated that this takes much more effort and has a negative influence on the child's ability to concentrate on other learning and skills.[95]

In reality, any compensatory skill could be labeled a splinter skill. For example, walking with crutches could imply insufficient foundation of equilibrium reactions and is an inefficient form of locomotion. However, there is a point in a child's life at which teaching skills, such as crutch walking, is both necessary and appropriate. Therapists should be aware of this need and provide adapted equipment or methods that allow performance of the skill but that prevent the development of maladaptive patterns.

It should be noted that, in some instances, the differences between direct and indirect approaches are more theoretical than practical. Both approaches may be developmental and the differences between, say, a developmental physical education program and an occupational or physical therapy program are in part a result of the stage of development that is being addressed. Neurodevelopmental therapy focuses primarily on the development of early motor functions, for example, equilibrium and righting reactions, and physical education historically focuses on higher-level skills, for example, standing balance and ball skills. However, when a developmental motor skills program begins with the early skills, there are fewer differences between direct and indirect therapy.

The distinction between these approaches was discussed at length by Ottenbacher,[227] who identified the direct approach with an educational model and the indirect approach with the medical model. Ottenbacher states that both models are needed and suggests that "The goal of therapists and educators working in the school system should be to create an atmosphere in which models can develop in a synergistic rather than an antagonistic fashion" (p. 84).

In conclusion, both direct and indirect approaches of remediation are necessary since the superiority of any one remedial method has not yet been demonstrated.[111] If we are to deal successfully with all learning-disabled children, we may need to draw on all existing procedures for the management of dysfunction, taking care that proportions of direct and indirect therapy are relevant to the child's age and the severity of his/her disability.[111]

The following sections address remedial approaches to the motor and perceptual-motor problems of the learning-disabled child. For the purposes of this chapter, approaches have been divided into those more commonly used by educators and those more commonly used by occupational and physical therapists.

Educational approaches to treatment. A number of educational models for learning-disabled children have advocated perceptual-motor and motor training as preparation for learning academic material. These approaches are included in this chapter since occupational and physical therapists have adapted many activities developed by the educational theorists, sometimes adopting the theoretical rationale as well and other times adapting the activities to a different rationale.

The theories of intervention that are discussed here include the perceptual-motor theories of Kephart,[98,163-165,243] Getman,[118] and Barsch,[33] the visual-perception theory of Frostig,[108-110] the physical education approach (motor learning theory) of Cratty,[74-76] and the neuroanatomically based patterning theory of Doman and Delacato.[84-86] Each of these theories of intervention is described and briefly evaluated. Theories that assume that sensorimotor and perceptual-motor training influence academic learning are critiqued on the basis of their theoretical rationale and on research into the effectiveness of therapy. All the theories are reviewed for evidence of the effectiveness of therapy on improved motor performance.

Perceptual-motor theorists. Intervention programs that involve perceptual-motor training have their roots in the work of Strauss and Lehtinen.[283] The basic assumption in this type of remediation is that a major consequence of some form of brain damage is a deficit in the recognition, organization, or integration of visual information. It is assumed that perceptual-motor training will remediate deficits in basic visual-perceptual skills and that the development of visual perception will enhance academic competence. Four theorists, Frostig, Kephart, Getman, and Barsch, based their programs on the premise that visual perception was critical for reading. Kephart, Getman, and Barsch made the additional assumption that the development of visual perception was dependent on total-body motor experiences.

Perceptual-motor theory of Kephart. Kephart[98,163-165] was the most influential and the most articulate educator advocating perceptual-motor training programs for children with learning disorders. In the development of his theory he cited Piaget and Hebb, but his postulates were based primarily on interpretations of infant development. Since the infant is observed to handle and mouth objects extensively during the first few months of life, it was proposed that the tactile sense was the most primitive and the first used to obtain information about the world. The child was thought to learn about the visual surroundings by integrating visual experiences with what he/she could touch and manipulate and to develop spatial perception by moving about within the environment. To Kephart, the first learnings of the infant were motor learnings; tactile-kinesthetic input was then matched to motor; finally, visual input was matched to tactile-kinesthetic-motor. Thus the sequence was motor-tactile-kinesthetic, motor-visual-motor, and finally visual. The end product of this development was the establishment of a stable perceptual-motor world within which solid percepts would develop. The highest level of learning, that of concept formation, could then occur through the manipulation of percepts.[100]

Thus the foundation of all learning was considered dependent on muscular activity—on basic motor learnings. Kephart[163] perceived motor learning as the acquisition of motor skills and of motor patterns and as the generalization of these motor patterns. A motor skill was defined as a highly specific group of movements designed to accomplish a specific purpose. If a skill was learned before a child had the physiological readiness to learn, it was considered a splinter skill, maladaptive, and not generalizable. Motor patterns, on the other hand, were defined as a broad range of movements, any one of which could be used to accomplish a purpose. For example, if walking consisted of putting one foot in front of another, that would be a motor skill that all learning-disabled children have. However, they did not all have the motor pattern that Kephart called

locomotion, in which attention is on the goal and could include running, changing direction, going around one obstacle, and stepping over another. Kephart's perceptual training program was directed toward the acquisition of motor patterns and their generalization into widely varied motor tasks.

Kephart[163,243] developed an evaluation of perceptual-motor skills and designed remedial exercises for each of the areas evaluated. Categories of training included (1) exercises to develop balance, posture, and laterality, (2) perceptual-motor matching, in which eye-hand activities were used, (3) ocular training that consisted of tracking objects with the eyes, (4) chalkboard training that was designed to help establish directionality, and (5) training in form perception, which was defined as matching forms or visual patterns.

Kephart strongly emphasized sensorimotor learning as the foundation for all learning and made recommendations about motor experiences for normal children and mentally retarded children as well as for learning-disabled children. His approach was to develop readiness to learn by remediation of impairments in basic motor skills and by developing generalizations on which higher learning could proceed.

Movigenic theory of Barsch. Barsch described a theory known as movigenics in which motor efficiency was considered critical to academic learning. The emphasis of this theory is on movement in space, and the learning difficulties of a child are considered inadequacies in spatially oriented movement.

> Perception is movement and movement is perception. According to this view, any effort to enrich perception and cognition must be initiated as a frank approach to attaining the highest possible state of efficiency in the fundamental patterns of physical movement.*

The movigenic approach suggests that once basic motor patterns have been learned, movement efficiency is achieved and the individual will easily learn academics. Barsch advocated the movigenic curriculum for children with, as well as without, specific learning difficulties.

The movigenic curriculum is based on 12 dimensions of the child's movement in space. Specific activities are selected for each of the categories. The first four categories involve the maintenance of body control and movement through space: they are termed muscular strength, dynamic balance, body awareness (labeling body parts), and spatial awareness (turn to left or right on command). The next four are concerned with information processing and include tactual dynamics (stereognosis), kinesthesia (e.g., cutting with scissors), auditory dynamics, and visual dynamics. The final four relate to the efficiency of the first eight categories and include bilaterality, rhythm, flexibility, and motor planning.

*Reference 33, p 229.

Visuomotor theory of Getman. The visuomotor complex model of Getman[118] is a visual development and learning model that stresses the role of visual perception. It is postulated that visual perception is based on developmental sequences of physiological actions of the child. The following developmental sequences are postulated:

1. Innate response systems
2. General movement patterns (whole-body movement)
3. Special movement patterns (eye-hand activities)
4. Eye movement patterns
5. Visual language patterns (language and concept formation)
6. Visualization patterns (form recognition and matching)
7. Visual-perceptual organization (the perceptual event)
8. Cognition—integration of perceptions, abstractions, higher symbolic activity

Getman was an optometrist, and his methods are widely used in optometric programs. An optometric program might include a broad array of perceptual-motor and direct academic remediation techniques, but the unique aspect involves specific eye exercises to improve visual tracking abilities, binocular functions, and visual-perceptual-motor skills. Laterality training, balance board, and perceptual training similar to Kephart's are also used.

Visual-perceptual training of Frostig. Frostig[108-110] considered visual-perceptual abilities as critical for academic learning and developed a highly structured program of evaluation and training in five subskills of visual-motor perception. The subskills, labeled eye-hand coordination, figure-ground, form constancy, position in space, and spatial relations, were evaluated with pencil and paper tests. Extensive paper and pencil training activities keyed to each subskill were also published.[108] Training manuals also described a series of gross motor activities that were recommended as supplements to the perceptual training program.

The Frostig Developmental Test of Vision Perception (DVPT)[108] and the Frostig-Horne worksheets to be used with the test provided an easy, structured training program that made it popular in education. One suspects, however, that the program has often been used in isolation, although Frostig recommends that the Illinois Test of Psycholinguistic Ability,[171] the Wepman Test of Auditory Discrimination, and the Wechsler Intelligence Scale for Children, as well as a survey of motor abilities be used with the DTVP in the evaluation of learning disability and that training in sensorimotor and language functions be integrated with the visual-perception training. Perceptual-motor training was recommended as an adjunct for education, not as a prerequisite or substitute. It was designed to be used when deficit visual perception was found.

CRITIQUE OF THE THEORIES OF KEPHART, BARSCH, GETMAN, AND FROSTIG. One of the premises of perceptual-motor training that is not supported by known facts is that perceptual and motor maturity are necessary prerequisites to higher-level learning. The validity of the theory of the motor basis of visual perception is poorly supported by the research of the last 20 years. Kephart's theory was based on the theories of Piaget and Hebb, both of which are controversial. Furthermore, studies of infants in the last 20 years using more sophisticated experimental techniques tend to disprove the motor-tactile, motor-visual-motor, visual sequence that Kephart hypothesized. Long before infants can manipulate objects or move around in space, they have well-developed visual-perceptual abilities, including form discrimination, size and shape constancy, and depth perception. Visual discrimination of forms precedes the visual-motor ability of copying forms by years (compare the age at which a child can successfully match a form to a form board with his or her ability to copy that form).

Visual perception is a highly complex function, some capacities of which are present at birth and others not fully developed until adolescence. Perhaps some visual-perceptual capacities are dependent on some kinds of motor abilities, but in the global use of the term and in the way in which it is operationally defined in measuring instruments and training activities, the relationships are not valid. Furthermore, children with athetoid cerebral palsy do not typically show visual, visual-motor, or reading deficits.[3] It has been reported that a child with congenital absence of all four limbs showed normal cognitive abilities at age 2, without any therapy.[175] Research findings do not support the idea of a causative relationship between motor development and perceptual and cognitive functions.

Another critique is of the postulated relationship of visual-perceptual abilities to reading. Visual-perceptual functions are certainly disrupted in some learning disorders, and it is reasonable to suppose that reading could be retarded as a result of visual-perceptual deficits. However, severe spatial disorientation, body image, and perceptual disorders can occur in children with normal reading skills.[34] Furthermore, some poor readers show visuospatial disorders and others do not.

Visual perception is unquestionably necessary for reading proficiency. However, the types of visual discrimination tasks and the levels of performance of these tasks, which are essential, is still a matter of controversy. Furthermore, visual perception is only one of many areas of performance in which skill development is necessary. A major criticism of visual-perception training is that it is used without an equal emphasis on other prerequisites for reading, for example, auditory discrimination and linguistic processes.

An additional criticism has been directed toward optometric training programs. Optometric training has been criticized for its use in isolation for a child with a reading problem and for its application to a wide variety of reading and associated learning disabilities. In 1973 the American Academy of Pediatrics and the American Academy of Opthalmology issued a joint organizational statement expressing reservations about the appropriateness of optometric training. The criticism is that many of the optometric procedures were related to peripheral eye defects and peripheral eye defects do not produce dyslexia and associated learning disabilities. The concern expressed was for the unwarranted expense and the delay of proper education for the young child using procedures whose effectiveness has not been documented.[186]

RESEARCH ON THE EFFECTS OF PERCEPTUAL-MOTOR AND VISUAL-PERCEPTUAL TRAINING ON ACADEMIC PERFORMANCE. Perceptual-motor training proliferated in the 1960s and became a popular subject of research studies, most of which were based on training programs patterned after Kephart, Barsh, Getman and Frostig. It is difficult to evaluate the research because a variety of subjects were used, including normal, disadvantaged, and mentally retarded individuals, unselected learning-disabled individuals and learning-disabled individuals with specific deficits. The variety of research designs, many of them poor, and the wide range in the length of remediation add to the problem. Some studies showed perceptual-motor training to affect academic performance and others did not. One of the better-designed studies that showed positive outcomes was conducted by Serwer and her associates.[261] These researchers compared the effectiveness of four methods of instruction on the achievement of 62 first-grade children at high risk for learning disabilities. The children were randomly assigned to one of four groups: (1) the direct group, receiving the Distar method for teaching reading; (2) the indirect group, receiving training in auditory, visual, and gross and fine motor areas; (3) a combined group, receiving both direct and indirect remediation; and (4) a control group, receiving no treatment. There was scattered support for the indirect method in word recognition, in arithmetic, and in one type of error in reading. The combined and indirect groups also did much better on the handwriting scale, as well as on gross and fine motor tasks.

This study showed some research support for the value of perceptual-motor training on academic performance. However, many studies show no effect of training.[159] Myers and Hamill[218] reviewed over 200 studies of perceptual and perceptual-motor training conducted between 1964 and 1974, and found little evidence supporting the effectiveness of perceptual-motor training in improving visual perception or academic performance. A meta-analysis of 180 studies of perceptual-motor training showed a similar result.[158] The lack of support for the value of perceptual and motor training in academic and cognitive areas has led many authors to dismiss perceptual-motor training as a viable approach to the education of learning-disabled children.[45,133,134,186,222] Other authors recognize the lack of

consistent evidence but recommend continued use and evaluation of these programs as an adjunct to other educational procedures.[111,128,183]

To keep the status of the educational merits of perceptual-motor training in perspective, it should be noted that no approach to the remediation of learning-disabled children has been demonstrated to be consistently more effective than another in promoting academic learning. There is no more empirical evidence supporting the value of language-based programs, task analysis, or psychological counseling with learning-disabled children than there is for perceptual-motor training.[133,134,222] The dismissal of perceptual-motor training and not these other techniques is therefore based on what seems relevant to the reviewer. Hallahan[133] concluded that there is a "lamentable lack of methodological sophistication which seems to be inherent in the learning disabilities field" (p. 47). Perceptual-motor training may be of academic value in selected learning-disabled children, but the benefits have little research support.

Motor learning theory of Cratty. Cratty[74-76] is a physical educator who advocates the use of gross motor activities for motor learning and physical fitness. His interest in perception is primarily as it affects motor activity, and he does not believe that motor training per se affects cognition or academic performance. However, he stresses the importance of motor proficiency to a child's general well-being. Participation in motor activities can enhance health, self-esteem, acceptance by peers and have an indirect influence on academic performance.[76] Cratty also suggests that some classroom learning could be enhanced by the use of gross motor activities and games to teach basic concepts. Such activities are motivating and might also lengthen a child's attention span. Cratty is a prolific writer and his books on motor development and motor learning can be of value to therapists.

Despite Cratty's pragmatic approach to the use of gross motor activities, his programs are often grouped with the perceptual-motor theorists. A few studies have been done with academics as a dependent variable with results similar to the perceptual-motor theorists.[218]

Patterning theory of Doman and Delacato. The method of treatment developed at the Institute for Achievement of Human Potential by Glen Doman and Carl Delacato,[84-86] as applied to children with cerebral palsy, has been widely publicized. Their patterning theory of neurological organization has also been applied to mentally retarded and reading-disabled children.[84-86] The theory proposes that full neurological organization requires that the individual pass through sequential developmental levels associated with progressively higher anatomic levels of the nervous system. The five early levels, anatomically identified as spinal cord, medulla, pons, midbrain, and early cortex, cover developmental patterns from reflex action through walking, usually achieved by around 1 year of age. The sixth level is cortical hemispheric dominance, which normally occurs by 8 years of age.

For the child with a learning problem, critical importance is placed on this sixth level.[84] The achievement of unilateral eye, hand, and foot preference consistent with the dominant hemisphere of the brain is considered a primary aim of treatment. It is believed that children with learning disability or hyperactivity can be "cured" if the appropriate neurological organization is promoted. Techniques for the facilitation of dominance include the forced restriction of the nondominant hand, active training of the dominant hand, patching to strengthen the dominant eye, and elimination of nonverbal music because it is presumed to stimulate the nondominant hemisphere.

Critique of patterning theory. A critique of the patterning theory by Chapanis[66] includes a comprehensive discussion of the theories on which it is based. Chapanis noted that there is no evidence that passive manipulation of the limbs and head will affect neurological organization. The accumulated evidence of neuropsychological research in hemispheric specialization during the 20 years since the theory was developed raises questions about the accuracy of the dominance theory. The need for congruent eye, hand, and foot dominance is questionable: 35% of the normal population have a mixed dominance in this respect. Furthermore, many of the unusual techniques are based on poorly substantiated premises, and questions have been raised about inaccuracies in these authors' calculation of developmental ages.[66]

Research on the effects of patterning therapy. There is no solid evidence to support the efficacy of patterning therapy. Studies with positive outcomes have been found to have serious flaws in methodology.[66] The effectiveness of patterning therapy for mild dysfunction has not been established. In addition, the practice of patterning therapy has been severely criticized in a statement used by 10 voluntary and professional organizations for what appears to be the excessive nature of undocumented claims for its effectiveness and for the extreme demands that are placed on parents.[5,66,186]

Occupational and physical therapy approaches to treatment. For convenience, occupational and physical therapy approaches to the remediation of motor deficits in children with learning disabilities are classified as sensory integration, neurodevelopmental, sensorimotor, developmental motor skill, and physical fitness. These categories are far from mutually exclusive, either in theory or in practice, and most therapists use a combination of two or more approaches.[11,207] However, the categories identify emphases in the management of children with minimal motor dysfunction. Sensory integration, as well as neurodevelopmental and sensorimotor therapy, relatively speaking, represent the indirect approach, and developmental motor skill and physical fitness represent a more direct approach.

Sensory integration theory of Ayres. The sensory integration theory has been developed and articulated by Ayres,[12-26,28,29] an occupational therapist and psychologist. It includes concepts drawn from neurophysiology, neuropsychology, and development. These concepts are unified by clinical observation. Sensory integration theory is based on the premise that higher cortical functions are dependent on adequate neural organization at subcortical brain levels. For example, the development of visual perception is believed to require integration with other sensory information, especially from somatosensory and vestibular processing mediated at the brainstem/midbrain. Ayres[16] suggests that the child with motor deficits and underlying sensory integration problems can be treated by influencing neurophysiological integration through controlling sensorimotor behavior. Emphasis is on the development of the capacity to perceive, remember, or plan motor movements. With such capacity, the mastery of academic and other tasks is facilitated. However, it must be emphasized that the motor deficits seen in the learning-disabled child with sensory integration dysfunction are the result of problems in processing sensory input. Thus sensory integration therapy is different from neurodevelopmental therapy in that the disorders treated by clinicians using neurodevelopmental therapy are primarily motor, and the types of problems addressed using sensory integration procedures are primarily disorders in sensory processing. In sensory integration, motor processes are considered significant because they are "observable and measurable."

Ayres states clearly that sensory integration procedures are designed for sensory integration dysfunction and that this dysfunction accounts for only some aspects of learning disorders. Research by Ayres[12-14,17,21] has been a continuous search to identify the kinds of deficits that respond to sensory integration procedures.

Types of sensory integration dysfunction. Through a series of factor analysis studies and cluster analyses, Ayres[12-14,17,21,28] has described certain characteristics that seem to occur together and relate to deficits in processing in certain sensory systems. These types of sensory integration dysfunction are often associated with deficits in tactile and/or vestibular processing. It must be emphasized that these patterns are not absolute. Considerable overlap exists and most children do not exclusively fit into one category. Therefore Ayres[20] prefers the term "disorder in the neural system." The five types of disorders that Ayres described as a result of the factor analysis studies are (1) disorders in vestibular function and in postural-ocular control and bilateral integration, (2) dyspraxia, (3) tactile defensiveness, (4) form and space perception problems, and (5) auditory-language problems. Recent cluster analyses with the Sensory Integration and Praxis Tests have further clarified the nature of praxic deficits and differentiated two types of praxis, visuo- and somatopraxis, and praxis to verbal command. The first two types of disorders will be elaborated because they are the disorders most closely associated with motor deficits. Although the motor deficits are being addressed, it is integration of sensory information within the CNS that is most important; the motor output is merely a means of assessing status and change in sensory integration (see Ayres[16,25,28] for a complete review of the types of sensory integration disorders).

DISORDERS IN VESTIBULAR FUNCTIONS AND IN POSTURAL-OCULAR CONTROL AND BILATERAL INTEGRATION. Children with learning problems often exhibit deficits in vestibular, postural, and ocular systems. Certain indicators of inadequate vestibular functions have been noted in the learning-disabled child. One of the most frequently used measures of vestibular function is the postrotary nystagmus response, the back and forth movements of the eyes following rotation. This response is a manifestation of the vestibular ocular reflex and is a normal adaptive response designed to reestablish the original fixation on a visual field.[19] Several studies have linked hyporesponsive (shortened) duration of nystagmus to learning disabilities. De-Quiros[95] and Ayres[19,24] found that more than 50% of the learning-disabled children they each studied had shortened duration of nystagmus. Frank and Levinson[105] found that almost 90% of their learning-disabled children had vestibulocerebellar deficits. Thus there seems to be a significant percentage of learning-disabled children with a reduced duration of postrotatory nystagmus. Several mechanisms have been suggested to explain this phenomenon.[19] An absence or decreased duration of nystagmus may be reflective of inadequate input being relayed by the vestibular nuclei. Another interpretation suggests that an adequate amount of sensory excitation is not reaching the vestibular nuclei. Another interpretation suggests that an adequate amount of sensory excitation is not reaching the vestibular nuclei. Nystagmus may be diminished as a result of overinhibition of the vestibular nuclei by the cerebellum. Alternatively, the general arousal (the reticular activating system) of the child may be diminished.

It should be emphasized that nystagmus is only one manifestation of vestibular functioning. Certain other problems, such as postural and ocular problems, have been associated with vestibular system dysfunction.[209] The vestibular system serves a primary role in the development of postural control and equilibrium. Many learning-disabled children have poorly integrated reflexes and immature or poorly developed equilibrium (e.g., a positive Romberg's sign). Standing balance is often impaired.[121] Standing balance with the eyes closed may be more impaired than standing balance with eyes open since when the eyes are closed the child cannot use vision and must rely on vestibular and proprioceptive input.[19,20] The child may also show an inability to assume and maintain the prone extension position (head, trunk, and leg extension against gravity). It has been suggested that this reflects inadequate vestibular processing.[20,24,57,225] Other indicators of vestibular

dysfunction may be inadequate muscle tone and inadequate cocontraction.[16,80,209,225] Adequate muscle tone enables the body to be readied for movement. Descending influences from the lateral vestibulospinal tract facilitate both alpha and gamma motor neurons.[244]

The vestibular system has also been implicated in ocular control. Through its interaction with the oculomotor mechanism, the vestibular system serves to stabilize the eyes during head and neck movements in order that a fixed visual image may be perceived.[16]

Ayres[18] has hypothesized that the vestibular system may be involved in some aspect of interhemispheric communication and lateralization of cerebral function. This hypothesis is based, in part, on the clinical observation of a group of children with vestibular disorders who also show problems in bilateral integration and lateralization of function.

The bilateral integration deficit is reflected by an impaired ability to use both sides of the body together in a coordinated way and to use one body side in the contralateral side of space.[16] Behavioral tasks demonstrating these difficulties may be problems in jumping with both feet together, reciprocal stair climbing, or skipping. The child may tend to avoid crossing the midline and may either shift his/her entire body to avoid crossing the midline or tend to use his/her right hand on the right body side and the left hand on the left body side. This interferes with the development of a preferred skilled hand.

DEVELOPMENTAL DYSPRAXIA. Developmental dyspraxia represents an impairment in the ability to plan skilled movements that are nonhabitual. Children with developmental dyspraxia can learn specific skills with practice, but they do not have the generalized ability to plan unfamiliar tasks. Gubbay[128-131] refers to the child with developmental dyspraxia as the "clumsy child." Movements are performed with an excessive expenditure of energy and with inaccurate judgement of the required force, tempo, and amplitude.[299] There is an inability to relate the sequence of motions to each other. Ayres[25,27] has suggested that praxis is more than just motor planning. Rather, it involves programming a course of action that includes the ability to organize behaviors and to develop strategies. Children with problems in programming a course of action are often disorganized and have poor work habits—characteristics that frequently accompany developmental dyspraxia.

According to Ayres,[16] motor planning ability is strongly dependent on an adequate body scheme and on understanding of one's relationship to the environment. "The body scheme which provides the substrate for praxis is a product of intersensory integration" (p. 165). Motor planning depends on the adequate integration of somatosensory, vestibuloproprioceptive, and visual information. As such, disorders in any of these senses may result in poor motor planning ability.

Both Ayres[12-14,17,21,28] and Kephart[165] have noted

problems in processing tactile-kinesthetic information in the dyspraxic child. Ayres[16] hypothesized a close relationship between problems in processing tactile information, problems in body scheme, and motor planning problems. Motor planning involves the development of a semiconscious motor scheme. The scheme is developed by sensory awareness initiated by the tactile system, which is a mature sensory system right at birth. During early development, the child experiences much of his/her environment through the tactile system and gains a diffuse awareness of his or her body. The child also learns and discovers the nature of objects through manipulation. Proprioceptive input from the muscles, tendons, joints, and vestibular system work with the tactile system to establish a child's awareness of his or her body and how it works. "Sensory input from the skin and joints, but especially from the skin, helps to develop in the brain the model or internal scheme of the body's design as a motor instrument" (p. 168).[16]

It is suggested that the dyspraxic child is receiving incorrect or an inadequate amount of tactile input. Consequently, the child's ability to plan adaptive responses is impaired. "If the information that the body receives from its somatosensory receptors is not precise, the brain has a poor basis on which to build its body scheme" (p. 170).[16]

Manifestations of poor motor planning ability are apparent in many daily tasks. Dressing is often difficult. The child is not able to plan where or how to move his/her limbs to put on clothes. Problems are often demonstrated in constructive manipulatory play, such as tinker toys, cutting, and pasting. Similarly, learning how to use utensils, such as a knife, fork, pencil, or scissors, is difficult. The dyspraxic child often has problems with handwriting. As was mentioned previously, dyspraxic children can learn through repetition of a task; however, there is limited generalization of the learned skill to similar tasks.

Principles of sensory integration procedures. A central principle in sensory integration procedures is providing planned and controlled sensory input with the eliciting of an adaptive response in order to enhance the organization of neural mechanisms. Provision of sensory input follows a developmental sequence, with a focus on input mediated at the brainstem or midbrain level since this is hypothesized to be the site of disorder.[16] Treatment focuses on sensory input and its continual interaction with motion. The goal is to elicit responses that better reflect sensory integration and more normal patterns of sensory input as opposed to improving motor skill for the sake of skill itself.

Another principle on which therapy is based is that lower parts of the brain develop before higher structures and that cortical functions are in some respect still dependent upon brainstem functions.[16] Both the tactile and vestibular systems send large quantities of input to the brainstem/reticular activating system and can exert influence on brain function.

While there are general principles for sensory integra-

tion procedures, each child's plan must be individualized based on the results of evaluation and observation in therapy. The general steps in sensory integration procedures are:

1. Improve sensory integration in general
2. Enhance maturation of postural responses and related proprioceptive mechanisms
3. Develop praxis or the capacity to motor plan
4. Encourage interaction of the two sides of the body and space
5. Develop form and space perception

The steps are detailed by Ayres,[16,18] and treatment principles and suggested activities are elaborated in a number of sources.*

It should be mentioned that the vestibular and tactile sensory input that are used in therapy are powerful types of input and must be used with caution. The autonomic as well as behavioral responses of the child must be carefully monitored. The therapist should be knowledgeable about sensory integration theory and treatment before using these procedures. Treatment precautions are elaborated in Ayres.[16]

Critique of sensory integration theory. Sensory integration theory is immensely complex since it is derived from neurophysiological and psychological knowledge, but it is shaped by ongoing research and is therefore changing and developing. Most critics of sensory integration theory are general in their criticism.[269] For example, Gottlieb[125] found the theoretical model to be inconclusive, noting that while a demonstration of an association between tactile-perceptual development, sensorimotor impairment, and high-level cognitive functioning has been made, application of tactile-perceptual training or sensorimotor training to improve cognitive and intellectual abilities remains a controversial issue. Sieben[265] questioned the theory based on the lack of clinical signs of brainstem malfunction in learning-disabled children and on the lack of clarity in the process by which sensory stimulation is supposed to foster integration in the brainstem. This criticism may result in part from the use of the term "brainstem" as a synonym for subcortical structures. However, the hypotheses about brain functioning are not directly testable. This criticism of the theory is directed at the lack of support rather than at evidence of contradiction with known facts. Although various individuals have criticized sensory integration because the research has not shown why it works,[10] it is clearly very difficult to substantiate why sensory integration is effective through the research tools and methodologies now available because these aspects are highly theoretical and difficult to observe. However, according to Tickle[286] it is not appropriate to conclude on the basis of this difficulty that the theory is not correct. Tickle[286] states that the pur-

*References 16, 25, 37, 69, 100, 123, 139, 267.

pose of early research in a field, particularly in a practice field, is to demonstrate whether the given treatment is or is not effective. As the research progresses, researchers start examining factors that influence the effectiveness of therapy. Later they examine why therapy works.

Research on the effects of sensory integration procedures on academic and motor performances. Since 1980 there have been seven articles that have reviewed the sensory integration effectiveness literature.* Examination of these reviews and other related literature indicates that, at present, there is not consistent agreement regarding the effectiveness of sensory integration. Clinicians who are using sensory integration procedures are convinced that it is effective. There are many testimonials from parents of children who have received occupational therapy using sensory integration procedures. However, empirical data is limited, and its interpretation is highly varied. For example, in a review of the sensory integration research with learning disabilities, Henderson[141] concluded that "the studies . . . provide preliminary evidence of the value of sensory integrative therapy for children with learning disabilities" (p. 45) and that "Certainly they provide sufficient evidence to warrant further investigation of the effects of sensory integrative therapy on academic learning as well as on perceptual and motor skills" (p. 45).

In a review of the effectiveness studies, Ottenbacher[227] categorized the outcome measures of the effects of sensory integration procedures into three groups: academic achievement, language, and motor performance. The only studies of sensory integration procedures for learning-disabled children that had academic learning as the dependent variable have been those conducted by Ayres.[15,24] The results of both studies indicate that sensory integration procedures have a positive effect on scores on academic tests. Gaddes[111] noted that the studies failed to control for the effects of different therapists/teachers in the experimental and control groups. However, this criticism can be partially countered by a finding of the second study that some learning-disabled children, specifically those with hyperactive nystagmus, benefitted more than other learning-disabled children receiving sensory integration procedures.[24]

The effectiveness of sensory integration on motor functions has also been examined. Following a program that emphasized gross motor planning and vestibular stimulation but that did not include training in eye-hand coordination, learning-disabled children with mild choreothetosis made significantly greater improvements in eye-hand coordination than a control group not receiving therapy.[23] DePauw[94] reported sensory integration procedures to be more effective than remedial physical education in improving scores on perceptual-motor and fine motor tests. In his analysis of the eight studies of sensory integration, Otten-

bacher[226] also found a moderate effect size for a motor-reflex variable.

In 1986, Clark and Pierce[68] presented a literature review on sensory integration and other relevant treatment effectiveness studies specifically carried out with pediatric populations by occupational therapy researchers. Twenty-six studies were found, including research with large samples as well as single-subject designs. Thirteen of the studies examined the effectiveness of sensory integration procedures as their independent variable, four examined the effect of systematically applied vestibular stimulation, four of multisensory input, and five of perceptual-motor training. Given these numbers of studies, it becomes apparent that useful research in this area is progressing, although slowly.

Ottenbacher[226] has performed a statistical analysis of effect size on the results of eight studies of sensory integration procedures with a total of 47 hypotheses. The subjects in these studies included learning-disabled, mentally retarded, aphasic, and at-risk children. The analysis found that the average child receiving sensory integration performed better on academic measures than three-fourths of control children, a moderate effect size.

In a summary of his meta-analysis, Ottenbacher[227] stated that "the meta-analysis of the SI research literature did provide suggestive support for the effects of SI therapy" (p. 319). However, the number of studies that met the criteria for inclusion (the research study had to have a control group, for example) was only eight, which, Ottenbacher emphasized, is quite small for a meta-analysis.

These studies provide preliminary evidence of the value of sensory integration in influencing the academic and motor performance of children with learning disabilities. Careful review of the studies shows that some children respond to therapy and others do not and that some academic abilities might be affected and others not. Additional research is needed to define the dimensions of disabilities relevant to sensory integration procedures.

Neurodevelopmental theory of Bobath. As is evident from the description of motor deficits, a maturational lag in the integration of primitive postural reflexes is often found in learning-disabled children. This has led clinicians to apply or adapt neurodevelopmental treatment to learning-disabled children. Neurodevelopmental treatment emphasizes the inhibition/integration of primitive postural patterns, promotes the development of normal postural reactions, and has an important goal—the normalization of abnormal tone.[47] Neurodevelopmental therapy is essentially a developmental approach and stresses the importance of early treatment. The techniques for developing postural and equilibrium reactions in learning-disabled children include the therapy ball and positioning in the classroom. Neurodevelopmental therapy is directed toward the improvement of motor function; influence of treatment

---

*References 10, 68, 141, 227, 228, 257, 286.

on academic performance is considered secondary to the reduction of postural stress.

Critique of neurodevelopmental theory. Neurodevelopmental theory is extensively reviewed in Chapters 3 and 6. The reader is also referred to the recent review of this theory by Keshner.[166] One criticism that Keshner offered is that Bobath's explanation of the CNS disorder and of intervention is based on a hierarchical unidirectional model of the nervous system that is not adequate for the understanding of motor control systems.

Research on the effects of neurodevelopmental therapy. Neurodevelopmental therapy is based on principles derived from research in motor development and neurophysiology. However, the techniques arise from careful and extensive clinical observations. The system of therapy is widely used with children with cerebral palsy, the group for which it was designed, but it has been subjected to little experimental verification. Two studies of this theory with children with cerebral palsy found a greater mean change in the motor development of the children in the experimental group.[61,258] A third study found differences in only one of several subgroups, that of spastic quadriplegic children.[307] Because each of these studies had methodological problems, the evidence for the effectiveness of the neurodevelopmental theory remains tentative. There are no studies of the use of this theory and related systems of therapy for learning-disabled children.

Sensorimotor therapy. Neurodevelopmental therapy may be used as a single treatment approach (as is often the case with children with cerebral palsy), but the systems of sensorimotor therapy that have been developed for learning-disabled children are commonly a combination of neurodevelopmental therapy and sensory integration procedures.[100,120,139,207,210]

Sensorimotor therapy, as used here, is therapy planned to enhance gross motor development as defined by Hoskins and Squires.[145] These authors operationally defined gross motor development as the sequential integration of automatic, stereotyped, reflex phenomena leading to the emergence of voluntary, discrete, nonobligatory motor behavior concerned with posture and locomotion. The emphasis in sensorimotor therapy is on functions mediated largely on a subcortical level. It includes integration of residual primitive postural reflexes, the development of efficient righting and equilibrium reactions, and the improvement of tone and cocontraction.

Miller and Goldberg described an illustrative program for a 6-year-old with residual primitive reflexes, immature, exaggerated righting reflexes, hypotonicity, and hypermobile joints.

Rolling, commando crawling, crawling, and knee walking were performed by the child, with the therapist administering rhythmic stabilization and contract-relax techniques in three positions. These activities, given in combination with therapeutic techniques, seemed to gradually improve his muscle strength, static balance, joint stability and kinesthetic awareness. The second half hour of treatment was aimed at improving his dynamic equilibrium and righting reactions, as well as inhibiting the residual primitive reflexes. The rocker board, scooter board and large beach ball were used to elicit dynamic equilibrium reactions. Bilateral arm and leg activities using such equipment as cage balls, rubber balls, and broom sticks were used to inhibit primitive reflexes and to strengthen his upper extremities (p. 502).[207]

Sensorimotor therapy is developmentally based. Reflex integration is approached in the sequence in which inhibition of primitive postural reflexes and the elicitation of equilibrium and righting reactions occur in the normal child. Although the learning-disabled child with motor dysfunction walks and runs, he/she may demonstrate inadequate postural reactions in lying, sitting, or kneeling positions. Therefore these functions are remediated.

In the development of postural reactions, attention is given to performance both with the eyes open and closed. Many children have a poor tactile, proprioceptive, and vestibular integration basis for movement and an overreliance on vision for equilibrium and righting reactions. Sensory integration techniques for stimulating the vestibular system are appropriate.[16,95] The improvement of tone through proprioceptive neuromuscular facilitation (PNF) and Rood techniques can be incorporated into the activities for reflex integration. Vestibular stimulation in the prone position has also been found to increase extensor tone of the neck and back musculature.

For further discussion of sensorimotor therapy, the reader is referred to Gilfoyle and Grady,[119,120] Heiniger and Randolph,[139] Knickerbocker,[179] Ayres,[16] and DeQuiros and Schrager.[95] These sources also describe many therapeutic activities for the development of postural functions in learning-disabled children.

Developmental motor skill training. Sensorimotor therapy includes training in motor skills that are basic, that is, those that develop in infancy and early preschool years. The skills taught in developmental motor skill training programs are usually, although not always, of a higher level. The real difference is in the approach used. Developmental motor skill training involves the learning of skills and subskills sequenced by the ages at which they are accomplished or by steps from less demanding to more demanding skills. Evaluation identifies the point at which a child fails; treatment involves a hierarchy of tasks from gross to fine.[129,130]

Abbie[1] described the developmental motor skills training approach: "One can . . . break down the skills into their simplest forms and give the child opportunities to practice each in as many varied ways as possible so that he does not learn one isolated splinter skill" (p. 200).[1] As an example, Abbie suggested that a child with poor balance in standing practice balance in all positions—kneeling, all fours, sitting, and prone—and on both stable and mobile surfaces. Abbie used multiple approaches, including neurodevelopmental theory, modern dance, and gymnastics.

Knickerbocker[174] has developed a structured approach for developing skills that span a progression from early postural functions to perceptual skills, noting that learning-disabled children are often exposed to learning experiences for which they are not developmentally ready. The development of postural skill is organized around the use of five basic pieces of therapeutic equipment: an indoor climber, a carpeted barrel, a scooter board, inflated equipment, and suspended equipment. Program plans are presented with activities given for three levels of accomplishment. Knickerbocker emphasizes the close relationship between diagnostic assessment and treatment procedures and presents an evaluation system that basically consists of qualitative descriptions of a child's response to the therapeutic equipment. Thus the overall plan provides a graded system that includes an ongoing evaluation of performance.

DeHaven and others[82] constructed a test that evaluates aspects of coordination and found that, in a group of 122 learning-disabled children, the primary deficits were in the alternate movements of distal joints and in static and dynamic balance. DeHaven and Mordock[81] found that exercises designed to improve fine motor skills were effective in the improvement of distal reciprocal movements. These authors suggested that the rationale for exercises for children with cerebral palsy also applied to learning-disabled children with motor dysfunction.[212] Accordingly, they recommended exercises that provide additional sensory stimulation. Other criteria suggested for exercises were as follows:

1. Each exercise should require voluntary reciprocal movements; this means that the child must initiate the movement on command without manual assistance from the instructor.
2. Each exercise should contain within it different stages of complexity; each stage should require greater concentration and neuromuscular control than the previous one.
3. The exercises should require movement of more than one extremity or joint at one time; thus the training takes place not just on the dominant side but also on the nondominant side.
4. Structure of activities should include sequential muscular involvement from proximal to distal, but with greater emphasis on distal segments.[212]

The writings of the perceptual-motor theorists include the description of a wealth of activities that can be used for the development of motor skills in learning-disabled children. The recommended activities of these theorists include indirect remediation as well as motor skill development.[139] However, much of the treatment is directed

*References 33, 74, 75, 76, 118, 163, 164, 192.

toward the acquisition of basic skills as described by Abbie.[1,2] A basic principle is to provide a great variety of motor activities at the child's developmental motor level to promote motor generalizations. The activities recommended include balance, locomotion, body awareness, and hand-eye coordination.

A final area of skill that should not be ignored is that of activities of daily living. Clumsy children are frequently delayed in the basic self-care skills of tying shoe laces, using a knife and fork, and blowing their nose, as well as a general inefficiency in dressing for school.[128,130] Inadequacy in self-care is a sensitive area for children whose peers have no such difficulty, and teachers and therapists should be aware of a child's need to learn these basic skills.

Physical fitness. In addition to the primary deficits in sensorimotor functions, motor skills, and sensory integration functions, a learning-disabled child is at risk for poor posture, body mechanics, and physical fitness. Physical fitness, as defined here, includes strength, endurance, speed, agility, flexibility and cardiorespiratory endurance.

Arnheim and Sinclair[11] pointed out that there is a vicious cycle in the relationship between motor ability and physical fitness. The child with poor motor ability avoids physical activity, and the poor fitness that develops through lack of exercise lessens motor ability.

The physiologically based poor posture and inefficient body use can be exaggerated by a secondary disability. The child's poor self-concept may be reflected in a hunched, withdrawn posture and the avoidance of any physical activity beyond that needed in everyday activities. This latter pattern can also be found in learning-disabled children without a primary motor disability.

The physical therapist should monitor and prevent or correct loss of movement in the joints of the neck and spine and work with the physical educator to ensure that a child receives sufficient exercise to maintain his/her physical fitness. Arnheim and Sinclair[11] presented graded levels of activities for fitness in the four levels of strength and muscular endurance, flexibility, agility and large muscle coordination, and cardiorespiratory endurance.

Summary. Many models of training emphasize the identification and training of deficit cognitive, perceptual, and/or motor skills as a preparation for learning academic material. This discussion has been limited primarily to the models that advocate whole-body motor activity as a prerequisite for, or as an adjunct to, traditional education for learning-disabled children.

Training programs that emphasize whole-body movement may appear similar to the layperson, and many specific training techniques are common in more than one program. The approaches also have some assumptions in common, although the rationale for an assumption may differ markedly. Many of the theories are developmental, postulating predictable developmental sequences and sharing the assumption that planned experiences can influence the nature and rate of development, but the theories of development may be very different. One major difference among the theories is the extent to which motor learning is considered to be reflected in later cognitive learning. Kephart, Getman, and Barsch considered that certain levels of perceptual-motor skills were necessary prerequisites to higher-level learning and that remediation should focus on the underlying deficits with academic and cognitive skills waiting until readiness was established. These theories were based on psychoeducational constructs, and they advocate the application of perceptual-motor training as an aid to learning for handicapped as well as normal children, suggesting that modern living deprives children of adequate gross motor activity and that this in turn affects academic learning. Doman and Delacato also applied their theory to the development of normal children, but their theoretical base was derived from concepts of phylogenetic as well as ontogenetic development of the nervous system. DeQuiros, Ayres, and Frostig believed that remediation of basic perceptual and sensory integration deficits facilitates academic learning but advocated training as an adjunct to regular remedial education. Neurodevelopmental therapy is primarily directed toward the remediation of motor deficits. Within the motor area, both Ayres and Bobath are developmentalists. Cratty makes no assumptions about academic learning except as it is indirectly affected by more efficient motor function and/or motivation.

Reviewers who support perceptual-motor and sensory integration programs primarily do so with the provision that the programs are planned within a context that includes special education. For example, on the basis of her review of perceptual-motor theories, Lerner came to this conclusion:

We cannot conclude that motor development is unimportant or that this aspect of learning should be discarded. Rather, these studies suggest that plans are needed for building the bridge between motor training and academic learning. Efficient motor movement may be a prerequisite but alone it is insufficient (p. 155).[183]

Silver[270] noted that research results suggest that sensory integration is valid, but that a child should always have a complete special education evaluation and that therapists should work as a part of a special education team in a school environment.

We agree that on the basis of known scientific theory and available research that motor training should not replace an academic program. Furthermore, in practice with children with deficits, training should be recommended on the basis of improving perceptual and motor functions, not only on hypothesized improvement in higher-level training. However, the academic performance of some children

appears to improve with perceptual, perceptual-motor and sensorimotor training, and we believe that research into the relationship of perceptual and motor performance and learning should continue.

Finally, this discussion of motor training has reflected controversy as it relates to the influence of motor training on cognitive learning capacity. Motor performance is an important aspect of the total development of the child, and training to maximize perceptual-motor and sensorimotor functions is necessary for learning-disabled children with motor deficits.

Organization of occupational and physical therapy services. Traditionally, occupational and physical therapy have been provided in clinics that were completely separated from educational services or in special schools or classes for orthopedically or multiply handicapped children. In special schools and classes, the therapists work with teachers but with a philosophy similar to that of a clinic. The service is optimal for interdisciplinary cooperation, teachers and therapists are readily accessible to one another, and the program has the potential for maximizing educational and therapeutic benefits for the child. In such a setting therapists provide direct "hands on" treatment for the child, as well as work with the teacher and the child's parents to facilitate motor functioning in the classroom and at home.

Although in some states occupational and physical therapists have provided services for multiply handicapped children in public schools for many years, therapy for children with minor motor deficits, such as the learning-disabled child, is more recent. During the last 10 years, occupational therapy services for learning-disabled children have become increasingly common; physical therapy for learning disabled children has been even more recently established and is still less common. However, the establishment of the Education for All Handicapped Act (PL 94-142) is rapidly changing the status of therapy in public school systems. The provision of related services, including occupational and physical therapy as well as special education, is now a mandated part of the educational process. As specialists in the evaluation of motor functions, therapists provide evaluation services for children with all levels of motor dysfunction, and therefore see children not referred for service formerly.

PL 94-142 has also changed the location and kinds of services provided to children with special needs. The educational and social disadvantages of segregating handicapped children from their age peers have been cited, and the concept of least restrictive placement has been articulated in the law. "Least restrictive" implies an appropriate education in an environment as close to that of the normal child as possible. For the learning-disabled child, this usually means mainstreaming by the placement of a child in a regular class. Supplemental special education instruction is provided by an itinerant teacher, a resource room,

*Reference 183, p 155.

or a consultant to the regular classroom teacher. Meeting the needs of these children requires a change both in occupational and physical therapy evaluation and treatment services and in the methods of delivery of those services.[155,178,184,216,259]

Kalish and Presseller[155] have identified five areas of function for the physical or occupational therapist in the educational environment. They include:

1. Screening and evaluating children with a wide variety of functional deficits
2. Program planning based on evaluation results and related to a child's ability to receive maximum benefit from his educational experiences
3. Treatment activities designed to meet program goals
4. Consultation to teachers, other school personnel, and parents around carry-over of services into the classroom and home programming
5. In-service training for individuals and/or group relative to the needs of handicapped children

Because each of these functions is usually required of the public school therapist, the time available for providing direct services to children is limited. Treatment service must be done, in part, through consultation to parents, classroom teachers, and physical educators. The child's motor development needs can sometimes be met, wholly or in part, through the physical education program. The therapist can evaluate the child and suggest therapeutic activities that could be incorporated into an adaptive physical education program.

Kalish and Presseller[155] point out the necessity of integrating therapy into the educational process, first by adapting therapy to reinforce educational goals and then by incorporating therapy into routine classroom activities. The therapist must be flexible and discover alternate methods of reaching therapy goals, such as positioning and using unobtrusive adaptive equipment. The teacher's responsibility for all of the children in his or her classroom must always be kept in mind. Before proposing the incorporation of a therapeutic activity into a classroom, its feasibility must be assured. In some classrooms a teacher's aide might be available for individual attention, but in all instances both the child's time and the teacher's time must be considered in relation to the total program requirements.

In the provision of direct services, learning-disabled children can often be treated effectively in small groups, and occupational therapy and physical therapy aides are often available. It is important to plan schedules carefully so that the child is not removed from the classroom at times critical to his or her academic education. It must be recognized that what may be considered "optimal therapy" within a medical model may not be possible in an educational model. It is important for therapists to understand that the public schools' principal concern is the educational rather than the medical well-being of the child.

The therapist should become a participant in the educational process.[184] It is essential for the therapist working in the public school to learn about the public school system as a social institution, about the educational philosophies that guide teachers, and about the legislative regulations governing programs for children with special needs, as well as about the legal responsibilities of public school therapists.[216] Within a specific setting the therapist needs to know which model of special education service delivery is being used. The therapist needs to translate medical information for educational personnel and must write evaluation and progress reports without using medical jargon. In short, the therapist must become a participant in the educational process.[184] Comprehensive discussions of occupational and physical therapy in public school systems are presented in a number of publications.*

BEHAVIORAL AND EMOTIONAL SEQUELAE OF LEARNING DISABILITIES

Although the majority of literature and work in learning disabilities has been addressed to the identification, analysis, and remediation of academic deficits, there are often behavioral and emotional sequelae that accompany a learning disability and that may sometimes become of even greater importance than the learning disability itself.[51,73,122,300] Ames[8] stressed that there is no single behavior pattern prevalent in all those who are learning disabled but that there are some commonalities, the most obvious of these being a poor self-image. Although the child with a learning disability may initially be an integral part of the social and educational milieu, because of poor academic progress, disruptive behaviors, and the necessity for special attention from the teacher, guidance counselor, or resource personnel, the learning-disabled child perceives himself and is perceived by others as being "different."[125] A self-defeating cycle may be established: the child experiences learning problems, the school and home environments become increasingly tense, and disruptive behaviors become more pronounced. These responses, in turn, further affect the child's abilities to learn. Lack of success generates more failure until the child anticipates defeat in almost every situation.[310] The learning-disabled child is often discouraged and fearful, attitudes are defensive and negativistic, and motivation may be lost. Self-concept, self-confidence, and peer relationships are often affected.† Research has confirmed that these children tend to be rejected more often and that they are less popular than "normal" peers in regular classrooms.[53,67,186] The child's behavior and impaired learning usually generate a state of perpetual anxiety for the entire family.[8,125]

---

*References 6, 7, 155, 157, 178, 292.
†References 36, 54, 99, 245, 272, 303.

Life-span learning disabilities

Research with learning-disabled adolescents and adults has indicated that, for the most part, children do not outgrow learning disabilities[35,58,78,161] and that these problems tend to persist in some or all of the following areas: attention and activity, neuromaturation, cognition and academic performance, emotional adjustment, and social interactions.

In fact, the definition of learning disabilities proposed by the Association of Children and Adults with Learning Disabilities (ACLD, 1985) emphasizes that the disability persists, stating "Throughout life, the condition can affect self-esteem, education, vocation, socialization, and/or daily living activities."[181]

Follow-up studies of hyperactive children indicate that while hyperactivity itself becomes less of a problem as children get older, many other problems exist. Routh and Mesibov[250] found that, of 83 teenagers who had been hyperactive as children, 58% had failed one or more grades in school, low self-esteem was common, and several had been involved in delinquent behavior. In a 5-year follow-up study of hyperactive children, Weiss and others[302] found that 70% had repeated at least one grade as compared to 15% of matched control subjects. The chief complaints of the children's mothers included distractibility and poor concentration, although the hyperactivity itself had declined. Hoy and others[146] did a 5-year follow-up study of hyperactive children and found that at adolescence, although the activity declined, the hyperactive children still had attentional and stimulus-processing difficulties that affected both their academic and social functioning. Overall, results indicated that childhood hyperactivity seems to be predictive of continued academic failure, poor concentration, impulsivity, low self-esteem, and poor conduct.

Research has also indicated that there are long-term academic effects of learning disabilities during the school years. In looking at whether or not children outgrow learning disabilities, Book[49] tested 472 Utah kindergarten children on standardized tests and assigned each student to one of three categories of presumed risk. Students were retested on academic achievement tests in first through fourth grades. Fewer than 11% of the students assigned to the high-risk group ever performed above the fiftieth percentile. Only 4% in the lowest-risk group ever performed below the twenty-fifth percentile.

Helper[140] reviewed follow-up studies of children with learning disabilities and found that, both emotionally and behaviorally, learning-disabled boys continued to have a much higher frequency of problems than did controls. In addition, persistent deficits in learning skills (e.g., reading achievement) along with deficits in attention and information processing were noted.

Even within the motor domain, there is increasing evidence that children do not outgrow their deficits.* despite some arguments to the contrary.[71] In fact, Denckla[91,93] pointed out that although many clumsy children do later master certain motor skills, they fail new age-appropriate ones. The same seems to be true in many domains.

Learning disabilities appear to have a persistent effect on self-concept. Of the adolescent populations with learning disabilities or hyperactivity studied, 40% to 60% have been found to have low self-esteem.[279] Depression, thoughts of suicide, and low expectations for the future also seemed to be more prevalent in the learning-disabled adolescent.[198]

The finding that learning disabilities are associated with behavioral problems has resulted, in recent years, in an interest in the relationship between learning disability and juvenile delinquency. A high rate of antisocial behavior in adolescence, "trouble with the law," or "police contact" are frequently found in follow-up studies of children with learning disabilities.[58] Learning or skill deficiencies are considered an element in a significant number of delinquents.[41] Several studies of delinquent, adolescent boys have shown that 25% to 30% have learning disabilities,[99] and Mauser[194] reported that 50% to 70% of juvenile delinquents in his sample exhibited evidence of learning disabilities. Rubin and Braun[251] found that the major deficits in juvenile delinquents were visual-spatial-orientational and visual-motor coordination deficits. It is recognized that not all children with learning disabilities become juvenile delinquents. Although there is not evidence for a causal link between juvenile delinquency and learning disabilities, there does seem to be a relationship.[177,310] Some clinicians believe that the learning-disabled child is at risk for developing deviant and antisocial behaviors and that educational and psychological trauma occurring in the classroom may be expressed as aberrant social functioning in the community.[310]

Study of the adult with learning disabilities is fairly recent, in part because "learning disabilities" were not diagnostic entities until the 1960s. Thus the children diagnosed in the 1960s are just now reaching adulthood. Many of the current reports on learning disabilities in adulthood are from persons who were diagnosed as learning disabled in their teenage or adult years. Thus they did not receive the early intervention services that learning-disabled children are currently receiving. Moreover, whereas the learning-disabled child of today is recognized as being bright with specific learning disabilities, those persons whose learning disabilities were recognized in their later years may have been considered lazy, unmotivated, or stupid in their formative educational years. Because of the recency of intervention services for learning disabilities, we cannot evaluate the effectiveness of treatment or its effect on long-term

---

*References 143, 182, 262, 276, 293, 303.

A letter from a learning disabled adult

I am 26 years old, a professional bassoonist with a master's degree in Music Performance. My name is Wendy. Through Jane, an occupational therapist, I discovered that I had learning problems and sensory integration problems when I was 24 years old.

I invert letters and especially numbers. When people speak English to me, I feel it's a foreign language. There's translation lag time. When learning new things, I either understand intuitively or never. I can't seem to go through step-by-step learning processes.

Physically, I'm extremely sensitive to motion. When I was little, we moved every year. I spent the first 5 years of my life feeling sick. It seems that I feel everything more strongly than most people. I have an extremely low threshold of pain and even pleasure tends to overload me. If I am touched unexpectedly it hurts; it's so jarring. This causes a lot of problems with interpersonal relationships. I can't stand to have people close to me; it produces an adrenalin reaction.

Motor activities are also a problem; my muscles don't seem to remember past motions. Despite the many times I've walked down steps and through doors, I still have to think about how high to lift my foot and about planning my movements. When eating, I have to think about chewing or I bite my tongue or mouth. I don't think other people think about these things. I'm physically inept; I can bump into the same table 10 times running. I'm always bruised, and as a child people constantly labeled me as clumsy. Physical education courses were hell as a child, especially gymnastics, where you are forced to leave the ground and swing or walk on balance beams or uneven bars. I cannot begin to explain the terror or disorientation.

Academically, I was labeled stupid or, more frequently, lazy. I was told that I was not trying. Actually, my I.Q. is very high and my coping mechanisms are very complex. If they only knew how hard I was trying. I was lucky because I taught myself to read at an early age. I would never have learned to read otherwise. Even so, my first grade teacher wouldn't believe that I could read so far past my age. She called me a liar when I said that I had finished each stupid "Dick-Jane" book. I was forced to read each one 50 times before she would give me a new one.

Not all teachers were so insensitive. My fourth grade teacher made very effort to let me go at my own pace, letting me read on a college level and do 2 years of math on my own. Left to my own devices, I can learn and love to do so. My fifth grade teacher forced me to do math the long way with steps. I just know the answer by looking at multiplication or division problems, even algebra problems, but to this day I cannot understand how one does it in steps. If a teacher didn't accept this, I was in for a year of hell. I cried a lot in school, from frustration mostly, and I pretended to be sick a lot.

I never had friends until college. I guess I was too different to be acceptable. I grew up in a very rigid, repressive, religious community which made it especially difficult to be accepted. My differences were labeled evil or, at best, I was ignored. I left high school at age 16 for college, where at least I could structure what I wanted to learn. It's never been easy for me to make friends, although it's better now. Music circles tend to be a bit crazy so I fit in more easily.

My learning disabilities still are problems. My motor and learning problems get in the way of my music, but my coping mechanisms are strong. I deal better with my clumsiness now. Just being diagnosed by Jane has made a big difference. To have things labeled, to be told and realize that it's not my fault, has given me a sense of peace. It's also allowed me to turn from inward depression to outward anger at those who labeled me stupid and clumsy. Just being able to admit anger allows one to let it go.

Other than my testing and subsequent conversations with Jane, I have not received treatment for my problems. I believe that adults with my problems can be helped. I wish programs were available in all areas of the country. At age 26, I feel much better about myself than I did even at age 24. It's a matter of growth and coping with major differences.

The greatest advice I would give to educators and therapists working with problem children is: accept. Accept what they can do well; don't make an issue of what they can't do. We all have are strengths and weaknesses. If a child can't do math, so what! Buy the child a calculator and the child will do a lot better with it than with a label of stupidity following her through life.

---

disability. For these reasons, it may not be possible to generalize from the learning-disabled adult of today to the learning-disabled adult of the future.

Much of our knowledge about the learning-disabled adult today is largely anecdotal and in the form of case histories. Documentation has clearly been lacking. Few research studies have systematically explored the continued effects of a learning disability in adulthood. In reviewing the current literature in learning disabilities in adulthood, it appears that among adults, as among children, learning disabilities can be expressed throughout the total personality—cognitively, perceptually, and emotionally.[9] Many individuals have developed good "cover up" strategies for their disabilities so that it is often difficult to recognize that learning disabilities are present. This can sometimes be a disadvantage to the person, for instead of his or her behavior being interpreted empathetically as the result of a learning disability, it is interpreted as, for example, the person's not being able to comprehend or being slow. The same cycle that the person experienced as a child may be repeated as an adult. Chronic anxiety and tension are often present. An example of this is Mrs. B., Paul's mother, who also had a learning disability but was not diagnosed as learning disabled until age 20. Nevertheless, she completed both college and a master's degree in counseling. Although the academic problems were no longer an issue, the learning disability interfered with her home and work performance. For example, Mrs. B. described her organizational problems and identified a continuous need to make lists in order to function in her job. Mrs. B. said she had to work hard to not look clumsy and that she was fearful that she would trip over things and look foolish. She said that it seemed as though it took a lot more effort for her to learn and accomplish things as compared to her peers. Mrs. B. also discussed how her learning disability interfered with her relationship with her husband and children. Because of her tactile defensiveness, she disliked it when her children would come up from behind and unexpectedly grab her, and she only felt comfortable being touched (hugged, caressed) on her own terms. Thus it is apparent that even in the adult the learning disability continued to present difficulty.

In the box on p. 313 is a letter from a woman with learning disabilities and sensory integration problems. She describes how her learning disability affects her current functioning and how it affected her when she was a child.

SUMMARY

Meeting the needs of the learning disabled child offers new challenges in occupational and physical therapy. As a result of the passage of PL 94-142, the treatment of children is moving from the clinical arena to the public school arena. Providing service for any handicapped child requires changes in patterns of service delivery, especially an increase in skills for consultation and in service education. In order to treat the learning disabled child with motor dysfunction, a therapist must also develop new skills in evaluation and treatment.

Occupational and physical therapists must assume responsibility for learning disabled children with motor problems and must make sure that motor problems and their import in the overall development of a child are recognized. It is important for therapists to understand that the principle concern of the public school is the educational rather than the medical well-being of the child. The role of the therapist must be kept in perspective. Occupational and physical therapists are specialists in abnormal motor behavior and can identify problems and possible underlying deficits better than psychologists or teachers. The therapist can help the teacher understand a child's limitations and can offer suggestions that can both facilitate the child's motor performance and reduce the stress of his/her everyday motor activities. Furthermore, it is the therapist who can best explain the child's need for a program to lessen his/her motor deficit.

On the other hand, the child's motor needs must be assessed in the context of his/her overall educational and emotional development. The question is often not whether the child would benefit from therapy but which types of remediation are the most essential for the child at a given time in his/her development. Some children with motor incoordination cope quite well as long as their problem is recognized. As Gubbay[14] says, "Bringing the child into focus by the recognition of his problem immediately reduces the pressures to conform."[p. 157] In an environment in which parents, teachers, peers, and the child recognize the nature of the deficit and set reasonable expectations, some children accept their motor disability, and academic skills and alternative forms of recreation assume greater importance.

As this review has indicated, evidence supporting the effectiveness of treatment of motor deficits in learning disabled children is as yet fragmentary. Learning disabled children present highly variable patterns of disability that make it difficult to predict or measure response to therapy. Both formal research and careful documentation of clinical outcomes are needed to explore and define the dimensions and significance of motor disorders in learning disabled children that are relevant to therapy. Only then can we better categorize children, improve the precision of treatment, and validate treatment theory.

REFERENCES

1. Abbie MH: Physical treatment for clumsy children—not enough? Physiotherapy 64:198, 1978.
2. Abbie MH and others: The clumsy child: observations in cases referred to the gymnasium of the Adelaide Children's Hospital over a three year period, Med J Aust 1:65, 1978.
3. Abercrombie MLJ: Perceptual and visuo-motor disorders in cerebral palsy, London, 1964, Spastics Society, Medical Education and Information Unit, in association with William Heinemann, Ltd.
4. Adelman HS and Taylor L: An introduction to learning disabilities Glenview, Ill, 1986, Scott Foresman & Co.
5. American Academy of Pediatrics, Committee on the Handicapped Child: The Doman Delacato treatment of neurologically handicapped children, J Pediatr 72:750, 1968.
6. American Occupational Therapy Association: Occupational therapy in the public school system, Rockville, Md, 1976, The Association.
7. American Physical Therapy Association Board of Directors: Physical therapy practice in an educational environment. In American physical therapy house of delegates handbook, Phoenix, 1980, The Association.
8. Ames TH: Post secondary problems: an optimistic approach. In Weber RE, editor: Handbook on learning disabilities: a prognosis for the child, the adolescent, the adult, Englewood Cliffs, NJ, 1974, Prentice-Hall, Inc.
9. Anderson CM: The brain-injured adult: an overlooked problem. In Weber RE, editor: Handbook on learning disabilities: a prognosis for the child, the adolescent, the adult, Englewood Cliffs, NJ, 1974, Prentice-Hall, Inc.
10. Arendt RE, MacLean WE, and Baumeister A: Critique of sensory integration theory and its application in mental retardation, Am J Ment Defic 92:401.
11. Arnheim DD and Sinclair WA: The clumsy child: a program of motor therapy, St Louis, 1979, The CV Mosby Co.
12. Ayres AJ: Patterns of perceptual motor dysfunction in children: a factor analytic study, Percept Mot Skills 20:335, 1965.

13. Ayres AJ: Deficits in sensory integration in educationally handicapped children, J Learning Dis 2:160, 1969.
14. Ayres AJ: Characteristics of types of sensory integrative dysfunction, Am J Occup Ther 25:329, 1971.
15. Ayres AJ: Improving academic scores through sensory integration, J Learning Dis 5:338, 1972.
16. Ayres AJ: Sensory integration and learning disorders, Los Angeles, 1972, Western Psychological Services.
17. Ayres AJ: Types of sensory integrative dysfunction among disabled learners, Am J Occup Ther 26:13, 1972.
18. Ayres AJ: Sensorimotor foundations of academic ability. In Cruickshank WM and Hallahan DP, editors: Perceptual and learning disabilities in children, vol 2, Research and theory, New York, 1975, Syracuse University Press.
19. Ayres AJ: Southern California Postrotary Nystagmus Test, Los Angeles, 1975, Western Psychological Services.
20. Ayres AJ: Interpreting the Southern California Sensory Integration Tests Los Angeles, 1976, Western Psychological Services.
21. Ayres AJ: Cluster analyses of measures of sensory integration, Am J Occup Ther 31:362, 1977.
22. Ayres AJ: Dichotic listening performance in learning disabled children, Am J Occup Ther 31:441, 1977.
23. Ayres AJ: Effects of sensory integrative therapy on the coordination of children with choreoathetoid movements, Am J Occup Ther 31:291, 1977.
24. Ayres AJ: Learning disabilities and the vestibular system, J Learning Dis 11:18, 1978.
25. Ayres AJ: Sensory integration and the child, Los Angeles, 1980, Western Psychological Services.
26. Ayres AJ: Southern California Sensory Integration Tests Manual, Revised, Los Angeles, 1980, Western Psychological Services.
27. Ayres AJ: Developmental dyspraxia and adult onset apraxia, Torrance, Calif, 1985, Sensory Integration International.
28. Ayres AJ: The Sensory Integration and Praxis Tests, Los Angeles, 1988, Western Psychological Services.
29. Ayres AJ, Mailloux Z, and Wendler C: Developmental dyspraxia: Is it a unitary function?, Occup Ther J Res 7(2):93, 1987.
30. Badian NA and Wolff PH: Manual asymmetries of motor sequencing in boys with reading disabilities, Cortex 13:343, 1977.
31. Bannatyne A: Language, reading and learning disabilities, Springfield, Ill, 1971, Charles C Thomas, Publisher.
32. Banus BS and others: The developmental therapist, ed 2, Thorofare, NJ, 1979, Charles B Slack, Inc.
33. Barsch RH: Enriching perception and cognition, vol 2, Seattle, 1968, Special Child Publications.
34. Bateman B: Learning disabilities—yesterday, today, and tomorrow. In Frierson EC and Barbe WB, editors: Educating children with learning disabilities, New York, 1967, Appleton-Century-Crofts.
35. Bax M and MacKeith R: Minimal cerebral dysfunction in the adolescent, Pediatr Clin North Am 27:79, 1980.
36. Beasley DS and others: Learning disabilities: a problem in communication? In Gottlieb MI and others, editors: Current issues in developmental pediatrics: the learning disabled child, New York, 1979, Grune & Stratton, Inc.
37. Becker M and Banus BS: Sensory-perceptual dysfunction and its management. In Banus BS and others, editors: The developmental therapist, ed 2, Thorofare, NJ, 1979, Charles B Slack, Inc.
38. Beery KE: Revised administration, scoring, and learning manual for the Developmental Test of Visual-Motor Integration, Cleveland, 1982, Modern Curriculum Press.
39. Belmont T: Perceptual organization and minimal brain dysfunctions. In Rie RH and Rie ED editors: Handbook of minimal brain dysfunctions: a critical view, New York, 1980, John Wiley & Sons, Inc.
40. Bender ML: The Bender-Perdue Reflex Test and Training Manual, San Rafael, Calif, 1976, Academic Therapy Publications.
41. Berman A and Siegal AW: Adaptive and learning skills in juvenile delinquents: a neuropsychological analysis, J Learning Dis 9:583, 1976.
42. Birch HG and Belmont L: Auditory-visual integration in normal and retarded readers, Am J Orthopsychiatry 35:852, 1964.
43. Birch HG and Belmont L: Auditory-visual integration, intelligence, and reading disability in school children, Percept Mot Skills 20:295, 1965.
44. Birch HG and Walker HA: Perceptual and perceptual-motor dissociation, Arch Gen Psychiatry 14:113, 1966.
45. Black PE: Brain dysfunction in children: etiology, diagnosis and management, New York, 1981, Raven Press.
46. Black PE: Introduction: changing concepts of "brain damage" and "brain dysfunction." In Black PE, editor: Brain dysfunction in children: etiology, diagnosis and management, New York, 1981, Raven Press.
47. Bobath K: The motor deficits in patients with cerebral palsy, Clinics in Developmental Medicine, no 23, London, 1966, The National Spastics Society Medical Education and Information Unit in association with William Heinemann Medical Books, Ltd.
48. Boder E: Developmental dyslexia: a new diagnostic approach based on the identification of three subtypes, J Sch Health 40:289, 1970.
49. Book RM: Identification of educationally at-risk children during the kindergarten year: a four-year follow-up study of group test performance, Psychol Schools 17:153, 1980.
50. Bortner M and others: Neurological signs and intelligence in brain damaged children, J Special Education 6:325, 1972.
51. Brown JS and Zinkus PW: Screening techniques for early intervention. In Gottlieb MI and others, editors: Current issues in developmental pediatrics; the learning-disabled child, New York, 1979, Grune & Stratton Inc.
52. Bruininks RH: Bruininks-Oseretsky Test of Motor Proficiency, Minnesota, 1978, American Guidance Service, Inc.
53. Bruininks VL: Actual and perceived peer status of learning disabled students in mainstream programs, J Special Educ 12:51, 1978.
54. Bryan TH and Pearl RA: Self concepts and locus of control of learning disabled children, Education Horizons 59:91, 1981.
55. Bryant PE: Comments on the design of developmental studies of cross-model matching and cross-modal transfer, Cortex 4:127, 1968.
56. Bryden MP: Auditory-visual and sequential-spatial matching in relation to reading ability, Child Dev 43:824, 1972.
57. Bundy AC and Fisher AG: The relationship of prone extension to other vestibular functions, Am J Occup Ther 35:782, 1981.
58. Cannon IP and Compton CL: School dysfunction in the adolescent, Pediatr Clin North Am 27:79, 1980.
59. Capute A and others: Primitive reflex profile, Baltimore, 1978, University Park Press.
60. Capute A and others: Primitive reflex profile, Phys Ther 9:1061, 1978.
61. Carlson P: Comparison of two occupational therapy approaches for treating the young cerebral palsied child, Am J Occup Ther 29:267, 1975.
62. Carmon A: The two human hemispheres acting as separate parallel and sequential processors. In Inbar GF, editor: Signal analysis and pattern recognition in biomedical engineering, New York, 1975, John Wiley & Sons, Inc.
63. Cermak SA and others: The effect of concurrent activity on dichotic listening in boys with learning disabilities, Am J Occup Ther 32:493, 1978.
64. Cermak S: Developmental dyspraxia. In Roy E, editor: Neuropsychological studies of apraxia and related disorders, New York, 1985, Elsevier Science Publishing Co Inc.

65. Cermak S, Ward E, and Ward L: The relationship between articulation disorders and motor coordination in children, Am J Occup Ther 40:546, 1986.

66. Chapanis NP: The patterning method of therapy: a critique. In Black P, editor: Brain dysfunction in children: etiology, diagnosis and management, New York, 1981, Raven Press.

67. Chapman JW and Boersma FJ: Affective correlates of learning disabilities, Lisse, Netherlands, 1980, Sets and Zeitlinger, B.V.

68. Clark FA and Pierce D: Synopsis of pediatric occupational therapy effectiveness: studies on sensory integrative procedures, controlled vestibular stimulation, other sensory stimulation approaches, and perceptual-motor training. Paper presented at the Occupational Therapy for Maternal and Child Health Conference, Santa Monica, Calif, 1986.

69. Clark F, Mailloux Z, and Parham D: Sensory integration and children with learning disabilities. In Clark PN and Allen AS: Occupational therapy for children, St Louis, 1985, The CV Mosby Co.

70. Clements SD: Minimal brain dysfunction in children: terminology and identification, NINDB Monograph no 3, Washington, DC, 1966, United States Department of Health, Education, and Welfare.

71. Committee on Children with Disabilities: School-aged children with motor disabilities, Pediatrics 76(4):648, 1985.

72. Conners CK and Barta F: Transfer of information from touch to vision in brain-injured and emotionally disturbed children, J Nerv Ment Dis 145:138, 1967.

73. Cook LD: The adolescent with a learning disability: a developmental perspective, Adolescence 14:697, 1979.

74. Cratty BJ: Perceptual and motor development in infants and children, New York, 1970, Macmillan Publishing Co, Inc.

75. Cratty BJ: Movement behavior and motor learning, ed 3, Philadelphia, 1973, Lea & Febiger.

76. Cratty BJ and Martin M: Perceptual-motor efficiency in children, Philadelphia, 1969, Lea & Febiger.

77. Crinella FM: Identification of brain dysfunction syndromes in children through profile analysis: patterns associated with so-called "minimal brain dysfunction," J Abnorm Psychol 82:33, 1973.

78. Cruickshank WM and others: Learning disabilities, the struggle from adolescence toward adulthood, Syracuse, New York, 1980, Syracuse University Press.

79. Cunningham DA and Goetzinger CP: Floor ataxia test battery, Arch Otolaryngol 96:559, 1972.

80. DeGangi GA and others: The measurement of vestibular based dysfunction in pre-school children, Am J Occup Ther 34:452, 1980.

81. DeHaven GE and Mordock JB: Coordination exercises for children with minimal cerebral dysfunction, Phys Ther 50:337, 1970.

82. DeHaven GE and others: Evaluation of coordination deficits in children with minimal brain dysfunction, Phys Ther 49:153, 1969.

83. DeHirsch K and others: Predicting reading failure: a preliminary study, New York, 1966, Harper & Row, Publishers, Inc.

84. Delacato CH: The treatment and prevention of reading problems: the neurological approach, Springfield, Ill, 1959, Charles C Thomas, Publisher.

85. Delacato CH: The diagnosis and treatment of speech and reading problems, Springfield, Ill, 1963, Charles C Thomas, Publisher.

86. Delacato CH: Neurological organization and reading, Springfield, Ill, 1966, Charles C Thomas, Publisher.

87. Deloria DJ: Review of Miller Assessment for Preschoolers. In Mitchell, JV Jr, editor: The ninth mental measurements yearbook, Lincoln, Neb, 1985, University of Nebraska Press.

88. Denckla MB: Development of speed in repetitive and successive finger movements in normal children, Dev Med Child Neurol 15:635, 1973.

89. Denckla MB: Development of motor coordination in normal children, Dev Med Child Neurol 16:729, 1974.

90. Denckla MB: MBD and dyslexia: beyond diagnosis by exclusion, Top Child Neurol 19:253, 1977.

91. Denckla MB: Developmental dyspraxia: the clumsy child. In Levine MD and Satz P, editors: Middle childhood development and dysfunction, Baltimore, Md, 1987, University Park Press.

92. Denckla MB and Rudel R: Rapid automatized naming (RAN): dyslexia different from other learning disabilities, Neuropsychologia 14:471, 1976.

93. Denckla MB and others: Motor proficiency in dyslexic children with and wihtout attentional disorders, Arch Neurol 42:228, 1985.

94. Depauw KP: Enhancing the sensory integration of aphasic students, J Learning Dis 11:142, 1978.

95. DeQuiros J and Schrager O: Neurophyschological fundamentals in learning disabilities, San Rafael, California, 1979, Academic Therapy Publications.

96. Doehring DG: Reading disability subtypes: interaction of reading and nonreading deficits. In Rourke BP, editor: Neuropsychology of learning disabilities: essentials of subtype analysis, New York, 1985, Guilford Press.

97. Dunn W: A guide to testing clinical observations, Rockland, Md, 1981, American Occupational Therapy Association.

98. Dunsing JD and Kephart NC: Motor generalizations in time and space. In Hellmuth J, editor: Learning disorders, vol 1, Seattle, Washington, 1965, Special Child Publications.

99. Faigel HC: The learning disabled adolescent. In Gottlieb MI and others, editors: Current issues in developmental pediatrics: the learning disabled child, New York, 1979, Grune & Stratton, Inc.

100. Farber SD: Neurorehabilitation: a multisensory approach, Philadelphia, 1982, WB Saunders Co.

101. Finucci MM: Genetic considerations in dyslexia. In Myklebust HR, editor: Progress in learning disabilities, vol 4, New York, 1978, Grune & Stratton, Inc.

102. Fiorentino MR: Reflex testing methods for evaluating CNS development, Springfield, Ill, 1963, Charles C Thomas, Publisher.

103. Folio MR and Fewell R: Peabody developmental motor scales (POMS): revised experimental edition, Allen, Tex, 1983, DLM Teaching Resources.

104. Ford FR: Diseases of the nervous system in infancy, childhood and adolescence, ed 5, Springfield, Ill, 1966, Charles C Thomas, Publisher.

105. Frank J and Levinson H: Dysmetric dyslexia and dyspraxia, J Am Acad Child Psychiatry 12:690, 1973.

106. Fregly AR: Vestibular ataxia and its measurement in man. In Kornhuber HH, editor: Vestibular system, part 2 (vol V 1/2), New York, 1974, Springer-Verlag New York, Inc.

107. Freides D: Human information processing and sensory modality: cross modal functions, information complexity, memory and deficit, Psychol Bull 81:284, 1974.

108. Frostig M: Developmental test of visual perception, Los Angeles, 1963, Consulting Psychologists' Press.

109. Frostig M: A treatment program for children with learning difficulties. In Bortner M, editor: Evaluation and education of children with brain damage, Springfiield, Ill, 1968, Charles C Thomas, Publisher.

110. Frostig M: The role of perception in the integration of psychological functions. In Cruickshank WM and Hallahan DP, editors: Perceptual and learning disorders in children, vol 1, Psychoeducational practices, Syracuse, New York, 1975, Syracuse University Press.

111. Gaddes WH: Learning disabilities and brain function: a neuropsychological approach, ed 2, New York, 1985, Springer-Verlag Publishing Co.

112. Galaburda A and Kemper TL: Cytoarchitectonic abnormalities in developmental dyslexia: a case study, Ann Neurol 6:94, 1979.

113. Galaburda AM and others: Developmental dyslexia: four consecutive cases with cortical anomalies, Ann Neurol 18:222, 1985.

114. Gardner RA and Broman M: The Purdue Pegboard: normative data on 1334 school children, J Clin Child Psychol 1:156, 1979.

114a. Gardner MF: TVMS test of visual-motor skills, San Francisco, 1986, Children's Hospital of San Francisco.

115. Gazzaniga MS: Brain theory and minimal brain dysfunction, Ann NY Acad Sci 205:89, 1973.

116. Geschwind N: Language and the brain, Scientific Am 226:76, 1972.

117. Geschwind N and Galaburda A: Cerebral lateralization: biological mechanisms, associations, and pathology: I, II, III, Arch Neurol 42:428, 521, 6, 1985.

118. Getman GN: The visuomotor complex in the acquisition of learning skills. In Hellmuth J, editor: Learning disorders, vol 1, Seattle, 1965, Special Child Publications.

119. Gilfoyle EM and Grady A: A developmental theory of somatosensory perception. In Henderson A and Coryell J, editors: The body senses and perceptual deficit, Proceedings of the Occupational Therapy Symposium on Somatosensory Aspects of Perceptual Deficit, Boston, 1972, Boston University.

120. Gilfoyle EM and others: Children adapt, Thorofare, NJ, 1981, Charles B Slack, Inc.

121. Gillberg IC: Children with minor neurodevelopmental disorders— III: Neurological and neurodevelopmental problems at age 10, Dev Med Child Neurol 27:3, 1985.

122. Goff JR: A neuropsychological approach to the learning disabled child. In Gottlieb MI and others, editors: Current issues in developmental pediatrics: the learning disabled child, New York, 1979, Grune & Stratton, Inc.

123. Goleta Union School District: Title III, Elementary and Secondary Education Act No 5127: the identification, diagnosis and remediation of sensorimotor dysfunction in primary school children, Goleta, Calif, 1971, Goleta Union School District.

124. Goodwin WL and Driscoll LA: Handbook for measurement and evaluation in early childhood education, San Francisco, 1900, Jossey-Bass, Inc, Publishers.

125. Gottlieb MI: The learning-disabled child: controversial issues revisited. In Gottlieb MI and others, editors: Current issues in developmental pediatrics: the learning disabled child, New York, 1979, Grune & Stratton, Inc.

126. Grant W and others: Developmental patterns of two motor functions, Dev Med Child Neurol 15:171, 1973.

127. Gross K and others: Duration thresholds for letter identification in left and right visual fields for normal and reading disabled children, Neuropsychologia 16:709, 1978.

128. Gubbay SS: The clumsy child, New York, 1975, WB Saunders Co.

129. Gubbay SS: The management of developmental apraxia, Dev Med Child Neurol 20:643, 1978.

130. Gubbay SS: The clumsy child. In Rose FC, editor: Pediatric neurology, London, 1979, Blackwell Scientific Publications, Inc.

131. Gubbay SS and others: Clumsy children: a study of apraxic and agnosic deficits in 21 children, Brain 85:295, 1963.

132. Hainesworth PK and Siqueland ML: Early identification of children with learning disabilities: the Meeting Street School screening test, Providence, RI, 1969, Crippled Children and Adults of Rhode Island, Inc.

133. Hallahan DP: Comparative research studies on the psychological characteristics of learning disabled children. In Cruickshank WM and Hallahan DP, editors: Perceptual and learning disabilities in children, vol 1, Psychoeducational practices, New York, 1975, Syracuse University Press.

134. Hammill D and Bartel N: Teaching children with learning and behavior problems: a resource book for preschool, elementary and special education teachers, Boston, 1975, Allyn & Bacon, Inc.

135. Hammill DD and others: A new definition of learning disabilities, Learning Disabilities Quarterly 4:336, 1981.

136. Hanson C: A study of the presence of the asymmetrical tonic neck reflex in fifth and seventh grade children, master's thesis, 1976, Sargent College, Boston University.

137. Hardy M and others: Developmental patterns in elemental reading skills: phoneme-grapheme and grapheme-phoneme correspondences, J Educ Psychol 63:433, 1972.

138. Harris NP: Duration and quality of prone extension position in four, six, and eight year old normal children, Am J Occup Ther 35:26, 1981.

139. Heiniger MC and Randolph SL: Neurophysiological concepts in human behavior, St Louis, 1981, The CV Mosby Co.

140. Helper MJ: Follow-up of children with minimal brain dysfunctions: outcomes and predictors. In Rie HE and Rie ED, editors: Handbook of minimal brain dysfunctions: a critical view, New York, 1980, John Wiley & Sons, Inc.

141. Henderson A: Research in occupational therapy and physical therapy with children. In Camp BW, editor: Advances in behavioral pediatrics, Greenwich, 1981, Jai Press.

142. Henderson SE and Hall D: Concomitants of clumsiness in young school children, Dev Med Child Neurol 24:448, 1982.

143. Hern A: Neurological signs in learning disabled children: persistence over time, and incidence in adulthood compared to normal learners, doctoral dissertation, Victoria, BC 1984, University of Victoria.

144. Hiscock M and Kinsbourne M: Specialization of the cerebral hemispheres: implications for learning, J Learning Dis 20(3):130, 1987.

145. Hoskins T and Squires J: Developmental assessment: a test for gross motor and reflex development, Phys Ther 53:117, 1973.

146. Hoy E and others: The hyperactive child at adolescence: cognitive, emotional and social functioning, J Abnorm Child Psychol 6:311, 1978.

147. Hughes JE and Riley A: Basic gross motor assessment, Phys Ther 61:503, 1981.

148. Hulme C and others: Visual, kinaesthetic and cross-modal judgements of length by normal and clumsy children, Dev Med Child Neurol 24:461, 1982.

149. Hulme C and Lord R: Review: clumsy children—a review of recent research, Child Care Health Dev 12:257, 1986.

150. Hulme C and others: Visual perceptual deficits in clumsy children, Neuropsychol 4:475, 1982.

151. Illingsworth RS: The clumsy child. In Bax M and MacKeith RM, editors: Minimal cerebral dysfunction, Clinics in Developmental Medicine, no 10, London, 1963, The National Spastics Society Medical Education and Information Unit in association with William Heinemann Medical Books, Ltd.

152. Johnson D: Paper presented at the 85th Convention of the American Psychological Association, Washington, DC, Sept, 1976.

153. Johnson DJ and Myklebust HR: Learning disabilities: educational practices and principles, New York, 1967, Grune & Stratton, Inc.

154. Joschko M and Rourke BP: Neuropsychological subtypes of learning-disabled children who exhibit the ACID pattern on the WISC. In Rourke BP, editor: Neuropsychology of learning disabilities: essentials of subtype analysis, New York, 1985, The Guilford Press.

155. Kalish R and Presseller S: Physical and occupational therapy, J Sch Health 50:264, 1980.

156. Kantner RM and others: Effects of vestibular stimulation on nystagmus response and motor performance in the developmentally delayed infant, Phys Ther 56:414, 1976.

157. Kauffman NA: Occupational therapy theory, assessment, and treatment in educational settings. In Hopkins, HL and Smith HD, editors: Willard and Spackman's occupational therapy, ed 5, Philadelphia, 1978, JB Lippincott Co.

158. Kavale K and Mattson PD: One jumped off the balance beam: meta-analysis of perceptual-motor training, J Learning Dis 16:165, 1983.

159. Keim RP: Visual motor training, readiness, and intelligence of kindergarten children, J Learning Dis 3:256, 1970.

160. Kendrick KA and Hanten WP: Differentiation of learning disabled children from normal children using four coordination tasks, Phys Ther 60:784, 1980.

161. Kenny TJ and Burka A: Coordinating multiple interventions. In Rie HE and Rie ED, editors: Handbook of minimal brain dysfunctions: a critical view, New York, 1980, John Wiley & Sons, Inc.

162. Keough K: A compensatory model for psychoeducational education of children with learning disorders, J Learning Dis 4:544, 1971.

163. Kephart NC: The slow learner in the classroom, Columbus, Ohio, 1960, Charles E Merrill Publishing Co.

164. Kephart NC: Teaching the child with a perceptual-motor handicap. In Bortner M, editor: Evaluation and education of children with brain damage, Springfield, Ill 1968, Charles C Thomas, Publisher.

165. Kephart NC: The perceptual motor match. In Cruickshank, WM and Hallahan, DP, editors: Perceptual and learning disabilities in children, vol 1, Psychoeducational practices, New York, 1975, Syracuse University Press.

166. Keshner EA: Re-evaluating the theoretical model underlying the neurodevelopmental theory, Phys Ther 61:1035, 1981.

167. King-Thomas L and Hacker B: A therapist's guide to pediatric assessment, Boston, 1987, Little, Brown & Co.

168. Kimball JG: Normative comparison of the Southern California Postrotary Nystagmus Test: Los Angeles vs Syracuse data, Am J Occup Ther 35:21, 1981.

169. Kinsbourne M: Minimal brain dysfunction as a neurodevelopmental lag, Ann NY Acad Sci 205:268, 1973.

170. Kinsbourne M: Editorials: MBD—a fuzzy concept misdirects therapeutic efforts, Postgrad Med 58:211, 1975.

171. Kirk S: Illinois Test of Psycholinguistic Abilities: its origin and implications. In Hellmuth J, editor: Learning disorders, vol 2, Seattle, 1966, Special Child Publications.

172. Kirk S: National Advisory Committee on Handicapped Children: special education for handicapped children, first annual report, Washington, DC, 1968, United States Department of Health, Education, and Welfare.

173. Klasen E: The syndrome of specific dyslexia, Baltimore, 1972, University Park Press.

174. Knickerbocker BM: A holistic approach to the treatment of learning disorders, Thorofare, NJ, 1980, Charles B Slack, Inc.

175. Kopp CB and Shaperman J: Cognitive development in the absence of object manipulation during infancy, Dev Psychol 9:430, 1973.

176. Koppitz EM: The Bender Gestalt Test for young children, New York, 1963, Grune & Stratton, Inc.

177. Lane BA: The relationship of learning disabilities to juvenile delinquency: current status, J Learning Dis 13:20, 1980.

178. Langdon HJ and Langdon LL: Initiating occupational therapy programs within public school systems: a guide for occupational therapists and public school administrators, Thorofare, NJ, 1983, Charles B Slack, Inc.

179. Lansdell H: Theories of brain mechanisms in minimal brain dysfunctions. In Rie HE and Rie Ed, editors: Handbook of minimal brain dysfunctions: a critical view, New York, 1980, John Wiley & Sons, Inc.

180. Laszlo JI and Bairstow PJ: Kinaesthesis: its measurement, training, and relationship to motor control, Q J Exp Pscyhol 35A:411, 1983.

181. Reference deleted in proofs.

182. Lebby M: Incidence of mirror and overflow movements in learning disabled and normal young adults, Master's thesis, 1988, Sargent College, Boston University.

183. Lerner J: Children with learning disorders, Boston, 1976, Houghton Mifflin Co.

184. Levangie PK: Public school physical therapists, Phys Ther 60:774, 1980.

185. Levine M: Pediatric examination of educational readiness at middle childhood, Cambridge, Mass, 1985, Educators Publishing Service.

186. Levine MD and others: A pediatric approach to learning disorders, New York, 1980, John Wiley & Sons Inc.

187. Levy J and others: Perception of bilateral chimeric figures following hemispheric deconnexion, Brain 95:61, 1972.

188. Lucas AR: Muscular control and coordination in minimal brain dysfunctions. In Rie HE and Rie ED, editors: Handbook of minimal brain dysfunctions: a critical view, New York, 1980, John Wiley & Sons, Inc.

189. MacKeith RM: Defining the concept of minimal brain damage. In Bax M and MacKeith RM, editors: Minimal cerebral dysfunction, London, 1963, The National Spastics Society Medical Education and Information Unit in association with William Heinemann Medical Books, Ltd.

190. Marcel T and others: Laterality and reading proficiency, Neuropsychologia 12:131, 1974.

191. Mathiowetz V and others: The Purdue Pegboard: norms for 14- to 19-year olds, Am J Occup Ther 40:174, 1986.

192. Mathis HJ and Harshman HW: Therapeutic program for the learning disabled, Phys Ther 57:823, 1977.

193. Mattis S and others: Dyslexia in children and young adults: three independent neuropsychological syndromes, Dev Med Child Neurol 17:150, 1975.

194. Mauser AJ: Learning disabilities and delinquent youth, Acad Ther 9:389, 1974.

195. McClanahan LJ: The effectiveness of perceptual training for slow learners, Dissertation Abstracts 28:2560A, 1967.

196. McGrady HL and Olson DA: Visual and auditory learning processes in normal children and children with specific learning disabilities, Except Child 36:581, 1970.

197. McReynolds LV: Operant conditioning for investigating speech sound discrimination in aphasic children, J Speech Hear 9:519, 1966.

198. Mendelson W and others: Hyperactive children as teenagers: a follow-up study, J Nerv Ment Dis 153:273, 1971.

199. Michaels WB: Review of Miller Assessment for preschoolers. In Mitchell JV Jr, editor: The ninth mental measurements yearbook, Lincoln, 1985, University of Nebraska Press.

200. Michael-Smith H: Reciprocal factors in the behavior syndrome of the neurologically impaired child. In Hellmuth J, editor: The special child in century 21, Seattle, 1964, Special Child Publications.

201. Miller LJ: Miller assessment for preschoolers, Littleton, Colorado, 1982, The Foundation for Knowledge in Development.

202. Miller LJ: Longitudinal validity of the Miller Assessment for preschoolers: study I, Percep Mot Skills 65:211, 1987.

203. Miller LJ: Differentiating children with school-related problems after four years using the Miller Assessment for preschoolers, Psychol in Schools 25:10, 1988.

204. Miller LJ: Longitudinal validity of the Miller Assessment for preschoolers: study II, Percept Mot Skills 66:811, 1988.

205. Miller LJ: Miller Assessment for Preschoolers: manual 1988 revision, San Antonio, Tex 1988, The Psychological Corporation.

206. Miller LJ and Schouten PGW: Age-related effects on the predictive validity of the Miller Assessment for Preschoolers, J Psycheducat Assess 6(2):99, 1988.

207. Miller TG and Goldberg MA: Sensorimotor integration, Phys Ther 55:501, 1975.

208. Montessori M: The Montessori Method: scientific pedagogy as applied to child education in the children's houses (translated by E George), New York, 1912, FA Stokes.

209. Montgomery P: Assessment of vestibular function in children, Phys Occup Ther Pediatr 5:33, 1985.

210. Montgomery P and Richter E: Effects of sensory integration train-

ing on neuromuscular development of retarded children, Phys Ther 57:799, 1977.

211. Mordock JB: Behavioral problems of the child with minimal cerebral dysfunction, Phys Ther 51:398, 1971.

212. Mordock JB and DeHaven GE: Movement skills of children with minimal cerebral dysfunction, Rehabil Lit 30:2, 1969.

213. Morrison DC, Hinshaw SP, and Carte E: Signs of neurobehavioral dysfunction in a sample of learning disabled children: stability and concurrent validity, Percept Mot Skills 61:863, 1985.

214. Mould RE: An evaluation of the effectiveness of a special program for retarded readers manifesting disturbed visual perception, doctoral dissertation, Washington State University, Ann Arbor, Mich 1965, University Microfilms, No 22-228A.

215. Muehl S and Kremenak S: Ability to match information within and between auditory and visual sense modalities and subsequent reading achievement, J Educ Psychol 57:230, 1966.

216. Mullins J: New challenges for physical therapy practitioners in educational settings, Phys Ther 61:496, 1981.

217. Mutti M and others: QNST: Quick Neurological Screening Test: revised edition, Novato, Calif, 1978, Academic Therapy Publications.

218. Myers PI and Hammill DD: Methods for learning disorders, New York, 1976, John Wiley & Sons, Inc.

219. Myklebust HR: Learning disabilities: definition and overview. In Myklebust HR, editor: Progress in learning disabilities, vol 1, New York, 1968, Grune & Stratton, Inc.

220. Myklebust HR: Learning disabilities and minimal brain dysfunction in children. In Tower DB, editor: The nervous system, vol 3, Human communication and its disorders, New York, 1975, Raven Press.

221. O'Brien V, Cermak S, and Murray E: The relationship between visual-perceptual motor abilities and clumsiness in children with and without learning disabilities, Am J Occup Ther 42:359, 1988.

222. Ohlson EL: Identification of specific learning disabilities, Champaign, Ill, 1978, Research Press.

223. Olson M: Laterality differences in tachistoscopic word recognition in normal and delayed readings in elementary school, Neuropsychologia 11:343, 1973.

224. Orton ST: Reading, writing and speech problems in children, New York, 1937, WW Norton & Co, Inc.

225. Ottenbacher K: Identifying vestibular processing dysfunction in learning disabled children, Am J Occup Ther 33:317, 1979.

226. Ottenbacher K: Sensory integration therapy: affect or effect? Am J Occup Ther 36:571, 1982.

227. Ottenbacher K: Occupational therapy and special education: some issues and concerns related to public law 94-142, Am J Occup Ther 36:81, 1982.

228. Ottenbacher K and Short MA: Sensory integrative dysfunction in children: a review of theory and treatment, Adv Devel Behav Pediatr 6:267, 1985.

229. Ottenbacher K and others: Nystagmus duration changes of learning disabled children during sensory integration therapy, Percept Mot Skills 48:1159, 1979.

230. Ottenbacher K and others: The use of selected clinical observations to predict postrotary nystagmus changes in learning disabled children, Phys Occup Ther Pediatr 1:31, 1980.

231. Ozols E and Rourke BP: Dimensions of social sensitivity in two types of learning-disabled children. In Rourke BP, editor: Neuropsychology of learning disabilities: essentials of subtype analysis, New York, 1985, The Guilford Press.

232. Parmenter C: The asymmetrical tonic neck reflex in normal first and third grade children, Am J Occup Ther 29:463, 1975.

233. Parr C and others: A developmental study of the asymmetrical tonic neck reflex, Dev Med Child Neurol 16:329, 1974.

234. Peck BB and Stackhouse T: Reading problems and family dynamics, J Learning Dis 6:506, 1973.

235. Pirozzola F and Rayner K: Hemispheric specialization in reading and word recognition, Brain Lang 4:248, 1977.

236. Porter JP and Rourke BP: Socioemotional functioning of learning disabled children: a subtypal analysis of personality patterns. In Rourke BP, editor: Neuropsychology of learning disabilities: essentials of subtype analysis, New York, 1985, The Guildford Press.

237. Prechtl HFR: Dyslexia as a neurological problem in childhood. In Money J, editor: Reading disability, Baltimore, 1968, Johns Hopkins University Press.

238. Prechtl HFR and Stemmer C: The choreiform syndrome in children, Dev Med Child Neurol 4:119, 1962.

239. Punwar A: Expanded normative data: Southern California Postrotary Nystagmus Test, Am J Occup Ther 36:183, 1982.

240. Reuben RN and Bakwin H: Developmental clumsiness, Pediatr Clin North Am 15:601, 1968.

241. Rie ED and others: An analysis of soft neurological signs in children with learning problems, Brain Lang 6:32, 1978.

242. Rie HE: Definitional problems. In Rie HE and Rie ED, editors: Handbook of minimal brain dysfunctions: a critical view, New York, 1980, John Wiley & Sons, Inc.

243. Roach EG and Kephart NC: The Purdue Perceptual Motor Survey, Columbus, Ohio, 1966, Charles E Merrill Publishing Co.

244. Roberts TDM: Neurophysiology of posture mechanisms, ed 2, Boston, 1978, Butterworth Publishers.

245. Rogers H and Saklofske DH: Self-concept, locus of control and performance expectations of learning disabled children, J Learning Dis 18:273, 1985.

246. Rourke BP: Brain-behavior relationships in children with learning disabilities: a research program, Am Psychol 30:911, 1975.

247. Rourke BP, editor: Neuropsychology of learning disabilities: essentials of subtype analysis, New York, 1985, The Guildford Press.

248. Rourke BP and Telegdy GA: Lateralizing significance of WISC verbal-performance discrepancies for older children with learning disabilities, Percept Mot Skills 33:875, 1975.

249. Rourke BP and others: The relationship between WISC verbal-performance discrepancies and selected verbal, auditory-perceptual, visual-perceptual and problem solving abilities in children with learning disabilities, J Clin Psychol 27:475, 1971.

250. Routh DK and Mesibov GB: Psychological and environmental intervention: toward social competence. In Rie HE and Rie ED, editors: Handbook of minimal brain dysfunctions: a critical view, New York, 1980, John Wiley & Sons, Inc.

251. Rubin E and Braun J: Behavioral and learning disabilities associated with cognitive motor dysfunction, Percept Mot Skills 26:171, 1968.

252. Rudel RG and Teuber HL: Pattern recognition within and across sensory modalities in normal and brain injured children, Neuropsychologia 9:389, 1971.

253. Rylander P: The ATNR in eight and twelve year old LD and normal boys, master's thesis, 1977, Sargent College, Boston University.

254. Sahler OJ and others: Learning disorders and the hyperactive child: the pediatrician's role. In Smith DH and Hoekelman RA, editors: Controversies in child health and pediatric practice, New York, 1981, McGraw-Hill, Inc.

255. Sapir SG: Educational intervention. In Rie HE and Rie ED, editors: Handbook of minimal brain dysfunction: a critical review, New York, 1980, John Wiley & Sons, Inc.

256. Satz P and others: An evaluation of a theory of specific developmental dyslexia, Child Dev 42:2009, 1971.

257. Schaffer R: Sensory integration therapy with learning disabled children: a critical review, Can J Occup Ther 51:73, 1984.

258. Scherzer A and others: Physical therapy as a determinant of change in the cerebral palsied infant, Pediatric 58:47, 1976.

259. Sellers JS: Professional cooperation in public school physical therapy, Phys Ther 60:1159, 1980.

260. Semmes J: Hemispheric specialization: a possible clue to mechanism, Neuropsychologia 6:11, 1968.

261. Serwer BL and others: The comparative effectiveness of four methods of instruction on the achievement of children with specific learning disabilities, J Special Educ 7:241, 1973.

262. Shafer S and others: Ten year consistency in neurological test performance of children without focal neurological deficit, Dev Med Child Neurol 28:417, 1986.

263. Shaw L, Levine M, and Belfer M: Developmental double jeopardy: a study of clumsiness and self-esteem in children with learning problems, J Dev Behav Pediatr 3:191, 1982.

264. Shaywitz SE and others: Current status of the neuromaturational examination as an index of learning disability, J Pediatr 104:819, 1984.

265. Sieben RL: Controversial medical treatment of learning disabilities, Academ Ther 13:133, 1977.

266. Sieg K and Shuster JJ: Comparison of three positions for evaluating the asymmetrical tonic neck reflex, Am J Occup Ther 33:240, 1979.

267. Silberzahn M: Sensory integrative theory. In Hopkins HL and Smith HD, editors: Willard and Spackman's occupational therapy, ed 5, Philadelphia, 1978, JB Lippincott Co.

268. Silver AA and Hagin R: Specific reading disability: delineation of the syndrome and relationship to cerebral dominance, Comp Psychiatry 1:126, 1960.

269. Silver LB: Acceptable and controversial approaches to treating the child with learning disabilities, Pediatrics 55:406, 1975.

270. Silver LB: Treatments for attention deficit disorders, Sensory Integration Special Interest Section Newsletter 4:1, 1981.

271. Silver S: Psychologic aspects of pediatrics: postural and righting responses in children, Pediatrics 41:493, 1952.

272. Silverman R and Zigmond N: Self-concept in learning disabled adolescents, J Learning Dis 16:478, 1983.

273. Sklar B, and others: An EEG experiment aimed toward identifying dyslexic children, Nature 240:414, 1972.

274. Sparrow S: Dyslexia and laterality: evidence for a developmental theory, Semin. Psychiatry 1:270, 1969.

275. Sparrow S, and Satz P: Dyslexia, laterality, and neuropsychological development. In Bakker BJ and Satz P, editors: Specific reading disabilities: advances in theory and method, Rotterdam, 1970, University of Rotterdam.

276. Spreen O: Learning disabled children growing up: a follow-up into adulthood, Victoria, BC, 1983, Department of Psychology, University of Victoria.

277. Steinberg M and Rendle-Short J: Vestibular dysfunction in young children with minor neurological impairment, Dev Med Child Neurol 19:639, 1977.

278. Sterrit GM and others: Auditory-visual and temporal-spatial integration as determinants of test difficulty, Psychonomic Sci 23:289, 1971.

279. Stewart MA and others: Hyperactive children as adolescents: how they describe themselves, Child Psychiatry Hum Dev 4:3, 1973.

280. Stott DH: A general test of motor impairment for children, Dev Med Child Neurol 8:523, 1966.

281. Stott DH and others: Test of motor impairment, rev ed, Guelph, Ontario, 1984, Brook Educational Publishing, Ltd.

282. Strang JD and Rourke BP: Adaptive behavior of children who exhibit specific arithmetic disabilities and associated neuropsychological abilities and deficits. In Rourke BP, editor: Neuropsychology of learning disabilities: essentials of subtype analysis, New York, 1985, The Guilford Press.

283. Strauss AA and Lehtinen LE: Psychopathology and education of the brain-injured child, New York, 1947, Grune & Stratton, Inc.

284. Sweeney JE and Rourke BP: Spelling disability subtypes. In Rourke BP, editor: Neuropsychology of learning disabilities: essentials of subtypes analysis, New York, 1985, The Guilford Press.

285. Tarnopol L and Tarnopol M: Brain function and reading disabilities, Baltimore, 1977, University Park Press.

286. Tickle-Degnen L: Perspectives on the status of sensory integration theory, Am J Occup Ther 42(7):427, 1988.

287. Tiffin J: Purdue Pegboard Test, Lafayette, Ind, 1968, Layfayette Instrument Co.

288. Touwen BCL: Examination of the child with minor neurological dysfunction, Clinics in Dev. Med., No. 71, London, 1979, William Heinemann Medical Books, Ltd.

289. Touwen BCL and Prechtl HFR: The neurological examination of the child with minor nervous dysfunction, Philadelphia, 1970, JB Lippincott Co.

290. Touwen BCL and Sporrel T: Soft signs and MBD, Dev Med Child Neurol 21:528, 1979.

291. Towbin A: Neuropathologic factors in minimal brain dysfunction. In Rie HE and Rie ED, editors: Handbook of minimal brain dysfunctions: a critical view, New York, 1980, John Wiley & Sons, Inc.

292. Training and management in occupational therapy (TOTEMS), Rockville, Md, 1980, American Occupational Therapy Association.

293. Trimble H: Comparison of bilateral motor coordination in older learning disabled and normal boys, master's thesis, 1988, Sargent College, Boston University.

294. Urbanowicz J: Balance abilities of learning disabled boys, master's thesis, 1979, Sargent College, Boston University.

295. Vande Voort L and others: Development of audio-visual integration in normal and retarded readers, Child Dev 43:1260, 1972.

296. Vellutino F: Dyslexia: theory and research, Cambridge, Mass, 1979, The MIT Press.

297. Vellutino F and others: Reading disability and the perceptual deficit hypothesis, Cortex 8:106, 1972.

298. Vellutino F and others: Inter- versus intra-hemispheric learning in dyslexic and normal readers, Dev Med Child Neurol 20:71, 1978.

299. Walton JN and others: Clumsy children: a study of developmental apraxia and agnosia, Brain 85:603, 1963.

300. Weber RE: Handbook on learning disabilities, Englewood Cliffs, NJ, 1974, Prentice-Hall, Inc.

301. Weiner BB: Curriculum development for children with brain damage. In Bortner M, editor: Evaluation and education of children with brain damage, Springfield, Ill, 1968, Charles C Thomas, Publisher.

302. Weiss G: MBD: critical diagnostic issues. In Rie HE and Rie ED, editors: Handbook of minimal brain dysfunctions: a critical view, New York, 1980, John Wiley & Sons, Inc.

303. Whyte L: Characteristics of learning disabilities persisting into adolescence, Alberta J Educ Research 30(1):14, 1984.

304. Witelson SF: Developmental dyslexia: two right hemispheres and none left, Science 195:309, 1977.

305. Wolff PH, Gunnoe CE, and Cohen C: Associated movement as a measure of developmental age, Dev Med Child Neurol 25:417, 1983.

306. Wolff PH and Hurwitz I: Functional implications of the minimal brain damage syndrome. In Walzer S and Wolff PH, editors: Minimal cerebral dysfunction in children, New York, 1973, Grune & Stratton, Inc.

307. Wright T and Nicholson J: Physiotherapy for the spastic child: an evaluation, Dev Med Child Neurol 15:146, 1973.

308. Yeni-Komshian GH and others: Cerebral dominance and reading disorders: left visual defect in poor readers, Neuropsychologia 13:83, 1975.

309. Younes R, Rosner B, and Webb G: Neuroimmaturity of learning disabled children: a controlled study, Dev Med Child Neurol 25:1152, 1978.

310. Zinkus PW: Behavior and emotional sequelae of learning disorders. In Gottlieb MI and others, editors: Current issues in developmental pediatrics: the learning disabled child, New York, 1979, Grune & Stratton, Inc.

311. Zurif E and Carson G: Dyslexia in relation to cerebral dominance and temporal analysis, Neuropsychologia 8:351, 1970.

APPENDIX—SUMMARY OF STANDARDIZED MOTOR TESTS

1. Bruininks-Oseretsky Test of Motor Proficiency
2. Purdue Perceptual-Motor-Survey Rating Scale
3. Test of Motor Impairment
4. Peabody Developmental Motor Scales
5. Quick Neurological Screening Test
6. Miller Assessment for Preschoolers
7. Tests for Motor Proficiency of Gubbay
8. Southern California Sensory Integration Tests
9. Sensory Integration and Praxis Tests
10. Meeting Street School Screening Test
11. Bender Gestalt Test for Young Children
12. Developmental Test of Visual Motor Integration
13. Test of Visual Motor Skills
14. Basic Motor Ability Tests—Revised
15. Purdue Pegboard Test

1. Bruininks-Oseretsky Test of Motor Proficiency (1978)[52]

Author: Robert H. Bruininks, Ph.D.
Source: American Guidance Service, Inc.
Circle Pines, Minn. 55014
Ages: 4½ to 14½ years
Administration: Individual; 45 minutes to 1 hour
Equipment: Test kit needed
Description: The Bruininks-Oseretsky Test of Motor Proficiency is the most recent revision of the Oseretsky Tests of Motor Proficiency first published in Russia in 1923. The Oseretsky Tests were first adapted by Doll in 1946 and then by Sloan in 1955 as the Lincoln-Oseretsky Motor Development Scale. As with the earlier versions, the Bruininks-Oseretsky Test yields an age equivalency score but standard scores, and percentile ranks are also available. The test assesses motor functioning in eight areas, each with standard score information. The areas are:

1. Running speed and agility	Runs 15 yards, picks up blocks, and returns
2. Balance	Eight items ranging in difficulty from standing on one leg to stepping over object on a balance beam
3. Bilateral coordination	Seven items that require use of upper and lower extremities simultaneously or in sequential movement, e.g., tapping feet and fingers, and jumping and clapping. Final item requires pencil use with both hands simultaneously
4. Strength	Three items: standing broad jumps, sit-ups, and push-ups
5. Upper-limb coordination	Five items that involve catching and throwing balls and an additional four items assessing precise finger movements
6. Response speed	Requires a quick catch of falling stick
7. Visual motor control	Eight pencil, paper, and scissor items
8. Upper-limb speed and dexterity	Eight items that range from putting pennies in a box to making dots in circles

Construction and reliability: The Bruininks-Oseretsky Test has been carefully standardized on 765 subjects from differing geographic regions and community size. Test-retest reliability coefficients for the subtests ranged from 0.50 to 0.89 and that of the total battery was 0.87 for second graders and 0.86 for sixth graders. With the exception of "response speed," the subtests differentiated significantly between normal and learning-disabled children.

Comment: The Bruininks-Oseretsky Test of Motor Proficiency appears to be one of the better standardized tests of motor performance. A short form, taking 15 to 20 minutes, can be used for screening. In testing children with motor dysfunction, careful attention must be paid to performance on individual items. For example, a child who compensates for poor proprioceptive postural control with vision can score in the normal range on the balance subtest, even though he/she fails the single item of balance with eyes closed. A problem with finger sequencing in the upper limb coordination subtest could be masked by good ball skills. These kinds of problems could result in not identifying a child's deficit. Another problem with the subtests is that a single item has a disproportionate effect on a child's age equivalence. Nevertheless, this is an excellent test for monitoring the motor development of a dysfunctioning child.

2. Purdue Perceptual-Motor Survey Rating Scale (1966)[243]

Authors: Eugene G. Roach and Newell C. Kephart
Source: Charles E. Merrill Books, Inc.
1300 Alum Creek Drive, Columbus, Ohio 43216

Ages: 6 to 10 years
Administration: Individual; 30 minutes to 1 hour
Equipment: Can be assembled from descriptions in manual

Description: The purpose of the Purdue Perceptual-Motor Survey Rating Scale is to identify children who lack the perceptual-motor abilities theorized to be necessary for acquiring academic skills and to designate problem areas for remediation. The test is made up of 30 items divided into five subtests.

1. Balance and postural flexibility	Includes board walking and jumping skills
2. Body image and differentiation	Includes identification of body parts, imitation of movements, obstacle course, the Krause-Weber subtest, and angels in the snow
3. Perceptual-motor match	Includes chalkboard activities and rhythmic writing
4. Ocular control	Assesses the ability to establish and maintain visual contact with a target
5. Visual achievement forms (also called developmental drawings)	Measures a child's ability to copy geometric forms. The test is rated both for the form of the figures copied and for their organization and size on the page

Construction and reliability: The normative sample of 200 children came from a single school, and although a test-retest reliability of 0.95 has been reported, it was based on only 30 children. Reliability of the subscales, and reliability for differing age groups have not been established. Overall, the standardization of the test is poor.

Comment: Hammill and Bartel[134] suggested that this test was never intended for use as a standardized instrument and that it is better employed as a structured informal device. As such, it can be used as a source of items for the evaluation of learning-disabled children. Its use as the major means of evaluation is questionable. Care must also be taken in the interpretation of performance. The rationale of the test is based on a perceptual-motor theory of development that has not been substantiated (see discussion of Kephart's theory).

3. Test of Motor Impairment—Henderson Revision (1984)[281]

Authors: D.H. Scott, F.A. Moyes, and S.E. Henderson
Source: Brook Educational Publishing, Ltd.
P.O. Box 1171, Guelph, Ontario, Canada N1H 6N3
Ages: 5 to 12 years
Administration: Individual; 20 to 40 minutes
Equipment: Test kit required

Description: The Test of Motor Impairment—Henderson Revision is a version of the Oseretsky Tests of Motor Proficiency. However, it does not result in a motor age, since its purpose is to differentiate children with motor impairment from normal children.[280] The test is divided into four age bands: for children 5 and 6 years; 7 and 8 years; 9 and 10 years; and 11 years and older. Testing is done in eight categories with a single item for each age band in each of the categories. The eight categories are as follows:

1. Manual dexterity 1	Speed and sureness of movement by each hand
2. Manual dexterity 2	Coordination of two hands for a single task
3. Manual dexterity 3	Hand-eye coordination using the preferred hand
4. Ball skills 1	Ball task emphasizing aiming at a target
5. Ball skills 2	Ball task emphasizing catching a ball
6. Static balance	Balance task
7. Dynamic balance 1	Balance task emphasizing spatial precision
8. Dynamic balance 2	Balance task emphasizing control of momentum

Construction and reliability: Normative data was gathered on 923 English-speaking children, 443 from one school district in Canada and 480 from one large city in the United States. Both urban and rural (mostly white) children were included. A number of studies of reliability and validity used the 1972 version as well as the current revision.

Comment: This revision is much clearer than the former version; moreover, cut-off scores for motor impairment are more easily interpretable. This test could be used for screening groups of children to identify motor impairment. Selected test tasks could also be used as a part of a therapist's evaluation. The test would not be useful to assess change except on an item-by-item basis.

4. Peabody Developmental Motor Scales (PDMS): Revised Experimental Edition (1983)[103]

Authors: M. Rhonda Folio and Rebecca R. Fewell
Source: DLM Teaching Resources
P.O. Box 4000, One DLM Park
Allen, Texas 55002
Ages: Birth to 7 years
Administration: Individual (birth to 3 years) or group (4 to 7 years); 40 to 60 minutes (test items may be scored by direct observation or by parent or teacher report)

Description: The Peabody Developmental Motor Scales were designed for use with children who show delay or disability in fine and gross motor skills. Test items are similar to those on other developmental scales but only motor items are included. Items are scored on a 3-point scale, 0 for unsuccessful, 1 for partial, and 2 for successful performance. Age-equivalent, motor quotients, percentile rankings and standard scores are provided. The following skill categories are tested in the gross motor scale (170 test times). These tasks are considered to require precise movements of large muscles of body.

1. Reflexes (12 items)	Includes items such as turning head in response to sound, aligning head on pull to sit, ATNR, protective reaction, and kicking
2. Balance (33 items)	Includes propping, levels of sitting and standing as well as higher-level items such as standing on one foot, beam walking, and walking on tiptoes
3. Non-locomotion (42 items)	Includes items such as head control, rolling, weight bearing as well as higher-level tasks such as jumping and sit ups
4. Locomotion (58 items)	Examples include creeping, cruising, walking, stairs, hopping, tricycle riding, running, and jumping hurdles
5. Receipt and propulsion (25 items)	Catching, throwing, and kicking balls

The fine motor scale has 112 test items considered to require precise movements of small muscles. The following skill categories are included:

1. Grasping (22 items)	Includes reflex grasping and voluntary grasping with the hands and with the fingers as well as crayon grasp
2. Hand use (26 items)	Includes a variety of items ranging from maintaining hands closed to hand preference and including the manipulation of cubes, pegs, and other objects
3. Eye-hand coordination (46 items)	Early items include visual fixation and tracking; later items—form boards, cube building, and copying forms
4. Manual dexterity (18 items)	This category begins with page turning and includes screwing, winding, lacing, and buttons

Construction and reliability: The 617 children making up the normative sample ranged in age from birth to 83 months, with samples beginning at 2-month intervals and increasing to 1-year intervals in older children with the result that subgroups are small, a majority having 30 or fewer children. Samples were selected to reflect socioeconomic status and rural-urban characteristics. A test-retest reliability of .95 for the gross motor scale and of .80 for the fine motor scale was reported based on a sample of 38 children. Validity was demonstrated by the significantly lower scores of 104 children with developmental deviations on all but the 0- to 5-month children. Another study of 43 children established a low but significant correlation (.37) between the PDMS gross motor scale and the Bayley Psychomotor Index and a moderately high correlation (.78) between the PDMS fine motor scale and the Bayley Mental Scale.

Comment: The PDMS are primarily useful for children with mild to moderate motor deficits, such as a learning-disabled child or a child with developmental delay. The test does not discriminate among children with moderate to severe motor disability as they fall far below the standard scores given. The standardization sample is small, especially in the age subgroups. The fine motor scale has a high cognitive element as demonstrated by the high correlation with the Bayley Mental Scale. The skill categories are unevenly distributed and have too few items at some age levels to be meaningful. Despite its drawbacks, the PDMS is probably the most valuable motor scale currently available for preschool children.

5. Quick Neurological Screening Test (1978)[217]

Authors: M.A. Mutti, H.M. Sterling, and N.V. Spalding
Source: Academic Therapy Publications
      20 Commercial Boulevard, Novato, Calif. 94947
Ages: 5 years and over
Administration: Individual; 20 minutes
Equipment: None
Description: The Quick Neurological Screening Test (QNST) was developed as a screening device to identify children who have possible learning disabilities. The tasks are adapted from pediatric neurological examina-

tions as well as from developmental assessments. The test is made up of the following fifteen subtests:

1. Hand skill	Writing his or her name and a sentence
2. Figure recognition and production	Naming, then drawing, five geometric forms
3. Palm form recognition	Recognizing numbers written on their palm by examiner with his finger
4. Eye tracking	Following pencil back and forth and up and down
5. Sound patterns	With hands on knees and eyes closed, imitating patterns demonstrated by the examiner
6. Finger to nose	Finger to nose test; includes observation
7. Thumb and finger circle	Forming circle with thumb and each of the fingers; laterality also observed
8. Double simultaneous stimulation of hand and cheek	With eyes closed, child must identify hands and cheeks touched by examiner in various combinations simultaneously
9. Rapid reversing, repetitive hand movements	Observation of diadochokinesis
10. Arm and leg extension	With eyes closed, extending legs, arms, and tongue for 1 to 15 seconds
11. Tandem walk	Walking straight line, heel to toe, forward and backward
12. Stand on one leg	Balancing first on one leg, then on other, 10 seconds each; eyes open, then closed; right-left differentiation observed
13. Skip	Skipping across the room
14. Left-right discrimination	Scored from subtests: 6, 7, and 12
15. Behavior irregularities	General observation for behaviors such as distractibility, perseveration, defensiveness, hyperactivity

The test is scored based on careful observation and requires a subjective evaluation of performance. The manual provides ages at which 75% of neurologically intact children pass each test as well as total scores indicative of probable neurological dysfunction.

Construction and reliability: The QNST has been used in numerous research studies of normal children and of children with suspected learning disabilities. Although the manual reported these studies, formal standardization of the test has not been done. Reliabilities on the whole test on learning-disabled children of 0.81 and 0.71 are reported, but the data are incomplete. Ages at which 25%, 50%, and 75% of normal children pass each subtest are given based on a compilation of subjects from many studies. Norms for the total test are not given.

Comment: The QNST is a screening device that identifies children with possible neurological dysfunction. It is not and should not be used as a standardized test but rather as an adjunct to clinical observation. It is important to realize that the test is primarily of motor function. It does not include language tests and, therefore, will not identify all children with learning disabilities. The test does screen for possible minimal brain dysfunction or motor deficits.

6. Miller Assessment for Preschoolers (MAP) (1988)[201,205]

Author: Lucy Jane Miller

Source: Psychological Corporation
555 Academic Court, San Antonio, Texas 78204-0952

Ages: 2 years 9 months to 5 years 8 months

Administration: Individual; 20 to 30 minutes including scoring

Equipment: The MAP Test Kit

Description: The Miller Assessment for Preschoolers was designed to identify children who exhibit mild to moderate developmental delays. The MAP was developed with two goals: to develop a short screening tool that could be used by educational and clinical personnel to identify those children in need of further evaluation and to provide a comprehensive, clinical framework that would be helpful in defining a child's strengths and weaknesses and that would indicate possible avenues of remediation. The test is made up of 27 items and a series of structured observations. The test items are divided into five performance indices:

1. Foundations	Items generally found on standard neurological examinations and sensory integrative and neurodevelopmental tests
2. Coordination	Gross, fine, and oral motor abilities and articulation

3. Verbal	Cognitive language abilities, including memory, sequencing, comprehension, association, following directions, and expression
4. Nonverbal	Cognitive abilities such as visual figure-ground, puzzles, memory, and sequencing
5. Complex tasks	Tasks requiring an interaction of sensory, motor, and cognitive abilities

Construction and reliability: The MAP has been well standardized on a random sample of 1200 preschool children. The sample was stratified by age, race, sex, size of residence, community, and socioeconomic factors. Data were collected nationwide in each of nine U.S. Census Bureau regions. Reported reliabilities are good. In a test-retest on 90 children, 81% of the children's scores remained stable. The coefficient of internal consistency on the total sample was 0.798. Interrater reliability on 40 children was reported as 0.98.

Comment: The MAP is a new test that shows promise as a useful screening instrument. It was developed by an occupational therapist and provides information that is of particular relevance to therapists. It is carefully standardized and fills a need for early identification of learning and motor deficits in children. Several articles have now been published supporting the validity of this test as a screening instrument.[202,203,204,206] Reviews of the MAP in the Ninth Mental Measurements Yearbook have described it as "the best available screening test for identifying preschool children with moderate 'preacademic problems' "[87] and "an extremely promising instrument which should find wide use among clinical psychologists, school psychologists, and occupational therapists in assessing mild to moderate learning disabilities in preschool children."[199] A more complete review of this test is provided by King-Thomas and Hacker.[167]

7. Tests of Motor Proficiency of Gubbay (1975)[128]

Author: Sasson S. Gubbay
Source: In Gubbay SS: *The Clumsy Child,* Philadelphia, 1975, W.B. Saunders Co.
Ages: 8 to 12 years
Administration: Individual; 2 to 5 minutes
Equipment: Described in book, must be purchased or constructed
Description: Gubbay's Tests of Motor Proficiency make up a quick screening instrument for the identification of developmental dyspraxia. The battery is made up of eight items that were found to best discriminate between clumsy and normal children in a study of 1000 school children. The test items are:

1. Whistle through pursed lips
2. Skip forward five steps
3. Roll ball with foot around objects
4. Throw tennis ball, clap hands, then catch tennis ball
5. Tie one shoelace with double bow
6. Thread 10 beads
7. Pierce 20 pinholes in graph paper
8. Posting box: fit six shapes in appropriate slots

The first two items are scored pass or fail; the score for the fourth item is the number of claps, and the other items are timed. Percentile values at each age level from 8 to 12 years are reported.

Comment: Gubbay's tests were devised as a rapid screening to be used together with teacher questionnaires to identify clumsy children in a school program. They are valuable if used as intended. One or more of the items could be incorporated into an evaluation protocol using a cutoff based on normative data given. However, this is not a fully standardized test, and further normative data as well as validity and reliability studies are required.

8. Southern California Sensory Integration Tests (SCSIT) (1980)[26]

Author: A. Jean Ayres
Source: Western Psychological Services
12031 Wilshire Boulevard, Los Angeles, Calif. 90025
Ages: 4 to 8 years
Administration: Individual; 1¼ to 1½ hours; examiner certification recommended
Equipment: Test kit required
Description: The Southern California Sensory Integration Tests are clinically oriented and designed to identify sensory integrative dysfunction in learning-disabled children. There are 17 tests; some were derived from neurological tests and others from psychological tests. The tests and their descriptions are as follows:

1. Space visualization	Select from two blocks the one that will fit into a form board; it is necessary to mentally manipulate the forms to arrive at the correct choice on the more difficult test items
2. Figure-ground perception	Select from six pictures the three that are superimposed or embedded with other forms on the test plates

3. Position in space — Sequences of from three to six geometric forms are presented in varying orientations; the design must be selected from a set of designs; in one of the three sections, selection is made from memory

4. Design copying — Copy a design by connecting dots on a dot grid

5. Motor accuracy—revised — Trace a printed, curved, black line with a red pen, first with the preferred hand and then with the nonpreferred hand

6. Kinesthesia — With vision occluded, the child attempts to place his or her finger on a point at which his or her finger had been placed previously by the examiner

7. Manual form perception — A geometric form is held in the hand and the counterpart is selected from a visual display

8. Finger identification — With hands screened from view, the examiner touches the child's finger; the child then points to the finger touched

9. Graphesthesia — The examiner draws a design on the back of the child's hand without the child looking; the child then reproduces the design

10. Localization of tactile stimuli — With vision occluded, the child touches the spot on his/her hand or arm that was touched by the examiner

11. Double tactile stimuli perception — One or two tactile stimuli are given by the examiner to the child's hands and/or cheeks; the child identifies where he/she was touched

12. Imitation of postures — The child imitates a series of positions or postures assumed by the examiner

13. Crossing the midline — The child imitates a series of movements in which the examiner points to his own ear or eye on the same or on opposite sides of the body

14. Bilateral motor coordination — The child imitates patterns and sequences of clapping the thighs or hands

15. Right-left discrimination — Discrimination of left and right on self and on examiner through the execution of verbal commands or answering questions

16. Standing balance—eyes open — The child stands on one foot for as long as possible without losing balance

17. Standing balance—eyes closed — Same as above, with eyes closed

In addition to these 17 tests, interpretation of the SCSIT requires the use of a test of postrotary nystagmus to assess vestibular function and a series of clinical observations. These clinical observations include the following:

1. Eye dominance
2. Eye movements
3. Muscle tone
4. Cocontraction
5. Postural background movements
6. Postural security
7. Equilibrium reactions and protective extension
8. Schilder's arm extension posture
9. Supine flexion
10. Prone extension
11. Asymmetrical tonic neck reflex
12. Hyperactivity, distractibility
13. Tactile defensiveness
14. Ability to perform slow motions
15. Thumb-finger touching
16. Diadochokinesis
17. Tongue-to-lip movements
18. Hopping, jumping, skipping

Construction and reliability: The construction of the Southern California Sensory Integration Tests was based on a theoretical model developed from observation of learning disabilities and supported by factor analytic studies. The tests follow a clinical model and interpretation is based on patterns of scores rather than on a poor score on any one test. Test-retest reliability is reported for each test at each age group. Generally, the coefficients show only moderate reliability. The tests have been criticized on this basis as well as on the lack of study of criterion related validity.[124] The SCSIT have recently been revised and restandardized (see below).

Comment: The SCSIT is a clinical tool; its value in the diagnosis of dysfunction in learning-disabled children is dependent on the level of clinical skill of the user. Appropriate use requires insight and experience as well as the understanding of the theory on which interpretation is based. Certification in administration and interpretation of these tests is essential for use. The tests are a vehicle by which a clinician can gain insight to a child's problems and plan a remediation program. They are not designed to be used in monitoring change with treatment.

9. The Sensory Integration and Praxis Tests (SIPT) (1988)[28]

Author: A. Jean Ayres

Source: Western Psychological Services
12031 Wilshire Boulevard, Los Angeles, Calif. 90025

Ages: 4 to 8 years

Administration: Individual; 1½ hours; examiner certification recommended

Equipment: Test kit required

Description: The Sensory Integration and Praxis Tests are a major revision and restandardization of the Southern California Sensory Integration Tests. Four new tests of praxis have been added, five tests have had major revisions, eight have had minor changes and four tests have been deleted. The tests are designed to identify sensory integration and praxic deficits in learning-disabled children. There are 17 tests described as follows:

1. Space visualization	Select from two blocks the one that will fit into a form board; it is necessary to mentally manipulate the forms to arrive at the correct choice on the more difficult test items
2. Figure-ground perception	The child select from six pictures the three that are superimposed or embedded with other forms on the test plates
3. Manual form perception	Part I: a geometric form is held in the hand and the counterpart is selected from a visual display
	Part II: a geometric form is felt with one hand while its match is selected from several choices with the other hand
4. Kinesthesia	With vision occluded, the child attempts to place his or her finger on a point at which his or her finger had been placed previously by the examiner; a separate recording sheet is provided for each child
5. Finger identification	With hands screened from view, the examiner touches the child's finger, the shield is removed and child then points to the finger touched
6. Graphesthesia	The examiner uses his or her finger to draw a design on the back of the child's hand, without the child looking; the child then reproduces the design
7. Localization of tactile stimuli	With vision occluded, the child touches the spot on his or her hand or arm that was touched by the examiner with a specially designed pen
8. Praxis on verbal command	The examiner verbally describes a series of body movements and the child executes them
9. Design copying	Part I: the child copies a design by connecting dots on a dot grid
	Part II: the child copies a design without the use of a dot grid; both process and product are scored
10. Constructional praxis	Working with blocks, the child attempts to duplicate two different block structures; in the first structure, the child observes the examiner building the model; the second structure is pre-assembled

11. Postural praxis	The child imitates unusual body positions demonstrated by the examiner
12. Oral praxis	The child imitates movements of the tongue, lips, and jaw demonstrated by the examiner
13. Sequencing praxis	The child imitates a series of simple arm and hand movements demonstrated by the examiner
14. Bilateral motor coordination	The child imitates a series of bilateral arm and foot movements demonstrated by the examiner
15. Standing and walking balance	The subtest consists of 15 items in which the child assumes various standing and walking postures
16. Motor accuracy	The child traces a printed, curved black line with a red, nylon-tipped pen, first with the preferred hand and then with the nonpreferred hand
17. Postrotary nystagmus	The child is rotated first counter-clockwise and then clockwise on a rotation board and the duration of postrotary nystagmus, a vestibulo-ocular reflex, is observed

Comment: SIPT subtests are computer scored, interpreted, and profiled. A full eight-color profile (WPS Chroma-Graph) is provided that summarizes major SIPT testing and statistical results in a clear manner.

10. Meeting Street School Screening Test (1969)[132]

Authors: P.K. Hainesworth and M.L. Siqueland
Source: Crippled Children and Adults of Rhode Island, Inc.
Meeting Street School
667 Waterman Avenue, East Providence, RI 02914
Ages: 4 to 7½ years
Administration: Individual; 20 minutes
Equipment: Test booklet and protocol sheets required
Description: The Meeting Street School Screening Test was developed to help identify children in kindergarten and first grade who have cerebral dysfunction or neuro-

logical impairment. The test consists of three subtests that survey the child's development in specific areas of information processing: whole body awareness and control, visual-perceptual-motor abilities, and speech and language. The total score reflects the overall efficiency in information processing, and the three subtest scores reflect skill in each of the modalities. Items for each of the subtests are as follows:

Motor patterning subtest

1. Gait patterns	Samples the child's effectiveness in learned unilateral and bilateral body movement patterns
2. Clap hands	Examines the child's
3. Hand patterns	ability to see, remember, and reproduce unlearned, sequential movement patterns in appropriate spatial relationship to his or her own body
4. Follow directions I	Assesses the child's ability to comprehend and retain verbal directions involving spatial concepts and to translate them into movements of his or her body in space
5. Touch fingers	Examines the child's skill in coordinating his/her hands and fingers in rapid bilateral patterned movement

Visual-perceptual-motor subtest

1. Block tapping	Measures the child's memory for place (spatial) sequences
2. Visual matching	Samples visual-perceptual discrimination of form
3. Visual memory	Samples the child's short-term memory for geometric and letter-like forms
4. Copy forms	Assesses the child's ability to coordinate hand and eye in the reproduction of geometric and letter-like forms in the correct shape, orientation, and spacing

5. Follow directions II — Samples the child's understanding of spatial and directional concepts when drawing on a piece of paper

Language subtest

1. Repeat words — Assesses the child's ability to listen to and repeat unknown and familiar speech sound sequences in their correct form, order, and rhythm

2. Repeat sentences — Assesses the child's ability to listen and repeat language material that is more complex, both in length and grammatical form, than the words and phrases above

3. Counting — Assesses the child's ability to sequence numbers in automatically learned and in interrupted sentences

4. Tell a story — Assesses the child's ability to formulate and express his or her thoughts in meaningful language about an abstract picture

5. Language sequencing — Assesses the child's ability to sequence time concepts and understand order and meaning of time units

Construction and reliability: The Meeting Street School Test was standardized on 500 children of varied socioeconomic backgrounds in a single geographical location. The reliability was reported to be about 0.85 for the whole test and between 0.75 and 0.85 for the subareas, but the specific data and numbers of subjects in the reliability studies were not given. Several studies of predictive validity were reviewed in the manual.

Comment: The test was designed for use in the early identification of learning disabilities and can be used for screening large numbers of children. The manual includes considerable information on the interpretation of children's performance. The test can be used diagnostically if supplemented by other tests, but its main value is in the identification of children who need further evaluation. Another version by the same authors, Early Identification in Preschool Children, can be used with children 4 to 4½ years of age.

11. Bender Gestalt Test for Young Children (1963)[176]

Author: E.M. Koppitz
Source: Grune and Stratton, Inc.
New York, NY
Ages: 5 to 10 years
Administration: Individual; 7 to 15 minutes; special training required
Description: The Bender Gestalt Test for Young Children is an adaptation of the Bender Visual Motor Gestalt Test, which is an individually administered test of performance in copying designs. The test consists of nine designs that are printed on separate cards and that are presented one at a time to the child. The child is given unlimited time to copy each successive design on a sheet of paper. The developmental scoring system for young children to age 10 was developed by Koppitz.[176] The Bender Gestalt is used by psychologists to assess visual motor functions and possible neuropsychological impairment, and it is also used with the Koppitz scoring system to evaluate perceptual-motor maturity and emotional adjustment. The reproduced design is scored for distortion, rotation, perseveration, method of reproduction, and other factors. The Koppitz scoring system yields an estimate of the child's developmental age.

Construction and reliability: The Bender Gestalt Test is a widely used and heavily researched test of neuropsychological impairment following brain injury in adults. The Koppitz version, standardized for children, makes possible similar diagnoses with children. Test-retest reliability for the Koppitz scoring of the Bender Visual Motor Gestalt test are moderate, ranging from 0.60 to 0.66. Interscorer agreement is given as 93%.

Comment: The Bender Gestalt Test yields more information about a child's deficit than simpler tests of geometric form reproduction, but it requires special skills for its interpretation. Inability to copy geometric forms may occur for several reasons: faulty visual-perceptual discrimination, poor motor ability, or, more likely, problems in the translations of the percept of the form to its reproduction.

12. Developmental Test of Visual Motor Integration (VMI)—Revised (1982)[38]

Author: K. Beery
Source: Modern Curriculum Press
13900 Prospect Rd., Cleveland, Ohio 44136
Age: 2 to 15 years
Administration: Individual or group; 10 to 15 minutes
Equipment: Forms or protocol books
Description: The Developmental Test of Visual Motor Integration tests the ability to copy geometric forms. A booklet is provided with 24 designs in an age-graded sequence. The child copies each design in a space directly below it. Items are judged pass or fail based on criteria

given in the manual. Age equivalency scores are based on the number of forms passed.

Construction and reliability: The Visual Motor Integration Manual contains information relating to ages at which forms are passed based on Gesell and other researchers as well as age equivalencies based on a sample of 3090 children. Data on reliability are incomplete, but test-retest reliability was reported for groups of children of all ages to range from 0.63 to 0.92. There were no reports of reliability at individual ages. Split, half reliability was reported to range from 0.66 to 0.93, and inter-scorer agreement was 0.93.

Comment: The Developmental Test of Visual Motor Integration provides a quick and easy method of assessing the development of a child's ability to copy geometric forms. It is useful as an adjunct to other assessments of the learning-disabled child. When the test is presented to the child, he/she is told that the booklet must remain parallel to the edge of the table. This prevents some of the problems of other tests, e.g., the child turning the individual paper on which designs are reproduced. But the structured format does not allow the assessment of overall organization of copying forms, as can be done when the child copies forms on a blank sheet of paper (e.g., Bender Gestalt Test). Therefore overall organization should also be tested.

13. Test of Visual-Motor Skills (TVMS) (1986)[114a]

Author: Morrison F. Gardner
Source: Children's Hospital of San Francisco
Publication Department OPR-110
P.O. Box 3805, San Francisco, Calif. 94119
Ages: 2 to 13 years
Administration: Individual or group; 3 to 6 patients
Equipment: Protocol booklet
Description: The TVMS consists of a series of 26 forms to be copied by the child. Each form is on a separate page of the booklet, which has some forms commonly used in visual-motor tests (lines and circles, for example), but many more forms are unique to this test. Care was taken to avoid forms with a resemblance to language symbols. The forms are scored from 0 to 2. A score of 0 indicates that the child is unable to copy the form with motor accuracy. A score of 2 demonstrates precision in execution. A score of 1 indicates poor coordination or control. Criteria for scoring at each level are given with examples for each form. Age equivalents and standard scores are provided.
Construction and reliability: The Test of Visual-Motor Skills was administered to 1009 children in the San Francisco Bay area at 11 age levels from 2 years to 12 years. The number of subjects in each age group ranged from 38 to 132, with about half male and half female children. Cronbach's coefficient *alpha* was used to determine the internal consistency of the test. These reli-

ability coefficients were lower for the younger children (0.31 at 2 years and 0.69 at 3 years) but otherwise good, ranging from 0.78 to 0.90 for older age groups and reaching 0.97 for the sample as a whole. Test-retest reliability was not reported in the manual, but the author noted the need for research in that area.

Comment: The TVMS is a companion test to the Test of Visual-Perceptual Skills (TVPS), which is a motor-free test of form perception. Using the tests together can be determine whether the child's form reproduction reflects incorrect visual perception or whether the problem is in motor execution. The TVMS places greater expectations on motor precision than other visual-motor tests. For example, a line must touch an intersecting line without crossing over it. Therefore it should be used only when motor control as well as constructive abilities are important.

14. Basic Motor Ability Tests—Revised (BMAT—Revised) (1979)[11]

Authors: D.D. Arnheim and W.A. Sinclair
Source: In D.D. Arnheim and W.A. Sinclair, *The Clumsy Child,* St. Louis, 1979, The C.V. Mosby Company
Ages: 4 to 12 years
Administration: Individual, 15 to 20 minutes; or group, 30 minutes
Equipment: Assembled from description
Description: The Basic Motor Ability Tests—Revised consists of eleven tests:

1. Bead stringing	Bilateral eye-hand coordination and dexterity
2. Target throwing	Eye-hand coordination in throwing
3. Marble transfer	Finger dexterity and speed of arm movement
4. Back and hamstring stretch	Flexibility of back and hamstring muscles
5. Standing long jump	Strength and power in thigh and lower legs
6. Face down to standing	Speed and ability in changing from prone to standing
7. Static balance	One foot standing with eyes open and eyes closed
8. Basketball throw for distance	Arm and shoulder girdle explosive strength
9. Ball striking	Coordination in striking dropped ball with hand
10. Target kicking	Eye-foot coordination
11. Agility run	Ability to rapidly move body and alter direction

Construction and reliability: The data on standardization presented in *The Clumsy Child* are fragmentary. The authors have tested 1563 children and report a test-retest reliability of 0.93, but no additional data are given on breakdown by ages. Normative information for each test is presented in percentiles at each age.

Comment: The structure of this test is such that one or more of the tests can be used individually with normative data providing an indication of expected performance. Use of the test as a whole or in part could be a valuable part of an evaluation program.

15. Purdue Pegboard Test (1948, 1968)[287]

Author: Joseph Tiffin, Ph.D.
Source: Lafayette Instrument Co.
P.O. Box 5728, Lafayette, Ind. 47903
Ages: 5 years through adult
Administration: Individual; 10 to 15 minutes
Equipment: Pegboard with pins, collars, and washers required
Description: This test of manual dexterity consists of four parts, each described below:

1. Right hand	Subject inserts small pegs into holes in pegboard using right hand for a 30-second trial
2. Left hand	Subject inserts pegs into pegboard with left hand for a 30-second trial
3. Both hands	Both hands pick up and insert pegs into board at same time for a 30-second trial
4. Assembly	Using hands cooperatively, subject assembles sequences of pens, collars, and washers for a 60-second trial

Construction and Reliability: This test has recently been standardized with 1334 normal school children, ages 5 to 16, from New Jersey. Means, standard deviations, and percentile scores are presented as a function of age (6-month intervals) and sex. Reliability data on children are not presented in the test manual, although reliability with college students ranged from 0.60 to 0.71. A number of validity studies indicate that learning-disabled subjects perform more poorly than normal controls on this test. Additional normative data are presented in the manual for various age and diagnostic groups.

Comment: This test was originally designed for adults to assist in the selection of employees for manual industrial jobs. It has recently been standardized with school-age children[114] and adolescents.[191]

Chapter 12

PERIPHERAL NEUROPATHIES

William K. Ogard and Bradley W. Stockert

The classification of peripheral neuropathies covers a wide range of etiological factors. An anatomic classification has been presented by Schaumberg and others[26] that describes two overall types: (1) symmetrical generalized neuropathies and (2) focal and multifocal neuropathies. Others have described neuropathies with regard to specific pathology, noting the agent's effect on the peripheral nervous system, but that information appears to be included in Schaumberg and others' anatomical classification.[26]

Traumatic peripheral neuropathies are classed as focal or multifocal neuropathies in the category of physical injuries, which includes severance, focal crush, compression, stretch or traction, and entrapment.[26] The physical therapy literature has not described peripheral neuropathies with regard to these categories, however, articles describing specific pathological entities have been presented.[21] Some of the specific problems discussed include thoracic outlet syndrome (TOS), specific entrapment syndromes (e.g., suprascapular nerve entrapment), traction injuries (e.g., brachial plexus), and acute compression syndromes (e.g., Saturday night palsy, casting and splinting). Although the treatment and the signs and symptoms of these syndromes and pathologies has been given much attention, less consideration has been afforded the specific pathophysiology of the peripheral nerve injury in traumatic peripheral neuropathies.

The purpose of this chapter is to discuss traumatic peripheral neuropathies with regard to classification, neuroanatomy, pathogenesis, degeneration, orthopedic implications, evaluation, and treatment of orthopedic problems relating to traumatic peripheral neuropathies. Although many similarities exist between traumatic and degenerative neuropathic problems and both have been included, the discussion will focus primarily on peripheral trauma because of its clinical link to orthopedic management.

NEUROANATOMY OF PERIPHERAL NERVOUS SYSTEM

The peripheral nervous system (PNS) may be generally described as that portion of the nervous system outside the central nervous system (CNS), which includes the brain and spinal cord.[16,26] Its major components include motor neurons, primary sensory neurons outside the CNS, and autonomic neurons. Specific components include dorsal and ventral spinal roots, spinal and cranial nerves, dorsal root and other sensory ganglia, sensory and motor terminals, and the bulk of the autonomic system (Fig. 12-1).

Pratt[21] describes three levels in the organization of a peripheral nerve or nerve trunk (Fig. 12-1). At the innermost level, the nerve fiber is a small conducting component of the trunk and a process of a neuron or nerve cell. It is surrounded by endoneurium consisting of connective tissue. The second level is a nerve bundle, the funiculus (fascicle), consisting of nerve fibers surrounded by perineurium.[21,26] The third level is the nerve trunk, formed by one to many funiculi enclosed by another connective tissue layer, the epineurium. Extensions from the epineurium extend into the nerve, separating the funiculi. The connective tissue is loose and irregular and contains cells, fibers, and ground substance.[20]

Microscopically, a nerve fiber consists of an axon, which may be myelinated or unmyelinated, a Schwann cell and its nucleus, and a surrounding basal or basement membrane. The nerve fiber is separated into segments defined by a single Schwann cell and the myelin sheath produced by that cell. Junctions of consecutive Schwann cells separated by the cell membrane are termed nodes of Ranvier. The basement membrane is not interrupted by the nodes of Ranvier. Although the nodes may interrupt the myelin sheath, the basement membrane remains consistent along the length of the axon. The axon itself is continuous, forming a tubular structure surrounded by an axolemma. The axon contains cytoplasm, mitochondria, neurofilaments, and neurotubules. Axoplasmic flow of cellular components to and from the neuron (nerve cell or cell body), termed retrograde and anterograde axoplasmic transport respectively, provides for metabolic needs of the nerve and end-organ tissue.[16] The substances exchanged through axoplasmic flow between axons and the tissues they innervate are termed trophic factors.[16] The neurotubules and neurofilaments are thought to be connected with the fast component of axoplasmic flow.[2,18,29]

CLASSIFICATION OF TRAUMATIC PERIPHERAL NEUROPATHIES

Seddon's clinical classification of nerve injury[28] is defined by mechanical trauma. Neurotmesis ("cutting of nerve") refers to severance of all essential structures, including the axon; a visible disruption may not be apparent and the epineurium may be intact. Axonotmesis is a lesion to the axon severe enough to cause degeneration of the axon distal to the lesion, but with no interruption of continuity of the endoneurium. Neurapraxia ("nonacting nerve") is injury to the nerve, causing some degree of paralysis but no peripheral degeneration. This classification is descriptive from the standpoint of morphology of regeneration, functional loss and recovery, and clinical prognosis.[10]

Schaumberg and others[26] utilize Seddon's classification, proposing an anatomical classification defining neuropraxia, axonotmesis, and neurotmesis as Class I, Class II, and Class III injuries (Table 12-1). Class I injuries result in a reversible blockade of nerve conduction that tends to be the result of mild or moderate focal compression. The following two types are described: (1) mild, rapidly reversible, resulting from transient ischemia with no anatomic changes; and (2) persistent conduction block resulting from paranodal demyelination.

Clinically, Class I injuries may result in decreased (or loss of) strength and absent tendon reflexes below the level of the lesion, slight sensory loss (confined to large diameter fibers), and no change in sympathetic function. There

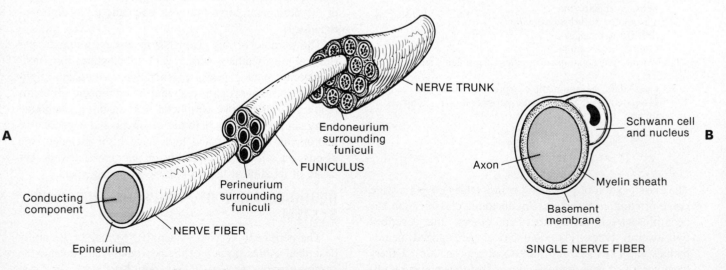

Fig. 12-1. Three levels of organization of a peripheral nerve or nerve trunk. **A,** Nerve trunk and components. **B,** Microscopic structure of nerve fiber.

Table 12-1. Classification of acute (traumatic) peripheral nerve injury

Anatomic classification	Class I	Class II	Class III
Previous nomenclature	Neurapraxia	Axonotmesis	Neurotmesis
Lesion	Conduction block resulting from ischemia demyelination	Axonal interruption	Nerve fiber interruption with connective tissue damage; nerve severance (complete)

Adapted from Schaumberg HH, and others: Disorders of peripheral nerves, Philadelphia, 1983, FA Davis Co.

is no damage to the axon itself. Recovery is generally spontaneous and occurs within 3 months.[26]

Class II injuries (axonotmesis) result in variable loss of sensory, motor, and sympathetic function.[26] Both myelinated and unmyelinated fibers may be involved. Muscle atrophy may occur and areflexia occurs consistently. These lesions generally occur as a result of closed-crush or per-

cussion injuries. The axon is damaged, but the Schwann cell basal lamina remains intact along with the endoneurial connective tissue. Although Wallerian degeneration occurs distal to the lesion, regeneration is generally effective, because Schwann cell integrity is maintained. Recovery is generally slow (several months to more than 1 year), with axonal regeneration occurring at a rate of 1 to 8 mm per day, depending on the specific nerve.[2,29]

Class III injuries (neurotmesis) commonly result from stab wounds, high-velocity projectiles, or nerve traction that disrupts the connective tissue components of the nerve along with complete transaction of the nerve trunk. Wallerian degeneration occurs distal to the lesion. Regeneration may occur, but because of damage to connective tissue and Schwann cells, sprouting may occur randomly. As a result, proper end-organ function may not be restored, and the formation of neuromas is not uncommon.[26]

PATHOGENESIS OF PERIPHERAL NEUROPATHIES

As described previously nerve degeneration is a salient feature of Class II and Class III traumatic neuropathies. Waller is credited with describing nerve degeneration that occurs distal to the site of injury; this process is called Wallerian degeneration (Fig. 12-2).[2] Primarily, the axon

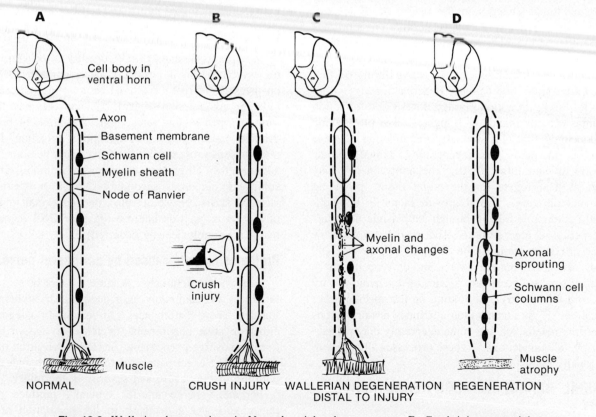

Fig. 12-2. Wallerian degeneration. **A,** Normal peripheral motor nerve. **B,** Crush injury to peripheral nerve. **C,** Wallerian degeneration distal to site of injury. **D,** Regeneration with axonal sprouting guided by Schwann cell columns. (Adapted from Schaumberg HH, Spencer PS, and Thomas PK: Disorders of peripheral nerves, Philadelphia, 1983, FA Davis Co.)

shrinks, fragments, and becomes irregular in shape. Secondarily, myelin, if present, breaks down and associated cells undergo change. This myelin breakdown involves chemical alteration of myelin lipids and is accompanied by retraction of the myelin sheath from the axon at the nodes of Ranvier and breakdown of the sheath into ellipsoid or digestive chambers.[2] Enzyme activity can be seen ultrastructurally. Fragments of axon and myelin debris are broken down by lysosomal vacuoles in Schwann cells and to some extent within macrophages that migrate into the nerve during early stages of degeneration. Loss of protein within the first 24 hours is the basic chemical change of axonal and myelin degeneration.[34] These changes reflect a cessation of normal axonal flow with disintegration of cell organelles. Organelles identified in this focal accumulation include mitochondria, microtubules, and dilated vesicles.[29,34] At the time of and shortly after injury, there is a proliferation of Schwann cells, which then form columns of cells (bands of Bungner) that serve to guide the regenerating axons to their termination. The entire process of Wallerian degeneration prepares the nerve stump for regeneration and may also cause the elaboration of neurotrophic factors that promote this goal.[19] Retrograde changes may also occur in the nerve proximal to the site of the injury. These may include retraction of the axon proximal to the lesion, chromatolysis (breakdown of Nissl substance), and other changes in the neuron itself (central chromatolysis or retrograde axon reaction).[29] This process may be followed by either cell death or the process of regeneration.

The Schwann cell continues to be active during the first 24 hours after injury and beyond. Reactive changes within the cell lead to proliferation through mitosis and formation of columns of cells (bands of Bungner) takes place along the endoneureal tube.[29] Essentially the function of these columns is to guide the regenerating axonal sprouts (filopodia) to their target tissue. The Schwann cell may also act as a surrogate for the target tissue, providing trophic material (e.g., neural growth factor in unmyelinated and autonomic fibers) through axoplasmic flow during the period of regeneration.[4] The axonal sprouts grow from the proximal stump to the distal stump, the rate and progress dependent on the extent and/or type of injury (i.e., crush versus severance).[29] Rates of regeneration vary from 1 to 8 mm per day, depending on the specific nerve and location.[2,29] As regeneration continues distally, axons may become myelinated and some eventually may reestablish peripheral connections.[34] These processes all appear to be neuronally regulated.[19]

SURGICAL REPAIR OF PERIPHERAL NERVE INJURY

Surgical repair of peripheral nerve injuries has historically been accomplished by either nerve suturing or use of a nerve graft. Although both procedures have been successful, nerve suturing appears to be the more effective.[27] End-to-end suturing of peripheral nerves is possible when the transected nerve ends can be closely approximated. If there is a considerable gap between the severed ends of the nerve, nerve suturing may not be effective and a graft may be considered.[17]

There are many factors influencing the success of a nerve suture procedure. Success of failure depends on the age of the patient, location and/or level of the injury, extent or size of the defect, delay time from injury to repair, the type of nerve (motor or sensory), extent of paralysis, and surgical or technical factors.[6]

Nerve graft procedures have used heterografts, homografts, and autografts as donor material. Autografts seem to have provided the best clinical and experimental results.[17] The factors that influence the success of the nerve graft procedure include graft survival (i.e., revascularization), length, caliber, shrinkage, delay in placement, and sources.[27]

TYPICAL CLINICAL SIGNS AND PROBLEMS

Primary and secondary clinical problems resulting from traumatic peripheral nerve injuries are found distal and, to a lesser extent, proximal to the lesion. Though pure motor and pure sensory disturbances are found in some pathological states (e.g. poliomyelitis), the pattern typically seen with trauma is mixed motor and sensory loss.[23]

Nonneurological injuries directly caused by trauma

Multiple tissue damage is frequently associated with the trauma that results in peripheral nerve damage. Depending on the specific type of trauma (e.g., gun shot, stabbing, falls, or compression injury), the damage may take the form of open wound sites, bone fractures, blood vessel damage, muscle tears, edema, and/or infection. Each of these lesions presents problems that must be addressed. In addition, they all prolong the period of immobilization, resulting in numerous secondary clinical problems (e.g., vascular stasis, disuse atrophy, and abnormal joint range of motion as well as internal organ or CNS damage that may have simultaneously occurred).

Problems directly caused by peripheral nerve injury

Sensory disturbances. A large number of sensory disturbances are commonly associated with peripheral nerve injuries. These disturbances can be grossly categorized as either negative phenomena (decrease or loss of a sensation) or positive phenomena (increased sensation or dysesthesia).[3] The exact pattern of the sensory change(s) varies with the specific cause and severity of the injury.

Peripheral nerve injuries typically produce negative phenomena and a decrease in the perception of touch, proprioception, and stereognosis. These sensations are associated with large-diameter fibers that are generally more vulnerable to compression than small-diameter fibers.

Small-diameter fibers are associated with temperature and pain sensation.[3] Any absence or decrease in the perception of noxious stimuli diminishes normal protective reactions and leads to further peripheral problems as a result of neglect.

In addition to the obvious difficulties found with these sensory disturbances, there is the problem of patient neglect associated with an "insensitive" area. The diminished protective reactions and poor hygiene habits commonly found with a neglected area often lead to an increased incidence of repeated trauma and secondary problems, such as swelling with dependent positioning. If the client's CNS has also been damaged as a result of trauma, degeneration, or substance abuse, these problems can become pronounced.

Positive phenomena associated with peripheral nerve injuries include contact dysesthesia, hyperalgesia, burning, and pins-and-needles sensation. An increased perception of pain is often associated with compression applied directly over the injury site, as well as just proximal and distal to the lesion. Hyperalgesia and pins-and-needles sensation are the most common positive phenomena found with peripheral nerve injuries.[3]

Weakness/paralysis of denervated muscle. The specific pattern of weakness and/or paralysis seen with traumatic peripheral nerve injuries is directly related to the site and severity of the injury. Sites that are particularly vulnerable to injury include the peroneal nerve near the proximal fibula and the radial and ulnar nerves as they respectively pass the radial groove and medial epicondyle on the humerus.[13]

In general, partially denervated muscle shows some degree of weakness, whereas completely denervated muscle becomes flaccid. In both cases, atrophy begins to appear shortly after denervation. Concomitant with denervation is the patient's complaint of rapid fatigue and diminished capacity to perform activities of daily living. Deep-tendon reflexes are diminished or absent, and electromyographic (EMG) readings are abnormal following nerve injury.[11]

Following muscle denervation, EMG readings remain electrically silent for 5 to 7 days, at which time fibrillation potentials begin to appear. Frequent fibrillation potentials are characteristic of denervated muscle and are present within 3 weeks after the injury. The EMG pattern after that time depends on the degree of nerve repair and regeneration. The appearance of low amplitude, short duration, highly polyphasic motor-unit potentials is evidence of repair and regeneration. Motor-unit potentials often occur before there is any palpable contraction. As regeneration continues, the fibrillation potentials diminish and the polyphasic motor-unit activity increases. Fibrillation potentials typically remain for 2 to 3 years and sometimes 4 to 5 years in severe injuries.[11]

Vasomotor disturbances. In some cases of peripheral nerve injury (e.g., complete transection), the peripheral sympathetic nerve fibers are cut. This loss decreases sympathetic vasomotor tone and results in vasodilation.[33] The vasomotor paralysis and resultant vasodilation increase the incidence of edema. This situation compounds the problem of swelling in an insensitive limb left in a dependent position.

Changes secondary to traumatic peripheral nerve injury

Soft tissue changes. Connective tissue changes occur secondary to disuse following paralysis and/or immobilization. Close examination and palpation frequently reveal thickening of tendon sheaths and fibrotic adhesions, especially in the periarticular areas. These soft tissue changes can decrease the available physiological and accessory range of motion (ROM) at a joint and ultimately limit a patient's functional recovery following reinnervation.

Joint weakness and instability develop initially from the weakness and/or paralysis of the muscles surrounding the joint. Over time, edema and disuse result in weakness of the joint capsule and ligaments, predisposing the joint to hypermobility. In all joints, hypermobility increases the probability that degenerative changes will occur. Hypermobility and instability make the joint more susceptible to subluxation, damage to articular surfaces, and further compromise of the joint integrity.[33] Additional joint deformities may appear secondary to the unopposed pull of an antagonist or from abnormal biomechanics in weight-bearing joints.

Bony changes. Studies have shown that the changes in bone after nerve section with motor paralysis are similar to the changes in bone following a similar period of immobilizations without nerve section.[1,8,33] The rate of onset and extent of bony changes are more directly related to the degree of disuse than the cause of the neural disturbance. In adults the changes include a decrease in cortical and trabecular thickness, concomitant with an increase in decalcification, porosity, and medullary canal diameter. These changes appear to be only partially reversible following reinnervation and mobilization.[25,33] These alterations in bone structure result in an overall decrease in bone strength and can lead to an increased incidence of fracture, especially in weight-bearing bones.

The pattern is somewhat different in growing bones. Immediately after the injury there is a period of hyperplasia followed by premature cessation of growth.[24,25] This results in a permanent decrease in the length and diameter of the bone as well as the size of the bony prominences.[33] This childhood injury is one of the causes of leg-length or arm-length discrepancies in adults.

EVALUATION
Patient history

A complete medical history should be taken for each patient. Even when the diagnosis is known, the history will give additional valuable information regarding the diagnosis, the prognosis, and the patient's perceptions of his or her condition. Relevant past medical history, treatment, and response should be discussed.

Observation

This portion of the evaluation is used to gain a gross overview of the patient. If the patient walks into the treatment area, the gait pattern should be observed to determine if further assessment of that activity is necessary. In addition, the examiner should observe the patient's general posture, integrity of the skin, and general willingness to move and cooperate. If the patient is seen at bedside, his or her overall appearance should be observed as the examiner enters the room. It is important to know whether the patient is being treated for any fractures, vascular compromise, or other problems that must be considered during evaluation and treatment. The patient's willingness to move the affected area and to move in general should also be assessed. In addition, the patient's overall disposition should be noted and its potential effect on the evaluation and treatment process determined.

Objective examination

A thorough, objective evaluation will help the therapist classify the extent of the peripheral nerve injury. Classification is useful in determining the prognosis, setting realistic goals, and developing an appropriate treatment plan. A good differential diagnosis is especially important in cases of multiple trauma to separate true peripheral nerve injuries from other possible sources of nerve injury (e.g., herniated nucleus pulposus or foramina entrapment).[13] Similarly, clients with other confounding problems, such as CNS involvement, must be assessed in their entirety with the peripheral system being one component of the whole.

Nerve conduction test

A thorough evaluation of a patient with a suspected peripheral nerve injury will require equipment and personnel not available in many physical therapy clinics. Nerve conduction velocity should be tested. In a peripheral nerve injury, this test will demonstrate a normal velocity proximal to the lesion, but a decreased velocity or loss of the signal at the injury site and distally. Following Wallerian degeneration, regenerated axonal tissue typically demonstrates a conduction velocity equal to only 60% to 80% of the value predicted for normal tissue.[33] (Refer to Chapter 26 for further discussion of electrodiagnosis.)

Electromyography

Electromyography (EMG) will demonstrate the presence or absence of normal innervation to a muscle. As denervated muscle becomes reinnervated, the EMG pattern changes in a characteristic fashion that suggests specific

stages of recovery have occurred. The time required for muscle reinnervation and normal muscle potentials to return depends upon the severity of the injury and the distance between the muscle and the site of injury.[11] (Refer to Chapter 26 for further discussion of electrodiagnosis.)

Sensory testing

Sensory testing can be performed in any physical therapy facility, and the results can give significant clues about the severity of the injury. Because large-diameter fibers are more vulnerable to injury than small-diameter fibers, the presence or absence of the various sensory modalities gives an indication of the extent of the nerve injury. Touch, proprioception, and stereognosis are senses transmitted along large-diameter fibers, whereas temperature is a sensation transmitted on small-diameter fibers. All of these sensory modalities are readily tested. The Tinel sign is a provocation test used on regenerating nerves to determine the leading edge of the regenerating axon. The test consists of tapping on the end of the regenerating nerve. A positive sign consists of pain or tingling in response to tapping over the distal end of the regenerating axon. The pain or tingling will occur in areas where the nerve has regenerated. No sensation will be perceived in those areas still lacking innervation.[15] Although Tinel's sign is commonly used to give an accurate indication of axonal regeneration, in some cases (e.g., Class III peripheral nerve injury) the sign can be extremely misleading and unreliable.[33] Sensory testing should be used in cases of multiple trauma to determine if the loss in sensation follows a true dermatomal pattern or a peripheral nerve distribution. Appropriate high-level functional sensory testing (e.g., balance and coordination) should be performed to develop a thorough picture of the patient's level of dysfunction and the progress of the rehabilitation program.

Range of motion testing

ROM testing is essential. Physiological and accessory motions need to be tested for hypomobility as well as hypermobility. All relevant end-feels (the sensation perceived by the therapist at the end of a passive ROM) should be assessed. This information is used to help determine the need for mobilization, stabilization, and/or protection of a given area.[5,15]

Manual muscle test

Thorough manual muscle testing should be done: (1) to determine the pattern (myotome versus peripheral nerve) of any weakness and/or paralysis, (2) to delineate if the nerve injury is unifocal or multifocal, and (3) to assess the severity of each lesion. Muscle testing provides a baseline to judge the patient's recovery and the effects of treatment. When appropriate, testing should include functional tests to determine a patient's ability to perform activities of daily living. An endurance factor should be included in testing, because partially denervated muscle may demonstrate near normal strength but fatigues very quickly.

Soft tissue palpation

Soft tissue palpation is often an overlooked technique, but it is an important part of this evaluation process. Layer palpation is typically begun superficially and then progresses to deeper tissues. During palpation care must be taken that the fingers move with the skin. If the fingers slide over the skin, the patient will experience discomfort and skin abrasions may occur. When skin integrity is poor, palpation must be done with precaution to avoid abrasion and tearing of the superficial skin layer. Initially the skin should be inspected for signs of neglect and then palpated for a determination of temperature and mobility. Palpation progresses to the subcutaneous layers to assess the pulses of relevant blood vessels, the mobility of subcutaneous fascia, and the presence of edematous tissue, especially in dependent, affected limbs. Thorough palpation should include some assessment of skin fat folds, which may mask muscular atrophy. Deep palpation is done to assess the status of fascial planes, ligaments, tendons, and tendinous sheaths. Careful soft tissue palpation can reveal abnormalities (e.g., adhesions or thickenings) in tissues that may impair joint and/or soft tissue function.[15,31]

TREATMENT PROCEDURES

One of the unfortunate realities of treating peripheral nerve injuries is that physical therapy treatment is directed only at the secondary consequences of the nerve injury. The nerve injury per se is not affected by traditional physical therapy treatment. Our approach eliminates or minimizes these secondary changes while we wait to see how much functional reinnervation will occur. This approach focuses on anticipating changes in an effort to minimize their impact. Patient education is essential to maximize functional return and avoid secondary conditions resulting from sensory neglect.

Weakness/paralysis

In denervated muscle the effectiveness of treatment with electrical stimulation remains unproven in humans.[7,30] The classic study by Gutmann and Gutmann[9] in 1942 showed that electrical stimulation was effective in retarding atrophy in denervated muscle of rabbits. Some studies using other animal models have confirmed these results and other studies found no effect.[20,30] At this time no controlled study has been done in humans that proves electrical stimulation will retard atrophy in denervated muscle. Rancho Los Amigos[22] has reported that electrical stimulation has assisted in "carryover" to voluntary movements in patients with partially denervated muscles.

Successful studies in animal models do suggest some guidelines for the application of electrical stimulation. Treatment should begin as soon as possible after the injury because the rate of atrophy is greatest immediately following the injury and declines exponentially. However, if the denervation period lasts less than 100 days, the recovery will not be significantly modified by the use of electrical stimulation.[30] Denervated muscle has no "motor point" and so the current must pass through the bulk of the muscle to cause a contraction. As a result, interrupted galvanic or sinusoidal current alternating at 25 to 60 cycles per second is recommended. Stimulation should be strong enough to produce 15 to 20 strong contractions per session and the sessions should be repeated three to four times per day.[29] This approach has helped to retard atrophy in the denervated muscle of rats[30] and rabbits[9] but not cats.[20]

In a partially denervated muscle the number of innervated muscle fibers remaining will determine if any increase in the strength of those fibers will be sufficient to create a clinically significant effect.[35] Strengthening exercises for partially denervated muscle generally follow one of two philosophies. Sister Kenny developed a series of exercises that attempts to isolate the effort to the affected muscle. This treatment strategy was originally developed for use on patients with poliomyelitis.

The second approach, proprioceptive neuromuscular facilitation (PNF), consists of therapeutic exercises that use a series of facilitation and synergy patterns in an effort to get muscle strengthening, neuromuscular reeducation, and "overflow" from the stronger muscle groups to the weaker muscle groups.[32] In this system the weaker muscles work with the stronger muscles and not in isolation. For example, consider a patient who has isolated weakness in the tibialis anterior muscle resulting in foot drop. The Sister Kenny approach would involve exercises specifically designed to isolate the effort to that muscle (e.g., resisted dorsiflexion with inversion). In contrast, a therapist using patterns of facilitation and synergy might involve the entire lower extremity in the exercise, employing hip flexion, adduction, and lateral rotation with the ankle dorsiflexion and inversion. This pattern would be done to combine the strengthening effort in the affected muscle with the effort in the unaffected muscles. This is an attempt to produce "overflow" from the stronger muscle groups to the affected muscle and adds an element of neuromuscular reeducation. In either case the results will be limited by the number of innervated muscle fibers. These exercises do have the additional benefit of assisting in maintenance of ROM and reduction of edema.

The patient should be taught an appropriate home exercise program as soon as possible. Again, if the patient has additional problems, application of either approach needs to be modified to the needs of the individual.

For example, if the patient is elderly and has cardiopulmonary problems, the response to motor output and overflow would need to be monitored carefully to avoid excessive stress on this and other systems. However, if the patient previously had a CVA that caused a fall with resultant peripheral nerve injury, then modification of the treatment approach would need to be considered. Maximal effort with "overflow" may not be the optimal choice of exercises because of the synergistic patterns often accompanying volitional movement in hemiplegia. Thus any treatment approach needs to be adapted to the individual patient's needs.

Sensory impairment

Physical therapy treatment of the sensory-impaired area should include extensive patient education about limb neglect. The patient should learn to regularly inspect the affected area in an attempt to reduce further trauma to the area. Monitoring the redevelopment and quality of returning sensations can be helpful in assessing the repair and regeneration of the injured nerve.

Vasomotor disturbances

Though vasoconstrictor paralysis cannot be directly altered, the edema produced by the paralysis can be addressed. Primary treatment consists of prevention through patient education about the causes of edema, such as dependent positioning and limb neglect. Reduction of edema can be accomplished through a variety of techniques, including pump massage, compression, and elevation. These techniques are means of assisting venous and lymphatic return from an extremity. For example, someone with swelling around the ankle and foot would benefit from having the distal extremity elevated above the level of the heart whenever possible. Reduction of the edema could be further enhanced with the use of an elastic wrap. This would apply a mild, constant compressive force over the swollen area. Pump massage is a technique that attempts to manually assist venous and lymph return. This is done, for example, in the anterior ankle by gently sliding one hand proximally over the swollen area while the other hand guides the foot and ankle into plantarflexion. This combines compression and lengthening of the edematous tissue in an attempt to manually "squeeze" the fluid out of the area. Patients with sensory neglect, whether as a result of peripheral nerve injury or not, will benefit from this type of treatment to eliminate edema associated with decreased muscle function and dependent positioning. This problem is often seen in head trauma. (For further information on vasomotor disturbance, see Chapter 16, inflammatory problems; Chapter 22, CVA; Chapter 23, the elderly.)

Soft tissue changes

Connective tissue and contractile tissue become progressively shorter when not stretched regularly.[14] Normal activities of daily living provide stretching and ROM to the soft tissues and joint structures. However, with flaccid or weak muscles the ability to perform those activities is diminished, and the potential for developing restrictions and contractures is increased. Again, this is true whether the disuse is a result of peripheral or central nervous system injury.

The most effective treatment program uses preventive measures, such as ROM exercises. These exercises may initially be done by the therapist as passive or active-assisted exercises. However, as soon as possible the patient is taught how to do the appropriate exercises independently. Basic to any "stretching" exercise is the premise that a slow, prolonged stretch will provide for a more plastic or permanent response than the elastic or temporary response of a ballistic stretch. Special care must be given to protect insensitive structures.

If a restriction to physiological or accessory ROM is found, the cause must be determined. The type of dysfunction can normally be accurately assessed by determining the quality of the end-feel in the restricted movement. The quality of the end-feel suggests a cause and prognosis as well as an appropriate treatment approach for the restriction. The end-feel may have a bony, hard quality similar to elbow extension. This suggests a poor prognosis when found in an abnormal position, such as less than 20 degrees of elbow extension, or in a joint whose end-feel is not normally bony, such as extension of the knee. Treatment will often have no beneficial effect in these cases because of the probable presence of a bony block. Tissue stretch is the end-feel often described as being the same feeling perceived with normal hamstring stretching. This end-feel suggests a soft tissue restriction is present. These restrictions should respond to stretching and soft tissue mobilization. A common restriction following immobilization results from adhesions and/or capsular tightness. These dysfunctions give an end-feel similar to the sensation perceived at the end of lateral rotation in the shoulder. The sensation is often described as leathery or capsular. The restriction can usually be successfully treated with soft tissue and joint mobilization techniques.[5,12,15]

For example, following a fracture of the humeral shaft, which may or may not include trauma to the radial nerve, the shoulder is often immobilized. Following this period of immobilization, the glenohumeral joint often lacks abduction and lateral rotation. Other movements may also be affected. Assessment of joint play motion will usually reveal a lack of such accessory movements as inferior glide (needed for normal abduction) and anterior glide (required for lateral rotation) of the humerus. Typically the end-feels of the restricted physiological and accessory motions in this example are leathery. This combination of findings suggests a capsular restriction that should respond well to joint mobilization.

Soft tissue restrictions may be found during the assessment of ROM or through the use of palpation. Many soft tissue dysfunctions respond to stretching programs, but others may require the use of soft tissue mobilization techniques, such as myofascial release. These techniques are particularly effective at removing restrictions in areas where various anatomical structures need to freely slide by one another (e.g., fascial planes between muscles). For example, the trauma that results in peripheral nerve injury will quite often cause soft tissue trauma. These lesions frequently produce scar tissue that may abnormally adhere the various soft tissue layers to other superficial or deep structures. As a result, motion may become limited or painful as these adhesions restrict the normal soft tissue movement that should occur. Transverse friction massage and myofascial release techniques have been found to be effective at removing soft tissue restrictions and promoting proper collagen fiber alignment. Myofascial release techniques are also effective at helping to restore mobility in soft tissues following prolonged periods of immobilization.[5,31] This immobilization may be the result external forces (e.g., casting) or internal forces (e.g., spasticity or rigidity).

Orthotic applications

Peripheral nerve injuries may necessitate the application of an orthotic appliance to protect an extremity, especially the weight-bearing lower extremity. Orthoses can be used to protect bony structures and articular surfaces, as well as muscles, ligaments, and nerves, during periods of rehabilitation. The orthotic appliance assists in preventing deformities and limiting pathological motor patterns that can develop with muscular weakness and aberrant sensory input. (See Chapter 28 for further discussion of orthotics.)

CASE STUDY PRESENTATIONS: EXAMPLES OF PROBLEMS AND TREATMENT

Two case studies are presented to illustrate general treatment approaches to peripheral neuropathic injuries. Case I describes a patient with a traumatic peripheral neuropathy, concomitant orthopedic problems, and specific intervention. Case II describes a patient with a nontraumatic (alcoholic) peripheral polyneuropathy with orthopedic and neurological implications and outlines a general approach to treatment with relevant references.

Case study #1: Traumatic compression injury

History. Mr. J.S. was seen as an outpatient 1 week after he had received a traumatic injury to the right lower extremity. The trauma resulted in a compression injury in the area of the common peroneal nerve, near the head of the fibula. Before coming to physical therapy, a nerve conduction study and electromyography were done. Based on these studies and other findings, the physician described the injury as a unifocal, class I neurapraxia of the common peroneal nerve.

Evaluation

Subjective findings. The patient's chief complaint at the time of our evaluation was weakness and a lack of coordination in the right foot. He reported significant difficulty walking, and he used a cane that a friend had given him. In addition, he reported that the right foot seemed to feel "asleep" or "not there" at times. He had no complaints of pain. Mr. J.S. was an office worker. He had no special outside interests that required specific advanced ambulatory skills.

Observations. When J.S. walked into the treatment area, he used a cane in the left hand. Gait deviations included (1) increased left lateral translation of the trunk and (2) a steppage gait to compensate for a right-foot drop. His posture in standing with the cane was normal. Without the assistive device, his standing posture was unsteady and unsafe. Mr. J.S. demonstrated a willingness to move the entire right lower extremity, but his ankle movements were laborious and done with substitutions. Mild pedal edema was noted on the right. Circumferential measurements of the lower extremities were essentially equal bilaterally, except where swelling was present in the ankle and foot.

Sensory testing. J.S. reported decreased sensation to light touch on the dorsum of the right foot and in the first web space. This pattern corresponds to the cutaneous distribution of the two terminal branches of the common peroneal nerve (i.e., the superficial and deep peroneal nerves). Cutaneous sensation was intact elsewhere.

Proprioceptive awareness was diminished in movements at the talocrural joint (dorsiflexion, plantarflexion), subtalar joint (eversion, inversion), and the phalanges (flexion, extension). Temperature sensation was intact throughout both lower extremities.

Strength and range of motion. Active ROM and manual muscle testing were performed. Strength and ROM were within normal limits in the left foot and bilaterally at the hips and knees. Strength in the distal right lower extremity was diminished. Anterior compartment muscles in the leg (tibialis anterior, extensor hallucis longus, extensor digitorum longus, and peroneus tertius) had $\frac{2}{5}$ strength. Lateral compartment muscles (peroneus longus and peroneus brevis) were found to have strength that measured $\frac{2}{5}$. Toe extensors as a group had less than $\frac{3}{5}$ strength. Posterior compartment muscles had normal strength.

Passive ROM tests were equal for all motions bilaterally. The end-feels had the same quality bilaterally with each movement tested.

Palpation. Superficial palpation found the temperature and the integrity of the skin were within normal limits in the distal right lower extremity. Pedal pulses were equal bilaterally. Palpation of deeper soft tissues was remarkable for the presence of edema throughout the ankle and dorsum of the foot. No significant adhesions nor hypomobility was noted in any of the soft tissues or joint play motions. Skin fat folds of the legs were equal bilaterally, confirming the lack of muscular atrophy suggested with circumferential measurements.

Stage I

Goals. Short-term goals included the following: (1) improving strength from 2/5 to 3/5, (2) decreasing and controlling the swelling, (3) teaching the patient to walk without gait deviations using appropriate assistive devices, and (4) developing a home program to help meet goals 1 through 3. Long-term goals included the following: (1) normalizing strength (5/5) and endurance, (2) elimination of swelling, (3) walking without assistive devices and without deviations, and (4) normal proprioception, balance, and coordination reactions.

Treatment. The obvious strength deficits in the anterior and lateral compartments were addressed. We chose to include proprioceptive neuromuscular facilitation (PNF). In our approach we used repeated contractions of the hip patterns combined with knee pivots in an effort to get overflow from the strong proximal musculature to the weaker distal muscle groups. This activity had the additional benefit of (1) assisting venous and lymphatic return from the foot and ankle and (2) providing sensory stimulation to those areas with impaired sensation. Stationary bicycling, with toe clips to hold the right foot safely in position, was done for strengthening, endurance, sensory stimulation, cardiovascular fitness, and to promote a sense of "wellness" in the patient.

Swelling in the right lower extremity was diminished through the combined use of pump massage and elevation. In addition, the edema was affected during the active exercise sessions by the action of the lower-extremity muscles, the muscular pump.

The patient was fitted with a plastic ankle-foot orthosis (AFO). This assistive device was used to help protect the weight-bearing joints and soft tissues in the right lower extremity. These areas are particularly susceptible to trauma during walking when weakness, decreased sensation, and instability are present in the lower extremity.

Home program. The patient's home program was designed to supplement the treatment sessions in the clinic. The home program focused on the same dysfunctions addressed in the clinic—weakness, decreased sensation, swelling, and instability in the distal right lower extremity. Initially, significant amounts of time were used for patient education rather than providing just "direct" treatment of the patient's dysfunctions.

Strengthening and ROM exercises were taught to the patient. J.S. was shown how to apply manual assistance and manual resistance with his exercises. This was done to provide tactile sensation and proprioceptive input. He was instructed to watch the body part move during the exercises while visualizing how normal movement should feel. Exercises focused on toe extension and ankle dorsiflexion, with and without eversion or inversion.

The patient was instructed in the proper use of the AFO and the cane. He was shown how to ambulate without the gait deviations he initially demonstrated. He was encouraged to ambulate as much as possible or until fatigue forced him to ambulate with deviations.

J.S. received extensive instruction on the care of an insensitive limb. He was taught to inspect the area for skin breakdown and swelling on a daily basis. The effects of prolonged dependent positioning and elevation were discussed. The patient was instructed in the use of ICE (*i*ce, *c*ompression, and *e*levation) to treat and control the edema.

Stage II

Reevaluation results. After approximately 6 weeks of treatment, J.S. had shown significant improvements in the dysfunctions assessed on initial evaluation. His strength had improved from 2/5 to 3^+/5 in the affected muscles. Light touch and proprioception were improved but still diminished in the distal right lower extremity. Passive range of motion in dorsiflexion and plantarflexion was slightly decreased 5 to 10 degrees on the right. The end-feels of those restricted motions were leathery, suggesting a mild capsular restriction. Swelling was a problem only with prolonged (longer than 3 hours) dependent positioning.

Goals. Short-term goals included: (1) improving strength from 3^+/5 to 5/5, (2) improving endurance with walking, (3) improving proprioception, (4) eliminating the motion restriction at the talocrural joint, and (5) eliminating swelling.

Long-term goals remained the same as stated in Stage I.

Treatment. Weakness (3^+/5) was still a problem with the toe extensors and in the anterior and lateral compartment. Strengthening exercises continued using lower-extremity PNF patterns with repeated contractions and knee pivots. Slow reversals and ankle pivots were added to further enhance strengthening and neuromuscular reeducation in the distal components. At this point (strength equal to or greater than 3/5), controlled weight-bearing activities were initiated without the cane and AFO. This was done to combine strengthening with functional proprioceptive input. Initially, weight transfers side-to-side and front-to-back provided the focus of our functional activities in a weight-bearing position. PNF gait activities emphasizing the swing phase of gait were utilized to provide additional training in functional patterns in a non-weight-bearing position. Stationary bicycling was continued for the reasons mentioned previously.

Over time, J.S. had developed a mild restriction to plantarflexion and dorsiflexion. The leathery end-feels suggested a capsular restriction that typically responds to joint mobilization procedures. Graded joint play movements were used to produce capsular stretching at the talocrural joint. This approach resolved the motion restrictions within a few treatment sessions. For an explanation of the guidelines, indications, and contra-indications to joint mobilization procedures, please review the suggested readings of Cyriax,[5] Kaltenborn,[12] and Magee.[15]

Home program. J.S. was instructed to walk without

the use of any assistive device when he could do so without any noticeable deviations. With the onset of fatigue and/or deviations in gait, the cane was required. Because swelling was still an intermittent problem, the guidelines regarding dependent positioning and ICE were reviewed. The adverse consequences of swelling, such as diminished balance reactions, were reviewed to emphasize the need to completely control the problem.

J.S. continued with his manually resisted home exercises, but he was encouraged to increase the amount of resistance. Home exercises in weight-bearing positions were added to his home program. He was encouraged to perform weight-shifts and single-leg stances to affect strength and proprioception in functional positions. To improve the safety of these activities, he was encouraged to perform the exercises on nonslippery surfaces, where he could hold onto a stable object for contact assistance (e.g., behind the couch or at the kitchen sink). J.S. was encouraged to begin bicycling as part of his home program.

Stage III

Reevaluation results. At approximately 10 weeks J.S. had shown further significant improvement in the dysfunctions seen on initial evaluation. Swelling was no longer present, even with prolonged sitting. Sensation to light touch was intact and normal throughout. Range of motion was within normal limits in both lower extremities. Strength had returned to normal (5/5) in all muscle groups, but endurance was less on the right. He was able to walk short distances (4 blocks) without assistive devices and with no gait deviations. However, proprioception, balance, and coordination reactions continued to be mildly decreased on the right.

Goals. Short-term goals included: (1) improving endurance in ambulation without assistive devices, (2) maintaining normal ROM in the distal right lower extremity, (3) improving proprioception, balance, and coordination reactions, and (4) discharging the patient with a thorough home program that would allow for continued improvement of his dysfunction. Long-term goals included: (1) ambulation without assistive devices, (2) normal endurance, balance, and coordination with ambulation, and (3) no residual dysfunction in the right lower extremity.

Treatment. We continued to work on strength, endurance, and neuromuscular reeducation of the right lower extremity through the use of PNF. Hip patterns were done with full integration and resistance of the distal components. Gait activities included work on the swing and stance phases. To improve diminished coordination and balance reactions, we added high-level functional activities, such as running agility tests and obstacle courses with figure 8s, angular turns, and uneven surfaces.

The patient was encouraged to continue the balance and coordination activities as part of his home program. J.S. was told to continue these activities until he could perform them faultlessly. He was shown how to increase the degree of difficulty in the activities so he could continue to progress independently at home. The patient was encouraged to continue bicycling to improve his endurance and his cardiovascular fitness.

Case study #2: nontraumatic peripheral neuropathy

History. R.A. is a 60-year-old male with a 40-year history of chronic alcoholism. Diagnosis is progressive, peripheral polyneuropathy, secondary to alcoholism and nutritional (dietary) deficiency and concomitant peripheral vascular compromise.

Evaluation. Findings on evaluation are as follows:

I. Weakness
  A. Bilateral lower extremities
    1. ³/₅ posterior compartment muscles
    2. ²⁺/₅ anterior compartment muscles
    3. ²⁺/₅ lateral compartment muscles
    4. Generalized weakness intrinsic muscles of both feet
  B. Bilateral upper extremities:
    1. ⁴/₅ strength wrist, hand, intrinsics
II. Sensation
  A. Bilateral lower extremities, localized below mid-calf
    1. Decreased superficial sensation with moderate impairment of touch, pain, and temperature
    2. Decreased deep sensation with mild impairment of deep pressure, vibration, and position sense (proprioception)
  B. Bilateral upper extremities: wrist and hand
    1. Decreased superficial with mild impairment of touch, pain, and temperature
III. Range of motion
  A. 5 degree flexion contracture at both knees
  B. dorsiflexion to neutral (passive) bilateral talocrural joints
IV. Gait: mild ataxia with steppage gait (resulting from anterior and lateral compartment muscle weakness) bilateral lower extremities

Patient also has several areas of skin ulceration on dorsum of the right foot, glossiness of the skin around the distal aspect of the leg, ankle, and foot bilaterally. Hyperhidrosis of feet and hands are noted bilaterally. There is also slight and occasional dysphagia and constant hoarseness.

Patient R.A. has relatively classic findings associated with peripheral polyneuropathy secondary to chronic alcoholism. The goal of treatment of the patient with a traumatic peripheral neuropathy may be to return to normal function, depending on the prognosis for regeneration. In this case the peripheral polyneuropathy is a progressive disease and the goal is one of maintenance.

Suggestions for treatment. Lower-extremity weakness may be addressed by the use of manual active-assisted and/or resisted exercises using linear patterns or proprioceptive neuromuscular facilitation (PNF) techniques. Manual contacts would provide proprioceptive and exteroceptive input and would address sensory deficits as well. PNF techniques, such as repeated contractions or slow reversal, would facilitate strength as well as rhythm and coordination. Upper-extremity weakness might be addressed in the same manner with the inclusion of activities to maintain fine motor skills and coordination.

Sensory deficits may be addressed in several ways. As mentioned above, manual contacts during exercise may subserve proprioceptive/exteroceptive function. Because this disease is progressive, patient education regarding sensory changes and sequelae (e.g., skin lesions) is critical. Cognitive changes may be a limiting factor in educating the patient. (For further information concerning memory/learning changes, please consult Chapter 4 on the Limbic System.)

Ataxia associated with alcoholism may be addressed in relation to cerebellar dysfunction and subsequent changes in coordination of motor function. Please consult Chapter 21 on cerebellar dysfunction.

Loss of range of motion as a result of weakness and/or contractures may be corrected by either maintaining strength or stretching. Orthotic devices may be helpful but must be used judiciously to prevent skin lesions from pressure. Please consult Chapter 28 on orthotics for further information. Dysphagia and hoarseness may be a result of progressive motor weakness. Please refer to Chapter 24 regarding speech pathology for further information.

The outcome of alcoholic neuropathy can be good if the disease is not advanced and the drug addiction is stopped. If the alcoholic continues drinking, the peripheral neuropathic outcome will become progressively worse as additional peripheral nerves become involved.

SUMMARY

This chapter has focused on the nature and clinical implications of traumatic peripheral neuropathy. Although involving the nervous system directly, the neurological and musculoskeletal effects of trauma to the peripheral nervous system (PNS) differ significantly from the effects of trauma to the central nervous system (CNS). Also, although traumatic peripheral injuries created by an external force are relatively well focused, peripheral neuropathy of a multifocal nature occurring from an internal mechanism (e.g., alcoholic neuropathy) can be quite traumatic as well. Classification of injuries, pathophysiology of degeneration, and regenerative processes are presented. Specific findings on evaluation with guidelines and prescriptions for specific treatment of possible orthopedic problems with reference to peripheral nerve injury are discussed. It is hoped that the information presented, along with case studies, will be valuable to physical therapists and other health professionals in the treatment of traumatic peripheral neuropathies.

REFERENCES

1. Allison N and Brooks B: Bone atrophy, Surg Gynec Obstet 33:250, 1921.
2. Allt G: Pathology of the peripheral nerve. In London DN, editor: The peripheral nerve, 1976, Chapman Hall.
3. Bradley WG: Disorders of peripheral nerves, London, 1974, Blackwell Scientific Publishing.
4. Bunge Richard P: Some observations on the role of the schwoann cell in peripheral nerve regeneration. In Jewitt DL and McCarrol HR Jr, editors: Nerve repair and regeneration: its clinical and experimental basis, St Louis, 1980, The CV Mosby Co.
5. Cyriax J: Textbook of orthopedic medicine, ed 8, vol 1, Diagnosis of soft tissue lesions, London, 1982, Bailliere Tindall.
6. Doyle James R: Factors affecting clinical results of nerve suture. In Jewitt DL and McCarrol HRJr, editors: Nerve repair and regeneration: its clinical and experimental basis, St Louis, 1980, The CV Mosby Co.
7. Forester R: Clayton's electrotherapy, ed 8, London, 1981, Bailliere Tindell.
8. Grey EG and Carr GL: An experimental study of factors responsible for noninfectious bone atrophy, Bull Johns Hopkins Hosp 26:381, 1915.
9. Gutmann E and Guttmann L: Effects of electrotherapy on denervated muscle in rabbits, Lancet 1:169, 1942.
10. Hall S: The myelinated nerve fibre. In London DN, editor, The peripheral nerve, 1976, Chapman Hall.
11. Jewett DL and McCarroll, HRJr, editors: Nerve repair and regeneration: its clinical and experimental basis, St Louis, 1980, The CV Mosby Co.
12. Kaltenborn F: Mobilization of the extremity joints: examination and basic treatment techniques, Oslo, 1980, Olof Norlis Bokhandel.
13. Kopell HP and Thompson WAL: Peripheral entrapment neuropathies, Baltimore, 1963, Williams & Wilkins.
14. Kottke FV and others: The rationale for prolonged stretching for correction of shortening of connective tissue, Arch Phys Med Rehab 47:345, 1966.
15. Magee D: Orthopedic physical assessment, Philadelphia, 1987, WB Saunders Co.
16. Mather LH: The peripheral nervous system: structure, function and clinical correlations, Reading, Mass, 1985, Addison-Wesley Publishing Co, Inc.
17. Miyamoto Y, Takashi S, and Tsuge K: Nerve grafting and nerve regeneration. In Sobue I, editor: Peripheral neuropathy, Oxford, England, 1983, Excerpta Medica.
18. Pleasure D: In Sumner AJ, editor: The physiology of peripheral nerve disease, Philadelphia, 1980, WB Saunders Co.
19. Politis MJ and others: The role of distal nerve stumps in guiding regenerating fibers. In Sobue I, editor: Peripheral neuropathy, Oxford, England, 1983, Excerpta Medica.
20. Pollock LV and others: Electrotherapy in experimentally induced lesions of peripheral nerves, Arch Phys Med Rehab 32:377, 1951.
21. Pratt NE: "Neurovascular entrapment" in the regions of the shoulder and posterior triangle of the neck, Phys Ther 66:12, 1986.
22. Rancho Los Amigos Rehabilitation Engineering Center: Annual report of progress to the rehabilitation services administration, No 8, Washington, DC, 1979, US Department of Health, Education and Welfare.
23. Refsum S:. In Refsom SA, Bolis CL, and Sonchez AP, editors: International conference on peripheral neuropathies, Oxford, England, 1982, Excerpta Medica.
24. Ring PA: The influence of the nervous system upon the growth of bones, J Bone Joint Surg 43B:121, 1961.

25. Ring PA: Paralytic bone lengthening following poliomyelitis, Lancet 2:551, 1958.
26. Schaumberg HH and others: Disorders of peripheral nerves, Philadelphia, 1983, FA Davis Co.
27. Seddon HJ: Surgical disorders of the peripheral nerves, New York, 1972, Churchill Livingstone, Inc.
28. Seddon HJ: Three types of nerve injury, Brain 66:237, 1943.
29. Seltzer ME: Regeneration of peripheral nerve. In Sumner AJ, editor: The physiology of peripheral nerve disease, Philadelphia, 1980, WB Saunders Co.
30. Stillwell G: In Dyck PV, editor: Peripheral neuropathy, ed 2, Philadelphia, 1984, WB Saunders Co.
31. Stoddard A: Manual of osteopathic techniques, ed 3, London, 1980, Hutchinson & Company.
32. Sullivan P: An integrated approach to therapeutic exercise, Reston, Va, 1982, Reston Publishing.
33. Sunderland S: Nerves and nerve injuries, ed 2, Baltimore, 1978, Williams & Wilkins.
34. Weller RO and Cervos-Navarro J: Pathology of peripheral nerves, Woburn, Mass, 1977, Butterworth.
35. Wolf SL: Electrotherapy: clinics in physical therapy, New York, 1981, Churchill Livingstone, Inc.

Chapter 13

TRAUMATIC HEAD INJURIES

Susan Snyder Smith and Patricia A. Winkler

□ Special thanks to Terry W. Elliott, M.B.A., P.T., Julie Rollin, and Donna J. El-Din, Ph.D., P.T. for their assistance with the preparation of the original manuscript; and, for their assistance with the photography, Ted Becker, Ph.D., P.T., Sharon Bezner, P.T., Laura Hunter, P.T., Laurie May, P.T., Cindy Alvis, P.T., Shirley Meissner, P.T., Lorraine Mojica, P.T., and the photographic subjects at the Dallas Rehabilitation Institute.

Although many experiences in rehabilitation are challenging, exciting, and rewarding, certainly none is more so than working with clients with traumatic head injuries. In few cases is the therapist faced with such disruption of cognitive, physical, psychosocial, emotional, and vocational functions. This disruption and a sense of hopelessness discourage many therapists from fully accepting the challenges presented by severe head trauma. Clients are not the only losers when hopelessness prevails. Therapists may be depriving themselves of a thrilling and rewarding experience because in no other area of rehabilitation is the potential for improvement so dramatic.

The National Head Injury Foundation provides the following definition of traumatic head injury:[60]

"Traumatic head injury is an insult to the brain, not of a degenerative or congenital nature but caused by an external physical force, that may produce a diminished or altered state of consciousness, which results in impairment of cognitive abilities or physical functioning. It can also result in the disturbance of behavioral or emotional functioning. These may be either temporary or permanent and cause partial or total functional disability or psychological maladjustment."

A combination of features distinguishes traumatic brain injury from other cerebral disorders. These features include the suddenness of onset, age group of the clients, potential extensiveness and patterns of brain damage, coma, and the possibility of concomitant injuries. While these features necessitate a unique management approach, the problems encountered in head trauma share similarities with those common to other conditions—not only neurological, but musculoskeletal and cardiopulmonary problems as well.

Head injury may occur without loss of consciousness or with a mild concussion. In the majority of cases cerebral injury is mild. The symptoms experienced by these clients gradually resolve. Prolongation of unconsciousness beyond 6 hours or any delay in improvement signifies a more severe head injury. This chapter focuses on management of adolescents and adults with severe brain trauma—that is, those having experienced prolonged alterations in consciousness.

AN OVERVIEW OF HEAD INJURY
Epidemiology of traumatic head injury

Industrialized countries have an appalling number of traumatic head injuries. Statistics on the incidence of head injury are difficult to compare, partly because of the lack of a standardized definition of what constitutes a head injury. However, Kraus and others[50] reported that there are 700,000 head injuries each year in the United States resulting in 140,000 deaths and in 50,000 to 70,000 permanently disabled persons.

Motor vehicle accidents are the major cause of these injuries, with industrial and domestic accidents, assaults, falls, irradiation, and injuries from sports, leisure activities, electricity, and birth also contributing to the statistics.[25,43] Some cases of cerebral palsy can be considered a form of pediatric head trauma.

Population of head-injured clients

The incidence of head injuries is higher for males than for females by more than 2:1. Over 50% of the population of head-injured clients are between the ages of 15 and 24 years.[43] Children are by no means spared head injuries. The number of children treated for head injuries has increased steadily. Traumatic brain injury is now a major cause of childhood disability. The majority of brain injuries in children are caused by falls.[39] The rehabilitation of brain-injured children is distinguished from that of brain-injured adults by many of the same characteristics that normally distinguish the two age groups. The differences include the maturation and plasticity of the central nervous system (CNS), cognitive and motor development, capacity for learning, psychosocial status, interests, and physical size.

The problem-solving approach to rehabilitation of clients with head trauma presented in this chapter is adaptable to children; however, the application of specific techniques requires modification for the special concerns associated with children. Chapters 8 through 11 in this text and pediatric literature may provide guidance for those involved in treating brain-injured children.

Mechanisms of injury

Acceleration, deceleration, and rotational forces can act on the head at the time of impact, resulting in a temporary deformation of the skull. Brain damage is caused by tissue compression, tension, shearing, or a combination of these mechanisms.[25] Injuries to the brain can be both coup (injuries at the site of impact) and contrecoup (injuries distant from the part of the brain sustaining the blow).

In acceleration injuries, the slower-moving cerebral contents can be damaged by impact with the bony irregularities at the base of the cranial vault. Coup and contrecoup injuries can result when there is rapid deceleration of the skull. This occurs when the head strikes a stationary object. For example, a fall on the back of the head can result in contusion of the frontal and temporal lobes. Shearing forces are a major cause of contrecoup injuries to the brain.[25] These forces result from rotation and movement of the brain within the cranial vault. Shearing can occur at any site in the brain and can be quite destructive.[25,43] Wherever the impact, brain lesions are frequently bilateral and symmetrical, and they tend to be most marked between tissues with different properties, such as between the tissue of the brain and blood vessels.[43] Although the lesions tend to be bilateral, the postinsult residual effects may be more devastating on one side of the body than on the other side.

Types of head injuries

To determine the medical treatment regime, it is necessary for the physician to distinguish between primary (impact) brain damage and secondary brain damage. Primary damage includes skull fractures, contusions of the gray matter, and diffuse white-matter lesions. Secondary damage includes brain swelling, intracranial hematoma, cerebral hypoxia, and ischemia. The objective, of course, is to prevent, or minimize, secondary brain damage. The secondary damage can develop as rapidly as within an hour of injury.[43] Thus by the time the therapist initiates treatment, a combination of primary and secondary sequelae has developed.

Gilroy and Meyer[25] describe different types of traumatic head injuries. Their list, discussed below, includes skull fractures, closed head injuries, penetrating wounds of the skull and brain, and traumatic injury to extracranial blood vessels.

Skull fractures. Linear or comminuted fractures generally result from low-velocity objects, and depressed fractures generally result from higher-velocity objects. Impact damage can be direct or remote. Linear fractures can produce contusions, lacerations, traumatic aneurysms, and cranial nerve damage. Depressed fractures decrease the volume of the cranial cavity and can produce uncal or lower-brainstem herniation, in addition to cranial nerve damage, contusions, and lacerations. Compound, depressed skull fractures are considered open head injuries. Skull fractures also can occur without subsequent brain damage.[25]

Closed head injuries. Persons sustaining closed head injuries without a fracture can experience minor injury, or they can experience severe and irreversible brain damage. Damage suffered from closed head injuries includes brainstem damage, contusions, diffuse white-matter lesions, injury to blood vessels, damage to cranial nerves, and traumatic cerebrospinal fluid rhinorrhea.

Brainstem damage can be primary or secondary. Primary damage can be the result of an acceleration or deceleration pressure wave causing a downward displacement of the brainstem through the foramen magnum.[25] However, it is doubtful that primary brainstem damage occurs except in conjunction with more extensive cortical and subcortical destruction.[43] Secondary damage can result from the development of brain swelling or intracranial hemorrhage, which increases the bilateral or unilateral volume of the supratentorial contents. Since the supratentorial contents are contained within a rigid structure, increased pressure can result in cingulate herniation, uncal herniation, and central (or transtentorial) herniation, with progressive brainstem dysfunction.[25]

Contusions of the gray matter can occur beneath the site of impact or remote from it. Occipital blows are more likely to produce contusions than are frontal or lateral blows. Contusions of the undersurface of the temporal and frontal lobes and on the anterior poles of the temporal lobes are common because of the irregular surface of the cranial vault in these areas. Cerebral contusions are not necessarily associated with a loss of consciousness, but they can initiate the processes of secondary brain damage.[43]

Diffuse damage to the white matter involves severance of axons because of shearing forces at the time of impact.[81] Lesions frequently occur in the splenium of the corpus callosum and diffusely in the white matter elsewhere in the brain.[25,43] Diffuse white-matter damage can result in a sudden loss of consciousness with bilateral extensor rigidity of the extremities and usually with some autonomic dysfunction. Clinically, these signs are frequently attributed to "primary brainstem damage." However, at autopsy the lesions are not confined to the brainstem.[43]

Traumatic injury to blood vessels can also occur with closed head injury. Examples of damage to blood vessels include weakening of and damage to arterial walls by contact with bony prominences (such as damage to the internal carotid artery at the point where it enters the skull through the carotid canal), torn cortical veins (resulting in hematoma), and ruptured capillaries (which produce hemorrhages).[25]

Direct trauma, brainstem damage, avulsion, contusion, or increased intracranial pressure can damage cranial nerves. All of the cranial nerves are susceptible to injury, but damage to the optic, vestibulocochlear, oculomotor, abducens, and facial nerves is more common. Lesions of the olfactory nerve may or may not be detected. Statistics on cranial nerve involvement, however, vary with the source.

Closed head injury is one cause of cerebrospinal fluid rhinorrhea. Shearing forces or a sudden increase of intracranial pressure can cause this complication. However, cerebrospinal fluid rhinorrhea more frequently occurs with fractures of the posterior wall of the frontal sinus, with tearing of the dura and arachnoid. A persistent or intermittent clear fluid discharge from the nose should be reported. This drainage is increased by neck flexion, coughing, or straining.[25]

Penetrating wounds of the skull and brain. A variety of both high- and low-velocity objects can penetrate the skull. High-velocity penetration, or missile injury, is likely the result of a gunshot wound. Metallic objects, sticks, and sharp toys are capable of puncture wounds. Bone fragments may penetrate the dura in nonmissile injuries. In an interesting case, damage was caused by a fall on a kite stick that penetrated the brain through the orbit. Location, pathway, depth of penetration, and the subsequent secondary complications determine the ensuing brain damage.[25] In addition, there is the risk of intracranial infection with open injuries.

Traumatic injury to extracranial blood vessels. Gunshot wounds, blows to the neck, injuries to the face, or cervical hyperextension can damage the internal carotid artery.[25] The vertebral artery can be injured during cervical manipulation,[56] cervical traction, or sudden hyperextension or rotation of the neck.[32] Insufficiency or infarction can occur in such cases. The consequences of any of these types of injuries vary, but they might include neuronal loss, axonal degeneration, diffuse brain atrophy, hydrocephalus, scar tissue formation, and abnormal neuronal activity.[25]

There are additional types of head injuries and other traumatic and disease entities involving the brain that can exhibit clinical manifestations approximating those found in severe head trauma. In some open injuries, portions of the skull and brain are actually abolished. Drug overdoses, tumors, certain cerebral hemorrhages, and a variety of hypoxic conditions, such as near-drownings, may clinically fall into the category of brain injuries.

Immediate clinical aspects

The immediate clinical aspects of traumatic head injury can include alterations in autonomic function, consciousness, motor function, pupillary responses, ocular movements, and other brainstem reflexes. Each of these aspects is briefly discussed here.

Alterations in autonomic function can occur, and one vital sign may change without affecting the others. The pulse and respiratory rates can be slow, normal, rapid, irregular, or otherwise abnormal. Temperature can be elevated. Blood pressure can be low, normal, or elevated. The variations and combinations of changes in vital signs assist the physician to determine the specific diagnosis in head injury and to prevent secondary damage. Other disturbances in autonomic function can also be present, including excessive sweating, salivation, lacrimation, and sebum secretion.[13]

Consciousness may or may not be altered. Plum and Posner[64] provide an in-depth account of this fascinating area. Conscious behavior is determined by content and arousal. Content is the sum of cognitive and affective functions. Arousal is associated with wakefulness and depends on an intact reticular formation and upper brainstem that function in collaboration with other parts of the brain. Content (or cognition) and arousal may be individually impaired, or a combination of impairments of both of these physiological components may be present. For example, arousal does not guarantee cognition, a circumstance that is clinically observable.

Alterations in consciousness result from conditions in which there is diffusely extensive and bilateral cerebral hemispheric depression of function, direct depression or destruction of the brainstem-activating mechanisms responsible for consciousness, or a combination of the two effects. Stupor and coma indicate advanced brain failure, and the more prolonged the failure, the more guarded the prognosis.[64]

In mild concussion the loss of consciousness lasts a relatively short time, and there is little or no retrograde amnesia. The client may be irritable or distractable and have difficulty with reading and memory. There may be complaints of headache, fatigue, dizziness, and changes in personality and emotional disposition. This group of symptoms constitute what is called *posttraumatic neurosis* or *syndrome*. Whether these symptoms are organic or psychogenic is unclear.[25]

In moderate or severe head injury, unconsciousness can be prolonged. A variety of terms are used to label gradations of consciousness; many of them are conflicting. There is agreement that clear-cut criteria for levels of consciousness are difficult to establish. As a result, it is probably more accurate and helpful to disregard the various labels and to describe the client's levels of arousal and cognition. Therefore in the interest of clarity, levels of consciousness are discussed below separately from levels of cognitive functioning.

Plum and Posner's definitions[64] of various stages of acutely altered consciousness are briefly presented, intermingled with some insights from the descriptions offered by Gilroy and Meyer.[25] One difference between these two continua is that Plum and Posner[64] do not equate the presence or absence of motor responses with the depth of coma. These authors point out that the neural structures regulating consciousness differ from and are more anatomically distant from those regulating motor function.

Coma is defined as a complete paralysis of cerebral function, a state of unresponsiveness. The eyes are closed, and there is no response to painful stimuli. Within 2 to 4 weeks, nearly all clients in coma begin to awaken. *Stupor* is a condition of general unresponsiveness. However, the client, who is usually mute, can be temporarily aroused by vigorous and repeated stimuli. *Obtundity* describes a client who sleeps a great deal and who, when aroused, exhibits reduced alertness, disinterest in the environment, and slow responses to stimulation. *Delirium* is often observed in recovery from unconsciousness after severe head injury.

This state is characterized by disorientation, fear, and misinterpretation of sensory stimuli. The client is frequently loud, agitated, and offensive. *Clouding of consciousness* is a state of quiet confusion, distractibility, faulty memory, and slowed responses to stimuli. Recovery to *consciousness,* if it occurs, includes a gradual recovery of orientation and recent memory.[64] The duration of each of these stages is variable and can be prolonged. Improvement can be arrested at any point.

Motor abnormalities after severe head trauma are common. Reflex motor responses in unconscious clients are tested by applying a noxious stimulus, such as pressure on a nail bed using a pencil or supraorbital pressure, and observing the response. Internal stimuli can also elicit tonic spasms. Motor responses generally fall into three categories: appropriate, inappropriate, or absent.[64] Dysfunction reflects either selective involvement of various motor neurons and their pathways, or functions that are "released" when higher-center control is disrupted. The extent and locations of the brain injury determine the patterns of motor disturbances.

The usual abnormalities include monoplegia or hemiplegia and abnormal reflexes. Great variance exists. Initial flaccidity can gradually become spasticity or rigidity. The terms *decorticate* or *decerebrate rigidity* are often used to denote abnormal posturing. However, as with other labels, these are not always well defined, and a description of the abnormalities is preferred. Examples of typical motor disturbances include abnormal flexor responses in the upper extremities and extensor responses in the lower extremities (decorticate), abnormal extensor responses in upper and lower extremities (decerebrate), abnormal extensor responses in the upper extremities with flaccid or weak flexor responses in the lower extremities, absence of motor responses (flaccid), or a mixture of these. Responses can be bilateral or unilateral. Furthermore, the same client can initially display flexor responses in the arms that can later change to extensor responses. These shifts possibly reflect the physiological effects of changes in the amount of tissue compression or irritation.[64]

Pupillary responses and ocular movements can become pathological signs in coma because the brainstem areas controlling consciousness are adjacent to those controlling the pupils and ocular motility. Abnormalities in pupil size, shape, and light reflexes can be manifested unilaterally or bilaterally. Eye movements in coma can be abnormal, as can the oculocephalic and oculovestibular reflexes. Oculomotor and pupillary signs are valuable in assisting with the diagnosis, localizing brainstem damage, and determining the depth of coma.[64] Interpretation can be difficult, partially because of the variety of influences on these signs.[43]

Other brainstem responses might include grimacing to pain, which is frequently associated with a flexor or localizing motor response. The pharyngeal reflex may also be absent; the implications of this are obvious. Absence of brainstem reflexes usually indicates a poorer prognosis, but this is not necessarily a predictor of ultimate outcome.[13]

Diagnostic monitoring procedures and medical management

In addition to the traditional neurological examination that the physician performs, a variety of diagnostic and monitoring procedures may be ordered for the recently injured client. The selection of the tests depends on the availability of the special equipment required for testing and on the perceived need for the tests. Although therapists are not educated in the interpretation of these procedures, a general understanding of their purposes is useful. In addition to the primary aim of guiding the physician, the results of some of these procedures may secondarily aid the therapist in the selection of intervention strategies. Conversely, other monitoring procedures may restrict the choice of therapeutic approaches.

A list of the more common procedures might include the Glasgow Coma Scale (GCS) and additional neurological assessments, radiographic examination, computed axial tomography (CT) scanning, cerebral angiography, radioisotope imaging, ventriculography, echoencephalography, monitoring of intracranial pressure and cardiorespiratory and cardiovascular function, measurement of cerebral blood flow and metabolism, electroencephalography (EEG), cerebral spinal fluid and other biochemical studies, and evoked potential studies of the visual, auditory, and somatosensory systems. A third of the clients hospitalized with head injuries have extracranial injuries, which are explored with a physical examination and appropriate special tests.[43]

It is neither our intent nor is it within the scope of this chapter to report on the potential diagnostic, monitoring, and prognostic capabilities of specific procedures. References on these techniques are abundant; for example, a brief overview is available in Jennett and Teasdale's *Management of Head Injuries*.[43] Three of these monitoring procedures, however, deserve mention here: the GCS, CT scanning, and evoked potential studies.

The GCS (see box), introduced in 1974, is designed to assess and monitor the level of consciousness. Three aspects of coma are observed independently: eye opening, best motor response, and verbal performance. Each of these components has a numerical scale. An overall coma score is obtained by adding the numerical value assigned to each of the three components. Coma scores range from 3 (least responsive) to 15.[43] According to Jennett and Teasdale's definition of coma ("not obeying commands, not uttering words, and not opening the eyes")[43], a Glasgow total score of 8 or less defines coma in 90% of the cases. Pupillary reactivity, spontaneous eye movements, and oculovestibular responses are additional neurological assessments used in conjunction with the GCS. Spontaneous eye movement classifications can include visual fixation, conjugate, roving dysconjugate, nystagmus and no

Glasgow Coma Scale	
Eye opening	**E**
Spontaneous	4
To speech	3
To pain	2
Nil	1
Best motor response	**M**
Obeys	6
Localizes	5
Withdraws	4
Abnormal flexion	3
Extensor response	2
Nil	1
Verbal Response	**V**
Orientated	5
Confused conversation	4
Inappropriate words	3
Incomprehensible sounds	2
Nil	1
Coma Score (E + M + V) = 3 to 15	

From Jennett B and Teasdale G: Management of head injuries, Philadelphia, 1981, FA Davis Co.

movement. The oculovestibular reflex is tested using ice water irrigation, and the responses can include conjugate eye movements, dysconjugate eye movements, nystagmus, or no response. One importance of the GCS is that both the coma score and the grades of response on each component of the scale have been demonstrated in some studies to correlate with outcome[34,43] (discussed later in this chapter). However, Van Den Berge and others[84] found difficulties with interrater reliability in assessing oculocephalic responses. Also, the relative value of each component of the scale differs according to the time interval elapsed.[55] Another concern is the practice of adding the scores on this scale, which is an ordinal-level scale.

CT scanning, a radiological technique that permits visualization of intracranial structures,[61] "makes it possible to observe the presence, evolution, and resolution of lesions that could previously only be presumed on the basis of clinical features or deduced indirectly. . ." (p. 114).[43] Sequential CT scanning is frequently used with head-injured clients to follow their course of recovery. CT scanning reveals the current status of the lesion. With the possible exception of the diagnosis and, hence, prognosis of diffuse white-matter impact damage,[91] the Glasgow study[76] and the other studies[51,91] reviewed by Jennett and Teasdale indicate that prediction of outcome should not be based on CT scanning alone. However, in our experience and in that of other therapists, outcome prediction has been attempted largely based on CT scanning.

Changes in electrocerebral potentials that occur in response to specific stimuli are also studied. Visual, auditory, and somatosensory evoked potential examinations are used with brain-injured clients. Evoked responses may yield more information than the clinical neurological examination alone and may also assist in localizing the structural damage. Evoked potential studies may aid in prognosis;[30,64] however, the usefulness and significance of evoked potential studies with these clients is still being investigated. (Refer to Chapter 26 for additional information.)

On admission to the hospital, a neurosurgeon usually assumes initial and primary responsibility for the client. The first priority in medical care is resuscitation, after which baseline assessments are made and a history obtained. Immediate surgery may or may not be indicated. Early concerns may include the management of respiratory dysfunction, cardiovascular monitoring, treatment of raised intracranial pressure by means of pharmacological, mechanical, or surgical procedures,[13] and general medical care. Examples of general medical care are familiar: maintenance of fluid and electrolyte balance, nutrition, eye and skin care, prevention of contractures, postural drainage, and possibly restraints.[43] This type of care gradually lessens as the client responds, or it may continue if unconsciousness persists.

Pharmaceutical agents are prescribed as an adjunct to care for a variety of reasons. Antibiotics may be used with respiratory complications or with compound fractures. Anticonvulsants may be prescribed for treatment or prophylaxis of seizures. Raised intracranial pressure might be treated with diuretics or barbiturates.[13,43] Traumatically acquired neuroendocrine dysfunctions, such as hyperphagia and thermal regulation, may be treated with pharmacological agents.[26]

Medications may also be prescribed to decrease spasticity. Diazepam (Valium) initially was the drug most commonly administered. However, diazepam also promotes drowsiness, decreased responsiveness, and can increase muscle weakness and ataxia.[90] These side effects actually hinder rather than assist in rehabilitation. Glenn[27] concludes that, "rarely, if ever, are the benefits of diazepam's antispasticity effect great enough to justify its use in the brain-injured population" (p. 71). Baclofen is now used more frequently with brain-injured clients; however, baclofen can also produce lethargy, confusion,[90] and reduction in attention span[27] in some clients. Dantrolene sodium is another medication used to decrease spasticity. This drug works directly at the muscle level and is therefore less likely to cause cognitive disturbances, but more likely to cause generalized weakness.[89] Therapists skilled with inhibition techniques rarely need pharmacological assistance to adequately exercise a client. Inhibition and facilitation techniques, combined with an early and consistent positioning program, are usually sufficient to prevent fixed myotatic contractures. If not, phenol nerve blocks are sometimes prescribed.

Sedative drugs ordered in an attempt to control delirium may add to the client's confusion[43] and may also contribute to a decreased responsiveness. Later in the rehabilitative process, various antidepressants may be used to treat aggressive and disruptive behaviors. These, too, may have deleterious side effects.

Thus although therapists are not directly concerned with drug therapy, awareness of the effects of drugs on a specific client is a necessity. If a drug is perceived as interfering with the goals of therapy, this can be discussed with the physician or nurse. Perhaps the dosage can be adjusted or an alternative drug prescribed, or perhaps the drug (or the therapy) can be administered at a different time of day.

Sequelae and complications

Roughly four categories of sequelae from the head injury itself can be identified: physical, cognitive, behavioral, and medical. These are not meant to diminish the significance of the social and economic sequelae, which are considered elsewhere. The types and frequencies of deficits in each category are largely a matter of speculation. Reports of sequelae are influenced by the time that has elapsed since the injury, the skill of the examiner, and the assessment equipment available.

Motor disturbances resulting from head injury generally have a good prognosis.[13] Of the physical deficits encountered, dysfunctions in the cerebral hemispheres and of the cranial nerves are the most common disorders, and these may partially resolve. In a Glasgow study some degree of hemiparesis was present 6 months after injury in 49% of the 150 clients who regained consciousness after severe head injury.[43] The specific manifestations of the hemiparesis can include a wide range of deficits, such as loss of selective motor control, balance, righting reactions, primitive reflexes and sensation as well as the presence of abnormal tone. Combinations of asymmetrical cerebellar and pyramidal signs and of bilateral pyramidal and extrapyramidal signs have been reported.[66] In at least two studies[43,66] a quarter of the cases had no neurophysical sequelae.

As already mentioned, damage to one or more cranial nerves is not uncommon. Recuperation tends to occur with the exception of the complete recovery of hearing, vestibular function, and smell. These losses can be more permanent.[13,43]

Aphasia, dysarthria, dysphagia, and visuospatial and perceptual motor difficulties can occur because of focal lesions. Posttraumatic epilepsy is also a possible sequela. More severe head injuries tend to manifest more persistent physical problems.[43]

Either temporary or permanent disorders of intellectual function and memory are frequent. Mental (cognitive and behavioral) sequelae can result from generalized or focal brain injuries. Decreased attention span, perseveration, reduced problem-solving ability, lack of initiation, and loss of reasoning and abstract thinking are signs commonly observed by therapists. Formal testing of intellectual function can be hampered by inadequate perceptual, visual, and motor performance.

Memory impairments are an aftermath of generalized lesions. Two types of amnesia are frequently associated with head injury. *Retrograde amnesia* is defined by Cartlidge and Shaw[13] as a "partial or total loss of the ability to recall events that have occurred during the period immediately preceding brain injury." The existence of a correlation between the severity of the injury and the length of retrograde amnesia is controversial. The duration of the retrograde amnesia may progressively decrease. *Posttraumatic amnesia* is defined "as the time lapse between the accident and the point at which the functions concerned with memory are judged to have been restored" (p. 55).[13] The duration of posttraumatic amnesia is considered a clinical indicator of the severity of the injury.[13] An additional deficit can be the inability to form new memory, referred to as *anterograde memory*. This could result in decreased attention or inaccurate perception. The capacity for anterograde memory is frequently the last function to return following recovery from loss of consciousness.[71] The client's inability to develop ongoing short-term memory can be quite frustrating for the rehabilitation team.

For the family, behavioral sequelae are perhaps the most devastating feature of head injury. Personality changes nearly defy measurement and may be apparent only to those closest to the client. Behavioral changes can be present even without cognitive and physical deficits. Frontal lobe lesions are a common cause of alterations in behavior. Irritability and aggressiveness are possible manifestations, as are losses of inhibition and judgment. A client may become anxious, euphoric, apathetic, or emotionally labile. Personal hygiene may be neglected. With some clients there is a general reluctance to change. This reluctance seems to parallel that found among the geriatric population. Although actual psychoses can be sequelae, they appear to be neither common nor definitively related to the head injury. The depression encountered seems to be reactive rather than endogenous in nature.[13,43]

The social consequences of inappropriate behavior can be disastrous and a stumbling block to achievement of therapy goals. A correlation between preinjury personality and postinjury changes has not been established.[43] It does seem reasonable, however, that factors within an individual's psychological makeup may affect reaction to the injury. Head trauma frequently happens to adolescents—an age group fraught with its own problems that may be aggravated by the injury.

Medical disorders in other bodily systems can be caused by damage to the brain. These disorders include metabolic, neuroendocrine, cardiovascular, gastrointestinal, respiratory, and hematological disorders. Headaches are also a postinjury complaint.[13]

Finally, no discussion of the sequelae of head injury would be complete without mention of those unfortunate enough to remain in a "persistent vegetative state" (PVS). This state is characterized by a wakeful, reduced responsiveness with no evident cerebral cortical function. The vegetative state can result from diffuse cerebral hypoxia or from severe, diffuse white-matter impact damage. The brainstem is usually relatively intact. Clients may track with their eyes and show minimal spontaneous motor activity, but they do not speak, nor do they respond to verbal stimulation.[41] Life expectancy can be weeks, months, or years.[43,70] Brain-injured clients who remain vegetative for 3 months rarely achieve an independent outcome. However, the term "persistent" should not be added to "vegetative state" until the injury has stabilized or lasted for approximately 1 year.[4]

In the early weeks after injury, certain behaviors exhibited may lead to what later turns out to be false optimism. For example, one young woman who has seemingly remained in a vegetative state for over 3 years has been known to pedal a bicycle when placed and held on it, to turn pages of a magazine, to flip the photographs in a picture-display caddy, and to pet a horse. Yet she has no head control, no balance, no definitive response to verbal stimulation, and no communication of any kind. The motor behaviors could be automatic, triggered by the stimulus, but are they completely subcortical? Perhaps she was too easily classified as "vegetative." In this case, however, the distinction between severely disabled and vegetative is subtle, since no intellectual contact has been established with this client.

A list of the complications that could accompany head injury would be limitless. In addition to any concomitant injuries, some of the diagnostic, monitoring, and therapeutic procedures themselves carry hazards. So does prolonged bed rest. Catheters, nasogastric tubes, and tracheostomies can cause iatrogenic injuries. Infections, contractures, skin breakdown, thrombophlebitis, pulmonary problems, heterotopic ossification, and surgical complications are but a few risks. Indeed, in one case a bone fragment from a client's skull fell to the floor during surgery and had to be autoclaved and returned!

EVALUATION PROCEDURES
Philosophy of the evaluation

The form and function of the examination of clients with head trauma can be viewed as are other neuromuscular and musculoskeletal examinations the therapist performs. The purpose of the evaluation is to identify problems that can be managed by therapy and those that influence or restrict the choice of therapeutic approaches. The therapist is also establishing a baseline on which to judge future improvement or lack of improvement. This baseline should be *quantified* to permit measurement of the effectiveness of the intervention strategies.

Treatment effectiveness is not only critically important for an individual client; it also helps to establish the efficacy of treatment regimes on populations of brain-injured clients. Third-party payers are increasingly demanding objective, quantitative data documenting progress. A system for obtaining quantitative measurements of human performance is discussed later in this section.

Some argue that a separate evaluation by a variety of health professionals is not cost effective. However, information needed by the therapist may not be found in an evaluation performed by another health professional, or the information may not be current. This is especially true in the acute care stages and with bedside evaluations. Furthermore, members of each discipline approach evaluations and make observations from a myriad of different backgrounds. The emphasis of the speech pathologist will differ from that of the physical therapist, but each must have a picture of the client as a whole. Observations of language or cognition by therapists in no way equal or replace formal testing by experts in those fields. As an example, the purpose of the therapist's examination of vision is to determine whether visual or auditory stimulation may be effective or whether compensatory or retraining methods must be used. The diagnostic and lesion-localizing purposes for testing the optic nerve are not the primary focus. These differences in purpose are not always distinct and can be misunderstood in the physician-therapist relationship and among the different health professionals. If current, accurate evaluation data are available, however, then they should, by all means, be used.

As technologically sophisticated measurement systems evolve, a measurement science may emerge.[47] Clients may be sent to performance measurement laboratories much as they are currently sent to radiology. In this case, measurements of a broad spectrum of human performance will be collected, and members of each discipline may pick and chose relevant data from the measures and plan treatment strategies according to their evaluation of the measures. *Measurement* here refers to the use of a standard (e.g., a ruler) to quantify an observation (e.g., length in number of centimeters). In contrast, *evaluation* involves determining the importance or worth of the numbers. Measurements are tools of evaluation. Computerized measurement systems may decrease redundancy in some formal examination procedures and may ultimately cause a change in discipline domain. If findings are not used in the process of goal setting and treatment, then the client's investment of time and money for examination procedures is unjustified.

Problem-solving approach to evaluation

Forms are available to guide in the examination of clients with neurological problems, including forms designed especially for clients with head trauma. Some are specific to individual facilities and reflect the needs of those evaluating clients at differing stages of their rehabilitation. Other forms reflect the local practice of a given discipline. For example, evaluation and treatment of oral motor dysfunction may customarily fall within the purview of physical therapy in some regions and occupational therapy in others. To avoid the pitfalls of dealing with these variables, the possible components, or content areas, for a physical therapy examination are presented. Construction and use of a suitable form based on these components may facilitate more thorough, systematic evaluations.

Possible examination areas are presented in the box on p. 355 on components of evaluation. The categories obviously overlap, and the inclusion of certain tests in a particular category is arbitrary and simplistic. Therapists are challenged by emphasizing and modifying traditional examination methods for use with head trauma clients, rather than by the examination content. The initial evaluation usually consists of gathering information from four general sources: the medical record, the nurses, the client and family, and the physician(s) and other team members.

Medical record data. After receiving a referral to treat a client with head injury, the therapist usually reads the medical record. This task may involve considerable time, since the chart can be quite thick. Demographic information, past medical and social history, diagnoses, present history, medical interventions (including surgeries and medications), course of recovery, and reports from other disciplines are noted. If the client has transferred from another facility, discharge summaries may be available. Review of the master problem list and management plan is suggested. The master problem list and diagnoses may alert the therapist to the need to examine particular areas more closely. The management plan may yield practical information, such as the method and schedule for feeding and medications. The client's current status can be previewed from the physician's progress notes, nursing notes, and vital sign charts. For various reasons charting may be sketchy in some areas, and it behooves the therapist to read test reports carefully. To illustrate, incomplete chart reading might have resulted in irreparable spinal cord damage to a client with a head injury whose x-ray report indicated a displaced third lumbar vertebral fracture. This information was not noted elsewhere in the chart, yet the fracture subsequently required Harrington rod stabilization.

Nursing observations. Before examining a client, it is often helpful to solicit impressions from the primary care nurse, especially if the client is in an intensive care unit. Even an experienced therapist may feel anxious when approaching a critically injured client. The nurse can provide up-to-the-minute observations of the client's medical stability, the family's participation, and a wealth of other information. The therapist should not be biased by the eval-

---

Components of evaluation

I. Medical record data
II. Nursing observations
III. Client/family data
    A. Subjective data: personal factors and goals
    B. Objective data
       1. General observations
       2. Screening of systems
          a. Respiratory
          b. Circulatory
          c. Integumentary
          d. Musculoskeletal
          e. Bowel and bladder
       3. Cerebral function
          a. General cerebral function (e.g., cognition)
          b. Specific cerebral function (e.g., language)
       4. Autonomic nervous system function
       5. Sensory function
          a. Primary sensations
          b. Cortical or integrative sensations
       6. Motor performance
          a. Composite motor activities
             (1) Developmental activity level (e.g., rolling, gait)
             (2) Type and quality of movement and movement pattern composition
             (3) Nonequilibrium coordination
             (4) Equilibrium (balance)
          b. Components, or basic elements, of motor performance
             (1) Tone
             (2) Threshold of abnormal responses
             (3) Postural reflex mechanism integration
             (4) Muscle strength
             (5) Muscle length/flexibility
             (6) Response speed
             (7) Movement speed
             (8) Muscular endurance
       7. Activities of daily living
       8. General cardiovascular endurance/fitness
       9. Social/economic/family factors
IV. Physician and other team member assessments

---

uations made by other professionals. Although input from others is valuable, personal evaluation of the client may ultimately differ from reports or discussions of colleagues. Recall that each health professional evaluates the client for different purposes and through different eyes. One evaluator may be relying on visual observations; one may be evoking responses. Differences simply accentuate the desirability of a team approach to the evaluation and management of head trauma clients.

Client/family data. Prepared with background information, the therapist is ready to safely examine the client. At this point the examination must be individualized. The order, emphasis, and adaptations of the examination are based on the diagnoses, the client's condition, and the therapist's time. The client may be unable to tolerate the entire examination in one session. Life-support and monitoring equipment, concomitant injuries, and the level of arousal and cognition may preclude various aspects of the examination. Furthermore, assessment of such factors as the client's level of arousal and motor responses may require several brief examinations. The infinite variety of potential problems prevents a definitive statement of *how* to evaluate clients with head trauma. This variety challenges the therapist to create individual adaptations!

The environment where the evaluation takes place may affect the client's responses. Environment should be considered in evaluation just as it is in treatment. The therapist may want to evaluate in different environments or to manipulate the environment. This is a concern especially when the client is agitated or easily distracted. Instructions may need to be simplified and time allowed for delayed responses.

An additional concern is conducting an unbiased evaluation of the client. One pitfall is making assumptions based on what seems to be apparent. For example, it cannot be assumed that the client who has no head control, who cannot speak, and who drools is unable to respond cognitively. Seeing what one expects or desires also can be an error. Interpreting a hand squeeze by a client as communication may be an example of wishful thinking.

Subjective data. Clients' participation in the subjective examination depends on their level of cognitive function. A therapist has little difficulty obtaining subjective information (pain, concerns, goals of treatment) from a fully conscious client. One should not be deterred just because a client is unconscious. The medical record and nurses may have already provided much of the historical and personal data. The family can relate the client's personality traits, education, occupation, interests, hobbies, likes, dislikes, and names of family, friends, and pets. All of this information becomes important in individualizing the program for the *person* who was injured. At first the client may be a passive participant in the process of expressing concerns and establishing treatment goals; the family can substitute as the active partner.

Pain, which the therapist assumes is present as a result of a client's grimacing or reactions to movement, is sometimes described as subjective data. The character of the pain remains questionable. (See Chapter 27 for additional information.)

More cognitively advanced clients can report their feelings, perhaps only nonverbally at first. Many clients will be able to assist in at least short-term goal setting, and if they are able to think abstractly, they can describe their long-term treatment expectations.

Objective data. Efforts should be made to gather and record measurable, reproducable objective information.

When this is not possible, the therapist should qualify the observations. Ongoing assessment of the effectiveness of treatment demands this discipline. The experienced therapist will gather and process much of the information simultaneously. Family members are also helpful in gathering objective data because they may spend the most time with the client and have valid observations.

General observations. An assortment of general observations can be made on entering the client's room. Included among these might be the presence and location of the catheter, life-support and monitoring equipment, and signs of family, friends, and personal belongings. The therapist should note if the client's eyes are open or closed, if the client is conscious and alert, and if he or she is lying still or moving. If the client is moving, the character of the movement should also be noted. Unstructured posturing should be observed in detail, as it will substantially determine the eventual positioning program. If the client comes to the therapy department, many of the same observations can be made: for example, sitting or standing posture, head control, and level of consciousness. These observations determine the structure of the examination and the examination environment. Introductions and explanations are in order, even if they are one-sided.

Screening of systems. Depending on the treatment setting, local convention, and the client's condition, the therapist's examination may include a screening of several systems. These include the respiratory, circulatory, integumentary, and musculoskeletal systems and the extent of the client's bowel and bladder control. The depth of the physical examination will vary with the problems of the individual client. Preexisting or concomitant injuries require more in-depth inspection. Important in this category is ascertaining passive range of motion, including specific joint mobility. To do so may require two people and the use of tone-inhibiting techniques. Limitations should be measured, and the type of restrictions (noncontractile, contractile, or both) should be determined. The type of restriction will dictate treatment. Hypermobility can also occur. Tone, skin condition, responses to movement and to pain, and even proprioception might be obtained simultaneously with range of motion. If touch or movement agitates the client, an idea of the range can be estimated during voluntary activities, provided the client has some selective motor control.

Cerebral function. This category includes both general cerebral functions and specific, or more focal, cerebral functions. General cerebral functions include cognition and behavior. These functions are observed by therapists. Definitive cognitive testing is performed by those more qualified.

Regardless of the level of consciousness, much of the general cerebral function can be determined during other aspects of the physical and neurological examination. If the client is conscious and able to speak, general behavior, (e.g., attitude, cooperation), emotional status (e.g., depression, euphoria, apathy), thought content (e.g., preoccupations, phobias), orientation (e.g., to time, place, person, self, and situation), intellectual performance, memory, and insight can be assessed throughout the examination process. In assessing some of these general processes, such as memory and orientation, therapists need to use some common sense. Hospitalized clients (even those without head trauma) cannot realistically be expected to recite the date. Many of us ask the date when we begin writing a report or a check! Additionally, it is foolish to ask questions of a client to test memory if the therapist does not know the answers. Asking a client what he or she ate for breakfast as a check for recent memory is not useful unless the therapist knows the correct response.

The therapist will have to work harder to determine the general mental status if the client is conscious but unable to speak, perhaps because of a tracheostomy. If the client is not fully conscious, note the level of consciousness, the response to stimulation, and general behavior. As discussed earlier, a description of the client's behavior and cognition is usually more precise than labeling the coma stage.

Numerous observations of clients with head injuries at Rancho Los Amigos Hospital[33] resulted in a descriptive categorization of various stages of "cognitive function":

   I. No response
  II. Generalized response
 III. Localized response
 IV. Confused-agitated
  V. Confused-inappropriate
 VI. Confused-appropriate
VII. Automatic-appropriate
VIII. Purposeful-appropriate

Although termed a cognitive scale, this scale actually includes both cognitive and behavioral components of general cerebral function. Even before this categorization was developed, therapists experienced with head trauma clients had observed that mental recovery was characterized by a progression through a series of stages. The publication of these observations by the Professional Staff Association at Rancho offers a more uniform assessment, documentation, and prediction of these stages. Scales such as this one serve as a common ground for communication. Perhaps as knowledge of the development and the redevelopment of cognitive and behavioral functions increases, so will sophistication of the scales. This would permit a more independent evaluation of these two related, yet separate, cortical functions. Fig. 13-1 depicts the close association of cognitive, behavioral, and physical functioning soon after injury. The three domains gradually become more distin-

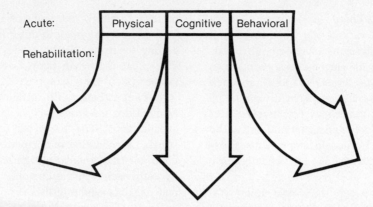

Fig. 13-1. Schema representing the close association of cognitive, behavioral, and physical functioning soon after injury. The three domains gradually become more distinguishable in the later stages of recovery.

guishable in later stages of recovery and can be assessed more independently; however, their interrelationships remain exceedingly complex.

Sensory integration, perceptual motor integration, and language are considered specific cerebral functions, and tests for agnosia, apraxia, and aphasia might be indicated. Of these, physical and occupational therapists are less concerned with definitive evaluation of aphasia. However, knowledge of a client's ability to communicate and to do so reliably is exceedingly important to the therapist. Communication is the window to the client's mental status and central processing capabilities. If the client can be aroused and responds with visual or auditory attention, try simple commands to establish communication. The client who cannot speak may be able to respond with facial expressions or gestures. Accuracy and reliability of any communication, including verbal communication, must be checked. Again, to check accuracy and reliability, the therapist must know the correct answers.

Motor planning activity might be assessed in lower cognitive stages by observing various activities, such as hand-to-mouth or reaching for an object. Perception is difficult to assess until the client can be evaluated through perceptual activities such as imitating, solving puzzles, overcoming obstacles, crossing midline, or identifying body parts. Later, formal tests for apraxia and perception may be helpful. Sensory integration is discussed in the section on evaluation of sensory function. Additional information can be found in Chapter 11, learning disabilities.

Autonomic nervous system function. Both the central and peripheral nervous systems can be influenced by the autonomic nervous system (ANS). Assessing this system consists of recognizing the sympathetic and parasympathetic responses in various organs. Understanding how a client is interpreting and thus reacting to sensory stimuli is important. For example, touch may inadvertently startle a

client, causing mass sympathetic reactions such as emotional excitement, increased blood pressure, and sweating.[20] The client's respiratory and heart rate may subtly increase with movement, even when the client is in a reduced state of consciousness.

Sensory function. The sensory system develops in a sequential manner, as does the motor system. Therapists spend hours in school learning the motor developmental sequence but spend comparatively little time on the developing sensory system. Brain injury can cause the sensory system to revert to a more primitive level.[20] Various sensations can be impaired. Problems in the sensory system are very often reflected in the motor system, creating a distorted feedback loop that perpetuates problems in both systems.

Two broad categories of sensations can be defined based on type of information: primary sensations and cortical (or integrative) sensations. This arbitrary division is useful functionally, but is not based on the anatomical divisions used to localize lesions. Primary sensations include exteroception and proprioception. The exteroceptors of smell, sight, and hearing are sometimes referred to as teloreceptors. Vision, hearing, olfaction, gustation, pain, touch, temperature, position sense, and kinesthesia are commonly checked primary sensations. Sensations cannot be definitively tested clinically without client cooperation, but some information can be ascertained. If the client is communicative and cooperative, these sensations can be tested in the usual ways. Suggestions for checking primary sensations while a client is in lower levels of consciousness are presented below. In addition, the therapist may review the results of the multimodality evoked potential studies.

Vision can be grossly checked by observing tracking or focusing. If necessary, a threatening movement toward the eyes may evoke a blinking response. A client's reaction to his or her name or to a loud noise may indicate auditory function. The introduction of various odors and tastes may evoke changes in facial expression, increased salivation, or tongue movements. With the unconscious client, tests for deep pain are the same as those used to elicit reflex motor responses, which have already been discussed. A tactile defensiveness to light touch may be observed. Reactions to different forms of vestibular stimulation can be appropriate or inappropriate. Purposeful movements or extremity postures may provide a clue as to the client's sense of position.

Primary sensations require cerebral cortex interpretation. Stereognosis, topognosis, and two-point, texture, and visual discrimination can be tested with traditional methods when the client can communicate and follow simple commands. Of these perhaps only topognosis, or localization, can be recognized in lower stages of consciousness and then only if the client responds by attending to the location of the stimulus.

Motor performance. The traditional medical neurological examination of motor function includes evaluation of muscle tone, size, strength, and type of movements. Cerebellar function is usually assessed separately and includes evaluation of coordination, equilibrium, and gait. The motor and cerebellar systems are tested by the physician in the attempt to localize lesions and to diagnose problems. The therapist dealing with clients with upper motor neuron deficits is primarily concerned with the integration of posture and movement; therefore, a different organizational structure for motor system evaluation is required. The organizational structure selected must directly relate to treatment concepts.

The organizational structure presented here represents aspects of both of the two major constructs used to evaluate human performance in any context, from back strength in low back pain clients to gait in head-injured clients. One construct consists of analyzing composite high-level activities, such as walking, dressing, and transferring. Activities of daily living, gait, and developmental-type evaluations are representative of this organizational structure. Tasks such as gait, however, are composed of *basic elements of performance*[48] such as strength, speed, range of motion, and so on, which are combined in a specific manner to create the high-level composite tasks. Hence, the second construct for viewing human performance consists of evaluating the basic elements, that is, the factors intrinsic to the high-level tasks. Although therapists have always used both of these approaches, we may have been doing so without recognizing the values and limitations of each approach. If a client has "normal" gait, he or she must by definition have all the necessary elements necessary for that task. Therefore, the therapist need not evaluate further. If, on the other hand, the gait is not normal, the therapist must look for those factors (decreased strength, abnormal reflexes, improper timing) that might

be responsible for the gait deviations. Treatment can then be focused on correcting those limiting factors and reintegrating them into the higher-level functions. These views of evaluating human performance are not limited to the motor system but encompass all domains involved in performance, including life-sustaining functions, environmental interface functions, and cerebral, or central processing capabilities.[48] The following discussion uses these constructs in evaluating motor performance because therapists have not traditionally recognized the differences in these two approaches in the context of motor performance. Recall that in evaluating the sensory system, therapists tend to evaluate the basic sensory elements (vision, position sense) and the secondary, or interpretative, sensations separately and distinctively. However, therapists more readily recognize that stereognosis is dependent on intact touch sensation and that if stereognosis is present, then touch must also be intact in the body sites tested.

Following brain injury, a phylogenetic regression of function takes place in many areas, including motor performance. This reversion presumably results from loss of higher-center control. There can be changes in muscle tone and in the normal postural reflex mechanism. Primitive postural reflexes, once integrated, reappear and can dominate. The client's physical progress is dependent on the normalization of postural tone, the reintegration of primitive reflexes, and the subsequent redevelopment, or rediscovery, of normal automatic movement reactions. Hence an adaptation of the pediatric model for evaluation of the motor system is one approach used to evaluate composite performance.

The physical and psychological modifications needed for evaluating adults from a neurodevelopmental perspective are obvious. In addition, the theoretical framework requires modification. Namely, in an adult, motor disabilities are superimposed on previously acquired motor skills. Although motor performance is impaired, previous skills are not necessarily extinguished. The difference with children, of course, is that a motor disability not only impairs existing motor performance but also the ability to *develop* new motor performance. For those therapists not inclined toward neurodevelopmental techniques, development can be viewed as a dynamic, hierarchical list of functional activities suggestive of a sequence for acquiring progressively more complex tasks.

In addition to the client's level of development, the other composite motor skills frequently evaluated include the type and quality of movement and movement pattern composition, nonequilibrium coordination, and equilibrium, or balance. The typical components, or basic elements, of motor performance are evaluated in an effort to determine *why* a client is exhibiting particular motor dysfunctions. The basic elements include tone, the threshold of abnormal responses, postural reflex mechanism integration, muscle strength, muscle length, or flexibility, response speed, movement speed, and muscular endurance. Each of these aspects of the motor evaluation is discussed below. Some of the motor testing does not require the client's conscious participation; however, if the client is agitated, an indirect assessment during activities may be needed. Hearing and visual deficits present additional challenges. Assessment of motor function can be impeded if the therapist continually moves the client passively into positions rather than providing stimuli and allowing the client a chance to respond motorically.

Although a variety of gross motor-development scales exists, most are age related, and the age equivalents for acquisition of motor skills are unnecessary and inappropriate with adults. It is the *sequence* of acquisition that later can become a guide to treatment. Evaluation should begin at the client's approximate level of controlled function. This can be anywhere from head control to skipping. Assuming, maintaining, and moving into and out of patterns is part of the motor skill appraisal. If the client is unable to perform the activity with the desired response, the missing components of the activity should be analyzed. Five components of movement have been described by Stone[79]: head control, trunk strength/rotation, extension/abduction of the limbs, midline orientation, and weight shift. Motor milestones can be described in terms of acquisition of these components in postures, in preparatory activities, and in movements. The components become important in relearning motor skills. Also important are Rood's concepts of levels of control throughout activities, that is, mobility, stability, controlled mobility, and skill.[78] Oral-motor function may require evaluation. Many references are available on this topic, including Winstein[86] and Chapter 24 of this text.

Type and quality of movement and movement pattern composition should be assessed. Type of movement refers to its character, that is, either voluntary or involuntary. Tremor is an example of involuntary movement. Both resting and intentional tremors have been reported as possible sequelae of head trauma. Frequently, there is a dissociation between voluntary and automatic movements. If there is voluntary movement, the quality of the movement can be assessed. Evidence of self-assertiveness, such as the client pulling at tubes while still semicomatose, is not only a cognitive sign; it gives the therapist an early view of motor performance. Observation of combined or selective limb and trunk movements that are controlled independently of abnormal, stereotyped patterns is useful, especially in the presence of hemiplegia. Bobath[6] and Brunnstrom[11] have both developed guides for this purpose. *Controlled movement implies that muscle contractions can be slow or rapid, can be held in various positions throughout the range, and can be relaxed quickly and reversed.* Videotaping a client performing various activities may be a useful way of recording the quality of movement.

Movement pattern composition is a concept related to, and in the view of some therapists the same as, the concept of quality of movement. *Quality of movement* is the term used more often with neurologically impaired clients, and *movement pattern composition* is the term used more frequently with musculoskeletally impaired clients. In either case, the client displays a faulty movement pattern. Sahrmann[72] describes active and passive muscle imbalances. Active muscle imbalances occur when one of a synergistic pair of muscles predominates during a movement, and passive muscle imbalances occur with either excessive or restricted muscle length. One or both types of imbalances could preexist in a client, or could occur as a result of abnormal movement patterns and muscle tone changes. For example, a client might be unable to adequately separate hip flexion from low back flexion: (1) because of excessive length of the back extensor muscles and concurrent hamstring tightness, or (2) because excessive extensor tone predominates, preventing hip flexion, and the client attempts to compensate with lumbar flexion. Both clients will demonstrate poor quality movement.

The order in which muscle groups are recruited in performing an activity is also part of movement composition. For example, the trunk muscles must be activated to provide postural stabilization immediately before various leg and arm movements. These movements are preparatory activities essential for successful motor performance. Head-injured clients typically maintain trunk flexion while attempting to elevate an arm overhead (see Fig. 13-5, *A*). The therapist will have to assess the basic elements to determine the cause(s) of motor dysfunctions.

Nonequilibrium coordination can be evaluated and viewed as an extension of the quality of movement assessment. Fine-motor scales may be helpful for this, or traditional cerebellar tests can be used, such as finger-to-nose and finger opposition. Movement capabilities are assessed bilaterally in four main areas: reciprocal motion, movement composition, movement accuracy, and fixation (or postural holding).[62] Tests for coordination assume that isolated, selective movements are possible and that there is adequate strength and range of motion.

Quiet standing in humans is maintained primarily by proprioception, with the visual and vestibular systems exercising important but secondary controls.[37] Head trauma clients often experience difficulty balancing in both sitting and standing positions. Proprioception can be altered or absent in these clients. Visual and vestibular balance systems can also be affected.[58]

Balance requires the coordination of many muscles, especially those of the hips, knees, and ankles, to maintain the body's center of gravity over its base of support. This complex coordination of muscle control is accomplished by sequences of stereotyped patterns mediated via the brainstem and cerebellum, often referred to as a "pattern generator."[59] Static and dynamic equilibrium coordination can be evaluated in several ways. Bobath[6] describes observational techniques for evaluating perturbed balance. Timed tests with the client's eyes either opened or closed are sometimes used for measuring static balance. Body sway can be measured on force plates. Sophisticated balance-testing equipment can be used if available. However, the therapist must not only assess whether balance reactions are present or limited but also identify the precise problems (such as timing and sensory input) that are affecting the balance response (see the review of balance mechanisms on p. 388).

The applicable aspects of these high-level composite movement tests reveal the client's motor abilities and disabilities. Again, the next step is to determine the basic mechanisms functionally responsible for the disabilities.

Muscle tone is classically evaluated by detecting the degree of resistance to passive stretch that is of sufficient velocity to elicit a response. Tone can be altered in any gradation from absence to hyperactivity. Abnormal tone manifests itself in patterns of movement, not in isolated muscles. Frequently, early abnormal tone is distributed throughout the entire body, with one side affected more than the other. The tone is not static but is influenced by a variety of circumstances, such as position, a full bladder, infection, anxiety, and transitional movements. Spasticity also changes in character with time. Statements reporting postural tone need qualification, if not quantification, as to the degree and manner in which the tone is altered. Inability to control abnormalities of tone can affect the components of movement during activities, the quality and composition of movements, and postural reflex mechanisms. Tone can be assessed through observation of movement and through handling the client. Use of electromyography (EMG) can yield a more objective measurement of tone. EMG is less readily available, but the need for definitive documentation is moving it out of the laboratory and into the hands of clinical therapists.

Analogous to determining the irritability of a painful joint is determining the threshold at which spasticity, or lower-level and abnormal reflexes and reactions, responds to stimuli. In other words, how much or how little effort, speed, or sensory stimulation might cause an increase in spasticity or associated reactions? This threshold level serves as a guide to treatment and to future improvement.

The postural reflex mechanism as described by Bobath[6] and Bobath[7] is the culmination of normal postural tone and normal reciprocal innervation, which combine with the three primary automatic movement reactions (righting, protective extension, and equilibrium reactions) and respond to sensory and perceptual input. The presence of abnormal postural reflexes, such as asymmetrical tonic neck reflexes and positive support reflexes, can impede movement and disturb this mechanism. Fiorentino,[21] Bobath,[6] and Brunnstrom,[11] among others, describe methods to either check postural reflexes or to examine the effects of

their presence. If automatic and voluntary movements are dissociated, the patterns of dissociation require evaluation. Some clients are better able to perform voluntary movements; others are better able to perform automatic movements. Distinguishing between these differences helps determine treatment. Charts combining developmental scales and postural reflex testing may further assist in determining the relationships of the reflexes with development of motor skills.

Strength, particularly of antigravity musculature, is a critical aspect of motor performance. In acquired upper motor neuron lesions, one problem may be an inability to direct and drive motor impulses.[6] Traditional manual muscle testing is based on the ability to perform isolated contractions in specific positions. In the presence of abnormal tone and primitive reflexes, isolated movements are not possible, and the effort exerted during the test makes the movements even less possible. Muscle testing is legitimate with lower motor neuron lesions, such as peripheral nerve injuries. The presence of spasticity renders the *traditional* manual muscle test inappropriate until tone and abnormal reflexes are normalized. However, this discussion does not suggest that there is no loss of strength, only that the loss may not be initially and reliably ascertained by traditional methods. Atrophy in spastic muscle groups is clinically observable in clients with long-standing upper motor neuron lesions.

Disuse, cast immobilization, joint dysfunction, improper nutrition, drugs, and aging (all potential problems with head-injured clients) can cause differential weakness with altered morphological, biochemical, and physiological characteristics within the muscle.[67] Shortened muscles tend to be strong in short ranges, and lengthened muscles are strong in lengthened ranges and weak in shortened ranges.[72] Electromyographical studies by numerous investigators[68,82] suggest that reduced activity alters motor unit properties, discharge frequency, and recruitment patterns. Controlled EMG studies of an individual client may be very helpful in determining the nature of the client's weakness. Strength can also be ascertained during the quality of movement assessment and by observing the client moving against gravity. Gravity is, after all, the primary resistance used developmentally in acquiring stretch sensitivity and adequate strength for function.

Muscle length, or flexibility, is an important evaluation component for therapists. Flexibility should be evaluated in a variety of positions such as prone lying, crossed-leg sitting, and all-fours positioning. Preexisting active or passive muscle imbalances can become exaggerated, and new muscle imbalances can be created. Muscle inflexibility can mechanically impede function. In a familiar example, tight heel cords restrict the body moving over the ankle during the stance phase of gait. When the ankle cannot dorsiflex in stance, the knee hyperextends. Alternately, perhaps the hip retracts because of increased tone, which hyperextends the knee, and the heel cords become tight secondarily. In such a case correction would require more than just heel cord stretching. The purpose of the movement analysis is to definitively identify the cause(s) of the dysfunction and to treat accordingly. Developmental and quality of movement evaluation forms commonly neglect the area of muscle length.

Response speed, or reaction time, is important in coordinating a number of both gross and fine movements. Response speed is defined as the time elapsed between a stimulus and the client's initiation of movement. Response speed involves receiving a stimulus, processing the stimulus (decision time), and initiating a movement. Reactions are obviously important when balance is threatened but can also be important in activities such as sitting from standing. Response speed can be measured by timing the lag between presenting a given stimulus and observing the response.

Movement speed begins where response speed ends. Movement speed is the time that elapses between the initiation of a movement and its completion. Weight shifting in all positions and during all activities must occur in a reasonable time. For example, during walking an individual must complete weight shifting onto one leg to lift and advance the opposite leg normally. Coordinated activities all involve movement speed. Finger tapping and alternating movements are typically checked as indexes of movement speed.

Endurance at the muscular level is the length of time a muscle, or group of muscles, can hold or perform repetitively. Muscular endurance is integral to the completion of innumerable tasks and can be examined by timing or observing performance degradation during a given task. EMG methods are also used to measure endurance.

Activities of daily living (ADL). A functional evaluation might encompass bed mobility, self-care activities, dressing, eating, management of appliances, wheelchair transfer skills, walking, household operations, and elevation activities such as stair climbing. ADL assessment forms may be helpful. Function is of utmost importance to the client and needs appropriate emphasis by the therapist.

General cardiovascular endurance/fitness. General endurance or cardiovascular fitness is a frequently neglected aspect of evaluation and treatment. Early evaluation of endurance may include tolerance to treatment or length of sitting time. Later, heart rate and blood pressure can be monitored during walking, upper or lower extremity cycling, or step testing. Fitness must be addressed because decreased fitness can interfere with achieving therapy goals. (Refer to Irwin S and Tecklin JS: *Cardiopulmonary Physical Therapy* for further information.)

Social/economic/family factors. To establish realistic goals, the client's socioeconomic background, occupation, family responsibilities, and the availability and extent of family participation should be assessed. Factors such as

the distance the family lives from the treatment facility and the presence of children also need consideration.

Physician and other team member assessments. When a client is seen soon after injury, it is helpful to contact the physician early after the evaluation—not only to exchange information but to inquire as to the presence of any medical precautions or contraindications. If the client has concomitant injuries, several physicians may need to be consulted. Much valuable time can be wasted if the therapist is unaware of the boundaries of treatment. Can the client sit, lie prone, invert the head, and be treated in the therapy department? Knowing the precautions and restrictions gives the therapist more confidence in considering treatment alternatives and generally permits a more aggressive program. In a less acute setting, such as the rehabilitation environment, precautions are usually more obvious: a team has already evaluated the client, and its members conduct regular staff meetings to share information and ideas.

The evaluative findings of other health professionals should be discussed. This may be informal, as in the acute stages, and more formal during the rehabilitation phase.

Computerized measurements of human performance

Although physical therapy remains high-touch, it is also becoming high-technology. Isokinetic dynamometers, EMGs, videotape and high-speed cinematography, force plates, hand-held force transducers, and computers—all formerly tools of research—are rapidly becoming indispensable tools of clinical practice. Smith and Kondraske[75] recently described an integrated system for measuring selected aspects of human sensory and motor performance, including measures of isometric strength, body stability, speed, reactions, muscle tone, and manual dexterity. Systems such as the one described above permit objective, reliable, and standardized methods for quantifying individual client performance, documenting disability, justifying reimbursement, assisting with vocational placement, and demonstrating the effectiveness of treatment. Although these high-technology instruments are not yet adequately enough developed to fully analyze the complexities of human performance, their sophistication is increasing at an astonishing rate, and they are becoming valuable adjuncts to therapy.

Ongoing evaluation

Evaluation is not over after the initial examination. It is a continuous processes intimately intertwined with treatment. Less formal evaluation takes place *during* treatment and at the *end of each* treatment session.

During handling techniques and with the introduction of various forms of stimuli, the client's reactions are observed. Immediate modification of input may be required to elicit the desired response. In this regard keen visual analytical skills are a tremendous asset for a therapist.

At the conclusion of each structured treatment session, the therapist asks self-directed questions such as, "Did the treatment make a difference? Is the client more relaxed or more responsive? Does the client have better control?" If the answer is no, perhaps a component of the treatment regime needs alteration.

At weekly or monthly intervals, a formal reevaluation measures progress toward achievement of each short-term goal. This reevaluation leads to revision of short-term and perhaps long-term goals, and of the treatment plan.

ASSESSMENT AND TREATMENT GOALS

As an identified step in the medical problem-solving model, *assessment* refers to the process whereby the client's problems are identified and appraised and realistic treatment goals are established. Problems are identified from the results of the subjective and objective examinations. The significance of the problems and assets is determined, and this information assists in setting the treatment goals.

Problem identification

Following examination of the client, the assets and problems for which there might be intervention are identi-

fied. Therapists deal most directly with problems in five systems: the musculoskeletal, circulatory, respiratory, integumentary, and nervous systems. The problems are analogous to the sequelae identified earlier in the chapter. Fig. 13-2 summarizes some of the more common problems for which therapy offers intervention strategies. Problems in any or all of these systems can lead to an interruption of function. The purpose of therapy is to restore or adapt function in each of the involved systems.

In an attempt to facilitate communication, some head injury teams have developed standardized problem lists to use in record keeping.[54] Although this is helpful for reporting, the therapist must be cognizant of the specific problems of an individual client.

With traumatic head injuries, evaluating the examination results entails familiarity with factors that have been shown or that are suspected to indicate a favorable or unfavorable prediction of outcome. These factors are considered when establishing realistic treatment goals.

Prognostic indicators or outcome predictors. Much has been published on the topic of prognosis following head injury. The correlation between outcome and numerous factors has been researched. Multimodality evoked potential studies, CT scan results, duration of coma, depth of

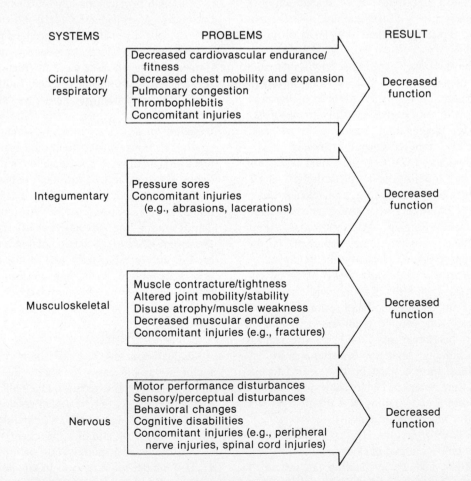

Fig. 13-2. Therapists develop intervention strategies to deal with functional deficits that may result from a variety of problems occurring primarily in one or more of the body systems depicted.

coma, age, intercranial pressures, and psychological factors are but a few of the variables on the basis of which prognosis has been attempted. The preoccupation with finding outcome predictors is based on an attempt to channel medical and rehabilitative resources to those clients who would realize the most benefit. This is an important practical concern. A second reason is to evaluate the efficacy of treatment intervention.

However, numerous problems are encountered in trying to predict outcome. Included among these problems are the accuracy and reliability of appraisal of factors by a number of different observers, the uniform implementation and interpretation of predictive factors, the percentage of error in prediction, the possible effects of intervention strategies and bias in treatment based on predictions, and, finally, the definition of what constitutes a "successful" outcome. Understanding these problems is imperative because the therapist can provide persuasive suggestions as to the type and intensity of rehabilitative care after injury. Consequently, the following discussion of prediction precedes a presentation of some possible prognostic indicators.

Accurate observations are important in predicting outcome and in assessing progress. Inaccuracy can result in improper decisions about continued care—as illustrated in the following dramatic example. Less than 10 minutes after his physician had examined him and reported in the medical record that he was still unresponsive and not progressing, a client not only sat unsupported at his bedside but walked approximately five feet with a walker and minimal assistance in spite of a tracheostomy and nasogastric and chest tubes. In actuality, the client had been following commands from his therapist for over a week and had demonstrated the endearing behavior of kissing the therapist's hand as thanks for treatment. Not only had the physician and therapist failed to communicate adequately with one another, but the two observers also interpreted the client's level of function in very different ways. Measures must be taken so that health professionals can make similar observations.

If indeed there are factors or tests that have predictive value, then they need to be administered, compared, and interpreted uniformly. The differences in operational definitions, types and sizes of populations, and length of time after injury when outcome assessment was made contribute to the lack of consistency in studies of predictive factors. For example, several authors have found that clients under age 20 usually recover;[2,43,77] however, even this has not been uniformly confirmed.[23] One study of the Glasgow Coma Scale[40] indicates that this scale is a simple and consistent outcome predictor. However, other studies[55,84] have not confirmed the scale's reliability and suggest that the criteria may not be standardly applied.

Another concern is the percentage of error in prediction. If prediction is 80%, or even 90%, accurate, there are still 10% to 20% of the clients with head trauma whose outcome may be incorrectly predicted. Even if the statistics are significant, one may feel very differently if the client whose future is misinterpreted is a family member.

One possible pitfall in prediction may be the interjection of bias, such as the Rosenthal effect identified in experimental design.[69] In this effect, demonstrated with rats and again with schoolchildren, the information given the unsuspecting subjects influenced the results. In the case of the rats, the trainers were told that they had a superior strain of rats although they did not. As a result, their rats learned faster than the rats in the control group. The so-called superior rats were handled and stimulated more than the control rats. In the case of clients perhaps the parental rejection that sometimes occurs and the reduced attention from nurses and therapists negatively influence outcome. Alternatively, a more optimistic prognosis may promote a stimulating therapeutic environment, which may positively affect outcome.

A potentially greater problem in prognosis is defining what constitutes a successful and worthwhile outcome. Therapists accustomed to working with children who may from birth be profoundly mentally retarded and multiply handicapped have perhaps learned to measure improvement in minute increments over a period of time. Perhaps through dealing with C2-3 quadriplegic clients, therapists have come to believe that life is more than independence in ADL and gainful employment. The definitions of "successful rehabilitation" and "severely disabled" are relative. Each element of disability, be it cognitive, behavioral, social, or physical, follows its own, but interrelated, course of recovery. Outcome for each area may be different and of differing significance to the client, family, and rehabilitation team members. Clarification of expectations is needed so that physicians, families, clients, and health professionals can better communicate.

Predicting outcome is an important goal for which research is beginning to supply possible answers. In general, however, these predictors are more reliable with *groups* of head-injured clients than with *individual* clients. For the individual client, predictors are best used as guidelines (see the textual discussion and the box on p. 362 on factors influencing management and recovery after a traumatic head injury). True assessment of outcome, as opposed to prediction, should occur 6 months to 1 year after injury.

Prognostic indicators may be divided into two major categories: preinjury characteristics and postinjury characteristics. Postinjury characteristics can be arbitrarily subdivided into static and dynamic characteristics. Many of the factors that may influence management and outcome are self-explanatory. Those that surface as being more indicative of outcome include pretraumatic intelligence and personality, age, cause and type of injury, immediacy of injury, length of retrograde amnesia, duration of posttraumatic amnesia, depth and duration of coma, posttraumatic cognitive and behavioral changes, family adjustment and

---

Factors that can influence management and recovery after a traumatic head injury

Preinjury characteristics

A. Cognitive factors
   1. Intelligence*
   2. Memory
   3. Level of education
B. Behavioral factors
   1. Personality*
   2. Psychological status
C. Social factors
   1. Vocational skills
   2. Avocational skills
   3. Interpersonal skills
   4. Family/friends support systems
D. Physical factors
   1. Age*
   2. General health and physical fitness
   3. Existing physical deficits
   4. Morphology
   5. Level of motor skill development and capacity for motor learning

Postinjury characteristics

A. Static factors
   1. Trauma factors (neurological)
      a. Location(s) and extent of injury
      b. Cause and type of injury*
      c. Immediacy of injury*
   2. Cognitive factors
      a. Ultimate duration of retrograde amnesia (RA)*
      b. Ultimate duration of posttraumatic amnesia (PTA)*
   3. Physical factors: extracranial injuries

B. Dynamic factors
   1. Trauma factors (neurological)
      a. Depth and duration of coma*
      b. Secondary brain damage
      c. Brainstem reflexes
      d. Special investigations (radiological and laboratory tests)
   2. Cognitive factors
      a. Rate of recovery of intellectual and memory functions*
      b. Quality of recovery of intellectual and memory functions*
      c. Communication disorders
   3. Behavioral factors
      a. Primary personality changes*
      b. Secondary personality changes
      c. Psychological status
   4. Social factors
      a. Opportunity to reenter occupation/school
      b. Avocational reintegration abilities
      c. Reaction to family/friends
      d. Family adjustment and support capabilities*
   5. Physical factors
      a. Pattern and quality of sensory/motor recovery*
      b. Rate of recovery of sensory/motor function*
      c. Range of motion and muscle flexibility
      d. Cranial nerve deficits
      e. Concomitant disabilities
   6. Environmental factors
      a. Staff/facilities/equipment available
      b. Attitude of health care providers
      c. Expertise of health care providers
      d. Room/housing and treatment settings

*Discussed in the text.

---

support, and pattern and quality of sensory/motor recovery. These factors are briefly discussed here.

Only under rare circumstances (usually in the military) are objective measures of the client's preexisting intellectual and behavioral characteristics available. Pre- and postinjury impressions of the client's personality are useful but certainly cannot be considered objective. Thus there is a paucity of studies linking outcome to the preexisting personality. However, preinjury mental characteristics are generally believed to contribute to outcome. That is, those persons with a history of low intellectual ability, difficulty with interpersonal relationships, and emotional disturbances have fewer resources with which to cope with injury than those who are more self-confident, ambitious, vital, well-educated, intelligent, and emotionally stable.

Numerous researchers[2,27,47] have reported age as an important factor influencing both mortality rate and functional recovery; it is a single factor with predictive power.

Generally, younger clients (under 20 years of age) make a better recovery even after deeper or more prolonged unconsciousness.[43] However, long-term follow-up to prove or disprove this hypothesis does not exist. Perhaps the immediate improvement is greater, but is the *capacity* for learning affected? Recent evidence suggests that although children may experience fewer cognitive and physical deficits, they may have more behavioral problems.

The cause and type of head injury is also indicative of prognosis. For example, clients with subdural hematomas have been demonstrated to have a poor outcome, whereas clients with epidural hematomas have demonstrated good to moderate recoveries.[22] Hypoxic or ischemic damage, such as occurs with near-drownings, late resuscitative efforts, and as a complication of the primary injury, suggests a poor outcome.[4]

Most recovery occurs within the first 6 months after injury—a finding of data bank study of more than 500 brain-injured survivors.[43] However, this does not imply that recovery does not continue after 6 months, only that the rate of improvement progressively slows. Therefore the time at which the client is assessed will influence the prognosis. It should also be noted that death as a direct result of the brain injury usually occurs within the first 2 to 3 days after injury.[12] An additional time-related factor in outcome may be the interval between the injury and the start of a rehabilitation program. Gogstad and Kjellman[28] in Sweden report that "continuous and rapid rehabilitation gives better responses than late introduced efforts, evidently through preventing social and psychological complications" (p. 283). Prevention of physical complications could be added to their list.

The duration of retrograde amnesia, defined earlier in this chapter, is considered an indicator of the severity of the injury in head trauma.[13,25] Posttraumatic amnesia marks the duration of altered consciousness[43] and also has been demonstrated to correlate with the severity of injury.[19,24] However, because these are retrospective indicators and because they are difficult to assess in clients with severe neurological deficits, their value in influencing management decisions is questionable.

The most important factor in determining prognosis is the degree of brain damage sustained. This is indicated by the depth and duration of coma, and it has been related to outcome.[12,23,80] The definition of what constitutes coma varies considerably, and as noted in a previous example, observer accuracy and reliability are not always optimal. Although coma duration cannot be determined initially, it can be a useful guide for prognosis relatively early during the course of recovery. Stover and Zeiger[80] report that coma lasting over 1 week is usually associated with either some permanent mental or physical disability or both.

The Glasgow Coma Scale, designed to reliably assess and monitor the degree of impairment of consciousness,[42] allows more objective observation of coma depth and duration.[43] When a client is assessed during the first week after trauma, the overall coma score and the best response grades on each component of the scale correlate with outcome at 6 months.[44] This scale may be a useful predictor because of its reported reliability and its availability. However, it is not without limitations. One problem is that data collection does not begin until 6 hours after trauma.

Outcome, as classified by Jennett and Bond[40] (see box on the Glasgow Outcome Scale), is used in statistically correlating early clinical features with outcome. An extended scale with more discriminating categories is needed for analyzing the rate and degree of recovery,[43] for assessing the efficacy of treatment strategies, and for justifying continued formal treatment. Also, for the purpose of further assessing outcome, it is useful to determine the component disabilities (cognitive, physical, behavioral, and social) that are present and the relationship of each to the overall outcome.[8] For example, a client may be dependent

---

Glasgow outcome scale

Vegetative state

A persistent state characterized by reduced responsiveness associated with wakefulness. The client may exhibit eye opening, sucking, yawning, and localized motor responses.

Severe disability

An outcome characterized by consciousness, but the client has 24-hour dependency because of cognitive, behavioral, or physical disabilities, including dysarthria and dysphasia.

Moderate disability

An outcome characterized by independence in ADL and in home and community activities but with disability. Clients in this category may have memory or personality changes, hemiparesis, dysphagia, ataxia, acquired epilepsy, or major cranial nerve deficits.

Good recovery

Client able to reintegrate into normal social life and could return to work. There may be mild persisting sequelae.

Modified from Jennett B and Bond M: Lancet 1:480, March 1975.

---

because of cognitive or behavioral (rather than physical) dysfunction. Rappaport's Disability Rating Scale[65] may be a more sensitive scale for clients in long-term rehabilitation programs; however, further study is indicated.[17]

Other aspects of coma, in addition to the response score and coma duration, are important in reflecting brain dysfunction.[34] Favorable clinical signs include pupillary reactivity, evidence of intact brainstem function, and reflexive and spontaneous eye movements. On the other hand, nonreactive pupils, absent eye movements, and abnormalities in brainstem function indicate greater brain dysfunction. These signs may signify a prognosis that is poorer than it is for those clients who do not exhibit these negative signs. However, negative signs per se do not necessarily indicate that the clients will be unable to successfully reintegrate into society, particularly if they are young and if these signs are interpreted early. Outcome predictions based on very early assessments can be excessively pessimistic.[44] Nonetheless, the pattern of posttraumatic consciousness remains an important variable for predicting the outcome after head injury and for judging progress.

The rate and quality of return of intellectual and memory function may also affect ultimate outcome and the occupational outlook. Generally, the faster and more complete the improvement in mental factors, the better the prognosis. In the Gilchrist and Wilkinson[23] study of 84 clients, the degree of mental involvement affected the capacity to return to work. Of their clients, 62% with no changes or mild mental changes returned to work, whereas only 23% of their clients with moderate or severe impairments returned to work. Cognitive disability can greatly interfere with recovery since independent function cannot occur when cognition remains greatly decreased. This is particularly true when there is an impaired rate and ability to learn. Observation of the speed with which a client moves through stages of consciousness may assist in ascertaining the rate of cognitive return. Communication of any kind is a positive sign, as are signs that the client is understanding communication, such as appropriate facial expression.

Lesions causing behavioral changes—such as loss of insight, disinhibition, aggression, depression, impaired judgment, apathy, or hyperactivity—can interfere with rehabilitation and social reentry. In one study the group of clients who were unaware of their own condition tended to be those who experienced the behavioral disturbances. This lack of insight persisted even at their 2-year followup. Interestingly, a substantial number of these clients also had posttraumatic epilepsy.[31] The fewer the personality changes, the easier for all involved. Early observations of the client progressing through various phases of consciousness may give clues as to the extent and persistence of personality changes.

There is little doubt that when the client is beyond the vegetative state, the level of family support and adjustment to the loved one affects outcome to some extent. The family can assist or hinder the client in the adjustment process. Work by Bond[9] in Glasgow suggests that positive reactions by families of clients with head injuries include insight, acceptance of rehabilitation goals, willingness to share responsibilities necessary to attain goals, resourcefulness, and tolerance of increased stress. Lack of insight, denial, nonacceptance of rehabilitation, dependence on professionals, hostility, overly ambitious expectations, overprotectiveness, depression, and a low level of intelligence are among the negative family factors. In most families there tends to be a mixture of both positive and negative factors in the members' reactions.[9] Fostering family interest, involvement, and concern is a critical part of the treatment.

The rate, pattern, and quality of sensory and motor recovery also affect management and outcome. Again, outcome is a relative term. For example, prolonged flaccidity as a result of brain trauma is a very poor sign. "Decerebrate rigidity," or a full extensor response of all four limbs, carries a higher mortality rate than that of a unilateral extensor response, a combined *decerebrate* and *decorticate-type* response, or a full *decorticate* response.[10] However, clients who have initially exhibited extensor responses have been known to recover and to resume many of their former activities. From a clinical point of view, it is probably safe to speculate that persistent flaccidity and prolonged severe spasticity are consistent with poor func-

tional return of the affected segments. Apart from those extremes, the location and degree of the tonal changes partially govern outcome and management decisions about motor function. For example, moderately severe extensor spasticity affecting both lower extremities may be incompatible with a goal for independent ambulation.

Sensory disturbances, of course, greatly affect motor responses. Absent sensation of a limb may be a greater deficit than a motor impairment alone. Sensory deficits occurring alone or in combination with motor deficits can be physically debilitating, depending on their distribution and extensiveness. The faster and more complete the normalization of sensorimotor integration, the better the quality of physical restoration.

Not only is each of the variables a consideration when the therapist determines goals of treatment, but the interplay among the variables is also important. Although it is tempting to search for the *one* reliable and accurate outcome predictor, prognosis most probably depends on multiple predictor variables. For example, a combination of the GCS score, oculocephalic response, and age predicted outcome with 80% accuracy.[14] Different predictive factors also may be more or less significant to each individual client. Perhaps Evans[18] still has the most accurate categories for depicting the outcome of the acute head injury: "death, rapid complete recovery, or anything else." Rehabilitation programs must select from the group of clients classified as "anything else." Recognition of prognostic indicators and the outcome predictors assists in directing clients to facilities that best meet their needs and serves as the background to develop realistic treatment goals.

General guidelines for establishing goals

The overall objective for rehabilitation of clients with head injuries is to return them as quickly and as fully as possible to the mainstream of their lives. This requires achieving maximal functional recovery and assisting the client in coping with residual disabilities. Because of the multiplicity of problems, accomplishing the overall objective demands setting priorities, sequencing, and teamwork.

Achieving goals by setting priorities is necessary in making the most effective use of time, money, and resources; sequencing is necessary for an organized, logical treatment approach; and teamwork is necessary for a comprehensive treatment program that incorporates adequate carryover during a variety of activities. True teamwork does not consist of each discipline working with the client toward achievement of its own goals. True team meetings do not consist of reporting on the extent to which the client has achieved the goals of that discipline. A better approach means that members of each discipline prepare a list of possible goals from their examinations and then establish and rank an overall list of long- and short-term goals. The members determine how the disciplines will coordinate and contribute to the attainment of the goals. Overlap is welcomed as reinforcement. That is, a client would be positioned, moved, and instructed consistently in every department from speech pathology to respiratory therapy. This sort of teamwork is important in the acute and rehabilitation phases of care. It involves cross-training among professionals in addition to improved communication and role flexibility. In some centers clients are treated simultaneously by two or more team members.

The specialists of a treatment team will differ from center to center and from one client to another. Frequently, a team consists of dietitians, nurses, occupational therapists, physical therapists, physicians, psychologists, respiratory therapists, social workers, and speech pathologists. Other members may include ministers, orthotists, recreational therapists, rehabilitation counselors, special educators, and vocational consultants.

Of course, any team effort is incomplete without the client's family and, when possible, the client. It is, after all, their problem, and they need to have input into the goal-setting process and in implementing the treatment plan. Friends may also be included on the team; they often want to help.

One additional point needs reiteration before a discussion of more specific goals. A client may simultaneously exhibit different levels of function cognitively, behaviorally, and physically, as depicted in Fig. 13-3. Therefore a sequence for each area of disability may be needed and their interplay carefully coordinated. Since a client may progress more rapidly in one area than in another, the balance of responsibility for care may shift periodically. For example, a client may make rapid physical gains and slower gains in cognitive function. At times full physical progress may be retarded until such time as the client has developed the judgment appropriate to match the physical status. Decisions such as this are certainly not to be made unilaterally.

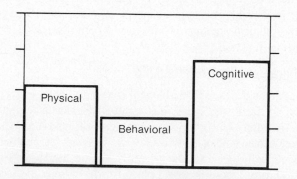

Fig. 13-3. Levels of functioning of a client with head trauma. A client with head injury may exhibit any combination of different levels of function. This client is functioning at a higher level cognitively than physically or behaviorally. The intervention strategies developed for the client must reflect this disparity of functional levels.

Long-term goals

Establishing long-term goals is very difficult in the early stages after injury since a long-term goal is really a prediction of outcome, or discharge, status. However, a month or so after a severe injury the team members need an overall direction. After they assess the prognostic indicators and the client's status, a few long-term goals can be determined. Long-term goals tend to be global, limited in number, functional, and open ended, and they evolve with time. Team members can ask themselves: "What would make the greatest difference in this client's life as it is right now?" Frequently, the answers will emphasize cognitive, behavioral, self-care, vocational, and mobility concerns.

Not only does establishing the long-term goals help to focus care, but the process of determining goals helps team members to become more proficient at doing so. That is, by comparing the actual outcome with the predicted outcome, the more important determinants may gradually emerge. Of course, long-term goals can and should be revised if the client's progress differs from what was expected.

Short-term goals

Short-term goals are the steps required to achieve the long-term goals. They identify what is to be relearned. Short-term goals can be remedial, prophylactic, or palliative. Again, the goals should be team goals, and they should be written in measurable terms.

Because physical therapists usually deal with problems in the systems depicted in Fig. 13-2, the goals with which therapists are most involved tend to be with those systems. Some potential areas for discipline overlap in treatment goals include family and client education, prevention of sensory deprivation and deficits, normalization of postural tone, enhancement of cognitive skills and memory, improved communication skills, passive range of motion, prevention or reduction of contractures, increased flexibility, social reentry, improved ADL, feeding, vocational and leisure-time pursuits, bowel and bladder retraining, skin care, increased endurance and physical fitness, breathing exercises, increased chest expansion, relief of pain, increased mobility, integration of postural reflexes, improved motor performance and balance, and behavior modification. The individual goals in any one of these areas may be quite modest. Once the specific goals have been developed and given priorities, the means of achieving the goals, or the treatment plan, can be devised.

GENERAL TREATMENT PROCEDURES

Any discussion of treatment is difficult because of the uniqueness of clients and their problems after traumatic head injury. There are no patent answers, no scientifically proven techniques, and no "cookbooks." To some therapists this uncertainty is a frustrating stumbling block. To others the uncertainty is a stimulus and a challenge.

Concepts of motor control

Treatment approaches depend on theories of motor control. The generally accepted developmental model, which is hierarchical and assumes a set unidirectional flow of information in the brain, has been challenged by the systems, or functional, model.[3] In the systems model circular interactions between brain structures enable each CNS level to change from dominant to subordinate in relation to any other level (i.e., heteroarchical). The systems model poses a flexible nervous system that can more readily accommodate to changes in the external environment. This is important because much of the development and growth of the brain's neuronal connections may result from external environmental stimuli.

The systems model of movement describes a pattern generator. The output of the pattern generator are motor patterns in the form of synergies. A synergy in this context is the functional organization of muscle groups that contract in a specific sequence and with fixed timing resulting in movement. The parameters of normal motor synergies are appropriate amplitude (magnitude), timing, sequencing, speed, and duration. The pattern generator determines which synergy will be used, but the synergy itself exhibits some flexibility. Peripheral and central inputs determine "when" and "how much" muscle contraction will be needed to result in a coordinated movement. The inputs are integrated and abstracted from environmental stimuli. Routine movements such as walking are fairly stereotyped and therefore minimize the necessity for much additional input, freeing higher centers for analysis of novel feedback.

An example of flexibility of the nervous system to meet environmental demands will illustrate this concept. A person is gently pushed forward. According to Nashner's work,[59] the upward rotation at the ankles as the man falls forward triggers a synergy in which the gastrocnemius, hip extensor, and paraspinous muscles contract in a distal to proximal pattern at an amplitude appropriate to the push and at a specific speed. This synergy restores the standing balance. If the same person stepped onto a backward tipping board, the stimulus of upward ankle rotation would be the same, but the usual synergy would cause a further backward loss of balance. The pattern generator in this case receives information from the visual and vestibular systems within milliseconds. The visual and vestibular input modifies the response, and the synergy now consists of dorsiflexion, hip flexion, and abdominal contraction, which nicely restores the person's balance. This change in synergy illustrates a switch from proprioceptive dominance of balance to dominance of the vestibular and visual information. Thus, the systems model provides an efficient method of responding with preprogrammed movement in the form of synergies to the normal environment, and yet is still flexible enough to adapt to novel stimuli. (Additional information on motor control may be found in Chapters 2, 3, and 4 with specific emphasis found in Chapter 4.)

Mechanisms of recovery

To discuss treatment, the mechanisms of recovery from brain lesions are important, and yet these mechanisms are poorly understood. Are alternative or redundant neural pathways responsible? How much of recovery is spontaneous? Johnson and Almi[45] identified eight possible mechanisms from their literature review: cerebral shock, equipotentiality, vicarious function, substitution, functional reorganization, denervation supersensitivity, collateral sprouting, and regeneration. These potential mechanisms of recovery are briefly discussed.

Some recovery is a spontaneous reemergence of function that was temporarily suppressed as a result of cerebral shock. Equipotentiality suggests that there may be latent motor pathways in several areas of the cortex or in the contralateral hemisphere that can be activated to assume the function of the damaged brain tissue. Another mechanism, vicarious function, demonstrated in humans when one hemisphere has been removed, suggests that the remaining hemisphere may assume functions, such as speech, originally controlled in the removed hemisphere. However, the quality of both the functions originally controlled and those recently acquired in the remaining hemisphere may be reduced. Substitutions are "tricks" used to replace an absent function, much like when a client attempts to substitute a stronger muscle for a weaker synergistic muscle. In the cortex, for example, a grasp reflex might be inhibited by using an avoidance reaction, such as active finger extension to inhibit grasp, that gives the illusion of normal control. Evidence also suggests that there may be a reorganization of function, or that the brain exhibits plasticity. The concept of denervation supersensitivity is defined as a situation where the postsynaptic membrane becomes more sensitive to less output so fewer neurotransmitter agents cross the synapse but have a stronger influence. Collateral sprouting and even regeneration may be responsible for some aspects of recovery. However, physiological attempts at recovery do not always result in normal function.

Therapist-client relationship

Although research by physiologists, psychologists, educators, therapists, sociologists, and physicians is beginning to shed light on the complex problems of head injury, science alone cannot provide all the answers to treatment. Continually pursuing the related scientific literature is important, but there is also a place for developing the *art* of physical therapy.

Most studies in therapy are directed toward the effectiveness of the procedures provided rather than focused on who is providing them. Yet not all therapists, even those with similar knowledge and treatment skills, are effective with all types of clients or even with the same client all the time. The reasons for this are not entirely clear, but superior knowledge is not the sole distinguishing factor.

If the prerequisite skills for effective management of clients with head trauma could be identified, perhaps they might be enhanced and developed where they are lacking. The specific personal qualities of the "master clinician" have not been established, but there seem to be certain skills in observation, analysis, and problem solving that are well-developed in those therapists successful with brain-injured clients. There also seems to be a desire for personal involvement, coupled with the sensitivity to empathize with the client emotionally and physically. Optimism, creativity, perseverance, patience, organization, and an enjoyment of working with clients with CNS dysfunction are also common traits. Of course, a knowledge of neurophysiology, normal and abnormal movement, learning theories, and an integrated approach to treatment of dysfunction are decidedly necessary.

Treatment techniques

Many of the techniques that therapists employ in the treatment of clients with neurological deficits have yet to be validated by research. Of those that have been substantiated, few have been studied specifically in clients with brain injury. Many techniques have been empirically developed. Others have been developed on the basis of generalizations from studies of animals, infants, and children, or they are merely consistent with the current knowledge of neurophysiology and motor control theories.

With those limitations and with the therapist's unique qualities in mind, some general guidelines to treatment are presented. Therapists working with adults who have sustained brain injury are primarily expected to contribute expertise in facilitating the acquisition and refinement of isolated limb manipulative skills, locomotor skills, and postural movements, all of which entails providing sensorimotor experiences, preventing and minimizing deformities, integrating the cognitive and behavioral aspects of motor learning, and educating the client, family, and other health professionals. These areas are emphasized in the section on treatment.

General philosophy underlying treatment

Acquiring motor skills implies learning or, in the case of clients with brain injury, relearning voluntary movements. The therapist is essentially a facilitator who guides the client in the efficient execution of solving motor tasks. Not only is the therapist interested in helping the client acquire the skill to accomplish a specific task at hand but also to acquire the skill to solve new motor problems. Learning motor skills and learning to learn the skills are the desired responses.

On at least an elementary level, the client must perceive the problem, be motivated to solve it, define the task, set the goal, weigh the alternatives, decide on a solution, implement the solution, and evaluate the consequences of the action. In short, the client must solve problems. At times the client may deliberately work through a problem, but usually problems are solved without knowledge of the process.

The therapist's responsibility is to help motivate the client, select and present motor tasks, present the proper stimuli, guide in achievement, provide feedback, encourage success, provide opportunities for practice and reinforcement, facilitate self-evaluation, and promote independence in each area. That is, the therapist must teach. (See Chapter 1 for additional information on problem solving, learning, and teaching.)

Teaching implies being able to adequately identify the component(s) of a skill that are missing or that are preventing the client from accomplishing the task. This refers to the therapist's continuous assessment of the client, which was already discussed in a more global manner. The missing component, for example, could be the inability to shift weight, or inadequate response speed.

Once the problems are appropriately identified, the therapist suggests a sequence, and the alternatives are assessed. Within the constraints of the client's morphological structure and certain biomechanical principles, the therapist must change the task, change the stimuli, change the environment, or facilitate a change in the client's attitude.

Consistent with the general philosophy of treatment is the idea that if sensorimotor experiences are not provided either inherently by the client or environmentally, the ability to learn and develop motor skills may be reduced. In other words, what is not used may be lost either temporarily or permanently. In addition, if inappropriate or nonfunctional movements are reinforced, those will be the skills learned. Psychomotor tasks are assumed to have cognitive and behavioral (or affective) components. Either of these components can purposefully or inadvertently alter the motor response, and motor skills cannot be accomplished independently of these two domains.

Acquisition of motor skills can take place formally in a therapy department, but much of the motor learning takes place informally in unstructured environments. Therefore other team members, including the client and family, need to reinforce proper learning throughout the client's day, not just in the structured environment.

In summary, the philosophy here is that the client needs to relearn motor skills and that the therapist facilitates the acquisition of these skills by providing the appropriate stimuli. The general sequence for the acquisition of motor skills is suggested from developmental sequence and from taxonomies developed for the psychomotor domain.[73] If opportunities for skill acquisition are not seized, then learning will not progress. Furthermore, those skills that are practiced and reinforced will be those that are learned.

Motor skills have inseparable cognitive and behavioral components that must be addressed. In addition, much of motor learning occurs outside the structured therapy setting.

Guidelines for treatment

Treatment generally consists of motivating clients, sequencing activities, providing the proper stimuli, having the clients practice the components of motor skills and the overall skills, planning for transfer of learning to new tasks, and incorporating cognitive and behavioral components into each of these aspects of the treatment plan.

Motivating the client. Although motivation is effected by external stimuli, it is an internal quality. Concrete, goal-directed, functional, and recreational activities that the client can perceive are highly motivating. Motivation is enhanced by immediate feedback, reinforcement (verbal and nonverbal praise, recognition, reward, success in achieving the goal), and activities that are personalized—that is, of particular interest to specific clients.

Treatment of the unconscious client is essentially passive in that the client is the intended recipient of the sensory input, whether it is proprioceptive, auditory, gustatory, or any other stimulus. The idea is to provide sensorimotor experiences because the client is unable to provide his or her own, and the input from the hospital environment tends to be undirected and monotonous. The responses come when the client perceives the stimuli. Until this time motivating the client is improbable. Even when perceiving the stimuli, the client may not do so accurately and may not be motivated when unattended. As the client gradually becomes less comatose, he or she may be confused, disoriented, and easily distracted. The individual may not recall the events that led to the hospitalization, thoughts in general may be disorganized, and memory gaps may exist. The reasons for discomfort—the tubes, the restraints, and the bed rails—are not clear. The client responds to the immediate experience of discomfort and confinement. At this stage the client cannot be expected to fully respond to a rational explanation of the reasons for being exercised, rolled, transferred, casted, stretched, or cooled. What motivates the client is removal of annoying, threatening, and uncomfortable stimuli and the fulfillment of basic physiological needs. Gratification must be immediate.

Motivating clients, particularly by assisting them to identify a goal, even if it is only to receive a cookie, *is an extremely important concept.* If clients cannot perceive some reason for their actions, no matter how small, they will not be motivated to perform. If they receive no reinforcement, they will be less likely to repeat the performance.

The concepts of motivation and reinforcement carry over into the cognitive and behavioral aspects of the treatment. When a client, unable to understand the ultimate goal, responds out of proportion to a stimulus, such as screaming during gentle positioning, immediate small goals can be provided. For example, the position can be held while the client counts to ten. Counting preoccupies the client, providing a goal (pain will stop at ten), a reward (removal of pain), reinforcement ("good"), an active role, and some control over treatment. At this stage the therapist may be viewed as an authoritarian figure who expects and demands compliance. Allowing the client not to comply when able to do so may lead to behavioral difficulties later. Also, the client who remains resistant may not receive adequate rehabilitation services. Time and money are wasted. The client needs to learn that the therapist cannot be manipulated. This may involve formal or informal behavior modification. The client will realize that it is easier to comply and "get it over with" than it is to fight compliance. A *client-therapist trust* also develops. "One more time" means only one more time. "You may go back to your room in 30 minutes" means that the client *will* be back in 30 minutes. A sense of trust is important in any therapeutic relationship, and it will be infinitely helpful throughout treatment. This client-therapist trust often becomes strong and enduring. Years after the formal rehabilitation process has ended, former clients may periodically consult or visit with their therapists.

A home visit or pass from the acute care setting, even when the client does not seem ready for such an adventure, is sometimes a remarkably useful treatment option. In addition to being a reward, the home visit is an orienting, behavior-modifying, motor-learning, and problem-identifying experience. As the client becomes less agitated and resistant, the therapist can rely less on immediate, concrete rewards and begin to use explanations, which are more abstract, to help the client achieve the goals they have set together. (Refer to Chapters 7 and 31 for additional information.)

Sequencing activities. A developmentally structured model may be useful in suggesting a sequence of activities in the early stages of management with clients functioning at lower levels. However, this model may be less useful with clients in the later stages of care who are functioning at higher levels. Generally, sequencing means that skills are taught in a simple to complex progression and that each skill can be broken down into its component parts, or basic elements. (See further discussion of this concept in a later subsection.)

Inappropriate sequencing can be detrimental to learning. If the activities selected are too difficult, the client may be unsuccessful. If the activities are too simple or perceived as condescending, the client may be bored and difficult to motivate. If the activities are random (that is, without sequence), the skills may be difficult to learn and to integrate into composite motor skills. Hence sequencing cannot be overemphasized, but neither can it be definitively determined. Numerous authors have suggested treatment sequences, including Bobath,[6] Farber,[20] and Rood.[78]

In addition to selecting activities appropriate to the client's function, *it is imperative that activities are introduced that are at least one to two stages beyond the present level of function.* Motor control within these postures is not anticipated, but in development, one activity is not fully mastered before the next activity is attempted. In fact, if an activity is not practiced, it cannot be learned. When babies cannot roll, parents roll them over. Long before infants learn to sit, they have experienced sitting in car seats, strollers, and carrier seats. They have been carried about by their parents and held in supported sitting. In addition, these activities take place frequently. Adults have previously learned these postures and have become oriented to the upright (vertical) position. Three points of this discussion should be reemphasized. First, activities selected in treatment must include those beyond the client's immediate level of function. Selecting experiences that are too basic is a common error in sequencing. The result is a nonaggressive program. Second, the new postures and activities may be initially passive or guided. Third, the activities should take place frequently throughout the client's day.

Providing proper stimuli. The most basic requirement in achieving an improved motor response is to use the proper stimuli. For example, in retraining walking, unless stimuli such as rotation of the ankle and hip joints and proper joint compression occur, swing and stance are not facilitated appropriately. Postural muscle tone may need to be normalized before normal movement can be imposed. *Proper input is prerequisite to proper output.* However, it should also be remembered that many activities are stimulated in a feed forward mode, rather than in a feed back mode.

Structured motor activities are facilitated by techniques such as approximation, brushing, slow stroking, tapping, and quick icing. A seemingly infinite number of possible treatment techniques and their combinations are at the therapist's disposal. (See Chapter 6 for specific treatment techniques and alternatives with their rationales.) In essence these techniques consist of a variety of stimuli—exteroceptive (including teleceptive), proprioceptive, and even interoceptive—that can be manipulated in frequency, duration, speed, variety, intensity, complexity, and quality according to the desired responses. These stimuli can be anything from inhibitive casting, which is proprioceptive input of long duration, to biofeedback, which can be brief visual and auditory stimuli provided as reinforcement for correct perceptual motor tasks.

Deciding on specific techniques requires a knowledge of the variety of techniques and their rationales, open-mindedness, skill in implementation, and a desire to create new options. The skill and ease with which one therapist works with given treatment techniques may be partially responsible for the success that therapist has using those techniques with clients. Implementing techniques is not only a cognitive but also a perceptual motor skill. The same principles of acquiring and retaining motor skills apply to therapists and clients alike.

Correcting and practicing component and composite motor skills. As alluded to previously, composite skills (e.g., rolling, balancing, walking) are composed of a number of components, or elements (e.g., normal tone, strength, speed). Missing or weaker components must be restored or relearned, the stronger components reinforced or inhibited, and then all components need to be reintegrated into the performance of composite motor tasks with proper central processing control.

When treating motor problems, it may be useful to think in terms of six, albeit rather arbitrary, aspects of the problem: (1) changing the basic elements of performance, that is, changing strength, muscular endurance, and flexibility, and matching morphological constraints; (2) accommodating to external environmental and biomechanical constraints of movement; (3) changing the internal central processing of movement, such as movement pattern composition; (4) sensory retraining; (5) increasing general cardiovascular fitness; and (6) combining the movements into functional tasks and ADL activities. Each of these six aspects of treatment is discussed below.

Changing the basic elements of motor performance. Tone may need to be normalized through positioning or with techniques such as weight bearing. EMG biofeedback using two screens, one for the agonist and one for the antagonist, is also useful in normalizing tone. With this technique, the therapist first facilitates an increased firing rate in the agonistic muscle and then, while maintaining that high level of firing, works on decreasing firing in the antagonistic muscle.

Loss of muscle strength acquired through disuse and muscle imbalances can be corrected with traditional methods or by using various proprioceptive neuromuscular facilitation (PNF) techniques.[85] If tone prohibits resistive strengthening, the client may need to learn movement without resistance and progress to controlling movement against the resistance of gravity.

Sustained active or passive stretching may increase flexibility, but care must be taken to avoid facilitating unwanted movement with positional and quick stretch. Retraining with very specific, controlled movements to separate, say, glenohumeral movement from scapulothoracic movement may be preferable to early stretching.[72] Splinting, bracing, and serial casting may be used to not only maintain proper length but to prevent length-associated changes in strength as well. Overstretched muscles become weaker in shortened ranges.[29] Some splints and braces are designed to increase independent motor control (Fig. 13-4). (Refer to Chapter 28 for additional resources.) Craniosacral techniques and soft tissue mobilization may be useful in achieving relaxation and restoring range when there are fascial restrictions.

Numerous studies demonstrate that strength gains are speed-specific, and most activities require the ability to change speeds. This implies that training must take place at different speeds as soon as the client is ready. Muscular

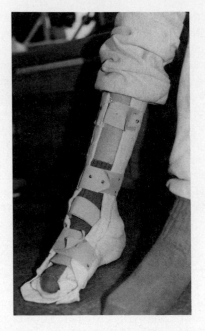

Fig. 13-4. The Thomas-Utley Dynamic Splint (TUDS) is a custom-made, tone-inhibiting, dynamic splint that allows minimal dorsiflexion and plantar flexion in a neutral position. The splint can be worn inside a shoe.

endurance can be enhanced through repetitive use of specific muscle groups during any selected activity. Response speed can improve as a result of practicing a specific act with emphasis on quickness. Abnormal postural reflexes need to be reintegrated using rotation and other activities as discussed in many chapters of this text.

Morphological constraints are those imposed by the individual's anatomical structure and perceptual processes. These include body weight and height, limb length and weight, sex, age, and receptor function.[35] Therapists are generally more aware of morphological constraints, and they tend to design and select tasks and equipment that match morphology or that compensate for these constraints.

Accommodating to external environmental and biomechanical constraints of movement. Environmental and biomechanical constraints must be understood. Therapists may choose to ignore learning about these principles, but these principles are operant in *all* movement on earth. Matching movements to these constraints will increase the client's capacity for motoric success. (The following discussion is taken in part from Higgins,[35] and the reader is referred to this reference for more information.)

Goal-directed movements are spatially and temporally regulated. Spatial elements of the environment are those relative to the position of objects in space. Temporal elements refer to the sequential relationship between events and objects. In some skills the environment is stable and predictable; in others the environment is unstable and unpredictable.

Spatial elements can vary from along one to three dimensions, or planes (frontal, sagittal, and transverse), of movement. Temporal elements are continuous in only one dimension. A ball tossed to a client can move through all three planes of movement. The time the ball takes to reach the client is the temporal element. Spatial elements refer to *where* an object or person will appear or an event will occur; temporal elements refer to *when* an event or movement will occur. The initiation and termination of movements, as well as their rhythmicity, are temporal elements.

To effectively retrain clients, the therapist needs to determine which elements are primary in a task or choose tasks that stress particular dimensions. Otherwise, the client may be in the wrong place, in the wrong position, or be there at the wrong time to accomplish the task. For example, kicking a stationary ball reduces the temporal element of the task. The client does not need to predict the movement of the ball in relationship to time, and the plane of movement can be restricted by the type of kick selected. By contrast, walking in a crowded area requires both spatial and temporal regulation, and the predictability of the environment is low. In the latter example, the client needs a larger repertoire of movements to match changing environmental conditions.

Biomechanical constraints are those imposed by physical forces such as gravity and inertia. To move, one must overcome these external biomechanical constraints. Various body positions are essential to generate adequate forces or speeds to complete coordinated movements. If the general goal of the movement requires accuracy, this is more easily accomplished with a stable base of support, stable proximal segments, and use of distal extremity segments. The distal extremities consist of longer muscles with increasingly larger CNS representation. If speed is important, then the radii of limb segments should be small at various ranges of the movement. For example, hip flexion can be more rapidly accelerated with the same amount of muscle force when the knee is flexed (note that sprinters have increased knee flexion). Also speed and force are facilitated if all the participating muscles and muscle groups initiate movement from a fully lengthened position, as also described in PNF.[84] Force can best be produced when movement begins near the midline, when force is transferred from large (trunk) to small (distal extremity) segments during the movement, when the base of support is wider and the center of gravity is lower, and when the application of the force being generated is in the desired direction.

The size of the base of support is important in activities that involve stopping rapidly and changing direction. The body's center of gravity is constantly shifting with movement and requires a constant shift in the base of support. For example, when moving from sitting to standing, a normal individual usually tilts the pelvis anteriorly, flexes the trunk forward at the hips, and flexes the knees bringing the feet back in preparation for weight bearing. The center of gravity is thus moved forward, and the base of support is ready to accept the weight transfer. The typical head-injured client tends to remain in a slumped posture with a posterior pelvic tilt, attempts to rise without sufficient hip flexion, and fails to bring the feet back under the body to prepare an adequate base of support. The client's center of gravity therefore remains behind the base of support. No one could stand independently given these circumstances. The biomechanical constraints must be accounted for in order to move.

Following a movement the body segments must decelerate and return to the original or to a new position in preparation for the next movement. Frequently, the head-injured client cannot decelerate or prepare for the next movement in a timely manner and is, in fact, in the wrong place, position, and time to accomplish the next movement, which may be simply taking the next step.

Changing the internal central processing of movement.
The central processing of movement presupposes adequate strength, length, and other elements, and includes movement pattern composition and movement coordination, such as proximal stability, sequencing, bilateral integration, processing speed, and preparatory movements. These concepts are highly interrelated and discussing them individually is somewhat misleading.

A client must be able to stabilize (hold) adequately at one joint and move at another. Proximally holding can be enhanced with techniques developed by Voss,[85] Bobath,[6] and Rood.[78]

Specific PNF techniques, such as "timing" and "timing for emphasis,"[85] can be used to reestablish sequencing, or small components of the task can be emphasized repeatedly as suggested by Bobath.[6] Functional electrical stimulation (FES) may be effective to reeducate timing problems. In addition, small, portable EMG biofeedback units are sometimes used to correct deficits in sequencing, timing, and strength of muscle firing. For example, in stance, a small unit attached to the gluteus medius provides the client with performance feedback. Electrical bracing can be used to enhance walking patterns. Repetition of correct patterns is important to reduce central processing speed, or lag time. Slowness is frustrating to clients, family members, and health professionals.

Coordinating both halves of the body is important. Midline activities as well as squatting and sliding begin to develop bilateral integration, as do bilateral, reciprocal activities. Jumping, minitrampoline activities, and moving boards can help refine this aspect of motor control.

Preparatory movements, discussed previously, place the body and limbs in an advantageous position for the movement itself. The head-injured client in Fig. 13-5, *A* maintained a slumped posture even when attempting to raise her arm overhead. In Fig. 13-5, *B* the therapist assists the client by facilitating an anterior pelvic tilt and upper back

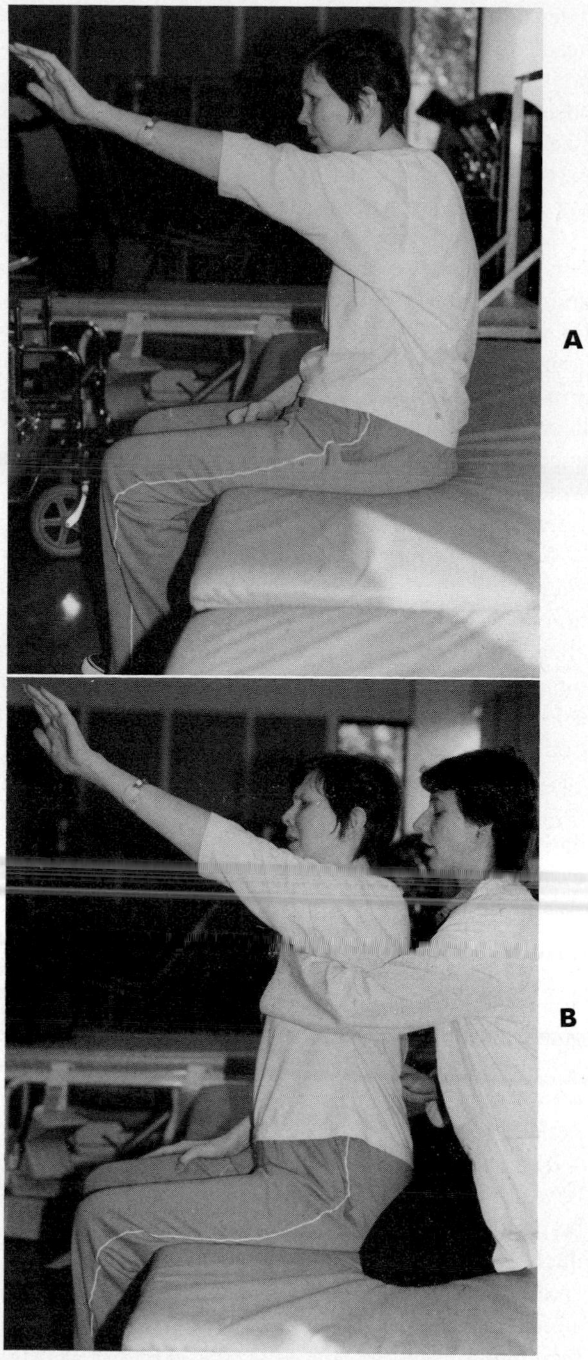

Fig. 13-5. A, Preparatory trunk movements are essential to provide postural stability immediately before some extremity movements. For example, spinal extension and an anterior pelvic tilt usually accompany elevating an arm overhead. However, head-injured clients frequently lack adequate preparatory movements and typically maintain trunk flexion while attempting this activity. **B,** The client maintained a slumped posture even when attempting to raise her arm overhead. The therapist can assist the client by facilitating an anterior pelvic tilt and upper back extension, which are preparatory movements for raising the arm overhead.

extension, which are preparatory for raising the arm over-head. Some preparatory movements can be practiced in a pool, where the movement can be supported and slowed adequately to allow the proper response without falling. Exercises that assist the client to learn and reestablish preparatory movements and patterns in sitting, rising to standing, and standing are important.

Muscle activation patterns, or selecting the proper pattern generator, is essential to movement. For example, when an individual who is standing reaches forward to turn on a light, the first muscle response is in the gastrocnemius to counteract the forward shift in the center of gravity as the arm moves forward. Again, providing the proper stimulus is critical. The therapist must realize that movements frequently require total body adjustments, that is, one cannot work on reaching the arm forward in standing without considering the required response in the trunk and legs.

Sensory retraining. The first sensory problem in the client with altered consciousness may be sensory deprivation. Sensory stimulation programs are used to increase client responsiveness. Sensory stimulation may increase input to the reticular activating system and may also avoid sensory deprivation, which adversely affects CNS function. When applying stimuli, the therapist should control environmental distractions and apply the stimuli in brief sessions one at a time to observe the response. Stimuli that the client can identify, such as familiar voices, may be more likely to evoke a response. Preferably, responses should be reinforced with verbal and nonverbal social interaction.[87] A variety of stimuli, including tactile, taste, smell, visual, auditory, vestibular, and kinesthetic sensations, should be presented and graded while allowing adequate time for a response. Once contact has been established with a client and sensation can be tested, sensory stimulation should be used only to achieve specific functional responses.[87]

Sensations may be distorted or intensified following head trauma. In such cases extraneous sensations should be minimized and directed stimuli can be introduced at reduced intensities. Lights can be lowered and touching decreased, for example. Desensitization procedures, designed to cause a client to accommodate to specific stimuli by administering the stimuli despite possible objections by the client, may or may not be effective in reducing hypersensitivity. Behavioral modification may be effective in some of these cases.

Sensations are likely to be reduced or absent. Reduced sensations, particularly cutaneous, proprioceptive, integrative, and special sensations, are frequently treated by "bombarding" a particular system with increased stimuli in an attempt to accommodate to a presumed higher threshold. The hope is that the threshold can be gradually changed. In addition to being a deficit itself, sensory damage profoundly affects motor function. For example, a client may rotate or tilt the head to suppress double vision.

This, in turn, may affect body alignment, postural tone, motor control, and coordination. The treatment consists of oculomotor exercises and corrective lenses, not necessarily improved head righting. Prism glasses might assist in cases of oculomotor dyskinesias (see Chapter 25). Retraining techniques may be useful—for example, in decreasing hypersalivation (see Chapter 24) and for improving olfaction.

Compensatory training, or substituting one system for another (such as visual for proprioceptive), may be necessary but may compromise the client's motor capabilities. Adaptive equipment may be used as compensation, such as the glasses mentioned above and augmented communication aids.

Increasing general cardiovascular fitness. Decreased general endurance or fitness is almost always a problem and can limit achievement of many therapy goals. The traditional methods for increasing aerobic fitness—a rhythmic activity using large muscle groups at the appropriate intensity as determined by a percentage of maximum predicted heart rate, sustained for an adequate duration (about 20 to 30 minutes) and performed with adequate frequency (3 to 5 days a week)—can be used or modified for head-injured clients. Stationary bicycles, upper-extremity ergometers, treadmills, restorators, rowing machines, swimming, or ordinary walking might all be as useful to the brain-injured person as they are to normal persons.

Combining movement components into composite functional tasks and ADL activities. The average client could care less if his or her gastrocnemius contracts at the proper time or if he or she achieves 180 degrees of shoulder flexion with or without participation of the trunk. The client *is* interested in being able to roll over, sit up, stand, walk, dress, groom, eat, communicate, and participate in leisure and work or school activities. In short, practicing and emphasizing only the components of motion will be unmotivating and unfulfilling to clients and families. *Therefore, it is exceptionally important that all work on components be integrated into meaningful activities and that meaningful activities be used to achieve progressively more challenging movement.* Overemphasis on components ignores the stimulus provided by previously overlearned activities. For example, continuing a mat exercise program until all the components of walking are achieved before having the client stand and attempt to walk probably will not be successful. The standing, weight-bearing, and weight-shifting activity is a stimulus for activating the sensations and patterns necessary for walking (note criterion *VBF* in the boxed material on page 376). The *specificity of training* principle applies here. Practicing gait components while side-lying on a mat may only enhance one's ability to perform gait-like movements while side-lying on a mat, and may not transfer to standing and walking patterns. Further aspects of transferring learning are discussed in the next section.

Transferring learning. It is noteworthy that the higher levels in Simpson's taxonomy of the psychomotor domain[73] include "adapting and originating responses." Too frequently, the client who can perform specified tasks in a formal setting in an automated way is discharged. Yet the client may be unable to function adequately in a different environment. There may be no carry-over if the client has not been taught the abilities to transfer and to create motor responses. Transfer of learning cannot be assumed to take place automatically. It, too, is a skill that can be taught by incorporating different environments and situations into the treatment. The same task may be presented under new conditions—for example, progressing from walking on level surfaces to walking upstairs creates the need for adaptation. Tasks not encountered before, such as stepping onto an escalator, can be presented to use previously learned components.

Not all clients can remaster the capacity to create original, or even adaptive, movements. Cognitive, behavioral, or physical disabilities or a combination of these disabilities may limit performance to rote, automatic movements. Other clients may always require guidance in motor performance. This relates to realistic determination of treatment goals.

Integrating the cognitive and behavioral aspects of human performance. The concept of sequencing is important in integrating the cognitive and behavioral elements of skills with the physical elements. Early activities may need to be structured and repetitive. The client may need to be asked to count, to repeat a series of warm-up exercises independently, or to sing songs or recall names, activities, or rationales while moving. Eventually, the client may be asked to suggest a game, analyze his or her own performance, "invent" a new exercise, "treat" the therapist, or teach another client or friend a skill. Involving clients in this manner not only assists them in learning and remembering the motor skills but also helps them develop their mental capabilities.

Cognitive or behavioral problems sometimes limit motor performance more than specific physical problems. Perhaps the client is apathetic and content to reap attention and secondary benefits. Perhaps the client is so aggressive that he or she is unable to receive adequate therapy. The treatment for these "motoric" problems is probably behavior modification.

An often overlooked aspect of physical care is using physical activity to affect changes in behavior rather than vice versa. Recreational therapists employ this concept, but other health professionals can use physical activity for this purpose as well. Williams,[63] one of the influential physical educators of the 1930s to the 1960s, advocated education *through* the physical, not just *by* the physical. He taught that recreational and sport activities enhanced self-esteem, individual responsibility, self-achievement, a sense of belonging, leadership, and acceptable standards of behavior. Games, group activities, and individual physical achievement could be goal-directed and structured to develop or modify specific behaviors.

The gist of this section can be summarized as follows: movements are exceedingly complex and involve numerous internal and external constraints. Efficient, effective treatment of motor skills depends on an accurate diagnosis of the specific problem or problems limiting the performance. Anything less is random treatment that may or may not lead to improved performance. Treatment by chance is tantamount to stealing money and time.

Selection of intervention strategies

The ability to select, evaluate, and revise a program and specific techniques is important in developing a successful, individualized treatment approach. Following are some of the criteria for analyzing intervention strategies (see the box on p. 376). If the plan has not been effective, perhaps the reason(s) can be identified. In this regard, criterion *IA* cannot be overlooked. Not all clients with traumatic head injury can improve even when provided with the best possible intervention.

Creation of an individualized treatment plan

This section of the chapter consists of two divisions: a discussion of the early management of clients and a discussion of the management of clients during later stages. Arbitrarily, the client who begins to respond appropriately is considered to be "recovering." Several sample cases with a mixture of problems are discussed in each section. The location of treatment during these stages can be the acute care hospital, rehabilitation center, private office, home, or combination of facilities.

The first case is developed in detail to demonstrate the problem-solving process of selecting intervention strategies. Additional cases are discussed more generally. These examples were selected to depict some of the possible management ideas for a variety of selected problems. The goals, plans, and problems used in the examples are not presented in their entirety. Only fairly discrete problems were selected for the purposes of this discussion.

Treatment planning may proceed either informally or formally, that is, in writing. Fig. 13-6, used in conjunction with the questions in the boxed material on p. 376, depicts a format for logically working through the process of developing a care plan. References are made to this information in the first sample case.

Early management

The flaccid and unresponsive client. An unidentified female client, injured 14 days ago in a motor vehicle accident, is in the intensive care unit of a large county hospital. She is being sustained with life-support equipment. A thorough and accurate evaluation was conducted, satisfying criteria *IIA* and *B* on p. 376. Following the initial evaluation the physician was contacted about specific treat-

Possible criteria for selecting, evaluating, and revising treatment programs, specific techniques, or both

I. Clinical/medical condition

Is the treatment program based on a clear understanding of the
A. Medical condition and extent of injury?
B. Precautions?
C. Extracranial injuries?
D. Endurance/physical condition?

II. Evaluation

Is the treatment plan based on
A. Accurate subjective and objective data?
B. A thorough evaluation?

III. Assessment/analysis of data

Is the treatment program based on
A. Specifically identified problems?
B. Consideration of prognostic indicators?

IV. Goal setting

Is the program based on goals that are
A. Appropriate for level of function?
B. Realistic according to positive and negative prognostic indicators?
C. Measurable?
D. Ranked by priority?
E. Developed by the rehabilitation team?
F. Consistent with recovery mechanisms?

V. Plan

Is/does the treatment program/technique
A. Selected to accomplish specific goals for problems in *each system?* For example, the goals for motor performance may be suggested by
  1. Mobility
  2. Stability
    a. Tonic holding
    b. Cocontraction
  3. Controlled mobility
  4. Skill
    a. Locomotion
    b. Manipulation[78]
  5. Postural reflex mechanism integration
  6. Flexibility
  7. Muscular endurance
  8. Strength
  9. Movement and response speeds
  10. Movement pattern composition
  11. Nonequilibrium coordination
  12. Balance
  13. Cardiovascular endurance/fitness
  14. Sensory retraining

B. Matched to environmental and biomechanical constraints?
C. Selected from among alternatives?
D. Based on current rationale?
E. Sequenced according to development of skill(s)?
F. Started at the appropriate level, including activities at least one (or two) levels beyond current function?
G. Age, status, and morphologically appropriate?
H. Based on learning principles?
  1. Optimal environment
  2. Motivating
  3. Functional or purposeful
  4. Active versus passive when possible
  5. Reinforced through repetition, reward, success
  6. Provision for transfer of learning
I. Involve the family?
J. Incorporate higher-level involvement?
  1. Perceptual motor activities
  2. Cognitive (memory, communication) activities
  3. Behavioral retraining
K. Based on administrative considerations?
  1. Economical for client and therapist
  2. Make best use of available time
L. Provide for carry-over throughout additional activities?

VI. Implementation

Is the treatment program/techniques implemented
A. Specifically consistent with the goals and plans?
B. In an optimal position for the client and therapist?
C. Such that stimuli presented is consistent with the desired response?
D. Consistent with patterns of movement (including preparatory movements)?
E. With specific criteria to control stimuli (for example, speed and intensity)?
F. Skillfully?

VII. Reevaluation

Is the program/technique
A. Modified in keeping with client responses?
B. Progressive?
C. Achieving the goals?

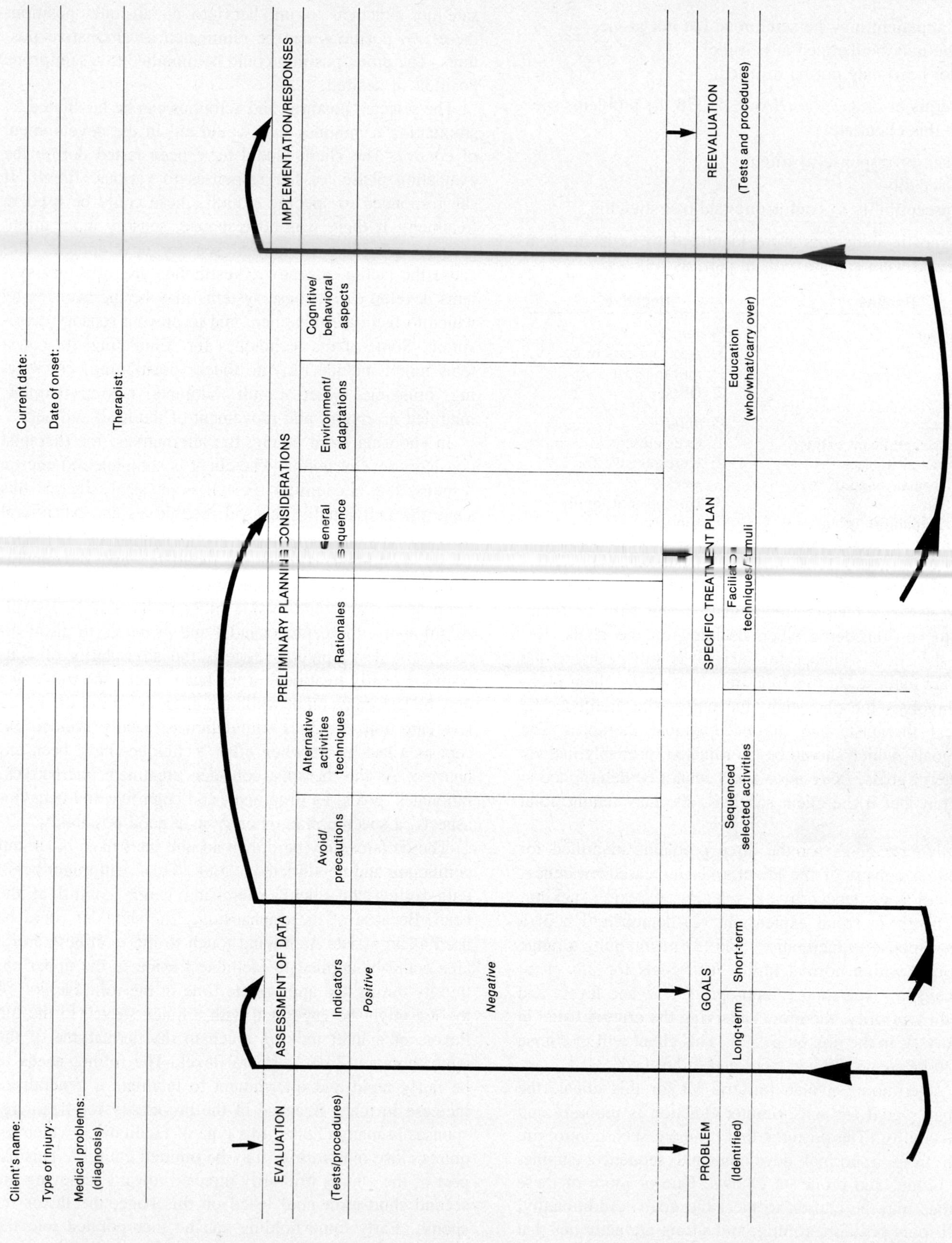

Client's name: _____

Type of injury: _____

Medical problems: _____
(diagnosis) _____

Current date: _____

Date of onset: _____

Therapist: _____

EVALUATION

(Tests/procedures)

ASSESSMENT OF DATA

Indicators	Avoid/ precautions	Alternative activities techniques
Positive		
Negative		

PRELIMINARY PLANNING CONSIDERATIONS

Rationales	General sequence	Environment/ adaptations	Cognitive/ behavioral aspects

IMPLEMENTATION/RESPONSES

PROBLEM

(Identified)

GOALS

Long-term	Short-term

SPECIFIC TREATMENT PLAN

Sequenced selected activities	Facilitation techniques/stimuli	Education (who/what/carry over)

REEVALUATION

(Tests and procedures)

Fig. 13-6. Treatment planning guide. Note the direction of the arrows when attempting to read or use guide.

ment precautions in regard to positions and movements. The following guidelines were given:

- The patient may lie semiprone but not prone.
- She may be dangled at bedside.
- Her head may not be inverted.

In terms of criteria on *IIIA* on p. 376 the problems specific to this client are

- Lack of response to stimuli
- Flaccidity
- Susceptibility to contracture and overstretching

Prognostic indicators were identified to assist in goal setting and were categorized, in part, as follows:

Positive	Negative
Preinjury	*Preinjury*
Unknown	1. Age (appears to be mid-thirties)
	2. Obese
Postinjury	*Postinjury*
1. No significant extracranial injuries	1. Eyes closed
2. Normal range of motion	2. Unresponsive for 2 weeks
3. Availability of equipment and expert care	3. No apparent family support
	4. No return of sensorimotor function
	5. Need for ventilator

The negative factors predominate in this case, and they need to be considered when deciding on the goals. Because the client's chance for survival is still in doubt, the goals are modest. At this time treatment of the client probably involves the physician, the nurse, the dietitian, the physical therapist, and the occupational therapist. The team goals, which should be coordinated, probably include short-term goals. *Long-term goals* cannot be determined at this time, but if the client survives, she may require total care.

Short-term goals for the three problems identified for discussion consist of the client's (1) increased awareness to stimuli as evidenced by eye opening, reflexing sucking, or a change in facial expression, (2) demonstration of a flexor response to facilitation, and (3) maintaining a range of motion within normal limits. The goals for this client are realistic, measurable, appropriate for her level, and ranked by priority, therefore satisfying the criteria listed in category *IV* in the box on p. 376. This client will of course need to be treated in her room and in her bed.

In determining a plan (criteria *V*) for this client, the therapist's goal for sensorimotor function is mobility and early stability. The postures that promote such control are drawn from a normal developmental sequence: supine, pivot prone, and prone on elbows. One or more of these activities may be chosen to meet the goals. Additionally, the all-fours position, rolling, and sitting are activities that might satisfy criterion *VF*, which suggests that activities

beyond the current level of function be initiated. However, because the client cannot lie prone and it would be neither safe nor practical to put her into an all-fours position, these two positions can be eliminated as alternative postures. The prone position could be modified to a semiprone position, if desired.

The selected postures and activities can be facilitated by stimulation techniques that would aid in the development of control. The client would have been tested during the evaluation phase for her responses to various stimuli. If she responded to specific stimuli, these could be used in treatment. If there was no response, sensory input might proceed according to normal sensory development. Because the tactile, gustatory, vestibular, and olfactory systems develop early, these systems may be the avenues by which to facilitate this client and to prevent sensory deprivation. Some of the techniques for stimulating these systems might include moving touch, positioning, quick icing, brushing, sweet stimuli, odorants, noxious stimuli, modified inversion, and movement of the head and neck.

In choosing from among the alternatives, the therapist considers several points. The client is stimulated to elicit a response that is cognitive as well as physical, since at this stage the individual's physical, cognitive, and behavioral activities are intertwined and nearly inseparable (see Fig. 13-1). Vestibular stimulation facilitates eye movement, tone, and arousal; therefore, modified inversion and anteroposterior and side-to-side movements may be useful. Additionally, the cephalocaudal and proximal to distal direction of development suggests the advisability of concentrating early treatment at the head, neck, and trunk. Ice may be less convenient while the client is still in the intensive care unit. Noxious stimulation is usually avoided except as a last resort when other techniques have been exhausted. As the therapist considers treatment alternatives, rationales, goals, environment, and cognitive and behavior aspects, a specific plan emerges as a good possibility.

The curtains may be drawn around the bed to block out conflicting and nondirected stimuli. Treatment might begin with rolling the client, exercising gentle control at the head. Because of the tracheostomy the shoulder could be used as an assist. A moving touch to the midline perioral area could be applied to facilitate flexion of the upper extremity during the appropriate time in the roll. Flexion of the leg might be expedited with a quick stretch to the hip flexors or a light moving touch to the dermatome of the tenth thoracic (T10) vertebral level. The rolling needs to be fairly rapid and intermittent to facilitate a generalized increase in tone. Because of the propensity for flexor responses in many clients, this type of facilitation, which requires close monitoring, may be omitted entirely. This aspect of the plan is primarily directed toward achieving the second short-term goal listed on this page, the flexor response. Early tonic holding can be incorporated into the next sequence.

For the first short-term goal, increased client awareness, cautious vestibular stimulation and an oral facilitation program are selected. The client might be rolled and brought to a sitting position with her legs over the side of the bed. Sitting would require the assistance of a second person, but the value of out of bed treatment cannot be overemphasized. The client's feet should be supported on the floor or a stool. Since her head cannot literally be inverted, the position can be modified by leaning her trunk forward while she is seated. Her arms can be supported on elbows using a bed-tray table. Thus there would be the facilitatory effect of weight bearing through the upper and lower extremities. Gentle approximation of the client's head can be provided by the supporting person while the therapist applies additional cautious stimulation to the vestibular system. The early treatments may use only one type of stimulation with a gradual buildup as each type of stimulation is tolerated. Again, if the vestibular stimulation is to be facilitating, it should be fairly rapid and intermittent rather than slow and rhythmical. Motion can at first be in the form of anteroposterior rocking or shaking and progress to a side-to-side movement, later incorporating head and trunk rotation. As with any vestibular stimulation, the effects need to be carefully monitored.

While the client is sitting, either in a chair or an elevated bed, pleasant gustatory and olfactory stimuli might be introduced. The client's favorite flavors and scents, if known, would be chosen. The therapist observes the client for changes in muscle tone, facial expression, or reflex sucking. The therapist might press on the client's eyelids to elicit eye opening, limb movement, or other adaptive responses.

The third short-term goal selected for this client would be partially met during the rolling and sitting activities, since they would simultaneously move the client's joints. If needed, slow and gentle stretch might be used as a supplement for areas susceptible to contracture, such as the heel cords and hamstrings. However, it is a positioning program that is critical to achieving this goal. Preferably, the client would be positioned in side lying to reduce the effects of the tonic labrythine reflexes and for skin care. The upward arm and leg would need support as would her wrists and hands. Her feet should be supported in a neutral ankle position with a splint or shoe that is cut off at the toes, exposing the ball of the foot to avoid stimulating a positive supporting reflex.

Activities stressed for carry-over with the nurses (and family when available) would be the positioning plan, segmental rolling, and frequent sitting in a semireclined high-backed chair or a specially modified wheelchair. The frequent sitting provides stimulation, and it will gradually build endurance. The nurses need to be aware of the importance of their role in providing cutaneous stimulation during bathing and mouth care. This realization may make their job more interesting and rewarding.

Because of the client's condition, the treatment sessions should be short and frequent. This may mean physical therapy twice a day and occupational therapy twice a day, appropriately spaced. Gustatory and olfactory stimuli may be more effective before the client has been fed and should be timed accordingly. The vestibular stimulation, on the other hand, might be better tolerated on an empty stomach. Consistency of the treatment time, the sequence of activities, and the care providers are important in laying the groundwork for trust. Of course the therapists and nurses should talk to the client before, during, and after the treatment. This client also needs a specific pulmonary toilet program and skin care, although moving and sitting are helpful in prevention of pneumonia and bed sores. When this client's family is located, more individualized information may be obtained. Fig. 13-7 shows the partially developed intervention plan for this client.

The remaining sample cases in this section are discussed less extensively, but the process for creating an individualized treatment plan is the same. These cases are not necessarily progressions of each other. Each represents examples of varying combinations of physical, cognitive, and behavioral problems that might be encountered, in full or in part, at any time during a client's recovery.

The bedridden client who exhibits severe extensor responses (decerebrate) and generalized responses to stimuli. Internal and external stimuli cause opisthotonos posturing. The problems and goals of treatment for such a client are in the areas of *tone* and *movement*. It is hoped that this type of client will be referred very early for therapy since contractures can develop rapidly and hinder rehabilitation during recovery stages. Therapists can facilitate early referral by acquainting themselves with the intensive care nurses, who are in daily contact with the physicians. This rapport can be developed formally through in-service education and informally on an individual basis. Maintaining respect and open communication with these nurses during the client's stay in the intensive care unit and then returning clients to the unit for a visit after substantial recovery may also assist in fostering rapport.

The key aspects of the physical management of this client include positioning, gentle handling, and facilitating movement. The initial position of choice for treatment may be side lying or semiprone to decrease the influence of the tonic labyrinthine reflex in supine. If the client must remain supine, flexion can be incorporated by elevating the head of the bed and flexing the hips and knees. Rolling may be an additional treatment activity.

The therapist will need to be sensitive to the client's responses to manual contacts and the speed of the movements. Rotation of the trunk and proximal parts of the extremities may assist with exercising the client, as may gentle shaking or rocking. Treatment may require two people. Precautions would be to handle the joints gently and to avoid overstretching. Facilitation of movement would pro-

Current date: 3/28
Date of onset: 3/14
Therapist: S. Smith, PT

Client's name: (Unidentified)
Type of injury: Traumatic head injury MVA
Medical problems: Comatose
(diagnoses): Tracheostomy
Abrasions

EVALUATION (Test/procedures)	ASSESSMENT Indicators	PRELIMINARY PLANNING CONSIDERATIONS — Avoid/precautions	Alternative activities/technique	Rationales	General sequence	Environment/adaptations	Cognitive/behavioral aspects	IMPLEMENTATION/RESPONSE

1. Screening systems
2. Cerebral function
  a. General
  b. Specific
3. ANS
4. Sensory function
  a. Pain reaction
5. Motor function
  a. Developmental level
  b. Tone
  c. Quality of movement
  d. Muscle length (ROM)
	Positive
	1. No significant extracranial injuries
	2. Normal ROM
	3. Availability of equipment/care
	
	Negative
	1. Age
	2. Obesity
	3. Eye closed
	4. Unresponsive for 2 weeks
	5. No family support
	6. No return of sensorimotor function
	7. Need for ventilation
		1. Prone lying
		2. Inversion
			1. Activity ideas:
			  a. Supine
			  b. Pivot
			  c. Prone on elbows
			  d. All fours
			  e. Rolling
			  f. Sitting
			2. Technique ideas:
			  a. Touch
			  b. Smell
			  c. Taste
			  d. Positioning
			  e. Noxious stimuli
			  f. Modified inversion
			  g. Movements of head and neck
			  h. Quick icing
			  i. Quick stretch
			  j. Weight bearing
			  k. Approximation
				1. Prone positioning eliminated. All fours impractical. Rolling stimulates motor and cognitive responses and sitting is the advanced posture indicated
				2. Cognitive and motor responses can be stimulated through vestibular system. Concentration on head/neck/trunk and early sensory stimulation. Icing less convenient and noxious stimuli used as a last resort. Therefore use: a, b, c, d, f, g, j, k, maybe i. Apply stimuli in facilitatory manner
					1. Cephalocaudal
					2. Proximal to distal (head/neck/trunk)
					3. Developmental sequence activities roll → sit → oral stimulation program
						1. Draw curtains around bed
						2. One aide/one therapist
						3. Consistent times, caregivers, activities
						4. Short frequent sessions
							1. Talk to client
							2. Facilitatory voice tones
							3. Facilitatory stimuli
							4. Vestibular stimuli
								1.
								
								2.

PROBLEM (Identified)	GOALS — Long-term	Short-term	SPECIFIC TREATMENT PLAN — Sequenced selected activities	Facilitation technique/stimuli	Education (who/what/carry over)	REEVALUATION (Tests and procedures)

1. Flaccid
 	
2. Unresponsive to stimuli
 	
3. Susceptibility to contracture and overstretching
	1. Undetermined 4/28	1. Increase awareness to stimuli as evidenced by eye opening, reflex sucking, or change in facial expression
		2. Demonstrate a flexor response to facilitation
		3. Have ROM maintained WNL
			1. Rolling → sitting, rolling in bed
			
			2. Rolling → sitting, oral facilitation
			
			3. Positioning and handling
				1. a. Control at head
				  b. Moving touch to perioral area
				  c. Quick stretch to hip flexors or lt. moving touch to T10 dermatons
				  d. Rapid and intermittent stimuli
				2. a. Modified inversion (sitting)
				  b. UE and LE weight bearing
				  c. Approximation of head
				  d. Pleasant gustatory and olfactory stimuli
				3. a. 1 and 2 above
				  b. Slow bentle stretch
				  c. Positioning aids
					1. Nurses:
					  Positioning
					  Handling
					  Segmental rolling
					  Increased sitting
					  Sensory stimulation
						1. Observation of eye opening, reflex sucking, change in facial expression with stimuli
						2. Motor function: Flexor response Tone change Quality of movement
						3. Muscle length (ROM)

Fig. 13-7. Partially completed sample treatment planning guide for the first case discussed in the chapter.

ceed cautiously to avoid also facilitating further muscle tone. Determining the threshold for abnormal reactions is important in this case.

In conjunction with the handling program, positioning is critical; positioning is generally in reflex-inhibiting patterns toward positions opposite those of the client's tendencies. Pads and wedges cut out of dense foam and then covered can be "custom-made" to assist in optimal positioning of the client. The neck and trunk positions are also considered. The client who continually rests with the head rotated to one side may develop unilateral trunk shortening. Positioning and movement can help prevent such a problem. Serial casts can be applied, especially to the feet, ankles, and elbows, if splints and ROM activities are insufficient to control contracture formation. Serial casts are applied with the extremity in functional, tone-inhibiting positions and are changed every 7 to 14 days. Alternatively, inflatable air splints could be used for some clients. Air splints provide some of the benefits of casting without many of its inconveniences. Cones can be placed in the client's hands and maintained with Velcro straps, or finger spreaders might be used. Photographs of proper positioning placed at bedside may aid in compliance with the positioning program.

Because spasticity of the neck and trunk and prolonged use of respiratory equipment reduce chest expansion, manual chest stretching and facilitation of involuntary respiration are important aspects of this client's care. Prevention of sensory deprivation, which was discussed previously in this chapter, is also crucial. This stage of injury, characterized by severe extensor responses and generalized responses to stimuli, can last for an extended period, and it is important that the therapists, physicians, family, and nurses not become discouraged.

The client who exhibits moderately severe flexor spasticity and lethargic responses. A female client (A.S.) demonstrates brainstem-level reflexes and moderately severe flexor responses of the head, neck, trunk, and extremities. A.S. should be dressed and treated in the therapy department in an environment uncomplicated in sights and sounds. The aspects of A.S.'s treatment plan addressed in this discussion are (1) normalizing her tone, (2) integrating the brainstem-level reflexes, (3) developing stability (primarily in her head, neck, and trunk), and (4) stimulating arousal.

The activities selected for A.S.'s level might include pivot prone, prone on elbows, prone on extended arms, and rolling. More advanced postures should also be initiated, including sitting, all fours, kneeling, half kneeling, and perhaps standing in a standing table. Unlike the first case, A.S. does have tone that permits more advanced postures. Of course, positions and activities that produce undesirable responses can be postponed or modified to include the important component parts.

Vestibular stimulation, particularly inversion, may reduce tone and facilitate trunk extension and cocontraction at the neck. Prone lying over a large ball or barrel could be used and A.S. moved in an anteroposterior direction. Because her neck flexors are overactive and because the extensors are postural muscles, the client's head should be supported in a mid-to-shortened position of postural neck extension. She would be unable to extend her neck from the extreme range. Pictures of family or pets could be placed low and used as visual stimuli to facilitate the head righting. Proprioceptive stimuli, such as approximation to the head and neck, might assist with the cocontraction, but they should be added gradually as previous responses are assessed.

Prone on elbows, perhaps using a wedge as illustrated with the male client in Fig. 13-8, would be another position from which to treat A.S. Prone on elbows would facilitate extension and also cocontraction of the shoulders. Again, visual stimuli and approximation might be useful adjuncts. Vibration with an electric vibrator may facilitate the neck and upper trunk extensors. A.S. could also be moved in an anteroposterior and side-to-side direction in this position. Segmental rolling can be facilitated in transitional movements between treatment postures. This client could be treated in sitting, all fours, and kneeling (Fig. 13-9) positions.

One dilemma in a lethargic yet spastic client such as A.S. is the intensity and speed at which the stimuli might best be applied. To relax the tone would require slow, rhythmical movements. However, this client needs to be cognitively aroused. It may be possible to determine a speed that is arousing but below the threshold for the undesired motor responses. Fig. 13-10 illustrates an activity that can be easily modified to achieve the desired level of stimulation. Perhaps some types of stimulation will cause arousal without changing muscle tone, or perhaps there are consistent times during the day when the client is more alert. Alertness may be evidenced by more eye tracking and a less glazed look. If so, treatment may be more beneficial at these times. Otherwise, the therapist may need to prioritize the goals and temporarily sacrifice one for the other during a phase of the treatment. For example, cognitive stimulation would likely be of primary importance should such a choice be required.

A prefeeding, positioning, and pulmonary program would be indicated for A.S., as would education of the family and nursing staff. Their education would include methods of stimulating this client visually (as with pictures and bright colors), through sound (by talking to her, playing tape recordings of familiar voices, and intermittently using television and radio), and by touch and movement. Some facilities even permit pet-client visitation privileges as a means of stimulation, or use specially trained dogs to facilitate client interaction.

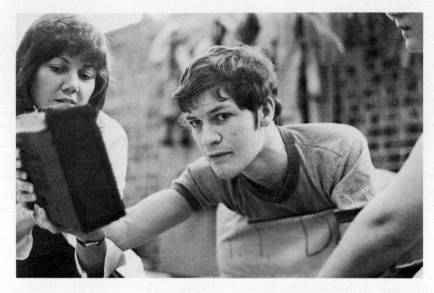

Fig. 13-8. Prone on elbows stimulates a contraction of the muscles of the head, neck, scapulae, and upper trunk and inhibits lower-extremity flexor spasticity. Weight bearing through the elbows may activate tonic shoulder musculature and promote proximal stability. A wedge to support the trunk and visual stimuli further assist in facilitating head control.

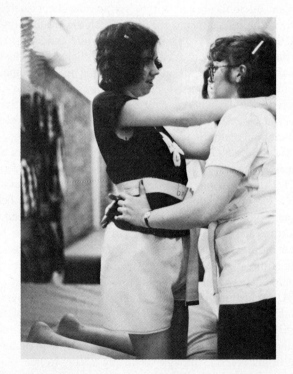

Fig. 13-9. The kneeling position places the lower extremities in a combination of hip extension with knee flexion and enhances trunk control and balance. This position can be assumed as the client gains adequate hamstring, quadriceps, and hip extensor tone. Initially, stability can be facilitated at the pelvis using manual approximation. A later progression would be controlled mobility activities in this position.

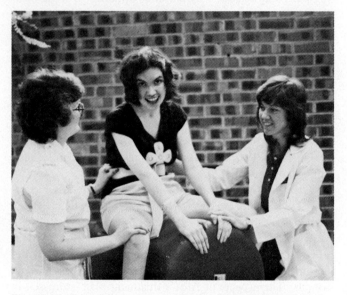

Fig. 13-10. Stimulation of the vestibular system can result in facilitatory or inhibitory motor and cognitive responses, depending on the speed, direction, and rhythmicity with which the labrythine mechanisms are activated. The side-to-side movements also facilitate weight shifting.

The apathetic client who has moderate extensor responses and responds inconsistently to stimuli and commands. Three basic aspects of a program are discussed: (1) motivating and increasing the consistency of responses, (2) facilitating head control in the presence of extensor responses, and (3) temporary wheelchair adaptations.

A male client, R.T., needs consistent and repetitive orienting explanations as to the reason for hospitalization, the name and location of the hospital, the whereabouts of his family, the season, dates, times, locations of treatments, names of therapists, and reasons for therapy. This sort of orienting, which may be a one-way conversation, needs to continue until the client is more capable of recalling these facts on his own.

R.T. seems apathetic. He has followed commands but does so inconsistently. Once again the client needs arousal without increasing tone. General body activities requiring active versus passive participation promote arousal and attending behaviors. During treatment, when the therapist observes that R.T. is more alert, he can be instructed to participate in goal directed and preferably "overlearned" functional activities. The therapist must select an activity that the client is capable of managing and must position him for doing so. The activity should also be interesting and motivating. Commands need to be simple (one-step), and extra time should be allotted for a delay in response. Once the command is given, the therapist must expect completion. The client will begin to understand the expectations and to recognize that the therapist cannot be manipulated. Once the task is completed, the performance is appropriately rewarded. The therapist is employing learning principles.

Another problem encountered with a client like R.T. is that many of the activities that would facilitate cocontraction of the neck also facilitate extensor tone. Therefore activities such as those selected for the client with flexor responses (A.S.) require modification. For example, the inverted position prone over a ball, as shown with the female client in Fig. 13-11, *A* and *B*, facilitates not only the trunk extensors but also the quadriceps and the gastrocnemius-soleus muscle groups. To reduce this effect and yet facilitate the upper back extensors and neck cocontraction, the legs may need to be flexed at the knees as demonstrated in Fig. 13-11, *C*. Or the client may sit with the knees flexed, ankles dorsiflexed, and feet supported (that is, weight bearing), and then lean forward from the waist. A low stool or bench is useful for this purpose. The client in Fig. 13-12, *A* is unable to sit independently. However, when his extensor tone is relaxed with trunk flexion and rotation (Fig. 13-12, *B*), abduction and rotation of the upper extremities (Fig. 13-12, *C*) and upper-extremity weight bearing using a table, the client is able to sit and control his head (Fig. 13-12, *D*). Gravity provides resistance and helps develop internal stretch sensitivity and strength.

The client is asked to perform an activity that not only reinforces the motor performance on a subcortical level but also incorporates the cognitive (e.g., attending, recalling, sequencing) and behavioral (e.g., cooperation, interest, initiative) aspects of care. For instance, while sitting, the client could turn the pages of a favorite magazine, flip through family photographs, or look at a camera and smile. As already mentioned, follow-through of the command by the client is expected, even if it takes several minutes to encourage the response.

The client with general extensor tone and positive supporting reactions tends to continually slide the hips forward out of chairs. Chair adaptations might be needed to counteract this. The modifications already suggested for facilitating the head and trunk provide clues. The hips need to be flexed. Placing wedges on the seat and foot pedals of the client's chair assist with positioning. Wedges of various sizes can be prefabricated and used as needed, or the thighs can be flexed with bolsters or firm towel rolls. The feet can be splinted or strapped onto the wedges with the balls of the feet left unsupported to avoid eliciting a positive supporting reaction. Toe spreaders can be used to reduce toe clawing. A firm hip abduction device might be needed if scissoring is a problem. A small lumbar roll and lateral trunk supports may aid in aligning the head and trunk, and a dynamic or static head-support system may be required. Use of head supports, knee spreaders, and similar devices should be closely monitored. If the client exerts spastic forces against the system, increased tone could develop. Keener and Sweigart[46] describe a temporary, reusable adaptive seat insert that can be individually fitted and easily readjusted as the client's needs change. A wheelchair tray table, which would promote upper-extremity weight bearing, symmetry, and bilateral activities, should also be used. If wrists and fingers are flexed, the client could grasp cones mounted onto the tray table, which are positioned with the shoulders protracted. Foam finger spreaders might be used in place of the cones and the arms left free.

Work with respiratory and abdominal muscles might be used to stimulate speech with this client. Additional aspects of care would include family instruction in positioning, wheelchair modifications, orienting explanations, and motivating the client.

The client who is hyperactive, confused, and nonaggressive. D.N. is restless and exhibits perseveration in activities and phrases. She is disoriented and has little recall of present events; she has no awareness of concurrent activities. Often D.N. will parrot words or phrases. She may speak incoherently but will occasionally "tune in" and respond appropriately to questions and commands in an automatic way. Frequently, clients like D.N. also demonstrate, in a tremor-like manner, perseveration in a motor activity, such as rapidly alternating elbow flexion and extension. The constant activity can be harmful if it is either "intentionally" self-abusive or if the client recklessly strikes against objects.

Two aspects of D.N.'s treatment plan deal with *hyperactivity* and *confusion*. Restraints and medication are sometimes used during this stage of recovery; however, neither is recommended unless they cannot be avoided since both can increase the agitation and confusion. As a substitute for restraints, the bed can be padded with foam

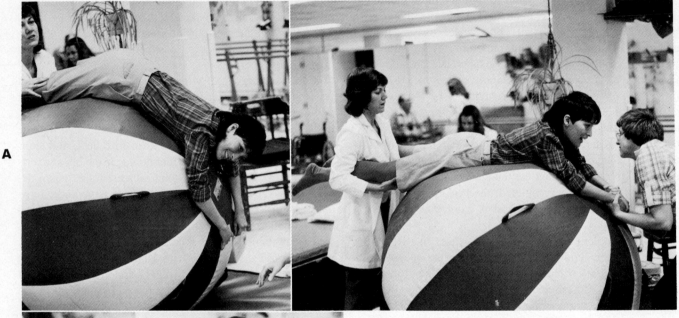

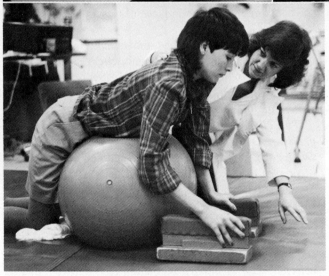

Fig. 13-11. A, The inverted position generally reduces hypertonicity. Gentle anteroposterior movement in this position promotes further relaxation. **B,** Inversion facilitates the neck and trunk extensors in addition to other extensor muscles such as the gluteus maximus, quadriceps, gastrocnemius, and soleus. **C,** To decrease the facilitatory effect of inversion on the lower extremity extensor musculature, the legs can be flexed at the hips and knees. The extremity weight bearing reduces extensor tone by placing pressure on the patellar tendons and by maintaining a prolonged stretch of the quadriceps. This position facilitates proximal stability of the hips and shoulders. Care is taken to avoid maintained stretch on the finger flexors.

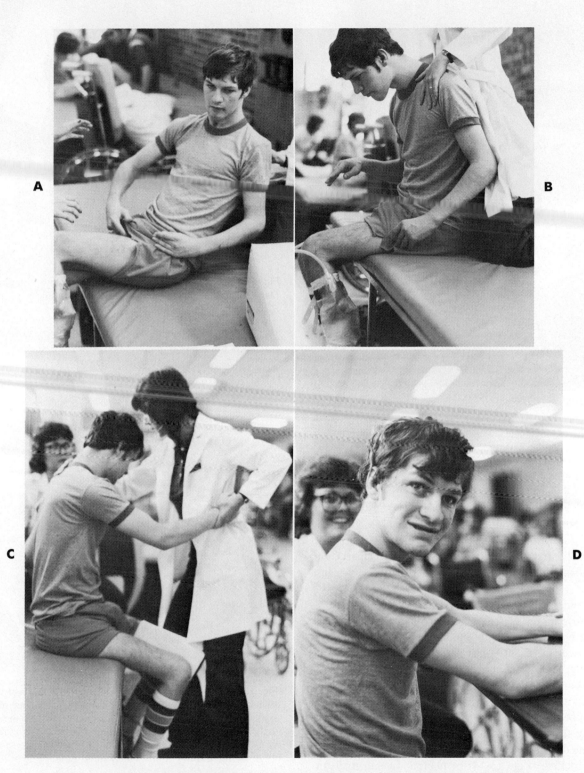

Fig. 13-12. A, This client is unable to sit independently because of extensor hypertonicity. **B,** The extensor hypertonicity can be reduced by rotating and flexing the trunk at the hips. Approximating at various points in the range promotes stability. **C,** Abduction and external rotation of the upper extremities further normalizes tone. **D,** These preparations, combined with upper- and lower-extremity weight bearing, permit independent sitting.

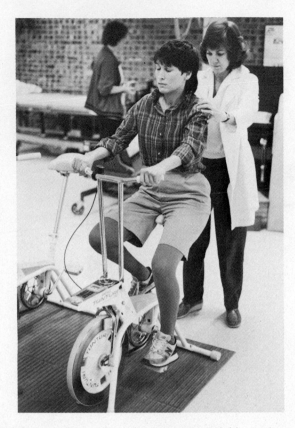

Fig. 13-13. Active, reciprocal, gross motor activities such as stationary cycling can calm agitated clients, foster muscular endurance, increase movement speed, promote cardiovascular fitness, and help prepare the lower extremities for ambulation.

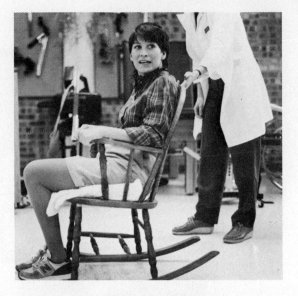

Fig. 13-14. Slow rocking, an adaptation of anteroposterior vestibular stimulation, promotes generalized inhibition.

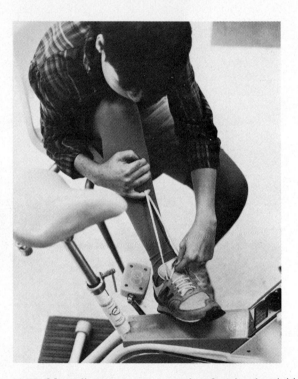

Fig. 13-15. Most clients seem to respond to functional activities such as dressing. Sitting, leaning forward (as to put on shoes) simulates the inverted position and actively involves the client in the treatment. This is also an example of integrating components of movement into a meaningful activity and using the same activity to further develop motor components.

and mittens can be used for the client who scratches, or air splints can be applied. Some facilities substitute floor mats for beds and furniture in the clients' rooms to avoid the need for restraints and to decrease the potential for injuries. Clients at this stage require constant supervision. For medication to be effective the dosage may cause lethargy.

Like hyperactive children, these clients may require directed gross motor activities before inhibitive techniques. These activities use clients' energy constructively and in essence wear them out. Active, reciprocal exercises, such as walking, stair climbing, or stationary cycling (Fig. 13-13), can be performed. If adequate balance or coordination for such activities is lacking, two people can assist the client. Weather permitting, the walk might take place outside and away from the hospital environment. Once the client has fatigued somewhat, general inhibitive techniques such as slow rocking (Fig. 13-14) or neutral warmth may further quiet the client. Weight bearing on the extremity exhibiting perseveration during the activity may decrease it, particularly if the client's attention is drawn elsewhere. Alternatively, engaging the client in an activity using the extremity may be effective. Few demands can be made of D.N., but she may respond better to functional activities such as dressing or drinking from a drinking fountain than

to specific exercises. With imagination these activities can be carefully selected to accomplish specific goals. For example, sitting and leaning forward to put on shoes as shown in Fig. 13-15 simulates the inverted position and thus the therapist can facilitate righting and equilibrium reactions. Frequently, this sequence of treatment precedes other treatments, such as speech therapy, that require a calmer, more responsive client. As the periods of calm increase, activities that demand increased attention and selective attention can be gradually added.

Because D.N. has difficulty with attending processes and with differentiating among stimuli, the treatment environment should control external stimuli. In a busy department this may entail treating a client at a time when the department is less busy or moving a floor mat into a private treatment area. Structure is provided both externally (treatments are scheduled at the same times each day) and internally (the treatment sequence is similar). The therapist, of course, uses a slow, calming voice, gives simple, concrete instructions, continually orients the client, makes references to familiar people and things, and explains what is going on during treatment. A brief home pass during this stage sometimes remarkably decreases confusion. Given the chance, families can be quite resourceful, and they may be more capable of handling the client than previously realized.

The client who is agitated, confused, hostile, and uncooperative. Uncooperative clients whose physical status permits may exhibit predictable or unpredictable combative behaviors. They may hit, bite, or punch those around them. They frequently repeat profanity and use abusive language. These reactions are governed behaviorally rather than cognitively. The client acts from the frightened, sympathetic "fight or flight" mode. These behaviors are recognized as a stage of recovery that usually passes in 2 to 3 weeks. Most clients never recall their actions during this stage of recovery. Clients' behaviors are organically induced, and they cannot be held accountable for their actions at this time any more than they can be blamed for being hemiplegic. Even though this is a stage, it is still a highly individualized period.

Several problems require attention in treating an agitated client. Those stimuli that seem to agitate the client are removed if possible. The therapist must be actively observant. For some clients a family member's presence during treatment is calming; for others, it is agitating. Some clients are intermittently agitated; others are more constantly agitated. Some are hypersensitive to touch; others appear reassured by touch. Placing demands on the client, however, seems almost universally agitating. The therapist cannot allow contractures to develop or to entirely waste rehabilitation time, even though the client's capacity for learning is diminished. The therapist must speak in a calm, controlled voice, and avoid sounding condescending when calming this client, because some individuals seem capable of responding to the therapist's tones and behaviors if not the intent. The client must still be treated with respect.

The importance of the environment, of orienting explanations and of structure has already been discussed. Unlike D.N., this client may be entirely calm unless provoked. Involving such a person in an activity requires patience. The therapist must gradually "warm up" to the client.

Sometimes the individual can be persuaded to perform functional-type activities for a reward such as food or perform activities of interest, such as shooting baskets (throwing a ball into a trash can). When the weather permits, being outdoors in a peaceful location seems soothing. The therapist needs to remain calm but firm and consistent. Otherwise, clients learn that they can have their own way and need not be cooperative.

Because a client in this stage can be cooperative and then turn suddenly hostile, the therapist needs readily available help. Merely reaching an arm across the client's face may elicit a bite. Fortunately for the therapist, these clients' attention can be diverted fairly easily since their attention span is short.

In more extreme cases of uncooperative or persisting hostile behavior, behavior modification can be instituted, and it may prevent persistent behavioral problems later. When the client is abusive, the therapist may simply leave (with the client in a safe situation). Wood[88] calls this *time-out-on-the-spot (TOOTS)*, the purpose of which is to deny attention. The therapist can then return with the same request when the individual has calmed down. Once this is begun, however, the client must comply, even if it takes a couple of hours. To be effective, all persons, including the family, need to adopt a similar attitude. Family education is very important for carry-over. The family is typically so delighted that their loved one is alive and beginning to respond that they have difficulty with disciplining the client and understanding this stage.

The client who exhibits a dissociation between voluntary and involuntary activities. C.L. has not reached a level where he can be more formally tested for apraxia, and the therapist may observe him using an extremity for activities—something he is unable to perform on request. C.L. may respond to activities that are directed yet automatic, such as rolling a ball, turning pages of a magazine, or holding an object as in preparation for use by the dominant hand. This observed dissociation of voluntary and automatic movement might also be true of other activities, although less apparent because of abnormal tone. Stationary cycling might trigger an automatic response in a client like C.L.; it could be tried, provided he could be situated and held safely on a bicycle. Modifying the cycle with C.L. seated in a chair and his feet strapped to the pedals might not trigger the same automatic response. C.L. might also assist with routine dressing activities. He may perform coordinated activities that appear beyond his overall level because these are automatic, overlearned activities. No new learning is required. These activities will actively involve the client in the treatment, which is important throughout recovery. (Concrete suggestions for management of clients with apraxia are discussed in Chapter 11.)

Management during later recovery stages. As the brain injury stabilizes, the client may have a variety of residual physical deficits, as noted in the section on sequelae. Hemiparesis is common. Therapists are familiar with most of the physical problems manifested in the later stages of physical recovery. Clients may require normalization of tone, facilitation of selective movements, integration of abnormal reflexes, restoration of normal postural reflex mechanisms, strengthening, flexibility, and retraining of gait: sensory, perceptual, endurance, balance, and functional). As usual, a definitive evaluation and therapy diagnosis is a *prerequisite* to selecting specific intervention strategies. Suggestions for alternative treatment techniques are available throughout this text, particularly in Chapters 6, 15, 16, 21, 22, 24, and 25. The normal postural reflex mechanism and an integrative working knowledge of the observations described by Rood,[78] Voss,[85] Bobath,[6] Brunnstrom,[11] and others assist in selecting appropriate treatment strategies.

When possible, motor problem-solving activities are incorporated into activities used in the recovery stages. The principles of learning psychomotor skills are especially useful in these later recovery stages. Practiced skills can be gradually performed in different environments and in new situations. At first one or two components of an activity can be manipulated; later, entirely new tasks can be presented. The learning principles outlined in the box (see criterion *VBH*) on p. 376 are important. The client needs to be provided with interesting, goal-directed, and functional activities that can be accomplished successfully. Thus the client appreciates the achievement and is moti-

vated toward self-evaluation. Activities during later stages of recovery usually involve increased emphasis on accommodating for the temporal and spatial elements of movement. Walking can lead to dribbling a ball, dancing, or braiding (Fig. 13-16), all of which stress more difficult spatial and temporal components. Games and recreational activities are not only useful for learning motor problem-solving skills but also for continuing development of strength, movement speed, coordination, flexibility, response speed, and endurance.

Frequently, the client with minimal physical deficits presents a greater challenge. This is because the therapist must have more sophisticated knowledge of motor pattern composition, pattern generators, sequencing, and appropriate stimuli selection. Typically, clients at more advanced levels lack or distort sensory input from the proprioceptive, visual, or vestibular systems, select the wrong sensory input system, lack timing, respond with a limited repertoire of strategies, cannot scale their responses based on expectations, and produce muscle contractions that are either too small or too large in amplitude. Also, many secondary behavioral problems surface at this time and present an additional, and often confounding, challenge. A sample case study is used to illustrate possible treatment ideas to refine motor control and to improve balance reactions. Strategies to accommodate or modify various behavior problems are discussed in general terms in a following subsection. Before reading the intervention strategies in the case study, it may help to review some of what has been reported about balance.

A brief review of balance reactions. As noted previously, the upright position on flat surfaces is primarily maintained by proprioception (mechanoreception) with the visual and vestibular systems exercising secondary controls.[37] Balance demands coordination of many muscles, especially those of the lower extremities, to maintain the body's center of gravity over its base of support. This sophisticated coordination of muscle control is accomplished by sequences of stereotyped patterns, or synergies. These synergies are mediated via the brainstem and cerebellum, often referred to as a "pattern generator."[59] These synergies are triggered (but may be modified by visual and vestibular input) by mechanoreceptor input in response to movement or body sway. In quiet standing, posture is stabilized by small changes in the angle between the foot and leg. For example, when length, force of contraction, or movement velocity of the calf muscles exceeds the threshold of mechanoreceptors in the muscles, skin, or joints, mechanoreceptor signals initiate rapid postural readjustments by triggering a synergistic response. For small center-of-gravity movements, these synergies are sequenced distal to proximal. The direction of body sway (anterior-posterior, lateral, or up and down) determines the particular synergy elicited to correct for the shift in the center of gravity. In forward sway, contraction of the stretching

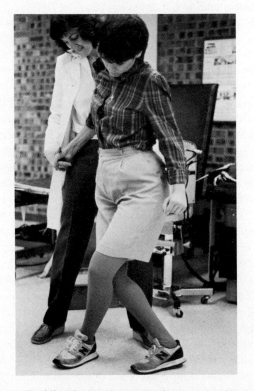

Fig. 13-16. Braiding is an advanced gait sequence that includes trunk rotation, crossing midline, extension/abduction of the lower extremities, and weight shifting.

posterior ankle muscles in unison with the hip and back extensors reduces motion. In backward sway, the muscles of the anterior compartment of the ankle, hip flexors, and abdominals contract. These smaller center-of-gravity movement corrections are called "ankle strategies." If the loss of balance is slightly greater, causing the center of gravity to move further, a "hip strategy" is used that involves hip and knee flexion. Finally, if the balance loss or shift in center of gravity is large and outside the foot base, then a third strategy, that of "stepping," is used to regain balance.[37] Because these synergies or strategies are "long loop" rather than spinal cord reflexes, flexibility in response is possible, providing a means of adapting to different modes of perturbation. Mechanoreception as well as visual and vestibular input are critical, not just in eliciting the response, but also in determining which synergies will be activated from the pattern generator in standing and walking.

The synergies elicited in normal standing are appropriate to restore balance regardless of unexpected changes in mode of perturbation. However, in conditions where the ankle angles are unusual, such as when standing on uneven terrain or on a movable platform, the mechanoreceptor system is not as effective.[52,53] In fact, mechanoreceptor system responses, while standing on a movable platform, are inappropriate and result in destabilization of the body. This destabilization occurs because, although motor synergy responses are appropriate in responding to movements of one part of the body relative to other parts, mechanoreceptor input cannot distinguish between body motions relative to a stable support and body motions in response to motion of external objects. Adaptation of balance reactions occurs slowly in these unusual situations and involves integration of inputs from the mechanoreceptor, visual, and vestibular systems.

Each of these three systems operates differently to provide sensory input for controlling balance. The mechanoreceptor system is ideally suited to be the dominant influence on balance during normal standing. It responds maximally to the low-frequency range of body sway (1 Hz and below) and can respond rapidly (100 to 110 msec latency) to perturbation.[1,57]

The three semicircular canals apparently provide most of the vestibular input to balance.[57] The canals monitor angular acceleration by deflection of the hairs of ampullar sensory cells during changes in the speed and direction of rotation. However, the semicircular canals' sensitivity (0.1 to 1.0 Hz) and response time (175 to 200 msec) make it more effective in correcting larger sway and balance losses.

In contrast to the vestibular system, retinal image motion produced by postural sway provides an ideal supplement to, or substitute for, the mechanoreceptor system's control of balance. The visual system is highly sensitive in the low-frequency range of 0.03 to 1.0 Hz, the range of normal postural sway.[16] The influence of vision on an adult's standing posture can easily be demonstrated by increased amplitudes of sway in standing subjects when their eyes are closed compared with when their eyes are opened. The decrease in postural sway amplitude with the eyes opened averages about 50% in normal adults.[15,83]

To summarize: vision is appropriate for balance reactions when proprioceptive input conflicts and visual-vestibular input agree; proprioceptive input is appropriate when vestibular and proprioceptive input agree and conflict with vision; and vestibular input is appropriate when vision and proprioception conflict.[38]

Therefore in treatment providing the appropriate sensory input is critical to stimulating the correct synergy or balance response. While treatment of mechanoreceptive balance problems requires using readily available flat, firm surfaces, visual and vestibular balance problems are best treated on moving, irregular, or compliant surfaces.

The client who demonstrates movement sequencing latency and unrefined gait and balance reactions. P.H. is an out-patient who comes to therapy once or twice a week. She has a home program that she performs in addition to her therapy sessions. P.H. has fairly good lower-extremity strength and some active, selective movement at the hips, knees, and ankles. However, she elicits the hip strategy with mild forward movement of the center of gravity (as seen with quick stops and turns) when she should be using the ankle strategy. She also has difficulty walking on ramps and grass.

Part of P.H.'s treatment consists of further refining her foot and ankle movements by working on heel walking, toe walking, and foot tapping in standing, keeping her hips and knees extended. Because standing and walking are "pattern generated," it is critical that clients work in the standing position so that sensory input from the visual, mechanoreceptive, and vestibular systems are integrated with balance and walking.

One of the client's home exercises to improve her ankle strategies consists of standing with her feet 6 inches away from and facing a wall or kitchen counter. She leans her hips onto the counter, then attempts to pull away from the counter using only ankle motion. She is instructed to avoid hip and knee flexion. Another of her home exercises consists of standing straight on the floor and swaying 1 to 2 inches forward and backwards without any movement except at the ankle. Her therapy sessions consist of FES to facilitate proper sequencing of distal to proximal muscle contractions.

As her ankle strategies develop and the motor sequencing of her lower extremities improves, P.H.'s therapy sessions consist of increasing her repertoire of situations that input to balance. To involve the vestibular and visual systems, she practices balancing on a square rocker board. At first she attempts small ankle motions progressing to larger motions that stimulate the hip strategy. She can practice

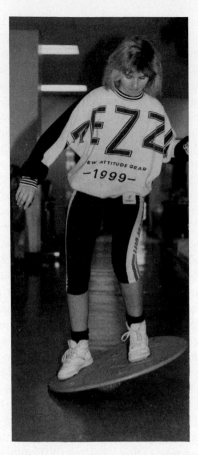

Fig. 13-17. Providing the appropriate sensory input is critical to stimulating the correct movement synergy or balance response. Although treatment of mechanoreceptive balance problems requires using flat, firm surfaces, visual and vestibular balance problems are best treated on irregular, compliant, or moving surfaces, such as the multidimensional balance disk shown. The client should not be permitted to hold onto the therapist or to assistive devices because use of the arms changes the balance responses.

this activity in both the frontal and sagittal planes. As she progresses, she can use a more advanced, multidimensional rocker disk that requires quicker responses and improves timing (see Fig. 13-17). Note that braces cannot be used during effective balance retraining; neither can clients be permitted to hold on or use their arms, your arms, or assistive devices (like parallel bars, canes) while working on balancing. Use of assistive devices appears to change the balance synergies.[36] Of course, the therapist may need to stand by or otherwise provide for safety.

As P.H. improves with rocker board activities, an even more difficult activity can provide visual and vestibular input to balance, increase response speed, and promote independent leg reactions (needed for walking). This activity involves using one-foot thick foam split in the middle three-quarters of the way down. The split permits independent leg motions. The client stands on the foam with one foot on each half and shifts her weight side-

to-side and fore and aft, alternating dorsiflexion and plantar flexion.

As a home activity during this time, the client can begin to learn one-leg stance. She could begin by standing with a narrow base, that is, with one leg in front of the other, heel-to-toe with her weight on her back leg (this should be practiced with each leg taking a turn in back). She can then progress to standing on one leg with her eyes opened for about 15 to 20 seconds and from there to performing the same activity with her eyes closed to eliminate visual input. If she also nods her head yes and no during this narrow-base standing activity, she can reduce both visual and vestibular input and practice relying primarily on proprioceptive input.

An effective way to equalize weight bearing on both limbs and to improve weight shifting, amplitude of movement, movement speed, and response time is to have the client stand on a force plate and use a visual computer monitor to provide feedback on controlling the center of pressure. Such systems are commercially available.

In addition, clients at this stage may also need advanced upper-extremity and manipulative skill retraining.

Strategies to address neurobehavioral and cognitive problems impacting physical management. Some problems encountered in the recovery stages are related to adapting the motor and sensory retraining strategies to the cognitive and behavioral problems that may still coexist. The therapist, while attempting to accomplish the physical goals, may be guided to deal directly or indirectly with some of these problems. Input from team members is perhaps even more crucial in recovery stages (see the next section on integrating the team approach).

Some of the problems commonly encountered during recovery stages that affect physical management include automatic, robot-like behavior, decreased initiative, decreased attention, poor concentration, lack of judgment and insight, selfishness, reluctance to change, delayed learning, and continued aggressive or otherwise socially maladaptive behaviors. The specific physical adaptations for these problems, of course, relate to their severity and to the extent of the physical deficits. Some of the behavioral and cognitive problems can be generally addressed. The psychologist can provide more specific suggestions.

The client with *decreased initiative* can be given a minimal number of activities to perform as a warm-up to each therapy session—for example, taking off shoes and lying down on a mat table, gathering equipment, or specific exercises. The verbal and visual cues and physical assistance for doing these activities can gradually be decreased. More complex expectations can be added and the structure gradually withdrawn. The family can provide a few similar expectations for the client, such as bed making, teeth brushing, or doing laundry. Appropriate disciplinary action, based on love and security, may be taken for neglected responsibilities after sufficient time for learning has passed. As clients become self-motivated, more activities can be added and the client reeducated and—on demonstration of interest—rewarded. Games and recreational activities are useful and well-adapted to adolescent clients with head trauma. Tape on the floor can serve as a handball court, an elevated wastebasket can become a basketball hoop, and sheets or string can become a volleyball net. Some departments include basketball hoops, trampolines, and tether balls as part of the therapeutic exercise equipment. Involving the client in these types of activities helps foster initiative. A ball tossed to a person tends to initiate motor activity. The speed, duration, quality, and intensity of the stimuli can be easily controlled, and the activities are adaptable to recumbent, wheelchair-bound, and ambulatory clients. When the client is ready, a friend may participate and help stimulate initiative and the desire of the client to perform well and to "look good." Friends in their innocence can have an almost remarkable effect on clients with brain injury—as can children on their brain-injured parents.

The problems of *delayed learning* and *memory disturbances* influence, and are influenced by, decreased initiative, decreased attention, and poor concentration. Structure, consistency, and repetition assist with recall. The same techniques of warm-up activities, counting repetitions, or keeping score are examples of actively incorporating the cognitive components into the physical management program. Games can also assist in increasing attention and memory. Memory logs are used in some centers. Further, cues can gradually be withdrawn, repetitions and duration increased, and remembering rewarded. (Identifying and managing learning disabilities are discussed in depth in Chapter 11.)

A client's *reluctance to change* is another management problem encountered by therapists when initiating new activities. The environment is less structured, and the client feels threatened. Even progressing from a wheelchair to a walker or from a walker to a cane may elicit a loud refusal. One such client would hurl his glasses across the room. Another client would refuse to stand up from the mat and would scream in protest. The therapists cannot allow themselves to be manipulated, but at the same time, they must remain flexible and empathize with the client about the threat that change represents. Preparing the person for the change several days in advance may help. During that time the therapist can attempt to increase the client's confidence in the proposed progression. Naturally, the therapist must select activities that the client can accomplish. The new activity can be initiated with remnants of the former activity, such as allowing the individual at first to use a cane in the parallel bars.

Not infrequently the client's willingness to progress can be misjudged, or the client may suddenly feel threatened and react without warning. The therapist might compromise, saying, for example, "Take two steps with the cane,

and then you can sit down." But the therapist cannot back down, even if it takes an hour! Once the client has performed the activity, the effort should be generously rewarded. It should be remembered that success cannot be experienced without risk. The little girl who cries on the first day of school each year for fear she may not succeed in her new grade still must attend school. The family needs to be well-informed and to collaborate with the therapists during this stressful and persistent period.

More serious *combative, aggressive,* and *uncooperative* behaviors that may have developed or persisted through this period are best treated by personnel at facilities equipped to handle these problems. This is certainly preferable to admitting individuals with brain injury to routine psychiatric wards where there may be little understanding of brain trauma, its resolution, and the nature of the dysfunction. Most centers specializing in management of neurobehavioral problems use behavioral modification approaches that might include a token economy system, time-out rooms, aversive stimulation, shaping procedures, and positive reinforcement.[88] Traditional as well as nontraditional psychotherapy may be required. On examination, many of these clients suffer memory deficits and residual—occasionally occult—perceptual deficits that require concomitant treatment.

Again, early and appropriate intervention may prevent some severe secondary behavioral problems. Behaviors can be learned, just as motor skills are learned. However, the location of the brain damage and preexisting behavioral problems certainly influence the persistence of problems. Parents need guidance from counselors and psychologists in dealing with behavioral problems. Older adolescents may have been on their own, and the parent is past disciplining or shaping their behavior. Sometimes the parents are so glad that their son or daughter is alive that they make concessions that they would not otherwise have permitted. Both parents and team members have difficulty dealing with the spontaneous changes in the client's levels of behavior—sometimes mature, other times immature. In a reaction to the more obvious physical deficits, family and staff may treat the client below his or her level of behavioral and intellectual capabilities. It is not unusual to find a client who can, for example, write and tell jokes but who has no head control.

Most therapists adjust "automatically" to cognitive and behavioral differences among their clients. Written instructions are given to some clients, simplified language is used with others, and words and activities are sought to help motivate certain individuals. This is part of physical management. The challenge and the difference in clients with head trauma are in the magnitude and multiplicity of their problems.

Group treatment sessions for clients are often begun in the rehabilitative stages. The group members both support and compete with each other in constructive ways. Group activities may take place in mat classes, wheelchair classes, or volleyball games. However, classes should be an adjunct to regularly scheduled treatment sessions. They cannot replace individualized treatment and the client's need for privacy, despite the attractiveness of groups to department and center administrators.

Creation of an individualized treatment plan involves imagination, respect, caring, empathy, communication, observational skills, problem-solving skills, and skill in selecting goal-oriented activities, motivating clients, reinforcing success, and providing proper stimuli, repetition, and transfer of learning. It also involves being a part of a team.

Integrating the team approach

The previous sections dealt with problems encountered in, but not unique to, physical management and with the team's role in goal selection. Multiple problems require the professional assistance of all team members working in concert. The team's role in treatment may be nontraditional, particularly in the early stages after trauma.

Cognition, speech, and behavior (just as sensory and motor systems) have developmental sequences. These sequences are as yet less consistently documented, but nonetheless a sequence exists. Erikson, for example, has described stages of personality development, and Piaget has described stages of intellectual development.[74] Taxonomies for the affective and cognitive domains have been developed.[5,49] Not only are psychologists, speech pathologists, social workers, and counselors invaluable to the client; they are also invaluable to therapists. In fact, the psychologist's value in the early stages after injury may be as consultant to the therapists. Because the motor development is generally a more primitive system than the development of personality and cognitive processes, it is expected to return earlier if both systems are affected. The psychologist may be a passive observer during the physical therapy. From this perspective the psychologist may be better able to identify problems and suggest alternatives for cognitive and behavioral intervention during physical management. The speech pathologist may do the same because early prespeech sounds are frequently elicited during physical activity. The speech pathologist might assist the therapists in communicating more effectively with the client. In both cases individualized, one-to-one, or group psychotherapy and speech therapy may be inappropriate. However, because the client is indirectly receiving the benefit of the professional services of these persons, billing the client for treatment is appropriate.

When direct speech and behavioral therapy sessions become appropriate, the therapist may be the consultant, for example, in properly positioning the client to generate speech, to maintain head control, or to normalize tone. If scheduling does not permit this sort of consultation time, a physical therapy treatment session might occasionally be omitted because, as emphasized previously, consistency and repetition of desired activities are critical to the success of the client's rehabilitation. Physical therapy does not take place only in physical therapy departments.

The therapist may have a role in the speech goals. One client, who was able to whisper and speak appropriately, was unable to produce volume. The therapist contributed by assisting the client to synchronize speech production with breathing and by increasing chest expansion. Because activities in therapy may arouse the client, the therapist might discover that the mute client can follow instructions and write. The therapist may also discover how to motivate the client. For example, one professional was timing an apparent motor lag in a client. The therapist was able to use a goal-directed activity (that is, "See if you can hand me all the bean bags in 30 seconds") to drastically reduce the supposed delay in response.

Unless the client has severe residual physical deficits, the physical goals, in time, may assume a secondary role to vocational, educational, and behavioral goals. Each discipline contributes in an interactive and almost hierarchical way to the total management of clients with severe head trauma.

Intensity, extent, and duration of treatment

Some important questions are still virtually unanswered: who should receive intensive rehabilitation, who should provide it, how should it be provided, and for how long? The ultimate question does not deal exclusively with whether the client will improve with continued rehabilitation; most will derive some benefit. The question is rather: are the rate and extent of progress sufficient to justify the cost?

It is generally accepted that a realistic expectation is 6 months of spontaneous recovery followed by slower progress the first year, with continued progress for at least 6 months to 5 years. Thus at least 6 months to a year of rehabilitation seems appropriate. However, not all clients continue recovery beyond 6 months, particularly those with hypoxic brain damage (e.g., near-drowning or late "successful" cardiac resuscitation), who seem to plateau early.

Gilchrist and Wilkinson[23] report that the length of coma can be related to the length of rehabilitation. They found that clients who were unconscious for 24 hours to 1 week required 6 months of treatment, while those who had been unconscious for 2 to 7 weeks required nearly 1 year. Those who were very severely injured and unconscious for 8 weeks or more required nearly 2 years of treatment (p. 359). Rosin[70] identified late neurological recovery (after 1 year or more) in six patients as demonstrated by their ability to swallow, improved head or trunk control, limb movement, and increased awareness. He reports the potential for focal recovery may extend beyond the second year after injury.

Usually rehabilitation potential and continued improvement are the prerequisites for rehabilitation. Yet these terms are ill-defined. Rosin[70] suggests that the objective ability to communicate should be the basic criterion for continuing care. However, should therapy for clients with minimal residual dysfunction be discontinued to make room for those with more severe problems? Or do clients with minimal residual dysfunction deserve the more intensive care because they may make the greatest gains? The reality is that economic factors usually determine the answer to most of the questions regarding who receives care, who provides it, how, and for how long, regardless of other factors. One way or another those who can afford it receive continued care.

And what about the client who has been "rehabilitated" but cannot return home? Fortunately, transitional and permanent living facilities, other than traditional nursing homes, are springing up. These facilities are equipped to handle the postrehabilitation, long-term management of individuals with severe brain injury. Unfortunately, these facilities are few, and they may be located far from the client's family. Further, even clients who are able to go home to their families should receive regular long-term, follow-up care. These clients will need updated home programs and evaluation for possible long-term effects or secondary problems that might develop.

Only research validation in all areas will identify appropriate candidates and will determine the most effective and most economical rehabilitation methods. Increased public awareness and interest in this problem of traumatic head injuries may spark research and subsequent funding. Therapists need to standardize terminology, to chart recovery curves, to effect linkup with computer data banks, and to perform controlled clinical studies with alternative treatment strategies. One of the goals of the National Head Injury Foundation is to facilitate specially designed programs and facilities. This organization serves to educate the public about head injury and to promote its prevention, which is, after all, the greatest resolution.

PSYCHOSOCIAL AND ADJUSTMENT CONSIDERATIONS

A 25-year-old man has a 25-year-old wife who has been unresponsive for 2 years. Three children have a mother who no longer has the skill and judgment to care for them. A widowed mother has a 17-year-old brain-injured daughter who demonstrates disinhibition. Parents close to retirement suddenly have a dependent child. Plans are ruined, dreams are shattered, roles are changed, families are disrupted. A brain injury produces many victims.

The family and the client

Family members frequently have difficulty accepting their loved one, who may be irritable, quick tempered, and lacking in spontaneity and judgment. The family may deny the problem and wait for normalcy. In any case, a great deal of stress falls on spouses and on parents, particularly mothers. The increased demands of caring for their loved one isolate them from friends and family, making them feel lonely.

Not only are the family members' feelings often detrimental to their own well-being, but they can affect the rehabilitation of the client. The mother who must drive her daughter to the center for therapy 3 days each week, wait there for 2 hours, initiate her daughter's self-care activities, and attend to her needs each day begins to feel resentful. The mother's feelings become counterproductive not only for the mother but also for the daughter. Therapists must be sensitive to the family's needs as well as to those of the client. Professional help may be sought, but additionally, the therapists may make alternative arrangements. Perhaps the therapy could be reduced to twice a week or day-care arrangements could be made. Family education and group therapy sessions have been organized at many head-injury rehabilitation centers to help families cope with their feelings. However, this kind of help may not be available in many treatment settings.

Clients themselves may lack insight into their own personality and intellectual changes, which compounds the problem. They can also be lonely because they may have lost contact with friends and have fewer opportunities to develop new friends. Group and individual counseling sessions may be appropriate while physical, occupational, and recreational therapists begin social and community reentry programs.

Clients need to relearn how to manage themselves and how to do so in a variety of environments, including home and community. Retraining programs need to begin while the client is still at the hospital or rehabilitation center. The team members can gradually assist the individual in managing time and in accepting responsibility. The client might make the hospital bed, select clothing, perform routine warm-up exercises, arrive at therapy at scheduled times, and make phone calls independently. Gradually, the client can be exposed to the community through outings that might involve making change, shopping, using public transportation, crossing the street, and interacting with people. The return to community, with professionals, with family, and with friends, can assist with reality training and also with learning new skills and adapting those previously learned.

Avocational and vocational counseling is frequently required. New interests may be cultivated, or modifications may be required for pursuit of previous interests. Educational evaluation and guidance are needed by those clients who have not finished high school or who desire training for new careers. Job retraining and placement are based on such factors as the client's physical ability, endurance, interest, motivation, communication skills, and rate of work. Sheltered workshops are sometimes an option. Clients with brain injury may perform better in familiar areas and where there is less responsibility. Returning to a job or to school usually boosts self-esteem and helps the client develop new friends.

The problems of psychosocial adjustment are great and require a team effort. Furthermore, these problems must be identified and managed throughout the rehabilitation process, not delayed until discharge is imminent. (See Chapter 7 for a more thorough discussion of the adjustment process of both the client and the family.)

Barriers to treatment

Even today many clients with brain injuries are treated in hospitals where physicians, therapists, and other medical personnel are virtually inexperienced in handling these cases. Families are misinformed. Clients receive little, if any, therapy, and it is started after contractures and sensory deprivation have developed. The potential for improvement may be misjudged, and even young clients may be transferred to traditional geriatric nursing homes without a legitimate trial of rehabilitation. Later attempts at rehabilitation may be less successful because valuable time is then spent on contracture reduction rather than on functional retraining and learning new skills. The time required to arouse from coma is sometimes underestimated, and clients are not given sufficient opportunity to "come around." Reports of potential are sometimes based on inappropriate and inaccurate tests and observations. Thus hopeless, pessimistic attitudes and lack of education are great barriers that can prevent a client from receiving even a chance. Additional barriers to treatment include lack of a scientific basis for treatment strategies, inadequate documentation, inconvenient location of treatment facilities, insufficient numbers of educated personnel, inadequate community resources for educational and vocational pursuits, and family stress and misunderstanding.

Unfortunately, clients are frequently discharged from care when they are physically improved. Insurance companies seem more reluctant to continue care for behavioral and cognitive retraining even though deficits in these areas may be more debilitating in the long run. There is a need for long-term follow-up care by the rehabilitation team. This serves both the client and the team, whose members need long-term studies to confirm or refute rehabilitation strategies and to identify late-developing problems.

Professional and public awareness about traumatic head injury has heightened in the last decade. There are now workshops, conferences, grants, research projects, journal articles, a dedicated journal, books, and newspaper accounts about individuals with head trauma. Professional schools are educating students about head trauma apart from stroke, mental retardation, and cerebral palsy. Acute care and rehabilitation centers are beginning to develop programs that are unique to the needs of clients with head injury. Transitional living facilities are being developed.

Therapists are better prepared in research methodology, and the opportunities for clinical research are increasing. Not only are therapists in an excellent position to implement qualitative and quantitative research studies with these clients, but in fact they bear a responsibility to do so.

The barriers to treatment, particularly those of attitude and lack of education, funds, resources, and methods, are breaking down. This should give each client with head trauma the opportunity for the best possible quality of life.

Quality of life

A life has been saved. The job of the rehabilitation team is to help improve the quality of that life. But what is quality of life? Family members knew the client before injury. The "rehabilitated" client may be dramatically different from their expectation. The rehabilitation team members, who can contrast the client's progress only since injury, may be quite pleased. Is quality measured by past performance, past potential, present performance, or future potential? Clients themselves may or may not have insight into past, present, or future performance and potential. What are the standards by which quality in life is measured? Is it income, reduction of dependency, contribution to society, or social interaction? Each of these indicators has been used as a standard. Ultimately, the determination of successful rehabilitation relies on the answer to these questions. Jennett and Teasdale[43] suggest that there are six aspects of living: ADL, mobility and life organization, social relationships, work or leisure activities, present satisfaction, and future prospects. Most of these factors, while helpful, cannot be quantitatively measured, and they do not entirely answer the question of quality of life. However one estimates the quality of life, those who have chosen to help rehabilitate clients with head injury continue to pursue an ideal of quality for each life that has been saved and may, by doing so, enhance the quality of their own.

REFERENCES

1. Adams J: Feedback theory of how joint receptors regulate the timing and positioning of a limb, Psychol Rev 84:504, 1977.
2. Berger MS and others: Outcome from severe head injury in children and adolescents, J Neurosurg 62:194, 1985.
3. Bernstein N: The coordination and regulation of movement, Oxford, 1967, Pergamon Press Ltd.
4. Berrol S: Evaluation and the persistent vegetative state, Head Trauma Rehabil 1:7, 1986.
5. Bloom BS, editor: Taxonomy of educational objectives, handbook 1, Cognitive domain, New York, 1956, David McKay Co, Inc.
6. Bobath B: Adult hemiplegia: evaluation and treatment, ed 2, London, 1978, William Heinemann Medical Books Ltd.
7. Bobath K: The motor deficit in patients with cerebral palsy, Clinics in Developmental Medicine, No 23, Lavenham, Suffolk, 1966, Spastics International Medical Publications in association with William Heinemann Medical Books Ltd.
8. Bond MR: Assessment of psychosocial outcome of severe head injury, Acta Neurochir 34:57, 1976.
9. Bond MR: Outcome as a reflection of the interaction of the brain-

injured and their families. Unpublished paper presented at the sixth annual postgraduate course on the rehabilitation of the brain-injured adult, Williamsburg, Va, June 10, 1982.

10. Bricolo A and others: Decerebrate rigidity in acute head injury, J Neurosurg 47:680, Nov 1977.

11. Brunnstrom S: Movement therapy in hemiplegia: a neurophysiological approach, New York, 1970, Harper & Row Publishers Inc.

12. Carlsson CA and others: Factors affecting the clinical course of patients with severe head injuries. I. Influence of biological factors; II. Significance of posttraumatic coma, J Neurosurg 29:242, Sept 1968.

13. Cartlidge NEF and Shaw DA: Head injury, London, 1981, WB Saunders Co Ltd.

14. Choi S and others: Chart or outcome prediction in severe head injury, J Neurosurg 59:294, 1983.

15. Dichgans J: Visual vestibular interaction. In Held R and others, editors: Handbook of sensory physiology, New York, 1978, Springer, Berlin, Heidelberg.

16. Diener H and others: Stabilization of human posture during induced oscillation of the body, Exp Brain Res 45:126, 1982.

17. Eliason MR and Topp BW: Predictive validity of Rappaport's disability rating scale in subjects with acute brain dysfunction, Phys Ther 64:1357, 1984.

18. Evans CD: Assessment of disability after head injury, Rheumatol Rehabil 15:168, Nov 1976.

19. Evans CD and others: Rehabilitation of the brain-damaged survivor, Injury 8:80, Nov 1976.

20. Farber SD: Neurorehabilitation: a multisensory approach, Philadelphia, 1982, WB Saunders Co.

21. Fiorentino MR: Reflex testing methods for evaluating C.N.S. development, ed 2, Springfield, Ill, 1973, Charles C Thomas Publisher.

22. Gennarelli TA and others: Influence of the type of intracranial lesion on the outcome from severe head injury, J Neurosurg 56:26, 1982.

23. Gilchrist E and Wilkinson M: Some factors determining prognosis in young people with severe head injuries, Arch Neurol 36:355, June 1979.

24. Gillingham FJ: The importance of rehabilitation, Injury 1:142, Oct 1969.

25. Gilroy J and Meyer JS: Medical neurology, ed 3, New York, 1979, Macmillan Inc.

26. Glenn MB: Update on pharmacology: pharmacologic interventions in neuroendocrine disorders following traumatic brain injury, Part I, J Head Trauma Rehabil 3:87, 1988.

27. Glenn MB and Wrobewski B: Update on pharmacology: antispasticity medications in the patient with traumatic brain injury, J Head Trauma Rehabil 1:71, 1986.

28. Gogstad AC and Kjellman AM: Rehabilitation prognosis related to clinical and social factors in brain injured of different etiology, Soc Sci Med 10:283, 1976.

29. Gossman MR and others: Review of length-associated changes in muscle: experimental evidence and clinical implications, Phys Ther 62:1799, 1982.

30. Greenberg R and others: Prognostic implications of early multimodality evoked potentials in severe head injury patients: a prospective study, J Neurosurg 55:227, 1981.

31. Groswasser Z and others: Re-evaluation of prognostic factors in rehabilitation after severe head injury: assessment thirty months after trauma, Scand J Rehabil Med 9:147, 1977.

32. Gurdjian ES and others: Closed cervical cranial trauma associated with involvement of the carotid and vertebral arteries, Laryngoscope 81:1381, 1971.

33. Hagen C and others: Levels of cognitive functioning. In Rehabilitation of the head injured adult: comprehensive physical management, Downey, Calif, 1979, Professional Staff Association of Rancho Los Amigos Hospital Inc.

34. Heiden JS and others: Severe head injury: clinical assessment and outcome, Phys Ther 63:1946, 1983.

35. Higgins JR: Human movement: an integrated approach, St Louis, 1977, The CV Mosby Co.

36. Horak F: Determinants of movement in central nervous system damage: implications for assessment and treatment of children and adults, Unpublished paper presented at Symposia, Denver, Colo, July 27-29, 1984.

37. Horak FB and Nashner LM: Central programming of postural movements: adaptations to altered support-surface configurations, J Neurophysiol 55:1369, 1986.

38. Horak FB and Shumway-Cook A: Balance deficits in neurologic patient, Unpublished paper, course notes, Denver, Colo, March 25, 1988.

39. Ivan LP and others: Head injuries in childhood: a two year study, Can Med Assoc J 128:281, 1983.

40. Jennett B and Bond M: Assessment of outcome after severe brain damage: a practical scale, Lancet 1:480, March 1975.

41. Jennett B and Plum F: Persistent vegetative state after brain damage: a syndrome in search of a name, Lancet 1:734, April 1972.

42. Jennett B and Teasdale G: Aspects of coma after severe head injury, Lancet 1:878, April 1977.

43. Jennett B and Teasdale G: Management of head injuries, Philadelphia, 1981, FA Davis Co.

44. Jennett B and others: Prognosis of patients with severe head injury, Neurosurgery 4:283, April 1979.

45. Johnson D and Almi CR: Age, brain damage, and performance. In Finger S, editor: Recovery from brain damage, New York, 1978, Plenum Press.

46. Keener SM and Sweigert JE: Early use of adaptable seating for patients with head trauma, Phys Ther 64:206, 1984.

47. Kondraske GV: Measurement science concepts and computerized methodology in the assessment of human performance. In Munsat TL editor: Quantification of neurologic deficit, Stoneham, Mass, 1989, Butterworth Publishers.

48. Kondraske GV and others: Human performance measurement: some perspectives, IEEE Eng Med and Biol Soc Mag 7:11, 1988.

49. Krathwohl DR and others: Taxonomy of educational objectives, vol 2, Affective domain, New York, 1964, David McKay Co Inc.

50. Kraus JF and others: The incidence of acute brain injury and serious impairment in a defined population, Am J Epidemiol 119:186, 1984.

51. Lanksch W and others: Correlations between clinical symptoms and computer tomography findings in closed head injuries. In Frowein RA and others, editors: Advances in neurosurgery 5, Berlin, 1978, Springer-Verlag.

52. Lee D and Aronson E: Visual proprioceptive control of standing in human infants, Percept Psychophysics 15:529, 1974.

53. Lee D and Lishman J: Visual proprioceptive control of stance, J Human Movement Studies 1:87, 1975.

54. Lynch WJ and Mauss NK: Brain injury rehabilitation: standard problem lists, Arch Phys Med Rehabil 62:223, May 1981.

55. Marrubini MB: Classification of coma, Intensive Care Med 10:217, 1984.

56. Mehalis T and Farhat SM: Vertebral artery injury from chiropractic manipulation of the neck, Surg Neurol 2:125, 1974.

57. Nashner LM: Organization and programming of motor activity during posture control, Prog Brain Res 50:177, 1979.

58. Nashner LM: Sensory and motor aspects of postural control throughout the life span, Unpublished paper presented at the Sensorimotor Integration Symposia, San Diego, Calif, July 25, 1986.

59. Nashner LM and Woollacott M: The organization of rapid postural adjustments of standing in humans. In Talbott R and Humphrey P, editors: Experimental conceptual model in posture and movement, New York, 1979, Raven Press.

60. National Head Injury Foundation, Annual Report, 1985-1986.

61. Oldendorf WH: The quest for an image of brain: a brief historical and technical review of brain imaging techniques, Neurology 28:517, June 1978.

62. O'Sullivan SB and others: Physical rehabilitation: evaluation and treatment procedures, Philadelphia, 1981, FA Davis Co.

63. Paterson A and Hallberg E: Background readings for physical education, New York, 1965, Holt, Rinehart & Winston.

64. Plum F and Posner JB: The diagnosis of stupor and coma, ed 3, Philadelphia, 1980, FA Davis Co.

65. Rappaport M and others: Disability rating scale for severe head trauma: coma to community, Arch Phys Med Rehabil 63:118, 1982.

66. Roberts AH: Long-term prognosis of severe accidental head injury, Proc R Soc Med 69:137, Feb 1976.

67. Rose SJ and Rothstein JM: Muscle mutability. I. General concepts and adaptations to altered patterns of use, Phys Ther 62:1773, 1982.

68. Rosenfalck A and Andreassen S: Impaired regulation and firing pattern of single motor units in patients with spasticity, J Neurol Neurosurg Psychiatry 43:907, 1980.

69. Rosenthal R: Experimenter effect in behavioral research, New York, 1966, Appleton-Century-Crofts.

70. Rosin AJ: Very prolonged unresponsive state following brain injury, Scand J Rehabil Med 10:33, 1978.

71. Russell WR: Cerebral involvement in head injury: a study based on the examination of two hundred cases, Brain 55:549, 1932.

72. Sahrmann S: Posture and muscle imbalance: faulty lumbar-pelvic alignment and associated musculoskeletal pain syndromes. In Postgraduate advances in physical therapy, a comprehensive independent learning office study course, Alexandria, Va, 1987, American Physical Therapy Association.

73. Simpson EJ: The psychomotor domain, Washington, DC, 1972, Gryphon House.

74. Smart MS and Smart RD: Children, ed 3, New York, 1977, Macmillan, Inc.

75. Smith SS and Kondraske GV: Computerized system for quantitative measurement of sensorimotor aspects of human performance, Phys Ther 67:1860, 1987.

76. Snoek J and others: Computerised tomography after recent severe head injury in patients without acute intracranial haematoma, J Neurol Neurosurg Psychiatry 42:215, March 1979.

77. Stewart WA and others: A prognostic model for head injury, Acta Neurochir 45:199, 1979.

78. Stockmeyer SA: An interpretation of the approach of Rood to the treatment of neuromuscular dysfunction. In Bouman HD, editor: Proceedings: an exploratory and analytical survey of therapeutic exercise, Northwestern University special therapeutic exercise project, July 25, 1966 to Aug 19, 1966, Am J Phys Med 46, Feb 1967.

79. Stone C: Evaluation and treatment of adult hemiplegia, Unpublished paper, Dallas, Texas, April 28, 1978, Texas Woman's University.

80. Stover SL and Zeiger HE: Head injury in children and teenagers: functional recovery correlated with the duration of coma, Arch Phys Med Rehabil 57:201, May 1976.

81. Strich SJ: Lesions in the cerebral hemispheres after blunt head injury, J Clin Pathol 23(suppl 4):154, 1970.

82. Tang A and Rymer WZ: Abnormal force—EMG relations in paretic limbs of hemiparetic human subjects, J Neurol Neurosurg Psychiatry 44:690, 1981.

83. Travis R: An experimental analysis of dynamic and static equilibrium, J Exp Psych 35:216, 1945.

84. Van Den Berge JH and others: Interobserver agreement in assessment of ocular signs in coma, J Neurol Neurosurg Psychiatry 42:1163, 1979.

85. Voss DE and others: Proprioceptive neuromuscular facilitation: patterns and techniques, ed 3, Philadelphia, 1985, Harper & Row Publishers.

86. Weinstein CJ: Neurogenic dysphagia: frequency, progression, and outcome in adults following head injury, Phys Ther 63:1992, 1983.

87. Whyte J and Glenn MB: The care and rehabilitation of the patient in a persistent vegetative state, J Head Trauma Rehabil 1:39, 1986.

88. Wood RIl: Brain injury rehabilitation: a neurobehavioral approach, Rockville, Md 1987, Aspen Publishers Inc.

89. Young RR and Delwaide PJ: Drug therapy: spasticity part 1, N Engl J Med 304:28, 1981.

90. Young RR and Delwaide PJ: Drug therapy: spasticity, part 2, N Engl J Med 304:96, 1981.

91. Zimmerman RA and others: Computed tomography of shearing injuries of the cerebral white matter, Radiology 127:393, May 1978.

Chapter 14

CONGENITAL SPINAL CORD INJURY

Jane W. Schneider and Kathryn L. Gabriel

A spinal cord injury is a complex disability. When a spinal cord lesion exists from birth, an additional complexity is added. This congenital condition predisposes that many areas of the CNS may not develop or function adequately. In addition, all areas of development (physical, cognitive, and psychosocial) that depend so heavily on central functioning will likely be impaired. The clinician therefore must be aware of the significant impact this neurological defect has not only on motor function but also on a variety of related human capacities.

A developmental framework has been used to aid in understanding the sequential problems of the child with spina bifida. The developmental model, however, must always stay in line with the functional model for adult trauma, since the problems of the congenitally involved child grow quickly into the disabilities of the injured adult. With concentration on the present but with an eye to the future, appropriate management goals can be achieved.

AN OVERVIEW OF CONGENITAL SPINAL CORD INJURY

A congenital spinal cord lesion is one that occurs in utero and is present at the time of birth. To understand how this malformation develops, one needs an appreciation of normal nervous system maturation.

The nervous system develops from a portion of embryonic ectoderm called the neural plate. During gestation, the neural plate develops folds that begin to close, forming the neural tube (Fig. 14-1). The neural tube differentiates into the CNS, which is composed of brain and spinal cord tissue.[66]

In the normal embryo, neural tube closure begins in the cervical region and proceeds cranially and caudally. Closure is generally complete by the 26th day.[66]

Types of spina bifida

In spina bifida there is a defect in the neural tube closure and the overlying posterior vertebral arches. The extent of the defect may result in one of two types of spina bifida—occulta or cystica.

In spina bifida occulta there is a failure of one or more of the vertebral arches to meet and fuse in the third month of development. The spinal cord and meninges are unharmed and remain within the vertebral canal (Fig. 14-2, A). The bony defect is covered with skin that may be marked by a dimple, pigmentation, or patch of hair.[81] The common site for this defect is the lumbosacral area, and it

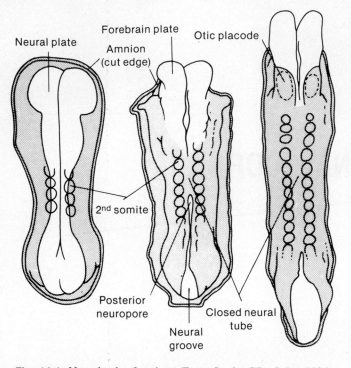

Fig. 14-1. Neural tube forming. (From Stark, GD: Spina bifida problems and management, London, 1977, Blackwell Scientific Publications Inc.)

is usually associated with no disturbance of neurological or musculoskeletal functioning.[60]

Spina bifida cystica results when the neural tube and overlying vertebral arches fail to close appropriately. There is a cystic protrusion of the meninges or of the spinal cord and meninges through the defective vertebral arches.

The milder form of spina bifida cystica, called meningocele, involves protrusion of the meninges and cerebrospinal fluid (CSF) only into the cystic sac (Fig. 14-2, *B*). The spinal cord remains within the vertebral canal, but it may exhibit abnormalities.[57] This is a relatively uncommon form of spina bifida cystica.

The more common and severe form of the defect is known as myelomeningocele in which both spinal cord and meninges are contained in the cystic sac (Fig. 14-2, *C*). Within the sac, the spinal cord and associated neural tissue show extensive abnormalities. Abnormal growth of the cord and a tortuous pathway of neural elements make normal transmission of nervous impulses impossible. The result is a sensory and motor impairment at the level of the lesion and below.[81]

A closed myelomeningocele is covered with a combination of skin and membranes. In an open myelomeningocele, nerve roots and spinal cord may be exposed with dura and skin evident at the margin of the lesion.

Although spina bifida cystica can occur at any level of the spinal cord, meningoceles and closed myelomeningoceles are most common in the thoracic and lumbosacral re-

gions. Two-thirds of open lesions involve the thoracolumbar junction.[81]

Since myelomeningocele occurs in 94% of the cases of spina bifida cystica and since these are the cases most often requiring rehabilitation, the terms *spina bifida* and *myelomeningocele* are frequently used interchangeably.[57]

Failure of fusion of the cranial end of the neural tube results in a condition know as anencephaly. In this condition, some brain tissue may be evident, but forebrain development is usually absent.[60] Since sustained life is not possible with this neural tube defect, anencephaly will not be discussed further.

Incidence and etiology

Figures on the incidence of spina bifida vary considerably in different parts of the world. In the United States the incidence is approximately 2 per 1000 births.[49] This is about midrange in world statistics, considering a spina bifida birth rate of 0.3 per 1000 in Japan and as high as 4.5 per 1000 in certain parts of the British Commonwealth.

There is some evidence of seasonal variation, suggesting a positive relationship between the occurrence of spina bifida and conceptions in March to May.[10,77,81]

Spina bifida is thought to be more common in females than in males, although some studies suggest no real sex difference.[39,57,81] The incidence of spina bifida is higher in those of Celtic origin; it is lower in those of the Negro and Mongolian races.[10,54] A significant relationship has also been noted between social class and spina bifida, such that the lower the social class, the higher the incidence.[61,62]

Genetic factors seem to influence the occurrence of spina bifida. The chances of having a second affected child are between 1% and 2%, whereas in the general population the percentage drops to one fifth of 1%.[46,49]

While the above factors have been shown to be related to the incidence of spina bifida, the cause of this defect remains in question. Environmental conditions, such as hyperthermia in the first weeks of pregnancy, or dietary factors, such as canned meats, potatoes, or tea, have been implicated but not substantiated.[10,37,38,81] In addition, nutritional deficiencies, such as folic acid and vitamin A, have been implicated as a cause of primary neural tube defect.[50,78] Genetic considerations, such as an Rh blood type, a specific gene type (HLA-B27), and an X-linked gene, have again been implicated, but not conclusively.[6,12,68] It appears that environmental factors, combined with genetic predisposition, may trigger the development of spina bifida, although definitive evidence is not available to support this claim.[54,81]

The incidence of spina bifida can be expected to decline with the advent of a procedure used to detect a variety of congenital abnormalities, amniocentesis. The presence of significant levels of alpha-fetoprotein (AFP) in the amniotic fluid has led to the detection of large numbers of af-

SAGITTAL VIEW   TRANSVERSE VIEW

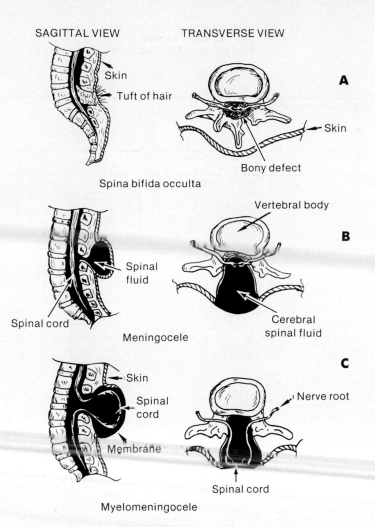

Spina bifida occulta

Meningocele

Myelomeningocele

Fig. 14-2. Types of spina bifida. **A,** Spina bifida occulta. **B,** Meningocele. **C,** Myelomeningocele. (From McClone, DG: An introduction to spina bifida, Chicago, 1980, Children's Memorial Hospital, Northwestern University.)

fected fetuses.[30] Currently, maternal serum AFP levels have been effective in detecting approximately 80% of neural tube defects.[24] Prenatal screening can be most effective when a combination of serum levels, amniocentesis/amniography, and ultrasonography are employed.[32] While this screening is not yet done routinely, it is suggested for those at risk for the defect. Knowledge of the defect allows for preparation for cesarean birth and immediate postnatal care. This includes mobilization of the interdisciplinary team who will continue to care for the child. For parents who decide to carry an involved fetus to term, their adjustment to their child's disability can begin before birth, which includes mobilizing their own support systems.

Other advances in the field of prenatal medicine include the in utero treatment of hydrocephalus. It can be expected that treatment such as this, in conjunction with prenatal diagnosis, will have a positive impact on the incidence and severity of complications of congenital abnormalities, such as spina bifida.

Clinical manifestations

The most obvious clinical manifestation of myelomeningocele is the loss of sensory and motor functions in the lower limbs. The extent of loss, while primarily dependent upon the degree of the spinal cord abnormality, is secondarily dependent upon a number of factors. These include the amount of traction or stretch resulting from the abnormally tethered spinal cord, the trauma to exposed neural tissue during delivery, and postnatal damage resulting from drying or infection of the neural plate.[81]

The above factors indicate that determining neurological involvement is not as straightforward as it would seem. At birth, two main types of motor dysfunction in the lower extremities have been identified. The first type involves a complete loss of function below the level of lesion, resulting in a flaccid paralysis, loss of sensation, and absent reflexes.[10,81] The extent of involvement can be determined by comparing the level of lesion with a chart delineating the segmental innervation of the lower limb muscles (Fig. 14-3). Orthopaedic deformities may result from the unop-

CHILDREN'S MEMORIAL HOSPITAL
MUSCLE EXAMINATION
PHYSICAL/OCCUPATIONAL THERAPY

Patient Name: _____   Medical Record #: _____

Attending Physician(s): _____   Patient Date of Birth: _____

The form has Left side columns (Comments, *+, *+) and Right side columns (*+, *+, Comments) flanking the central nerve-root grid.

Region	Action	Muscle	(C1)2,3	T1,2,3,4	T5,6	T7,8	T9,10,11	T12	L1	L2	L3	L4	L5	S1	S2	S3
Neck	Flexors	Sternocleidomastoid	•													
	Extensor Group	C1,2,3,4,5,6,7,8,T1														
Truck	Extensors	Thoracic Group		•	•	•	•	•								
		Lumbar Group		•	•	•	•	•								
	Flexors	Rectus Abdominis			•	•	•									
		Lt. Int. Obl. Rt. Int. Obl.				•	•	(•)								
	Rotators	Rt. Ext. Obl. Lt. Ext. Obl.				•	•	•	1	(2)						
	Pelvic Elev.	Quadratus Abdom.						•	1	2	3					
Hip	Flexors	Iliopsoas							1	2	3	4				
		Sartorius								2	3	(4)				
	ADDuctor Group									2	3	4				
Knee	Extensors	Quadriceps								2	3	4				
Hip	ABDuctors	Gluteus Medius											5	1		
		Tensor Fasciae Latae										4	5	1		
	IR Group											4	5	1		
Foot	Inv. Dorsfl.	Tibialis Anterior										4	5	1		
	Evertors	Peroneus Brevis										4	5	1		
		Peroneus Longus										4	5	1		
Hallux	M.P. Ext.	Ext. Hall. Br.										4	5	1		
	I.P. Ext.	Ext. Hall. L.										4	5	1		
	M.P. Flexor	Flex. Hall. Br.										4	5	1		
Toes	I.P. Flexors	Flex. Digit. Br. — 1										4	5	1		
		Flex. Digit. Br. — 2										4	5	1		
		Flex. Digit. Br. — 3										4	5	1		
		Flex. Digit. Br. — 4										4	5	1		
	M.P. Extensors	Ext. Digit. Br. — 1										4	5	1		
		Ext. Digit. Br. — 2										4	5	1		
		Ext. Digit. Br. — 3										4	5	1		
		Ext. Digit. Br. — 4										4	5	1		
	I.P. Extensors	Ext. Digit. L. — 1										4	5	1		
		Ext. Digit. L. — 2										4	5	1		
		Ext. Digit. L. — 3										4	5	1		
		Ext. Digit. L. — 4										4	5	1		
Hip	E.R. Group											4	5	1	2	(3)
Foot	Invertor	Tibialis Posterior										(4)	5	1		
Hip	Extensor	Gluteus Maximus											5	1	2	
Ankle	Plantar Flexors	Soleus											5	1	2	
		Gastrocnemius												1	2	
Hallux	I.P. Flexors	Flex. Hall. L.											5	1	2	
Knee	L. Flexor	Biceps Femoris											5	1	2	3
Knee	M. Flexors	Inner Hamstrings										(4)	(5)	1	2	
Toes	I.P. Flexors	Flex. Digit. L. — 1											5	1	(2)	
		Flex. Digit. L. — 2											5	1	(2)	
		Flex. Digit. L. — 3											5	1	(2)	
		Flex. Digit. L. — 4											5	1	(2)	
Toes	M.P. Flexors	Lumbricales — 1										4	5	1		
		Lumbricales — 2										(4)	(5)	1	2	
		Lumbricales — 3										(4)	(5)	1	2	
		Lumbricales — 4										(4)	(5)	1	2	

* Enter initials of examiner
+ Enter date of examination

Code	Grade	Definition
X	Present	Unable to be graded
N	Normal	Complete range of motion against gravity with full resistance
G	Good	Complete range of motion against gravity with moderate resistance
F+	Fair Plus	Complete range of motion against gravity with slight resistance
F	Fair	Complete range of motion against gravity
F−	Fair Minus	Incomplete range of motion against gravity
P	Poor	Complete range of motion with gravity eliminated
P−	Poor Minus	Incomplete range of motion with gravity eliminated
T	Trace	Contraction is felt but there is no visible joint movement
0	Zero	No contraction felt in the muscle
R	Reflexive	Contraction is a stereotypic movement in response to one specific stimulus
S	Spasticity	Increased tone noted during active or passive movement

Form No. 77053

Fig. 14-3. Muscle examination form. (Courtesy Josefina Briceno, PT, Children's Memorial Hospital, Chicago.)

Patient Name: _____   Medical Record #: _____

Comments (Left)	* +	* +					C_1	C_2	C_3	C_4	C_5	C_6	C_7	C_8	T_1	* +	* +	Comments (Right)
			Scapula	Elevator	Upper Trapezius			2	3	4								
				Depressor	Lower Trapezius			2	3	4								
				ADDuctors	Middle Trapezius			2	3	4								
					Rhomboids					4	5							
			Shoulder	ABDuctors	Middle Deltoid					4	5	6						
					Supraspinatus					4	5	6						
				Ext. Rotator	Infraspinatus					(4)	5	6						
					Teres Minor					(4)	5	6						
				Flexor	Anterior Deltoid						5	6						
					Posterior Deltoid						5	6						
			Elbow	Flexors	Biceps Brachii						5	6						
					Brachioradialis						5	6						
			Shoulder	Extensor	Teres Major						5	6	7					
				Horiz. Add.	Pectoralis Major						5	6	7					
				Internal Rotator	Subscapularis						5	6	7					
			Forearm	Supinator	Supinator						5	6	7					
			Scapula	ABDuctor	Serratus Anterior						5	6	(7)	8				
			Wrist	Extensor	Ext. Carpi Rad. L. & Br.						5	6	(7)	8				
			Forearm	Pronation	Pronator Group							6	7					
			Shoulder	Extensor	Latissimus Dorsi							6	7	8				
			Wrist	Flexors	Flex. Carp. Rad.							6	7	8				
				Extensor	Ext. Carp. Uln.							6	7	8				
			Finger	M.P. Extensor	Ext. Digit. Com.	1						6	7	8				
						2						6	7	8				
						3						6	7	8				
						4						6	7	8				
			Thumb	M.P. Extensor	Ext. Poll. Br.							6	7	8				
				I.P. Extensor	Ext. Poll. L.							6	7	8				
				ABDuctor	ABD. Poll. L.							6	7	8				
			Elbow	Extensor	Triceps							6	7	8				
			Wrist	Flexors	Palmaris Longus							(6)	7	8				
			Fingers	M.P. Flexors	Lumbricales	1						(6)	7	8	1			
						2												
			Thumb	M.P. Flexor	Flex. Poll Br.							6	7	8	1			
				I.P. Flexor	Flex. Poll. L.							(6)	7	8	1			
				ABDuctor	ABD. Poll. Br.							6	7	8	1			
				Opponens	Opponens Poll.							6	7	8	1			
			Wrist	Flexor	Flex. Carpi Uln.								7	8	1			
			Fingers	M.P. Flexors	Lumbricales	3							(7)	8	1			
						4							(7)	8	1			
				I.P. Flexors (1st)	Flex. Digit. Sub.	1							7	8	1			
						2							7	8	1			
						3							7	8	1			
						4							7	8	1			
				I.P. Flexors (2nd)	Flex. Digit. Prof.	1							7	8	1			
						2							7	8	1			
						3							7	8	1			
						4							7	8	1			
				ABDuctors	Palmer Interossei	1								8	1			
						2								8	1			
						3								8	1			
						4								8	1			
				ADDuctors	Dorsal Interossei	1								8	1			
						2								8	1			
						3								8	1			
						4								8	1			
			Thumb	ABDuctors	ABDuctor Pollicis									8	1			

* Enter initials of examiner
+ Enter date of examination

Fig. 14-3, cont'd. For legend see opposite page.

posed action of muscles above the level of lesion. This unopposed pull leads commonly to hip flexion, knee extension, and ankle dorsiflexion contractures.

When the spinal cord remains intact below the level of lesion, the effect is an area of flaccid paralysis immediately below the lesion and possible hyperactive spinal reflexes distal to that.[10,81] This is very similar to the neurological state of the severed cord seen in traumatic injury. This second type of neurological involvement again results in orthopaedic deformities, depending upon the level of the lesion, the spasticity present, and the muscle groups involved.

The orthopaedic problems seen in myelomeningocele may be the result of (1) the imbalance between muscle groups; (2) the effect of stress, posture, and gravity; and (3) associated congenital malformations.[10]

Besides the obvious malformation of vertebrae at the site of the lesion, hemivertebrae and deformities of other vertebral bodies and their corresponding ribs may also be present.[10] A lumbar kyphosis may be present as a result of the original deformity. In addition, as a result of the bifid vertebral bodies, the misaligned pull of the extensor muscles surrounding the deformity as well as the unopposed flexor muscles contribute further to the lumbar kyphosis. As the child grows, the weight of the trunk in the upright position my also be a contributing factor.[10,57] A scoliosis may be present at birth because of vertebral abnormalities or may become evident as the child grows older. There is a low incidence of scolisis in low lumbar or sacral-level deformities.[75] A scoliosis at these levels may be indicative of a tethered cord and require further investigation. A lordosis or lordoscoliosis is often seen in the adolescent and is usually associated with hip flexion deformities and a large spinal defect.[10,57]

Many of these trunk and postural deformities exist at birth but are exacerbated by the effects of gravity as the child grows. They can lead to compromise of vital functions (cardiac and respiratory) and should therefore be closely monitored by the therapist and the family.

As has been alluded to previously, the type and extent of deformity in the lower extremities will depend on the muscles that are active or inactive. In a total flaccid paralysis, in utero deformities may be present at birth, resulting from passive positioning within the womb. Other common deformities are hip flexion, adduction, and internal rotation, usually leading to subluxed or dislocated hips.[10] Equinovarus deformity or "rocker-bottom" deformity are two of the most common foot abnormalities. Although many of these problems may be present at birth, it is of utmost importance to prevent positional deformity (such as the frog-leg position), which may result from improper positioning of flaccid extremities.[23]

Since the paralyzed limbs of the child with spina bifida have increased amounts of unmineralized osteoid tissue, they are prone to fractures, particularly after periods of immobilization.[20,70] Fortunately these fractures heal quickly with appropriate medical management.

Hydrocephalus develops in 80% to 90% of children with myelomeningocele.[54,49] Hydrocephalus is often associated with the Arnold-Chiari malformation, where the brainstem and cerebellum are herniated through the foramen magnum.[10] This results in a blockage of the normal flow of CSF between the ventricles and spinal canal, resulting in hydrocephalus.

The most obvious effect of the buildup of CSF is abnormal increase in head size. This may be present at birth because of the great compliance of the cranial sutures in the fetus, or may develop postnatally. Internally, there is usually a concomitant dilation of the lateral ventricles and thinning of the cerebral white matter. Without reduction of the buildup of CSF, increased brain damage and death may result.

Secondary to the brainstem malformation, problems with respiratory and bulbar function may be evident in the child with spina bifida.[10,54,81] Paralysis of the vocal cords occurs in a small percentage of cases and is associated with respiratory stridor. Apneic episodes may also be evident, although their direct cause remains in question. Children with spina bifida may also exhibit difficulty in swallowing and have an abnormal gag reflex.[81] Thus, depending on the orthopaedic deformities present and the neurological involvement, there is a potential from both sources for severe respiratory involvement in the affected child.

Because of the usual involvement of the sacral plexus, the child with spina bifida must commonly deals with some form of bowel and bladder dysfunction. Besides various forms of incontinence, incomplete emptying of the bladder remains a constant concern because infection of the urinary tract and possible kidney damage may result.[2] Regulation of bowel evacuation must be established so that neither constipation nor diarrhea occur. (For a more thorough understanding of neurogenic bowel and bladder dysfunction, please refer to Chapter 29).

The last major clinical manifestation resulting from the neurological involvement of myelomeningocele is that of impaired intellectual function. Although spina bifida children without hydrocephalus may show normal intellectual potential, children with hydrocephalus, particularly those who have shunt infections, are likely to have below-average intelligence.[10,11,52,69,81]

These children often demonstrate learning disabilities and poor academic achievement. Even those with a normal IQ show moderate to severe visual-motor perceptual deficits.[54] This inability to coordinate eye and hand movements not only affects learning but also may interfere with activities of daily living, such as buttoning a shirt or opening a lunch box.[29] Difficulties with spatial relations, body image, and development of hand dominance may also be evident.[29,81] (Chapter 11 should be of great assistance when dealing with these problems in the child with spina bifida.)

The impairment of intellectual and perceptual abilities has been linked to the damage to the white matter caused by ventricular enlargement.[10,81] This damage to association tracts, particularly in the frontal, occipital, and parietal areas, could account for the often severe perceptual-cognitive deficits noted in the child with spina bifida. Lesser involvement of the temporal areas may account for the preservation of speech, while the semantics of speech, dependent on association areas, is impaired. It is easy to be fooled by the "cocktail party speech" of children with spina bifida, since they generally use well-constructed sentences and precocious vocabulary.[10] A closer look, however, reveals a repetitive, inappropriate, and often meaning-less use of language certainly not associated with higher intellectual functioning.

Considering all the above clinical manifestations resulting from this congenital neurological defect, there is no doubt that social and emotional difficulties will arise for these children and their families. These will be considered as appropriate when discussing the stages of recovery and rehabilitation from birth through adolescence.

The preceding discussion concerning the clinical problems of the child with spina bifida was intended to inform, not overwhelm, the clinician. With a firm understanding of the difficulties to be faced, evaluation and intervention can be more efficient and effective.

Medical management

Before surgical closure of myelomeningocele. At birth, the myelomeningocele sac presents a dynamic rather than static disability. The residual neurological damage will be contingent upon the early medical management that the newborn receives.

Since the early 1960s the presence of a myelomeningocele has been treated as a life-threatening situation, and sac closure now takes place within the first 24 to 48 hours of life.[67,81] The aim of this surgery is to replace the nervous tissue into the vertebral canal, cover the spinal defect, and achieve a water-tight sac closure.[52] This early management has decreased the possibility of infection and further injury to the exposed neural cord.[51,54]

After surgery, during hospitalization. Progressive hydrocephalus may be evident at birth in a small percentage of children born with myelomeningocele. A greater majority, however, develop hydrocephalus 5 to 10 days after the back lesion is closed.[54,82] With the advent of the computed axial tomography (CT) scan, early diagnosis of hydrocephalus can be made in the newborn without dependence on clinical examination.

While clinical signs are not always definitive, hydrocephalus may be suspected if (1) the fontanels become full, bulging, or tense; (2) the head circumference increases rapidly; (3) there is a palpable separation of the coronal and sagittal sutures; (4) the infant's eyes appear to look downward only, with the cornea prominent over the iris (sun-setting sign); and (5) the infant becomes irritable or lethargic and has a high-pitched cry, persistent vomiting, difficult feeding, or seizures.[35,49]

If the results of the CT scan confirm hydrocephalus, a ventricular shunt is indicated. This procedure involves diverting the excess CSF from the ventricles to some site for absorption. In general, two types of procedures—the ventriculoatrial (VA) and ventriculoperitoneal (VP) shunt—are currently used, the latter being the most common[77] (Fig. 14-4). The shunt apparatus consists of tubing made of a rubber-silicone polymer and a pumping chamber with one-way valves. The two most commonly used shunt systems are the Spitz-Holter and the Pudenz-Heyer. As CSF is pumped from the ventricles toward its final destination, back flow is prevented by the valve system. In this manner intercranial pressure is controlled, CSF is regulated, and hydrocephalus is prevented from causing damage to brain structures.

Unfortunately for children with spina bifida, their problems do not end after the back is closed and a shunt is in place. Shunt complications occur frequently and require an average of two revisions before age 10.[54] The most common causes of complications are shunt obstruction and infection.[10,81] Obstructions can be cleared by revising the blocked end of the shunt. Infections may be handled by external ventricular drainage and courses of antibiotic therapy followed by insertion of a new shunting system.[81] The problem of separation of shunt components has been largely overcome by the use of a one-piece shunting system. The single-piece shunt has been found to decrease the complications of shunting procedures.

Prophylactic antibiotic therapy 6 to 12 hours before surgery and 1 to 2 days postoperatively has been found to be effective in controlling infection for both sac repair and shunt insertion.[54] This brief course of antibiotics has not led to resistant organisms. The main cause of death in children with myelomeningoceles remains increased intercranial pressure and infections of the CNS.[54] With the use of antibiotics, shunting, and early sac closure, the survival rate has increased from 20% to 85%.[52]

Following the sac closure and possible shunting, a urological assessment should be completed as soon as possible. Kidney damage is not usually present at birth, and it is the aim of the urology team to preserve renal function and to promote efficient bladder management.[49] Initially a renal and bladder ultrasound is done to assess those structures.[40] Intravenous pyelography (IVP), a procedure in which dye is injected into the blood and then followed by radiogram through the kidneys and bladder, is often chosen to evaluate kidney function.[10,49,81] As the dye is voided, radiograms can be taken (voiding cystourethrograms) to determine any blockage in the lower urinary

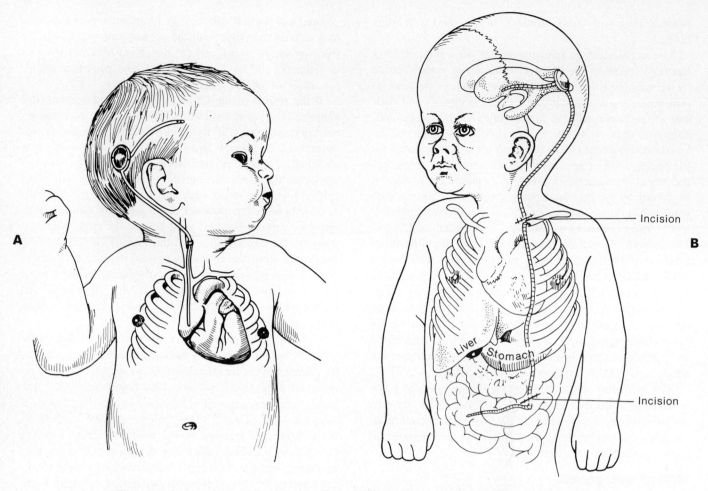

Fig. 14-4. A, Ventriculoatrial shunt *(VA).* **B,** Ventriculoperitoneal shunt *(VP).* (From Stark, GD: Spina bifida problems and management, London, 1977, Blackwell Scientific Publications.)

tract. Functioning of the bladder outlet and sphincters, as well as ureteric reflex, can also be evaluated.[10,49,81]

These tests, plus clinical observations of voiding patterns, help the urologist to classify the infant's bladder function. If the bladder has neither sensory nor motor supply, there will be a constant flow of urine. In this case infection is rare, because the bladder does not store urine and the sphincters are always open.[14]

If there is no sensation but some involuntary muscle control of the sphincter, the bladder will fill, but emptying will not occur properly. Overflow or stress incontinence results in dribbling urine until the pressure is relieved. Because of constant residual urine, infection is a potential problem and kidney damage may be the sequela.[14]

When some voluntary muscle control but no sensation is present, the bladder will fill and empty automatically. The child can eventually be taught to empty the bladder at regular intervals to avoid unnecessary accidents.

Regardless of the type of bladder functioning, urine specimens are taken to check for infection, and blood samples are taken to determine the kidney's ability to filter the body's fluids.

Based on clinical findings, the urologist will suggest the appropriate intervention. The Credé method of bladder emptying may be recommended when the bladder empties easily and residual urine is negligible.[2] This method requires manual expression of urine by direct pressure over the bladder. Because of possible reflux when pressure is applied, which may result in kidney damage, this is not the current method of choice.

A program of clean intermittent catheterization (CIC) to be done every 4 hours has been shown to produce good results in preventing infection and maintaining the urological system.[2,19] Parents are taught this method and can then begin[19] to take on their aspect of their child's care.

At the age of 4 or 5, children with spina bifida can be taught CIC. By doing so, they have become independent in bladder care at a young age. Achieving this form of independence adds to the normal psychological development of these children.

Some children may require urinary diversion through the abdominal wall (ileostomies) or other less common methods such as intravesical transurethral bladder stimulation to handle their urinary problems.[2] Although CIC is

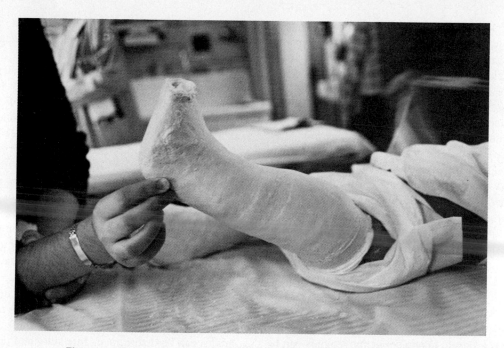

Fig. 14-5. Plaster cast of the foot and ankle to reduce club foot deformities.

not possible for all children with spina bifida, it remains the method of choice for bladder management.

Orthopaedic management of the newborn with a myelomeningocele will generally concentrate on the feet and hips. Soft tissue releases of the feet may take place during surgery for sac closure. Casting the feet has also been effective in reducing clubfoot deformities (Fig. 14-5). Short-leg posterior splints may be utilized to maintain and prevent foot deformities.

The orthopaedist will also evaluate the stability of the hips. In children with lower-level lesions, attempts to prevent dislocation are made by utilizing a hip abductor brace for a few months after birth (Fig. 14-6). With higher-level lesions, dislocated hips are no longer treated because they appear to have no effect on later rehabilitation efforts.[2,22,35,44]

PHYSICAL THERAPY EVALUATIONS

In attempting to evaluate the child with spina bifida, there are any number of evaluations from which to choose, each designed to test specific, yet perhaps unrelated, components of function. The following section has attempted to discuss those test procedures or specific standardized tests that would best serve to further define the complexity of the problem.

Manual muscle testing (MMT)

The first and most obvious request for evaluation may be to determine the extent of motor paralysis. In the newborn, testing may be done in the first 24 to 48 hours before the back is surgically closed. In this case, care must be taken not to injure the exposed neural tissue during testing.

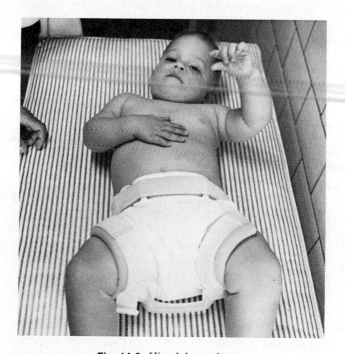

Fig. 14-6. Hip abductor brace.

Prone and sidelying to either side offers the most convenient and safe position for evaluation during this time. Subsequent testing is done soon after the back is closed and as indicated throughout childhood.

The traditional form of MMT is not appropriate or possible for the infant or young child. The following is a discussion of how muscle testing can and must be adapted for this age group.

In evaluating the newborn, the importance of state is paramount. A sleeping or drowsy baby will hardly respond appropriately during the evaluation. It is essential that the infant be in the alert or crying state to elicit the appropriate responses. There is an advantage to testing hungry or crying babies, since they are likely to demonstrate more spontaneous movements in these behavioral states.

Also, the cumulative effect of a variety of sensory stimuli may be more effective than using one mode in isolation. For example, the infant may be picked up and rocked vertically to allow maximum stimulation to the vestibular system and to help bring the child to an alert state. In addition, the therapist may talk to the child to help him fixate visually on the therapist's face. Tactile stimuli above the level of the lesion further add to the child's level of arousal, thus contributing to more conclusive test results. In this way, the CNS receives an accumulation of information from a variety of sensory systems, rather than relying on transmission from one system that may be weak or inefficient.

As the child is aroused, spontaneous movements can be observed and muscle groups palpated. Additional methods to stimulate movement may be necessary. For example, "tickling" the baby generally produces a variety of spontaneous movements in the upper and lower extremities. Passive positioning of children in adverse positions may stimulate them to move. For example, if the legs are held in marked hip and knee flexion, the baby may attempt to use extensor musculature to move out of that position. If the legs are held in adduction, the child may abduct to get free. Lastly, holding a limb in an antigravity position may elicit an automatic "holding" response from a muscle group when spontaneous movements cannot be obtained in any other way.[86]

Although none of these methods are fail-safe, they may prove helpful in adapting a muscle test to a newborn or young infant. Repeated evaluation may be necessary to get an accurate picture of muscle function.

In grading muscle strength, it is important to differentiate between spontaneous, voluntary movement and reflexive movement. Following severing of a spinal cord, distal segments of the cord may respond to stimuli in a reflexive manner. This results from the preservation of the spinal reflex arc and is known as "distal sparing." If distal sparing of the spinal cord is present, the muscles may respond to stimulation or muscular stretch with reflexive, stereotypical movement patterns. The quality of this reflexive movement will be different from that of spontaneous movement and must be distinguished when testing for level of voluntary muscle functioning.

Muscle strength is generally graded for groups of muscles and can be graded by using either a numerical or alphabetical designation (Table 14-1) or simply by noting presence or absence of muscular contraction. Initially, this latter method may be sufficient, but as the child matures a more definitive muscle grade should be determined.

By using an MMT form that lists the spinal segmental level for each muscle group, one can determine the level of lesion from the test results (Fig. 14-3). If reflex activity is also noted on the form, the presence of distal sparing of the spinal cord can be determined. Muscle testing of the newborn gives the clinician not only an appreciation of muscle function and possible potential for later ambulation but also an awareness of possible deforming forces. For example, if no hip extensors or abductors are functioning, then the action of hip flexors and adductors must be countered to prevent future deformities.

Muscle testing of the toddler or young child may require some of the techniques described previously. In addition, developmental positions can be used to assess muscle strength in an uncooperative youngster. For example, strength of hip extensors and abductors can be assessed as a child attempts to creep up steps or onto a low mat table. By adding resistance to movements, fairly accurate muscle grades can be determined. Ingenuity and creativity are certainly prerequisites for muscle testing the young child.

By the age of 4 or 5, muscle grades can generally be determined through traditional testing techniques, although the reliability of the test results will increase with the age of the child.

Muscle testing is indicated before and after any surgical procedure and at periodic intervals of 6 months to 1 year to detect any change in muscle function. In the growing child or adolescent, an increasing weakness resulting from tethering of the spinal cord can frequently be substantiated by a muscle test of the lower extremities.

Range of motion (ROM) evaluation

A complete range of motion evaluation of the lower extremities is indicated for the newborn with spina bifida. The therapist must be aware of normal physiological flexion that is greatest at the hip and knees. In the normal newborn these apparent "contractures" of up to 35 degrees are eliminated as the child gains more control of extensor musculature and kicks more frequently into extension.

In the child with spina bifida, contractures may be evident at birth because of unopposed musculature. Hip adduction should not be tested beyond the neutral position to avoid dislocation of hips that are often unstable. Range should be done slowly and without excessive force to avoid fractures so often experienced in paralytic lower extremities. Range of motion should be checked with the same frequency as muscle testing.

Active ROM of the upper extremities can be assessed by observation and handling the infant. A formal ROM evaluation for the upper extremities is not usually indicated. A baseline ROM and tone assessment of the upper extremities should be completed.

Table 14-1. Key to muscle grading*

Test performance	Kendalls Percent	Lovett Word & letter		Abbrev. of percent	Nat. Found. for Inf. Par., & a Study Percent	Aids to Invest. of Per. N. Inj. Numerals	Neurolog. Rating
The ability to hold the test position against gravity and maximum pressure, or the ability to move the part into test position and hold against gravity and maximum pressure	100 95	Normal Normal−	N N−	10 −	100	5 5−	++++
Same as above, except holding against moderate pressure	90 80	Good+ Good	G+ G	9 8	75	4+ 4	+++
Same as above except holding against minimum pressure	70	Good−	G−	7		4−	
The ability to hold the test position against gravity, or the ability to move the part into test position and hold against gravity	60 50	Fair+ Fair	F+ F	6 5	50	3+ 3	++
The gradual release from test position against gravity; or, the ability to move the part toward test position against gravity almost to completion, or to completion with slight assistance; or, the ability to complete the arc of motion with gravity lessened	40	Fair−	F−	4		3−	
The ability to move the part through partial arc of motion with gravity lessened: moderate arc, 30% or poor +; small arc, 20% or poor	30	Poor+	P+	3		2+	
To avoid moving a patient into gravity lessened position, these grades may be estimated on the basis of the amount of assistance given during anti-gravity test movements: a 30% or poor+ muscle requires moderate assistance, a 20% or poor muscle requires more assistance	20	Poor	P	2	25	2	+
In muscles that can be seen or palpated, a feeble contraction may be felt in the muscle, or the tendon may become prominent during the muscle contraction, but there is no visible movement of the part	10 5	Poor− Trace	P− T	− 1		2− 1	
No contraction felt in the muscle	0	Zero	0	0	0	0	0

From Kendall HO, Kendall FP, and Wadsworth GE: Muscles testing and function, ed 2, Baltimore, 1971, Williams & Wilkins.
*Restriction of range of motion may be denoted by putting the grade in parentheses.

Sensory testing

Sensory testing of the infant and young child is simplified in order to determine the level of sensation as accurately as possible, with a minimum amount of testing. Full sensory tests are not possible until the child has acquired sufficient cognitive and language abilities to respond appropriately to testing.

In the newborn, sensory testing can best be done if the child is in a quiet state.* Beginning at the lowest level of sacral innervation, the skin is stroked with a pin or other sharp object until a reaction to pain is noted. Because of dermatome innervation the pin is usually drawn from the anal area, across the buttocks, down the posterior thigh and leg, then to the anterior surface of the leg and thigh, and finally across the abdominal muscles. Reactions to be noted are a facial grimace or cry, which indicates that the painful sensation has reached a cortical level. Care must be taken to see that each sensory dermatome has been evaluated. Results can be recorded by shading in the dermatomes where sensation is present (Fig. 14-7).

The physical therapist may be called upon to evaluate the newborn before surgical closure of the spinal meningocele. Although sensory and motor levels can be determined as previously described, it is important to consider the infant's general condition when interpreting test findings. Any medication taken by the mother during labor and delivery may influence the neonate's performance and thus should be noted. In addition, the physiological disor-

*If the infant is initially quiet, evaluation should begin with a sensory test. This test usually brings the child to an alert or crying state, which is optimal for muscle testing.

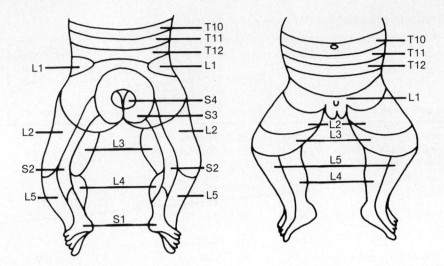

Fig. 14-7. Lower limb dermatomes. (From Brocklehurst, G: Spina bifida for the clinician, Clin Dev Med 57:53, 1976.)

ganization, normally seen in all infants during the first few days after birth, may also affect testing.[9] At best, this presurgical evaluation establishes a tentative baseline, and significant changes in the infant's neurological status in the first few weeks of life should not be surprising to the clinician.

In the young child from 2 to 7 years of age, light touch sensation and position sense can be tested in addition to pain sensation. Again, the ingenuity of the therapist will be called forth in order to elicit an appropriate response and reliable test results. Using games, such as "Tell me when the puppet touches you," or behavior modification techniques, like "Put your hand out for candy when I touch you," may be more effective for the young child than traditional testing methods.

From 7 years through adolescence, additional sensory tests of temperature and two-point discrimination may be added. Usually, traditional methods are sufficient to ensure reliable testing, but a more behavioral approach may again be indicated, depending upon the individual's cognitive functioning.

Following testing, a survey of the sensory dermatome chart should indicate where sensation is normal, absent, or impaired.

Reflex testing

The purpose of reflex testing is twofold: first to check for the presence of *normal* reflex activity and second to check for the integration of primitive reflexes and the establishment of more mature reactions. In the newborn, for example, one would expect strong rooting and sucking reflexes. In the child with spina bifida, because of possible involvement of the CNS as described previously, these reflexes may be depressed or absent. Since these reflexes play an integral part in obtaining nutrients for the infant, their value is obvious.

On the other hand, primitive reflexes, which persist past their expected span, may also indicate abnormality. For example, if the asymmetrical tonic neck reflex persists past 4 months, it will limit the infant's ability to bring the hands to midline for visual and tactile exploration.

As the primitive reflexes (initially needed for survival and to experience movement) become integrated, they are replaced by more mature and functional reactions. The righting and equilibrium reactions help the child attain the erect position and counteract changes in the center of gravity. Since these reactions depend on an intact CNS, as well as a certain level of postural control, they may be delayed, incomplete, or absent in the child with spina bifida. For example, a child with a low thoracic spinal cord lesion may show an incomplete equilibrium reaction in sitting. This may be caused by the lack of a stable postural base or by lack of initiation of the reaction centrally. Both the neurological and muscular components of these reactions must be considered.

Reflex testing for the child with spina bifida may not be as intensive as that for a child with cerebral palsy. It may, however, provide a check on the progress of normal development and as such reflect the integrity of the CNS.

Developmental/functional evaluations

Besides being aware of a child's sensory and motor levels, it is also important to assess the functional level. Two important questions need to be asked—"Does the child show normal components of posture and movement patterns?" and "What is the child's level of mobility?"

There are any number of developmental and/or functional evaluations that can be adapted for the child with spina bifida. The following are some suggestions for evaluation approaches or specifically designed tests to assist in assessment of this area.

Initially, a developmental sequence may be used to assess how a child is functioning. In each position used, both posture and movement will be evaluated. The goals in using this type of assessment are to determine what a child can and cannot do, the quality of the action, and what is limiting the child. If possible, the child should first be passively taken through the entire developmental sequence and then through active movements. The progression would begin in the supine position, rolling to prone, prone-on-elbows, prone-on-hands, up-to-sitting, hands-knees, kneeling, half-kneeling, standing, and walking. Both the ability to obtain and the ability to maintain the positions should be assessed.

It is not merely the accomplishment of the task that must be evaluated but, simultaneously, the *way* in which it is accomplished. For example, in rolling, is head righting sufficient to keep the head off the supporting surface? From the hands-knees position, can reciprocal crawling be initiated without the lower extremities being held in wide abduction? Can the child pull to stand easily by using trunk rotation? Assessing the quality of the child's abilities will assist the clinician in determining where therapeutic measures should begin and what the goals of such intervention will be.*

The Milani-Comparetti motor development screening test may prove useful in assessing the functional level of the child with spina bifida. This screening examination is designed to evaluate motor development from birth to 2 years of age (Fig. 14-8).[58] It requires no special equipment and can be administered in 4 to 8 minutes. The test evaluates both spontaneous behavior and evoked responses. Spontaneous behavior includes postural control of the head and body in various positions, as well as a sequence of active movement patterns. Primitive reflexes, righting, and equilibrium reactions comprise the evoked responses. The Milani-Comparetti test should assist the clinician in evaluating each child's underlying postural mechanisms and his or her ability to attain the erect position. Refer to the test manual for special examination procedures and scoring.[58]

The Peabody Developmental Motor Scales (PDMS)[28] is a recently standardized assessment that may prove helpful in evaluating a child with congenital spinal-cord injury. The PDMS consists of gross and fine motor scales from birth through 83 months. The two scales allow a comparison of the child's motor performance with a normative sample of children at various age levels. Although the disabled child would not be expected to pass many of the gross motor items at the later age levels, the scale still serves as a reminder of expected gross motor performance at each age. The fine motor scale offers a chance to assess fine motor performance of children with congenital spinal-cord injury. This area has been frequently overlooked with children with myelomeningocele. Fine motor develop-

ment, however, may be affected because of congenital abnormalities in brain development associated with myelomeningocele, or related to tethering of the spinal cord that can result in fine motor paresis. In addition, the PDMS offers guidelines for administering the test to handicapped children.[28]

Finally, a developmental activities inventory has been designed to assess the current functional status of the child with spina bifida and to compare the child's rate of achievement with that of others with the same level of lesion.[79] The inventory consists of 166 items listed in developmental sequence and grouped in the following categories: personal-social, eating, dressing, grooming, toileting, gross motor activities and locomotion. (The inventory and predetermined criteria for passing each item are available from the authors.) Results are available for four motor-level groups showing ages of routine performance of functional activities for the 173 children tested. These developmental guidelines should provide a reasonable estimate concerning the appropriateness of a developmental task. This information has been condensed into a self-care assessment tool that should assist parents, educators, and clinicians in setting realistic goals and expectations for each client.[85]

Perceptual/cognitive evaluations

In evaluating these children, it is important to include some assessment of perceptual/cognitive status. The appropriate assessment will depend largely upon the age of the child.

For the newborn from 3 to 30 days old, the Brazelton Neonatal Behavioral Assessment scale may be adapted to assess the infant's organization in terms of physiological response to stress, state control, motoric control, and social interaction. Ideally, the infant should be medically stable and free from CNS-depressant drugs before evaluation. Generally, this evaluation will occur after the back lesion is closed, and a shunt is positioned to relieve the hydrocephalic condition.

While test results may not have prognostic value because of the plasticity of the nervous system at this young age, they supply the clinician with information concerning the current status of the child. This information can be conveyed to the infant's caregivers—both medical personnel and parents—so that strengths can be appreciated and weaknesses anticipated and handled appropriately. Helping parents to identify that their infant has his or her own unique characteristics and assisting them in dealing with these characteristics does a great deal to strengthen already precarious parent-infant bonding.

Repeated administration of the Brazelton Neonatal Behavioral Assessment scale in the first month of life may help monitor the infant's progress in organization and reflect the curve of recovery. Although the manual for this behavioral assessment is quite complete, proper adminis-

*An excellent reference for the developmental sequence is Colangelo C and others: A normal baby: the sensory processes of the first year, Valhalla, NY, 1976, Blythdale Children's Hospital.

MILANI-COMPARETTI MOTOR DEVELOPMENT SCREENING TEST

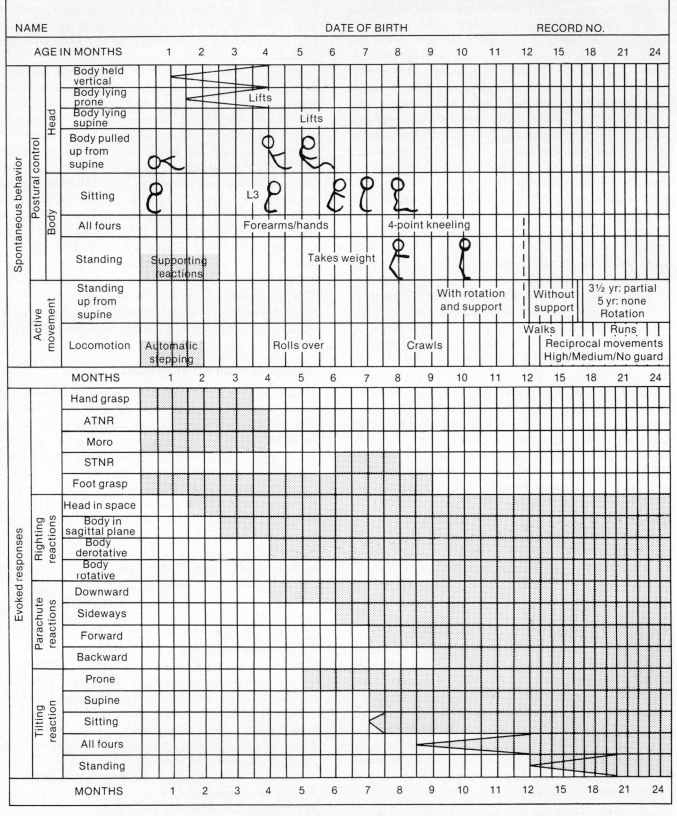

Fig. 14-8. Milani-Comparetti Motor Development Screening Test. (From Trembath J: The Milani-Comparetti Motor Development Screening Test, Meyers Children's Rehabilitation Institute, University of Nebraska Medical Center, Omaha, 1977.)

tration scoring and interpretation require direct training with someone already proficient in using the scale.[9] Excellent training films for the Brazelton Neonatal Behavioral Assessment scale are available for purchase or through your local university's learning resource center (see the appendix at the end of the chapter).

Two full developmental evaluations, appropriate for the infant and toddler with spina bifida, are the Bayley Scales of Infant Development[8] and the Revised Gesell Developmental Assessment.[42] Each evaluation contains information on gross motor, fine motor, language, personal-social, and cognitive development.

The Bayley Scales, consisting of a mental and motor scale and a behavioral record, can be used to test children from birth to 30 months. The recommended testing range is 2 months to 2 years of age. The Bayley is well standardized and reliable and takes about 45 minutes to administer. It is not an easy test to learn and would initially require supervision of an experienced tester. Two excellent videotapes are available to assist in this learning process (see the Appendix 1 at the end of the chapter).

The revised Gesell can be used to evaluate an infant from 4 weeks to 36 months and requires 20 to 40 minutes to administer. It has recently been restandardized and in its present form is a fully reliable and valid instrument. The manual accompanying this assessment is complete, although somewhat complicated. The novice examiner is advised to seek assistance in learning to use this tool.

Either the Bayley or the revised Gesell will provide the clinician with a broader view of the child's total development. The gross motor information from these developmental assessments will not be specific enough for a therapist evaluating a child with spina bifida. The additional information on fine motor, language, personal-social, and cognitive development, however, is sufficient and will be most important in planning an effective intervention program.

For the older child, the Purdue Perceptual-Motor Survey can be used to detect errors in perceptual-motor development.[71] Although this test was not designed for use with children having known deficits, it can still be adapted to give information about the spina bifida child's perceptual-motor status. The test was standardized on 6- to 10-year-olds but could be used with older children who are within that cognitive age range. The motor items on the test will be invalid because of the child's physical involvement. Items testing laterality, directionality, or perceptual-motor matching should prove valuable in program planning, however, since these areas are often found to be deficient in the child with spina bifida.[30] The test manual is straightforward, and test mechanics can be easily learned. The Sensory Integration and Praxis Tests (SIPT),[5] formerly the Southern California Sensory Integration Tests (SCSIT), may be used to assess the older child's sensorimotor function. Although these tests were designed to detect the presence of learning disabilities, they can be used with the spina bifida child to document learning difficulties and the extent of impairment of the sensory systems. They can often be used to reassure the classroom teacher and parents that learning problems do indeed exist and have a suspected neurological base. These tests were standardized on the 4- to 10-year-olds and will have limited value if used on children much older or those with severe perceptual or fine motor involvement. The SIPT battery can be given only by certified examiners, usually occupational or physical therapists.

With a firm data base provided by a thorough physical/occupational therapy evaluation and referrals to other professionals as appropriate, a reasonable treatment plan can be established and updated as necessary.

TREATMENT PLANNING AND REHABILITATION RELATED TO SIGNIFICANT STAGES OF RECOVERY
Newborn to toddler (preambulatory phase)

Stage 1: before closure of myelomeningocele — newborn. Physical therapy management of the infant in Stage 1 is limited by his or her medical condition (Table 14-2). Attempts can be made, however, to prevent deformity and to maintain ROM while giving stimulation to provide as normal an environment as possible.

In addition to evaluation, the therapist may begin some early intervention measures that can be continued and expanded postsurgically. Range of motion and positioning in prone or sidelying may be initiated to prevent or decrease contractures in the lower extremities. If club feet are present, soft tissue stretching may be indicated. Stretching begins distally on the soft tissue of the forefoot and proceeds proximally toward the calcaneus. This is done to take advantage of the pliability of soft tissue structures and to minimize fixed deformity later. When treating the newborn before surgery, great care must be taken to avoid contaminating an open sac, which is usually covered with a sterile dressing and kept moist with a saline solution.[54]

Stage 2: after surgery, during hospitalization — newborn to infant. Therapeutic intervention during Stage 2 will be more aggressive than before surgery but will often be limited by the infant's neurological and orthopaedic status. A major goal during this stage is to prevent contracture and to maintain range of motion.

Traditional range of motion can be taught to nursing staff and family. Range of motion can also be carried out while the child is being held at the adult's shoulder or prone over the adult's lap. These positions allow closeness between the caregiver and infant, thus encouraging maximum relaxation and interaction between them.

Because of their medical conditions, hospitalized infants often experience early separation from their parents. Teaching the family to handle the child as described above may enhance parent-infant bonding. Adequate

Table 14-2. Summary of treatment planning and rehabilitation related to significant stages of recovery

Stage of recovery	Major physical therapy goals	Physical therapy management
Stage 1: before surgical closure of sac	Prevent contractures and deformity	ROM, positioning
	Encourage normal sensorimotor development	Graded auditory and visual stimuli
Stage 2: after surgery during hospitalization	Prevent contracture and deformity	ROM taught to hospital personnel and family
		Positioning in prone and side-lying
	Encourage normal sensorimotor development	Providing toys of various colors, textures, and shapes
		Graded auditory and visual stimuli—music boxes, squeaky toys, brightly colored objects
		Therapeutic handling to encourage good head and trunk control
Stage 3: condition stabilized, preambulatory	Encourage normal development sequence	Work in sitting on head righting and equilibrium reactions
		Eye-hand coordination activities
		Early weight bearing on lower extremities
		Encourage prone progression
		Weight shifting in standing frame
		Comprehensive home program
Stage 4: toddler through preschool	Begin ambulation	Choose appropriate orthotic device
		Gait training
		Development and strengthening of righting and equilibrium reactions
	Continue development in cognitive and psychosocial areas	Consider placement in 0-3 stimulation group
		Public preschool program
		Continue home program
	Collaborate goals with other team members	Open communication with other team members
Stage 5: primary school through adolescence	Reevaluate ambulation potential	Replace orthotic devices as necessary
		Wheelchair prescriptions as necessary
	Maintain present level of functioning	Teach locomotion activities
		Maintain strength in trunk and extremities
	Prevent skin breakdown as child becomes more sedentary	Teach skin care
	Promote independence in self-care skills	Work with team members to teach dressing, feeding, hygiene, and bowel and bladder care
	Remediate any perceptual-motor problems	Provide program/activities for sensorimotor integration
	Provide appropriate adaptive devices	Check for fit and proper use of adaptive devices
	Promote self-esteem and social-sexual adjustment	Collaborate with other team members in counseling efforts

bonding is essential for normal psychosocial development to occur.

When the child is not being handled, resting positions can be used to maintain ROM and enhance development. The prone position is the most advantageous, because it prevents hip flexion contractures and encourages development of extensor musculature as the child lifts his or her head. Side-lying, which allows the hands to come to midline and generally encourages symmetrical posture, can be used for alternating positioning. As much as possible, the supine position should be avoided because the child is most dominated by primitive reflexes and the effects of gravity in this position. For example, for the spina bifida child with CNS involvement in addition to the spinal cord lesion, the effects of the tonic labyrinthine reflex combined with paralytic lower extremities make movement from the supine position extremely difficult.

A normal sensory experience should be presented to the child in spite of the hospital setting. Toys of various colors, textures, and shapes should be available. Musical mobiles held low enough for the child to reach provide a variety of sensory experiences. Stimuli such as squeaky toys or the human face and voice can be used to encourage visual and auditory tracking. Controlled stimulation relevant to the infant's neurological state, rather than overstimulation, should be the rule. Depending on the age of the child, appropriate learning situations must be presented in order to provide the child with as normal an environment as possible for perceptual and cognitive growth.

A major physical therapy goal will be to guide the child through the developmental sequence, ultimately preparing him or her for assumption of the upright posture. In this immediate postsurgical stage, primary emphasis will be on attaining good head and trunk control and eliciting appropriate righting reactions. For example, the child can be seated on the therapist's lap, facing the therapist, and alternately lowered slowly backwards and side-to-side. This will help to stimulate head righting and strengthen neck and abdominal muscles. Weight shifting in the prone-on-elbows position is another good activity for enhancing development of head and trunk control.

Developmental handling may be limited by frequent shunt revisions that require the infant to be kept flat for a period of days. Increased muscle tone caused by CNS involvement must also be normalized before appropriate developmental steps can be achieved. For example, when increased tone is evidenced by shoulder girdle retraction, inhibitory techniques must be applied before normal head control can be established. The arms must be moved forward, out of the abnormal retracted position, while rotation of the shoulder girdle on the pelvis is initiated. (For additional information on normalization of tone, refer to Chapters 6, 8, and 9.)

This second stage ends as the child is discharged from the hospital. The child will be followed closely by the rehabilitation team, which may include a neurosurgeon, an orthopaedist, a urologist, a nurse clinician, a physical therapy/occupational therapy (PT/OT) team, and a social worker. Before discharge, a definitive home program should be given to the family, and the child will most likely require therapy on an ongoing basis.

Stage 3: condition stabilized—infant to toddler. In this stage of rehabilitation, the major emphasis is on preparing the child mentally and physically for walking. Goals of preventing contractures and maintaining ROM will remain throughout the life of the child. Unless this is done, ambulation not only becomes more difficult but often impossible. If possible, prone positioning during play and sleeping assists greatly in stretching tight musculature. Resting splints for the lower extremities can be used as necessary.

Assuming that the child has previously gained good head and trunk control, the next step would be development of sitting equilibrium reactions. As sitting balance improves, fine motor and eye-hand coordination activities should be introduced. Upper-extremity functioning is often

overlooked in the child with spina bifida, whose problems appear to be concentrated in the lower extremities. Since most spina bifida children show decreased fine motor coordination,[54] this problem should be addressed as is developmentally appropriate. The normal infant begins to reach and grasp by 6 months of age[16]; therefore the child with spina bifida must be given ample opportunities to practice and to perfect these skills at an early age.

Early weight bearing is also of utmost importance, both physiologically and psychologically.[76] The upright position has beneficial effects on circulation and renal and bladder functioning, as well as on the promotion of bone growth[33] and density.[74] Psychologically, weight bearing in an upright posture allows a normal view of the world and contributes to more normal perceptual, cognitive, and emotional growth. One way to achieve this weight bearing is in the kneeling position. This is developmentally appropriate, since children 8 to 10 months old frequently use kneeling as a transition from all fours to standing.

Since young infants are frequently held in the standing position and bounced on their parents' laps, it is appropriate to introduce this form of weight bearing on the lower extremities from birth onward. To fail to do so will deprive the spina bifida child of the normal experience of standing at a very early age. When standing these children, however, care must be taken to see that the lower extremities are in good alignment and that undue pressure is not exerted on them (Fig. 14-9). In this way the risk of fractures is minimized, and a normal weight-bearing experience is provided.

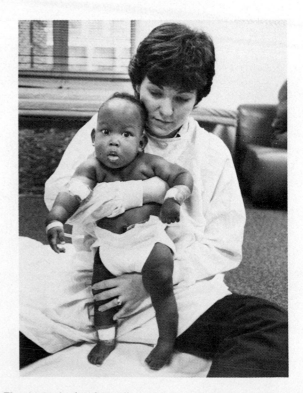

Fig. 14-9. Assisted standing with normal postural alignment.

Following a normal developmental sequence, the child with spina bifida will usually begin some form of prone progression as trunk and upper-extremity stability improve. This is a significant phase of development, since it allows for the development of a sensorimotor base, as the child expands environmental horizons.[43] During this phase of high mobility, anesthetic skin must be checked for injury frequently and often protected by heavier clothing. This may help to prevent any major skin breakdown, which could significantly delay the rehabilitation process.

For some children with high-level lesions where prone mobility is not safe or practical for long distances, a caster cart (Fig. 14-10) may be used.[43] This provides the child with a means of exploring the environment safely but independently.

When the child attempts to pull to a standing position or would be expected to do so normally (at 10 to 12 months of age), the use of a standing device is indicated. Generally, a standing frame is the first orthosis chosen.[43] This is a relatively inexpensive tubular frame to which adjustable parts are attached (Fig. 14-11). Because it is not custom made, it can be fitted fairly quickly, although adjustments may be necessary to accommodate spinal deformities. This standing device offers support of the trunk, hips, and knees and leaves the hands free for other activities. Time spent in the standing frame should be increased gradually. This will allow the child to adjust to the upright position in terms of muscle strength, endurance, blood pressure, and pressure on skin surfaces.

After children have built up a tolerance for standing,

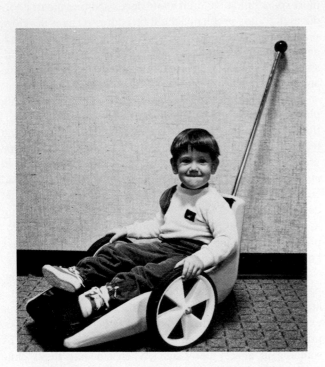

Fig. 14-10. Caster cart used for independent mobility.

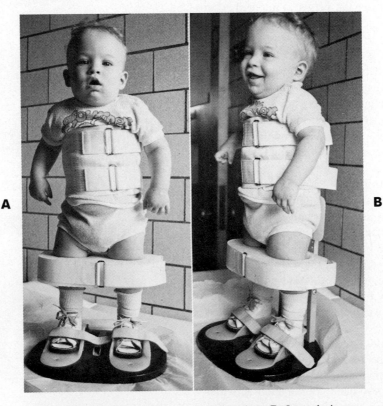

Fig. 14-11. Standing frame. **A,** Anterior view. **B,** Lateral view.

they may be taught to move in the device by shifting their weight from side to side. Initial shifting of weight onto one side of the body is necessary to allow the other side to move forward. This preliminary weight shift is also a prerequisite for developing equilibrium reactions in the standing position and thus will prepare the child for later ambulation. As the child shifts weight, the trunk musculature on the weight-bearing side should elongate and shorten on the non–weight-bearing side as muscle strength allows. This normal reaction to weight shifting also includes righting of the head and should be monitored closely by the therapist for completeness.

During this preambulatory stage therapy goals may be accomplished through a comprehensive home program, with frequent checks to note progress or problems and to change the program accordingly.

Often the program must be reevaluated and goals changed, if conditions such as shunt malfunctions or fractures occur. The warning signs for shunt dysfunctions are generally those previously described for suspected hydrocephalus. In addition, swelling along the shunt site may indicate a malfunction. Swelling and local heat or redness of a limb are the usual signs of a fracture. The limb may also look out of alignment. Fever may accompany a fracture. As mentioned previously, these fractures generally heal quickly with proper medical intervention and interrupt rehabilitation efforts minimally.

Toddler through adolescent (ambulatory phase)

Stage 4: toddler through preschool. This period in development marks the end of infancy and the beginning of childhood. For the normal child who has developed a strong sensorimotor foundation, physical development will be marked by increased coordination and refinement of movement patterns. In addition, a great variety of motor skills will be achieved as the normal child learns to throw, catch, run, hop, and jump. This is also a period of great cognitive growth, as children's use of mental imagery and physical knowledge of their environments expand. Concepts of size, number, color, form, and space are all developing. Emotionally, most children are becoming more independent and begin to break away from the sheltered environment of the home. They are now more interested in interacting with others and become social beings to a greater extent.

All of these changes in physical, cognitive, and emotional development will be evident in the child with spina bifida, although the degree will be dependent upon the extent of the disability. It is of utmost importance to be aware of the characteristics of normal development, so that they can be nurtured and enhanced in the disabled child.*

Goals for this, as for any other, stage must address not

*An excellent reference on developmental changes occuring during childhood is Papalia DE and Olds SW: Human development, New York, 1981, McGraw-Hill Inc.

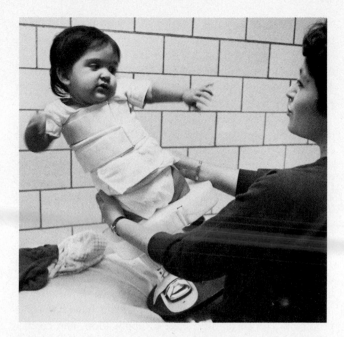

Fig. 14-12. Weight shift and forward rotation in standing frame.

only physical but cognitive and emotional development. The most obvious goal at this stage is to progress the child who is already standing to an ambulatory status. Even the child with a low thoracic lesion will usually manage some form of ambulation.

Thus far, the child has learned to shift weight in the standing frame. By rotating the trunk toward the weighted side, the non—weight-bearing side can be shifted forward (Fig. 14-12). By reversing the weight shift, the opposite side can be moved forward and a type of "pivoting-forward" progression can be accomplished. To maintain balance while shifting, the child may initially use a two-wheeled walker or a tripod cane. The therapist may help initiate weight shift and trunk rotation by alternately pulling the arms forward.[31]

Once the child has gained this form of mobility, the type of permanent bracing chosen will depend upon the level of the lesion. For thoracic and high-level lumbar lesions, a parapodium is often chosen. The parapodium was developed by the Ontario Crippled Children's Center in 1970 and is similar to the standing frame, except that hinges at the hips and knees allow for sitting and standing.[31] It too can be adjusted for growth and can accommodate orthopaedic deformities. As with the standing frame, proper alignment of the parapodium is critical. The therapist, in conjunction with the orthotist, should check for correct standing alignment. The prevention of additional orthopaedic deformities, development of good muscular control, and normal body image are dependent upon a good-fitting orthosis.

After a pivoting gait is learned with the parapodium, a swing-to or swing-through gait can be attempted. By 4 to

5 years of age, a swing-through gait, with the child using Lofstrand crutches, can usually be accomplished.[31]

Variations of the parapodium are appearing that allow for easier locking and unlocking of hip and knee joints.[11] Also, a swivel or pivot walker may be attached to the foot plate to allow for crutchless walking.

Another type of orthosis for the child with a high thoracic or low lumbar lesion is the Orlau swivel walker. It consists of modular design similar to the standing frame, with a chest strap and knee blocks attached to swiveling foot plates.[13] Rather than the whole base moving forward, as when weight is shifted in the parapodium, in the swivel walker each foot plate is spring loaded and is able to swivel forward independently. This allows for independent balance on one foot and, therefore, crutchless ambulation. The Orlau swivel walker is manufactured in Shrewsbury in the United Kingdom, and kits to be assembled may be obtained from there (see Appendix 2).[80]

Both the parapodium and swivel walker have had some problems with instability, ease of application, and cosmesis. New designs are appearing that attempt to correct these problems. Despite the attempts, existing limitations in the parapodium and swivel walker, particularly energy cost of walking, slow rate of locomotion, and cosmesis, have limited their use, primarily to the younger child.[73] These devices, however, remain an effective means of preventing musculoskeletal deformities caused by wheelchair positioning. They also enhance social-emotional development gained from the upright position.[13] Another option for the higher-level child with good sitting balance is the reciprocating gait orthosis. (RGO)[21] The brace consists of bilateral long-leg braces with a pelvic band and thoracic extension if necessary. The hip joints are connected by a cable system that can work in two ways. If the child has active hip flexors, he can activate the cable system by shifting his weight and flexing the non-weight-bearing extremity. This acts to bring the weight-bearing extremity into relative extension in preparation for the next step. Without hip flexors, the child extends his trunk over one extremity, thus positioning it in relative extension. By virtue of the cable system, the non-weight-bearing extremity moves into flexion, thus initiating a step.[48]

A more common means of maintaining the upright position has been through the use of long- or short-leg metal braces. In the 1970s conventional metal bracing was largely replaced by polypropylene braces. These plastic orthoses are considerably lighter than metal bracing and therefore reduce the energy cost of walking for the child with spina bifida.[45] They allow close contact and can be slipped into the shoe rather than being worn externally, thus affording the patient a better-fitting, more cosmetic orthosis. These polypropylene braces are generally most effective with lower lumbar lesions where only short-leg bracing is required (Fig. 14-13). While these braces cannot

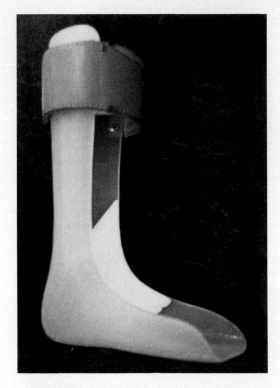

Fig. 14-13. Polypropylene ankle-foot orthosis.

be worn by everyone, they have greatly improved the rehabilitation potential of those able to use them.

The type of orthosis chosen (long-leg, with or without pelvic band, or short-leg) will depend upon the level of the myelomeningocele and the muscle power within that level. Because lesions are frequently incomplete, muscle strength must be assessed accurately before bracing is prescribed. Even children with L3 lesions, who demonstrate incomplete knee extension, may be able to use a short-leg brace with an anterior shell rather than requiring long-leg bracing.[17] The physical therapist must work in conjunction with the orthopaedist and orthotist to have each child fitted with the minimum amount of bracing, which allows for joint stability and a good gait pattern. (See Chapter 28, Therapeutic Application of Orthotics.)

Children ambulating with ankle-foot orthoses often show excessive rotation at the knee because of the lack of functioning lateral hamstrings. Rather than going to a higher level of bracing, a twister cable can be added, which often decreases the rotary component during gait.[17]

For children with a low lumbar or sacral lesion, often a polypropylene shoe insert to control foot position is the only bracing needed. These inserts fit snugly inside the shoe and help to control calcaneal and forefoot instabilities.[43]

Gait training, begun as the child first started to stand, can now continue in a more formalized manner. Using the appropriate orthosis and assistive devices (walker, crutches, or cane), each child must be helped to achieve

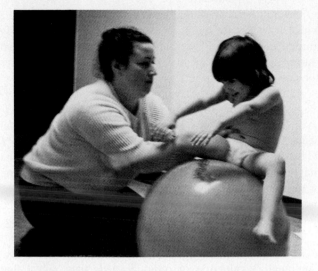

Fig. 14-14. Balance and strengthening exercises done on a movable surface.

the most efficient and effective gait pattern possible. As a part of gait training, the child should be taken out of the bracing and "challenged" so that righting and equilibrium reactions can be developed to their maximum. For example, having a child maintain balance while sitting on a ball or other movable surface (tilt board, trampoline) requires the participation of all available musculature (Fig. 14-14). These unconventional "gait-training" techniques can be used to improve muscle strength in general and to improve the gait pattern when bracing is reapplied.

Various forms of therapeutic exercise can be used with the spina bifida child to strengthen existing musculature. The work of Sullivan and others[83] can assist the therapist in this regard. These authors approach exercise from a developmental proprioceptive neuromuscular facilitation (PNF) point of view. A more traditional approach to therapeutic exercise can be found in Basmajian's work.[7] It includes a chapter on exercises in water, which may add an interesting adjunct to the therapeutic program for the child with spina bifida. Pearson and Williams[66] give the therapist a variety of therapeutic approaches that could be applied to the child with spina bifida. Finally, Williamson[84] provides a comprehensive overview of children with spina bifida. Especially pertinent is the chapter on sensorimotor assessment and intervention.

Regardless of the strengthening program chosen, the pediatric therapist has the special task of using creativity to involve the child in therapeutic "play activities." For example, when doing resisted rolling, a child could pretend to be trying to get away from attacking alligators. The ideas for creative activities are limitless, but essential, for combining therapy with age-appropriate cognitive abilities.

Gait training and muscle strengthening are not the only consideration of the physical therapist. How cognitive and psychosocial development can be enhanced during this stage of the child's development is also an important concern. One appropriate solution is to place the child in a 0- to 3-year stimulation group. While these groups may vary in the services they provide, most usually include age-appropriate play activities and some type of parental counseling. In addition, many offer therapeutic intervention from physical, occupational, and speech therapists. This intervention may be in groups or on an individual basis.

Besides the socialization that 0- to 3-year groups provide for the disabled child, they also teach the child age-appropriate activities of daily living (ADL), such as dressing and undressing. At this age ADL skills are more appropriately taught in a group setting than on an individual basis. For many children the 0-to-3 program, along with individualized physical therapy, is sufficient to enhance development in the physical, cognitive, and psychosocial realms.

Presently, when the children reach age 3, public school education becomes available to them. The preschool program provided continues to offer the same fundamental benefits as the 0-to-3 program. It is the role of the hospital-based therapist to communicate the specific needs of each child entering the public school system. In this way continuity in the child's rehabilitation program is preserved.

The rehabilitation team, usually headed by a pediatrician or clinical nurse specialist, continues to follow the child closely during this stage. The neurosurgeon will check shunt functioning and perform revisions as necessary. The orthopaedist will supervise bracing efforts to prevent and correct deformities in the spine and lower extremities. Well-child care and general medical treatment is the responsibility of the pediatrician on the team. The urologist continues to monitor renal functioning while keeping the child dry and free of infection. At this stage, bowel and bladder training will usually be taught to the child and family by the clinical nurse specialist. This clinician generally initiates this training when the child is 2½ years old.

Bladder training usually consists of transferring the job of intermittent catheterization from the parents to the child. Children as young as 3 years, but certainly by the age of 5,[1] can learn CIC in a short period of time.[1] The children may first practice on dolls with male and female genitalia. Next, using mirrors to magnify their own genitalia, they are able to accomplish the technique on themselves. CIC in conjunction with pharmacotherapy has proven useful in achieving continence in spina bifida children with overflow incontinence.[7] Another method of bladder training, recently being used in the United States is intravesical transurethral bladder stimulation. This technique has allowed children with neurogenic bladder to rehabilitate their bladder function so that they can detect bladder fullness and generate effective destrusor contractions leading to improved continence.[40,41]

Bowel training can be achieved through proper diet,

regular evacuation times, and appropriate use of stool softeners and suppositories.[40,49] Constipation (and resulting bypass diarrhea) can be prevented by a diet including brans, fruit, and lots of fluids. Large amounts of milk, apple sauce, bananas, or rice cereal should be avoided. Stool softeners (not laxatives and enemas) and suppositories should be used to keep the stools soft and to help stimulate evacuation. Last, toilet training, which amounts to scheduled toileting in time with the stool stimulants, usually achieves bowel continence. Consistency at each step along the way is the key to successful bowel training. A therapist may be called upon to assist the parents and child in obtaining independence in this ADL activity. See Chapter 29 for additional information on bowel and bladder care.

Other members of the team, such as a psychologist, a pedodontist, a social worker, and a dietician, continue to function in their appropriate roles, interacting with the child and family as necessary. Physical therapists, as members of the team, must be sure that their treatment plans collaborate with the efforts of other team members.

Stage 5: primary school through adolescence. This stage of development is marked by less rapid growth than earlier childhood but ends with a period of rapid physiological growth.[64] Children in the 6-to-10 age group are interested in a wider variety of physical activities as they challenge their bodies to perform. The adolescent, however, is going through a period of great sexual differentiation as primary and secondary sexual characteristics develop more fully.

Cognitively, children are able to solve problems in a more sophisticated manner, although they revert to illogical thinking with complex problems. As they reach adolescence, they become capable of hypothetical reasoning, and their thought processes approach that of adults.[64]

Emotionally, the 6- to 10-year-old is in a period of relative calm. Children are very interested in school work and are eager to produce. During this period, they are building the skills of the future, preparing them for adult work.

Adolescence is a stormy emotional period. Adolescents remain in turmoil as they seek their identities through sexual, social, and vocational activities. As their value systems develop, they feel less ambivalence between remaining as children or striving for independence.

A therapy program must be designed to meet the individual's needs in each area. Age alone does not determine the appropriate therapeutic goals. Goals that are not suited for the child's cognitive and emotional needs, in addition to physical needs, will be doomed to failure before they are attempted. For example, an 18-month-old may have the physical capabilities to ambulate independently with crutches and braces. The child may not, however, have the cognitive skills necessary to learn a 4-point gait or be ready emotionally to separate from his or her mother for intensive therapy sessions. A more realistic goal may be to let the child walk, holding onto furniture (cruising) while a wheeled walker for more independent ambulation is slowly introduced. Another alternative to using a conventional walker is to encourage the child to play with push-toys such as grocery carts and baby buggies.

As the energy cost of walking becomes too high, it often becomes appropriate for the adolescent to use a wheelchair for locomotion. To a teenager whose emotional needs include a strong peer identity, being confined to a wheelchair may be devastating. Appropriate alternatives may be to delay the decision to use a wheelchair full-time or to limit ambulation to short distances or to those places most important to the child. Again, goals must be tailored to the child's needs and encompass his or her whole being.

In accordance with the child's growth spurts, frequent adjustment or reordering of bracing will be necessary. Continual reevaluation of orthotic needs may reveal that the level of bracing may decrease as the child grows and becomes stronger. The opposite corollary is also a possibility.

Usually during this stage, if it has not occurred previously, the evaluation of future ambulation potential will occur. This evaluation is frequently requested by the child whose larger size and limited abilities make ambulation more difficult each day. It must be remembered that strength does not increase in the same proportion as body weight.[67] Ambulation, although possible for the young child, may be impossible for that same person as a young adult.

While no guidelines will include every patient, generally children with thoracic-level lesions are rarely ambulators by the late teens.[22,43,54] Those with upper lumbar lesions may be household ambulators with long-leg bracing but will require wheelchairs for quick mobility as adults. With low lumbar lesions, most adults can become community ambulators. Patients with sacral-level lesions are usually able to ambulate freely within the community. Many require minimal bracing and ambulate without assistive devices.[22,43,54] It must be remembered that ambulatory status is not determined by level of the lesion alone. The muscle power available, degree of orthopaedic deformity, age, height, weight of the patient, and of course motivation are also determining factors.[17,25,43,44,76]

Because a large number of older spina bifida children will become wheelchair dependent, potential problems connected with a sedentary existence must be explored. Skin care, always a concern for the child with spina bifida, becomes a priority for the constant sitter. Mirrors may be used for self-inspection of the skin twice daily.[35] Well-constructed foam seat cushions are essential for distributing pressure evenly. Children should be taught frequent weight shifting within the chair to relieve pressure areas. Clothing should not be constricting but heavy enough to protect sensitive skin from wheelchair parts. Children must also be taught to avoid extremes of temperature and environmental hazards such as radiators, sharp objects, and abrasive surfaces.[35] The therapist must reinforce the importance of skin care to prevent setbacks in the rehabilitation process that may result when skin breakdown develops.

Children with higher-level lesions may need spinal support to prevent deformities. Polyethylene body jackets can be used to provide this support and, hopefully, prevent the progression of any paralytic deformities.[43] Whatever type of device or wheelchair padding is used, the therapist must check to see that weight is distributed equally through both buttocks and that the spine is supported as necessary.

Part of the therapeutic intervention will be to provide strengthening exercises or activities to be done out of the supporting orthosis. This is necessary to maintain existing trunk strength and to preserve the child's present level of functioning.

Generally, in late childhood or early adolescence, orthopaedic deformities that have been gradually developing require surgical intervention. Progressive scoliosis or kyphosis may require internal fixation when conservative methods fail.[56] Often sectioning of contracted muscles at the hip and knee is required.[22] The iliopsoas, adductors, and hamstrings are frequently the offending muscles. These surgeries, followed by strengthening exercises and gait training, often add to the ambulatory life of the child with spina bifida. For example, in a child who displays an extreme lordotic posture, hip flexors may be contractured and require surgery to lengthen them. A postoperative therapeutic program might include periods of prone lying to prevent future contractures and strengthening of hip extensors and abdominals that were previously overstretched by the lordotic position.

Of primary importance during this stage is preparing the child for independence in activities of daily living (ADL), which may be broken down into self-care, locomotion-related, and social interaction activities.[79]

In conjunction with the nurse and occupational therapist, self-care skills of dressing, eating and food preparation, general hygiene, and bowel and bladder care can be addressed. Because the adolescent is so concerned with achieving independence, he or she is more likely to comply with a regime of strengthening exercises, if shown how they relate to functional independence. A creative therapist may, for example, incorporate trunk stability and upper-extremity strengthening work in activities such as gourmet cooking or getting ready for a dance.

Locomotion activities should include all gait-related skills, such as falling down, getting up, or ambulation on various terrains. Transfers of all types are also included in locomotion activities. Again, a creative therapeutic program helps to make achievement of skills more palatable. For example, school-age children may enjoy a competitive relay race situation, where each child falls, gets up, walks across the room, and sits down in a chair safely. This type of activity combines gait-training activities with group socialization and may meet a variety of goals (motor and psychosocial) at the same time.

It has been shown that achievement of independence in ADL for the child and adult with spina bifida is not solely dependent upon the level of paralysis.[79] Also important are psychosocial and environmental factors. Mean ages for the achievement of various ADL activities have been developed and may assist the therapist in establishing realistic therapeutic goals in this area.[79]

Often during this stage of recovery, the therapist may be asked to assist in assessing cognitive functioning. The perceptual/cognitive evaluations referred to earlier may be administered and the results interpreted for parents and school personnel.

As previously discussed, children with spina bifida have been found to have a general perceptual deficit.[19] This deficit can be manifested in a variety of ways. First, the child may have difficulty recognizing objects and the relationships that they have to each other. They may therefore perceive their world in a distorted manner, thus making their reactions unstable and unpredictable. These perceptual difficulties will most likely affect academic learning and may associate failure with the learning process. Difficulties in attaining independence in ADL activities are also linked to perceptual problems. Lastly, emotional disturbances may be attributed in part to the perceptual difficulties of the child with spina bifida.[29]

Remedial programs, such as the Frostig Program for the Development of Visual Perception, have been effective in improving the visual perception of spina bifida children.[29] Programs of this type are most effective when remediation begins early, preferably at or before the time the child enters school.

Children requiring programs for sensorimotor integration should be referred to a therapist certified in this area. If one is not available, many appropriate activities for sensorimotor integration may be adapted from Ayres[4] or Montgomery and Richter.[59]

Regardless of the school setting chosen for the child, the therapist should be able to serve the classroom teacher as a consultant. Advice on adaptive seating and therapeutic goals appropriate for the classroom will help to ensure that the rehabilitation process will continue in the classroom, as well as promoting optimal conditions for learning.

When a child is going from a special to a regular school setting, the support of the therapeutic team is essential and invaluable. Often, teachers in the public school setting have had little exposure to handicapped children.[36] The teacher's expectations, as created by the therapist regarding the spina bifida child's special needs and abilities, often spell the difference between success and failure of this attempt at integration both academically and psychosocially. Even though the child may no longer require direct therapeutic intervention, periodic checks, including site classroom visits, are recommended to prevent minor problems from erupting into major ones. For example, bowel and bladder accidents can be avoided by scheduling regular times for toileting. The teacher may be able to make minor adjustments in the teaching schedule to accommodate for this. Also, full-control braces (from hip to ankles) may seem overwhelming to the lay-person. If the teacher is shown how the braces lock and unlock to allow the child to sit or stand to walk, he or she may feel more at ease if ever called upon to assist the child.

The physical therapy goals in this stage will all be colored by the psychological perspective of the child. As the child nears adolescence, these psychosocial aspects become of paramount importance. While the physical therapist should not take on the role of the psychologist, collaborative efforts in the area of counseling will be necessary. Questions will arise many times during the physical/occupational therapy sessions, requiring factual answers that the therapist can and should provide.

Adolescents with spina bifida show great concern about self-esteem and social-sexual adjustment.[34] These concerns appear directly related to efficient bowel and bladder management.[47] Strategies to cope with bowel and bladder difficulties, as previously outlined, combined with appropriate emotional support from family and medical personnel will help to alleviate this concern.

Questions about sexuality may be brought up by either the parents or the child. Parents of children with spina bifida realize the need to teach their children about sexuality, feel inadequate about doing so, and are often reluctant to bring up questions to health professionals.[65] The therapist must be open, informed, and able to provide resources to both parents and children.

Generally, the sexual capacity of the female with spina bifida is near normal, that is, she has potential for a normal orgasmic response, is fertile, and can bear children.[15,35,54] The pregnancy, however, may be considered high risk, depending upon existing orthopaedic abnormalities. Affected males are frequently sterile and have small testicles and penises. Their potential for erection and ejaculation will depend upon the level of the lesion.

In many cases psychological problems may be a primary cause of sexual failure.[54] It must be remembered that sexuality is not merely a process involving the genitals but depends upon a positive body image and a feeling of self-esteem that is nurtured from birth.[18,35]

PSYCHOSOCIAL ADJUSTMENT TO CONGENITAL CORD LESIONS

The previous sections on goal setting and rehabilitation of the child with spina bifida have covered birth through adolescence. After adolescence, rehabilitation can be handled in much the same manner as an adult spinal cord injury. It will be important, however, to keep in mind the global effects of spina bifida on the growing child as he or she approaches adulthood.

Because of the congenital nature of spina bifida, psychological adjustment will be somewhat different than adjustment to a traumatic spinal cord injury. The psychological adjustment to this congenital disability must be considered from the perspective of the parents, the family, and of course the child.

A longitudinal study concerning the psychological aspects of spina bifida shows that the parents go through a series of steps in the adjustment process. From birth to about 6 months of age, the parents experience shock and bewilderment. Information given during this time may be rejected or misinterpreted. Health professionals therefore must be ready to repeat the same information to parents on a number of occasions during the first few years of the rehabilitation process.

The period of 6 to 18 months of the child's life may be the most stressful on parents. Frequent hospitalizations during this time place increased pressure upon the whole family unit. Parents, now able to fully comprehend the implications of their child's disability, begin to worry about the future and the impact of the disability on the rest of the family structure.

The period from age 2 through the preschool years is a relatively peaceful one. The parents are more concerned with toilet training, social acceptability, and general information on child rearing. They seem less aware of their child's mental limitations as he or she continues to develop into a relatively happy, well-adjusted child.

By the age of 6 children are becoming more aware of their disabilities, and parents are concerned about problems that may arise as their children enter primary school. The child's psychological adjustment will depend, not on the severity of the disability, but primarily upon the attitude of the parents and family and on the environmental conditions to which he or she is exposed.[47,63,72]

There is some evidence indicating that children with spina bifida may grow up in extreme social isolation.[67] Being placed in special schools, they have little interaction with normal children their own age. Because of their disabilities, they are often denied small tasks or chores that promote a sense of responsibility in the growing child.[34,67] To promote emotional growth and psychological well-being, caregivers must be persuaded to "let go." Children with spina bifida must develop responsibility and independence by being given the chance to interact and even compete with their peers. As they approach adulthood, concerns of independent living situations and vocational placement must be addressed. With a foundation of strong support systems fostering emotional maturity, the future can be bright for the child with congenital spinal cord injury.

REFERENCES

1. Altshuler A and others: Even children can learn to do clean self-catheterization, Amer J Nursing 77:97-101, 1977.
2. American Academy of Pediatrics, Action Committee on Myelodysplasia, Section on Urology. Current approaches to evaluation and management of children with myelomeningocele, Pediatrics 63(4):663-667, 1979.
3. Ayres AJ: Southern California Sensory Integration Tests Manual, Los Angeles, 1972, Western Psychological Services.
4. Ayres AJ: Sensory integration and the child, Los Angeles, 1979, Western Psychological Services.
5. Ayres AJ and Mailloux Z: The Sensory Integration and Praxis Tests manual, Los Angeles, 1988, Western Psychological Services.
6. Baker DA and Olurny CJ: Spina Bifida and maternal Rh blood type, Arch Dis Child 54(7):567, 1979 (letter).
7. Basmajian JV: Therapeutic exercise, ed 3, Baltimore, 1978, Williams & Wilkins.
8. Bayley N: Manual for the Bayley Scales of Infant Development, New York, 1969, The Psychological Corp.
9. Brazelton TB: Neonatal Behavioral Assessment. In Clinics in developmental medicine, vol 88, Philadelphia, 1984, JB Lippincott Co.
10. Brocklehurst G: Spina bifida for the clinician. In Clinics in developmental medicine, vol 57, Philadelphia, 1976, JB Lippincott Co.
11. Brown JT and McClone DG: The effect of complications on intellectual function in 167 children with myelomeningocele, Z Kinderchir 34(2):117-120, 1981.
12. Burn J and Gibben D: May spina bifida result from an X-linked defect in a selective abortion method, J Med Genet 16(3):210-214, 1979.
13. Butler PB and others: Use of the Orlau Swivel Walker for the severely handicapped patient, Physiotherapy 88(11):324-326, 1982.
14. Cash J: Neurology for physiotherapists, ed 2, Philadelphia, 1977, JB Lippincott Co.
15. Cass AS and others: Sexual function in adults with myelomenigocele, J Urol 136:425-426, August 1986.
16. Colangelo C and others: A normal baby; the sensory-motor processes of the first year, Valhalla, NY, 1976, Blythdale Children's Hospital.
17. De Souza LJ and Carroll N: Ambulation of the braced myelomeningocele patient, J Bone Joint Surg 58A(8):1112-1118, 1976.
18. Dorner S: Sexual interest and activity in adolescents with spina bifida, J Child Psychiat 18:229-237, 1977.
19. Drago JR and others: The role of intermittent catheterization in the management of children with myelomeningocele, J of Urol 118:92-94, July 1977.
20. Drummond DS and others: Post-operative neuropathic fractures in patients with myelomeningocele, Dev Med Child Neurol 23:147-150, 1981.
21. Durr-Fillaver Medical, Inc—Orthopedic Division: LSU Reciprocating Gait Orthosis: a pictoral description and application model, Chattanooga, Tenn, 1983.
22. Feiwell E: Surgery of the hip in myelomeningocele as related to adult goals, Clin Orthop 148:87-93, May 1980.
23. Feiwell E and others: The effects of hip reduction on function in patients with myelomeningocele, J Bone Joint Surg 60A(2):169-173, 1978.
24. Ferguson-Smith MA and others: Avoidance of anencephalic and spina bifida births by maternal serum-alphafetoprotein screening, Lancet 1(8078):1330-1333, 1978.
25. Findley TW and others: Ambulation in the adolescent with myelomeningocele. I. Early childhood predictors, Arch Phys Med Rehabil 68:518-522, August 1987.
26. Fiorentino MR: Normal and abnormal development: the influence of primitive reflexes on motor development, Springfield, Ill, 1972, Charles C Thomas Publisher.
27. Fiorentino MR: Normal and abnormal development: the influence of primitive reflexes on motor development, ed 2, Springfield, Ill, 1980, Charles C Thomas Publisher.
28. Folio MR and Fewell RR: Peabody Developmental Motor Scales and Activity Cards, Allen, Tex, 1983, DLM Teaching Resources.
29. Gluckman S and Barling J: Effects of a remedial program on visual-motor perception in spina bifida children, J Genet Psychol 136:195-202, June 1980.
30. Goldberg MF and Oakley GP Jr: Interpreting elevated amniotic fluid alpha-fetoprotein levels in clinical practice: use of the predictive value positive concept, Am J Obstet Gynecol 133(2):126-132, 1979.
31. Gram MC: Using the parapodium: a manual of training techniques, Rochester, NY, Eterna Press.
32. Griscom NT and others: Amniography in second trimester diagnosis of myelomeningocele, AJR 133(6):1151-1156, 1979.
33. Guttman L: Spinal cord injuries: comprehensive management and research, ed 2, Oxford, 1976, Blackwell Publisher.
34. Hayden PW and others: Adolescents with myelodysplasia: impact of physical disability on emotional maturation, Pediatrics 64(1):53-59, 1979.
35. Hendry J and Geddes N: Living with a congenital anomaly, Can Nurse 74(6):29-33, 1978.
36. Hunt GM: Spina bifida: implications for 100 children at school, Dev Med Child Neurol 23:160-172, 1981.
37. Hyperthermia and meningomyelocele and anencephaly, Lancet 1(8067):769-770, 1978 (letter).
38. Hyperthermia and the neural tube, Lancet 2(8089):560-561, 1978, (editorial).
39. James WH: The sex ratio in spina bifida, J Med Genet 16(5):384-388, 1979.
40. Kaplan WE: Management of the urinary tract in myelomeningocele, Problems in Urol 2(1):121-131, 1988.
41. Katona F and Berényi M: Intravesical Transurethral Electrotherapy in meningomyelocele patients, Acta Paediatr S Hung 16(3-4):363-374, 1975.
42. Knobloch H and others: Manual of developmental diagnosis, Hagerstown, Md, 1980, Harper & Row Publishers Inc.
43. Kupka J and others: Comprehensive management in the child with spina bifida, Orthop Clin North Am 9(1):97-113, 1978.
44. Lee EH and Carroll NC: Hip stability and ambulatory status in myelomeningocele, J Pediatr Orthop 5:522-527, 1985.
45. Lindseth RE and Glancy J: Polypropylene lower extremity braces for paraplegia due to myelomeningocele J Bone Joint Surg 56A:556-563, 1974.
46. Lippman-Hand A and others: Indications for prenatal diagnosis in relatives of patients with neural tube defects, Obstet Gynecol 51(1):72-76, 1978.
47. McAndrew I: Adolescents and young people with spina bifida, Dev Med Child Neurol 21(5):619-629, 1979.
48. McCall RE and Schmidt WT: Clinical experience with reciprocal gait orthosis in myelodysplasia, J Pediatr Orthop 6:157-161, 1986.
49. McClone DG: An introduction to spina bifida, Chicago, 1980, Children's Memorial Hospital Myelomeningocele Service.
50. McClone DG: Results of treatment of children born with a myelomeningocele, Clin Neurosurg 30:407-412, 1983.
51. McClone DG: Treatment of myelomeningocele: arguments against selection, Clin Neurosurg 33:359-370, 1986.
52. McClone DG and others: Neurolation: biochemical and morphological studies on primary and secondary neural tube defects, Concepts Pediat Neurosurg 4:15-29, 1983.
53. McClone DG and others: Central nervous system infections as a limiting factor in the intelligence of children with myelomeningocele, Pediatrics 70(3):338-342, 1982.

54. McLaughlin JF and Shurtleff DB: Management of the newborn with myelodysplasia, Clin Pediatr 18(8):463-476, 1979.

55. McLaurin RL: Myelomeningocele, New York, 1977, Grune & Stratton Inc.

56. Menelaus MB: orthopaedic management of children with myelomeningocele: a plea for realistic goals, Dev Med Child Neurol 6(suppl 37):3-11, 1976.

57. Menelaus MB: The Orthopedic management of spina bifida cystica, ed 2, New York, 1980, Churchill Livingstone, Inc.

58. The Milani-Comparetti Motor Development Screening Test, Meyer Children's Rehabilitation Institute, Omaha, Neb, 1977, University of Nebraska Medical Center.

59. Montgomery MA and Richter E: Sensorimotor integration for developmentally delayed children: a handbook, Los Angeles, 1977, Western Psychological Services.

60. Moore KL: Before we are born: basic embryological and birth defects, revised reprint, Philadelphia, 1974, WB Saunders Co.

61. Nesbit DE and Ziter FA: Epidemiology of myelomeningocele in Utah, Dev Med Child Neurol 21(6):54-57, 1979.

62. Nevin NC and others: Influence of social class on the risk of recurrence of anencephalus and spina bifida, Dev Med Child Neurol 23:155-159, 1981.

63. Nielsen HH: A longitudinal study of the psychological aspects of myelomeningocele, Scand J Psychol 21:45-54, 1980.

64. Papalia DE and Olds SW: Human development, New York, 1981, McGraw-Hill, Inc.

65. Passo S: Parents' perceptions, attitudes and needs regarding sex education for the child with myelomeningocele, Res Nurs Health 1(2):53-59, 1978.

66. Pearson PN and Williams CE: Physical therapy services in developmental disabilities, Springfield, Ill, 1976, Charles C Thomas, Publisher.

67. Perspectives in spina bifida, Br Med J 2(6142):909-910, 1978 (editorial).

68. Pietrzyk JJ and Turowski G: Immunogenetic bases and congenital malformations: association of HLA-B27 with spina bifida, Pediatr Res 13(8):879-883, 1979.

69. Raimondi AJ and Soare P: Intellectual development in shunted hydrocephalic children, Am J Dis Child 127:664-671, 1974.

70. Ralis ZA and others: Changes in shape, ossification and quality of bones in children with spina bifida, Dev Med Child Neurol 18(6; suppl 37):29-41, 1976.

71. Roach EG and Kephart NC: The Purdue Perceptual-Motor Survey, Columbus, Ohio, 1966, Charles E Merrill Publishing Co.

72. Rogers BM: Comprehensive care for the child with a chronic disability, Am J Nurs 79(6):1106-1108, 1979.

73. Rose GK and Henshaw JT: Swivel walkers for paraplegics—considerations and problems in their design and application, Bull Prosthet Res 10(20):62-74, 1973.

74. Rosenstein BD and others: Bone density in myelomeningocele: the effects of ambulatory status and other factors, Dev Med Child Neurol 29:486-494, 1987.

75. Schaffer MF and Dias LS: Myelomeningocele: orthopedic treatment, Baltimore, Md, 1983, Williams & Wilkins Co.

76. Schopler SA and Menelaus MB: Significance of the strength of the quadriceps muscles in children with myelomeningocele, J Pediatr Orthop 7(5):507-512, 1987.

77. Singer HA and others: Spina bifida and anencephaly in the cape, S Afr Med J 53(16):626-627, 1978.

78. Smithells RW and others: Apparent prevention of neural tube defects by periconceptional vitamin supplementation, Arch Dis Child 56:911-918, 1981.

79. Sousa JC and others: Developmental guidelines for children with myelodysplasia, Phys Ther 63(1):21-29, 1983.

80. Stallard J and others: Engineering design considerations of the Orlau Swivel Walker, Eng Med 15(1):3-8, 1986.

81. Stark GD: Spina bifida: problems and management, Boston, 1977, Blackwell Scientific Publications Inc.

82. Stein SC and Schut L: Hydrocephalus in myelomeningocele, Childs Brain 5(4):413-419, 1979.

83. Sullivan PE and others: An integrated approach to therapeutic exercise, Reston, Va, 1982, Reston Publishing Co., Inc.

84. Williamson GG: Children with spina bifida: early intervention and preschool programing, Baltimore, Md, 1987, Paul H Brooks Co.

85. Wolf L: Development of Self-Care Assessment Tool for children with meningomyelocele, Developmental Disabilities 10(2):2-6, 1987.

86. Zausmer E: Evaluation of strength and motor development in infants, Phys Ther Review 33(12):621-628, 1953.

APPENDIX 1—AUDIOVISUAL RESOURCES

Brazelton Neonatal Behavioral Assessment (16 mm films)

Part 1 Introduction

Part 2 Self-scoring exam

Part 3 Variations in Normal Behavior

Educational Development Center
55 Chapel Street
Newton, MA 02160

The Bayley Scales of Infant Development (videotapes)

The Mental Scale Parts 1 and 2

J. Hunt Institute of Human Development
University of California at Berkley
Psychological Corporation, 1975

APPENDIX 2—ORLAU SWIVEL ROCKER DISTRIBUTORS

UK

J Stallard
Technical Director
ORLAU
Orthopaedic Hospital
Oswestry
Shropshire, SY107AG
UK

US

Mopac Ltd
206 Chestnut St.
Eau Claire, WI 54703
715-832-1685

Chapter 15

TRAUMATIC SPINAL CORD INJURY

Frederick J. Schneider

OVERVIEW OF TRAUMATIC SPINAL CORD INJURY

Before considering the physical therapy and rehabilitation management of the client with a spinal cord injury, it might be advantageous to delve into the etiological and demographic figures to more accurately define the problem. The statistics that will be cited are taken primarily from the recent (1986) report of the National Spinal Cord Injury Data Base (NSCIDB). This organization receives data from the 19 regional model Spinal Cord Injury Care Systems. The NSCIDB report is extrapolated data based on its current estimate that the 19 model systems are treating approximately 14% of the nations newly injured cases[227] and is currently considered the most comprehensive and accurate source of published statistics on spinal cord injury.

Demographic information

Incidence. Approximately 11,000 new cases of spinal cord injury that result in some degree of functional impairment occur in the United States each year. Of this total, 7000 to 8000 are the result of trauma to the spinal cord; the rest are spinal cord injury impairments that result from disease and congenital anomalies.[264] This relates to an incidence for acute hospitalized traumatic spinal cord injuries of from 40 to 50 per million population in the United States.[21,260] The ratio of high-level lesions (quadriplegia) to low-level lesions (paraplegia) is about equal, although paraplegic clients have a higher incidence of complete lesions (60%) than do quadriplegic clients (48%).[265] Based on very rough estimates, there are approximately 200,000 individuals presently living in the United States with some degree of impairment from spinal cord injury resulting from trauma, disease, or congenital anomalies.[264]

Of all cases of traumatic spinal cord injury reported to the NSCIDB between 1973 and 1985 (N = 9674), 82% of those injured were male, and 61.1% of the injuries occurred in the 16- to 30-year age range. Of all clients with these injuries, 85.4% were under the age of 45, 58.8% were single, and only 59.9% were employed at time of injury. In this population, an overwhelming 47.7% of the injuries were the result of automobile, motorcycle, and other vehicle accidents. This was followed by falls (20.8%), sports injuries (14.2%), and acts of violence (14.6%). Two thirds of the sports-related injuries were caused by diving accidents. Vehicular accidents caused approximately an equal percentage of quadriplegia and paraplegia, acts of violence most often resulted in paraplegia, and sports injuries most often resulted in quadriplegia. The incidence of spinal cord injury in children is poorly documented. A study by Burke[33] in 1976 showed that 4% of all clients with spinal cord injuries admitted to the Spinal Cord Injuries Unit of the Austin Hospital in Heidelberg, Australia were children. Gehrig and Michaelis[87] studied the annual incidence of spinal cord injuries in Switzerland and found that 5% of these were children under the age of 14. Kewalramani and others[126] conducted an epidemiological study of cord injuries in 18 counties of Northern California for the years 1970 and 1971 and showed 58 out of 617 cases (9.4%) to be children. Of these, 28 (4.6%) died before arrival at a hospital, and 30 (4.8%) were hospital admitted cases. A more recent study by this same group found that of 733 clients with spinal cord injuries admitted to the Institute for Rehabilitation and Research in Houston from 1970 to 1977 97 (14%) were children.[128] The authors hypothesized that this increase was the result of (1) an increase in the number of motor vehicle accidents and more violent outdoor recreational activities for children, (2) decreased fatalities as a result of better quality acute medical care, and (3) selective referral of children with spinal cord injuries to this center. In summary, disability resulting from insult to the spinal cord occurs most often in the young of our society and is most commonly the result of forceful trauma.

This is a devastating problem, not only to the injured person and his or her family, but to society, which has to bear, in most instances, the economic cost of attempting to restore the individual to a functional and meaningful life. These costs are staggering, both in terms of money and time invested. The National Spinal Cord Injury Data Research report[264] in 1979 cited the initial hospitalization and rehabilitation period (injury to home) for 2123 clients admitted to the model systems from 1975 through 1977. The mean period for incomplete paraplegic clients was 3.87 months, 4.25 months for complete paraplegic clients, 4.74 months for incomplete quadriplegic clients, and 6.60 months for complete quadriplegic clients. The mean total cost in 1977 for the initial hospitalization and rehabilitation periods for all of the 355 clients reported on was $37,373. Figures from one center for 1979 showed the average cost of hospitalization for the first year after injury to have risen to $57,683.[157]

These are only the initial costs encountered by the client and family following a spinal injury. The lifetime care costs for an average quadriplegic client in 1978 were $350,000 to $400,000.[265] This figure was based on an average age of 31 years at time of injury, with an additional conservative life expectancy of 20 years (50% of the normal additional life expectancy). The lifetime costs for a paraplegic client, using the same studies figures, were estimated to be $180,000 to $225,000. This study extrapolated these costs to the annual cost of all persons in the United States with spinal cord injuries. That figure was estimated at $2.4 billion. With continually improving initial, rehabilitative, and long-term follow-up care, the life expectancy of persons with spinal cord injuries is increasing. This, hopefully, provides the reader with some recognition of the tremendous economic and social impact made on society by persons having incurred a spinal cord lesion.

Clinical etiology

Traumatic mechanisms. Trauma, the most common cause of spinal cord injuries, occurs most often as the result of high-velocity impact forces. With the exception of gunshot and stab penetrating wounds, most injuries to the spine result from indirect forces generated by movement of the head and trunk, and only rarely are these injuries a result of direct forces at a vertebra.[207] Various areas of the spine are biomechanically more susceptible to the fractures and dislocations that result in spinal cord injury. In 1928 a study of 2006 cases by Jefferson[117] initially identified craniovertebral (C1 to C2), cervical (C5 to C7), and thoracolumbar (T12 to L2) as the three peaks of incidence for spinal fractures and dislocations. Approximately 10% to 14% of spinal fractures and dislocations result in injury to the spinal cord.[202] As a result of its biomechanical instability in relation to other areas of the spine, the cervical spine has a 40% chance of cord injury with fracture and/or dislocation. This incidence is 4% in the thoracic spine and 10% at the thoracolumbar junction.[207]

Another important consideration is the incidence of cord injury that results from mishandling of the client immediately after injury. Calenoff[207] sets the figure for all levels of injury at 5% to 10%; in 1966 Guttman[97] showed a 25% incidence in a survey of a large number of cervical injuries treated at the Edinburgh Royal Infirmary. With the recent improvement in training of emergency personnel and transportation techniques, these figures have decreased significantly.[157]

Trauma to the spine usually involves forceful flexion or extension in combination with rotation, compression, shearing, or distraction of the vertebrae. These forces usually result in vertebral fracture, dislocation, or a combination of both. Flexion with slight rotation is the most common mechanism of injury in the cervical spine.[54] This usually occurs through forced flexion of the head on the trunk with maximal forces occurring on the vertebral bodies of C4 through C7. Forceful flexion of the trunk on itself focuses on the thoracolumbar junction and accounts for a high incidence of fracture at the T12 to L2 level.[207] These flexion forces, if of a sufficient magnitude, can cause comminuted fractures of the vertebral bodies that are often designated as "bursting or explosion fractures," which can displace fragments into the spinal canal resulting in cord injury.[110] Extension injuries occur most often at the cervical level and usually result in rupture of the anterior longitudinal ligament and fracture of the posterior elements of the cervical spine.[31] These hyperextension injuries occur most commonly in the elderly as the result forward falls in which the head or chin strikes an object or the floor.[54,247] Shearing results when one segment of the spine receives a horizontal force in relation to an adjoining segment. Shearing occurs most frequently in the thoracic and lumbar spine, causes ligament tearing, and results in fracture dislocations.[207] Distraction forces are least common and can occur, for example, when the head undergoes greatly increased momentum ("whiplash") as in the common automobile rear-end collisions. This momentum is translated into tensile forces within the cervical spine. Another traction-type injury can occur during the birth process. For example, too forceful use of forceps distraction to the head can result in a cervical injury. During breech delivery it can result in fracture dislocation in the thoracic and lumbar regions.[37,109,133] With the advent of automobile lap-type seat belts in the 1960s, another type of spinal fracture appeared—the transverse or Chance fracture.[176] These are fractures of the lumbar spine; the seat belt acts as a fulcrum that is anterior to the spine. During the usual hyperflexion of the spine found in automobile accidents, forces cause the disruption of the posterior ligaments of the spine with the vertebral body often being split transversely into two parts or displaced anteriorly. This seat belt injury is often accompanied by rupture of the anterior abdominal wall and laceration of the visceral organs.[67,206] Depending on the spinal level, injuries occur to either the spinal cord or the cauda equina.

All professionals who interact with clients with spinal cord injuries should keep in mind the issue of the multiple noncontiguous vertebral injury, where the primary lesion causing the neurological deficit is identified and where additional secondary fractures proximal or distal to the primary lesion may or may not be identified.[235] Numerous surveys of large populations have isolated from 3.2% to 4.5% of persons with spinal cord injuries having multiple noncontiguous fractures of their vertebral column.[38,93,127] Without scrutiny of total spine radiograms, some of the secondary fractures may go undetected. The Calenoff[38] series found 42.9% of the secondary fractures occurring at the extremes of the spine, 14.3% occurring at C1 and C2, and 28.6% occurring at L4 and L5. Therefore undetected secondary lesions proximal to the primary lesion may subsequently lead to an extension of the neurological deficit. Undetected distal lesions may lead to spinal instability and subsequent deformity. It is extremely important that therapists and other professionals who interact daily with the client with a cord injury during the postacute mobilization period carefully monitor for any changes in the client's neurological signs and that they immediately report these signs to the referring physician for further study.

Nontraumatic mechanisms. Although the focus of this chapter is on the physical therapy management of the person with a traumatic cord injury, a comprehensive overview of the clinical cause should include a brief discussion of the nontraumatic causes. *Circulatory embarrassment* in the form of embolism, thrombosis, or hemorrhage causes neurological dysfunction at and below the involved cord area. *Compression* of the cord can be caused by a variety of pathological states. Among these are (1) vertebral subluxation from degenerative or rheumatoid arthritis, as well as vertebral spondylosis from ankylosing spondylitis, (2)

cord compression from primary and secondary neoplasms, (3) vertebral degeneration and subluxation from various infective states, such as staphylococcus and syphilis, (4) Paget's disease, and (5) prolapse of an intervertebral disk into the spinal canal and cord.

Symptoms of spinal cord dysfunction can also be caused by a variety of *demyelinating diseases,* such as multiple sclerosis and amyotrophic lateral sclerosis (these will be discussed in Chapter 18). Various *inflammatory processes* can affect the brain, spinal cord, and their associated coverings (these clinical problems will be discussed in Chapter 16). *Congenital malformations* of the spinal column with their resulting functional losses caused by cord and/or brainstem involvement were discussed in Chapter 14.

Hysterical paralysis, with either a conscious or subconscious motivation, may result in a clinical picture of loss of normal voluntary movement similar to that expressed by a spinal cord injury.[245]

Associated injuries and medical complications. Because injury to the spinal cord occurs most frequently as the result of high-velocity trauma, the rehabilitation of these clients often also involves the management of associated major injuries and subsequent medical complications. Young[265] reported on 615 clients with traumatic spinal cord injury admitted within 24 hours of injury to the regional spinal cord injury centers. The incidence of the major associated injuries found with this large group is reported in Table 15-1.

A more recent study by Davidoff and others[62] (reported on in 1988) found that 49% of all traumatic spinal cord injuries in their sample (N = 82) suffered some form of closed head injury that resulted in varying degrees of post-traumatic amnesia. All clients therefore need to be screened for memory loss, attention span problems, and other cognitive deficits that may affect their success at rehabilitation.

It is important to note that associated injuries, in particular major head injuries, are more prevalent in paraplegia than in quadriplegia. Young's study also found that the incidence of initial medical complications occurring with this group during their initial treatment period (onset to discharge home—an average of 145 days) showed urinary tract infections to lead the list in both paraplegia and quadriplegia (see Table 15-2). This was substantiated by the 1985 NSCIDB findings.

It was also found that these initial medical complications occur more frequently in quadriplegia than in paraplegia. Subsequent chronic medical complications differ in frequency and nature and will be discussed later in this chapter.

Classification of injuries—levels of lesions. Confusion can exist in literature, in the client's medical records, and in verbal communication between team members, if a clear understanding of the client's "level of le-

Table 15-1. Incidence of selected major associated injuries

Diagnoses	Paraplegia (N=281)		Quadriplegia (N=334)	
	Patients	%	Patients	%
Closed fracture ribs, sternum	79	28	12	4
Girdle and major long bone fracture	67	24	29	9
Open wounds and lacerations	64	23	52	16
Major head injuries	45	16	25	7
Pneumothorax, hemothorax	31	11	7	2
Injury to visceral organs	26	9	3	1
Injury to intrathoracic organs	23	8	9	3
Facial fractures	10	4	4	1

From Young JS: Spinal cord injury: associated general trauma and medical complications, Adv Neurol 22:255, 1979. Reprinted with permission of Raven Press, New York.

sion" is not established. The most common and internationally recommended[160] means of describing a spinal cord lesion is to state whether it is a complete or an incomplete lesion at a given level of the spinal column. This given level is defined as the vertebral level injured followed by the most distal uninvolved cord segment; for example, a fracture dislocation of C5 over C6 with a C7 complete quadriplegia (complete below C7). An oblique transection of the cord could result in the designation of complete paralysis of C5 on the right and C7 on the left. Incomplete cord lesions may have motor and sensory function present below the level of injury and are usually described in terms of the most distal uninvolved cord segment and the last segment providing any function. For example, incomplete lesion below T9 and complete below T11 as a result of fracture dislocation of T9 to T10 vertebrae.

Neuroanatomical types of traumatic lesions and syndromes

Trauma to the spinal column can result in complete or incomplete injury to the spinal cord, cauda equina, or peripheral nerve roots. Depending on the nature and location of the injury, it is possible to classify certain clinical pictures or syndromes that can aid the therapist and team to solve future management problems of the client.

Transitory abnormal neurological signs—cord concussion. An injury to the vertebral column may result in a transient disturbance of function of the spinal cord that shows initial signs of either complete or partial interruption of the function of the spinal cord or cauda equina but that usually results in full recovery within a few hours after injury. This state is often described by the term *concus-*

Table 15-2. Incidence of selected major medical complications

Diagnoses	Quadriplegia (N=334)		Paraplegia (N=281)	
	Patients	%	Patients	%
Urinary tract infection	203	61	152	54
Pressure sores	99	30	50	18
DVT, phlebitis, thrombophlebitis	44	13	43	15
Pneumonia	43	13	8	3
Anemia	41	12	32	11
Atelectasis	34	10	22	8
Respiratory arrest	30	9	3	1
Heterotopic ossification	22	7	20	7
Pleural effusion	18	5	24	9
Gastrointestinal bleeding	17	5	4	1
Pulmonary embolus	16	5	11	4
Cardiac arrest	16	5	6	2
Septicemia	14	4	6	2
Gastrointestinal ulcer	14	4	6	2
Calculus, kidney, ureter	3	0	4	1

From Young JS: Spinal cord injury: associated general trauma and medical complications, Adv Neurol 22:255, 1979. Reprinted with permission of Raven Press, New York.

sion of the cord [258] and is related to such factors as very transient compression from fluid build-up in the spinal column or slight bony or soft tissue pressure—both of which are rapidly relieved. The client may be admitted with symptoms that vary from slight parasthesias or tingling in the extremities to a generalized loss of neurological function below the level of injury; this is known as *spinal shock*. Hyperreflexia without spasticity usually occurs with this type of injury.[34] The client may recover without treatment or may require rapid surgical decompression to avoid secondary neurological destruction. This type of transient injury may be contrasted with an initial contusion-type injury often found in the cervical and thoracic spine.[154] Here the client may have no sign of initial neurological injury but, in the hours after injury, may develop profound signs of neurological damage resulting from progressive hemorrhage or edema at the level at which the cord is contused. Even with emergency medical care, the contusion may result in a permanent incomplete or complete paralysis.

Classification of spinal cord lesions

Complete cord lesions. A complete cord lesion is one in which no motor or sensory function exists below the level of injury. The cord may be completely transected, severely compressed as a result of bony/soft tissue impingement and/or hemorrhagic edema, or compromised by impaired cord circulation. The client is areflexive. A diagnosis of a complete lesion can usually be made 24 to 48 hours after the injury when the client shows no neurological improvement—especially when the client lacks reappearing sacral reflexes, which are the usual initial signs of an *incomplete* lesion.[237] An occasional rare case has been documented where progressive recovery begins after several days or weeks,[226] but total areflexia 24 hours following injury is usually considered a sign of a complete lesion.

Incomplete lesions and syndromes. Incomplete injuries to the spinal cord tend to preserve a mixture of motor and sensory function. The majority of incomplete lesions have no definite patterns of recovery and no distinct clinical pictures.[92] However, some partial injuries to the spinal cord do result in a distinct clinical picture or syndrome. The therapist needs to be aware that when the syndromes have been diagnosed, they will present a somewhat predictable course of recovery around which goals and subsequent treatment can be planned. These syndromes are outlined in this section.

Brown-Séquard's syndrome. This syndrome is named after the French physician who originally described it in 1869.[28] Its traumatic origin is usually a result of a stab wound, and it involves a hemisection of the cord. The classic picture of hemisection is rare, but partial hemisections are relatively common.[140] The clinical picture is usually as follows[258]: at the level of the lesion there is an ipsilateral, segmental, lower motor neuron paralysis as well as complete sensory loss in the level's dermatomal area.

Below the level of the lesion, there is ipsilateral destruction of the corticospinal tract resulting in a variable loss of motor function, increased tone, hyperactive deep tendon reflexes, absence of superficial reflexes, and a positive Babinski's sign on the same side. Because of posterior column loss, there is also ipsilateral proprioceptive and vibratory loss below the lesion. There is contralateral loss of pain and temperature sensation beginning a few segments below the level of lesion. This discrepancy in levels is caused by the distance that the lateral spinothalamic tracts ascend on the same side of the cord (usually two to four segments) before crossing. Tactile sensation may or may not be intact as a result of the many crossed and uncrossed fibers involved with this sense.

Anterior cord syndrome. The syndrome of acute anterior spinal cord injury is usually related to injury of the cervical cord. It involves compression of the anterior cervical cord from either a fracture dislocation or a cervical disk protrusion. It may involve the anterior spinal artery and the anterior horn cells. It is characterized by loss of motor function (corticospinal tracts) and pain and temperature (spinothalamic tracts) at and below the level of injury. The posterior columns are spared with the preservation of motion, position, and vibratory senses. Diffuse (light) touch sensation may or may not be involved.[216] The client with an anterior cord syndrome who is treated with anterior spinal decompression and fusion may have a significant return of motor function.[20]

Central cord syndrome. This cervical cord syndrome involves anterior and posterior cord compression from either an acute hyperextension injury or a chronic or congenital condition causing progressive stenosis. Damage is primarily the result of microvascular compromise of the central cord. With cord compression, the central gray matter of the cord is involved first because its metabolic needs and perfusion demands are greater than those of the surrounding white matter.[216] Central white matter may also be compromised. Therefore the syndrome is characterized by a disproportionately greater loss of motor power in the upper extremities than in the lower extremities with varying degrees of sensory loss (i.e., loss of motor horn cells in the gray matter and central long tracts of the white matter). Early sensory loss will involve pain and temperature, and further compressive damage may cause impairment of touch, motion, position, and vibration sensation.[268] Bladder dysfunction, in the form of urinary retention, may also occur.[207] With surgical decompression, the prognosis for significant functional recovery can be quite good. Surgery with traumatic injuries can be delayed until the client has stabilized into the subacute phase in 7 to 14 days.[20,26] The client usually recovers function in the lower extremities first; this is followed by upper-extremity functional gains and, lastly, by improvement of hand function. What is often a complete quadriplegia with only trace toe and other lower-extremity movements may, in some instances, progress to complete or near complete motor recovery. On rare occasions,[20] central cord syndromes occur more distally in the thoracic and lumbar segments. Here, for example, the client may have marked weakness in muscles innervated by the upper lumbar cord; he or she may be unable to flex and abduct at the hip but able to move his or her toes.

Sacral sparing. Another descriptive term that is used often is *sacral sparing.* This refers to an incomplete cord lesion that has degrees of intact sacral segment function, usually with sparing of the central long tracts. Sacral sparing is often the only early evidence of incomplete quadriplegia because the long tracts serving the sacral enlargement of the cord are relatively more protected from injury. The primary criteria for sacral sparing is proprioception in the rectum. Depending on the involvement of the lesion, other clinical signs of sacral sparing are intact perianal sensation, voluntary rectal sphincter contraction, active toe flexion, and an intact "saddle" pattern of cutaneous sensation. Persons with a central cord syndrome quadriplegia with complete sacral sparing may have near normal sexual, bladder, and bowel function.[56]

These are the primary incomplete cord syndromes and terms most often discussed in the literature; they are also the ones a therapist is most likely to encounter in a client's records. There are other syndromes and descriptive terms found in the literature that are based primarily on describing various combinations of involved tracts and cord areas. Because of their rarity and because of the conflicting definitions among sources, they are of little clinical use. Accurate serial motor, sensory, and reflex examinations by the team can best demonstrate the patterns and progress of incomplete cord lesions.

Cauda equina lesions. The spinal cord terminates distally at the conus medullaris, which extends into the cauda equina. This usually occurs at the vertebral level of L1, although considerable variation does exist. The cord may end as high as the middle of the twelfth thoracic vertebra and as low as the inferior border of the second lumbar vertebra.[258] *Complete* lesions of the cauda equina, which consists of anterior and posterior nerve roots, result in a lower motor neuron clinical picture. As a result of the interruption of the reflex arc, these nerve root lesions result in flaccid paralysis with loss of reflex activity and sensation. Because of the mobility of the nerve roots of the cauda equina within the neural canal, lesions of the cauda equina are most often *incomplete.* The injury is usually the result of direct trauma from fracture dislocations.[34] The clinical picture in incomplete injuries at this level is unpredictable and varied. Roots above and below the fracture site may be involved either unilaterally or bilaterally. Some roots may be severed; others may develop a neurapraxia, with potential for recovery. The client will demonstrate various states of motor imbalance; management is similar to dealing with a spectrum or peripheral nerve injuries. In addi-

tion, clients with complete and incomplete lesions of the cauda equina may show flaccid bowel and bladder paralysis and loss of sexual function.

Damage to the conus medullaris and to the cauda equina is often found in trauma to the thoracolumbar spine. Here a picture of upper and lower motor neuron damage results.

Nerve root lesions. The therapist must keep in mind that injury to nerve roots proximal to and surrounding the spinal cord at the level of injury can also occur. As with incomplete lesions of the cauda equina, recovery can occur through nerve regeneration. This recovery of nerve roots at or slightly above the level of cord lesion may cause one to incorrectly conclude that cord recovery is responsible for the improved sensorimotor picture. This is sometimes referred to as "root escape."[34]

Typical clinical signs and problems

Primary and secondary clinical problems involving virtually all systems of the body occur with injury to the spinal cord. This section discusses the most significant of these problems by system and analyzes briefly their effects and current medical and surgical efforts at prevention and treatment. Later in this chapter the physical therapy management appropriate to some of these problems is outlined.

Orthopaedic signs and problems

Potential for contracture. Connective tissues and muscle tissues show the property of progressive shortening when not stretched regularly by an opposing force.[135] These opposing forces occur at all joints with normal daily movement. With flaccid paralysis or hypertonicity as a result of cord injury, the opportunity for maintaining normal range of motion is threatened. The effects of gravity on flaccid joints and the lack of opposing forces to a joint, for example with flexor spasticity, may rapidly progress that joint structure toward development of a contracture. These contractures may initially involve changes in the muscle tissue but progress rapidly to capsular and pericapsular changes at the joint. If not managed effectively by the treatment team through an aggressive program of passive range of motion exercises along with effective positioning of the extremities and trunk, the contracture can rapidly progress to an ankylosed joint.[250] Contractures occur most frequently in flexor muscle groups and usually combine with adduction and internal rotation in the shoulder and hip joints. They can lead to secondary complications: for example, flexion contractures of the hip joint could lead to an asymmetrical sitting posture with a secondary potential for both scoliosis and ischial pressure sore formation.[106]

The most effective treatment is prevention through a program of passive and self range of motion exercises. Once contractures occur, management depends on the duration and severity of the contracture and ranges from mild stretching to surgical intervention for capsular releases and tendon lengthening procedures. The most effective stretch is one that is mild and sustained for a long period of time, allowing the collagen fibers to progressively lengthen.[135] Stretching that is too vigorous results in muscle and joint microtrauma and leads to further scarring and connective tissue proliferation with subsequent worsening of the contracture. Therefore many contractures can efficiently be managed through a sustained stretch program of serial casting or splinting.[70]

Joint ankylosis. As mentioned earlier, joint contractures that are left unmanaged may eventually lead to ankylosis of the joint. Ankylosis also occurs in approximately 20% of clients with ectopic bone formation.[108] Approximately 75% of ankylosed joints involve the hip; the shoulder, elbow, and spine may also become ankylosed.[250]

Osteoporosis, hypercalcemia, and fractures. Soon after the client incurs an injury to the spinal cord, he or she begins to experience a progressive loss in bone mass, osteoporosis, that primarily involves the bones below the level of the lesion. This loss of bone mass consists of both a loss of bone matrix and bone mineral. The cause of osteoporosis is not known.[107] It is acknowledged that disuse through immobilization plays a role in the development of osteoporosis, but the importance of this role is debated by investigators.[107] A current major theory posits a disruption of the normal mechanism by which bone is constantly undergoing formation of new bone by osteoblasts and a resorption by osteoclasts. This disruption may be the result of vascular modifications caused by damage to the autonomic nervous system.[45]

The initial sign of osteoporosis is an increase of calcium in the urine. Osteoporosis may be detected radiographically 2 to 6 months after the injury.[107] This bone mass loss progresses rapidly during the first year and then remains at a fairly constant state after 1 year.[102] Therefore it is believed that during this first year the rate of bone loss can be decreased, primarily through intensive mobilization with weight bearing.[102] Controversy exists as to what degree of weight bearing is effective in decreasing bone mass loss.[18,253] Some studies advocate that only ambulation has any effect on decreasing the amount of calcium secreted into the urine.[190] Sitting, standing through the use of a tilt table or a strap-standing set-up, and ambulating activities do have some therapeutic effect on decreasing the early rate of osteoporosis development, and they may have some long-term effects on the eventual degree of osteoporosis present beyond 1 year. Another interesting hypothesis is that the stress placed on the supporting bone by electrically stimulated paralyzed muscles decreases the amount of bone reabsorption.[88,125] Further study is needed in this area.

Primary complications of osteoporosis are bladder and kidney stone formation secondary to hypercalciuria and fractures that result from weakened bone. Another occasional complication of osteoporosis is elevated blood serum levels of calcium or hypercalcemia. This problem is rarely found in adults, but it is found in children and the incidence may be as high as 23%.[236] The severity of hypercalcemia has no relation to the severity of the paralysis. Hypercalcemia usually occurs during the first 3 months and is rarely found beyond 18 months after the injury.[125] It is managed through a controlled diet, drugs and, most importantly, increased wheelchair sitting time.[52]

Pathological fracture secondary to severe osteoporosis is not uncommon and can provide a major setback to a client's rehabilitation process or cause a regression in the functional level of a person who has been discharged. Reported incidence ranges from 1.45% to 4%, although the actual incidence is thought to be higher since many fractures are treated in local emergency rooms and not reported to the initial rehabilitation or spinal cord injury center.[195] In addition, because of the often anesthetic lower extremity, minor fractures may go unnoticed (Fig. 15-1). Fractures typically occur as a result of a relatively low-intensity movement, such as transferring from a wheelchair,

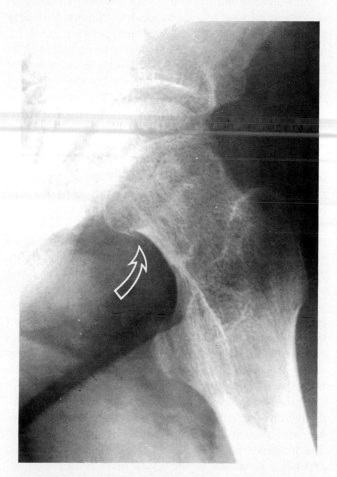

Fig. 15-1. Subtle femoral neck fracture *(arrow)* in 15-year-old incomplete paraplegic girl as a result of range of motion exercises. Client complained of pain for 4 days before radiological examination. Few fractures in clients with spinal cord injuries are this subtle, but they can occur. (From Hendrix RW: Skeletal changes after spinal cord injury. In Calenoff L, editor: Radiology of spinal cord injury, St Louis, 1981, The CV Mosby Co.)

or in the performance of passive or active range of motion exercises. They are usually closed fractures involving the long bones of the lower extremities, and they are best treated conservatively with soft splinting and early return to wheelchair mobility to avoid additional complications.[81] Surgical internal fixation may be necessary depending on the type, severity, and location of the fracture. Because these fractures are the result of minor trauma and because the client often has no sensory feedback from the fracture site, it is very important that the client be instructed to monitor his or her body for physical signs of a fracture.

Another potentially hazardous complication of osteoporosis involves marginal rib erosion. It is found in quadriplegic clients, and it occurs because the paralysis of the intercostal muscles no longer allows for normal stress and strain on the ribs, leading to resorption of the superior margin of the rib.[107] Since many quadriplegic clients are on active chest physical therapy programs, the hazards from this complication are obvious.

Spontaneous and stress fractures are rare but do occasionally occur with severe osteoporosis. Reports have been documented of a spontaneous fracture occurring during removal of orthoses,[123] and there have been reports of bilateral acetabular stress fractures occurring from prolonged transmission of forces through the femurs during swing-through ambulation with crutches.[193] With the increased incorporation of sports and other vigorous physical activities into the life-style of the person with a spinal cord injury, these types of fractures may become more common.

Spinal deformity. Spinal vertebral deformity is a long-term complication found with lesions above the thoracolumbar area. The deformity can take the form of a scoliosis, abnormal kyphosis, or lordosis, or it may involve any combination of these three. It may develop as a result of the long-term effects of the vertebral deformity at the site of injury or, more frequently, as a result of long-term abnormal sitting postures. Asymmetrical lesions can cause spinal muscular imbalances that necessitate compensatory postures needed to maintain sitting balance. In addition, hip flexor tightness, hip flexor spasticity with either abduction with external rotation or adduction with internal rotation, or hip dislocations can cause pelvic obliquities during sitting that also result in compensation of the spinal column.

Spinal deformities can occur in adults and children, although this problem is more common in children since spinal bone growth adds an additional complicating factor. The incidence in children is high over a long period and depends a great deal on the age of onset and on the level of injury.[125] Bedbrook[14] stated that children under the age of 11 who have complete or incomplete lesions above the T10 level will all eventually develop some degree of scoliosis.

The development of spinal deformities can add serious secondary complications; impaired respiratory function is of primary concern to therapists. Further secondary decreases in the symmetry of sitting can lead to pressure sore development.

Long-term monitoring of the client by the treating team is the key to preventing spinal deformity. Maintenance of a good sitting posture through correction of muscle imbalances or tightness is essential. This may involve a home exercise program, drug therapy, or phenol injections to decrease hypertonic musculature; use of a molded orthosis or wheelchair seat insert may help to manage slight developing deformities (Fig. 15-2).

Treatment of paralytic scoliosis in children with curves less than 40 degrees can be attempted through the use of a Milwaukee brace, Boston bucket, or other plaster or plastic jackets.[125] In children and adults with scoliosis beyond 40 degrees, surgical stabilization may become necessary. Two methods are commonly used.[107,125] A Dwyer compression device, which is inserted through an anterior approach and which is useful for stabilizing curves between T10 and L5, or Harrington rods, which are distracting stabilizers established through a posterior approach between T1 and the sacrum, may be used. A combination of both devices can also be used.

Heterotopic ossification (ectopic bone formation). Metaplastic osteogenesis in soft tissues is a complication that occurs in clients having neurological insults such as spinal cord injuries, cerebrovascular accidents, poliomyelitis, and head trauma; its cause is unknown.[118] It is not to be confused with myositis ossificans, which occurs after trauma to the muscle. Ectopic bone formation is always extra-articular and develops not within a muscle mass but in the connective tissue between muscle planes, in aponeurotic tissue, and in tendon.[108] There is no clear incidence of ectopic bone formation in the literature with reports varying between 4% and 49%.[108] No correlation has been found between the formation of ectopic bone in spinal cord injuries and the level of lesion, presence of spasticity or flaccidity, or presence or absence of passive range of motion to the area.[108] Although neurological deficit seems to be a predisposing factor, ectopic bone formation is not found in children with paraplegia as a result of spina bifida.[228] Ectopic bone formation does occur as a complication in children who have incurred a traumatic spinal cord injury.[125] There are many current theories regarding cause, including tissue hypoxia from poor circulation,[228] the presence of abnormal calcium metabolism,[1] and microtrauma resulting from too vigorous range of motion.[112,211,223]

Its location in spinal cord injury is usually adjacent to the large joints such as the anterior hip, knee, inferior to the shoulder joint—scapular complex—(Fig. 15-3), and near the elbow.[108] It is always found below the level of lesion. Occasionally, it occurs near the small joints, such as the wrist and fingers.[77,141] Affected clients usually have more than one area involved. It can appear on radiograms as early as 19 to 20 days after the injury, and its occur-

"Music You Can Trust To Be Good"

Inspire Productions, Inc.

Record Production & Jingles

WILLIE HILL
(919) 688-8563
Fax (919) 688-8565

302 E. Pettigrew Street
Suite 101
Durham, NC 27701

Barbara Ford

525-8901

BRE conf.

6/8/96

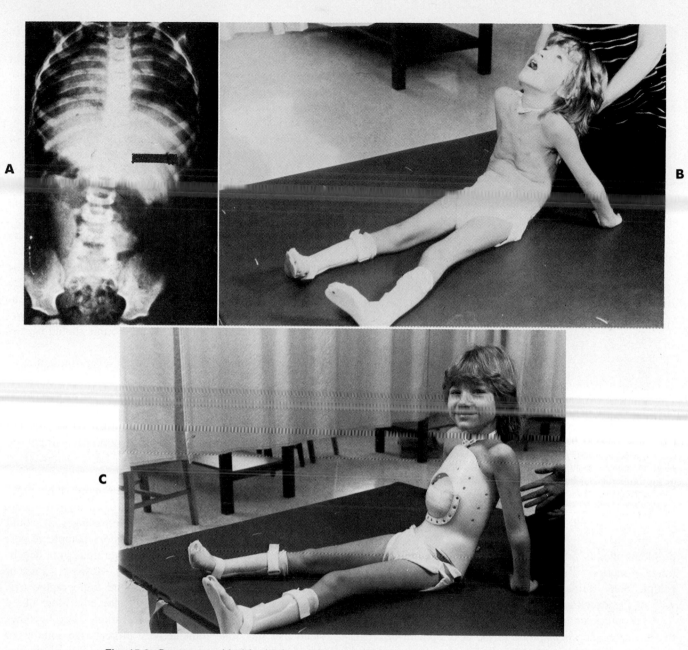

Fig. 15-2. Seven-year-old girl with incomplete traction cord lesion at C4 to C6. **A,** A slight scoliosis detected at age 4 has stabilized with the use of a body jacket. In addition to the scoliotic deformity, the body jacket assists with trunk stability and allows improved diaphragm expansion by restraining viscera with elastic binder support across hole in jacket, **B** and **C.**

rence is usually always within the first 6 to 12 months after injury.[108]

Ectopic bone formation develops over a period of weeks. Nicholas[175] described four stages. The initial signs are often confused with thrombophlebitis, septic arthritis, cellulitis, or a fracture. They include soft tissue swelling, pain, local warmth, and erythema near a large joint. Serum and alkaline phosphatase levels are elevated. No evidence is present on radiograms. In this initial stage, the swelling is firm to palpation and may cause some initial limitation of motion at the adjoining joint. In the second

stage swelling remains, there are continued high-alkaline phosphatase levels, and the formation is apparent on the radiogram. The third stage shows the initial swelling and erythema subsiding. In the last stage, which occurs 2 to 4 weeks after onset, extensive calcification has developed, and there may be initial signs of ankylosing of the adjacent joint.

Ankylosis is the primary complication in client function. Most clients experience no loss of function or problems with ectopic bone formation. The hip is the area that presents the most problems; one third of the clients with

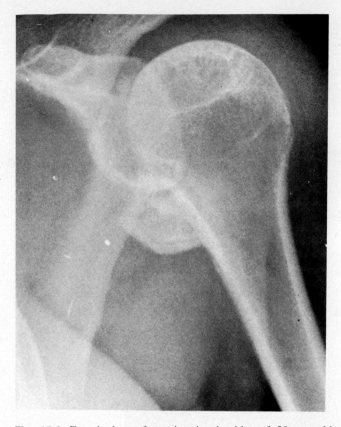

Fig. 15-3. Ectopic bone formation in shoulder of 30-year-old quadriplegic woman. Ectopic bone has formed in a characteristic position inferior to joint. It is continuous with the surgical neck of the humerus but has not fused with the neck of the scapula. (From Hendrix RW: Skeletal changes after spinal cord injury. In Calenoff L, editor: Radiology of spinal cord injury, St Louis, 1981, The CV Mosby Co.)

problems in this area have decreased active and passive range of motion.[250] Approximately 20% of the clients with ectopic bone formation progress to joint ankylosis, and 75% of the ankylosed joints involve the hip.[108]

A secondary complication of ectopic bone formation is that it makes the client prone to the development of pressure sores.[108] It can do this indirectly, for example, through a hip flexion contracture from ectopic bone causing a pressure area over the ischial tuberosity, or directly, when the bone formation itself becomes prominent in an area prone to pressure. Management of ectopic bone formation focuses on drug therapy, passive and active range of motion, and, as a last resort, surgery.

Diphosphonates (Etidronate disodium) are drugs that can be used to prevent the crystallization of calcium phosphate and thereby prevent ectopic bone formation. They have been shown to have some use before radiographic evidence of bone formation and to prevent ectopic bone recurrence after surgical resection.[229] These drugs have no effect on mature ectopic bone. Considerable controversy has existed over whether passive and active range of motion contributes to or helps prevent ectopic bone forma-

tion. Early studies[60,223] suggest that range of motion contributed to increased quantities of bone formation. More recent studies[228,249,250] have advocated vigorous range of motion during the early stages of development. These studies were not able to show any increase in quantity of bone formation developing from range of motion. It therefore seems logical that consistent range of motion combined with drug therapy during the early "plastic" stage of ectopic bone formation will aid in retaining functional range. If the formation of ectopic bone is so rapid and severe that ankylosis cannot be avoided, then it is the therapist's responsibility to see that the involved joint fuses in the most functional position.

Vigorous range of motion can fracture an ossified ectopic bone formation, and the fracture may form a pseudarthrosis. This is not advocated since recurrence of the ectopic bone will most likely occur with a good chance for further functional loss in motion. Clients have intentionally fractured an ectopic bone formation while performing self-range of motion exercises; this should be discouraged.

When ankylosing of a joint causes severe limitation of client function, surgical intervention is often necessary. The surgical goal is to resect enough of the mature bone formation to restore adequate joint function. The primary complication to surgery is the recurrence of the ectopic bone postoperatively.[108] This can be minimized if surgery is delayed until the ectopic bone is fully mature (Fig. 15-4).[234,258]

Degenerative joint abnormalities. Finally, with time, ambulatory and nonambulatory spinal cord injured clients are prone to severe degeneratative joint changes. It would seem that the active long-term ambulatory paraplegic person would be more prone to hip and sacroiliac joint degeneration than the nonambulatory person. However, a recent study by Wylie and Chakera[252] found radiographic evidence that the higher the level of lesion, the more likely the client is to develop joint degeneration. They hypothesized that moderate joint activity protects the joint from degenerative change by maintaining synovial fluid circulation and production necessary for sustaining articular cartilage. This is an important consideration during rehabilitation when consideration is given to goals of prolonged standing and/or ambulation.

Neurological signs and problems

Paralysis and tonal changes. Two primary descending motor pathways in the spinal cord are the pyramidal or corticospinal tract and an extrapyramidal pathway, the reticulospinal tract. The pyramidal tract carries impulses from the premotor, primary motor, and primary somatosensory cortical areas, and the reticulospinal tract carries descending impulses from the extrapyramidal and cerebellar motor control systems. Depending on the spinal level of injury and on the degree of cord damage to these tracts, the client will be faced with a clinical picture of motor pa-

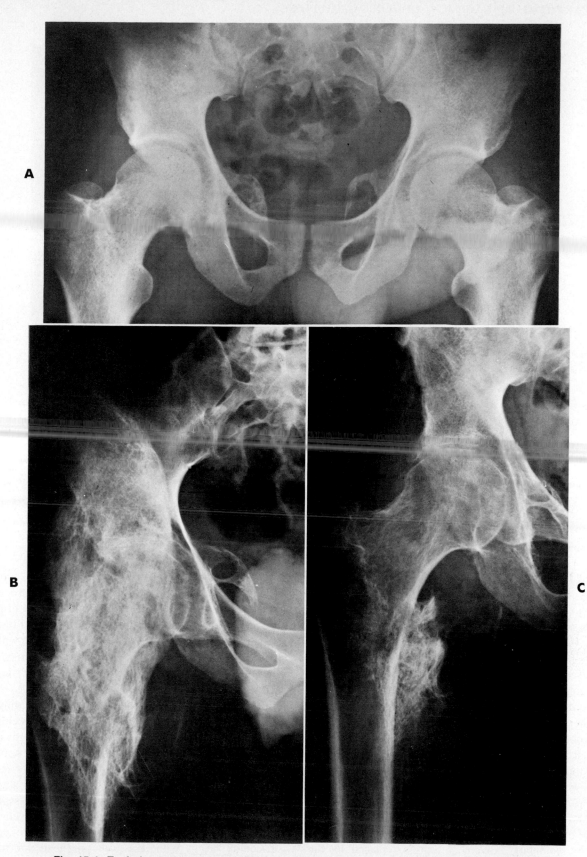

Fig. 15-4. Evolution and surgical resection of ectopic bone in C6 quadriplegic man. **A,** Ectopic ossification is present adjacent to left greater trochanter. Bilateral ossification adjacent to and continuous with posteroinferior iliac spines is unusual and has appeared within 1 year of client's injury. **B,** Six years after injury, extensive ectopic bone has formed anterior to right hip, resulting in extra-articular ankylosis of joint. There is narrowing of joint space superiorly. **C,** One month later, most of the ectopic bone has been surgically removed with restoration of joint motion. Narrowing of hip joint superiorly can be better appreciated.

Continued.

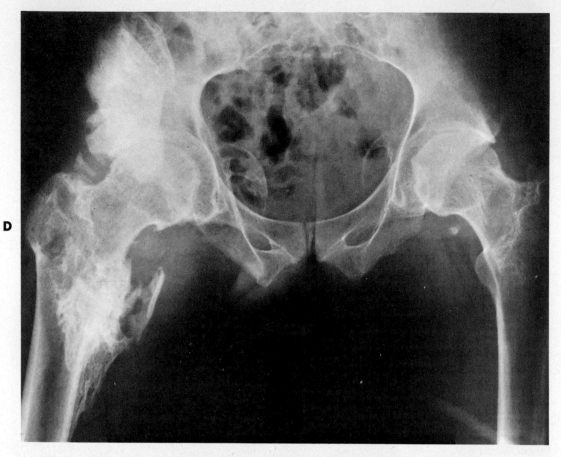

Fig. 15-4, cont'd. D, Three years and six months later, as is always true even after resection of mature ectopic bone, there is at least a small amount of recurrence, which is seen here superior to and anterior to the joint. (From Hendrix RW: Skeletal changes after spinal cord injury. In Calenoff L, editor: Radiology of spinal cord injury, St Louis, 1981, The CV Mosby Co.)

ralysis with either upper motor neuron hyper-reflexive spasticity or lower motor neuron hyporeflexive flaccidity.

Chapter 2 of this text presents insights into both the neurophysiological and neuroanatomical aspects of tonal changes from insult to the CNS. Chapter 6 presents the common physical therapy inhibitory and facilitory techniques used in the management of tonal problems. In this section some aspects of tonal changes that are unique to spinal cord injury are presented along with an overview of the medical and surgical techniques used in dealing with tonal problems. Also in this section the most common functional problems for the person with a spinal cord injury dealing with paralysis with an abnormal state of tone are reviewed.

Hypertonicity (spasticity) in spinal cord injury can cause (1) a decrease in joint range that may ultimately lead to a state of muscle/joint contracture, (2) a decrease in isolated joint voluntary movement that is replaced by the emergence of mass movement patterns of muscles (i.e., synergies) that are neurophysiologically linked, (3) abnormal sensory feedback that may impair the relearning of motor skills, and (4) the loss of reciprocal inhibition, which is one strong underlying basis for coordinated movement. Hypotonicity (flaccidity) can cause (1) joint hypermobility and instability that might result in pain and possible joint damage leading to deformity, (2) insufficient postural tonal support, and (3) muscle atrophy with resultant appearance of bony prominences that increase the number of potential pressure areas at risk for skin breakdown. Whereas spasticity can contribute to function through, for example, a client using it for bearing weight on the lower extremities during a transfer, flaccidity itself contributes nothing to the function of an individual.

Spasticity is characterized not only by hypertonicity but also by hyperreflexia and clonus. A state of flaccidity is without reflex responses and reaction to rapid stretch. Although spasticity is a changing neuromuscular phenomenon that is responsive to internal and external stimuli, flaccidity is not responsive to stimuli; therefore prolonged flaccidity brings with it a poor prognosis for functional change.

This discussion focuses on spasticity, which has therapeutic importance. Spasticity can be of cerebral or spinal origin. Both types develop slowly over a period of weeks or months after the insult. An exception would be the immediate state of hypertonicity known as decerebrate rigidity, which is found in high-brainstem lesions. As stated earlier, spasticity is a "plastic" phenomenon that changes constantly in response to internal and external stimuli. At any point in the recovery process, spasticity may be flexor or extensor dominant, either within a limb or over the whole body. Some clinical patterns of tone are believed to exist. In spasticity due to cerebral insult, tone is predominant in the antigravity muscles, that is, the flexors in the upper extremities and the extensors in the lower extremities. In spinal spasticity the clinical picture is more often associated with flexor muscle spasticity.[46]

With spinal cord injury some controversy exists as to what patterns of spasticity are seen, when they are seen in the recovery process, and whether these patterns can be predicted. Merritt[152] believes that there exists a predictable "crescendo of spasticity" during the client's recovery, with mass flexor responses predominating during the first 3 to 6 months that then "evolve" into mass extensor spasticity. Other observers state that early positioning of the paralyzed limbs will predict the pattern of spasticity that will eventually develop after the initial period of spinal shock.[63,98] Most authorities tend to agree that every client with a complete cord lesion and spasticity will have an underlying "base" tonal predominance into either flexion or extension and that this tonal state can be modulated by a wide variety of stimuli. The tonal state in incomplete lesions is affected by the magnitude and direction of remaining superspinal influences. Therapy (physical, chemical, and surgical) is then directed at modulating this constantly varying tonal state toward a level that allows maximal client function.

Spasticity may exist at a level that does not interfere with function or that contributes to function. When spasticity exists as, or changes toward, an interference with function, the physician, treatment team, and the client have to decide what internal and external stimuli can possibly be added, eliminated, or changed. Nociceptive internal stimuli that often cause increased spasticity include urinary tract infections, bladder or kidney stones, pressure sores, bowel impactions, painful joint contractures, deep vein thrombosis, and the level of mental stress. External stimuli that are often responsible for tonal changes include environmental temperature, noxious skin stimuli from tight clothing, catheter blockage or twisting, tight leg bag straps, and the position of the body parts.

Management of spasticity in cord injuries through physical therapy procedures will be discussed later in this chapter. Medical or drug management includes such medications as diazepam (Valium) and chlordiazepoxide (Librium) (benzodiazepines), dantrolene sodium (Dantrium), baclofen (Lioresal), and aminoacetic acid (Glycine), a new experimental drug currently in the animal testing stage.[152] These drugs are useful for controlling spasticity in certain clients with complete or incomplete lesions. However, they are not without their side effects. These side effects include drowsiness, fatigue, malaise, and weakness, all of which are clinically apparent.[152]

Percutaneous epidural neurostimulation has been successful in modulating spasticity in clients with spinal cord injury.[11,198] Chemical neurolytic procedures are sometimes useful when drug therapy has failed to promote the desired response. These procedures involve injections of chemicals into areas of the reflex arc to interrupt it and therefore reduce spasticity. These procedures include (1) phenol motor point injections,[101] (2) phenol nerve blocks,[129] and (3) intrathecal or extradural injections of alcohol or phenol into the spine.[63,152] Phenol-motor point injections and phenol nerve blocks are both useful for selectively decreasing tone in muscle(s), but they may be only temporarily effective. Intrathecal or extradural injections of alcohol or phenol are more permanent although also sometimes transient modulators of spasticity. Lioresal may also be infused into the subarachnoid space over a long time by using an implantable pump. This system consists of a catheter inserted into the subarachnoid space and connected to a pump surgically placed into a subcutaneous abdominal pocket. The pump is refilled every 2 to 4 weeks and allows delivery of a small, predictable dosage compared with oral administration.[186]

As a last resort, surgical intervention may prove useful. Orthopaedic surgery offers tenotomies, myotomies, tendon lengthening and transplant procedures, and neurosurgery can provide severance of the nerve roots (rhizotomy), nerves (neurectomy), and portions of the spinal cord (myelotomy, cordotomy, and cordectomy). Surgery may offer dramatic and permanent changes in spasticity. The postoperative functional capacity of the client is what is important; therefore careful client selection coupled with concerted preoperative and postoperative care by the managing team of surgeons and others is paramount.

The application of a topical anesthetic that appears to possibly interrupt the alpha gamma motor neuron excitability for approximately 4 hours is another modality that may temporarily control tone over a short period in order to allow performance of therapeutic exercises.[214]

Sensory loss, proprioception, and pressure sores. The person with a spinal cord injury is faced with two primary potential functional deficits as a result of having lost deep and cutaneous sensation. These are awareness of the position of body parts and awareness of pressure on the skin. Deep sensory loss involves joint receptors that provide the normal individual with proprioceptive feedback regarding awareness of static limb position and limb movement. Because controlled functional movement depends heavily on this deep proprioceptive feedback, the client who may have active voluntary movement without the presence of deep sensation is most likely going to lack functional movement. This sensory loss may affect the client's overall perceptual awareness of body image. This issue is addressed later in this chapter.

Diminished sensory function also often involves nociceptive stimuli from prolonged skin pressure. These stimuli are normally involved in producing weight shifting, which prevents the tissue ischemia and anoxia that lead to the development of pressure sores or pressure ulcers. These sores are a constant threat to the functional and financial stability of all persons with cord injuries. They are best dealt with through an aggressive program of team and client education aimed at identifying factors causing their development and through comprehensive preventative programs that explore all factors of pressure distribution during the client's initial hospitalization, rehabilitation, and life-style and environment after discharge.[71,177,179]

The causes of pressure sores are both intrinsic and extrinsic. In addition to loss of cutaneous sensation, intrinsic factors include the loss of vasomotor control, disturbances in the person's metabolic capacity from prolonged illness and/or poor nutrition, systemic infection, advanced age, and poor skin condition.[108] There is also recent evidence that underlying muscle might be more sensitive to pressure than is the skin and that it is here that initial pathological changes begin that then progress toward the skin.[61] Because subjective observation of skin color cannot detect this damage occurring in underlying muscle, recent attempts have been made to develop various quantitative tests to detect early biochemical changes indicating pressure ischemia and muscle breakdown.[100,205] Additionally, some clients who have been discharged have extensive histories of repetitive pressure sores that do not relate to the level of injury or other common predisposing factors. Therefore psychosocial issues have begun to be examined as possible predetermining factors.[5,263]

The primary extrinsic factor is the amount and duration of pressure applied to the skin. This pressure may take the form of direct compression, shearing forces that can cause stretch damage to subcutaneous tissue, and pressure combined with friction to the epidermis as caused by sheet burns. The amount of pressure needed to cause skin breakdown is determined by many variables, and there are no firm guidelines for determining what measurable amount of pressure can be tolerated by a given client without causing skin breakdown. Exposure of the skin to moisture can cause skin maceration, and local heat can cause increased tissue metabolism leading to the development of pressure ulcers.

The incidence and distribution of pressure sores have been studied extensively—most recently by Young and Burnst,[263] in a major study of 3030 cases reported to the NSCIDRC from 1975 to 1980,[263] and Stover,[228] who reported on the distribution and severity of pressure sores found in the 9647 clients admitted to the National SCI database from 1973 to 1985. Young and Burnst[263] found that complete and high-level lesions did have a greater inci-

dence during the initial medical/rehabilitation period than incomplete and low-level lesions. This incidence ranged from 57% in complete quadriplegic clients during this period to 22% in incomplete paraplegic clients. However, when they removed minor sores, those that did not penetrate the dermis, the whole population's incidence dropped to 5.8%. An interesting finding was that the completeness of the injury was a much more powerful determinant of sore occurrence than the level of lesion. Quadriplegic clients in general fared almost as well as paraplegic clients. The authors concluded that the quadriplegic client's impaired weight-shifting ability was offset by the paraplegic client's higher level of activity and subsequent exposure to tissue trauma.

In terms of distribution, this study found the most commonly involved body area was the sacrum; this was followed by the heels, ischium, trochanteric areas, and scapular areas. The establishment of major spinal cord injury centers, which admit client's with cord injuries immediately after injury into a system highly skilled in preventing skin breakdown, has brought about a significant decrease in the incidence of pressure sores among its clients.[263]

To facilitate precise communication among professionals in identifying the extent of involvement of a pressure sore, systems of grading the severity have replaced such vague terms as "superficial" and "extensive."[74,222] Pressure sores range in severity from erythema that lasts longer than 2 hours to massive lesions involving joint structures that can lead to profound osteomyelitis with subsequent amputation. They can be remarkably deceiving in that the visible skin wound may be small while the subcutaneous tissue destruction may be extensive. They may be associated with sinus tracts that connect with a large abscess cavity or an adjacent joint. A primary problem in treating this type of lesion is to identify its size. Two new methods used to determine the full extent of a sinus tract associated with a pressure sore are sinography, in which a radiopaque material is injected and radiographically viewed,[192] and computed tomography.[78]

Treatment ranges from local wound care with debridement of necrotic tissue to operative measures involving wound closure through the use of skin grafts, skin flaps, and muscle flaps.[3] As stated earlier, prevention through skin care and pressure relief and client education are the keys to dealing with this problem. Skin care is primarily a nursing responsibility during the initial acute phase of treatment, but after that it is a team effort that has to include the client. The long-term identification of risk factors for skin breakdown focuses on educating the client toward a goal of full responsibility for prevention. Pressure relief equipment and skills are discussed later in this chapter.

Autonomic dysreflexia. The loss of supraspinal control of the sympathetic and sacral parasympathetic systems found in cervical and high thoracic lesions forces the recently injured client to undergo a number of adjustments to this altered physiological state. There are a number of altered autonomic nervous system responses that the client with a spinal cord injury can demonstrate.[17] Those that are of primary importance are discussed.

Autonomic dysreflexia and autonomic hyperreflexia are acute syndromes of disordered autonomic homeostasis found in complete and incomplete lesions above T6. They occur as a result of the traumatic sympathectomy secondary to a lesion at this level and above and are primarily manifested by uninhibited mass autonomic reflexes. In general, it is triggered by noxious afferent stimuli to the skin and viscera below the level of the cord lesion. These stimuli, because of the loss of higher-level control mechanisms, result in a wide range of sympathetic and parasympathetic responses. A summary of the most common stimuli for autonomic dysreflexia and a list of its systemic effects and treatment alternatives are found in Table 15-3. For a detailed discussion of the pathophysiology and medical management of this clinical problem see the references at the end of this chapter.[75,124,139] The physical therapist needs to be aware of the origin of the noxious stimuli common to a physical therapy setting and of the established protocols for medical management of this problem within that setting.

Bladder distention and spasms and catheter irrigation are the primary causes of autonomic dysreflexia. These are followed by bowel impactions and rectal stimulation.[139] The therapist needs to watch for blockage or twisting of a urinary catheter. In addition, traction on a catheter or pressure on the glans penis, scrotum, or urethra during activities can promote an automatic dysreflexive response. On the occurrence of initial symptoms, the first place to focus would be inspection of the urinary drainage system along with palpation of the bladder and lower bowel for distention. Other common causes that might be inferred by a therapist are painful cutaneous stimuli below the level of the lesion. Careful inspection needs to be made for restrictive clothing, leg bag straps, shoes, abdominal supports, and orthoses. A less common cause may lie with muscle stretching, either from range of motion exercises or from passive stretching precipitated by tilt table or strap-standing activities. Unless contraindicated by spinal instability, the client's head should be elevated to assist in controlling the hypertensive response. The client's blood pressure and pulse should be monitored. This syndrome needs to be managed as a medical emergency. Severe complications, although rare, include retinal hemorrhage, convulsions, periods of unresponsiveness, and death as a result of massive intracranial bleeding.[75,124]

Certain clients are prone to recurrent episodes. All personnel should be aware of each occurrence, of the usual stimulus, and of the measures that have been effective with this client. Clients who are prone to recurrence may be effectively managed through drug therapy. In addition, a recent report discussed the use of percutaneous epidural electrical stimulation for the prophylaxis of autonomic dysreflexia.[200] Past attempts at surgical procedures to reduce or abolish autonomic dysreflexia, such as ganglionic blocks and bilateral rhizotomies, have proved to have a

Table 15-3. Autonomic dysreflexia

Stimuli	Systemic effects	Treatment
Bladder distention	Paroxysmal hypertension	Treat as a medical emergency
Bladder infection	Bradycardia	Identify and remove irritating stimulus
Urethral/bladder irritation	Tachycardia	Elevate head
Bowel impaction	Pounding headaches	Possible pharmacological intervention
Rectal stimulation	Vasoconstriction (below the level of	(primary sympathetic blocking
Cutaneous noxious stimuli	lesion)	agents)
Gastric irritation	Vasodilation—flushing, blotching of	
Uterus contraction (pregnancy)	skin, cold sweating (above the level	
Muscle joint receptor irritation	of lesion)	With recurrent episodes: possible pro-
Environmental temperature variations	Piloerection (goose bumps)	phylactic drug therapy and client
Extensive infected pressure sores	Pupillary dilation	education regarding self-
	Blurring of vision	management
	Horner's syndrome	
	Anxiety, apprehension	
	Nasal congestion	
	Nausea, congestion	
	Nausea, vomiting	
	Syncope	
	Cardiac arrhythmia	
	Increased spasticity	
	Parasthesias	
	Penile erection	
	Dyspnea (secondary to bronchospasm)	

high level of side effects and unwarranted secondary tissue destruction.[124,200] Clients who are prone to episodes of autonomic dysreflexia should be educated as to what stimuli precipitate the symptoms and what actions should be taken. This is particularly important after discharge, and certain clients may have to wear medical alert identification.

Of adult clients with lesions above T6, 48% to 85% experience autonomic dysreflexia.[124,139,258] The incidence in children is lower; one series reported that 24% of children with lesions above T6 developed this problem.[128] In very young children, restlessness, nausea, vomiting, thrashing of the head and neck, facial flushing, sweating, tightening of the abdominal muscles, and penile erections should arouse suspicion of autonomic dysreflexia.[125]

There is no way to predict which clients will incur an episode of autonomic dysreflexia.[139] Most occurrences are within the first year following injury.

Postural hypotension. In clients with lesions above the midthoracic level, the loss of sympathetic control of peripheral vasoconstrictor activity leads to the problem of hypotension. The loss of muscle tone also adds to peripheral venous and splanchnic bed pooling of blood. This "baseline" hypotension is further aggravated when the client begins the process of acclimating to vertical positions. With this postural change, further pooling of blood in the lower extremities and gut can occur, resulting in reduced venous return to the heart, further drops in blood pressure, and decreased cerebral blood flow. The process of gradually progressing the client toward vertical sitting is usually coordinated by the physical therapy staff in conjunction with the nursing staff. By closely monitoring the client's blood pressure and subjective responses, the therapist can gradually assist the client toward the vertical posture. For some unknown reason, the cardiovascular system adapts over time, and vasomotor tone is partially reestablished. The therapist can start the process by elevating the head of the bed and by switching to a reclining wheelchair when longer periods of vertical positioning are tolerated. Some therapists prefer to use a tilt table. However, some clients experience syncope, which appears extraneous to the cardiovascular hypotension, when the tilt table is elevated beyond 60 degrees vertical. Elastic, pressure gradient stockings and abdominal binders can retard venous pooling and assist in this acclimation process. Drug therapy may also be instituted. Elastic stockings are also helpful in controlling the pitting edema that occurs in the lower extremities secondary to both of the factors mentioned previously and the added decreased lymphatic return present in clients with spinal cord injuries. This edema reduction may also be assisted with the use of diuretic drugs. A last important point to remember is that this gradual compensatory process requires the full functioning of many systems and is usually very fatiguing in itself to the client. The inability

of the autonomic nervous system to cope with daily stress is very real, and clients and their families need to be educated regarding these systemic reactions.[17]

Deep vein thrombosis. The client with a spinal cord injury that is the result of trauma has a predisposition to the development of deep vein thrombosis in the lower extremities with possible secondary development of pulmonary embolism. This predisposition is primarily related to age and to the absence of the pumping action of the lower-extremity musculature, which precipitates venous stasis. In addition, trauma clients, especially those who have undergone surgery, have changes in blood factors toward a hypercoagulable state; this has been found to be common in spinal cord injuries.[210] Another predisposing factor is found in clients with high cervical lesions who, because of flaccid paralysis of the intercostal muscles, have a diminution of the negative intrathoracic pressure that assists venous flow to the heart.[258]

Deep vein thrombosis usually occurs within days after injury and can occur up to 2 to 3 months following injury. Medical management has focused on prophylactic anticoagulant drug therapy up to 6 months after injury.[73] Others have suggested the use of passive range of motion exercises during the acute stages as possibly being prophylactic for deep vein thrombosis.[79,83,241] In addition, pressure gradient elastic stockings, which were mentioned previously, may also serve as a preventive measure.

Clinically, apparent deep vein thrombosis has an incidence as high as 40%[241] in clients with acute spinal cord injury. However, a recent study found that the incidence of subclinical deep vein thrombosis may be much higher (72%) with the incidence increasing with the age of the client.[210] Therefore therapists need to be aware of the clinical signs (localized swelling, erythema, heat), test for deep vein thrombosis (Homans' sign), and carefully monitor clients on passive range of motion and early programs of mobilization. These clinical signs may be confused with early ectopic bone formation or long bone fracture.

Impaired temperature regulation. Clients with spinal cord injuries with lesions above T1 have impaired temperature regulation, especially during the acute stages of recovery.[189] This inability to regulate body temperature in response to environmental temperature extremes occurs in two ways. With a lesion at this level, the connection between the temperature-regulating centers in the hypothalamus and the sympathetic outflow from the cord, which causes vasoconstriction and sweating, is prevented. Second, damage to the motor tracts may prevent shivering. Temperature-regulating mechanisms appear to improve with time, although quadriplegic persons will usually retain an impaired ability to control the body temperature when confronted by environmental extremes.

Pain. In the client with a traumatic spinal cord injury, pain may be of organic origin with or without an emotional overlay. Organic pain can be grouped into four categories according to the site of origin.

Pain from precipitating trauma. Pain from precipitating trauma involves bony and soft tissue damage to the vertebral column and secondary injuries that lie within sensory innervated areas. This type of pain also arises from surgical procedures, such as laminectomies and spinal fusions, performed immediately after injury. It is considered acute somatic pain that gradually subsides with healing, generally within 1 to 3 months. It can have secondary chronic residual components when the involved joints incur long term arthritic changes. This is especially true in clients who have undergone a spinal fusion where the vertebral joints above and below the fused segments undergo increased stress, which precipitates degenerative changes. The acute somatic pain is usually managed conservatively with analgesic drugs. Chronic pain can be helped with local injections of steroids in, for instance, the facet joints.[64] The use of transcutaneous electrical nerve stimulators (TENS) has proved more successful with this type of acute and chronic soft tissue pain in clients with spinal cord injury than with the following types of pain.[65,201]

Radicular pain. Radicular pain occurs when vertebral damage causes acute compression or tearing of the nerve roots. Irritation and compression can also slowly involve the nerve roots through spinal instability or adhesion formation. In the cervical and thoracic areas, the number of nerve roots involved corresponds to the number of vertebral levels damaged. However, beginning with the thoracolumbar junction, many more roots become involved through the cauda equina. It is this client, the one with severe pain spreading diffusely through the lumbosacral trunk and lower extremities, who becomes debilitated with possible reliance on narcotic analgesics.

Typical nerve root pain usually follows a dermatomal distribution and can be described as a sharp, stabbing, shooting, or burning pain. Many cauda equina injuries are partial, and with some afferent input is still present. The increased pain may also indicate pathology in other areas, such as in the genitourinary and gastrointestinal systems. Treatment of nerve root pain, especially that involving the cauda equina, is difficult in the client with a spinal cord injury. Drug therapy, TENS, implantation of dorsal column stimulators, surgical neurectomies, and posterior rhizotomies have all proved useful, especially in conjunction with supportive psychotherapy.[64,258]

Spinal cord dysesthesias. Spinal cord dysesthesias are somewhat bizarre sensations of numbness, tingling, burning, and pain felt below the level of the lesion. They are diffuse and do not conform to any dermatomal distribution. These sensations are found in some form in most persons with spinal cord injury; documented incidences range from 82% to 94%.[64] Most dysesthetic feeling is present initially after injury and most is consistent; the intensity of dysesthesia declines with time and with increased activity of the client. The cause of dysesthesia is unknown; scarring of the distal stump of the severed spinal cord provides one theory[209,258] and persistence of a sympathetic nerve pathway another.[64] The feelings on occasion take the form of proprioceptive sensations with the client expressing that the lower extremities are in positions other than what actually exist. They have even been referred to as "phantom spinal pains,"[64,258] being analogous to those found with limb amputation. Dysesthesias are influenced by many factors, including depression, anxiety, inclement weather, cigarette smoking (including marijuana), excessive alcohol consumption, exercise and fatigue.[64] As with cauda equina nerve root pain, dysesthesia pain can be severely incapacitating. Two drugs, carbamazepine (Tegretol) and phenytoin (Dilantin), have been advocated in reducing dysesthesia pain.[64,258] Narcotic agents, dorsal column stimulators, TENS, and surgical interventions have shown little success.[64,258] In a small sample of clients suffering from this type of chronic pain, Grzesiak[95] had success using a combination of muscle relaxation techniques aimed at intact muscles below the level of lesion coupled with cognitive alterations in the attentiveness to pain.

Nonspinal somatic pain. Nonspinal somatic pain exists when sensation is intact or pathology is present above the level of the lesion. This type of pain is typically of musculoskeletal origin. One common problem is the painful shoulder joint complex often found in quadriplegic clients during the rehabilitation phase of treatment.[219] Its origin is usually the result of a combination of factors, including lack of full range of motion exercises and proper positioning during the acute phase with subsequent limitation of motion, especially toward hyperextension and external rotation. This is coupled with the increased stress on the kinematics of this complex found during the increased activity of rehabilitation, for example, during wheelchair propulsion and when assuming the prone on elbows position or the supine on elbows position. This pain usually subsides when full range of motion is regained and when strength is increased. Other examples of somatic pain are pain originating from severe upper motor neuron spasticity and from pressure sores found in incomplete lesions.

Because pain is so difficult to measure and has different meanings to different individuals, there is a lack of data regarding the incidence of pain in persons with spinal cord injury. However, one study by Nepomuceno in 1979[174] involved a survey-questionnaire of 200 clients following discharge. Eighty percent reported continued abnormal sensations, and 48% called this discomfort painful. A second study by Burke[32] examined a large difference in the incidence of perceived pain found among clients in two rehabilitation hospitals. He concluded that the difference resulted from two factors found in the hospital that contributed to clients reporting more pain. These factors were (1) a higher incidence of spinal surgery and (2) a delay in the period from injury to active involvement by the client in the rehabilitation process.

Since so much of what we currently know as pain has an emotional overlay, it is this active involvement in the rehabilitation process that may help the client to deal effectively with many of the problems of pain. Inherent in this active process is the client's ability to communicate to a receptive team feelings regarding awareness of pain and its relation to adjustment to injury.

Perceptual/body image dysfunction. Another clinical sign that may pose psychological problems is the body-image disorders that are found in persons with incomplete spinal cord injury. These have been documented most recently by Conomy.[57] Conomy studied 18 clients with traumatic cord injuries and 10 clients with various types of nontraumatic cord dysfunction. He found that all clients with traumatic injuries related somewhat stereotyped hallucinatory disturbances involving their perception of limb position and movement below the level of the cord lesion. These perceptions fell into three categories. The first is disorders of perception of static limb positions and relationships (these were the most common and lasted up to 25 years after the injury in one client). These disorders of perception typically involved perceptions of the lower extremities being in positions other than what actually existed. The second category is disordered perception of both static posture and kinetic limb movement. This often occurred early after the injury and consisted of hallucinations that joints were involved in rapid movements that were often perceived as strenuous work. These were again episodic and were often experienced during the period of spinal shock. As with all these hallucinations, gazing at the extremities corrected the illusion. The third and least common of these disorders involves disturbances in the perception of the size, somatic bulk, and continuity of body parts. The greatest incidence is an hallucinated increase in the size of the feet and legs. The group with nontraumatic injuries experienced very few disorders of body image; of those who did, most were brief and nonrecurrent. Based on his and other studies, Conomy[57] believes that all clients with spinal cord injury show at least some disruption of body scheme, although such disruption was very rarely found in clients with proven complete cord severance. Clients in his study experienced these disturbances periodically: they were predictable, and they were unique to each client. No anatomical basis for these disorders of body image has been explained, but Conomy reviewed current theories. This phenomenon is similar to the postamputation syndrome called "phantom limb sensation" with the exception that the limb is still present. The importance of being aware of this phenomenon is that the studies found that clients were reluctant to discuss these disorders and many in-

terpreted them as psychological in origin. Because they are fairly common and, if kept internalized, may be very disturbing to the client's psychological well-being, it would seem appropriate that therapists, who spend large amounts of time with clients, be aware of this clinical sign and be willing to intelligently discuss it with their clients.

Bowel and bladder dysfunction. Damage to the spinal cord results in functional changes in the genitourinary and gastrointestinal systems. Secondary complications involving these systems can include kidney and bladder stone formation, kidney and bladder infections, gastric stress ulcers, and reflex autonomic dysfunctions secondary to bowel impaction. Successful rehabilitation must take into account efforts aimed at retraining these systems toward a level of function that, although altered from what existed before injury, is medically safe and prophylactic and that efficiently fits into a person's life-style after discharge. Although programs of bladder and bowel rehabilitation typically are coordinated by a nursing staff, the therapist and other professionals who interact with a client for any time need detailed insight into that client's program. They need to understand the functional, anatomical, and neurophysiological similarities and differences among clients in order to intelligently answer a client's basic questions. In addition, bowel and bladder management programs involve special diets and scheduled routines that may directly involve the therapist.

For detailed insight into the applied physiology and clinical management of the bowel and bladder the reader is referred to Chapter 30 and to the work of Gore and Mintzer.[91]

Sexual readjustment. Damage at any level of the spinal cord brings with it alterations in sexual function (this topic is discussed at length in Chapter 30). Generally, females redevelop normal menses 1 to 3 months following injury and can give natural birth to children. Females typically have decreased sensation in the genital areas but heightened sexual arousal is possible with most every woman. The ability to achieve orgasm is difficult but possible either with incomplete lesions or through tactile stimulation above the level of a complete lesion—especially around the breasts and other intact erogenous zones. In the male, fertility is often decreased because of atrophy of the testicles and the resulting reduction in number and quality of sperm. The ability to achieve erection, to experience orgasm, and to ejaculate varies. Men with higher-level lesions can often achieve a reflexive erection but typically do not ejaculate. Those with lower lesions can more easily ejaculate, but the ability to facilitate an erection is more difficult. With cauda equina lesions erection and ejaculation are usually not possible. What was once a topic seldom if ever discussed even in the most progressive settings is today considered an important facet of the rehabilitation process. Most rehabilitation centers and hospital-based units recognize the importance of having a specialist on this topic who is responsible for supportively interacting at any level with clients and their family and for educating the other members of the team in this area.[164]

Therapists often field the initial inquiries regarding sexual issues simply because of the time they spend with their clients. The therapist who is comfortable responding to these questions needs to have accurate insight into the client's altered physiological state and potential sexual function. Therapists also need to refer the client to other support systems when the issues are beyond their abilities. In contrast, the therapist who is not comfortable in discussing sexual issues needs to openly and honestly communicate this to the client and offer to assist the client in finding another source of information.

The physical therapist can also be helpful in assisting clients with positioning and joint motion problems as they relate to sexual activities. They also often interact with the pregnant woman with spinal cord injury regarding prepartum and postpartum exercises and in developing strategies and adaptive equipment that will assist in early infant care.

This complex clinical problem involves not only the neural and endocrine physical changes but has a large impact on clients' self-image and emotional feelings regarding their sexuality. A positive premorbid self-image and feelings of self-worth are also important in overcoming the physiological, psychological, and technical problems. Problems with sexual activity need to be carefully worked out with the person with spinal cord injury and his or her partner. Any person who so chooses can, with proper counseling, lead a satisfying and meaningful sexual life that includes marriage, child-bearing,[119] and parenting.[7,131] In addition to Chapter 7 of this text, the reader is also referred to the work of Trieschmann[238] and Bedbrook.[16]

Metabolic and endocrine changes. Spinal cord injury involves partial or total removal of the sympathetic nervous system and partial removal of the parasympathetic nervous systems from brain integration. This results in a large number of metabolic and endocrine changes, some of which have been covered here. Most of these alterations have potential effects on a client's ability to perform in a physical therapy setting, and therapists need to be aware of the clinical implications of these changes. For a complete overview, the reader is referred to the references at the end of this chapter.[48-52]

Cardiorespiratory signs and problems. Most high-level paraplegic clients and all quadriplegic clients have to cope with a decrease in respiratory function from time of injury that eventually leads to a long-term level of cardiorespiratory function that is significantly altered from its premorbid state. This altered state corresponds in severity to the level of injury; clients with high-level spinal injuries also incur a high incidence of mortality from pulmonary causes, namely bronchopneumonia and pulmonary embolism.

In addition to the decrease in respiratory function that results from the paralysis of cord injury, clients often have to deal with other primary and secondary problems that impact on acute and long-term pulmonary function. Musculoskeletal trauma with or without fractures to the thoracic and lumbar spine, rib cage, sternum, and shoulder joint complex can obviously compromise respiratory function during the acute stage of care; it can also cause secondary long-term complications in the form of decreased mobility of the chest cage and scapulothoracic joint complex. Other acute injuries, such as pulmonary contusion, pulmonary hematoma, pneumonthorax, hemothorax, and esophygeal trauma, can complicate the early medical management and leave residual lung and intrathoracic scarring that can compromise long-term ventilatory efficiency.[165] The presence of premorbid pulmonary problems, such as pulmonary disease, allergies, the effects of smoking, and the aging process, can also complicate rehabilitation.

Depending on the level of lesion, the respiratory inefficiency of the quadriplegic client and high-level paraplegic client can be viewed as representing two primary problems. The first problem is *decreased inspiratory ventilation*. As the level of lesion rises, the two primary muscle groups responsible for inspiration (the diaphragm and external intercostals)[9] are progressively lost, beginning with the intercostals at the T11 level. The client's ability to ventilate the lungs becomes uncoordinated, and the accessory muscles of respiration progressively come into play. The second problem is *decreased expiratory pressure*. Again, with an ascending lesion, the two primary muscle groups of expiration (the abdominals and the internal intercostals)[9] are progressively lost, beginning with the abdominals at the T12 level. Although normal resting expiration is a passive process caused by the elastic properties of the lungs and thorax, beginning with lesions at the T12 level and above, expiration becomes an increasingly active and eventually labored process. This is the result of two factors. The abdominal muscles are progressively lost as the level of injury rises, and they no longer hold the viscera up against the diaphragm. The diaphragm then assumes an abnormally low resting or relaxed position within the thoracic cavity. Since the diaphragm's role in expiration is to be passively pushed upward by the contracting abdominals to assist in forced expiration, this lower resting state precipitates a decrease in the client's expiratory reserve volume. The second factor is that, with the loss of the internal intercostals whose active role in expiration is the depression of the rib cage, the client's ability to force air from the lungs during breathing and coughing is further compromised. Decreased cough results in the inability to remove normal bronchial secretions. This, combined with the overall poor ventilation of the lungs, puts the client at risk for segmental lung collapse (atelectasis), aspiration, and infection.

Poor ventilation of the lungs combined with the increased use of the accessory muscles of breathing results in a number of acute and chronic systemic problems. A very immediate result is decreased oxygenation of the blood with subsequent overall decreases in metabolic and functional efficiency. This is further compounded by the work involved in uncoordinated patterns of breathing. The end result is a significantly decreased ability to enter into the activities involved in the rehabilitation process.

Another acute complication is the client's predisposition to pulmonary embolism. Because the viscera assist diaphragmatic superior excursion in the supine position, the work of breathing is less in the supine position than in the sitting position.[99] However, long periods in recumbent positions combined with the decreased venous return from paralysis in the lower extremities precipitate the development of deep vein thrombosis and pulmonary embolism.[172]

Chronic problems include recurrent episodes of possible acute problems, for example, aspiration pneumonia, migratory atelectasis, and other respiratory infections. In addition, the motor paralysis results in the establishment of new breathing patterns. As the client increasingly relies on accessory muscles of breathing, a pattern of an increased superior excursion of the upper rib cage and a decreased anterior and posterior excursion of the lower rib cage develops. If left unmanaged, this can result in long-term postural changes and in a significant decrease in chest mobility (Fig. 15-5). This decreased chest mobility, uncoordinated breathing, and general decrease in total lung capacity result in voice quality changes with decreased volume and rate (words per breath).

As the level of cord lesion rises, the ability to achieve spontaneous functional respiration, even at rest, becomes compromised. This usually begins to occur at the C4 level. The client then may be taught the technique of glossopharyngeal breathing (GPB), which may improve respiratory reserve and the ability to assist with coughing. With the loss of the phrenic nerve at the C3 level, spontaneous respiration using the diaphragm is no longer possible and glossopharyngeal breathing along with the few remaining accessory muscles is usually no longer sufficient to maintain spontaneous respiration. The use of a mechanical respirator combined with a reclining wheelchair and an abdominal binder may allow assisted respiration and wheelchair mobility.[41] Victims of high-level (C1-2) traumatic injuries are surviving through improved emergency care; those with nondamaged phrenic nerves may become candidates for the use of an implanted electrical stimulator of the phrenic nerve[42,240] (Fig. 15-6).

The only primary cardiac problem with this client population is bradycardia in many quadriplegic clients. This may be severe during the early stages and results from the loss of sympathetic control of the vagovagal reflex.[41] Pulmonary dysfunction, with its often abnormal blood gas levels, may also cause cardiac abnormalities. Evaluation and treatment of cardiopulmonary problems in the physical therapy setting are discussed later in this chapter.

This concludes the overview of the clinical signs and/or problems that have impact on the rehabilitation process. Before discussing the physical therapist's role in this pro-

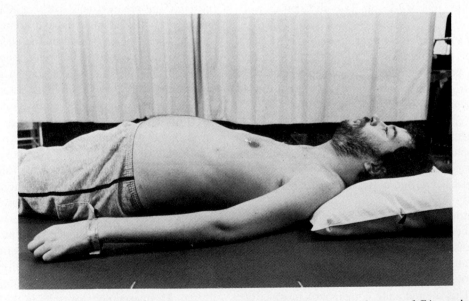

Fig. 15-5. Long-term postural changes in chest. The client is 2-years post-fracture of C4 vertebra with a complete lesion at the C5 cord level. Superior chest posture shows flattening with tight neck flexor muscle groups. Loss of abdominal and intercostal muscles results in protuberant viscera and an abnormally low resting position of the diaphragm.

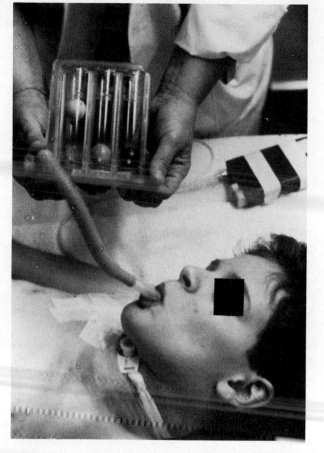

Fig. 15-6. Client with a complete cord lesion at the C1 level uses incentive spirometer during respiratory training. Note the battery power pack over the right shoulder for implanted phrenic nerve stimulator.

cess, insight needs to be gained into what factors and considerations have impact on the success of rehabilitation.

Prognosis for recovery

There are many factors inherent in, and external to, the client that influence the final outcome of rehabilitation efforts. To plan an effective and efficient course of treatment, the physical therapist needs to seek insight into these factors. This encompasses a complete and on-going review of the client's medical records as well as on-going communication with the physician, rehabilitation team, client, and family.

Spinal cord status. The primary factor in determining a prognosis for functional recovery of the client is gaining insight into the extent of damage to the spinal cord and determining what degree of recovery of cord function can be expected. This degree of cord recovery depends on the extent of the pathological changes incurred in the cord from the initial trauma. It also depends on preventing further trauma during rescue and evacuation of the client and on preventing additional neural damage from hypoxia and hy-

potension during initial stabilization in the acute care environment.[68] The initial reaction of the spinal cord to trauma is an inflammatory response that may further neural damage. Trauma also brings bleeding and edema into the spinal column that can compromise the metabolic demands of the neural tissue and subsequently decrease cord function. These reactions are dealt with by the initial medical team within the first 24 to 48 hours.[103] Decompression laminectomy can relieve the edema and allow the extent of visible cord damage to be viewed. However, viewing the cord during surgery is a poor prognosticator because, as mentioned earlier, severe damage may be present in the central gray matter even though the spinal column injury is mild and the cord appears normal. Fusion and surgical stabilization with devices can prevent further cord damage when mobility of the client is increased. These techniques are discussed later in this chapter. There have also been a number of nonsurgical treatments that have been used in animal studies and that have been used clinically during the very acute stages that are aimed at preventing further cord degeneration.[103,187] These include the use of steroids, hypothermia,[23] hypertonic agents to control edema, and hyperbaric oxygen.[86] Many of these treatments are advocated in conjunction with surgical decompression and myelotomy.

Much of this work is still in the animal study stages, and each treatment has its proponents and opponents as to its value in promoting retention of motor function in the immediate period following cord injury.

The clinical examination performed by the physician during the initial diagnostic process also impacts heavily on the prognosis. As mentioned earlier, sacral segments are examined for signs of sacral reflex sparing. These signs would include perianal sensation, voluntary toe flexion, reappearance of sacral reflexes (such as the bulbocavernosus reflex), and the presence of rectal tone. Absence of any of the signs beyond the initial period of spinal shock (a transient period where no reflex, sensory, or voluntary motor activity can occur distal to the level of the lesion) is usually indicative of a complete lesion.[110,226,237]

Tests such as myelography, electromyographic and H-reflex studies, and computed tomography (CT) can assist in determining the initial extent of cord damage without surgery.[122] These tests can also be useful in determining the effects of skeletal traction and of surgical and orthotic spinal stabilization.

Another test that has increasing significance in predicting functional outcome is the examination of somatosensory evoked potentials.[212] This noninvasive technique involves distal electrical stimulation of peripheral nerves below the level of injury with recording of the afferent evoked potentials over the primary sensory cortex. These potentials are absent in clients with complete motor and sensory loss below the level of spinal cord injury. Therefore they are useful in determining presence of recovery in incomplete lesions. Serial changes toward normalization of the evoked potential waveform have been shown to precede clinically observed changes in motor and sensory function. Because the majority of clients do not have complete transection of the cord,[158,159,265] somatosensory evoked potential responses will be increasingly used to determine rehabilitation outcomes.[266] They can be done by physical therapists[136] and should prove to be a more widely used evaluation tool during the rehabilitation phase of treatment. Finally, the extent of damage to the cord and surrounding nerve roots will determine the client's final clinical picture and chances for recovery. As noted earlier, lesions of the cauda equina and nerve roots show a greater propensity to improve. In a recent review of neurological recovery statistics from a number of different settings, Bedbrook[15] found that 65% of the clients reported on with cervical dorsal injury with neurological change were incomplete on admission and that 5% to 50% of lumbodorsal neurological injuries will manifest root sparing. Bedbrook's[15] review reported on studies that correlated postmortem findings to functional outcome and concluded that Brown-Séquard and central cord syndromes had a better prognosis than the anterior and posterior cord syndromes.[15]

After the process of acute stabilization, which occurs in the first 24 to 48 hours, it was believed that nothing further could be done to improve the function of the damaged part of the spinal cord. However, Naftchi recently reported on the use of clonidine, an adrenergic receptor agonist, that has a therapeutic effect at the distal stump of the tramatically injured cord in animal studies and in preliminary studies with humans during the subacute and chronic stages.[171] This orally administered drug has been used to control autonomic dysreflexia and minimize spasticity. Naftchi postulated that, because autonomic dysreflexia and spasticity may be caused by noxious stimuli arising from afferent somatic and visceral inputs conducted by the spinal cord below the level of the lesion, clonidine acts to block these stimuli from being transmitted over the adrenergic descending tracts. This study suggests that biochemical and pharmacological manipulation of receptors at the lesion site may prove to be the "breakthrough" needed to ameliorate paralysis and restore function to the person suffering a traumatic spinal cord injury.

The prospects for structural and functional restitution in the traumatically injured spinal cord have improved as a result of research in the last decade. These research efforts include: (1) facilitation of axonal sprouting around the collagenous scar tissue that forms at the lesion site and thereby improves chances for spinal cord regeneration, (2) the use of enzyme therapy to eliminate the scar tissue barrier, and (3) surgical reconstruction and nerve grafts in the spinal cord.[130,191] The long-held belief that nothing can be done to reverse the effects of spinal cord injury is giving way to increased research efforts that point toward effective treatment of the traumatically injured individual.

Client status. There are other factors inherent in the client that are external to the extent of the cord lesion but that affect the short- and long-term prognosis. The first factor is the age of the client. The older client may have difficulty in tolerating the high levels of stress placed on the body systems during the acute phase of care as well as the very large amounts of energy required during the rehabilitation stages. The older person may also be more likely to be dealing with premorbid health problems that will have varying degrees of adverse effects on rehabilitation outcomes. Because most older persons have achieved many of life's goals, they may be willing to settle for a more dependent long-term goal in rehabilitation. Lastly, the older person with spinal cord injury may have decreased ability to learn new tasks and to problem-solve many of the functional outcomes of the rehabilitation process.

The child who undergoes a traumatic spinal cord injury has added problems that will impact on the long-term prognosis.[40] Because physical growth is not complete, added problems related to potential for long-term altered body proportions and secondary deformities such as scoliosis need to be addressed and monitored throughout life. A child's immature strength and coordination will have an impact on his or her ability to perform in therapy. The infant who suffers a traumatic cord lesion, such as the traction injury mentioned earlier, does not have the experience of normal sensorimotor development with which to relate. Special attention also needs to be given to avoiding potential problems with a child's ongoing cognitive and social development.

Regardless of age, a person's body structure will impact on the outcome of rehabilitation. The very tall or very short person may need specially adapted equipment. The overweight person will have increased problems with mobility and may also require special equipment, such as an oversize wheelchair. Their decreased mobility may precipitate the need for additional assistance with functional activities after discharge. The very thin person may have problems with skin integrity as a result of increased bony prominences. Finally, a person's body proportions may influence his or her ability to perform functional tasks. A prime example is the person whose arms are long in relation to trunk length, who will more easily learn mobility activities in the sitting position because of the increased leverage and ability to raise and move the hips.

Motor learning abilities vary among individuals; those who had good premorbid coordination and possibly athletic prowess may learn mobility skills more easily and may progress farther in their rehabilitation efforts. Many athletes also have superior cardiorespiratory capacities that will improve their endurance during wheelchair and/or ambulation activities.

Closely related to motor learning ability is the ability to solve problems. Much of the rehabilitation process depends on an ongoing need to seek solutions to problems that interfere with a client's independence. The client has the rehabilitation team to assist with this process early on, but the need to be an effective problem solver continues throughout a disabled person's life. This ability varies between individuals and is not necessarily related to one's level of education.

One factor inherent in the effects of the lesion that greatly influences long-term function is the degree of residual spasticity. In spite of the many intervention strategies mentioned earlier that can be used to decrease excessive neuromuscular tone, there still exists a significant number of clients who are left with a level of spasticity that hinders their ability to achieve functional goals.

A client's premorbid occupation and level of education can influence the achievement of successful vocational rehabilitation. It can also affect the ability to teach others skills needed to assist the client in daily care.

The last, and probably the most important, factor is the client's ability to adapt and cope with his or her disability. Bracken and Shepard[22] analyzed this ability and concluded that premorbid personality and the influence of significant others were the two most important factors that partly explained why some clients were able to cope better with equally serious disability than others.[22] The ability to assume responsibility for one's self and one's level of assertiveness are other important factors.

In conclusion, all of these factors need to be considered on an on-going basis by the therapist and team when establishing realistic goals and functional outcomes for a client. It is these factors, combined with a sufficient level of economic funding, that lead to treatment planning that is efficient and feasible in achieving independence.

EVALUATION AND TREATMENT

Now that the clinical problems of the person with spinal cord injury have been defined, the remainder of this chapter will focus on the management of the systemic problems and on the achievement of functional goals as they relate to the practice of physical therapy. Because effective rehabilitation depends on a team effort in which all members of the clinical team have sufficient insight into each other's roles, appropriate references will continue to be made to other facets of clinical management that relate directly to the role of the physical therapist.

This discussion focuses on three phases of clinical management—the acute, rehabilitation, and community phases—with the primary emphasis on the subacute or rehabilitation phase. It is acknowledged that rehabilitation is an ongoing restorative and maintenance process that starts

at the time of injury and continues long after the person has been integrated back into the community. It is also ideal to have the same team manage this process through all three stages. However, the majority of clients have to interact with two or three different teams during this process, and it is for this pragmatic reason that these phases of care will be discussed separately.

Acute phase of management

The functional outcome of a person who suffers a traumatic injury to the spinal column with possible cord damage depends heavily on the quality and amount of care provided during the first 24 to 48 hours after injury.[92] The scene of injury is where this care must begin. As mentioned earlier in this chapter, a significant number of cord injuries are worsened by inappropriate emergency care at the scene of the accident. Emergency personnel need to be trained to question and/or inspect the injured person for any signs of spinal damage before attempting to evacuate the victim from the area. If any suspicion exists as to a spinal injury, then attempts must be made to prevent any active or passive movement of the spine. Cervical collars, rolled towels, tape, and back boards should be available to maintain the entire spine in a neutral anatomical position before attempting to transport the victim to a medical facility.

On arrival at the nearest medical emergency facility, attempts are made to stabilize the victim medically. Neurological physical examinations combined with tests such as a complete radiographic examination, tomography, and myelography are used to ascertain whether a cord injury exists and to possibly determine the extent of injury. Associated injuries also need to be identified and treated.

An important facet of the initial assessment is careful questioning of the client regarding the injury. This may provide some information helpful to the physician in establishing the degree of injury and in gaining some insight into a prognosis. For example, if the client remembers a complete loss of all sensation and movement during the initial minutes after the accident, then the outlook is poorer than if the paralysis gradually occurred over a period of many minutes or hours. This delayed onset of paralysis may be the result of the build-up of edema, which may brighten the prognosis for recovery through release of the edematous compression on the cord through surgical decompression.

Once the client is medically stable and the need for immediate surgical care has been dealt with, the client should be transported to either a major trauma center experienced in the care of spinal cord injuries or to one of the regional spinal cord injury centers. These centers have medical and ancillary personnel and the equipment capable of providing comprehensive services geared to this client population. They can coordinate care by radio from the scene of

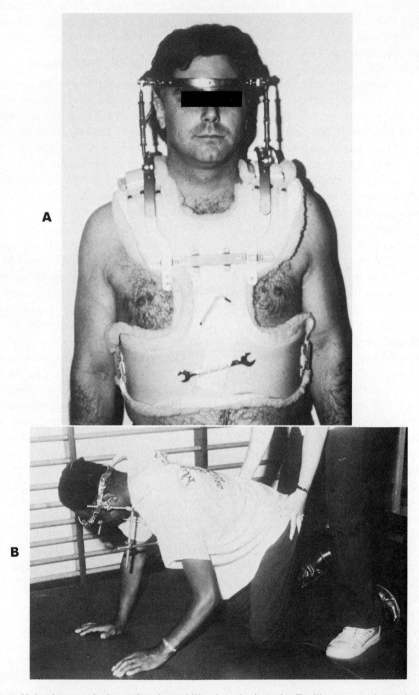

Fig. 15-7. Halo-ring cervical traction immobilization device. **A,** Facility protocol requires that tools needed to adjust the halo mechanism be taped to the body jacket. **B,** This and other spinal orthoses allow early initiation of activity while spinal stability is being achieved.

injury through the initial emergency facility stabilization period and subsequent transportation by ground or air to the spinal cord center. These centers are often affiliated with or administratively part of a comprehensive rehabilitation facility that enhances the potential for coordinated transfer to and through the rehabilitation facility and for long-term follow-up. The primary advantage of this coordinated care from the scene of the accident to and through acute stabilization at a spinal cord center is a dramatic decrease in the number of neurologically complete lesions. In one major center the number of clients admitted to the acute spinal injury service with complete irreversible neurological loss below the level of injury decreased from 72% in 1972 to 45% in 1978.[158,159] This was attributed to both the improved prehospital care plus the use of newer drugs, such as steroids and other drugs mentioned earlier, that have helped in controlling edema and inflammation toward improving the integrity of neural tissue.

Disadvantages or deterrents to the transfer to a regional spinal cord center include the potential lack of funding if the transfer is to another state, the occasional reluctance of the primary care physician in a client's community hospital to refer a client to a spinal cord injury center, and the client's loss of close ongoing contact with family and other support systems if the regional center is far from his or her home environment.

Once the client is admitted to the acute care or regional center, the use of other tests, such as computed tomography and monitoring of somatosensory evoked potentials, can further define the extent of damage to the cord.[154] Other clinical examinations, neuroradiological assessments, and nonsurgical treatments during this acute phase were discussed earlier in this chapter in the section on the status of the spinal cord and its relation to prognosis.

In the United States two major changes have occurred in the management of spinal cord injuries over the last 10 years that have significantly altered both the course and length of treatment and the survival and average level of injury of the client. The first change in care is the advent of regional spinal cord injury care centers that are capable of providing a broad team of specialists dedicated solely to the initial emergency through the rehabilitative care of the spinal cord injured person.[156] In addition, general trauma centers have been established locally. These centers are capable of coordinating the injured person's emergency care and safe evacuation from the scene of the accident. They then can effectively triage and transport that client to the closest regional spinal cord center. The second change in care has been the trend toward earlier mobilization of the client. This has been made possible by the introduction and increased use of spinal orthoses,[169] which allow the client to be out of bed and actively involved in the early stages of rehabilitation before the injured spine is medically and/or surgically stable.[19] These orthoses may be used with the client who has and the client who has not

had, surgery to explore and/or stabilize the spinal vertebral injury. The orthoses differ in the degree of stability needed and in the level of injury for which they are used. The halo device (Fig. 15-7, A and B) is used for complete and incomplete cervical lesions that require complete immobilization. It consists of a skeletal/skull immobilization halo with four pins screwed into the skull. This halo is then attached by four metal rods to a plaster or plastic body jacket. Halo rings provide initial traction reduction of the spinal injury and long-term immobilization. They may be used immediately after injury and are indicated for surgical and nonsurgical candidates. Before these devices were introduced, skeletal tongs were inserted into the client's skull and the client was confined to bed under traction for 8 to 12 weeks until cervical realignment and stability were achieved. Initial rehabilitation attempts were then aimed at undoing the negative effects of the prolonged bed rest. Recent studies have documented the use of the halo device as a primary factor in decreasing length of overall hospital stays by allowing this early start of rehabilitation.[217,232] Other advantages of the halo device are that they allow delayed decisions on whether surgery will be needed for stabilization and, if indicated, allow easy anterior or posterior access during surgery. Complications include (1) infections at pin sites, (2) loosening of pins, (3) pressure sore development from the plastic or plaster vest, and (4) redislocation of the vertebrae while the client is in the vest. To minimize these complications there must be written protocols and procedures outlining responsibilities for managing the halo device and vest along with appropriate limitations for each client regarding the positions and activities considered safe.[72] All team members interacting with a client who is in a halo device must be aware of that client's limitations. Skin integrity needs to be monitored by all members of the team. Adjustments and trimming of the vest by the orthotist are sometimes indicated, especially when the client initially assumes the sitting position. Assuming different positions and levels of activity during therapy sessions are possible but should be individualized to each client. Two other types of spinal orthoses are the SOMI jacket (Fig. 15-8) and the trunk body cast or jacket (Fig. 15-9). The SOMI (sterno-occipital-mandibular-immobilizer) provides less stringent three-point immobilization of the cervical spine than the halo device, and it may or may not be attached to a body jacket. Because the SOMI allows more movement and greater ability for adjustment, clients wearing the device need to be closely monitored for correct fit and degree of immobility of the cervical spine during activity in all positions. Clients wearing both the SOMI and the halo-type cervical immobilizers need to be monitored and instructed in the potential decrease in dynamic balance and equilibrium that has been clinically observed when cervical motion is restricted.[27]

The plaster body cast or jacket is used to immobilize

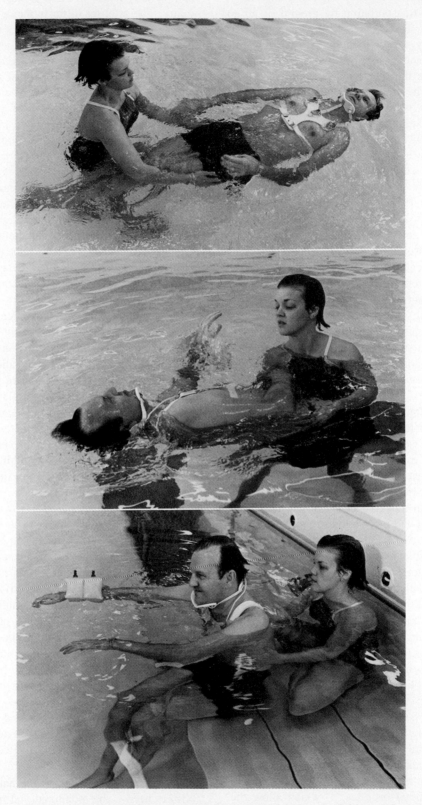

Fig. 15-8. SOMI cervical immobilizer. Client with a cervical lesion can initiate early trunk and chest mobility exercises, respiratory and kinesthetic awareness training, and upper-extremity strengthening (as well as relearning swimming skills) using the physical properties of water.

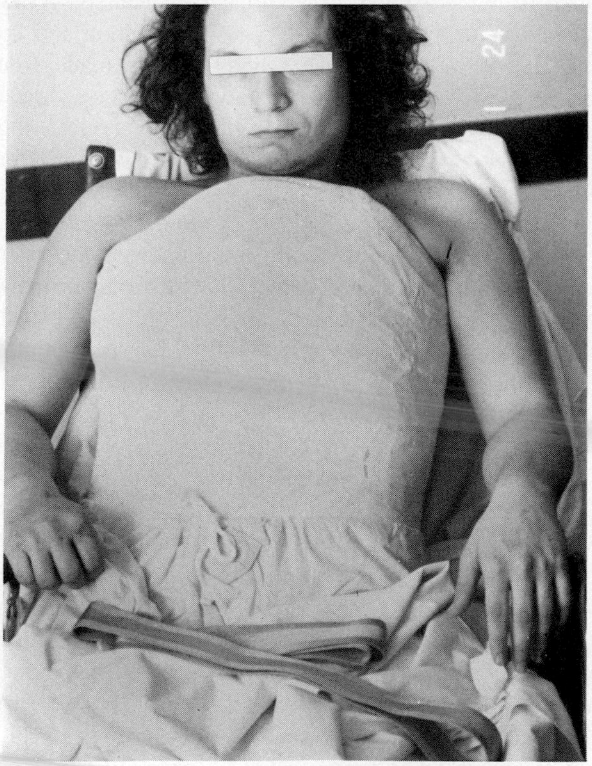

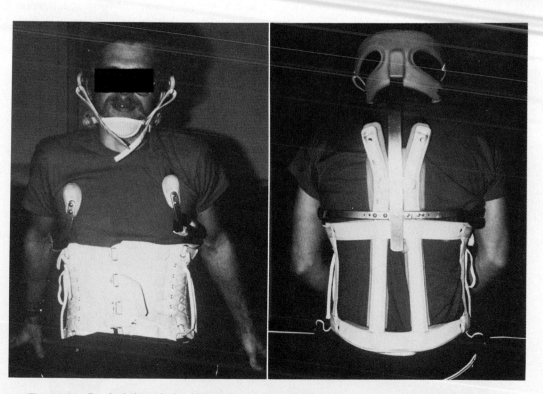

Fig. 15-9. Plaster of paris body jacket. This type of external immobilization is used when rigid stabilization of the thoracolumbar junction is required. If protective sensation is absent, care must be taken to pad the iliac crest well. This orthosis can be interchanged with a laminated plastic thoracolumbar jacket, which is removable. (From Meyer PR: Thoracic and lumbar spine stabilization in spinal cord injury. In Calenoff L, editor: Radiology of spinal cord injury, St Louis, 1981, The CV Mosby Co.)

Fig. 15-10. Cervical-thoracic-lumbosacral orthosis (CTLSO). This client had multiple-level spinal injuries involving cervical, thoracic, and lumbar vertebrae. He was fitted with a lumbosacral orthosis with an anterior corset panel, posterior thoracic extensions, subclavicular extensions, and a posterior cervical immobilizer extension with an adjustable mandibular strap were added.

fractures of the thoracic and lumbar spine, and it is usually applied from the sternum to the greater trochanters. It may be bivalved to allow removal for skin inspection and hygiene. In addition, removable body jackets made from plastics, plastizote, and other materials and corset braces (Fig. 15-10) are available to immobilize the cervical, thoracic, or thoracolumbar spine. Other types of spinal orthoses are popular in various parts of the country. They are all based on concepts and guidelines similar to those presented here. As cervical stability is achieved, the client may wear a plastic or soft foam collar before returning to restriction-free movement and activities.

Some centers choose to immobilize cervical injuries through the use of Crutchfield or Gardner-Wells tongs, which are inserted in the bony skull and to which traction is applied to reduce the fracture and/or dislocation. The client is then placed on a special bed, such as the Rotobed (Fig. 15-11), or on a Stryker frame (Fig. 15-12). These devices assist the nursing staff in maintaining the integrity of the desensitized skin to avoid pressure sores; they also assist in maintaining alignment of the spine. Some centers choose to use regular beds with water, gel, or foam pressure-relief mattresses and logroll the client every 2 hours. One type of turning frame used in the 1960s and early 1970s was the circular electric frame (Fig. 15-13), which allowed clients to be turned from the prone to the supine position through a full circle on their short axis versus the long axis turn (as in a "logroll") found with a Stryker frame. This circular frame is no longer advocated because of the loading of weight on the fracture site caused by being moved through the vertical position during turning[203] and because of the exacerbation of systemic effects of pos-

tural hypotension that can also result from this transient vertical positioning.[225] The decision to use spinal orthoses, traction, pressure-relief beds, or turning frames is dependent on the level and type of spinal injury and on the philosophy of the managing physician and team.

In conjunction with appropriate immobilization of the spine, other body systems need attention. The urinary system may require insertion of an indwelling catheter. Careful attention is given to maintaining respiratory and cardiovascular homeostasis. Gastrointestinal and bowel functions are maintained. Initial attempts to deal with the psychological disruption of the client and family are also made early in treatment. Contact with members of the rehabilitation team should also be made as early as possible. Social workers and therapists from the rehabilitation setting can begin preliminary planning for the client and can evaluate the existing factors that will effect long-term discharge planning. Before discussing the role of the physical therapist during this acute stage, some pertinent aspects of surgical intervention in the period after traumatic injury are examined.

There are two major indications for surgery following spinal cord injury. The first indication is decompression of the spinal column to preserve neural function; the other is correction of bony abnormalities following trauma in order to stabilize the vertebral column and prevent further damage to the cord. Surgical bony stabilization has a secondary benefit in that, in conjunction with the use of external spinal orthoses, it allows early mobilization of the client and thereby shortens the initial rehabilitation period.

Controversy still exists among physicians as to whether or not surgery is indicated in the acute phase. Those who

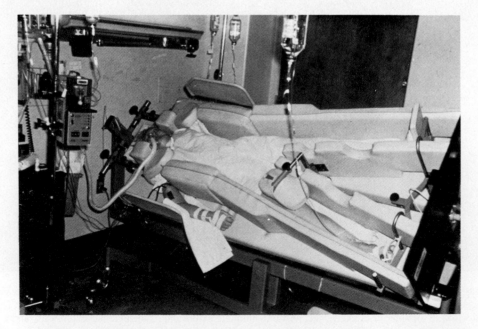

Fig. 15-11. A Roto-Bed slowly rotates the client on a longitudinal axis from side to side to provide pressure relief sufficient to prevent the onset of pressure sores.

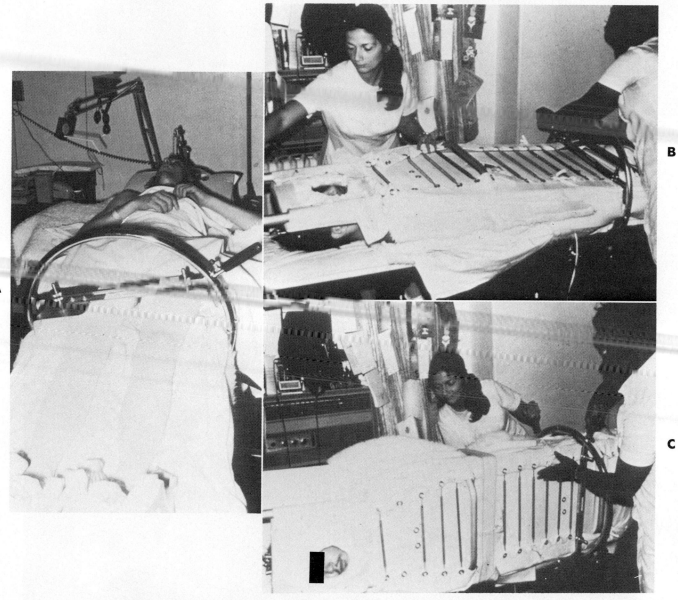

Fig. 15-12. Stryker frame. **A,** The client is lying supine on sheet-covered sheepskin and has on full-length elastic stockings. The client is turned on his longitudinal axis to the prone position, according to an established schedule. Turning is accomplished by securing a similar frame over the client. **B,** and then rotating him from the supine position to the prone position. **C.** Skeletal cervical traction can be constantly maintained with this method of pressure relief.

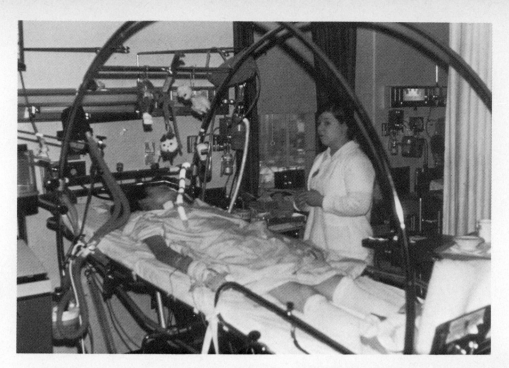

Fig. 15-13. Circular electric frame. Before turning the client a frame is secured over him in a manner similar to that used with the Stryker frame.

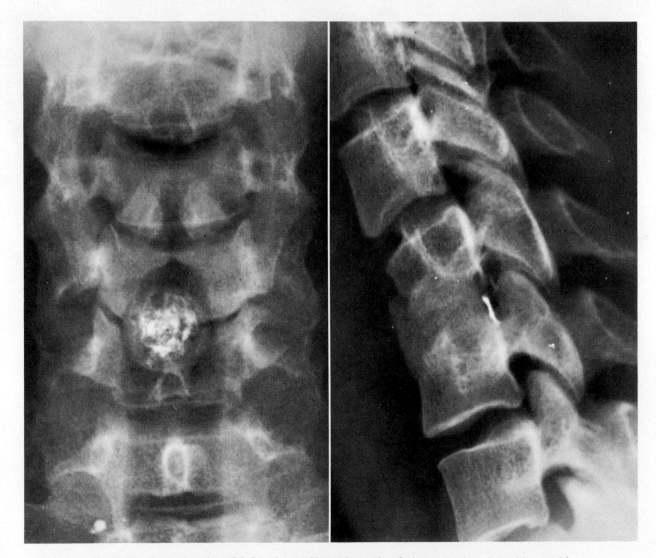

Fig. 15-14. Bone dowel at C5-C6 after a Cloward anterior fusion procedure in a 46-year-old woman injured in an automobile accident. Note opaque tantalum power marking Kiel bone (Kiel surgibone is a registered trade name for a specially cleaned cancellous bovine bone). (Cerullo LJ: Cervical spine stabilization in spinal cord injury. In Calenoff L, editor: Radiology of spinal cord injury, St Louis, 1981, The CV Mosby Co.)

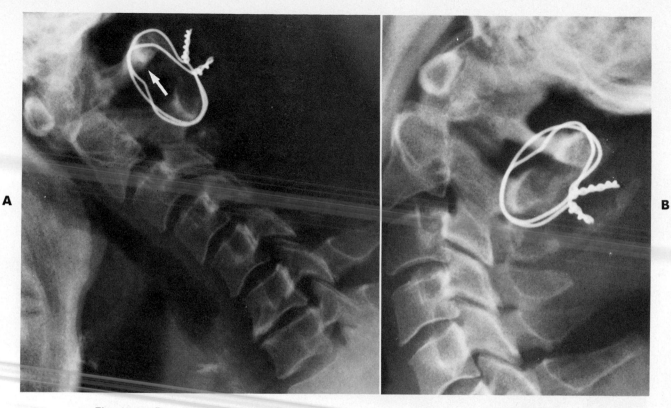

Fig. 15-15. Posterior fusion with wiring of spinous processes. Flexion-extension lateral radiograms taken after posterior fusion of C1-C2 in a 46-year-old man with an old odontoid fracture showing persistent instability. **A,** Flexion view shows good position of odontoid process but separation of spinous process *(arrow)* despite wiring. **B,** Extension view shows approximation of spinous processes and posterior displacement of odontoid process. (From Cerullo LJ: Cervical spine stabilization in spinal cord injury. In Calenoff L, editor: Radiology of spinal cord injury, St Louis, 1981, The CV Mosby Co.)

do not advocate surgery believe in a conservative program of traction and manipulation followed by a period of immobilization and bed rest to allow fracture healing. It is beyond the scope of this discussion to explore these two philosophies except to state that the majority of orthopaedic surgeons and neurosurgeons in the United States advocate surgical intervention when indicated. The type of procedure depends on many factors, including the level of lesion, the type of injury (including the amount of associated bony and ligamentous damage), and the remaining integrity of spinal cord and local nerve root tissue. Some general statements can be made regarding types of procedures usually indicated for different levels of injury.

Injuries of the cervical spine usually require anterior or posterior decompression and interbody spinal fusion either with bone grafts and/or through the wiring together of the spinous processes (Figs. 15-14 and 15-15).[44] Use of the anterior or posterior route during surgery depends on the level and type of injury: the posterior route is used more commonly with injuries to the upper cervical levels, and the anterior fusion is used more commonly at other cervical levels. The posterior approach involves more extensive disection of soft tissue, which will result in a greater chance for significant long-term limitation of motion.

Bony grafts are usually taken from cortical iliac bone or from the tibia. Healing at both of these graft sites may delay initial attempts at mobilizing the client.

The thoracic spine has greater stability as a result of the presence of the rib cage and the biomechanics of the vertebral bodies. Therefore the thoracic spine and the lumbar spine may be amenable to closed manipulation and reduction of fracture.[153] Again, the degree and the type of fracture are major factors in deciding on a closed versus surgical reduction in thoracic and lumbar spine injuries.[155] Anterior, posterior, or anterior-posterior approaches may be used. Because of the difficulty in reducing fracture dislocations and maintaining vertebral alignment in the thoracolumbar area, internal fixation devices may have to be used in addition to bone graft fusions. The four most commonly used devices are Harrington distraction rods (Fig. 15-16), Harrington compression rods (Fig. 15-17), and Weiss compression springs (Fig. 15-18),[155] and the Luque rod instrumentation.[156] The Harrington rods limit long-term spinal motion; they may fracture or they may result in a scoliotic deformity as a result of lateral angulation forces secondary to their being placed on one side of the posterior vertebral elements. Weiss compression springs also exert these same unilateral forces and may also precipitate scoli-

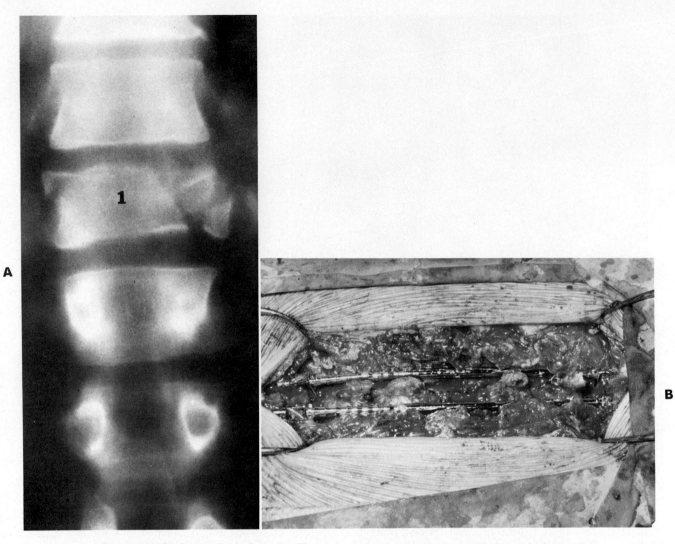

Fig. 15-16. Harrington distraction rods. These are used to support the vertebral column in fracture of L1 vertebral body and left pedicle. **A,** Open reduction and insertion of Harrington rods. **B,** Note hooks at proximal and distal ends attached to laminae. Spinous processes lie between the Harrington rods. **C** and **D,** Postoperative radiograms show satisfactory stabilization of spine. (From Meyer PR: Thoracic and lumbar spine stabilization in spinal cord injury. In Calenoff L, editor: Radiology of spinal cord injury, St Louis, 1981, The CV Mosby Co.)

osis. The primary advantage to the Weiss compression springs is that they are dynamic and that they allow more rapid mobilization of the client.[248]

Regardless of the type of surgical or conservative approach used to stabilize a spinal injury, the trend is for the client to use one of the types of spinal orthoses or body casts/jackets mentioned earlier to immobilize the client while bony and ligamentous healing takes place. Surgical management of spinal injuries is a very individualized process, and it is incumbent on the therapist to be totally familiar with the philosophies and strategies of surgical and postoperative care followed by each surgeon referring clients for rehabilitative management.

The physical therapist who functions as a member of the acute care team has a primary goal of facilitating a rapid and efficient transition into the rehabilitation pro-

cess.[116] This would include preventing contracture deformities, maximizing available muscular and respiratory function, and achieving a gradual acclimation to the vertical position. The client with an incomplete lesion who has significant returning muscle function and who is medically and surgically stable can enter into a more active rehabilitation process during this early stage.

Prevention of contracture deformities. Prevention of contracture deformities in this acute phase is achieved through a coordinated program of positioning, possible splinting, and range of motion exercises. These activities should begin as early as possible. Attaining a successful outcome depends heavily on the therapist's ability to plan activities that avoid compromising surgical stability and healing of associated bony and soft tissue secondary injuries. Positioning, turning schedules, and maintaining pos-

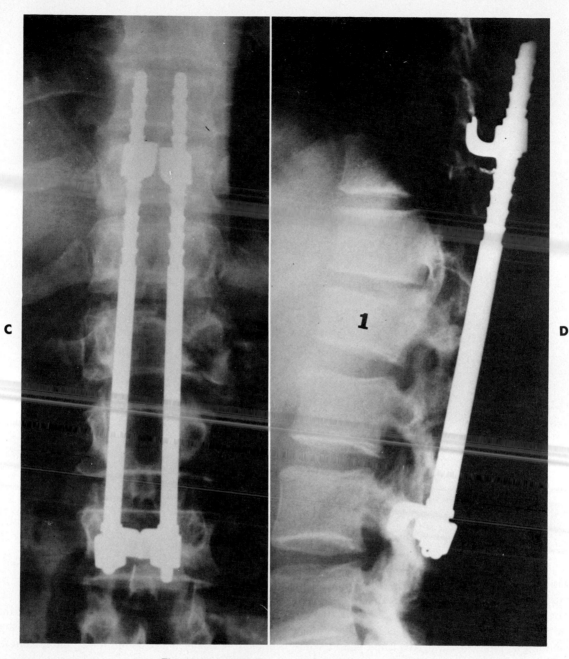

Fig. 15-16, cont'd. For legend see opposite page.

tural alignment are primarily ongoing nursing management functions to which the therapist contributes. Significant problem areas during this early stage are hip flexion, knee flexion, ankle plantar flexion tightness, and shoulder pain with tightness toward adduction and internal rotation. Prone positioning, if possible, can assist in preventing hip and knee flexor deformity, and splinting the ankle in neutral with pressure relief boots and daily range of motion exercises can prevent plantar flexion tightness. Caution should be used in performing range of motion to the lower extremities during this stage because of the significant incidence of subclinical thrombophlebitis in the acute client (this was mentioned earlier in this chapter). Also, when in-

creased neuromuscular tone is present and when passive stretching is indicated, care must be taken to avoid an autonomic hyperreflexive response, which has been noted to occur with passive stretch.[149] This can be avoided by positioning the lower extremity in a reflex inhibiting posture while performing range of motion activities.

Clients with cord lesions that involve muscles of the shoulder girdle complex are known to develop shoulder pain and stiffness during the acute stage. This often occurs in spite of daily range of movement exercises and can result in contractures that will severely limit the client's long-term functional activities. This painful syndrome can often be avoided by taking the shoulder to full abduction

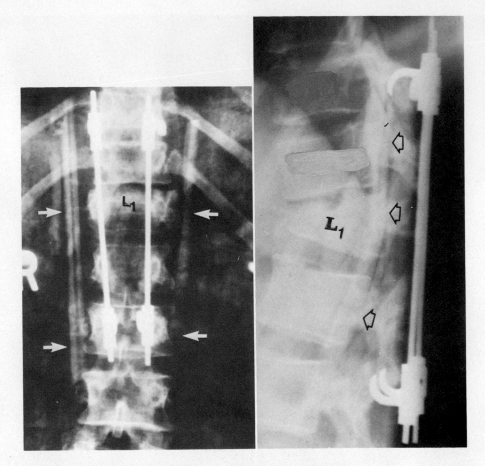

Fig. 15-17. Harrington compression rods. Comminuted fracture of L1 6 months after operative laminectomy, requiring insertion of Harrington compression rods. Because of posterior instability, kyphosis has occurred. Note posterolateral fibular bone grafts *(arrows).* (From Meyer PR: Thoracic and lumbar spine stabilization in spinal cord injury. In Calenoff L, editor: Radiology of spinal cord injury, St Louis, 1981, The CV Mosby Co.)

and external rotation in spite of the pain. When this is performed with the client in the supine position, care should be taken to assure free scapular movement, which can be hindered by the client's weight inhibiting scapular mobility. The following positioning techniques have been helpful in avoiding this problem during the acute phase of immobilization: (1) positioning both shoulders in 90 degrees of abduction and external rotation when the client is in the supine position and (2) propping the upper arm on pillows in abduction and 45 degrees of extension when the client is in the sidelying position while avoiding weight on the lower shoulder by placing an axillary pillow under the upper chest.[219]

Full motion in the other extremity joints during the early stage can be maintained with daily range of motion exercises. With high-cervical lesions, the wrist and hands may benefit from being supported in resting pan splints. Recording joint range of motion is helpful during this stage and establishes a baseline for the client's premorbid postural motion. This may become important in treatment planning during the rehabilitation stage. For example, approximately 110 degrees of passive straight-leg raising is considered minimal in order for paraplegic persons and low-level quadriplegic persons to perform activities of daily living in the long-sitting position. Many normal males have postural hamstring tightness that is going to be more resistant to stretching during the rehabilitation phase than if it were tightness acquired during the acute phase.

Maximizing available muscular and respiratory function. Available muscular and respiratory function is maximized through a selective program of muscle strengthening and, if indicated, chest physical therapy. An accurate baseline manual muscle test needs to be established within the limitations imposed by surgery, spinal stability precautions, spinal orthoses, possible casts or splints from secondary injuries, and the client's tolerance level, for example, to the prone position. When applying resistance to functioning muscles, extreme care must be taken to monitor the effect on spinal instability. It takes experience to accurately assess muscle strength during the acute and early rehabilitation phases. Therefore it is important to note any deviations from standard procedures that were used during a test in order to assure a reasonable degree of reliable and valid information on which to plan long-term treatment. During the acute phase, when a client's neurological status may be changing, it is common practice to perform gross motor and sensory tests hourly. These tests are performed by the nursing staff and physicians, and they assist in determining a definitive level of cord function.

Active and resistive exercises may be performed manually or with weights during this early stage. Maintaining spinal alignment is critical; this is usually achieved with closely monitored bilateral symmetrical activities that pre-

clude chances of spinal rotation. A recent study found that the use of belts to fixate the unstable thoracic and lumbar spinal fracture allowed a more active bilateral upper extremity strengthening program. This was determined through the measurement of pressure within the disk with and without fixation. It was also found that forward flexion shoulder exercises produced a greater increase in pressure within the disk than did bilateral shoulder abduction exercises both in the supine position and during elevation on a tilt table.[105] Finally, isometric exercises may be used when joint motion is not advisable.

All quadriplegic persons and most high-level paraplegic

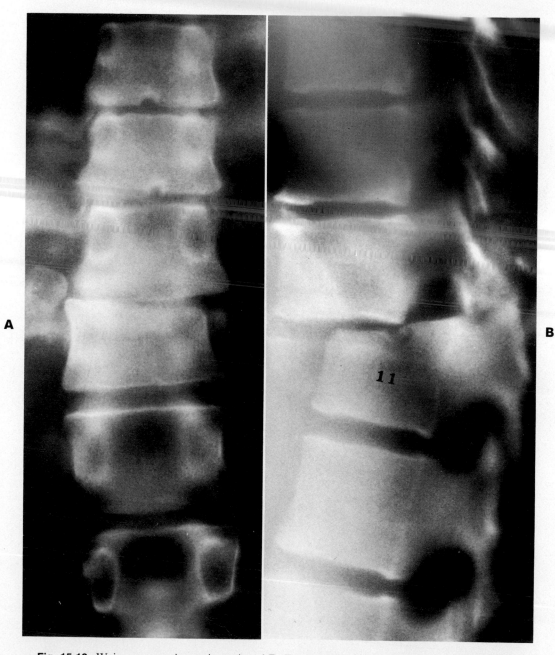

Fig. 15-18. Weiss compression springs. **A** and **B,** Fracture-dislocation of vertebral bodies at T10-T11 with fracture of posterior elements and dislocation of facets. *Continued.*

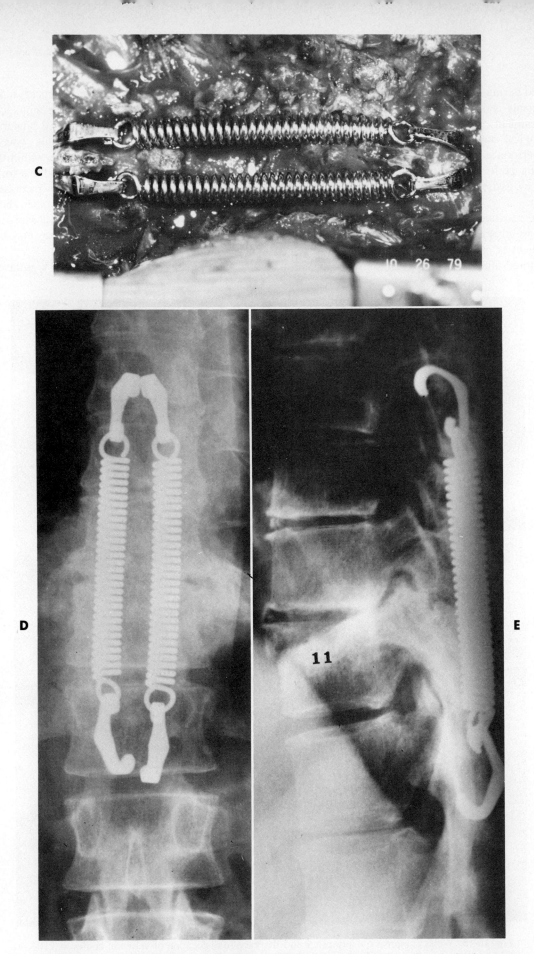

Fig. 15-18, cont'd. C, Open reduction; Weiss springs internal fixation is used to maintain compression across previously dislocated facets. **D** and **E,** Postoperative radiograms reveal reduction of spine and internal fixation. (From Meyer PR: Thoracic and lumbar spine stabilization in spinal cord injury. In Calenoff L, editor: Radiology of spinal cord injury, St Louis, 1981, The CV Mosby Co.)

persons will require some form of rehabilitation of the respiratory system,[53] this should start as early as possible. Early assessments include chest radiograms, blood gas measurements, vital capacity, and chest expansion measurements. Treatment is focused on stabilizing the respiratory system through the improvement of bronchial hygiene with intermittent positive pressure breathing (IPPB), chest percussion, assisted coughing,[147] and postural drainage. Instruction in segmental and diaphragmatic breathing will also assist the client to improve the efficiency of breathing. Training may begin on improving the effectiveness of coughing, which focuses on such factors as timing the cough with accessory movements that can increase the force of the cough and improve clearing of bronchial secretions. Strengthening of remaining primary and accessory respiratory muscles can begin to focus on obtaining long-term improved efficiency and coordination of breathing. Clients with very high-level lesions (C1 to 4) may be initially instructed in glossopharyngeal breathing to aid in pulmonary ventilation and cough production. When the client begins to assume the upright position, an elastic abdominal binder will be needed to assist the diaphram and the accessory muscles of respiration with breathing.

For the high-level client who is not successful at GPB respiration, either a phrenic nerve stimulator (as mentioned earlier) may be implanted or the client may be trained in using a pneumobelt.[163] It is a corset-like device that is used sitting or reclining, that allows a battery-operated pump attached to the wheelchair to inflate a bladder over the abdomen within the corset. The pneumobelt improves tidal volume by assisting expiration upon inflation and allowing inspiration upon deflation and subsequent passive falling of the abdominal contents and diaphragm. It is cosmetically more appealing because tubing does not have to be connected to a tracheostomy tube (as with other mechanical respirators) and the corset can be worn under clothing. A disadvantage is that it is effective in sitting but not supine, therefore forcing the client to use another means of mechanical respiration, such as the rocker bed,[163] at night. Finally, it is important to continue attempts at training in glossopharyngeal breathing[267] as a back-up in the event that a mechanical respirator malfunctions.

With more individuals surviving high-level cord lesions, the needs of these clients must be increasingly examined in relation to new technology, cost of rehabilitation, quality of life issues, and problems of discharge planning toward a safe and functional environment.

Achieving a gradual acclimation to the vertical position. Gradual acclimation to the vertical position is started when serial radiograms have shown sufficient spinal stability with or without a spinal orthosis. As mentioned earlier, injuries above the T6 to T12 sympathetic outflow will result in a generalized cardiovascular insufficiency when assuming the upright position. This is manifested by profound hypotension, vertigo, diaphoresis, and possible vi-

sual disturbances. In addition, most clients, whatever the level of spinal injury, will incur a more transient period of hypotension when assuming the vertical position after being recumbent for a prolonged time. Again, this postural response, as mentioned earlier, is not to be confused with the more sudden and critical response of autonomic dysreflexia. Gradually assuming the vertical position can be accomplished in three ways. If the client is in a regular hospital bed, the elevating head control may be used. A reclining wheelchair with elevating leg rests or a tilt table can also be used to elevate the client to the vertical position in small increments. This author prefers to use the reclining wheelchair because it allows the client the added benefit of experiencing his or her initial attempts at achieving mobility within his or her environment. In addition, as mentioned earlier, some clients occasionally experience a claustrophobic reaction when strapped to a tilt table, and other clients have expressed a "feeling of falling forward" when elevation goes beyond 60 degrees toward vertical. Blood pressure should be monitored during these activities because a sudden drop may precede the onset of symptoms. An abdominal binder and elastic stockings should be used to assist with venous return and help retard postural venous pooling.

During this acute stage, initial attempts to establish a bowel and bladder program are often begun, and the physical therapist, depending on the clinical setting, may be involved in these activities. Initial education of the client regarding skin care may be started. Finally, the initial development of long-range functional goals may be started depending on the client's psychological readiness. Clients who do not have problems with spinal stability, such as those incurring cord damages as a result of a gunshot or stab wound and those who have incomplete or lower-level lesions may achieve many more functional goals while in the acute setting.

Rehabilitation phase of management

Establishment of realistic goals. Rehabilitating any physically disabled person to the maximal level of independence is a highly individualized process. This process is based on full evaluation of all parameters and capabilities unique to that person and on the establishment of feasible and individualized short- and long-term goals that the client and his or her support systems (professionals, family, and funding sources) can work toward.

The physical therapy management of the person with a spinal cord injury has traditionally based the establishment of goals on absolute parameters related to the level of cord injury. Most texts that focus on the rehabilitation of spinal cord injury have contained charts that list functional goals for each level of complete cord injury. These charts are usually accompanied by statements that acknowledge that they are only general guidelines that are affected by the many variables within and external to the client. These guidelines are also replete with statements such as "possibly able to ambulate for short distances with knee-anklefoot orthoses," "may be able to transfer independently," and "wheelchair independence possible except in the presence of deformities, weakness, obesity, and other medical problems." In addition, close comparison of these charts shows that there exists significant variation between charts in projected functional expectations for each level of cord injury.

There are several reasons why these functional expectation charts are useless as general guidelines and why they may not be reasonable for use by students or therapists who are attempting to solidify their philosophies and principles of effective client management. The most obvious reason is that they are charts based on complete lesions, and, as mentioned earlier, approximately one half of spinal cord injuries are incomplete cord lesions.[159,265] In addition, there sometimes exists anatomical variation regarding what muscles are innervated by what nerve roots. It has been this author's experience that these charts have often "locked" students and practicing therapists into a set way of thinking in regard to the goals for a level of lesion. For example, for years it was believed that only clients with function at the C7 level and below had the ability to transfer from one surface to another independently. Today it is commonly acknowledged that many clients with higher lesions can independently transfer and accomplish many activities of daily living. Another widely disseminated chart stated that few clients with lesions above T12 will achieve any form of ambulation when, in fact, many extremely motivated younger clients with complete lesions as high as T6 can achieve some form of limited ambulation, be it as limited as physiological standing with a few steps in the parallel bars.[69]

Finally, with increased technical developments, such as lighter types of orthoses for ambulation, and with research into more efficient means of achieving mobility activities, it is highly probable that in the future persons with spinal cord injuries will be achieving levels of function that are well beyond what is considered at the "front edge" of client management today. Several recent outcome studies of large samples of clients who have undergone rehabilitation at a major United States regional spinal cord injury center[255,256,257] examined functional status at discharge in relation to spinal level of injury. Statistically significant increases were found in the number of patients able to perform higher levels of independent functional tasks compared to levels found in similar past studies. These findings further demonstrate the need to establish highly individualized client goals toward rehabilitation outcomes that are not guided or restricted by universal and sometimes outdated outcome charts.

To develop an inclusive understanding of physical therapy practice as it relates to this clinical problem (which is well beyond the scope of this chapter), the author recommends a text that clinically describes the neurological levels of spinal lesions[111] and a reference guidebook that presents in-depth processes for analyzing all the components and considerations necessary for the achievement of functional outcomes in spinal cord injury.[178] References such as these used in conjunction with a well-referenced text, such as this volume, should provide the inexperienced therapist sufficient resources to develop a process for achieving a problem-solving approach to physical therapy care for the client with spinal cord injury.

The remainder of this chapter presents an overview of physical therapy evaluation procedures appropriate during the rehabilitation phase. General considerations and concepts of physical therapy management related to the systemic problems and functional goals needed for success in rehabilitation are also discussed. Finally, a brief discussion presents factors that contribute to the health of this client population following discharge.

Evaluation factors and procedures

Subjective evaluations. It is often stated in discussions among experienced physical therapy clinicians that the most important factor in describing what constitutes a good clinician is the ability to observe—both visually and tactilely. Physical therapy is a field that has few objective evaluation tools when compared to other areas of medicine. Therefore it seems logical that successful clinicians are those who can observe and analyze a client performing a skill that is leading toward attainment of a short- or long-term functional goal and then make a decision as to whether that performance or response is adequate. This subjective aspect of ongoing evaluation is a key element in the "art of physical therapy."

Another key element to adequate treatment is sufficient insight into all aspects of a client's status, including the premorbid history, the course of treatment, and the present clinical state. This includes insight into the client's status relative to the myriad of clinical problems of spinal cord injury already mentioned in this chapter as well as ongoing reading of the client's medical records and communication with the client, family, and other members of the treatment team. Efficient and effective treatment and discharge planning depends on evaluation that is ongoing and comprehensive.

Objective evaluations. This chapter assumes that the reader is familiar with basic evaluation tools, such as muscle testing, range of motion analysis, reflex and sensory testing, and evaluations of activities of daily living. A brief discussion is therefore offered of pertinent aspects of the evaluation tools relative to this clinical problem.

Motor function. A standard, graded, manual muscle test that is related to spinal segments is most useful in developing a baseline for selective muscle strengthening and in charting any change in the client's neuromuscular status. Depending on the time available and on the skill of the tester, it is sometimes adequate and easier to test only one accessible muscle that clearly represents each spinal segment. There are a number of factors that affect the validity and reliability of manual muscle testing of the person with a spinal cord injury, and these must be considered. Interrater reliability is a problem with all manual muscle testing, and every effort should be made to confine serial testing to the primary therapist. Pain and limitation of joint motion limit accuracy and client compliance. Precautions regarding spinal stability and the continued wearing of spinal orthoses will limit access to a muscle and comprimise stabilizing body segments and positioning of the client. The presence of increased neuromuscular tone virtually invalidates the standard muscle test. Mass movement patterns prohibit isolated joint function. The deep and cutaneous sensory loss that is often present with increased tone can interfere with the client's ability to demonstrate accurate motor strength, and, as mentioned earlier, tone fluctuates in relation to numerous changes within and outside of the client. When increased tone is present, it is sufficient to make a general statement as to the degree of tone present at a joint segment, to note how the increased tone affects function, and to note significant changes in tone since a previous examination.

Another major problem with performing muscle tests on the person with a spinal cord injury, especially those clients with high-level lesions, is difficulty in positioning and stabilizing body segments. This is combined with the client's ability to substitute functioning muscles to mimic the movement of the muscle being tested. This can be a source of frustration to students and less experienced therapists. Validity can be increased by making compromises in positioning the body segment and noting them on the record and by paying close attention to palpating the muscle's contraction and comparing it with the tested muscle's origin, insertion, and the direction in which its fibers would pull.

When the client is recovering from the early stages of spinal shock, very weak muscles that cannot be observed contracting visually or through palpation can often be identified by using electomyogram (EMG) biofeedback with surface electrodes.[220] EMG biofeedback is also useful in determining the level of a thoracic lesion through the monitoring of intercostal muscles.

Evaluation of motor function in the person with a spinal cord injury might also encompass significant observations regarding the person's coordination and balance as they relate to functional status. Coordination relates to the achievement of quality of movement and can be described in terms of control ability, reaction time, accuracy, and speed of movement. Balance has two components—the ability to maintain static balance and the ability to achieve dynamic balance.

Sensory function. Although sensory testing is routinely done by physicians to diagnose the level of lesion or cord compression and to ascertain through serial testing return

of cord function, physical therapists will need access to this evaluative information because decreased cutaneous and proprioceptive sensation can interfere with motor learning and achieving kinesthetic awareness. Decreased cutaneous sensation also has an impact on skin care and on the precautions needed in performing activities of daily living.

Sensory testing in a physical therapy setting consists of evaluating light touch, pain, and proprioception according to dermatomal levels. Because these sensations are carried over different spinal tracts, incomplete lesions will present clinical pictures that vary between surface and deep sensations. Pain is representative of the spinothalamic system and it relates functionally to skin pressure relief as well as to trauma and thermal damage, possibly incurred during daily activities. Proprioception is representative of the posterior column system, and it is measured according to two variables—passive and dynamic position sense. Impaired sensation should be listed as increased (hyper) or decreased (hypo) from normal. For example, decreased sensation to pain should be stated as hypoalgesia at a given dermatomal level, and exaggerated light touch should be listed as hyperesthesia at a given dermatomal level.

Range of motion. A complete evaluation of joint motion in a client with spinal cord injury should include, if indicated and if possible, assessment of chest mobility and notation of any spinal postural deficits in addition to range of motion of the extremity joints (Fig. 15-19). Care should be taken to state whether the measurement was obtained actively or passively and to list the possible cause of any detected limitation. Depending on the needs of the clinical situation, range of motion can be classified in two ways. Movement can be classified in degrees of joint motion, or it can be classified more broadly by stating whether the joint motion is "normal" (N), "within functional limitations" (WFL), or "interferes with function" (IF).

Respiratory function. An evaluation of respiratory status is necessary for the high-level paraplegic client and for the quadriplegic client. For all levels of spinal cord injury, a baseline measurement of cardiorespiratory status according to one or more variables is very helpful in planning treatment activities that improve endurance.

A respiratory evaluation should include an assessment of which primary muscles of respiration are functioning. This should be compared to the client's breathing pattern in various positions. Observation of the client's breathing pattern will include an evaluation of how much and how efficiently the client is using the accessory muscles of respiration and the rate of respiration. An effective and efficient breathing pattern is dependent on the client's ability to coordinate breathing with the exertion of functional activities, coughing, and phonation. Objective measurements useful in treatment planning include the measurement of chest expansion, vital capacity (VC), tidal volume (TV), and forced expiratory volume (FEV). The reader is re-

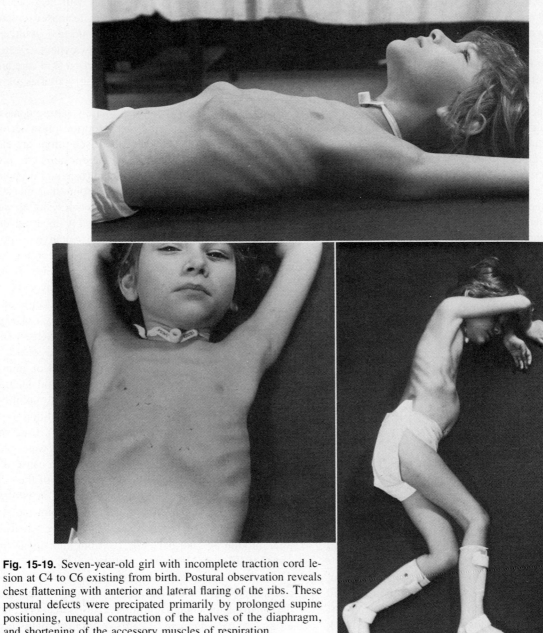

Fig. 15-19. Seven-year-old girl with incomplete traction cord lesion at C4 to C6 existing from birth. Postural observation reveals chest flattening with anterior and lateral flaring of the ribs. These postural defects were precipitated primarily by prolonged supine positioning, unequal contraction of the halves of the diaphragm, and shortening of the accessory muscles of respiration.

ferred to Cardiopulmonary Physical Therapy, volume one of this series, for procedures and values for normal persons. To my knowledge, there exists no normal values for any of these tests based on various levels of cord injury in relation to the usual variables of age, weight, and height. Adequate bronchial hygiene is dependent on an efficient and effective cough. A cough can be described as productive, impaired, or nonproductive. With the high-level and ventilator-dependent client, these tests may be compared with blood gas analysis to determine when the client can

be weaned off a ventilator or can begin training in glossopharyngeal breathing.

Vasomotor function. Subjective comments regarding a client's tolerance to the vertical position should be part of an evaluation during the acute phase of treatment. This tolerance can be described by comparing the client's pallor, blood pressure, and pulse to various degrees of vertical alignment and to the length of time that the position can be maintained. Cutaneous circulation and trophic skin change should be noted in any spinal cord evaluation.

Other evaluations. All of the tests mentioned previously can be incorporated into one printed form. Other information that might be included in this form would be comments on the client's problem-solving abilities and apparent cognitive abilities, or significant statements regarding the client's affect and apparent level of motivation, and any pertinent socioeconomic factors needed for discharge planning. Discharge planning is heavily based on home evaluations. Clients in a rehabilitation setting need to go home on "weekend passes" to delineate potential problems regarding architectural barriers and the need for adaptive equipment. The therapist can also visit the home to perform a more formal evaluation, which may be in the form of a written checklist.

Finally, a comprehensive measurement of the client's overall activities of daily living or functional status is needed. This comprehensive measurement should (1) be valid, reliable, and objective, (2) be useful to all professionals, and (3) not be limited to a specific diagnosis. Tools such as these can quantify a client's degree of disability, can improve communication between professionals, facilities, and third-party payers, and can serve as a basis for the validation and effectiveness of various client treatment regimes. Examples of this type of comprehensive measurement tool include the Barthel Index,[144] the Pulses Profile,[168] the Patient Evaluation Conference System (PECS),[104] and the Klein-Bell ADL Scale.[132]

Evaluation in the physical therapy setting also depends on an ongoing process of problem-solving feedback between the client and therapist. This has typically been verbal feedback that is complemented by demonstration by the therapist. The use of videotapes has proved to be a useful evaluative and educational feedback tool that assists the client in learning mobility and functional skills. It can be used in two ways. The client can view his or her own performance of a skill with the therapist and problem-solve improvement. Departments can also maintain a collection of videotapes of past clients who correctly performed various activities. These tapes can then be used by future clients.

Concepts of functional independence. This section presents significant concepts of client management in a physical therapy setting that lead toward the achievement of independence in each of the functional problem areas inherent in the rehabilitation of a client with a spinal cord injury. Concepts will not focus on specific facilitation and inhibition treatment techniques because these have been presented and analyzed in Chapter 6, but this section further analyzes the clinical problem and presents rationales for treatment.

The physical therapist's role in treating a client with a spinal cord injury involves developing an individualized treatment program that is problem-oriented, that is based on short- and long-term goals, and that is reasonable and realistic. It includes helping the client to solve problem situations that are timely and relevant to that client's future needs. It involves educating the client to the reasoning behind performing certain activities and to the relationship of these activities to functional independence. Finally, it involves educating the client, family, and funding sources as to what resources are needed and available regarding equipment, environmental adaptions, and possible community support systems.

The client's primary role is to be committed to the established goals. This is a particular problem with the person with a traumatic spinal cord injury who may not actively engage in the rehabilitation process until the second admission to a rehabilitation facility. Time is often needed to both accept the permanence of the functional losses and to reenter society to identify problems and goals that could not be identified or accepted earlier.

Systemic problems

Prevention of deformity. The primary goal regarding joint motion is to obtain pain-free functional range and mobility in all affected joints, including the rib cage and spinal column. The causes of contractual limitations of motion and their treatment were discussed earlier. Prevention is based on the ability to teach the client and/or caregivers to monitor involved joints daily for limitation of motion. During the acute and early rehabilitation stages, the maintenance of joint range is the responsibility of the therapy and nursing staffs. This responsibility is transferred to the client as soon as possible. Problem joints, such as those with increased tone, are identified, and the client is taught either to self-range that joint daily and/or to use positioning (such as sleeping or lying prone for a period of time to prevent hip flexion contractures) to prevent limitations. Some clients with lesions as high as the C6 level can develop ability to perform or assist in self-range of motion. Deterrents to this ability include excessive tone, obesity, advanced age, or internal rod or bony spinal fixation. Clients who cannot perform self-range of motion need to be taught to instruct others in this task. In the presence of excessive tone they also need to be taught to inhibit tone through the use of reflex inhibiting postures and maneuvers (see Chapter 6). Clients with high-level lesions need to be taught to monitor spinal alignment and rib cage mobility for early prevention of scoliosis. This is especially important in the child whose bone growth will increase the risk of this deformity.

Some patterns of joint limitation are encouraged because they enhance function. For example, in the client who has wrist extension but no active motion distally, some contracture of the long finger flexors is allowed to develop. This strengthens the client's ability to develop a tenodesis grasp between the thumb and the second and third fingers (three-point palmar prehension). This grasp can be further strengthened by the use of a tenodesis spring-loaded orthosis. Another example of selective functional tightness is the quadriplegic client who is allowed to develop tight low-back extensors that will provide posterior trunk stability on which to balance while performing activities in the long-sitting position. Stability in this long-sitting position can also be provided by tight hamstring musculature.

Precautions to range of motion activities include the presence of thrombophlebitis, joint ligament damage, healing fractures, and the long-term presence of osteoporosis. Because many clients are unable to feel pain, the client and the therapist are deprived of an important mechanism of protection during range of motion activities. Fractures, including spinal fracture that extends the cord lesion, have been reported as a result of too vigorous ranging[39] (Fig. 15-20).

Hypermobility of affected joints may occur from prolonged stress to joint ligamentous and capsular support and can result in pain and deformity that impairs function. The client who has little or no hip or pelvic active motion and therefore maintains standing balance by assuming a "C-curve" posture and "hanging" on the anterior iliofemoral and anterior capsule ligaments of the hip joint complex is an example. Another example is the quadriplegic client who, during rehabilitation mat activities, spends a great deal of time in the supine on elbows position. This position requires shoulder hyperextension that can place stress on the anterior shoulder complex and that has been shown to cause pain and other complications.[182]

Strengthening functional muscles. As soon as spinal stability is achieved or protected by orthoses, traction, or other precautionary measures mentioned earlier, the strengthening of available musculature should begin. Particular attention needs to be given early on to those muscles and movement patterns that are innervated by the most distal functioning segment of the spinal cord.

There are two philosophies for accomplishing this goal. The first is to plan specific strengthening exercises and progressions of activities aimed at the eventual achievement of functional activities. Another approach is to focus on functional activities to achieve gains in strength. This second approach is based on the pragmatic fact that time is a limiting factor in any rehabilitation program and that it is therefore more efficient to achieve strength and function concurrently. Moe[167] presented a very complete program for the client with a C6 lesion based on this function-activity related strengthening concept. Specific exercise regimes based on mat activities performed in various developmental postures relative to the client's level of function represents another philosophy. Sullivan[230] presented a series of mat activities for clients with different levels of lesions that relate developmental treatment progressions based primarily on concepts of proprioceptive neuromuscular facilitation (PNF) and that are geared toward the eventual accomplishment of functional goals. Bromley[25] and O'Sullivan[183] also presented examples of mat activity progressions within stages of the developmental sequence.

Traditional exercise activities that use weights, wall pulleys, sling suspension techniques, skate boards, and other resistive exercise regimes may be found in Basmajian.[12] Class or group exercise programs can provide an efficient means of strengthening functioning musculature in a cost-effective manner and with the added benefit of motivation through peer stimulation.

The gradation of treatment procedures from the initiation of very weak voluntary muscle activity to functional skill can be achieved by various techniques. Muscles that cannot be palpated can be monitored by EMG biofeedback,[170] and facilitation techniques such as tapping, icing, and quick stretch may be used (see Chapter 6) to achieve mobility and stability within a posture, controlled mobility, and eventual skill in movement. Another treatment procedure that can be used to facilitate motor activity is electrical stimulation of the muscle.[244] With the loss of cutaneous sensation and/or proprioception, electrical stimulation of a muscle may assist the client in achieving "awareness" of minimal voluntary motor control present. Electrical stimulation can also be used to provide or augment function at a selected joint segment.[118] Also, with weak, partially innervated muscles, electrical stimulation can assist a client in motor recruitment.

Considerable success has been achieved recently with using implantable wire electrodes in multiple muscle sites in the upper extremities of high-level quadriplegics.[185] Multichannel computer-controlled electrical stimulators have allowed selected patients to achieve significant functional grasp, as well as elbow and forearm motion. However, great caution must be exercised in introducing a patient to the fact that electrical stimulation can cause paralyzed muscles to contract. A myriad of expectations can be raised. The key question is: can a significant functional improvement occur with using this modality, one that cannot be achieved through less costly or more simple methods? A recent study has hypothesized, for example, that electrically stimulating paralyzed muscles of the lower extremities attached to a computer-controlled cycle ergometer can result in improved cardiovascular endurance, retardation of muscle atrophy, and concurrent increased muscle girth.[196] Questions have to be asked: is atrophy bad? Do permanently paralyzed muscles need long-term electrical stimulation to maintain some muscle bulk, possibly for cosmetic reasons? Can long-term cardiovascular endurance and wellness be achieved by wheelchair sports or the use of functioning musculature on simple ergometers?[66] Can it be achieved through active weight training,[58] rather than through a device that costs thousands of dollars and has unproven efficacy? There is also evidence that long-term use of surface-electrode electrical stimulation of paralyzed muscles causes a tendency toward increased spasticity in subjects with spinal cord injury.[204]

Finally, surgical transfer of tendons can provide motor control at a joint without innervated muscles. These techniques have been primarily limited to the upper extremity in clients with quadriplegia. For example, active elbow ex

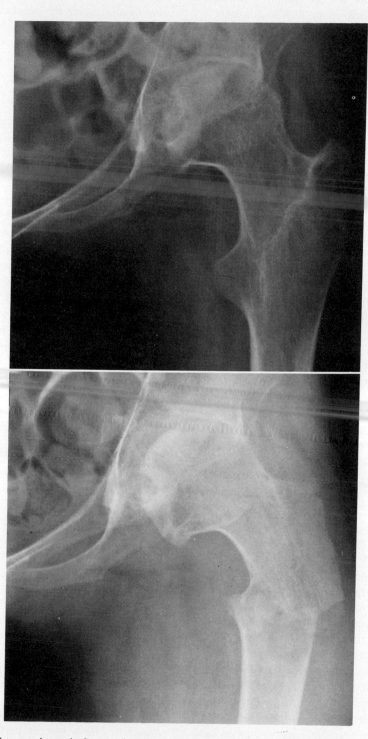

Fig. 15-20. Intertrochanteric fracture in a 24-year-old woman with C5 quadriplegia from a diving accident 9 years earlier. The fracture occurred during physical therapy range of motion exercises. Fracture was internally fixated with a Jewett hip nail and plate. (From Hendrix RW: Skeletal changes after spinal cord injury. In Calenoff L, editor: Radiology of spinal cord injury, St Louis, 1981, The CV Mosby Co.)

tension can be achieved by transferring the posterior portion of the deltoid muscle to the triceps tendon.[166] Because many persons with spinal cord injury lack tactile gnosis and proprioception, the "feedback" needed for controlled motor function is often limited to vision, which poses a major limitation to these types of surgery. These tendon transfers are often accompanied by arthrodesis of a distal joint, such as the fingers, to provide stability and improved function for the transplanted muscle.[55,120]

Kinesthetic reawareness and tolerance to vertical positioning

VASOMOTOR. Tolerance to vertical sitting and, when appropriate, supported standing is not always achieved during the early stages of rehabilitation. Clients who experience persistent symptoms of postural hypotension (decreased blood pressure, increased pulse, pallor, and dizziness) can be helped immediately by either tilting the wheelchair backward to lower the head and upper trunk below the lower extremities or by having the client lie recumbent on a mat or bed until the symptoms subside. These symptoms will usually decrease through repetitive attempts at sitting or standing in conjunction with continued use of pressure gradient stockings, abdominal binders, and drug therapy, although they may occasionally persist following discharge from the rehabilitation facility. The client and family need to be educated to this problem and to the means of alleviating the symptoms. Brucker and Ince[29] reported on a man who had severe postural hypotension of 3 years duration with a lesion at the T3 level and who was trained to adjust his blood pressure to alleviate his symptoms through the use of biofeedback training. As mentioned earlier, in many clients with high-level cord damage, the vasomotor system does not allow normal compensation to major environmental temperature changes. Again, the client and family must be aware of this potential problem.

PROPRIOCEPTIVE. The loss of proprioceptive sensation combined with decreased motor control and/or cutaneous sensation leaves many clients with the need to redevelop their ability to control and stabilize their movements. This leads to a new sense of kinesthetic awareness that is a basic prerequisite for learning subsequent functional skills such as bed mobility, transfer ability, and possibly ambulation. This relearning of postural responses can be accomplished in many ways. Mat activities allow the therapist to assist the client in learning new movement progressions. They also challenge the client's ability to stabilize in various positions using, for example, approximation and rhythmic stabilization techniques to facilitate postural control.

Sensory and vestibular stimulation can be provided by the use of swiss balls, by the use of a mirror to practice balancing activities, and by taking the client into a pool.[76] Veer[243] presented a varied program of using sling suspension activities to achieve trunk vestibular stimulation. The reader is referred to Gerhart,[89] who presented a program of kinesthetic reawareness training for a client with a C5 lesion; he also makes the excellent point of the added benefit of these activities to the person's psychological sense of body image.

The therapist should attempt to develop key muscles that underlie postural stability for the client with a high lesion. For example, the latissimus dorsi (C6-C8 innervation) can serve as a source of trunk control in the long-sitting position or braced standing in the parallel bars. This is accomplished by fixating its insertion on the humerus and by reversing its normal action to allow it to pull its origin on the lower spine and pelvis toward its insertion. Other key muscles are the trapezius (cranial nerve XI, C1-6), which extends to T12, and the other shoulder girdle muscles with origins on the upper rib cage.

Hypertonicity. The rationales and techniques for the facilitory and inhibitory methods of managing tonal problems were discussed in Chapter 6. Tonal changes with spinal cord injury were discussed earlier in this chapter, where the clinical pictures, factors that cause tonal changes, and the clinical and surgical treatments relative to managing tone in spinal cord injury were presented. It was also mentioned that lack of tone, as in spinal shock, was unchangable through treatment and did not contribute to function. This discussion will therefore be limited to managing problems of increased tone. When spinal shock ceases and when the client begins to demonstrate tone and reflex activity with or without voluntary motor control, this state will be defined here as mild hypertonicity, which the clinician has to decide whether or not to facilitate in conjunction with improving motor control. Some techniques for facilitating tone were mentioned earlier in this section on strengthening functioning muscles (see also Chapter 6). This section therefore addresses concepts relevant to the physical therapy management of increased tone in spinal cord injury that interferes with functional motor control. The two most important concepts regarding spasticity management in physical therapy are (1) that the physical therapy procedures used to change a tonal state are transient and that pretreatment inhibition is used to promote function or to facilitate client comfort and (2) that a primary goal of the therapist is to teach the person with a spinal cord injury to recognize his or her reflex patterns of spasticity, identify what stimuli within his or her body and environment can exacerbate this spasticity, and then to learn compensatory reflex-inhibiting or modulating techniques that he or she can perform or instruct others to perform to allow maximal function and comfort.

Reduction of tone can be achieved through prolonged stretch[152,181] that is obtained slowly so as not to elicit a stretch reflex and that is maintained for a long period of time. This can be achieved by positioning of the client or extremity and by the use of serial casts or orthoses.[188] Prolonged cooling of the spastic muscle is another technique mentioned in Chapter 6 that is useful for achieving a transient decrease in tone.

Electrical stimulation of the antagonist to a spastic muscle can temporarily decrease tone through reciprocal inhibition.[138,244] Long-term stimulation, as mentioned earlier, may increase spasticity.[204] However, Shindo and Jones[224] in England applied electrical stimulation alternately to agonist and antagonist muscle groups in regular treatment given to 32 patients with severe spasticity from complete and incomplete spinal cord lesions. In 90% of their subjects, they noted increasing periods of relaxation measured by change in passive range of motion and the patient's subjective analysis of how stimulation increased or decreased their functional abilities. Interestingly, a number of patients noted longer periods of relaxation after the same duration of stimulation. It was unclear why reduction of spasticity occurred with this protocol. Replicating studies need to be performed. EMG biofeedback training has proved useful in decreasing tone by having the client concentrate on decreasing tone by having the client concentrate on decreasing the electric signals from the spastic muscle or through the use of reciprocal inhibition by increasing the signals from the antagonist.[10] Finally, clients who use pool therapy for obtaining other goals, such as cardiorespiratory endurance, will find that the warmth of the water will decrease their spasticity for up to 1 to 2 hours after leaving the pool. It was mentioned earlier in this chapter that increased tone can be used for functional activities, for example, pinching the calf muscle can initiate a flexor response to assist in dressing. This is an important concept involved in management of activities of daily living with this clinical problem.

It is also important to teach the client as much as possible about the nature of spasticity because many clients relate a spastic reflex response to the return of function.

Skin protection. The incidence, types, cause, and medical and surgical management of pressure sores was discussed earlier. The prevention of pressure sores and trauma to desensitized skin is dependent on client/family education. The client is ultimately responsible for his or her care, and the ability to deal with this responsibility is paramount. The client must be trained by the nursing and physical therapy staff in pressure relief skills, in frequent skin inspections, and in avoiding trauma while transferring in and out of chairs, beds, tubs, and cars and on and off of the commode.

The process of teaching these skills varies widely between and within institutions, and this is an area in need of research. Behavior modification techniques have been tried by some facilities,[145] but long-term studies are needed to assess the effectiveness of this technique of training. What is important is that these skills be taught to *every* client and that some form of ongoing skin inspection be performed by the individual. The client must have a readily available support system, so that any potential sore can be

reported and inspected. Many clients do not have to perform pressure relief activities on a regular basis. There exists no valid criteria for selecting which client will or will not be prone to skin breakdown. In addition to the level of injury, there are numerous etiological factors. Some, like motivational status, can change quickly, and this precludes an easy way of identifying clients at risk.

Pressure relief skills for paraplegic clients that can be done in the wheelchair include push-ups. Forward and lateral leans can be done by quadriplegic clients while in the wheelchair; some of these clients may need the assistance of a web-belt loop to lean.[2] High-level quadriplegic clients recline in an electric recliner wheelchair for pressure relief and for assistance with diaphragmatic excursion. Some clients will need to teach caregivers to perform pressure relief lifts and to reposition them in the wheelchair. There are no definitive and validated parameters available on how long a push-up or lean should be maintained. Obviously this varies among clients in relation to the weight of the patient, the level of injury, the wetness of skin, the amount of adipose tissue over bony prominences, and other possible factors that have not yet been identified. Positioning and turning schedules need to be worked out while the client is in the rehabilitation facility and established during weekend visits home. Some people will require a pressure relief cushion placed in a cut-out in a foam bed mattress, and others will use positioning in various postures with the use of pillows and a regular mattress. Clients should be taught to inspect their skin every morning and evening and to use a mirror to examine the buttocks and ischial areas.

Over the last 20 years there have been many types of pressure relief cushions developed, and it would be tempting, but clinically unwise, to solely rely on the "best" of these for wheelchair and bed pressure relief. Over 12 different pressure relief cushions are currently on the market. The reader is referred to Nixon[178] and Noble[179] for insight into prescription parameters and discussions of types and designs of pressure relief cushions.

Attention also needs to be given to teaching skin protection from sources of extreme heat or cold. Burns can easily occur during bathing, from cigarettes, from hot water pipes under a sink, or from being too close to a car heater.

Respiratory/cardiovascular function. As mentioned earlier, all quadriplegic clients and most paraplegic clients should be evaluated and treated for some degree of respiratory insufficiency. This section presents an overview of respiratory management in a physical therapy rehabilitation setting. For an in-depth analysis of management, the reader is referred to Cardiopulmonary Physical Therapy, volume one in this series, and to the references at the end of this chapter.[4,41,84,142]

The two primary problems with respiration experienced by the person with a spinal cord injury are a decreased inspiratory ventilation and a decreased expiratory pressure.

The goals of treatment will depend on the level of cord lesion and on the clinical status of the client. In general, these goals include (1) training in more efficient and coordinated breathing patterns, (2) maintaining chest mobility, which can be decreased from paralysis of the intercostal and abdominal musculature, lack of trunk rotation, and uncoordinated chest expansion, and (3) maintaining bronchial hygiene.

Inefficient and uncoordinated breathing results in poor lung ventilation, decreased overall endurance in functional activities, and poor cough production. The high-level client may require long-term diaphragm pacing and a mechanical respirator to promote lung ventilation.[240] Glossopharyngeal breathing is a technique that is not easily taught but that can be learned by a highly motivated client and that can also be used when a client is off a mechanical respirator.[267] It results in decreased client apprehension and increased breathing efficiency, and it can increase vital capacity by as much as 1000 ml.[4] Van Steen[242] presented a summary of the problems of the high-level client in an article on the management of a complete lesion at C1.

The goal of improved lung ventilation can be measured by improved vital capacity, tidal volume, and inspiratory force. Methods of achieving this include the use of the incentive respirometer or spirometer one to two times a day; this can promote inspiratory and expiratory volume improvement. Also, the client can enter into respiratory group games that include sipping through straws and blowing bubbles and that can also improve motivation through peer stimulation, especially with the younger client.

Chesire and Flack[47] combined the use of incentive spirometry with behavioristic psychology operant conditioning technique.

In the client with diaphragm function, strengthening of the diaphragm by means of resisted inspiration has been shown to improve endurance and to protect against fatigue[94] (Fig. 15-21). Improved lung ventilation is also achieved by teaching the client to coordinate and pace the use of the accessory muscles of respiration (including the sternocleidomastoid, trapezius, levator scapula and scaleni) with inspiration and exhalation. Fig. 15-22 shows a child with an incomplete traction lesion at C4-C5-C6 using a rocking chair to learn this coordinated breathing task.

An elastic abdominal corset applied between the tenth rib and the iliac crest supports the abdominal contents while sitting and improves diaphragm function; therefore it has been shown to improve lung ventilation when the client is sitting but not when in the supine position.[146] A final comment regarding lung ventilation is the need to monitor high-level quadriplegic clients during the acute and early rehabilitation stages. It has been shown that many high-level quadriplegic persons have no sense of breathlessness during periods of apnea.[208] Also, even low-level quadriplegic clients may not have established enough proficiency with a trigger call device, such as a puff and sip call mechanism, to alert staff to their respiratory distress.

Maintaining and improving chest mobility is the second primary goal with the quadriplegic client. In addition to muscle paralysis, chest mobility can be decreased during the acute phase of treatment by spinal immobilization tech-

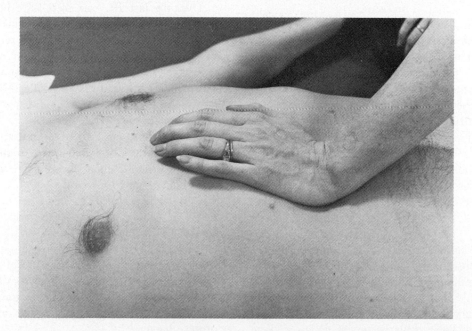

Fig. 15-21. Monitoring diaphragm excursion. Placing the heel of the hand just inferior to the xyphoid process of the sternum allows proprioceptive feedback to diaphragm contraction and cough coordination in a client with a C5 lesion. Gentle pressure can also assist the client to inhibit the diaphragm when learning use of the accessory muscles of respiration.

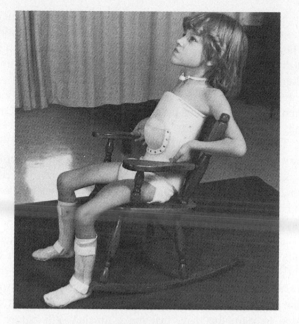

Fig. 15-22. Coordination of accessory muscle function with diaphragmatic function during inspiration and exhalation can be accomplished through rhythmic rocking.

niques, such as the halo and SOMI orthoses; surgical insertion of spinal fixating rods decreases long-term chest mobility. Poor chest mobility also has an impact on lung ventilization and drainage and needs to be effectively and aggressively managed. Mobility can be improved early, for example, the client who is still on a Stryker frame, can be taught segmental chest expansion and segmental breathing. The use of intermittent positive pressure breathing (IPPB) can improve chest expansion by gradually increasing the inspiratory pressure. EMG and other biofeedback techniques are also useful in teaching segmental breathing and in assisting with chest expansion.[215] During the rehabilitation phase, more aggressive exercises and mobilization techniques can be used. The client in Fig. 15-23 is using counter-rotation trunk exercises to not only improve chest mobility but to coordinate cough production with assisted expiration and to work on total chest expansion. Proprioceptive neuromuscular facilitation techniques used during mat activities are particularly effective for improving chest expansion and for resisted breathing to improve ventilation to a lung segment.

Maintaining bronchial hygiene is the third and final pri-

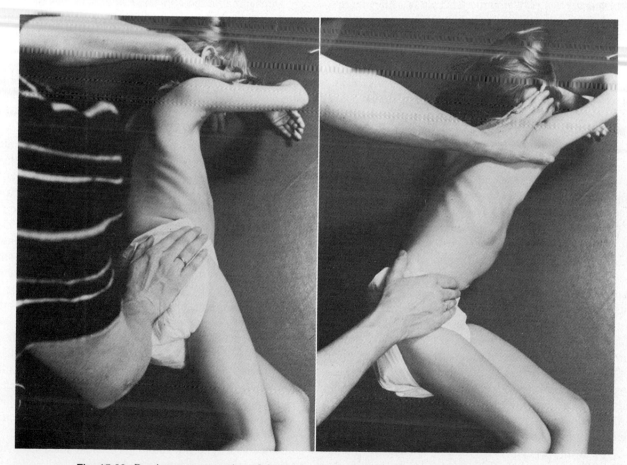

Fig. 15-23. Passive counterrotation of the trunk aids maintenance of chest/shoulder girdle mobility and should be coordinated with the client's breathing pattern.

mary goal. In the early stages, this may be primarily accomplished by suctioning through a tracheostomy, if the client is in traction. Very high-level clients will need bulbar training to improve swallowing and to decrease aspirations.[242] As the client is mobilized, assisted and resisted cough should be taught, and, if indicated, postural drainage using percussion and vibration techniques may be initiated. Teaching the client to coordinate accessory respiratory muscles with coughing is a key to maintaining lung ventilation and improving expiratory pressure. One of the few controlled studies in this area was done by McMichan and others.[151] They showed in a prospective study that assisted coughing, postural drainage, and deep breathing exercises performed by quadriplegic clients in an acute setting resulted in increased survival, decreased incidence of pulmonary complications, and decreased need for ventilatory support when compared to a retrospective group who did not receive vigorous chest physical therapy.

Client and family education in this area is very important before discharge. The client must be taught to request assistance with drainage or coughing when needed, and the family, when it is indicated, must be taught postural drainage, assisted coughing, suctioning, and chest mobilization/strengthening exercises.

Pool therapy can play an important role in achieving the goals of respiratory rehabilitation. Swimming and resistance exercise training have also been shown to improve cardiorespiratory function following discharge.[58,66,184]

Functional goals. Success in the management of the systemic problems lays the foundation for the accomplishment of functional activities. The four functional goals most common to the rehabilitation of any person with a spinal cord injury within a physical therapy setting are addressed again in terms of significant concepts. The attainment of independence in these activities is a highly individualized process of teaching that occurs between the therapist and client. It involves their being able to analyze a functional goal, break it down into its components, and then decide what tasks, adaptive equipment, and assistance from others is needed to achieve success. Strategies devised for the attainment of any functional goal are as numerous and as different as the differences that exist between clients and their eventual home and work environments. The therapist must be skilled in the problem-solving approach to achieving a functional goal, must be aware of the available equipment and possible home/work environmental adaptations, and must be willing, as must the client, to seek the advice of more experienced colleagues and to make use of printed and video resource materials that present options that have worked for others. An excellent printed reference is Ford and Duckworth[80]; this source is a good place to start problem-solving with a client because it goes into many options pictorially for all significant activities of daily living for clients with high-level lesions. Also, as mentioned earlier, with the advent of more affordable videotape equipment, departments should develop a collection of tapes for client education. Clients who develop a successful outcome to a problem skill are usually more than willing to be filmed for future client use. It is also most helpful to have a taping and playback unit in the treatment area so that clients can view themselves attempting tasks that can facilitate their learning.

The teaching of functional skills should always be relevant to the client's future home environment. Therapists need to be cognizant of the tremendous exertion needed for attaining many activities of daily living. Clients need to be taught to compromise at times and to try to plan each day in terms of possible pacing of their activities. Therapists also need to be aware of differences in the way clients learn. For example, one client might view another client's successful performance of a bathtub transfer and then be able to quickly devise the strategies needed to perform that task. Another client may view the same scene and still need to learn the parts that make up that skill before attempting to solve the problems involved and learn the necessary skills. Finally, cultural and social differences need to be considered in teaching and making decisions regarding future function.

Depending on the clinical setting, activities of daily living are taught by the physical therapy and/or occupational therapy departments. Skills usually unique to an occupational therapy setting, such as dressing, bathing, feeding, and grooming, are not covered in this chapter. Bowel and bladder retraining and functional skills relating to sexuality are covered in Chapter 29.

Bed mobility. The client needs to use the skills of momentum and leverage incorporated in relearning kinesthetic awareness during mat activities to achieve the ability to move in bed. Depending on the level of injury, the client can start to learn rolling, moving toward the head and foot of the bed, and assuming a sitting position in bed with the bed at the rehabilitation facility. Then, on weekend visits, the client can practice these skills in bed at home. Decisions may have to be made regarding changing the height of the bed, stabilizing the bed, adding loops, straps, and bed rails, and possibly changing the type of mattress. Also, nylon or silk sheets may be used to decrease friction. Depending on the type of transfer used, an overhead frame with a trapeze or loop may have to be attached, if possible, to the existing bed. Pressure relief adaptions may be made with the use of a foam covering with or without a gel or other pressure relief inserts. The client with a high-level lesion may need a hospital-type bed with an electric elevating head for respiratory and pressure relief. Various adaptions can be made to control the elevating head mechanism including the use of a puff and sip unit.

Transfers. The nonambulatory client must learn transfers from the wheelchair to and from the bed, toilet, bath, car, and possibly the floor. Teaching transfer techniques incorporates the widest variety of strategies, adaptions, and techniques needed in spinal cord injury rehabilitation. This is especially true for the client with a low-level cervical lesion, who has a number of transfer options including the roll-out, pivot, forward, looping, and back-out techniques. Solving the problems involved with the equipment and techniques needed for this level client will take full advantage of the strategies mentioned in the opening remarks of this section. For an in-depth analysis of transfer training, the reader is referred to the references at the end of the chapter.[80,134,150,178,243]

Wheelchair mobility. It is important for the client to learn mobility within the chair, including what factors and strategies are needed for weight shifting, pressure relief and, for the high-level client, wheelchair adaptive equipment for trunk support. The client who needs assistance must learn to instruct others in techniques of repositioning for pressure relief and to adjust clothing or a catheter.

The client also needs to learn mobility with whatever definitive chair is finally prescribed. The client with high cervical lesions will require an electric wheelchair with various control devices. This may range from a puff-and-sip unit to various types of "joystick" hand controls. The person in Fig. 15-24 has a motorized reclining wheelchair. Control of the joystick is through a hole punched in her wrist-hand orthosis (WHO). She controls the joystick/splint arrangement with shoulder and scapular motions and is independent in wheelchair mobility on most flat surfaces. This wheelchair is also equipped with an electric respirator, which she uses when the exertion of breathing becomes too exhausting and when lack of oxygen decreases her mental alertness in school.

In addition to controlling the mobility and reclining of a motorized wheelchair, puff-and-sip control units can also control electronic devices external to the wheelchair (extra-environmental electronic device control). These units can detect radio frequencies or infrared light to control devices for turning on a light, dialing a telephone, or using a computer. The person in Fig. 15-25 has a long-standing bulbar-level polio lesion that left no active movement below the neck. She is a glossopharyngeal breather who uses a puff-and-sip controlled computer-based system to carry out the responsibilities of a research associate/consumer advocate with a research and development center. This system allows her many capabilities, including handling a multi-functioning telephone switchboard, entering and bringing up information on the computer screen, and building, editing, and storing textual materials.

Some clients with only shoulder function and active elbow flexion can use a manual chair with wheel rim vertical or oblique projections. These clients can usually achieve independent wheelchair mobility on most smooth, flat surfaces, but they may need assistance on other types of terrain and on inclines.

If the client also has radial wrist extensor function, he

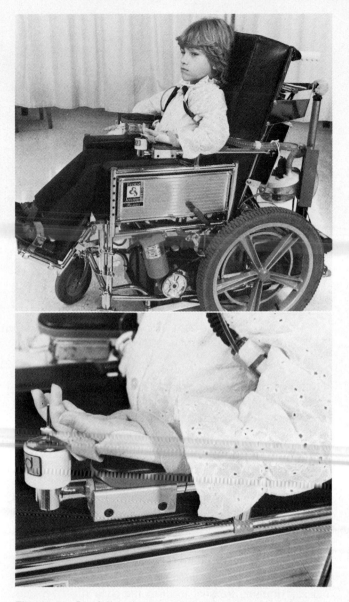

Fig. 15-24. Specially adapted motorized wheelchair with a battery-operated respirator (attached to tracheostomy) allows mobility for the child with a high-level cord lesion.

or she can trade the rim projections for plastic or rubber-coated rims and use a leather hand mitt to allow palmar pressure and friction with the mitt on the rim to achieve mobility on most smooth surfaces. These clients will also require assistance on other surfaces and inclines. Both of these previous client examples may trade manual wheelchair mobility for an electric chair when great distances or speed are required or when the energy demands of manual wheelchair propulsion leave little endurance for other physical and mental activities.

With the addition of some hand function, a regular wheelchair can allow achievement of independent mobility on level surfaces, but assistance may be needed on rough

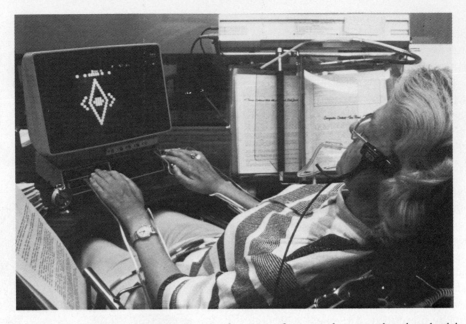

Fig. 15-25. Puff and sip control units allow performance of many tasks external to the wheelchair environment.

terrain. Most paraplegic clients with good arm, shoulder girdle, and upper trunk strength will achieve independent wheelchair mobility, including ramp and curb access.

These are very general guidelines and are affected by the many considerations inherent in the client that have been mentioned often in this chapter.

Training in wheelchair mobility skills can often be accomplished in group or class sessions and should include indoor and outdoor practice. Departments and therapists should have protocols and checklists specifying what constitutes independent basic, intermediate, and advanced wheelchair mobility. Wheelchair mobility training should not only include wheelchair propulsion skills but also training in what to do if the chair tips over and, if appropriate, how to transfer from the floor to the chair and from the chair to the floor. One advanced wheelchair skill is the "wheelie," which is necessary for jumping a curb. The client in Fig. 15-26 uses a rope to practice this skill without the need of close supervision. Another outcome of class wheelchair skills training can be activities that improve endurance and cardiorespiratory function.

One complication of wheelchair propulsion is shoulder pain, especially if the client has less than full shoulder girdle function or strength. Nichols and others[176] surveyed 708 members of a spinal cord injury association and found that 51.4% of the 79.5% who responded to a questionnaire suffered from shoulder pain that was particularly related to wheelchair usage as well as to other factors, such as transfer function.

A definitive wheelchair order should be delayed as long as possible to ensure that the chair meets the long-term needs of the client. New types of lighter and more durable chairs and accessories have finally been developed by an industry that, primarily because of a lack of competition, made few significant changes in the design of wheelchairs from the post World War II era until the mid-1970s.

Ambulation. The desire to "return to walking" is the most often heard desire of the client with spinal cord injury; this is especially true during the early stages after injury.

There are no precise guidelines based on the level of complete cord section that will indicate success at ambulation. The variables that affect success in rehabilitation were mentioned earlier in this chapter, and they need to be repeated and expanded on here. They include the client's completeness of cord lesion, age, endurance, weight, body build, general health status, amount of spasticity, amount of proprioceptive and other sensory loss (for incomplete lesions), joint range of motion, occupational and other special needs, financial funding, outlook regarding the energy and time requirements involved in ambulation with orthoses and in donning and doffing the orthoses, and finally motivation. The rehabilitation team needs to consider all these variables and provide this information when discussing potential ambulation with a client. The team also needs to have a consistent philosophy on what they see as the physiological and psychological benefits of ambulation and some general criteria for assessing the potential of a client to achieve some level of ambulation.

Philosophies have changed over the last 30 to 40 years and, with new technology and research, will hopefully change in the future. In 1964 Rusk[213] advocated that clients with complete lesions at or above T10 be provided

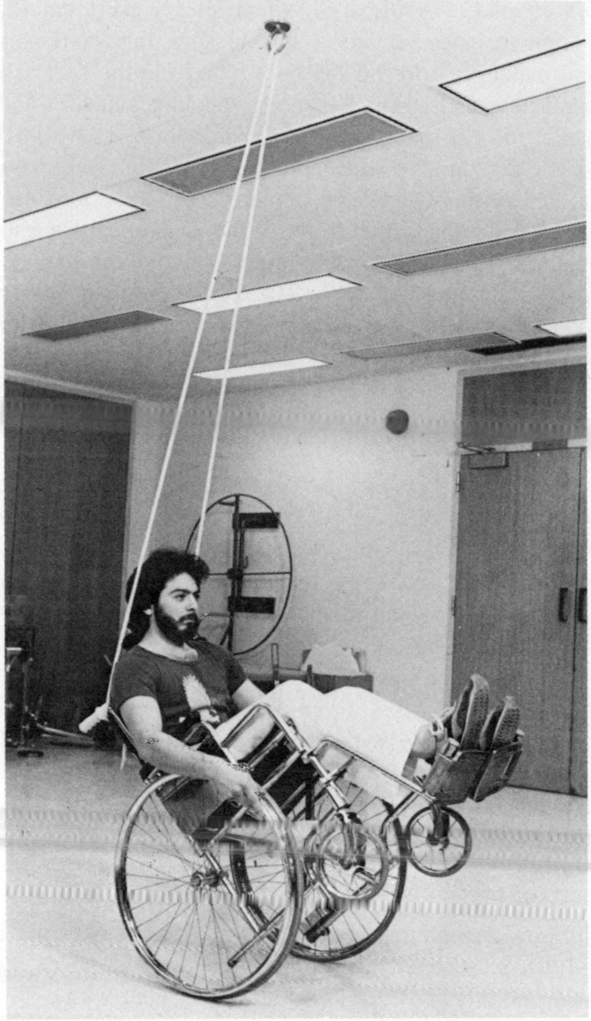

Fig. 15-26. Unsupervised practice in performance of a "wheelie."

with bilateral metal knee-ankle-foot-orthoses (KAFO) with a pelvic band and Knight spinal attachment. Rusk[213] advocated that those clients with lesions below T10 be fitted with bilateral metal KAFOs. The pelvic bands and spinal attachments were found to be simply too heavy, were difficult to get off and on, and at best allowed for only supervised ambulation for physiological reasons. Many clients also required assistance with sitting and standing as a result of their limited flexibility. Most clients simply discarded those orthoses upon discharge. In a follow-up study in 1973 of 164 clients who were discharged with some ambulatory function, Hussey and Stauffer[115] found that clients with pelvic control usually ambulated for exercise purposes only and that those without pelvic control were eventually nonambulatory and had reverted to wheelchair use. Of this sample, 82 (or 50%) were functional community ambulators. Only two of these community ambulators used bilateral KAFOs. Hussey and Stauffer[115] concluded

that "two long leg braces with locked knees seemed to be a limiting factor in ambulatory function." A more recent follow-up study on lower extremity orthotic KAFO usage following discharge was conducted by Mikelberg and Reid[161] in 1981. They questioned 60 people who had been discharged with lower-extremity orthoses in the 5-year period between 1973 and 1977. Of the 35 clients who responded, 60% used their wheelchair as their primary means of mobility. Thirty-one percent did not use their lower-extremity orthoses at all, and the majority who did use them did so only for standing and exercise. The authors questioned, based on their observation and experience, whether KAFOs should be prescribed on the first admission to a rehabilitation facility and also suggested that, since many of the clients used their KAFOs only for standing, less expensive standing devices should be considered as alternatives.

Another factor that should be considered in developing a philosophy on ambulation criteria is a social or cultural difference in the emphasis placed on ambulation. McAdam and Natvig,[148] in a recent 16-year follow-up study at the Oslo Norway State Rehabilitation Institute of 61 persons with complete lesions between T1 and L3, found that 69% used their orthoses regularly, that 64% were able to walk 100 meters indoors, and that 59% were able to climb up and down 20 stairs. Also, 59% were fully employed. They presented one client with a T6 complete lesion who was able to negotiate spiral stairs without handrails. Of their clients with complete lesions between T1 and T5, 16% had achieved the ability to climb up and down 20 stairs. They attributed the success of their program, which was presented in an earlier article,[173] to instituting very intense programs of physical training aimed solely at ambulation and to philosophically and psychologically deemphasizing the use of wheelchairs. They claim that their success at vocational rehabilitation is based on their client's ability to climb stairs and walk small distances indoors, as well as their ability to maintain close, ongoing follow-up with their clients.

Sensation, particularly proprioception, is very important to the client with an incomplete lesion in the achievement of functional ambulation. The Hussey and Stauffer[115] study found that in their group of community ambulators (n=82), only one person did not have proprioception in any of the major joints of the lower extremities. Kaplan and others[121] found that clients with polio accomplished greater levels of ambulation than did clients with spinal cord injuries with the same degree of motor loss. This further indicates the essential role that sensation, and more notably proprioception, plays in the achievement of functional ambulation.

A major consideration for the client and team is the energy requirement involved in ambulating with orthoses. This was pointed out in a study by Cerny and others,[43] who compared the energy requirements of propelling a wheelchair and ambulating with bilateral KAFOs of 10 clients with spinal cord injury. The clients had lesions between T11 and L2, had all been trained to use conventional KAFOs, and had all used either a swing-through or a swing-to-gait. Of these 10 clients, eight customarily used a wheelchair as their primary means of mobility and the other two had discontinued use of their wheelchairs. The study found that walking was significantly more inefficient than wheelchair propulsion, even in those who customarily ambulated with KAFOs. Their study found that swing-through stride length and heart rate were the best clinical indicators of ability to ambulate with bilateral KAFOs. Subjects who walked successfully had a long-gait stride, a minimal gait velocity of 54 m/minute, and had to be willing to work under anaerobic conditions while ambulating. Persons with less bracing, for example, those using one KAFO with one ankle-foot-orthoses (AFO) or those with bilateral AFOs, have a much better success rate at functional community ambulation.[115]

Some very general comments can be made regarding projected levels of ambulation for persons with complete spinal cord lesions, keeping in mind the many variables that have impact on these comments. These comments are based primarily on the author's clinical experience and are focused on the young, more athletic person who may be willing to incur the energy requirements mentioned in the Cerny study to achieve success.

The person with a mid-thoracic level (T6 to T9) lesion can usually achieve supervised ambulation for short distances using a swing-to-gait with bilateral KAFOs. The average client may require assistance with standing and sitting. The person with a lower thoracic level (T9 to T12) lesion can usually achieve independent ambulation on smooth surfaces using a swing-to or swing-through gait with bilateral KAFOs. The average client should be able to learn to fall correctly and to return to a standing position but may need supervision with ramps and rough or uneven surfaces and with ascending and descending stairs.

The person with a high lumbar level (T12 to L3) lesion should be independent in ambulation on all surfaces, including stairs, using a swing-through or alternating four-point gait with bilateral KAFOs or a combination of AFOs and KAFOs. The person with a lower lumbar level (L4 to L5) lesion can usually achieve independent ambulation with bilateral AFOs.

Only a brief discussion of orthoses will be presented here. The reader is referred to Chapter 28 as well as to Gould: *Orthopaedic and Sports Physical Therapy* for a more detailed presentation.

The author recommends the Scott-Craig orthosis[218] over more conventional metal KAFOs (Fig. 15-27). It has a simplicity of design that affords greater ease in donning and doffing. Its unique features include the ability to fixate but adjust the ankle joints, which may be either a single- or double-action joint. This provides adjustment of the degree of ankle dorsiflexion, which allows achievement of standing balance. It has a special shoe that combines a solid metal plate in the sole that runs from the heel to the metatarsel heads, which aids in standing balance, and a cushioned heel that eases force distribution at heel strike. It has one complete adjustable thigh band but only a solid pretibial band, which aids donning. The knee joint is set 1.5 cm posterior to the center of the anatomical knee joint for improved biomechanical alignment, and the knee joint has an automatic bail lock. There have been no objective studies comparing the efficacy of the Scott-Craig orthosis to conventional metal KAFOs. However, Huitt and Gwyer[114] had six clients try both types of orthoses, and all six preferred the Scott-Craig as they subjectively felt these orthoses provided increased hip stability. A recent follow-up study[155] showed better long-term usage than the previously cited studies on usage of more conventional orthoses.[115,161] The energy cost of ambulating with Scott-Craig orthoses was presented in a recent study by Huang and others.[100] Polypropylene KAFOs with metal uprights are another alternative KAFO.

Depending on the amount of knee stability needed, the client may use a polypropylene AFO or a conventional metal-upright AFO with a double-action ankle joint. The polypropylene AFO provides better cosmesis, and can be interchanged easily with different shoes; however, it provides less ankle and no knee control when compared to the double-action AFO, which can provide both ankle medial-lateral stability and control of knee extension.

There are alternative orthoses that are less expensive and that may better meet a client's individual needs. Seymour and others[221] discussed an adult client with a T7 lesion who used the Orlau swivel walker (originally developed for children with thoracic level myelomeningocele paraplegia.) This walker allows the client to ambulate with free hands and provides him stability for standing and working for up to 1 to 2 hours at a work bench. It is more awkward to use and requires greater energy but is an example of attempting to meet the individual's social and vocational needs. Recent orthotic advances in using lighter metals combined with polypropylene have resulted in orthoses that provide support above the hips but that do not have the weight and absence of hip control found in the older bilateral KAFOs with pelvic bands and various spinal attachments. Hip guidance orthosis (HGOs)[35] (also known as the Para Walker[36,246]) are one example of these new orthotic systems. These types of orthoses have allowed patients with complete lesions as high as T3 in adults and T1 in children to achieve some level of limited ambulation using a reciprocal gait pattern.[36,246] The HGO is fabricated to inhibit hip adduction on swing-through during ambulation. In addition, emphasis in training is placed on utilizing the latissimus dorsi (innervation at C6 to 8) to stabilize its insertion upon upper-extremity weight bearing through the forearm crutch and therefore acting as

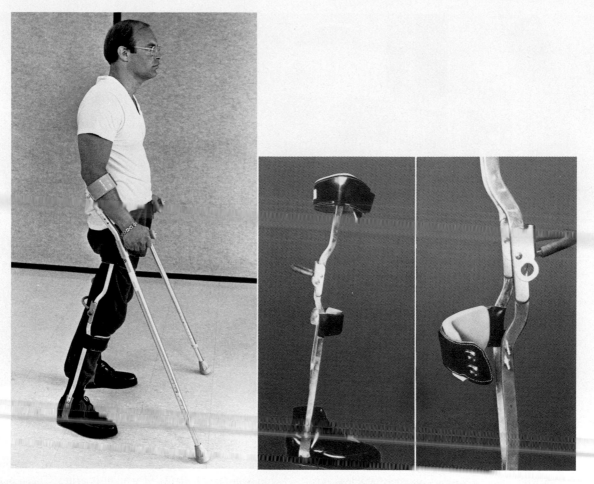

Fig. 15-27. Scott-Craig orthosis.

a stabilizer of the pelvis during lower-extremity swing-through. Also, hip abduction can be augmented during swing-through by electrically stimulating the gluteal muscles with a hand-triggered FES unit. Reciprocal gait is significantly lower in energy consumption than a swing-to or swing-through gait and is also more acceptable cosmetically.

A similar type of reciprocating gait orthosis (RGO) was developed at Louisiana State University and was initially reported on in 1984[259] as an ambulation device for children with myelomeningocele. The LSU RGO has been subsequently modified for use both by adults having spinal cord injury and those having weakness from other neuromuscular disorders.[13] The patient in Fig. 12-28 is using a modified LSU reciprocating gait orthosis. The primary features of this system, as noted in these pictures, are a molded pelvic girdles support with anterior velcro strap closure, polypropylene posterior thigh supports, and AFOs that extend along the plantar surface of the foot. The knees utilize droplocks for extension. The hip joints lock into extension and are unlocked by the small button seen posterior to the upright and inferior to the attachment of the

posterior cable. The two cables control bilateral hip extension (anterior cable) and flexion (posterior cable). These cables achieve this assistance to reciprocal gait during the patient's lateral weight shifts, thereby decreasing the energy requirements of ambulation. The patient seen in Fig. 15-28 is somewhat atypical. He has a complete T-11 lesion and was nonambulatory for a number of years postinjury. He returned to physical therapy with a strong goal of achieving ambulation. A complication was his having developed bilateral hip flexion contractures that did not respond to stretching. He therefore could not utilize bilateral KAFOs and a swing-to or swing-through gait pattern because this requires full hip extension and the ability to balance by hanging forward onto the anterior hip-Y ligaments as demonstrated by the patient in Fig. 15-27. However, he subsequently attained ambulation for moderate distances using a reciprocal walker. A high level of motivation and strong upper-extremity strength were key factors in his success.

As with the HGOs, patients with higher-level lesions than the person shown in Fig. 15-28 can also utilize FES to help with decreasing the fatigue factor in achieving am-

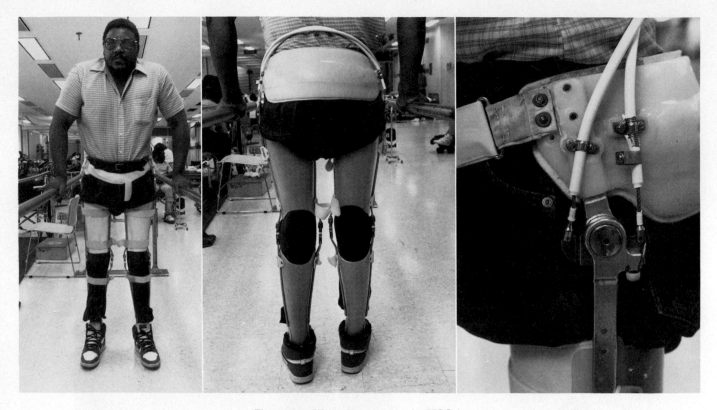

Fig. 15-28. Hip guidance orthosis (HGOs).

bulation. Bale locks can also be utilized at the knee joints for allowing greater ease in sitting, but they are less cosmetically pleasing under trousers because of the posterior bulge at the level of the knee. In summary, HGOs and RGOs offer to the appropriate patient a way of achieving ambulation with less energy consumption than with more conventional KAFOs, with or without pelvic and spinal attachments. They are, however, complex and costly systems that require coordinated efforts of the physical therapist and orthotist to prepare the patient for success in using these systems over a significant period of time.

There has been one recent follow-up study on the successful use of HGOs. Summers and colleagues[231] surveyed 20 adult paraplegics who were using HGOs (Para Walkers) independently at home for periods ranging from 6 to 44 months (average, 20 months). Seventeen (85%) were still regularly using their Para Walkers for independent ambulation both indoors and outdoors on a variety of surfaces. None in this sample utilized FES to augment the orthosis. All 20 had neurologically complete cord lesions between C8 and T12. More follow-up studies are needed to validate why these two systems achieve a higher long-term usage rate than that found with heavier conventional KAFOs.

Finally, there are also numerous mobile and immobile standing devices[85,194] that allow both paraplegic and quadriplegic persons to stand for long periods of time. These devices provide significant alternatives to ambulation with orthoses or mobility in a wheelchair, and they provide, in addition to the psychological benefits of standing,[6] the physiological benefits of weight bearing. These benefits include decreased contracture potential, possible decreased tone from prolonged stretch, a decreased level of osteoporosis, and improved urinary function from decreased hypercalciuria.

Use of electrical stimulation to the knee extensors has been advocated to achieve and maintain a standing position. This can be accomplished by placing surface electrodes over the quadriceps[8] or through implanted electrodes to stimulate nerves that control the muscles needed for hip and knee extension.[201] The problems with this means of achieving the standing position are muscle fatigue from the electrical stimulation and the extra cost, time, and gadgetry involved when compared to using a simple strap standing frame.

There has also been recent renewed interest in the use of electrical stimulation to augment ambulation with and without orthotic support.[244] Using electrical stimulation to assist in the control of a functional gait dates back to 1961 with the work of Liberson,[138] who studied stimulation of the peroneal muscles to achieve dorsiflexion and eversion during the swing-phase of gait in hemiplegic clients. Both surface and implanted electrodes have been used in studies over the years. With the use of small computers, more channels have been added. However, to date only a very primitive gait has been achieved for short distances with very close guarding of the client. Problems include the eventual rejection of implanted electrodes, poor client compliance with ongoing application of surface electrodes, skin irritation from prolonged use of surface electrodes, and muscle fatigue from electrical stimulation. The future may hold improved technology that will allow safe, efficient, and economically feasible ambulation using this modality.

In this section, an attempt has been made to identify some concepts, ideas, and approaches around which a physical therapist can develop a philosophy regarding ambulation and the person with a spinal cord injury. With the advent of cost-effective temporary orthoses that can be fitted universally to all clients, no client should be denied the opportunity to attempt ambulation. All members of the rehabilitation team should be utilized so that patients can achieve assistance in attaining personal goals that go beyond what is considered a normal outcome for a given level of injury.[254]

Psychosocial factors. In a major work on the psychosocial factors inherent in spinal cord injury rehabilitation, Treischmann[238] states that "Rehabilitation is the process of learning to live with one's own disability in one's own environment." Rehabilitation is indeed a "learning process" in which the physical therapist is one of the primary "teachers." The other important concept in Treischmann's statement is that the client has a commitment, a sense of feeling, that this process called rehabilitation involves goals and outcomes that are determined by the client and that depend on who, what, and where the client wants to be at any given point in this process. Most therapists would very readily agree with that statement, and most therapists agree that they know what outcomes should be achieved in "rehabilitating" a person with a spinal cord injury. Many therapists would also agree that they know that their goals and those of a client typically are in agreement.

This was disputed by Taylor,[233] who found a vast difference between the goals that occupational therapists set for persons with quadriplegia and the goals that the persons with quadriplegia had established for themselves. Quadriplegic clients identified work tolerance, muscle strengthening, bowel and bladder control, wheelchair mobility, and transfer ability as their most important goals. Occupational therapists rated development of adapted equipment and devices as most important, followed by eating skills, socialization, wheelchair mobility, and writing/typing skills. The persons with quadriplegia ranked the development of assistive devices thirteenth in importance to them. Taylor concluded that therapists may not be communicating goals to clients or soliciting feedback from clients regarding their goals and needs as often as they should to ensure the active involvement of the client in this process. Curtis also discussed conflicts between physical therapists' goals to promote patient independence and the therapist's ability to achieve role satisfaction.[59]

Treischmann[238] makes the point that aides and orderlies often spend the most time with clients and yet probably have the least developed personal interactive skills. A similar point can be made for physical therapists. We spend large amounts of time with our clients, yet our educational curricula typically provides little training in the psychological and counseling skills necessary to effectively interact with a client in a rehabilitation setting. Few students graduating in physical therapy today have even a moderate insight into such areas as listening skills, interviewing techniques, the complex concepts that constitute motivation, and how motivation is facilitated. More pragmatically, they often have little knowledge regarding the current theories on both a person's possible emotional reaction to the onset of a major injury and what factors are associated with adjusting to and coping with spinal cord injury or other major disabling injuries or illnesses. Most major rehabilitation facilities have staffs that consist of young physical therapists who are trying to develop their concepts and techniques of treatment. In this process they are trying to gain insight into a client's psychological coping and into their own reactions to this process called rehabilitation. The result is often "burnout," and the perpetuation of young staff again going through this process with less than adequate skills.

This problem was addressed by Gunther,[96] who, after many years of working as a consulting psychiatrist in a major rehabilitation hospital, concluded that staff members who work with clients with spinal cord injuries and with other massive physical disabilities have more frequent and more intense personal distress in their lives than do staff members who work with less seriously ill clients. Gunther concluded that the key to this problem is improved education of staff to better understand and formulate methods and skills to deal with these often unrecognized anxieties. For physical therapists this education can start earlier in their basic curricula by increasing the level of psychological training to equal that of other professionals working in a rehabilitation setting.

Much has been written about the psychology of spinal cord injury. What, if any, are the stages that a person with a spinal cord injury goes through in "adjusting" to the situation? Is there such a thing as a "spinal cord personality?" What are strategies for dealing with prognosis decisions and communications? Can we identify clients who will be more successful at rehabilitation early on?[197] These, and many other issues, are beyond the scope of this chapter. The reader is referred to a well-referenced text, such as Treischmann.[238] The author also encourages the reader to actively interact with the psychologists and psychiatrists working with them in their rehabilitation setting.

This section provides some "hints" on how to be more effective in interacting in the rehabilitation of a client with a spinal cord injury. (See also Chapter 7.)

1. Try to gain an understanding of what it feels like to have a spinal cord injury. Talk to your clients and try to get "inside of their skins." Get a sense of how they must feel or gain some insight into what they are going through.

Theodore Cole, a psychologist, had a client describe himself as "a head and shoulders floating in space." Read some of the available written reactions of persons with spinal cord injuries.[30,90,239]

2. Get to know your client as a normal human being. Read his or her chart and talk to family and friends. It is difficult to relate to people you know nothing about. Take the time to ask your client to "tell me about yourself."

3. Be cognizant of the timing involved in the rehabilitation process. Select tasks that your client can succeed at. Be aware that a client has to be ready to learn a skill or attain a goal. Remember that problem-solving is the art of what is possible, not the art of what is perfect. Closely monitor the frustration and fatigue level of your client.

4. Summarize achievement periodically: "Here is where we are and here is where I think we should go next." Then confirm agreement with your client. This process is especially important at the beginning and end of treatment sessions.

5. Establish an ongoing communication and problem-solving process with your client. Give reasons for tasks, explain how they relate to established goals, and, most importantly, facilitate self-responsibility and gradually increasing autonomy within the rehabilitation process. A client has to feel that what he or she is going through belongs to him or her, that he or she has control and not being manipulated by the rehabilitation team.

6. Finally, be in touch with your own feelings about your client. Be aware of any negative feelings you may be having toward a client and be willing to seek advice and help from your support systems in dealing with these feelings.

A final comment needs to be made regarding the client following discharge from the rehabilitation facility. The therapist and the team have the responsibility to prepare the client for this period and to instill insight as to what factors will need to be considered and dealt with to achieve and maintain a state of good, and hopefully improving, "postdischarge wellness." There are many things to consider outside of independence in functional skills. Issues of maintaining and improving physical fitness, nutrition, finances, housing, transportation needs and issues, advocacy for disabled person's rights, ongoing educational needs, and social support systems are a few facets of "doing well." There has also been a recent trend to establish independent living centers around the country. These centers are typically staffed by people who have physical disabilities and who can provide peer counseling and appropriate referrals for many of these issues. Many clients with spinal cord injuries and many other physically disabled clients are "lost" after discharge. Others assume a self-defeating lifestyle as confirmed by MacCleod,[143] who sampled 400 patients postdischarge and found 9% exhibited self-neglecting behavior. Therapists and other professionals in a rehabilitation setting need to take responsibility for establishing some strategies and means of communication for assuring the maintained and improved well-being of their clients long after discharge.

REFERENCES

1. Abramson AS: Bone disturbances in injuries to spinal cord and cauda equina (paraplegia): their prevention by ambulation, J Bone Joint Surg (Am) 30:982, 1948.
2. Agrawal BK and others: Webbelt loop for relief of pressure on buttocks, Arch Phys Med Rehabil 59:346, 1978.
3. Agris J and Spira M: Pressure ulcers: prevention and treatment, Ciba Clin Symp 31:1, 1979.
4. Alvarez SE and others: Respiratory treatment of the adult patient with spinal cord injury, Phys Ther 61:1737, 1981.
5. Anderson TP and Andberg MM: Psychosocial factors associated with pressure sores, Arch Phys Med Rehabil 60:341, 1979.
6. Antler L and others: Attitudes of rehabilitation patients toward the wheelchair, J Psychol 73:45, 1969.
7. Asael W: An approach to motherhood for disabled women, Rehabil Lit 43:214, 1982.
8. Bajd T and others: Use of a two-channel functional electrical stimulator to stand paraplegic patients, Phys Ther 61:526, 1981.
9. Bake B and others: Breathing patterns and regional ventilation distribution in tetraplegic patients and in normal subjects, Clin Sci 42:117, 1972.
10. Baker M and others: Developing strategies for biofeedback, Phys Ther 4:402, 1977.
11. Barolat G and others: Immediate effects of spinal cord stimulation on spinal spasticity, J Neurosurg 62:558, 1985.
12. Basmajian JA: Therapeutic exercise, ed 5, Baltimore, 1988, The Williams & Wilkins Co.
13. Beckman J: The Louisiana State University Reciprocating Gait Orthosis, Physiotherapy 73:386, 1987.
14. Bedbrook GM: Correction of scoliosis due to paraplegia sustained in pediatric age group, Paraplegia 15:90, 1977.
15. Bedbrook GM: Recovery of spinal cord function, Paraplegia 18:315, 1980.
16. Bedbrook GM: The care and management of spinal cord injuries, New York, 1981, Springer-Verlag New York, Inc.
17. Belson P: Autonomic nervous system dysfunction in recent spinal cord injured patients: a physical therapist's perspective. In Eisenberg MG and Falconer JA, editors: Treatment of the spinal cord injured, Springfield, Ill, 1978, Charles C Thomas Publisher.
18. Biering-Sorenson F and others: Bone mineral content of the lumbar spine and lower extremities years after spinal cord lesion, Paraplegia 26:293, 1988.
19. Black KS and Ferris E: Progressive rehabilitation of the patient in a spinal orthotics, Top Acute Care Trauma Rehabil 1:62, 1987.
20. Bohlman HH and others: Spine and spinal cord injuries. In Rothman RH and Simeone FA, editors: The spine, vol 2, ed 2, Philadelphia, 1982, WB Saunders Co.
21. Bracken MB and Shepard MJ: Coping and adaptation following acute spinal cord injury: a theoretical analysis, Paraplegia 18:74, 1980.
22. Bracken MB and others: Incidence of acute traumatic hospitalized spinal cord injury in the United States, 1970-1977, Am J Epidemiol 113:615, 1981.
23. Bricolo A and others: Local cooling in spinal cord injuries, Surg Neurol 6:101, 1976.
24. Brindley GS and others: Electrical splinting of the knee in paraplegia, Paraplegia 16:428, 1979.
25. Bromley I: Tetraplegia and paraplegia: a guide for physiotherapists, ed 3, New York, 1988, Churchill Livingstone, Inc.
26. Brookey JS and others: The syndrome of acute central cervical spinal cord injury revisited, Surg Neurol 14:251, 1980.

27. Brooks GS: Effects of a cervical orthosis and visual occlusion on dynamic balance, master's thesis, Boston University, 1981.

28. Brown-Sequard CE: Lectures on the physiology and pathology of the nervous system, Lancet 1:219, 1869.

29. Brucker BS and Ince LP: Biofeedback as an experimental treatment for postural hypotension in a patient with a spinal cord lesion, Arch Phys Med Rehabil 58:49, 1977.

30. Bucy PC: Sitting on a basketball: how it feels to be a paraplegic, Prospect Biol Med 17:151, 1974.

31. Burke DC: Hyperextension injuries of the spine, J Bone Joint Surg (B) 53:3, 1971.

32. Burke DC: Pain in paraplegia, Paraplegia 10:297, 1973.

33. Burke DC: Injuries of the spinal cord in children. In Vinken, PJ and Bruyn GW, editors: Handbook of clinical neurology, vol 25, New York, 1976, American Elsevier Publishers, Inc.

34. Burke DC and Murray DD: Handbook of spinal cord injuries, New York, 1975, Raven Press.

35. Butler PB and others: The technique of reciprocal walking using the Hip Guidance Orthosis (HGO) with crutches, Prosthet Orthot Int 8:33, 1984.

36. Butler PB and Major R: The Para Walker: a rational approach to the provisions of reciprocal ambulation for paraplegic patients, Physiotherapy 73:393, 1987.

37. Byers RK: Spinal cord injuries during birth, Dev Med Child Neurol 17:103, 1975.

38. Calenoff L and others: Multiple level spinal injuries: importance of early recognition, Am J Roentgenol 130:665, 1978.

39. Calenoff L and others: Lumbar fracture dislocation related to range-of-motion exercises, Arch Phys Med Rehabil 60:183, 1979.

40. Campbell J and Bonnett C: Spinal cord injury in children, Clin Orthop 112:114, 1975.

41. Carter RE: Medical management of pulmonary complications of spinal cord injury, Adv Neurol 22:261, 1979.

42. Carter RE and Donovan WM: Reflections of impact of electrophrenic respiration in the management of high quadriplegics, Sci Digest 3:37, 1981.

43. Cerney K and others: Walking and wheelchair energetics in persons with paraplegia, Phys Ther 60:1133, 1980.

44. Cerullo LJ: Cervical spine stabilization in spinal cord injury. In Calenoff L, editor: Radiology of spinal cord injury, St Louis, 1981, The CV Mosby Co.

45. Chantraine A: Actual concept of osteoporosis in paraplegia, Paraplegia 16:51, 1978.

46. Chapman CE and Weisendanger M: The physiological and anatomical basis of spasticity: a review, Physiotherapy (Canada) 34:125, 1982.

47. Chesire DJ and Flack WJ: The use of operant conditioning techniques in the respiratory rehabilitation of the tetraplegic, Paraplegia 16:162, 1978.

48. Claus-Walker J and Halstead LS: Metabolic and endocrine changes in spinal cord injury. I. The nervous system before and after transection of the spinal cord, Arch Phys Med Rehabil 62:595, 1981.

49. Claus-Walker J and Halstead LS: Metabolic and endocrine changes in spinal cord injury. II. Consequences of partial decentralization of the autonomic nervous system, Arch Phys Med Rehabil 63:569, 1982.

50. Claus-Walker J and Halsted LS: Metabolic and endocrine changes in spinal cord injury. III. Less quanta of sensory input plus bedrest and illness, Arch Phys Med Rehabil 63:628, 1982.

51. Claus-Walker J and Halstead LS: Metabolic and endocrine changes in spinal cord injury. IV. Compounded neurological dysfunctions, Arch Phys Med Rehabil 63:632, 1982.

52. Claus-Walker J and others: Spinal cord injury hypercalcemia: therapeutic profile, Arch Phys Med Rehabil 63:108, 1982.

53. Clough P and others: Guidelines for routine respiratory care of patients with spinal cord injury, Phys Ther 66:1395, 1986.

54. Cloward RB: Acute cervical spine injuries, Ciba Clin Symp 32:15, 1980.

55. Colyer RA and Kappelman B: Flexor pollicis longus tenodesis in tetraplegia at the sixth cervical level: a prospective evaluation of functional gain, J Bone Joint Surg (A) 63:376, 1981.

56. Comarr AE: Sexual function in patients with spinal cord injury. In Pierce DS and Nickel VH editors: The total care of spinal cord injuries, Boston, 1977, Little, Brown & Company.

57. Conomy JP: Disorders of body image after spinal cord injury, Neurology (NY) 23:842, 1973.

58. Cooney MM and Walker JB: Hydraulic resistance exercise benefits cardiovascular fitness of spinal cord injured, Med Sci Sports Exerc 18:522, 1986.

59. Curtis KA: Physical therapist role satisfaction in the treatment of the spinal cord injured person, Phys Ther 65:197, 1985.

60. Damanski M: Heterotopic ossification in paraplegia: a clinical study, J Bone Joint Surg (B) 43:286, 1961.

61. Daniel RK and others: Etiologic factors in pressure sores: an experimental model, Arch Phys Med Rehabil 62:492, 1981.

62. Davidoff G and others: Closed head injury in acute traumatic spinal cord injury: incidence and risk factors, Arch Phys Med Rehabil 69:869, 1988.

63. Davis R: Spasticity following spinal cord injury, Clin Orthop 112:66, 1975.

64. Davis R: Pain and suffering following spinal cord injury, Clin Orthop 112:76, 1975.

65. Davis R and Lentini R: Transcutaneous nerve stimulation for treatment of pain in patients with spinal cord injury, Surg Neurol 4:100, 1975.

66. Dehn ODM: Effect of arm ergometry training on wheelchair propulsion endurance of individuals with quadriplegia, Phys Ther 68:40, 1988.

67. Dehner JR: Seatbelt injuries of the spine and abdomen, Am J Roentgenol 111:833, 1971.

68. Donovan WH and Bedbrook G: Comprehensive management of spinal cord injury, Ciba Clin Symp, vol 34, no 2, 1982.

69. Duffus A and Wood J: Standing and walking for the T6 paraplegic, Physiotherapy 69:45, 1983.

70. Duttarer J and Edberg E: Quadriplegia after spinal cord injury: a treatment guide for physical therapists, Thorofare, NJ, 1972, Charles B Slack, Inc.

71. Edberg EL and others: Prevention and treatment of pressure sores, Phys Ther 53:246, 1973.

72. Edmonds VE and Tator CH: Coordination of a halo program for an acute spinal cord injury unit. In Tator CH editor: Early management of acute spinal cord injury, New York, 1982, Raven Press.

73. El Masri WS and Silver JR: Prophylactic anticoagulant therapy in patients with spinal cord injury, Paraplegia 19:334, 1981.

74. Enis JE and Sarmiento A: The pathophysiology and management of pressure sores, Orthop Rev 11:25, 1973.

75. Erickson RP: Autonomic hyperreflexia: pathophysiology and medical management, Arch Phys Med Rehabil 61:431, 1980.

76. Farrell RJ: A hydrotherapy program for high cervical cord lesion, Physiotherapy (Canada) 28:8, 1976.

77. Fett HC and Yost JG: Neurogenic ossifying fibromyopathies, Am J Surg 82:517, 1951.

78. Firooznia H and others: Computed tomography of pressure sores, pelvic abscess, and osteomyelitis in patients with spinal cord injury, Arch Phys Med Rehabil 63:545, 1982.

79. Flanc C and others: Postoperative deep-vein thrombosis, effect of intensive prophylaxis, Lancet 1:477, 1969.

80. Ford JR and Duckworth B: Physical management for the quadriplegic patient, ed 2, Philadelphia, 1987, FA Davis Co.

81. Freehafer AA and others: Lower extremity fractures in patients with spinal cord injury, Paraplegia 19:367, 1981.

82. Reference deleted in proofs.

83. Frisbie JH and Sasahara AA: Low dose heparin prophylaxis for deep vein thrombosis in acute spinal cord injury patients: a controlled study, Paraplegia 19:343, 1981.

84. Frownfelter DL, editor: Chest physical therapy and pulmonary rehabilitation, ed 2, Chicago, 1987, Year Book Medical Publishers, Inc.

85. Gaddy J: A standing device for paraplegics, Arch Phys Med Rehabil 58:86, 1977.

86. Gamache FW Jr and others: The clinical application of hyperbaric oxygen therapy in spinal cord injury: a preliminary report, Surg Neurol 15:85, 1981.

87. Gehrig R and Michaelis LS: Statistics of acute paraplegia and tetraplegia on a national scale, Paraplegia 10:232, 1976.

88. Geiser M and Trueta J: Muscle action, bone rarefaction and bone formation: experimental study, J Bone Joint Surg (B) 40:282, 1958.

89. Gerhart KA: Increasing sensory and motor stimulation for the patient with quadriplegia, Phys Ther 59:1518, 1979.

90. Goldiamond I: A diary of self-modification, Psychology Today 7:95, 1973.

91. Gore RM and Mintzer RA: Gastrointestinal complications. In Calenoff L, editor: Radiology of spinal cord injury, St Louis, 1981, The CV Mosby Co.

92. Green BA and others: Acute spinal cord injury: current concepts, Clin Orthop 154:125, 1981.

93. Griffith HB and others: Changing patterns of fracture in the dorsal and lumbar spine, Br Med J 1:891, 1966.

94. Gross D and others: The effect of training on strength and endurance of the diaphragm in quadriplegia, Am J Med 68:27, 1980.

95. Grzesiak RC: Relaxation techniques in treatment of chronic pain, Arch Phys Med Rehabil 58:270, 1977.

96. Gunther MS: The threatened staff: a psychoanalytic contribution to medical psychology, Compr Psychiatry 18:385, 1977.

97. Guttman L: Initial treatment of traumatic paraplegia and tetraplegia. In Guttman L, editor: Spinal injuries, Edinburgh, 1966, The Royal College of Surgeons.

98. Guttman L: Spinal shock and reflex behavior in man, Paraplegia 8:100, 1970.

99. Haas F and others: Time related, posturally induced changes in pulmonary function in spinal cord injured man, Am Rev Respir Dis 117:344, 1978.

100. Hagisawa S and others: Pressure sores: a biochemical test for early detection of tissue damage, Arch Phys Med Rehabil 69:668, 1988.

101. Halpren D and Meelhuysen FE: Phenol motor point block in management of muscular hypertonia, Arch Phys Med Rehabil 47:659, 1966.

102. Hancock DA and others: Bone and soft tissue changes in paraplegic patients, Paraplegia 17:267, 1979.

103. Hansebout RR: A comprehensive review of methods of improving cord recovery after acute spinal cord injury. In Tator CH, editor: Early management of acute spinal cord injury, New York, 1982, Raven Press.

104. Harvey RF and Jellinek HM: Functional performance assessment: a program approach, Arch Phys Med Rehabil 62:456, 1981.

105. Hein-Sorenson O and others: Disc pressure measurements in para- and tetraplegic patients: a study of mobilization and exercise in para- and tetraplegic patients, Scand J Rehabil Med 11:1, 1979.

106. Hendrix RW: Joint changes after spinal cord injury. In Calenoff L, editor: Radiology of spinal cord injury, St Louis, 1981, The CV Mosby Co.

107. Hendrix RW: Skeletal changes after spinal cord injury. In Calenoff L, editor: Radiology of spinal cord injury, St Louis, 1981, The CV Mosby Co.

108. Hendrix RW: Soft tissue changes after spinal cord injury. In Calenoff L, editor: Radiology of spinal cord injury, St Louis, 1981, The CV Mosby Co.

109. Henry's P and others: Clinical review of cervical spine injuries in children, Clin Orthop 129:172, 1977.

110. Holdsworth FW: Fractures, dislocations and fracture-dislocations of the spine, J Bone Joint Surg (A) 52:1534, 1970.

111. Hoppenfeld S: Orthopaedic neurology: a diagnostic guide to neurological levels, Philadelphia, 1977, JB Lippincott Co.

112. Hossack DW and King A: Neurogenic heterotopic ossification, Med J Aust 1:326, 1967.

113. Huang CT and others: Energy cost of ambulation in paraplegic patients using Craig-Scott braces, Arch Phys Med Rehabil 60:595, 1979.

114. Huitt CT and Gwyer JL: Paraplegic ambulatory training using Craig-Scott orthoses, Phys Ther 58:976, 1978.

115. Hussey RW and Stauffer ES: Spinal cord injury: requirements for ambulation, Arch Phys Med Rehabil 54:544, 1973.

116. Imle PC and Boughton AC: The physical therapist's role in the early management of acute spinal cord injury, Top Acute Care Trauma Rehabil 1:32, 1987.

117. Jefferson G: Discussion on spinal injuries, Proc R Soc Med 21:625, 1927.

118. Jensen LL and others: Neurogenic heterotopic ossification, Am J Phys Med 66:351, 1988.

119. Johnston B: Pregnancy and childbirth in women with spinal cord injuries: a review of the literature, Maternal-Child Nursing Journal 11:41, 1982.

120. Johnstone BR and others: A review of surgical rehabilitation of the upper extremity in quadriplegia, Paraplegia 26:317, 1988.

121. Kaplan LI and others: Reappraisal of braces and other mechanical aids in patients with spinal cord dysfunction: results of follow-up study, Arch Phys Med Rehabil 47:393, 1966.

122. Kassel EE: Myelography and computerized tomography for diagnosis in acute cervical cord injury. In Tator CH, editor: Early management of acute spinal cord injury, New York, 1982, Raven Press.

123. Katz JF: Spontaneous fractures in paraplegic children, J Bone Joint Surg (A) 35:220, 1953.

124. Kewalramani LS: Autonomic dysreflexia in traumatic myelopathy, Am J Phys Med 59:1, 1980.

125. Kewalramani LS: Spinal cord injury in children. In Calenoff L, editor: Radiology of spinal cord injury, St Louis, 1981, The CV Mosby Co.

126. Kewalramani LS and Taylor RG: Multiple noncontiguous injuries to the spine, Acta Orthop Scand 47:52, 1976.

127. Kewalramani LS and Tori JA: Spinal cord trauma in children—neurological patterns, radiological features and pathomechanics of injury, Spine 5:11, 1980.

128. Kewalramani LS and others: Acute spinal cord lesions in a pediatric population—epidemiological and clinical features, Paraplegia 18:206, 1980.

129. Khalili AA and others: Management of spasticity by selective phen-phenol nerve block with dilute phenol solutions in clinical rehabilitation, Arch Phys Med Rehabil 45:513, 1964.

130. Khalili AH and Hamash MH: Spinal cord regeneration: new experimental approach, Paraplegia 26:310, 1985.

131. Kopala B and Egenes KH: The physically disabled parent: assessment and intervention, Top Clin Nurs 24:10, 1984.

132. Klein RM and Bell B: Self-care skills: behavioral measurement with Klein-Bell ADL scale, Arch Phys Med Rehabil 63:335, 1982.

133. Koch BM and Eng GM: Neonatal spinal cord injury, Arch Phys Med Rehabil 60:378, 1979.

134. Kogl J and Loe ML: Sliding board modification for persons with C6-7 quadriplegia, Phys Ther 61:1291, 1981.

135. Kottke FJ and others: The rationale for prolonged stretching for cor-

rection of shortening of connective tissue, Arch Phys Med Rehabil 47:345, 1966.

136. Lehmkuhl DL: Evoked spinal, brain stem and cerebral potentials. In Wolf SL, editor: Clinics in physical therapy, vol 2, Electrotherapy, New York, 1981, Churchill Livingstone, Inc.

137. Liberson WT: Experiment concerning reciprocal inhibition of antagonists elicited by electrical stimulation of agonists in normal individuals, Am J Phys Med 36:306, 1965.

138. Liberson WT and others: Functional electrotherapy: stimulation of the peroneal nerve synchronized with the swing phase of the gait of hemiplegic patients, Arch Phys Med Rehabil 42:101, 1961.

139. Lindan R and others: Incidence and clinical features of autonomic dysreflexia in patients with spinal cord injury, Paraplegia 18:285, 1980.

140. Lipschitz R: Associated injuries and complications of stab wounds in the spinal cord, Paraplegia 5:75, 1967.

141. Lynch C and others: Heterotopic ossification in the hand of a patient with spinal cord injury, Arch Phys Med Rehabil 62:291, 1981.

142. Mackenzie CF and others: Chest physiotherapy in the intensive care unit, Baltimore, 1981, The Williams & Wilkins Co.

143. MacLeod AD: Self-neglect of spinal injured patients, Paraplegia 26:340, 1988.

144. Mahoney FI and Barthel BA: Functional evaluation: the Barthel index, Md State Med J 14:61, 1965.

145. Malament IR and others: Pressure sores: an operant conditioning approach to prevention, Arch Phys Med Rehabil 56:161, 1975.

146. Maloney FP: Pulmonary function in quadriplegia: effects of a corset, Arch Phys Med Rehabil 60:261, 1979.

147. Massery M: An innovative approach to assistive cough techniques, Top Acute Care Trauma Rehabil 1;1, 1987.

148. McAdam R and Natvig H: Stair climbing and ability to work for paraplegics with complete lesions—a sixteen year follow-up, Paraplegia 18:197, 1980.

149. McGarry J and others: Autonomic hyperreflexia following passive stretching to the hip joint, Phys Ther 62:30, 1982.

150. McGee M and Hertling D: Equipment and transfer techniques used by C6 quadriplegic patients, Phys Ther 57:1372, 1977.

151. McMichan JC and others: Pulmonary dysfunction following traumatic quadriplegia: recognition, prevention and treatment, JAMA 243:528, 1980.

152. Merritt JL: Management of spasticity in spinal cord injury, Mayo Clin Proc 56614, 1981.

153. Meyer PR: Closed reduction of spinal fracture and dislocations. In Calenoff L, editor: Radiology of spinal cord injury, St Louis, 1981, The CV Mosby Co.

154. Meyer PR: Emergency care of spinal cord injury. In Calenoff L, editor: Radiology of spinal cord injury, St Louis, 1981, The CV Mosby Co.

155. Meyer PR: Thoracic and lumbar spine stabilization in spinal cord injury. In Calenoff L, editor: Radiology of spinal cord injury, St Louis, 1981, The CV Mosby Co.

156. Meyer PR and Gireesan GT: Management of acute spinal cord injury Carr system, Top Acute Care Trauma Rehabil 1:1, 1987.

157. Meyer PR and others: Annual Progress Report IX (1981), Midwest Regional Spinal Cord Injury Care System, OHD-RSA-DHEW Grant No 13-P-55864.

158. Meyer PR and others: Annual Progress Report I (1972), Midwest Regional Spinal Cord Injury Care System, OHD-RSA-DHEW Grant No 13-P-55864.

159. Meyer PR and others: Annual Progress Report VII (1978), Midwest Regional Spinal Cord Injury Care System, OHD-RSA-DHEW-Grant No 13P-55864.

160. Michaelis LS: International inquiry on neurological terminology and prognosis in paraplegia and tetraplegia, Paraplegia 7:1, 1969.

161. Mikelberg R and Reid S: Spinal cord lesions and lower extremity bracing: an overview and follow-up study, Paraplegia 19:379, 1981.

162. Miller HJ and others: Pneumobelt use among high quadriplegics population, Arch Phys Med Rehabil 69:369, 1988.

163. Miller SL and Sperling KB: Evaluation and respiratory management of C_3 quadriplegia lacking diaphragm function, Arch Phys Med Rehabil 64:496, 1983.

164. Miller S and others: Sexual health care clinician in an acute spinal cord unit, Arch Phys Med Rehabil 62:315, 1981.

165. Mintzer RA and Gore RM: Pulmonary and other chest complications. In Calenoff L, editor: Radiology of spinal cord injury, St Louis, 1981, The CV Mosby Co.

166. Reference deleted in proofs.

167. Moe P: An approach for the physical therapy management of the individual with C6 quadriplegia, Houston, 1979, The Institute for Rehabilitation and Research.

168. Moskowitz E and McCann CB: Classification of disability in the chronically ill and aged, J Chronic Dis 5:342, 1957.

169. Mueller DG: Clinical applications in spinal orthotics, Top Acute Care Trauma Rehabil 1:48, 1987.

170. Nacht MB and others: Use of electromyographic biofeedback during the acute phase of spinal cord injury: a case report, Phys Ther 62:290, 1982.

171. Naftchi NE: Functional restoration of the traumatically injured spinal cord in cats by clonidine, Science 217:1042, 1982.

172. Naso F: Pulmonary embolism in acute spinal cord injury, Arch Phys Med Rehabil 55:275, 1974.

173. Natvig H and McAdam R: Ambulation without wheelchairs for paraplegics with complete lesions, Paraplegia 16:142, 1978.

174. Nepomuceno C and others: Pain in patients with spinal cord injuries, Arch Phys Med Rehabil 60:605, 1979.

175. Nicholas JJ: Ectopic bone formation in patients with spinal cord injury, Arch Phys Med Rehabil 54:354, 1973.

176. Nichols PJ and others: Wheelchair user's shoulder? Shoulder pain in patients with spinal cord lesions, Scand J Rehabil Med 11:29, 1979.

177. Nickel LD and others: Pressure ulceration: a philosophy of management, Sci Digest 4:36:, 1982.

178. Nixon V: Spinal cord injury: a guide to functional outcomes in physical therapy management, Rockville, Md, 1985, Aspen Systems Corp.

179. Noble PC: The prevention of pressure sores in persons with spinal cord injuries, Monograph no 11, World Rehabilitation Fund, Inc, (400 East 34th St, New York, NY 10016), 1981.

180. O'Daniel WE and Hahn HR: Follow-up usage of the Scott-Craig orthosis in paraplegia, Paraplegia 19:373, 1981.

181. Odéen I: Reduction of muscular hypertonus by long-term muscle stretch, Scand J Rehabil Med 13:93, 1981.

182. Ohry A and others: Shoulder complications as a cause of delay in rehabilitation of spinal cord patients, Paraplegia 16:310, 1978.

183. O'Sullivan SB and others: Physical rehabilitation: assessment and treatment, ed 2, Philadelphia, 1988 FA Davis Co.

184. Pachalski A and others: Effects of swimming on increasing cardiorespiratory capacity in paraplegics, Paraplegia 18:190, 1980.

185. Peckham PH and others: Restoration of functional control by electrical stimulation in the upper extremity of the quadriplegic patient, J Bone Joint Surg (A)70:144, 1988.

186. Penn RD and Kroin JS: Long-term intrathecal baclofen infusion for treatment of spasticity, J Neurosurg 66:181, 1987.

187. Perlman SG: Spinal cord injury: a review of experimental implications for clinical prognosis and treatment, Arch Phys Med Rehabil 55:81, 1974.

188. Perry J: Prescription principles. In American Academy of Orthopaedic Surgeons, Atlas of orthotics: biomechanical principles and applications, St Louis, 1975, The CV Mosby Co.

189. Pledger HG: Disorders of temperature regulation in acute traumatic tetraplegia, J Bone Joint Surg (B) 44:110, 1962.

190. Plum F and Dunning MF: Effect of therapeutic mobilization on hypercalciuria following acute poliomyelitis, Arch Intern Med 101:528, 1958.

191. Pochala E and Windle WF: The possibility of structural and functional restitution after spinal cord injury: a review, Exp Neurol 55:1, 1977.

192. Putnam T and others: Sinography in management of decubitus ulcers, Arch Phys Med Rehabil 59:243, 1978.

193. Rafii M and others: Bilateral acetabular stress fractures in a paraplegic patient, Arch Phys Med Rehabil 63:240, 1982.

194. Ragnarsson KT: Standing devices for paraplegics: an alternative to bracing, Sci Digest 3:5, 1981.

195. Ragnarsson KT and Sell GH: Lower extremity fractures after spinal cord injury: a retrospective study, Arch Phys Med Rehabil 62:418, 1981.

196. Ragnarsson KT and others: Clinical evaluation of computerized functional electrical stimulation after spinal cord injury: a multicentral pilot study, Arch Phys Med Rehabil 69:672, 1988

197. Richards JS: Psychological adjustment to spinal cord injury during first post-discharge year, Arch Phys Med Rehabil 67:362, 1986.

198. Richardson RR and McLone DG: Percutaneous epidural neurostimulation of paraplegic spasticity, Surg Neurol 9:153, 1978.

199. Richardson RR and Meyer PR: Prevalence and incidence of pressure sores in acute spinal cord injuries, Paraplegia 19:235, 1981.

200. Reference deleted in proofs.

201. Richardson RR and others: Transcutaneous electrical neurostimulation in musculoskeletal pain in acute spinal cord injuries, Spine 5:42, 1980.

202. Riggins RS and Kraus JF: The risk of neurologic damage with fractures of the vertebrae, J Trauma 17:126, 1977.

203. Roberts JB and Curtiss PH Jr: Stability of the thoracic and lumbar spine in traumatic paraplegia following fracture or fracture dislocation, J Bone Joint Surg (A) 52:1115, 1970.

204. Robinson CJ and others: Spasticity in spinal cord injured patients. II. Initial measures and long-term effects of surface electrical stimulation, Arch Phys Med Rehabil 69:862, 1988.

205. Rodriguez GP and Claus-Walker J: Biochemical changes in skin composition in spinal injury: a possible contribution to decubitus ulcers, Paraplegia 26:302, 1988.

206. Rogers LF: The roentgenographic appearance of transverse or chance fractures of the spine: the seat belt fracture, Am J Roentgenol 111:844, 1971.

207. Rogers LF; Fractures and dislocations of the spine. In Calenoff L, editor: Radiology of spinal cord injury, St Louis, 1981, The CV Mosby Co.

208. Roncorani AJ: Lack of breathlessness during apnea in a patient with high spinal cord transection, Chest 62:514, 1972.

209. Rosen JS: Rehabilitation process. In Calenoff L, editor: Radiology of spinal cord injury, St Louis, 1981, The CV Mosby Co.

210. Rossi EC and others: Sequential changes in factor VIII and platelets preceding deep vein thrombosis in patients with spinal cord injury, Br J Haematol 45:143, 1980.

211. Rossier AB and others: Current facts on para-osteo-arthroplasty (PAO), Paraplegia 11:36, 1973.

212. Rowed DW and others: Somatosensory evoked potentials in acute spinal cord injury: prognostic value, Surg Neurol 9:203, 1978.

213. Rusk H: Rehabilitation medicine, ed 4, St Louis, 1977, The CV Mosby Co.

214. Sabbahi MA and others: Topical anesthesia: a possible treatment method for spasticity, Arch Phys Med Rehabil 62:310, 1981.

215. Sadowsky S and others: Use of myoelectric and volume-linked feedback techniques for breathing training in patients with spinal cord injuries, Resp Care 26:130, 1981.

216. Schneider RC and others: Traumatic spinal cord syndromes and their management, Clin Neurosurg 20:367, 1973.

217. Schweigel JF: Halo devices for cervical spine injuries without neurological deficit. In Tator CH, editor: Early management of acute spinal cord injury, New York, 1982, Raven Press.

218. Scott B: Engineering principles and fabrication techniques for the Scott-Craig long leg braces for paraplegics, Orth Pros 25:14, 1971.

219. Scott JA and Donovan WH: The prevention of shoulder pain and contracture in the acute tetraplegic patient, Paraplegia 19:313, 1981.

220. Seymour RJ and Bassler CR: Electromyographic biofeedback in the treatment of incomplete paraplegia, Phys Ther 57:1148, 1977.

221. Seymour RJ and others: Paraplegic use of the Orlau swivel walker: case report, Arch Phys Med Rehabil 63:490, 1982.

222. Shea JD: Pressure sores: classification and management, Clin Orthop 112:91, 1975.

223. Silver JR: Heterotopic ossification: clinical study of its possible relationship to trauma, Paraplegia 7:220, 1969.

224. Sindo N and Jones R: Reciprocal patterned electrical stimulation of the lower limbs in severe spasticity, Physiotherapy 73:580, 1987.

225. Smith TK and others: Complications associated with the use of the circular electric turning frame, J Bone Joint Surg (A) 57:711, 1975.

226. Stauffer ES: Diagnosis and prognosis of acute cervical spinal cord injury, Clin Orthop 112:9, 1975.

227. Stover SL: Spinal cord injuries: the facts and figures, Birmingham, 1986, University of Alabama.

228. Stover SL and others: Heterotopic ossification in spinal cord injured patients, Arch Phys Med Rehabil 56:199, 1975.

229. Stover SL and others: Disodium etioronate in the prevention of postoperative recurrance of heterotopic ossification in spinal cord injured patients, J Bone Joint Surg (A) 58:683, 1976.

230. Sullivan PE and others: An integrated approach to therapeutic exercise, Reston Va, 1982, Reston Publishing Co, Inc.

231. Summers BN and others: A clinical review of the Adult Hip Guidance Orthosis (Para Walker) in traumatic paraplegics, Paraplegia 26:19, 1988.

232. Tator CH and others: Halo devices for the treatment of acute cervical spinal cord injury. In Tator CH, editor: Early management of acute spinal cord injury, New York, 1982, Raven Press.

233. Taylor D: Treatment goals for quadriplegic and paraplegic patients, Am J Occup Ther 28:22, 1974.

234. Tibone J and others: Heterotopic ossification around the hip in spinal cord injured patients, J Bone Joint Surg (A) 60:769, 1978.

235. Toerge J and others: Secondary spinal lesions in spinal cord injury patients, Arch Phys Med Rehabil 59:343, 1978.

236. Tori JA and Hill LL: Hypercalcemia in children with spinal cord injury, Arch Phys Med Rehabil 59:443, 1978.

237. Trafton PG: Spinal cord injuries, Surg Clin North Am 62:61, 1982.

238. Trieschmann RB: Spinal cord injury: psychological social and vocational adjustment, Elmsford, NY, 1980, Pergamon Press, Inc.

239. Valens E: A long way up: the story of Jill Kinmont, New York, 1966, Harper & Row Publishers, Inc.

240. Vanderlinden RG: The long term management of respiratory paralysis by diaphragm pacing in upper cervical cord injuries. In Tator CH, editor: Early management of acute spinal cord injury, New York, 1982, Raven Press.

241. Van Hove E: Prevention of thrombophlebitis in spinal injury patients, Paraplegia 16:332, 1978.

242. Van Steen H: Treatment of a patient with a complete C1 quadriplegia, Phys Ther 55:35, 1975.

243. Veer C: Physiotherapy for tetraplegics and paraplegics, Christchurch, New Zealand, 1978, Paraplegic Assn (CANTY), Inc.

244. Vodovnik L and others: Functional electrical stimulation for control of locomotor systems, CRC Crit Rev Bioeng 6:63, 1981.

245. Walton JN: Brain's diseases of the nervous system, ed 8, Oxford, England, 1977, Oxford University Press, Inc.

246. Watkins EM and others: Para Walker paraplegic walking, Physiotherapy 73:99, 1987.
247. Watson N: Patterns of spinal cord injury in the elderly, Paraplegia 14:36, 1976.
248. Weiss M: Dynamic spine alloplasty (spring-loading corrective devices) after fracture and spinal cord injury, Clin Orthop 112:150, 1975.
249. Wharton GW: Heterotopic ossification, Clin Orthop 112:142, 1975.
250. Wharton GW and Morgan TH: Ankylosis in the paralyzed patient, J Bone Joint Surg (A) 52:105, 1970.
251. Reference deleted in proofs.
252. Wylie EJ and Chakera TMH: Degenerative joint abnormalities in patients with paraplegia of duration greater than 20 years, Paraplegia 26:101, 1988.
253. Wyse DM and Pattee CJ: Effect of oscillating bed and tilt table on calcium, phosphorus and nitrogen metabolism in paraplegia, Am J Med 17:645, 1954.
254. Yarkony G and others: "Jones-Hedman Walker modification for C7 quadriplegic patient: case study in team cooperation, Arch Phys Med Rehabil 67:54, 1986.
255. Yarkony GM and others: Rehabilitation outcomes in C6 tetraplegia, Paraplegia 26:177, 1988.
256. Yarkony GM and others: Benefits of rehabilitation in spinal cord injury: multivariate analysis of 711 patients, Arch of Neurol 44:93, 1987.
257. Yarkony GM and others: Rehabilitation outcomes in 120 patients with C5 quadriplegia, Arch Phys Med Rehabil 68:672, 1987 (abstract).
258. Yashon D: Spinal injury, New York, 1978, Appleton-Century Crofts.
259. Yngve DA and others: The Reciprocating Gait Orthosis in myelomeningocele, J Ped Ortho 4:304, 1984.
260. Young JS: Initial hospitalization and rehabilitation costs of spinal cord injury, Orthop Clin North Am 9:263, 1978.
261. Young JS: Spinal cord injury: associated general trauma and medical complications. Adv Neurol 22:255, 1979.
262. Reference deleted in proofs.
263. Young JS and Burnst PE: Pressure sores and the spinal cord injured, parts I, II, III, Sci Digest, vol 3, 4, 1981-1982.
264. Young JS and Northrup NE: Statistical information pertaining to some of the most commonly asked questions about SCI, (monograph) Phoenix, 1979, National Spinal Cord Injury Data Research Center.
265. Young JS and others: Spinal cord injury statistics: experience of the regional spinal cord injury systems, Phoenix, 1982, Good Samaritan Medical Center.
266. Young W: Correlation of somatosensory evoked potentials and neurological findings in spinal cord injury. In Tator CH, editor: Early management of acute spinal cord injury, New York, 1982, Raven Press.
267. Zumwalt M and others: Glossopharyngeal Breathing, Phys Ther Review 36:455, 1956.

APPENDIX
Audiovisual resources
1. Physical Therapy Management of the Patient with Quadriplegia—Therapeutic Exercises (34 minute, color, ¾ inch U-Matic videotape)
Rehabilitation Institute of Chicago
Physical Therapy Education
345 East Superior Street
Chicago, IL 60611
2. Balancing and Gaiting Using Scott-Craig Long Leg Brace (45 minute, black and white, ¾ inch U-Matic videotape)
Craig Hospital
3425 South Clarkson
Inglewood, CO 80110
3. Ball Gymnastics for Postural Control (28 minute, color/sound, 16 mm film)
Bluehill Educational Systems
52 South Main Street
Spring Valley, NY 10977
4. Glossopharyngeal Breathing (10 minute, color, 16mm film)
Professional Staff Association of Ranchos Los Amigos Hospital
7413 Golondrinas Street
Downey, CA 90242
5. Consequences—Spinal Cord Injury (10 minute, color, 16 mm film)
Educational Services Department
University of Washington Press
Seattle, WA 98105

Chapter 16

THERAPEUTIC MANAGEMENT OF THE CLIENT WITH INFLAMMATORY AND INFECTIOUS DISORDERS WITHIN THE BRAIN

Rebecca E. Porter

The therapeutic management of the client with neurological sequelae that result from an inflammatory disorder within the brain (brain abscesses, encephalitis, or meningitis) challenges the therapist to deal with diverse problems and to creatively design an intervention program. Each client presents a combination of problems unique to that client only. Discussion of the therapeutic management of these clients as a diagnostic category therefore cannot focus on dealing with a set of "typical" problems, but rather will focus on the process of designing an intervention plan to deal with the specific dysfunctions of a specific client.

AN OVERVIEW OF INFLAMMATORY DISORDERS WITHIN THE BRAIN
Categorization of inflammatory disorders

Inflammatory disorders of the brain are categorized based on the anatomical location of the inflammatory process and the cause of the infection, as shown below.

A. Brain abscess
B. Meningitis (leptomeningitis)
    1. Bacterial meningitis
    2. Aseptic meningitis (viral)
C. Encephalitis
    1. Acute viral
    2. Parainfectious encephalomyelitis
    3. Acute toxic encephalopathy
    4. Progressive viral encephalitis
    5. "Slow virus" encephalitis

The inflammatory process may be a localized, circumscribed collection of pus, may involve primarily the leptomeninges, may involve the brain substance, or may involve both the meninges and the brain substance. The infecting agents may be bacterial, fungal, viral, protozoan, or parasitic. The most common agents producing meningitis are bacterial; the most common agents producing encephalitis are viral. However, bacterial encephalitis and viral meningitis also are disease entities. The following discussion of the inflammatory process within the brain will be organized based on the anatomical location of the infection.

Brain abscess

Brain abscesses occur when organisms such as pyogenic bacteria, colon bacilli, or *Pseudomonas aeruginosa* reach the brain tissue. The abscess may be a sequela to a penetrating wound to the brain, or more commonly, may manifest as a secondary infection as the result of an inflammatory process that involves the lungs, heart, cranial sinuses, or ear. The most frequent sites of involvement are the frontal and parietal lobes with the white matter more extensively involved than the gray matter. The initial symptoms of a brain abscess are those of a generalized infection and increased intracranial pressure. As the inflammatory process progresses, neurological symptoms appear that are specific to the area of involvement.

Meningitis

Definition. Meningitis (synonymous with leptomeningitis) denotes an infection spread through the cerebrospinal fluid with the inflammatory process involving the pia and arachnoid maters, the subarachnoid space, and to a lesser extent the superficial tissues of the brain and spinal cord.[19] Pachymeningitis denotes an inflammatory process involving the dura mater. Meningitis can be caused by a wide variety of organisms, some of which cross the blood-brain barrier and the blood–cerebrospinal-fluid (CSF) barrier. The CSF can also become contaminated by a wound that penetrates the meninges as a result of trauma or a medical procedure such as implantment of a ventriculoperitoneal shunt. Once the organism compromises the blood-brain and blood-CSF barriers, the CSF provides an ideal medium for growth, since the CSF has minimal or no capacity to produce antibodies and the immunoglobulins in the blood do not have access to the CSF.[14] The infecting organism is disseminated throughout the subarachnoid space as the contaminated CSF bathes the brain. The spread of the organism via the CSF circulation accounts for the differences in the variety and the extent of the neurological sequelae that can result from meningitis.

Bacterial meningitis

Clinical problems. The diagnostic categorization of meningitis depends on the infecting agent (e.g., *Haemophilus influenzae* meningitis, *Streptococcus pneumoniae* meningitis, and viral meningitis) and on the acute or chronic nature of the meningitis (acute, subacute, or chronic meningitis). The terms *acute bacterial meningitis* and *acute purulent meningitis* are used interchangeably in the literature and denote infections produced by any of a wide variety of bacterial organisms. The most common infecting organism producing acute bacterial meningitis varies according to the age of the population. During the neonatal period, infections by Gram-negative enterobacilli, especially *Escherichia coli,* are the most frequently occurring. In the population older than 2 months, *H. influenzae, Neisseria meningitidis,* and *S. pneumoniae* produce the majority of the cases.[15,28] In children and adults typical infecting agents are *Neisseria meningitidis* and *S. pneumoniae,* particularly in individuals with suppressed immune responses.[19,28] *H. influenzae* frequently is the organism responsible for bacterial meningitis in children.[16,19,28] The common causes of acute bacterial meningitis can be summarized as follows:

> Neonatal period—*E. coli*
> Childhood—*H. influenzae*
> Adolescence—*N. meningitidis*
> Adulthood—*S. pneumoniae*

An example of an organism that uses a typical systemic route of bacterial infection is a *H. influenzae* organism that is a normal flora of the nose and throat. During an upper respiratory tract infection, the organism may gain entry to the blood. Transmission of the organism from the blood to the CSF probably occurs via the choroid plexus, which is responsible for filtering organisms out of the blood during septicemia. The circulation of CSF spreads the infecting organism through the ventricular system and the subarachnoid spaces. The pia and arachnoid maters become acutely inflamed, and as part of the inflammatory response, a polymorphic and fibrinous exudate is formed. The exudate may undergo organization resulting in an obstruction of the foramen of Monro, the aqueduct of Sylvius, or the exit foramen of the fourth ventricle. The supracortical subarachnoid spaces proximal to the arachnoid villi may be obliterated, resulting in a noncommunicating or obstructive hydrocephalus as a result of the accumulation of CSF. As the CSF accumulates, the intracranial pressure rises. The increased intracranial pressure produces venous obstruction precipitating a further increase in the intracranial pressure. The rise in the CSF pressure compromises the cerebral blood flow, which activates reflex mechanisms to counteract the decreased cerebral blood flow by raising the systemic blood pressure. An increased systemic blood pressure accompanies increased CSF pressure.

The mechanism producing the headaches that accompany increased intracranial pressure may be the stretching of the meninges and pain fibers associated with blood vessels. Vomiting may occur as a result of stimulation of the medullary emetic centers. Papilledema may occur as pressure occludes the veins returning blood from the retina.

Other routes of bacterial infection may involve a local spread as the result of an infection of the middle ear or mastoid air cells. Meningitis may occur as a complication of a skull fracture, which exposes CNS tissue to the external environment or to the nasal cavity. Fractures of the cribriform plate of the ethmoid bone producing cerebrospinal rhinorrhea provide another route for infection. Meningitis may be a further complication to the clinical problems of the traumatic head injury (see Chapter 13).

Clinical features of bacterial meningitis include fever, severe headache, altered consciousness, convulsions (particularly in children), and nuchal rigidity. Nuchal rigidity is indicative of an irritative lesion of the subarachnoid space. Cervical flexion is painful as it stretches the inflamed meninges, nerve roots, and spinal cord. The pain triggers a reflex spasm of the neck extensors to splint the area against further cervical flexion; however, cervical rotation and extension movements remain relatively free.

Several clinical tests are utilized to demonstrate nuchal rigidity. Kernig's test consists of flexion of the cervical area with the client supine. Signs of pain indicate a positive test.[12] Kernig's sign refers to a test performed with the client supine in which the thigh is flexed on the abdomen and the knee extended. This pulls on the sciatic nerve, which pulls on the spinal cord, causing pain in the presence of meningeal irritation. The same results are achieved with passive hip flexion with the knee remaining in extension. This is the same procedure described by Hoppenfeld[12] as the straight leg raising test for determining pathology of the sciatic nerve or tightness of the hamstrings. Passive hip flexion with knee extension can be painful because of meningeal irritation, spinal root impingement, sciatic nerve pathology, or hamstring tightness. Brudzinski's sign refers to the adduction only and flexion of the legs elicited when cervical flexion (Kernig's test) is performed.[6] These signs will not be present in the deeply comatose client who has decreased muscle tone and absence of muscle reflexes. The signs may also be absent in infancy and senility.

The diagnosis of bacterial meningitis can be established based on blood cultures and a sample of CSF obtained by a lumbar puncture.[7,27] Depending on the age of the client and the type of organism involved, blood cultures are positive in 40% to 90% of the cases.[7] The decision to use a lumbar puncture to obtain the sample must be made judiciously because a lumbar puncture carries the risk of transtentorial herniation in the presence of increased intracranial pressure.[27] The CSF sample in bacterial meningitis typically reveals an increased protein count and a decreased glucose level because the bacterial organisms ferment sugar.

The type and severity of the neurological sequelae of acute bacterial meningitis relate directly to the area af-

fected, the extent of CNS infection, the level of consciousness at the initiation of pharmalogical therapy, and the pathological agent involved. Some of the common CNS complications include subdural effusions, altered levels of consciousness, seizures, involvement of the cranial nerves, increased intracranial pressure, and water intoxication (syndrome of inappropriate antidiuretic hormone secretion). Some clients demonstrate an opisthotonic posture. The posture may occur in conditions of meningeal irritation, decerebrate rigidity as discussed in Chapter 13, tetanus, or strychnine intoxication. In the presence of meningeal irritation, the opisthotonic posture may be an expansion of the same protective reflex mechanism that produces nuchal rigidity. This differs from the mechanism responsible for an opisthotonic posture in decerebrate rigidity. When a transecting mesencephalic lesion occurs, the antigravity supporting mechanism driven by the vestibular system is released from the inhibitory influences of the higher centers of the CNS. The increased level of tone will be expressed not only in the trunk extensors, as in meningeal irritation, but also as increased extension, adduction, and internal rotation tone in the extremities. These differences in the origin of the opisthotonic posture must be considered when developing the appropriate intervention strategies for each problem.

Medical management of bacterial meningitis. Medical management of bacterial meningitis consists of the initiation of the antimicrobial regimen appropriate to the infecting organism and procedures to manage the signs and symptoms of meningitis that have been described in the preceding paragraphs. Medical intervention strategies in both these areas change with the development of new pharmacological agents. The reader is encouraged to review recent literature if additional information is sought on current aspects of the medical management of the client with meningitis.

Potential neurological sequalae. Studies of the long-term outcome of children with bacterial meningitis indicate that 30% to 50% of the individuals have long-term neurological sequalae.[22] The neurological sequelae that must be considered by the therapist in developing an intervention plan will differ in each client. The sequelae may be the result of the acute infectious pathological condition, subacute or chronic pathological changes, or late pathological changes. The acute infectious pathological condition could result in sequalae such as inflammatory or vascular involvement of the cranial nerves or thrombosis of the meningeal veins. Subacute or chronic pathological changes include obstructive or communicating hydrocephalus, subdural effusion, and venous or arterial infarction. Late pathological sequelae may develop, such as meningeal fibrosis around the optic nerve or spinal roots or persistent hydrocephalus in children.

Damage to the cerebral cortex can result in numerous expressions of its dysfunction. Motor system dysfunction may be the observable expression of the damage within the CNS, but the location of the damage may include sensory and processing areas as well as those areas typically categorized as belonging to the motor system. Perceptual deficits or regression in cognitive skills may present residual problems. Cranial nerve involvement is most frequently expressed as impairment of ocular mobility or dysfunction of the eighth cranial nerve complex.

Aseptic meningitis. Aseptic meningitis refers to a nonpurulent inflammatory process confined to the meninges and choroid plexus usually triggered by contamination of the CSF with a viral agent. The symptoms, similar to acute bacterial meningitis but typically less severe, usually begin as a viremia that then localizes to the meninges.[19] Aseptic meningitis primarily affects children and young adults.[7]

Any neurotopic virus except rabies can produce aseptic (viral) meningitis. The most common ones are Coxsackie B, mumps, ECHO, and lymphocytic choriomeningitis viruses. The primary nonviral agent producing aseptic meningitis is *Leptospira*. The diagnosis of this type of aseptic meningitis may be established by isolation of the infecting agent within the CSF or by other techniques. While the glucose level of the CSF in bacterial meningitis is usually depressed, the glucose level in viral meningitis is normal.[15]

Treatment of aseptic meningitis consists of management of the symptoms. The condition does not typically produce residual neurological sequelae, and full recovery is anticipated within a few days to a few weeks.[7,15]

Encephalitis

Clinical problems. Encephalitis refers to a group of diseases characterized by inflammation of the parenchyma of the brain and its surrounding meninges. Although a variety of agents can produce an encephalitis, the term usually denotes a viral invasion of the cells of the brain and spinal cord. Viral encephalitis presents a syndrome of elevated temperature, headache, nuchal rigidity, vomiting, and general malaise (symptoms of asceptic or viral meningitis) with the addition of evidence of more extensive cerebral damage such as coma, cranial nerve palsy, or hemiplegia. The pathological condition includes destruction or damage to neurons and glial cells resulting from invasion of the cells by the virus, the presence of intranuclear inclusion bodies, edema, and inflammation of the brain and spinal cord. Perivascular cuffing by polymorphonuclear leukocytes and lymphocytes may occur as well as angiitis of small blood vessels. Widespread destruction of the white matter by the inflammatory process and by the thrombosis of the perforating vessels can occur. Increased intracranial pressure, which can result from the cerebral edema and vascular damage, presents the potential for a transtentorial herniation. Residual impairment of neurological functions is common. As the number of individuals who are immunosuppressed as a result lymphoma, leukemia, organ transplantation, and AIDS increases, it is likely that the incidence of encephalitis will increase.[21]

Plum and Posner[20] discuss viral encephalitis in terms of five pathological syndromes. *Acute viral encephalitis* is a primary or exclusively CNS infection. An example would be herpes simplex encephalitis, in which the virus shows a predilection for the gray matter of the temporal lobe, insula, cingulate gyrus, and inferior frontal lobe. *Parainfectious encephalomyelitis* is associated with viral infections such as measles, mumps, or varicella. *Acute toxic encephalopathy* denotes an encephalitis that occurs during the course of a systemic infection with a common virus. The clinical symptoms are produced by the cerebral edema in acute toxic encephalopathy, which results in increased intracranial pressure and the risk of transtentorial herniation. Reye's syndrome is an example. Global neurological signs such as hemiplegia or aphasia are usually present rather than focal signs. The clinical symptoms of the previous three syndromes may be very similar. Specific diagnosis may only be established by biopsy or autopsy.

Progressive viral infections occur from common viruses invading susceptible individuals, such as those who are immunosuppressed or during the perinatal to early childhood period. Slow, progressive destruction of the CNS occurs as in subacute sclerosing panencephalitis. The final category of encephalitis syndromes are *"slow virus" infections* by unconventional agents that produce progressive dementing diseases such as Creutzfeldt-Jakob disease and kuru.

Medical management of encephalitis. The medical management of virally induced encephalitis has been, and with many infecting agents remains, primarily symptomatic, at times necessitating intensive, aggressive care to sustain life. Pharmacological interventions are being developed to treat some viral infections, such as herpes encephalitis. The probability of neurological sequelae differs according to the infecting agent. Further information concerning the clinical features, medical management, and potential for neurological sequelae of a specific type of encephalitis should be sought in the literature based on the infecting agent.

EVALUATION PROCEDURES

Just as the medical intervention with clients who have an inflammatory disorder of the CNS is, to a large extent, symptomatic, so is the intervention by therapists. Designing an intervention program based on the client's problems necessitates a comprehensive initial and ongoing evaluation to define the symptoms and to note changes in them. Although the discussion of evaluation procedures is separated from the discussion of intervention strategies, it must be recognized that the separation is artificial and does not reflect the image of practice. Evaluation of the level of consciousness of a client on day one of intervention will provide a starting line for calculation of the distance spanned at the time of discharge. Perhaps more critical to the final outcome is evaluation of the level of consciousness before, during, and after a particular intervention technique to determine its benefit or detriment to the client. The evaluation process is a constant activity intertwined with intervention. The observations and data from the process are periodically recorded to establish the course of the disease process and the success of the therapeutic management of the client.

Observation of current functional status

The evaluation process to be described has numerous components that may lead to the appearance of an approach that is too time consuming to be practical. The first step in the process, however—observation of the current functional status of the client—is designed to allow the therapist to begin the decision-making process of the components to be included in a detailed observation and the components that can be eliminated or deferred. If the client is comatose and nonmobile, the focus of the initial session might be an assessment of the status of the vital functions, level of consciousness, and responses to sensory input. If the client is an outpatient with motor control deficits, the initial session might focus on defining motor abilities and the intactness of the sensory channels with a more superficial assessment of vital function status and level of consciousness. The therapist must be alert to indications of the need for a more detailed evaluation of perceptual and cognitive function (e.g., the client cannot follow two-step commands, indicating the necessity of an assessment of cognitive skills).

Some of the components discussed in the evaluation process may be assessment skills that are more typically possessed by other professions (e.g., assessment of emotional/psychological status). The inclusion of these items is not meant to suggest that the formal testing be completed by the physical therapist. The items are included to indicate factors that will affect goal setting for the client and that will impact on the intervention strategy. Although the physical therapist may not be the health team member who has primary responsibility for evaluation of these areas, the therapist should recognize these areas as potential sources of movement dysfunctions.

Observation of the current functional status of the client provides the therapist with an initial overview of the client's assets and deficits. This provides the framework into which the pieces of information from the evaluation of specific aspects of function can be fit. The therapist must not allow assumptions made during the initial observation to bias later observations. The therapist might note that the client is able to roll from the supine to the side lying position in order to interact with visitors in the room. When the same activity is not repeated on the mat table in the treatment area, the therapist, knowing the client has the motor skill to roll, might conclude that the client is uncooperative, or apraxic, or has perceptual deficits. The therapist may have failed to consider that the difference between the two situations is the presence or absence of side rails, which may have enabled the client to roll in bed by pulling over to the side lying position. It is characteristic of human observation skills that we tend to "see" what we expect to see. The therapist must attempt to observe behaviors and note potential explanations for deviations from normal without biasing the results of the subsequent observations.

The following discussion of the specific considerations within the evaluation process does not necessarily represent the temporal sequence to be used during the evaluation process. As different items are discussed, suggestions for potential combinations of items will be made. The sequence of the process is best determined by the interaction of therapist and client. Fig. 16-1 presents the components of the evaluation process to be discussed in the following paragraphs.

Evaluation of vital function/autonomic nervous system status

It is assumed that the therapist enters the initial interaction with a client after reviewing the available background information. This may provide the therapist with information on the baseline status of the client's vital functions. Any control problems in these areas should be particularly noted. Until the therapist determines that the vital functions such as respiration, heart rate, and blood pressure vary appropriately with the demands of the intervention process, these factors should be monitored. The monitoring process should include consideration of the baseline rate, rate during exercise, and time to return to baseline. The pattern of respiration and changes in that pattern should also be noted.

Clients with depressed levels of consciousness may display temperature regulation dysfunctions. One mechanism for assessing the client's ability to maintain a homeostatic temperature is to review the nursing notes. The events surrounding any periods of diaphoresis should be examined. If no causative factors have been identified, then interventions, which involve thermal agents as discussed in Chapter 6, should be used judiciously.

In addition to focusing on the specific vital functions previously discussed, the therapist should recognize them as functions controlled by the autonomic nervous system. Observation of functions under the control of the autonomic nervous system allows the therapist to make some assumptions concerning the client's set point on the continuum between sympathetic and parasympathetic responses. An understanding of the client's autonomic nervous system set point is critical because the set point will determine how the client interprets and therefore acts upon incoming sensory stimuli. For example, the caring gesture

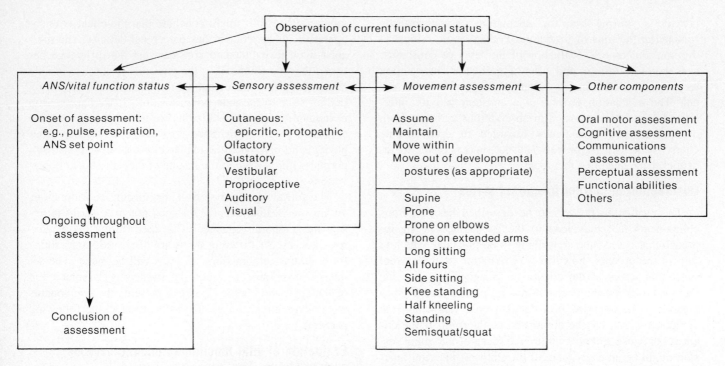

Fig. 16-1. Flow chart of components of the evaluation process.

of placing one's hand on the shoulder of a friend will elicit a much different response than will placing one's hand on the shoulder of a stranger in a dark alley. The tactile stimulation may be the same, but the interpretation of that sensory input, and therefore the motor response, will differ. If the client is functioning toward the sympathetic end of the continuum, sensory input that might be considered innocuous by the therapist may elicit a withdrawal response because the client interprets it as threatening. Fluctuations in the autonomic set point can also account for variations in the client's response to a particular intervention technique. Quick ice (see Chapter 6) may facilitate the desired muscle group during one session and may elicit an unwanted adversive withdrawal pattern during another session. A more comprehensive discussion of the assessment of the status of the autonomic nervous system can be found in the texts by Farber,[9] which describes an inventory for assessment of autonomic nervous system function, and by Heiniger and Randolph.[11]

The eating sequence is a vital function that should be observed. If the client is being fed via a nasogastric tube or a gastrostomy, the client may need intervention in the form of gustatory stimulation. The client who is self-feeding may be using inappropriate motor patterns, reinforcing the problems that are the focus of intervention during therapy sessions. The reverse situation should also be examined. Movement patterns executed during intervention sessions may be performed with adverse overflow to the oral musculature, thereby interfering with correct execution of the eating sequence. At the minimum, a gross assessment of the function of the oral musculature should be incorporated with the assessment of the client's head con-

trol in various postures. This may provide useful information when intervention strategies are being designed to focus on speech. Farber[9] describes evaluation of oral motor function in greater detail. Additional information may be found in Chapter 24.

Problems the client has with the elimination processes should be noted because therapeutic intervention strategies exist to deal with some of them. If elimination is triggered during an intervention session, the prior events should be recorded. Repetition of the series of events can be performed during other sessions to determine if a cause-effect relationship exists. If a relationship is present, the activities can be used to trigger elimination at appropriate times and can be avoided during intervention sessions. See Chapter 29 for additional evaluation and treatment techniques.

Evaluation of level of consciousness

Acute bacterial meningitis and various forms of viral encephalitis may result in changes in the client's level of consciousness. Consciousness is a state of awareness of one's self and one's environment.[20] Coma can be defined as a state in which one does not open the eyes, obey commands, or utter recognizable words.[13] The individual does not respond to external stimuli or to internal needs. The term *vegetative state* is sometimes used to indicate the status of individuals who open their eyes and display a sleep-wake cycle but who do not obey commands or utter recognizable words. DeMeyer[6] presents a succinct description of the neuroanatomy of consciousness and the neurological examination of the unconscious patient. Plum and Posner[20] also provide extensive information in this area.

Several scales have been developed to provide objective guidelines in assessing alterations in the state of consciousness. Jennett and Teasdale[13] developed the Glasgow Coma Scale, which assesses three independent items—eye opening, motor performance, and verbal performance. The scale yields a figure between 3 (lowest) and 15 (highest) that can be used to indicate changes in the individual's state of consciousness. The evaluation format is simple and the scale demonstrates both inter- and intra-rater reliability. The therapist can use assessment tools such as the Glasgow Coma Scale to determine if the intervention program has resulted in any recordable changes in the client's level of consciousness. Ideally, the client will be monitored continuously at consistent intervals to determine changes in status. Any carry-over or delayed effects of the intervention could then be noted. A constant record of the client's level of consciousness might also display a pattern of peak awareness at a particular point in the day. Scheduling an intervention session during the client's peak awareness time may maximize the benefit of the therapy. For additional information on levels of consciousness refer to Chapter 15.

In consort with the assessment of the client's state of consciousness is the assessment of his or her ability to communicate—both the expressive and receptive aspects of the process. If a dysfunction is present in the client's ability to communicate, the client should be evaluated by an individual with expertise in this area so that strategies for dealing with the communication deficit can be developed. Evaluation of the movement abilities of the client with communication deficits requires creative planning on the part of the therapist but can usually be accomplished if generalized movement tasks are used. With the client who cannot comprehend a verbal command to roll, the therapist could use an alternate form of communication as discussed in Chapter 24. The therapist could structure the situation to elicit the desired behavior by activities such as placing the client in an uncomfortable position or positioning a desired object so that it can only be reached by rolling.

The emotional and psychological aspects of the client as discussed in Chapter 6 and the cognitive and retention skills of the client should be evaluated informally by the therapist with referral to appropriate professionals if dysfunction in these areas is suspected. A coordinated team approach is a necessity with clients with emotional and psychological, cognitive, or communication problems or a combination of these problems. A consistent strategy used by all team members eliminates the necessity of the client to try to cope with different approaches by different people in an area in which he or she already has a deficit.

Evaluation of sensory channels

The evaluation process must include a thorough assessment of all channels for sensory input. The knowledge gained in the assessment of the sensory systems will be utilized in the program-planning process to select the inter-

vention strategies that have the highest probability of success. The therapist assesses both the client's ability to perceive the sensory stimulus and the appropriateness of the response to the stimulus. Tactile input could result in an appropriate activation of underlying muscles or a maladaptive increase of muscle activity in a stereotyped distribution. During the evaluation process, the therapist must note the sensory inputs that produce the adaptive behaviors so that these can be utilized as components of the intervention sequence.

The status of the individual's autonomic system as a variable in the client's (and therapist's) interpretation of sensory input has been discussed. The bias of the client toward a sympathetic or parasympathetic state must be evaluated before sensory testing is performed. If the client is sympathetically biased, the therapist should intervene to normalize the state of the autonomic nervous system before introducing sensory input because the sympathetic state may result in an interpretation of the input as adversive.

The therapist should develop a systematic approach to the initial cursory evaluation of the sensory systems. Deficits identified in the initial evaluation will provide structure for scheduling more comprehensive evaluation of deficits in specific systems. The therapist must also monitor changes in the status of the vital functions during sensory input, especially if the client has a history of instability of heart rate, blood pressure, or rate of respiration.

Cutaneous input has several aspects that must be assessed. Some of the inflammatory diseases of the brain may result in cutaneous distributions in which sensation is absent or diminished. These areas should be routinely evaluated for changes in distribution of level of sensation. Tests of light touch, pressure, sharpness, and dullness can be utilized if the client can communicate reliably. A gross assessment of the intactness of the touch system can be made in the noncommunicative client by introducing a mildly adversive (not painful) stimulus, such as a light scratch while monitoring the client for changes in facial expression, posture, or tonus. The possibility of a spinal-level reflex response should be kept in mind when interpreting the results of such a gross assessment.

Besides the traditional assessment tools to evaluate the function of the epicritic and protopathic pathways, the therapist should examine the client's response to maintained tactile input. Maintained manual contact with the face, palms, abdomen, or soles of the feet may have a calming effect on the client. Maintained manual contacts on the skin overlying a muscle may facilitate the muscle and its agonists while inhibiting its antagonists.[9]

The response of various muscle groups to light, moving touch should be assessed to determine adaptive and non-adaptive movement responses. Quick phasic cutaneous inputs, such as light, moving touch, can stimulate the ascending reticular system to elicit an arousal response. The therapist should continuously monitor the client for signs of changes in the level of consciousness. If an alerting response is elicited, the therapist must be aware of the potential for the client to rebound to a state of less awareness than before the stimulus was applied. Changes in poststimulus level of consciousness can best be detected in a situation in which the client's level of consciousness is monitored at regular intervals by all health team members.

The client's response to various types of temperature inputs (Chapter 6) can be assessed. Thermal applications that result in small deviations from the baseline temperature of the skin should be processed through epicritic pathways as fine discriminative information and therefore result in adaptive behaviors. Thermal applications that cause large fluctuations in the baseline skin temperature may be mediated via the protopathic pathways. If a large enough fluctuation occurs, the input will register as pain rather than temperature sensation. Thermal applications that travel in the protopathic pathways may produce adversive withdrawal motor responses by the client and reinforce primitive or stereotyped motor patterns.

The sensation of temperature changes (warmth or coolness) depends on the transfer of heat to or from the skin. The adequate stimulus therefore is a change in temperature. Although the normal baseline temperature for skin is 33° C (91.4° F), the baseline temperature for a particular skin area of the client at a point in time should be established if the "dose" of the heat or cold application is to be quantified. If neutral warmth (Chapter 6) produces the desired effect of normalization of muscle tonus, a record of the quantity of temperature change will provide a more reproducible guideline for repeating the desired result than a record of duration of the application.

The olfactory channels are unique among the sensory input routes because the primary olfactory pathway directly synapses with the olfactory cortex within the limbic system prior to going to the thalamus. Olfactory inputs may provide a mechanism to elicit arousal in an otherwise unresponsive individual. Farber[8,9] discusses the procedure to be utilized in administering olfactory input as well as the appropriate concentrations of a variety of substances that can be used in evaluation and intervention regimens.

Gustatory sensory information is not typically an input channel utilized by physical therapists. In the client who is not receiving any gustatory stimulation because of prolonged tube feeding or in the client who demonstrates dysfunction of the oral musculature, the gustatory avenue of sensory input should not be overlooked. Various tastes can be incorporated in the evaluation of the effects of sensory inputs on clients with depressed levels of consciousness. Farber[9] has defined a protocol for using gustatory stimuli with clients as well as for identifying precautions to be considered. Gustatory input can also be incorporated into an intervention plan with the goal of facilitating movement of the oral and facial musculature. The gustatory/tactile input of a small amount of peanut butter placed on the cor-

ner of the client's mouth may elicit tongue protraction with lateral deviation to remove the morsel. Introduction of a slightly sour taste may facilitate a pucker response of the orbicularis oris. The possibility of achieving desired goals through the inclusion of gustatory input should be considered during the evaluation process.

The complex functions of the vestibular system can be assessed through a variety of avenues. The integrity of the connections underlying a vestibularly induced nystagmus response are assessed by physicians through the caloric test (warm and cold water or air introduced into the ear channel to induce nystagmus). Therapists have used the Ayres Post-Rotatory Nystagmus Test[1,2] and variations of the test to gain information on the postrotatory nystagmus response.

Located in the utriculus and sacculus are the maculae, which record changes in the relationship of the head to the pull of gravity (position detectors) and changes in linear acceleration. It is this end organ that is responsible for the tonic labyrinthine reflexes. By manipulating the position of the client's head in relation to the pull of gravity, the therapist can evaluate this aspect of the vestibular system by noting changes in the distribution of muscle tone. The effect of rapid linear accelerations and decelerations can be evaluated as potential activating mechanisms increasing the level of consciousness or level of muscle activity. Slow, rhythmical reversals of linear movements may have a calming effect on the client's behavior or level of tone. Linear movements in all planes and diagonals should be explored. Evaluation of the influence of linear movements should follow the developmental sequence of movement within a posture. An infant mastering the all-fours position rocks first in an anteroposterior direction, proceeds to weight shifting from side to side, then proceeds to progression that incorporates diagonal movements. Because the desired therapeutic effect of vestibular input is a reflection of its influence in normal development, it is logical to use the developmental sequence to provide the guidelines for utilization of vestibular input.

Assessment of the client's response to proprioceptive input is incorporated within the assessment of the client's movement abilities and is intertwined with the intervention process because a variety of intervention techniques are based on proprioceptive input (Chapter 6). Evaluation of the proprioceptive channels can be conducted through assessment of the client's static position sense and dynamic kinesthesis. These tests allow the therapist to make inferences concerning the client's cognitive abilities to interpret proprioceptive information. Inherent in the successful completion of these tests is the necessity for the client to be able to understand directions and to be able to communicate data to the therapist. Because information input, processing, and output are involved in these tests, failure to comply with the test instructions cannot be definitively attributed to dysfunction of the proprioceptive system. The therapist should also consider information obtained from watching the client move before drawing a conclusion concerning the intactness of the proprioceptive channels. Some of the factors to consider include disregard of an extremity and variations in quality of performance between visually directed and nonvisually directed movements. Although tests of position sense and kinesthetics provide one aspect of the evaluation of the proprioceptive system, the therapist must also constantly be involved in assessing the client's response to the intervention techniques that are part of the treatment plan. This again illustrates the intermingling of assessment and intervention. During intervention, a demand for movement is placed on the client. As the movement occurs, the therapist assesses the quality of the movement. If the quality is not appropriate, the therapist initiates intervention to improve the quality. If the technique is assessed not to produce the desired result, a second technique can be tried and the cyclic process continues.

Auditory and visual channels can be grossly assessed by the therapist. More detailed information on the intactness of the sensory channels can be obtained from other health team members. The types of information available from other health team members can vary from the assessment of brainstem evoked potentials in response to auditory and visual inputs in the comatose individual to the identification of visual or auditory acuity deficits. Because the auditory and visual systems provide the therapists with a primary means of communicating with the client and because they can be used to augment performance in the event of deficits in other sensory channels, these systems should be incorporated in the therapist's evaluation process. Simple visual system tests, such as identification of field deficits, assessment of tracking abilities, and a gross evaluation of visual acuity, can be performed quickly. Texts such as De-Meyer[6] can be consulted on the techniques for administering these tests. Simple tests for assessing auditory thresholds can include such techniques as rubbing fingers by the individual's ear, placing a ticking watch to the client's ear, or assessing the presence of a startle response to sounds in the client with altered states of consciousness. Although these quick tests of the visual and auditory systems will not yield quantifiable information, they should provide the therapist with the necessary data to design an intervention plan that accounts for the presence of the deficits or that can use the intact system to compensate for input missing from an impaired system. Refer to Chapter 25 for additional information regarding the visual-perceptual system.

During the evaluation of the client as well as during intervention with the client, the therapist must be aware of the potential to bombard the client with sensory input and overload his or her ability to discriminatively respond to it. If the therapist detects indications that the client has difficulty in appropriately responding to sensory input, such as the client in a lowered, state of consciousness or an agi-

tated state or the client demonstrating tactile defensiveness, only one type of sensory input should be utilized during the initial evaluation or intervention sessions. If multiple sensory inputs are used, the positive or negative effects cannot be attributed to a specific input or necessarily to the series of inputs. Evaluation as well as intervention with sensory inputs should proceed in a controlled fashion. Inclusion of additional sensory modalities in the intervention plan should occur systematically.

Evaluation of movement abilities

Assessment of the individual's movement abilities is performed as he or she moves through the sequence of developmental postures from prone and supine to upright ambulation. The assessment focuses on both the quantity and quality of the motor performance. The extent of the progression through these developmental sequence postures is one component of the assessment. In each developmental posture as well as in the process of moving between the postures, a number of additional items relating to the client's movement abilities can be assessed. Indications of abnormal ranges of movement of all joints can be obtained. The range may show a limitation of movement or an indication of joint instability. Once the gross deviations are identified, these joints can be examined to determine the source of the problem—joint capsular, ligamentous, bony, skin, or muscular and fascial dysfunction. Conducting the gross assessment of range while the client is moving eliminates the time spent in performing a joint-by-joint goniometric evaluation on articulations with normal excursions.

As the individual is moving (either independently or with the therapist assisting), an assessment of tone distribution and fluctuations can be made. The therapist can identify the postures that will be the most conducive to optimal motor performances and those that should be avoided because they elicit inappropriate tone. Along with the assessment of the distribution of tone, the therapist can identify the reflexes and reactions influencing each posture. The reflexes and reactions should be categorized as supporting or interfering with the posture and movement patterns. Assessing the influence of the reflexes and reactions in each of the developmental postures provides a more realistic picture of their influence than conducting a reflex inventory test, which considers only one posture. Integration of the more primitive reflexes may appear to have occurred in the lower-level postures, while the reflex continues to influence movement at higher-level postures. Monitoring the influence of the reflexes and reactions as the client progresses through a sequence of postures provides the more comprehensive assessment of the problems to be dealt with in therapy.

Within each developmental posture, the therapist must examine the control the client displays over the posture. Because the assessment takes place as a part of a dynamic sequence, the therapist can assess the client's ability to assume the posture. If the posture cannot be achieved independently, the therapist assesses the factors interfering with achieving the position, the type of assistance necessary to facilitate assumption of the posture, and the effect of the various intervention techniques used to assist the client in achieving the position. Once the client is in the posture, his or her ability to maintain the posture is examined. Factors that have been previously discussed are examined, such as range of movement of joints, tone distribution, influence of reflexes and reactions, and vital functions status. The client's ability to move within the posture is identified. Movement demands placed on the client should include aspects of both static and dynamic equilibrium. Static equilibrium in the all-fours position could be demonstrated by clients matching the strength of a force attempting to displace them backwards. The presence of dynamic equilibrium of the upper torso in the all-fours position could be demonstrated by the client reacting to a quick sideways displacement force administered to the shoulder by crossing one arm over the other to maintain balance.

The final stage in examining control of developmental posture concerns the ability to move out of the posture. The client should have the ability to move out of the posture to a lower-level posture and to a higher-level posture before mastery of the posture is considered to have been achieved.

As the client is moving through the developmental postures, the function of specific musculature can be examined. Muscle groups should be examined concerning their ability to function in stability (distal segment fixed) situations and in mobility (distal segment free) situations. Because numerous demands are being placed on each muscle group, therapists can assess their ability to perform isometric and isotonic (concentric and eccentric) contractions. Each different posture introduces a new set of variables; therefore the performance of a muscle group must be reexamined as each new movement pattern is performed.

As indicated previously, the evaluation process is not compartmentalized. Many aspects of the client's performance are analyzed simultaneously. When the therapist assists the client in moving to a new posture, an analysis of the influence of facilitation and inhibition techniques is being conducted. The individual's response to these handling techniques cues the therapist in projecting the client's response to an intervention program. The therapist is constantly monitoring the client for changes in vital function rates or changes in the level of consciousness. Anything that results in expressions of pain by the client should be noted. Intervention programs should be a learning experience for clients. If they are attending to pain, they cannot attend to learning. The factor(s) producing the pain should be identified and measures instituted to eliminate the factor(s). If the factors producing the pain cannot be re-solved, the intervention program should be designed to avoid triggering the pain. (Refer to Chapter 27 on Pain Management.)

The presence of motor planning dysfunctions can also be noted as the client attempts a movement sequence. The therapist may have to physically cue the client to initiate the sequence, which then flows smoothly. The therapist may observe that the client has the correct components to a movement sequence but that the sequence of the components is incorrect. Or the client may demonstrate the ability to produce a movement sequence under one set of conditions but not another. Indications of these types of motor planning problems can be observed during the initial interactions with the client. The therapist should also be aware of any signs of cerebellar dysfunctions (see Chapter 21).

Having observed the client move through the developmental sequence postures, the therapist will have a baseline knowledge of the client's functional abilities. Whether the assessment of the client's skills in this area is performed by the physical therapist or other health team members, the results of the assessment are important to add to the data base from which the intervention plan will be formulated. Assessment of the client's functional abilities can provide more detailed information on the fine movement skills required of the upper extremity than the developmental posture assessment. Evaluation of functional abilities provides the therapist with the opportunity to compare the variety of observations as have been discussed previously, including range of movement, tone distribution, and function of specific muscles.

The final aspect of the evaluation process to be discussed, but once again an aspect that can be integrated in the observations of movement abilities, is identification of perceptual deficits. Aspects of the client's motor performance can provide indications for detailed perceptual testing to classify the deficits. This testing should be conducted by the health team member qualified in the area of perceptual testing. During the general evaluation procedures, the therapist can screen the client for signs of perceptual deficits. Clients' abilities to cross their midlines with their upper extremities can be demonstrated in movement sequences such as moving from the supine to the side sitting to the sitting position (Fig. 16-2). The quality of the integration of information from the two sides of the body can be indicated by the symmetry or asymmetry of posture in positions that should be symmetrical. The therapist may suspect that the client has a deficit in body awareness or body image by the poor quality of movement patterns that are within the motor capability of the individual. Spontaneous comments by the client verbalizing how he or she feels when moving ("my leg feels so heavy") also add to the therapist's assessment of the client's body image. Problems with verticality can be seen with the client who lists to one side when in an upright posture. When the therapist corrects the list to a vertical posture, clients may

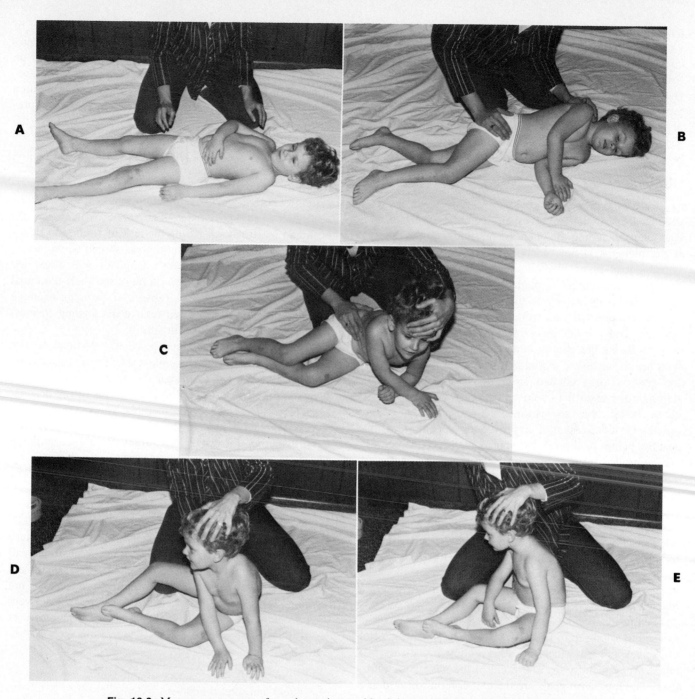

Fig. 16-2. Movement sequence from the supine to side sitting to sitting positions. **A,** Supine position. **B,** Handling to side lying. **C,** Handling toward side sitting; arm positions are important. **D,** Side sitting; note propping patterns with arms. **E,** Handling to symmetrical sitting.

express that they now feel that they are leaning to one side. Individuals who cannot appropriately relate their positions to the position of objects in their environments may have a figure-ground deficit or a problem with the concept of their position in space. When approaching stairs, these clients may fail to step up or may attempt to step up too soon. These examples should provide an indication of the observations that can indicate the need for detailed perceptual testing. See Chapters 11

and 25 for additional discussion of perceptual deficits.

The general philosophy that has been expressed in discussing the evaluation of the client with neurological deficits as a result of brain inflammation is that of a whole-part-whole approach. General observations of the client's performance provide a general description of the client's abilities while indicating deficits in his or her performance. The cause(s) of the deficits are explored to provide the pieces of data defining his or her performance. These pieces of data are then arranged within the framework provided by the general observation to define the whole of the client's assets and deficits. As the whole picture is established (with the realization that it will be constantly adjusted), the process of goal setting is initiated. The process presented for refining evaluation data into an intervention plan is applicable whether the client's neurological dysfunction is the result of a bacterial or viral infection, cerebral vascular accident, trauma, or other factors.

GOAL SETTING

Ideally, the process of goal setting for a client is a coordinated effort that involves all members of the health care team, including the client (if feasible) and the family. If the therapist is not functioning in a setting where involvement of many disciplines is a viable approach, the therapist can progress through the goal-setting process in relation to his or her role in the client's care.

Having collected data from the evaluation process, the first steps are to establish two lists—one dealing with specific problems the client is encountering and one dealing with his or her assets. Formulating an asset list focuses on the positive data elicited from the evaluation process. Items on the asset list could be observations, such as the client being able to assume the position of prone-on-elbows independently, improved head control in this posture being facilitated by approximation (Chapter 6), and controlled weight shifting being elicited by alternated tapping (Chapter 6). The asset list provides a reference defining the postures and intervention techniques that have been evaluated to be effective. This reference is utilized in developing the intervention plan. Formulating and recording a problem list and an asset list can be completed relatively quickly as one gains familiarity with the process. Just as the evaluation process is ongoing, so are the steps involved in goal setting. The asset and problem lists are redefined as the client's status changes.

Having identified assets and problems, the next step is to establish long-term goals. These goals are the general objectives toward which the intervention process is oriented. They identify the end point of the intervention process. The long-term goals are the exit criteria for terminating the intervention. If one of the client's problems was the interference of spasticity in the assumption and maintenance of several postures, a long-term goal for that client could be maintenance of appropriate muscle tone levels while moving through the developmental sequence postures.

Measurable, objective, short-term goals are established from the long-term goals. The goal should be measurable either in terms of producing a numerical indicator of performance, such as time span, number of repetitions, or distance covered, or in terms of an accurate description of the target motor behavior. The appropriate objective indicator must be carefully selected. Performing a movement more quickly may indicate that the individual is performing it with more normal tone and therefore greater ease of movement, or it may indicate that the individual has become more skilled in using an abnormal pattern based on inappropriate tone. If it is not appropriate to write the goal in terms of a numerical indicator, the goal can be written in terms of an observable behavior. The therapist can precisely describe body segment movements based on the component method of movement analysis presented by Van Sant.[25] For example, the task of coming to standing from supine can be described in terms of the upper-extremity component, axial component, and lower-extremity component. Formulation of an appropriate short-term goal could specify use of the upper extremities in a push and reach pattern during the task of coming to standing from supine. The short-term goals should be written so that observation of the client's behavior will allow the therapist to state whether the criteria of the short-term goal were or were not achieved. Table 16-1 gives an example of some components of short-term goals leading to mastery of functional activities in sitting.

The long-term goals define the client's destination. The short-term goals define the mileposts. The therapist then utilizes the asset list to design the intervention program, which is the vehicle to get the client to his or her destination. From the asset list, the therapist knows the intervention techniques that have the highest probability of success. Adopting this process simplifies the task of outlining the strategy for intervention.

The goal-setting process results in specification of the outcome objectives for a specific client; however, general goals of the intervention process can be stated. These goals cover the spectrum of problems typically dealt with in a physical therapy intervention program. Because of the broad nature of the goals, other professions will also be contributing to meeting them. The goals are written as outcomes of the intervention process and not as goals for a client. The general goals for the intervention program for clients with inflammatory CNS disorders as well as other neurological dysfunctions are as follows:

1. Promoting homeostasis of autonomic nervous system and vital functions
2. Promoting optimalization of postural set
3. Promoting integration of sensory input
4. Promoting integration of primitive reflexes to achieve the normal postural reflex mechanism
5. Enhancing progression through the developmental sequence activities
6. Promoting optimalization of movement patterns
7. Promoting optimalization of psychosocial and cognitive responses

Each of these goals will be discussed in conjunction with the general therapeutic intervention procedures that can be utilized to achieve the goal.

Table 16-1. Examples of short-term goals relating to mastery of functional activities in sitting*

Condition variables†		Activity	Criteria
1. When sitting on a mat	a. Using the upper extremities for support	The client will maintain the posture	for ___ seconds.
2. When sitting on the edge of a mat table	b. Using one upper extremity for support		
	c. Without using the upper extremities for support		
3. When sitting in a chair	d. With the therapist displacing the position of the: Pelvis Shoulders Head Lower extremities	The client will make postural adjustments of the head and trunk	appropriate to the degree of displacement.
		The client will bring right foot to left knee (as if to put on a shoe)	without losing balance.

*Long-term goal: The client will master functional activities in sitting. Short-term goals: Select one phrase from each column.
†Therapist needs to consider all aspects of each variable, i.e., 1—a, b, c, d; 2—a, b, c, d; 3—a, b, c, d.

GENERAL THERAPEUTIC INTERVENTION PROCEDURES IN RELATION TO INTERVENTION GOALS
Promoting homeostasis of ANS and vital functions

Promoting homeostasis of autonomic nervous system and vital functions is based upon an assessment of the client's current status and consideration of the optimal state to perform the desired activity. A calm, parasympathetic state would be appropriate if the intervention activity were a feeding program. If a movement program is the focus of the intervention, a more alert, action-oriented state would be appropriate. Once the therapist decides the direction in which the client should be moved on the continuum from sympathetic to parasympathetic states, numerous sensory inputs can be used to achieve the move.

To move the client to a more sympathetic state of arousal, brief bursts of sensory input either singly or in a rapid, repetitive, irregular sequence are effective. Cutaneous input such as a light, moving touch or quick ice (see Chapter 6) will facilitate the desired arousal. The response may be expressed as a movement response or as an increased attendance to the presence of sensory input. The olfactory channels can stimulate a sympathetic response when a noxious odor is introduced. The precautions discussed in Chapter 6 should be reviewed before odors in the noxious category are added to an intervention plan. Rapid alternating vestibular input, such as rapid rocking on an equilibrium board with stops and starts or an irregular rhythm of bouncing on an inflatable ball, can be effective in eliciting signs of an increased level of consciousness, such as eye-opening or increased vocalization. The therapist should add vestibular activities to the intervention protocol in a gradual manner because clients who have in-creased intracranial pressure may have increased sensitivity of the emetic centers of the brainstem and therefore a decreased tolerance to vestibular input.

Gustatory inputs that are sour (Chapter 6) may elicit an alerting response. Proprioceptive inputs such as an intermittent approximation force applied through the head can cue attending and provide the therapist with a mechanism to position the client for appropriate visual inputs. Bright colors and presentation of different objects into the visual field are examples of methods of using the visual channels for eliciting arousal. Establishment of eye contact between the client and therapist may also elicit signs that the client is more alert and therefore better able to participate in the intervention process. The type of auditory input the client is receiving should be considered. The client may have a more alert response to the therapist who speaks in a crisp, clear voice with fluctuating tone level than to monotone, monotonous repetition of movement commands. The background noise input should be considered. The sounds from slowly beeping monitors may override other types of input and counteract arousal inputs. Auditory inputs should not be constant. If a radio is played in the room of a comatose client, it should be turned on intermittently and not be a constant factor to which the client can accommodate.

When the therapist is utilizing sensory inputs to move a client toward the sympathetic end of the continuum, care must be taken so as not to cross the threshold that would elicit a sympathetic fight-or-flight response. The therapist is attempting to manipulate the autonomic nervous system set point so that appropriate adaptive behaviors can occur. Triggering a fight-or-flight response results in the client reacting to incoming sensory stimuli as threatening and therefore will not elicit the appropriate adaptive responses to the therapeutic intervention techniques. Similarly, as the client is reacting in a defensive mode, the client will be less likely to trust the therapist, thus limiting the latter's effectiveness.

The therapist may decide that the client should be functioning in a more parasympathetic state if, for example, the client is agitated or the intervention program is focusing on feeding. Cutaneous inputs such as neutral warmth or maintained manual contacts with the perioral region, abdomen, palms, or soles of the feet will produce a calming response. Olfactory and gustatory inputs that have pleasant past associations (favorite foods or special perfume or after-shave used by a parent or loved one) may calm the agitated client or alert the unresponsive individual. As with all types of sensory input, a single odor or taste should be introduced and the results evaluated before introducing a second stimulus.

Vestibular inputs that are sustained or that are rhythmical and repetitive provide for parasympathetic responses. Slow rocking of an individual combined with neutral warmth can be effective in calming.[9] Proprioceptive inputs such as approximation through the cervical vertebrae or through the extremity joints can be added to the above combination. At the same time, the auditory and visual inputs can be controlled so that the sensory input from all channels is appropriately directed to achieve a specific goal. (See Chapter 6 for additional examples.)

If the client has dysfunctions in the vital function areas of respiration, eating sequence, or elimination, the therapist can initiate an intervention program to address components of the problems. Because of the decreased activity level of these clients, respiratory patterns tend to be shallow and excursion of the rib cage limited. These problems should be addressed both to improve ventilation and to promote the rib cage expansion, which is interrelated with the vertebral column extension necessary for upright posture. Resisted breathing techniques as originated by Knott and Voss[23,26] can be implemented to achieve these goals. Mobilization techniques that maintain the accessory motions available at the articulations involved in respiration (such as the costovertebral joints) should be considered with clients who are unable to achieve rib cage expansion with techniques such as resisted breathing. Mobilization techniques maintain the mobility of the articulations so that limitations do not develop that will present additional difficulties at a later time.

Depending on the division of responsibilities within the health care team, the physical therapist may be responsible for providing postural drainage and percussion techniques as a treatment regimen or for designing a prophylactic positioning program to improve pulmonary drainage in the nonmobile client. As the client is able to move through the developmental sequence activities, with or without assistance, the changing postures and work load should elicit improved respiratory patterns. The therapist must contin-

uously monitor the client for indications of respiratory compromise in postures such as prone. If the prone position cannot be tolerated, the goals that were to be achieved in prone can still be reached by selecting an alternate posture. The weight bearing for the upper extremities in a prone-on-elbows position can also be achieved in the sitting position by leaning on a table of appropriate height. Respiratory function can also be augmented by including cervical and thoracic vertebral column flexion and extension patterns in various developmental postures. Timing breathing with the flexion and extension patterns will facilitate an improved pattern of respiration as well as elicit a better postural response to the demands of gravity.

Disorders in the function of the oral musculature caused by underlying problems such as hypotonicity, hypertonicity, or tactile defensiveness are usually seen in the difficulties the client has in eating, drinking, and producing speech. The setting in which one is treating a client as well as the expertise areas of the members of the health care team are determining factors as to whether it is the physical therapist, the occupational therapist, or the speech pathologist who directs intervention for oral-motor dysfunction. The professional label of the person providing the intervention is not as important as the inclusion of the intervention in the overall care plan. Once the evaluation process establishes the type of oral-motor dysfunction present, many of the same principles utilized in dealing with motor dysfunctions of the trunk and extremities can be implemented. The proprioceptive neuromuscular facilitation (PNF) approach of resisted diagonal movements can be applied to facilitate jaw opening and closure as well as tongue mobility. Cutaneous inputs can facilitate or inhibit the response of the masseters. Stretch pressure (Chapter 6) can be applied to the orbicularis oris to elicit lip closure. Discussion of specific techniques to deal with oral-motor problems can be found in Chapters 6 and 24 and in the works of Farber,[9] Gallender,[10] Knott and Voss,[26] Levitt,[17] and Sullivan, Markos, and Minor.[23]

Clients who are inactive and spend the majority of their day recumbent may experience difficulty with defecation. Although these problems are usually managed with medication, the therapist can add interventions that may augment the effectiveness of the medication or that may be useful in a transition period when medication is discontinued. Wood and Becker[29] discuss the influence of the mechanical pressure of massage as a reflex stimulus to increase peristalsis of the large intestine. Massage techniques such as stroking and kneading the pathway of the ascending, transverse, and descending colon may facilitate movement of the feces to the rectum. Elimination may then be stimulated by positioning the client in the lengthened range for the lower-extremity pattern of extension, adduction, and external rotation. The client attempts to pull his or her lower extremities down and together while

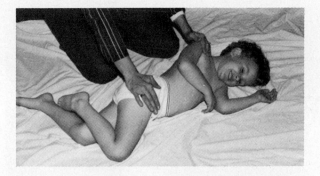

Fig. 16-3. Counterrotation of shoulder girdle backward (retraction) and the pelvis forward. Hand placement of therapist is important so that shoulder and hip movements can occur freely.

the therapist resists all motion except external rotation.[26] Repetitive bilateral asymmetrical lower-extremity flexion patterns to the right and to the left that press the thighs against the abdomen may also trigger elimination. If the client has spasticity of the trunk musculature, techniques should be implemented to normalize the trunk tone before focusing on elimination. One way to achieve this is by side-lying rhythmical movements in which the therapist gently moves the client's pelvis in one direction around the body axis while moving the shoulder girdle in the opposite direction and then reversing the movements (Fig. 16-3).

If possible, an individual who has previously had bowel control should be placed in an upright sitting posture for defecation. Adaptations to the toilet device should be made to ensure that the individual feels secure in the posture. The lower extremities should be positioned so that the hips are flexed at an angle greater than 90 degrees. The position should incorporate flexion, abduction, and slight neutral to slight internal rotation—the lengthened position for the extension, adduction, and external pattern mentioned previously. This position places the muscles used in defecation in a more appropriate position to contract. The therapist should also attend to the environment in which the toileting activity is to occur. An environment to which the client reacts with a stress or sympathetic response will be counterproductive to the desired result of defecation. See Chapter 29 for additional information.

Promoting optimalization of postural set

The intervention goal of promoting optimalization of postural set underlies the rest of the intervention goals. Optimalization of postural set includes the concepts of decreasing muscle tone that is too high to allow performance of an activity as well as augmenting tone that is too low to support the performance of an activity. The postural set of a client can fluctuate between degrees of hypertonicity and hypotonicity; the term *optimalization* allows the goal to be stated indicating that the optimal postural set for a particular movement is the desired outcome. Intervention tech-

niques to achieve this goal demand that the therapist constantly monitor the client's performance so that appropriate interventions are added when needed and continued only as long as they are needed.

Hypertonicity. If the client displays hypertonicity in a muscle group or groups that limits the performance of a movement as a result of an inappropriate postural set, the therapist can select intervention techniques that are mediated through any of the sensory channels functional for that client. The selection of which channel or combination of channels to use for the input will be based on the therapist's initial and continuing evaluation of the client's response to specific types of sensory input. Hypertonicity of the muscle group may be triggered by stimulation of an area of skin that is hypersensitive to cutaneous input. Cutaneous stimulation has strong facilitory polysynaptic input to the gamma motor neurons of muscles underlying the area of skin stimulation. Continuous application of a stimulus may produce accommodation to the input, thereby decreasing the facilitation of the gamma motor neurons.

The therapist can attempt to decrease hypertonicity of muscles by maintaining a continuous pressure to the skin overlying spastic muscles. This approach seems particularly effective in dealing with hypertonicity of the facial muscles. However, when the client is performing a movement pattern, it becomes very difficult for the therapist to maintain a constant level of input from the hand contacts with the client. The therapist should consider using hand placements that contact the client's skin overlying bony prominences (no facilitation to muscles) or skin overlying the antagonist of the hypertonic muscle group. Manual contact over the antagonist may facilitate the response of these muscles and provide reciprocal inhibitory input to the spastic muscles. The therapist must remember that the state of the muscle depends on a summation of the facilitory and inhibitory influences on that muscle (Chapter 6). The therapist is attempting to add facilitory or inhibitory inputs to alter the muscle tonus in the desired direction.

Vestibular input that is slow and rhythmical (as described in discussion of homeostasis of the autonomic system) promotes a generalized decrease in skeletal muscle tone. The therapist can create numerous methods for delivering vestibular input in a variety of developmental postures. Rood introduced utilization of a head-down position (tonic labyrinthine inverted position) to capitalize on the influence of the baroreceptors of the carotid sinus to produce a generalized decrease in muscle tone. Vestibular input in the inverted position may result in facilitation to postural extensors in the distribution described by Tokizane and others.[24] The inverted position can provide for a normalization of tone while preparing the midline neck and trunk extensors in particular to respond to the demands of gravity. McGraw[18] describes four stages in a maturational response to inversion. Initially the neonate responds with flexion of the extremities and signs of emotional dis-

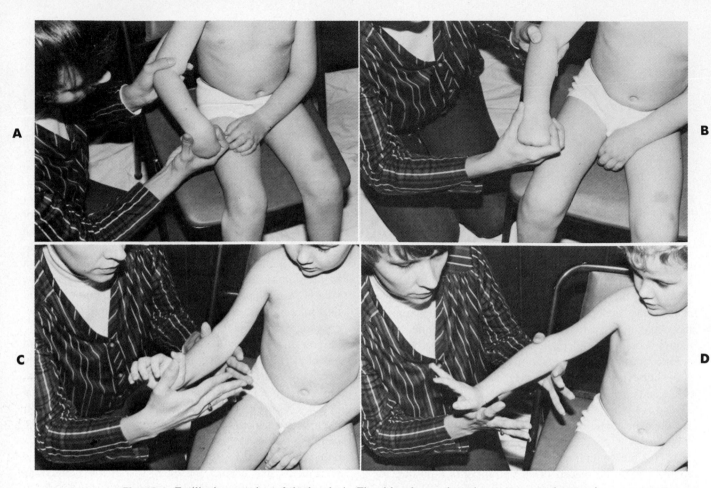

Fig. 16-4. Facilitating opening of the hand. **A,** Fisted hand; stretch to the extensors and approximation through hand, wrist, and elbow is applied. **B,** Approximation is continued, some resistance to the extensors may be applied. **C,** Approximation is applied to thenar eminence to further facilitate extensor tone. **D,** Full extension is achieved, approximation is maintained.

tress. In the second stage, the response is similar to the muscle activation pattern sought by Rood. The infant is not distressed by the inversion. As the righting reflexes develop, the infant attempts to orient to the upright posture. Emotional indications of frustration at the inability to reverse the inverted position occur in this third stage. Finally, the infant progresses to a stage of relaxed hanging in the inverted position. The research indicates that the progressions through these stages appear to have a maturational rather than an experiential basis. It is possible that individuals with CNS dysfunctions in the processing of vestibular input progress through similar stages.

The therapist must deal with hypertonicity influencing postural set as a generalized problem before focusing on the dysfunction of specific muscle groups. The tone of the trunk and shoulder girdles must be adjusted to the appropriate set before specific discreet movements of the upper extremity can be expected to occur. Once the overall level of the postural set has been addressed, techniques can be selected that deal with specific muscle groups.

The therapist may select from a variety of propriocep-

tive inputs to achieve the goal of reducing hypertonicity. Hypertonicity of an extremity may be released by applying approximation through the long axis of the extremity. The therapist's manual contacts for the application of the approximation force should be with the weight-bearing surface of the client's extremity (heel of the foot or heel of the palm). If the flexed position of the wrist prohibits application of the force to the heel of the palm, the approximation can be applied gradually through the fisted hand. As tone becomes more appropriate, the wrist can be moved toward the neutral position so that the therapist can then apply the approximation through the heel of the palm (Fig. 16-4). If the client tends to posture with his or her head rotated to one side, an approximation force should be applied through the head to the cervical vertebrae and maintained while attempting to correct the position of the head (Fig. 16-5). The approximation force may normalize the tone of the hypertonic muscles, allowing the correct posture to be assumed without inappropriately stretching the spastic muscles.

Proprioceptive techniques such as approximation are

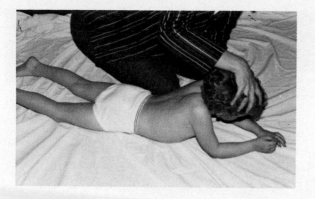

Fig. 16-5. Approximation applied through cervical vertebrae to reposition head to midline.

used to reduce inappropriate tone in specific muscles or muscle groups. Techniques such as vibration and tapping (Chapter 6) can be applied to the antagonist to reciprocally inhibit the spastic muscle and facilitate the antagonist. The therapist must monitor the response to vibration carefully because the mechanical vibration may be conducted through the muscle mass and bone of the extremity and elicit the tonic vibratory reflex in the antagonist to the muscle vibrated (Chapter 6).

Chapter 6 discusses some of the principal combinations of techniques that can summate to produce the desired response. Auditory and visual input must be controlled because the influence of the autonomic nervous system is interrelated to the tone level of skeletal muscle (Chapter 4). Since hypertonicity indicates a dysfunction in the balance of facilitory and inhibitory inputs, the therapist may need to provide inhibitory input via numerous channels to achieve the correct summation for an appropriate postural set. Sensory inputs should be added in a systematic fashion until the desired response is achieved. The inputs should also be withdrawn systematically to shape the client toward responding appropriately to the demands of a situation without the necessity of intervention.

Hypotonicity. Development of an appropriate postural set in the presence of hypotonicity follows the same general principles presented in discussing intervention in the presence of hypertonicity; however, the application of the techniques is usually reversed. Cutaneous input should be introduced in such a way that accommodation does not occur. Manual contacts on the skin over the belly of a muscle can increase the sensitivity of the reflex arc and CNS interactions and thus have the ultimate potential of increasing the sensitivity of the muscle spindle and preparing the muscle to respond to demands placed upon it. The manual contacts during movement sequences should be maintained in such a manner that accommodation to the continuous input does not occur. The therapist can offset accommodation by providing slight variations in the pressure utilized or skin areas touched. This can be achieved by the thera-

pist rolling his or her fingers on the client's skin while guiding a movement of sequence. Cutaneous input is also an adjunct to the response to proprioceptive techniques such as tapping or finger vibration.

Approximation can be effective in developing appropriate tone from a state of either hypertonicity or hypotonicity. Empirically, it seems that a greater amount of force is applied to increase tone than when the goal is to decrease tone. Approximation appears to elicit a response in all the muscles surrounding a joint as a preparation for responding to the demands of weight bearing. Approximation also lends itself to combination with other proprioceptive techniques, such as quick stretch or tapping.

Vestibular input in the presence of generalized hypotonicity should be rapid and irregular. The labyrinths should be stimulated by quick stops and starts with changes in direction. The program should include movements in all planes with the introduction of the planes presented in a developmental sequence. Rapid rotatory vestibular input (spinning) in a vertical posture does not appear as a component of the normal developmental sequence until the child has mastered walking sufficiently to begin spinning while in the standing position or on playground equipment. If the developmental sequence is providing a guideline for the direction sequence of application of vestibular input, the therapist should consider delaying spinning input until the client has mastered skills comparable to the stage described above.

Although the inverted position may initially augment the low tone level, the tonic labyrinthine reflex input, which increases tone in postural extensors, can be used to prepare the client to respond to proprioceptive and cutaneous inputs. A client who lacks head control could be inverted to facilitate the neck and midline trunk extensors. Sweep tapping (cutaneous and proprioceptive input) to the paravertebral muscles could be added while the client is verbally directed to look at an appropriately placed object to achieve the desired amount of cervical extension.

Promoting integration of sensory input

At the same time that the therapist is addressing the intervention goal of optimalization of postural set, the goal of promoting integration of sensory input must be considered. Unless the therapist has advanced knowledge of sensory integration theories, this goal may be a secondary rather than a primary one; however, it cannot be ignored. Before the therapist expects the client to exhibit adaptive behavior to the potential bombardment of input from combinations of cutaneous, proprioceptive, auditory, and visual input, the therapist must assess the ability of the client to respond to multisensory inputs. The ability to respond adaptively progresses from a response to a single sensory system input, to a response to the input in the presence of multiple system input, and then to an adaptive response based on inputs from two or more sources. The therapist must be sure that adding additional sensory inputs augments an adaptive response rather than detract from it. The client may respond to handling techniques providing proprioceptive and cutaneous cues but demonstrate a deterioration of performance when auditory input is added. When verbal cues are added, the therapist should follow the philosophy expressed in Proprioceptive Neuromuscular Facilitation[23,21] that verbal commands should be concise, sparse, and appropriately timed.

All sensory inputs should evoke the correct response on the part of the client rather than cause him or her to sift through the jumble of inputs to recognize the appropriate inputs to which a response should be made. At the highest level, the client will demonstrate cross-modal learning in which input from one sensory system will evoke a response based on input previously obtained via a different system. Recognition of a comb by touch is based on the precept of "combness" usually obtained initially by visual input. If the therapist recognizes the hierarchy in the process of integrating sensory input, intervention situations that require too high a level of performance from the client can be avoided. The client who can respond adaptively to input from only one source will not be expected to perform in a crowded treatment area that presents extraneous visual and auditory input. The therapist will also recognize the need to include in the intervention plan situations that involve the controlled introduction of sensory inputs so that the client progresses toward the ability to deal with multiple inputs. The reader should explore the writings of Jean Ayres[1,2] to expand these concepts.

Dysfunctions in perceptual integration are addressed as the client moves through developmental sequence activities. Although developmental sequence activities would not provide the total program for an individual with a specific perceptual integration dysfunction, goals in this area can be addressed if the therapist is aware of indications of dysfunctions. The therapist must critically observe the performance of a movement sequence to identify substitute actions to compensate for problems such as inability to cross the midline. The therapist must then attempt to redesign the demands of the situation to elicit the desired behavior. The client who moves from the supine to the side sitting to the long sitting positions without the upper extremities crossing the midline could be required to side sit to the left and transfer objects with the right hand from the left side of the body to the right side (Fig. 16-6). The therapist must determine if the client is truly crossing the midline or rotating the midline of the body to continue to avoid crossing it.

Promoting integration of primitive reflexes to achieve the normal postural reflex mechanism

Many of the clients recovering from brain infections who have residual dysfunction of the motor system exhibit the release of primitive reflexes as a component of the

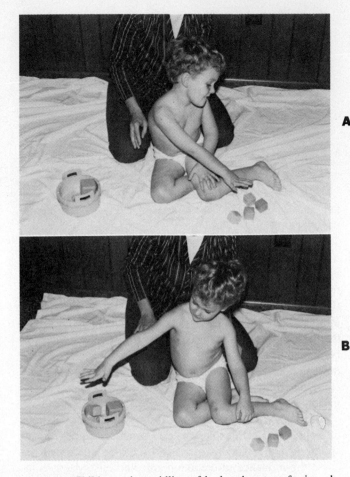

A

B

Fig. 16-6. Child crossing midline of body when transferring objects from left to right. **A,** Beginning active on contralateral side. **B,** Ending sequence by crossing midline and placing objects on ipsilateral side.

motor dysfunction. For these clients a goal of the intervention process is to promote integration of the primitive reflexes to achieve the normal postural reflex mechanism. The term *normal postural reflex mechanism* is used by the Bobaths[4,5] to refer to the automatic movements that can be grouped as righting reactions, equilibrium reactions, and adaptations of muscle tone to postural demands. The normal postural reflex mechanism develops with maturation of the CNS and can be used as an indicator of level of function (degree of maturation) of the CNS. The presence of the normal posture reflex mechanism underlies the ability to perform normal movement patterns. Primitive reflexes refer to those reflexes that are present in the process of normal development but whose influence is suppressed as maturation proceeds (e.g., asymmetrical tonic neck reflex—ATNR). Clients with neurological sequelae may exhibit a reappearance of the primitive reflexes with the influence of the reflexes augmented beyond the degree seen in the normal developmental process. The intervention process attempts to decrease the influence of the primitive reflexes while evoking the presence of the normal postural reflex mechanism so that appropriate movement patterns are possible.

A controversy exists concerning the utilization of primitive reflexes as part of the intervention techniques for clients who have a limited ability to perform motor responses. Primitive reflexes can be used to augment a response such as turning the head to the right (ATNR) to augment an extension response of the right upper extremity. The potential problem with this approach is that the client may be learning a behavior that reinforces the presence of a primitive reflex and blocks development of the normal postural reflex mechanism. Primitive reflexes can serve as a useful adjunct to elicit a response but should be reserved for those situations in which no other tool is effective. If the response is elicited via a primitive reflex, the therapist should immediately attempt to elicit the response without the reflex input. Shaping the sequence in this manner promotes the learning of the desired response and not reinforcement of an undesired stimulus to achieve the response. If the ATNR is used to elicit triceps function, the head should then be returned to the neutral position and function augmented by tapping, vibration, or other proprioceptive inputs. Once the triceps' response is achieved with the head in the neutral position, the head should be rotated away from the side of the triceps. This final stage promotes a functional response against the influence of a reflex, thus promoting its integration. Basing a decision on the needs of the client, the therapist must decide whether or not to use reflexes to augment the initial response in spite of the potential negative effects. Regardless of whether or not the primitive reflex is initially incorporated in the treatment plan, the intervention should progress from movement with neutral input from primitive reflexes to movement against the influences of those reflexes.

Integration of a primitive reflex cannot be categorically regarded as having occurred until it has disappeared as a negative factor in all developmental postures. Each higher developmental posture to which the client progresses may elicit signs of the influence of one or more primitive reflexes. Influence of the ATNR may be manifest in postures from prone and supine to upright progression. The integration process typically must recur at each level.

Inhibition of the influence of the primitive reflexes can occur by imposing control over the body segment that elicits the response (cervical vertebrae for the symmetrical tonic neck reflex) or controlling a body segment that is influenced by the reflex (maintain lower-extremity flexion against the influence of the tonic labyrinthine reflex supine). Bobath[3,5] discusses the utilization of proximal keypoints of control to influence the client's distribution of tone. The therapist must remember that the static imposition of control will not assist the client in learning to move. The therapist imposes control so that the client can move. As the client moves and gains control of the move-

ment, the therapist lessens the amount of control of the client. The therapist's goal should be to remove his or her hands from controlling the client's responses.

Facilitation of the normal postural reflex mechanism occurs as movement demands are placed on the client simultaneously with the inhibition of the influence of the primitive reflexes. The therapist has the dual task of preventing unwanted motions and facilitating the desired responses. The therapist is concerned not only with the presence of the primitive reflexes, eliciting righting and equilibrium reactions, but also with the level and distribution of tone, autonomic nervous system status, and ease and quality of the movement response. Although these are presented as separate intervention goals, the separation is artificial. During treatment the intervention techniques addressing these areas are intertwined. Facilitation of the normal postural reflex mechanism occurs as the client moves through the developmental sequence activities, which is the next item to be discussed.

Enhancing progression through the developmental sequence activities

The intervention goal of enhancing progression through the developmental sequence activities must be examined first in terms of demands that must be met in each posture. These are the same demands that were examined in the evaluation. The intervention process must focus on the quality of the client's ability to assume the posture, maintain the posture, move within the posture (static and dynamic equilibrium), and move out of the posture. The therapist will resequence this progression of activities to meet the needs of the client. The client may achieve independence in maintaining a posture while still requiring assistance in assuming the posture. Using guidelines from the normal developmental sequence, the therapist should progress the client to increased levels of demand before expecting a posture or a component of the posture to be perfected. An infant can maintain a sitting position when placed and display some components of equilibrium reactions before the position can be obtained independently. The movement in the all-fours position is being attempted before mastery of the sitting position occurs.

The therapist must regard the focus on the developmental sequence as a progression—a dynamic process. Intervention should incorporate movement both within a posture and between postures. Samplings of handling techniques to achieve this goal can be found in the works by Bobath,[3,5] Knott and Voss,[26] Levitt,[17] and Sullivan, Markos and Minor,[23] and others.

Promoting normalization of movement patterns

As the client is performing developmental sequence activities, the intervention goal of optimalization of movement patterns is also being addressed. Movement patterns are the building blocks that add up to the ability to move through a developmental posture. The client must have the ability to perform mobility patterns with the extremities. These are patterns in which the distal segment is free (open kinetic chain). These patterns are the necessary components for placing the extremities (e.g., swing phase of gait or reaching for a doorknob). These movement patterns are facilitated by phasic cutaneous inputs and proprioceptive inputs such as traction.

Electrical stimulation can be used as an adjunct to facilitate performance of a particular component of a mobility pattern. The wrist extension component of the PNF pattern of flexion, abduction, and external rotation can be reinforced by using a portable electrical stimulation unit with an adjustable surge duration. The electrical stimulation elicits the correct movement so that the client could learn from the feel of the correct pattern. By spacing performance of the pattern with and without the electrical stimulation device, the potential problem of reliance on the device to produce the movement can be avoided. Electromyography biofeedback also serves as a useful adjunct to achieve activation of specific muscle groups or to guide the client's attempts to reduce the level of tone of a muscle group.

Mobility patterns in the upper extremity have as their foundation the freedom of the scapula to appropriately adjust to the position of the humerus. The mobility of the scapula can be addressed through techniques that result in a general decrease in tone (such as neutral warmth) and diagonal movement patterns of the scapula. The scapular stabilizers, such as the rhomboids, trapezius, and serratus anterior, must be capable of allowing appropriate adjustment of the scapula as well as providing the fixation base upon which humeral elevation can occur.

Stability patterns are those in which the distal segment of the extremity is fixed (closed kinetic chain). These are the patterns utilized in the weight-bearing activities of the developmental sequence, such as the stance phase of gait and creeping. The components of the stability patterns are enhanced by proprioceptive input such as approximation and vibration, both of which provide muscle responses for the duration of the stimulus. During the performance of both stability and mobility patterns, the therapist should control the situation so that the client learns from the sensation of appropriate movement patterns and not patterns imposed by inappropriate tone.

As the client performs mobility and stability patterns as components of developmental sequence postures, all types of muscle contractions should be elicited from each muscle group. If a particular type of contraction poses a problem for a muscle group, the therapist can select an alternate posture in which to build in the ability of the muscle group to perform that type of contraction. For example, if the client has problems with eccentric hamstring control during the swing phase of gait, the pattern can be worked on as a component of the rolling sequence from the supine to the prone position (Fig. 16-7). Once the client gains control of the pattern within one movement context, the therapist must design activities to promote generalization of the pattern to other movement contexts. The client who has difficulty with the cocontraction stability pattern of the upper extremity in the all-fours position may have more success with a forward propping position in sitting, which may allow more control of the amount of weight being supported by the upper extremity. After gaining control in forward propped sitting, attempts can be made to generalize the response to such positions as side sitting and all fours.

Performance of movement patterns should progress toward the ability to easily reverse the direction of the movement. This can be promoted by incorporating rhythmical movements within a posture or between postures as early in the intervention sequence as is possible. The end point at which the reversal is required should vary. The client might be asked to move from the sitting position to all fours, and back to sitting; then the client could move from the sitting position to the half-way position to all fours, then reverse to sitting. Incorporating reversal of movement patterns within the intervention program prepares the client to deal with situations that mandate unexpected adjustments in the movement sequence.

Clients who demonstrate problems with the sequencing of movements, such as those with motor dyspraxia, frequently perform better if the movement is performed at a speed that is close to normal. Clients who, previous to the brain infection, had normal movement sequences seem to be able to trigger better movement responses at normal speeds than at slower speeds, which disrupt the normal flow of the movement. In working with clients with sequencing problems, all team members should provide the same, consistent sensory cues to elicit a movement pattern. For example, the therapist may establish a coupling of the verbal cue "roll" with a quick stretch to the ankle dorsiflexors to elicit a rolling pattern. These same cues can be used by other team members to assist the client in changing positions in bed or in performing dressing activities. The consistency of cues may elicit a consistent response from the client. Once the pattern is well established, the intervention program can be designed to include an extinction process for the cues progressing toward the ability of the client to perform the activity in response to the demands of the situation rather than to externally imposed cues.

The flow of a movement pattern may be disrupted by problems categorized as incoordination. The origin of the coordination problems could be dysfunction of the visual-perceptual system (see Chapter 25), or vestibular systems (see Chapter 11), dyspraxia (see Chapter 11), or dysfunction caused by cerebellar damage (see Chapter 21). If possible, the factors involved in producing a lack of coordination should be identified.

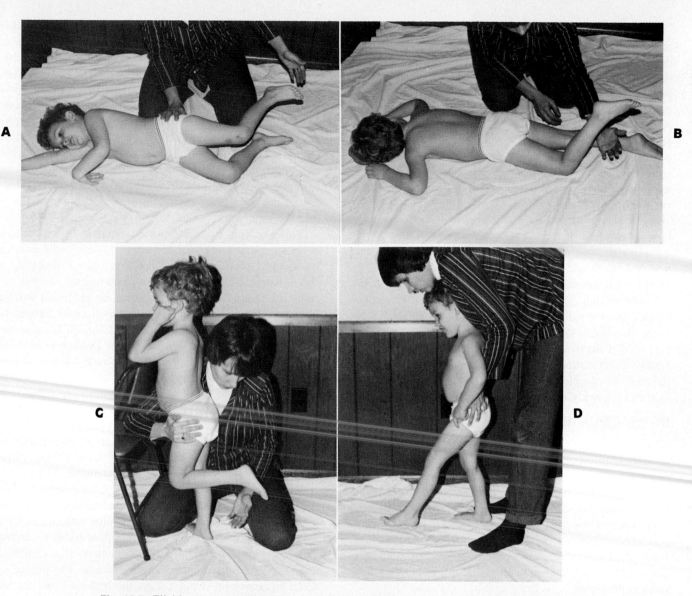

Fig. 16-7. Eliciting eccentric hamstring control within different movement contexts. **A,** Roll from the supine to side-lying position (beginning sequence). **B,** Roll from the side-lying to prone position with controlled lengthening of the hamstrings. **C,** Standing eccentric hamstring contraction. **D,** Controlled hamstring activity during swing phase of gait.

Promoting optimalization of psychosocial and cognitive responses

In addition to attending to the factors that are directly related to motor performance, the therapist must also attend to the psychosocial and cognitive responses of the client. Although the physical therapist does not have primary responsibility in this area, a goal of the intervention process should be to promote optimalization of psychosocial and cognitive responses. In Chapter 7 Burton discusses the psychosocial adjustment that occurs in the process of recovering from a neurological disability. The therapist must be aware of how the client's regression in affective and cognitive domains impacts on the intervention process. The therapist should seek assistance from the health care team members responsible for intervention in these areas in order to deal with the client in the most constructive fashion. The therapist must remember that both the family members and the client are in the process of adjusting to the client's changed and, hopefully, changing status. The family members may be an asset or a liability to the client's recovery process. During the therapist's interactions with the family members in activities such as instructions in the client's home program, the therapist should be prepared to deal with expressions of the individual's difficulty in adjusting to the situation. The therapist should be prepared to assist family members in identifying appropriate sources of assistance to help them in dealing with their problems.

As the therapist works with the client on an intervention program, situations arise that require problem-solving to determine a way or the best way to accomplish a task. If the task is to accomplish an independent transfer from a wheelchair into a bathtub, decisions have to be made concerning the sequence of movements. Therapists can approach this in two ways. They can instruct clients step-by-step in what to do, or they can involve clients to the extent possible in the process of deciding what to do. If the therapist instructs the client step-by-step, the client may master the task but may not be able to perform it under different conditions. If the therapist involves the client in the decision-making process, the client may be learning not only how to accomplish the specific task, but also how to accomplish the task under varied conditions. The intervention process should lead to the ability to respond to the demands of a situation, and involvement of clients in the problem-solving process helps prepare them for independence. The therapist must structure the client's role in decision making to the level of the client's ability to participate so that the experience is not frustrating. Although the client's participation may initially increase the time period required to complete a task, it promotes skills that may lead more quickly to independence of function.

INTERACTION WITH OTHER PROFESSIONALS

The necessity of the physical therapist to design an intervention program that is articulated with that of other members of the health care team has been mentioned in several areas of this chapter. The recovery process of the client should be facilitated by a care plan in which each team member reinforces the goals of the other team members. The care of the person must be a collaborative effort. Each client deserves an intervention process that considers him or her as a whole individual and not as a set of fragmented problems.

SUMMARY

The problem-solving process presented within this chapter for assessment, goal identification, and treatment planning is not limited to clients with inflammatory supraspinal disorders and can easily be applied to other neurological disabilities. In the overview of the inflammatory disorders within the brain, the variability of neurological sequelae is discussed based on the anatomical location of the inflammatory process and the cause of the infection. The response of the CNS to the inflammatory process must also be considered in the development of the intervention plan.

A client with meningitis or encephalitis may demonstrate signs similar to generalized head trauma, tumor disorder, or other identified abnormal neurological states. Yet a client with an inflammatory disorder has additional pathological complications unique to the dysfunction that may make the response to treatment very different. Because of the inflammatory process, his or her CNS is in an irritated state. Because of the irritation the client is frequently agitated. The specific level of agitation will vary from mild to severe depending both upon the client's unique CNS characteristics and upon the degree of inflammation. The agitated state may be the result of inappropriate or augmented response to sensory input. The client may respond to normal audible sound as though it were unbearably loud. Dull artificial light may be perceived as extremely bright. The clinician must be extremely sensitive to the client's interpretation of sensory input and gradate the input appropriately.

This agitation may also present itself in hypersensitive or exaggerated emotional responses to seemingly normal interactions. For example, when upset about dropping a spoon on the floor, a client may throw the tray across the room. In another example, when told his girlfriend will be a little late this afternoon, a client may become extremely upset and state that he is going to kill himself because his girlfriend does not love him anymore. Dealing with these emotional instabilities can become a major factor in goal attainment in other areas of clinical performance. Maintaining a positive, nonthreatening interaction allows the client to use the therapist as a reference for judging whether emotional responses are appropriate.

Because of the variety of pathological problems following acute inflammation, the client may have residual problems manifested as generalized brain damage. The specifics of these problems cannot be generalized because they are extremely dependent on the individual client.

Whether the meningitis or encephalitis was caused by a viral or bacterial infection is an important factor regarding potential recovery. Bacterial inflammation often results in more severe and permanent brain damage. The degree of CNS inflammation is not always the best indicator for the degree of recovery. For example, a client with a generalized viral meningitis may exhibit severe neurological dysfunction. That state may exist for an extended period of time. Once the client's acute inflammation has subsided, severe dysfunction may persist. Unlike a client with a progressive disease, such as an active growing tumor, the person who has survived the acute inflammatory disorder will stabilize and begin to regain function. This process can take extended periods of time, and the client may be discharged from a rehabilitation center before full recovery has occurred.

The perceptual cognitive processes are also affected following inflammation within the CNS. Thus clients often have distortions in perception as well as memory problems. As their memories return, accuracy of time and events may be distorted. This in itself can cause frustration and anxiety both for the client and those family and friends who are interacting within the environment. Repetition will help reorder past knowledge. This is best done in a nonstressful environment where attention and memory are not overshadowed by emotional pressure.

Although the neurological disorders discussed within this chapter are life threatening and often fatal, many clients recover and return to their previous life-style. These clinical problems can incorporate clinical signs seen in almost all neurological conditions. Clients will fall within the spectrum of minimal to severe involvement, specific to generalized CNS dysfunction, and little to full recovery following the acute distress. The clinician must remain flexible and willing to adjust every aspect of therapeutic intervention to meet the specific needs of each client.

The client who has or is recovering from an inflammatory disorder within the brain may have a variety of neurological problems. Prognosis for recovery depends on the type of infecting organism and the extent of the client's involvement. Thus the clinical picture for each individual will be composed of varied symptoms. This chapter has presented a brief discussion of the pathology and medical management of the various inflammatory process that affect the brain. The process of assessment, the role of assessment in designing an intervention program, and goals and techniques of the intervention process were presented to assist the reader in more effective management of these clients.

REFERENCES

1. Ayres JA: Sensory integration and learning disorder, Los Angeles, 1972, Wester Psychological Services.
2. Ayres JA: Southern California Postrotatory Nystagmus Test, Los Angeles, 1975, Western Psychological Services.
3. Bobath B: The treatment of neuromuscular disorders by improving patterns of coordination, Physiotherapy 55:18-22, 1969.
4. Bobath B: Abnormal postural reflex activity caused by brain lesions, ed 2, London, 1971, William Heinemann Medical Books, Ltd.
5. Bobath B: Adult hemiplegia: evaluation and treatment, ed 2, London, 1978, William Heinemann Medical Books, Ltd.
6. DeMeyer W: Technique of the Neurological examination, ed 4, New York, 1981, McGraw-Hill Book Co.
7. Ellner JJ: Central nervous system infections in the intensive care unit. In Henning RJ and Jackson DL, editors: Handbook of critical care neurology and neurosurgery, New York, 1985, Praeger Publishers.
8. Farber SD: Olfaction in health and disease, Am J Occup Ther 32(3):155-160, 1978.
9. Farber SD: Neurorehabilitation: a multi-sensory approach, Philadelphia, 1981, WB Saunders Co.
10. Gallender D: Eating handicaps, Springfield, Ill, 1979, Charles C Thomas, Publisher.
11. Heiniger MC and Randolph SL: Neurophysiological concepts in human behavior: the tree of learning, St Louis, 1981, The CV Mosby Co.
12. Hoppenfeld S: Physical examination of the spine and extremities, New York, 1976, Appleton-Century-Crofts.
13. Jennett B and Teasdale G: Management of head injuries, Philadelphia, 1981, FA Davis Co.
14. Johnson RT: Responses of the nervous system to infection. In Asbury AK, Khann GM, and McDonald WI, editors: Diseases of the nervous system, vol 2, Philadelphia, 1986, WB Saunders Co.
15. Kritchevsky M: Infection of the nervous system. In Wiederholt WC, editor: Neurology for non-neurologists, Philadelphia, 1988, Grune & Stratton Inc.
16. Kroll JS and Moxon ER: Bacterial meningitis in children. In Asbury AK, Khann GM, and McDonald WI, editors: Diseases of the nervous system, vol 2, Philadelphia, 1986, WB Saunders Co.
17. Levitt S: Treatment of cerebral palsy and motor delay, ed 2, London, 1982, Blackwell Scientific Publications, Inc.
18. McGraw MB: Neuromuscular mechanisms of the infant, Am J Dis Child 60(5):1031-1042, 1940.
19. Parker JC and Dyer ML: Neurological infections due to bacteria, fungi, and parasites. In Davis RL and Robertson DM, editors: Textbook of neuropathology, Baltimore, 1985, Williams & Wilkins.
20. Plum F and Posner JB: The diagnosis of stupor and coma, ed 3, Philadelphia, 1980, FA Davis Co.
21. Schooley RT: Encephalitis. In Roper AH and Kennedy SF, editors: Neurological and neurosurgical intensive care, ed 2, Rockwell, Md, 1988, Aspen Publishers Inc.
22. Stutman HR and Marks MI: Bacterial meningitis in children: diagnosis and therapy, Clin Ped 26(9):431-438, 1987.
23. Sullivan PE and others: An integrated approach to therapeutic exercise, Reston, Va, 1982, Reston Publishing Co, Inc.
24. Tokizane T and others: Electromyographic studies on tonic neck, lumbar, and labyrinthine reflexes in normal persons, Jpn J Physiol 2:130-146, 1951.
25. Van Sant AF: Rising from a supine position to erect stance—description of adult movement and a developmental hypothesis, Phys Ther 68(2):185-192, 1988.
26. Voss DE, Ionta MK, and Myers BJ: Proprioceptive neuromuscular facilitation, ed 3, Philadelphia, 1985, Harper & Row Publishers Inc.
27. Weisberg LA: Acute bacterial meningitis in adulthood. In Weisberg LA, Strub RL, and Garcia CA, editors: Decision making in adult neurology, Toronto, 1987, BC Decker Inc.
28. Weisberg LA, Strub RL, and Garcia CA: Essentials of clinical neurology, Baltimore, 1983, University Park Press.
29. Wood EC and Becker PD: Beard's massage, ed 3, Philadelphia, 1981, WB Saunders Co.

Chapter 17

CURRENT ISSUES IN NEUROLOGICAL REHABILITATION

Laura K. Smith (Part I)
Johnny Bonck and Anne MacRae (Part II)

An entire book could be written discussing the pathology, etiology, progression, and treatment procedures for infectious diseases that might affect the CNS. Some of those diseases have been discussed in other chapters (see Chapters 16, 18, and 19). In those discussions the specific pathogen may or may not have been clearly identified, but the common procedures have been. This chapter's purpose is to focus on two identifiable disease processes that originate through viral infection and are relatively new with regard to therapeutic treatment, but are being presented within the clinical setting in larger and larger numbers. Both disease processes have a dramatic effect upon the function of the CNS.

The first disease, postpolio syndrome, has been identified as a new problem that, if treated with strengthening or aerobic exercises as used in the postacute and chronic phases of polio, may have potentially harmful effects on the patient. As the last large epidemic of clients with acute polio is approaching its third to fourth decade postinsult, the clients' remaining intact motor units are responding negatively to their overuse between the time of onset of the disease and present day. If a therapist identifies weakness in a muscle group, a natural response is to develop a strengthening program. With this syndrome, however, that philosophy may cause further damage to the client. A confounding variable is the socialization of the survivors of acute polio. These people are used to being independent: they work to overcome their physical problems and are very resistant to accepting new physical limitations. The discussion of the multitudinous problems encountered in postpolio begins with an overview of acute and postacute problems and treatment. The focus of the polio section of this chapter is on the postpolio syndrome, its physiological manifestations, potential problems, and treatment suggestions. The author highly recommends that any therapist who is considering treating a client with postpolio problems develop the clinical knowledge base of the pathology of acute poliomyelitis, physiology of the recovery process, and the effects of long-term overcompensation on the neuromuscular and skeletal systems. This knowledge is necessary to implement a safe and effective treatment procedure.

The second section of this chapter deals with a more recently identified infectious disease, human immunodeficiency virus (HIV) illness, which in its latter phases causes the socially feared disease acquired immunodeficiency syndrome (AIDS). The understanding of the HIV, its destructive progression throughout the course of the disease process, and the alternative treatment procedures available are still in the beginning phases of evolution. Research is being reported daily that slightly alters the focus of how best to deal with all aspects of this disease. Thus, the reader must be cautioned that what is written in 1988 may seem very elementary in 1992.

Within this chapter the reader is introduced to the anatomy and physiology as well as to the possible pathogenic progression and outcome of an individual contracting HIV. The discussion focuses on the multitudinous health problems encountered throughout the progression of this illness and the possible role a therapist might play in helping to maintain a high quality of life for an infected individual. The myth that contact with AIDS victims will potentially lead to infection is discussed to help alleviate some of the fears encountered within the general public. The newness of this clinical problem and the social stigma placed on so many clients who have contracted the disease creates a dynamic clinical problem. Solutions to problems therapists have or will have in the future remain unknown, but ignoring the problem is certainly not the solution. The student is encouraged to read this section and develop an understanding of the disease process. If confronted with clients suffering the latter phases of HIV infection, a therapist should find ideas and treatment suggestions in this chapter that will help in development of a comprehensive therapeutic program.

Part I Poliomyelitis and the postpolio syndrome

Laura K. Smith

OVERVIEW

Poliomyelitis or infantile paralysis is an endemic disease of humans first recorded in paralytic form in 1300 BC.[44] It is an acute infectious disease caused by an enteric virus with worldwide distribution. Transmission is by human contact, and most of the people ingest the virus. Few persons, however, develop the paralytic form because they have developed immunity from breast-feeding, subclinical

infections, clinical infections without paralysis, and now vaccines. In the paralytic form, the virus selectively attacks the motor neuron cell bodies with resulting flaccid muscle paresis or paralysis.

As sanitation levels increased in industrialized countries in the first half of this century and formula-feeding was advocated, acute poliomyelitis escalated to epidemic proportions. Frightening epidemics swept across North America and Europe from 1910 to 1959. In 1921 New York City recorded 9000 cases with 2000 deaths. Franklin Roosevelt contracted poliomyelitis at this time. In 1937, when he was President of the United States, he founded the March of Dimes (The National Foundation for Infantile Paralysis). An unprecedented outpouring of public funds occurred to provide treatment, research, and professional education. The results were spectacular. In just 20 years the "War on Polio" was won with the introduction of the inactivated vaccine (Salk, 1955) and the live attenuated oral vaccine (Sabin, 1960). Polio was promptly forgotten as medicine and rehabilitation turned attention to other pressing disabilities. The March of Dimes changed focus to birth defects, and the surviving polio victims went on with their lives to compensate, compete, and become productive citizens.

Acute poliomyelitis and its sequelae, however, did not stop but rather continued on in its many phases. Currently there are an estimated 250,000 to 300,000 postpolio individuals in the United States. These people have all of the diseases and injuries found in an adult population. Evaluation and treatment is complicated by the previous paresis and by the poor or altered response to medical, surgical, and rehabilitation procedures. Over 25% of the postpolio individuals are experiencing new symptoms of fatigue, weakness, pain, and decreased functional ability of the postpolio syndrome.[14] Although the virus is still prevalent within industrialized countries, infection is prevented by immunization. There are 10 or more new cases of acute poliomyelitis per year in the United States, mostly vaccine related. The World Health Organization has calculated that there is an average of 275,000 new cases per year in the developing countries.[49]

IDENTIFICATION OF THE CLINICAL PROBLEM: PATHOLOGY

In most instances the widely prevalent polio viruses are destroyed in the stomach or excreted via the intestinal tract without clinical infection, or they may enter the bloodstream and produce a flulike infection with recovery and development of immunity. If the virus crosses the blood-brain barrier, it attacks almost all of the motor nerve cells in the brain, brainstem, and spinal cord. Symptoms during this 2-week febrile illness include headache, sore throat, elevated temperature, severe meningismus, severe muscle pain to touch and stretch, and flaccid muscle paresis or paralysis (signs and symptoms of severe life-threatening poliomyelitis are outlined by Spencer[44]). Many motor neurons fought off the virus and recovered, but many were destroyed. Bodian[2] in animal studies found only 4% of the anterior horn cells histologically normal at 2 to 6 days from onset, but by 14 days the neurons were either destroyed or of normal appearance.

Following the febrile illness a motor neuron with its 5 to 1500 muscle fibers could be unaffected, recovered, or destroyed with resulting denervation of the muscle fibers (Fig. 17-1). The 100 to 1000 motor neurons to a particular muscle might be unaffected or recovered, all of the motor neurons to a muscle could be destroyed, or the muscle could be partially denervated with combinations of recovered and destroyed motor neurons. Diagnostic EMG at this time would show fibrillation potentials indicating recent denervation of muscle fibers.

Physiological processes of recovery of muscle strength

In convalescent poliomyelitis, muscle strength in partially denervated muscles increases to a maximum over a 2-year period with 50% of the muscle strength recovery occurring in the first 3 months after onset and 75% in the first 6 months (Fig. 17-2). The rate and magnitude of the recovery, however, can be compromised by injudicious treatment, activity, and excessive exercise.[1,25,41]

Muscle strength recovery and increase in functional ability occurs by several physiological processes. Recovered neurons develop terminal axon sprouts to reinnervate orphaned muscle fibers[15,45,48] (Fig. 17-1). It is estimated that a single motor neuron can reinnervate up to 5 times its normal complement of muscle fibers. Electromyographi-

cally the action potentials of the single motor units are polyphasic with large amplitudes and are called giant motor units. The innervated muscle fibers can be hypertrophied by exercise and activity during the rehabilitation phase. This has been referred to as denervation hypertrophy. The third process provides an increase in functional ability and an apparent increase of strength by neuromuscular learning whereby practice of an exercise or an activity leads to increased skill and performance without necessarily increasing muscle strength.[38] The fourth process is the increased recruitment of the giant motor units with use of the muscle at high levels of its capacity.

Such extensive compensatory physiological processes mask the profound neurological deficits caused by the disease. This was demonstrated by Sharrard,[39] who counted the number of anterior horn cells in the spinal cords of postpolio individuals who died from other causes. He compared the percentage of cells present with previous muscle test grades. Sharrard found that muscles graded 5 (N) could have lost up to 60% of their anterior horn cells. Muscles previously graded 4 (G) had lost 60% to 90% of their motor neurons and muscles of grades 3, 2, and 1 (F, P, T) lost 90% to 98%.

Functional compensation

The body possesses a number of compensatory mechanisms to maintain function in the presence of residual paralysis (Fig. 17-3). These compensations include use of weak muscles at high levels of their capacity, substitution of strong muscles with increased energy expenditure for the task, and use of ligaments for stability with resulting hypermobility. Many convalescent polio clients in the

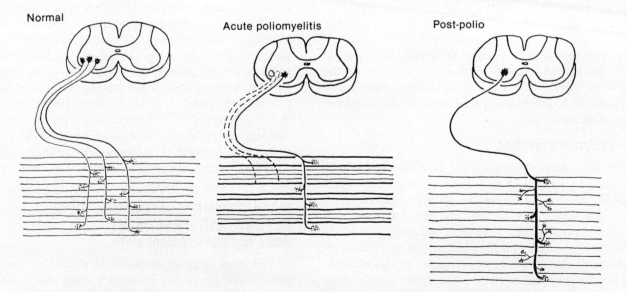

Fig. 17-1. Schematic representation of motor units to a muscle. *Normal* represents the 100 to 1000 motor neurons of a muscle and the 5 to 1500 muscle fibers each axon innervates. *Acute poliomyelitis* depicts viral destruction of some of the anterior horn cells with atrophy of denervated muscle fibers. *Postpolio* represents axon sprouting by recovered nerve cells with reinnervation of the orphaned muscle fibers and subsequent hypertrophy.

Percent chance of severely involved muscles recovering to "good" or "normal" eventual strength:

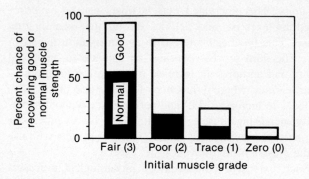

Rate of muscle recovery irrespective of the initial or final strength:

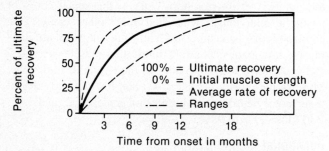

Fig. 17-2. The rate and extent of increase in manual muscle test scores in postacute poliomyelitis. Muscles showing some strength on initial examination will increase in strength unless they are overworked, in which case they may plateau or lose strength. The grade of Normal (5) is a clinical definition and not an indication of preillness strength. This grade can be recorded with loss of 60% of the anterior horn cells to a muscle.[39] (Adapted from Spencer, WA: Treatment of acute poliomyelitis, Springfield, 1956, Charles C Thomas, with permission).

early epidemics were encouraged to exercise for years and to use heroic compensatory methods for function. In the long term, however, such overcompensation leads to microtrauma of ligaments and joint structures and exhaustion of neuromuscular units.

The postpolio syndrome

The late effects of poliomyelitis have been recorded in the literature since 1875 by various authors.* These new problems occur at an average of 35 years after the acute onset, and thus it was not until the 1980s that the large number of survivors from the great epidemics of 1940 to 1957 made an impact on the medical system.[30] The syndrome is a combination of neurological, musculoskeletal, and psychosocial manifestations. The most common physical problems are profound fatigue, pain, and new weakness with decreased function, safety, and quality of life (Table 17-1). Other physical problems include muscle fas-

*References 3, 5, 16, 17, 22, 34.

Table 17-1. Most common new health problems in 132 confirmed postpolio individuals with a diagnosis of postpolio syndrome

	N	%
Health problems		
Fatigue	117	89
Muscle pain	93	71
Joint pain	93	71
Weakness		
Previously affected muscles	91	69
Previously unaffected muscles	66	50
Cold intolerance	38	29
Atrophy	37	28
ADL problems		
Walking	84	64
Climbing stairs	80	61
Dressing	23	17

Adapted with permission from Halstead L and Wiechers D, editors: Research and clinical aspects of the late effects of poliomyelitis, White Plains, NY, 1987, March of Dimes, p 17.

ciculations and cramps, hypoventilation, swallowing difficulties, and sleep disturbances.

The etiology of the new weakness and atrophy is unknown because few autopsy studies have been made. Several causes have been proposed and are reviewed in detail by Jubelt and Cashman.[20] There is little current evidence to implicate reactivation of the polio virus or an autoimmune response. Normal aging, with loss of neurons occurring after age 60,[46] may be a factor in the older postpolio individuals because the loss of a few neurons from an already markedly depleted neuronal pool could result in a significant decrease in strength. It has been suggested that the neurons that showed histological recovery from the virus may not have been physiologically normal and may be subject to premature aging and failure.[22,27] Most evidence points to an increased metabolic demand on the giant motor units with remodeling and pruning of the axon sprouts to reduce the number of muscle fibers innervated by the motor nerve cell.[28,29,35,36] Single-fiber EMG studies show instability or failure of transmission of the nerve impulse at the axon terminal or neuromuscular junction (jitter or blocking)[48] and some muscle biopsies are suggestive of new denervation of muscle fibers.[7,8]

MANAGEMENT: EVALUATION, GOAL SETTING AND TREATMENT
Acute and convalescent polio

Treatment in all of the stages of poliomyelitis is complex because the disease produces a spotty and asymmetrical paralysis with no two clients alike. Treatment needs will differ according to the stage of the disease, age of the person, time from onset, severity of involvement, amount of recovery, presence of joint hypermobility or hypomobility, previous treatment, and level of activity. Effective

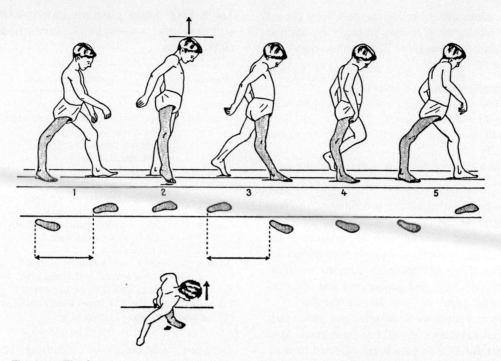

Fig. 17-3. The functional compensations of a boy with paralysis of the right lower extremity show increased energy expenditure and progressive ligamentous laxity. (Adapted from Ducroquet R and others: Walking and limping—a study of normal and pathological walking, Philadelphia, 1968, JB Lippincott Co, with permission of the copyright holder.)

treatment is based on pathology and is individualized by evaluation of the person. During the febrile illness the goal of treatment is to preserve and protect life and physiological functions. Rest and anticipatory medical and nursing care are obligatory. Physical measures other than positioning to relieve pain and pain-free passive range of motion are contraindicated. In the convalescent phase the goal is to develop useful function compatible with the patient's residual capacity. Physical and occupational therapy predominate with emphasis on pain relief, exercise, and independent function with major modifications for those with respiratory muscle paralysis. The following references provide details of the principles and methods of treatment of acute and convalescent poliomyelitis.[19,23,44]

Postpolio evaluation

The manifestations of the late effects of polio are nonspecific and similar to symptoms of many other conditions. A comprehensive interdisciplinary evaluation is essential to (1) confirm the original diagnosis of poliomyelitis because approximately 10% to 15% of people who thought or were told they had polio did not,[16,44] (2) identify all other physical-psychosocial health problems that may occur in the age ranges of 20 to 90 years, and (3) establish current diagnoses. The differential diagnosis of postpolio syndrome is made by exclusion.[14,30]

Physical therapy evaluation in postpolio syndrome differs markedly from that needed in the postacute and con-

valescent stages, where definitive manual muscle testing and goniometry form the basis of the treatment plan. In postpolio syndrome selective gross group testing is sufficient to provide information to help in the diagnosis of polio and direction of treatment needs. Time need not be spent searching for nonfunctional contractions (P+ to T or 2+ to 1) or to belabor the narrow range of grades from N− to P+ (5− to 2+), because these grades will vary markedly with previous activity. Comparisons with old muscle tests are interesting but are reliable only when the ability of the examiners and the criteria used for each muscle are known. Major aspects of the physical therapy evaluation include:

1. History and analysis of physical activity by type, time, and intensity in the home, at work, in travel, in community activities, in avocations, and in recreation and exercise
2. Detailed evaluation of habitual sleeping, sitting, standing, and walking postures
3. Modified spinal and upper-lower quarter evaluations according to problems presented
4. Evaluation of current orthoses and needs for orthotic interventions

Management of postpolio syndrome

The general goal at this stage is to provide the person with principles and methods for self-management of his or her body. The most important aspect of the program is patient and family education regarding the pathology caused by acute poliomyelitis, the processes of recovery, and the effects of long-term compensation. Specific musculoskeletal objectives are to:

1. Alleviate and prevent the causes of pain
2. Decrease the abnormally high work load of muscles relative to their limited capacity
3. Correct and minimize postural and gait deviations mechanically
4. Maintain and increase function, safety, and the quality of life

Pain. Pain was found to be the predominant problem of reporting postpolio individuals, with an incidence of 85% in those walking without orthotic assistance and 100% in those using crutches or manual wheelchairs for locomotion.[42] The types and causes of pain are multiple. One type of pain is diffuse and generalized and often described as as "bone pain" or "like having the flu." This pain occurs both in known weak muscles and particularly in extremities that have been thought to be normal. Most people report that this type of pain is not affected by medications or physical modalities and that it is increased by physical activity and decreased by rest. The pain or fatigue is unusual because it usually does not occur at the time of the activity but rather 1 or 2 days after the activity. Such findings point towards overuse of muscles for their capacity. Treatment should be directed to decreasing energy expenditure and the work load on the muscle.

Joint pains are more localized and caused by injuries and long-term microtrauma. Common conditions include osteoarthritis (particularly in the vertebrae), neck, back, and sacroiliac dysfunction, trochanteric bursitis, ligamentous laxity of the knee and ankle and patellar-femoral tracking problems, rotator cuff injuries, tennis elbow, carpal tunnel syndrome, and carpal-metacarpal injuries of the thumb. These conditions can be treated as athletic injuries. They are slow to respond, because rest of the part may be difficult if the polio survivor must continue to use the extremity for function.

Neck, shoulder, and back pain radiating to the hip and leg are reported by over 65% of postpolio individuals.[42] This pain is not unexpected because the incidence of major postural abnormalities and gait deviations is also high (Table 17-2). In the absence of radiculopathies or nerve entrapments, treatment should be directed to mechanical and orthotic correction of postures and locomotion accompanied by methods of pain relief and control. Nonsteroidal antiinflammatory medications may be useful for control of joint and postural type pain.

Many persons who had poliomyelitis underwent extensive orthopedic surgery, and some are experiencing pain or hypersensitivities at these sites. Orthotic supports can be helpful and are most successful in malalignment and pain in the ankle and foot. When the causes of pain cannot be

Table 17-2. Major postural abnormalities in sitting, standing, and walking in 111 confirmed postpolio clinic clients

Posture (N)	Abnormal deviation	No.	Percent
Sitting (N = 111)	Absent lumbar curve	64	54
	Forward head (loss of cervical curve)	50	45
	Uneven pelvic base*	29	26
	Structural scoliosis	38	34
Standing (N = 76)	Absent lumbar curve	52	68
	Uneven pelvic base*	40	53
	Weight bearing on stronger leg	29	38
Walking (N = 76)	Abnormal gait deviations	76	100
	Major lateral trunk oscillations	33	43
	Obvious forward lean	40	53

Adapted from Smith L and McDermott K: Pain in post-poliomyelitis: addressing causes versus effects. In Halstead L and Wiechers D, (editors): Research and clinical aspects of the late effects of poliomyelitis, White Plains, NY, 1987, March of Dimes (with permission).
*Pelvic asymmetry was ½ inch or more.

corrected, transcutaneous electrical nerve stimulation (TENS) and local cold should be considered to provide pain relief.

Temporary alleviation of pain is not particularly difficult, but correction of the causes and prevention of pain is indeed a challenge.

Abnormal fatigue. Abnormal fatigue is reported by almost 90% of the postpolio clients as a new problem (Table 17-1). Some will describe the phenomenon as a sudden and total wipeout that may include headaches and sweating suggestive of autonomic system overload.[41] Prevention can be attained by decreasing energy expenditure, breaking activities up into parts with frequent rest or change of activity, and by daily rest periods or a nap as necessary.

New muscle weakness. Abnormal muscle activity or atrophy occurs in extremities with previous paresis as well as in strong extremities not thought to have been affected by polio. The weakness is more noticeable with repetitive activities and stabilizing contractions than with single maximum efforts. Fasciculations may be seen at rest or during contraction and muscle cramps are common. New atrophy of muscles is sometimes reported and is most noticeable when it occurs in the gastrocnemius-soleus muscle group.[11]

These signs point to overuse of muscles for their limited capacity with encroachment on reserves. Treatment is directed toward decreasing the work load of the muscles and building a reserve by instituting energy conservation techniques, activity modification, and orthotic assistance.

Environmental cold intolerance. Cold intolerance is thought to result from sympathetic neuron involvement with loss of vasoconstriction and veno-constriction. Heat loss to the environment can be reduced with clothing. This problem causes most postpolio individuals to use heating pads and hot water for pain relief. Local cold, however, is usually more effective and longer lasting for pain caused by microtrauma and injuries.

Sleep disturbances. Sleep disturbances have been found in over 50% of reporting postpolio individuals.[12] These disturbances may be caused by pain, stress, under-ventilation, or obstructive apnea.[1,18,40] The role of the physical therapist is primarily in the area of pain. A history of pain or numbness that is worse at night or on rising points to sleeping surfaces that are too firm or sleeping with joints in closed packed positions—usually the neck and shoulders. These problems are correctable with foam mattress covers or waterbeds, cervical pillows, and modification of sleeping postures.

Life-threatening conditions. Life-threatening conditions such as hypoventilation, dysphagia, and cardiopulmonary insufficiency require management by medical specialists.[1,43,44] These problems occur in people with previous bulbar poliomyelitis who may or may not be using ventilatory assistance and in those with severe kyphosis or scoliosis. The role of the physical therapist is to modify activities and teach glossopharyngeal breathing, manually assisted coughing, or bronchial drainage as indicated.[6,10] If trunk supports are considered, vital capacity should be checked with and without an abdominal binder to determine the effect on breathing.

Decreasing the work load of muscles

Energy conservation techniques. Energy conservation techniques provide the easiest way to decrease the work of muscles without loss of function. An occupational therapy program to assist the person in analysis of all activity by type, time, distance, and intensity is valuable. Such an inventory forms the basis for setting priorities and determining where and how individuals wish to use their limited neuromuscular capacity. Questions to be addressed include:

1. Can one trip do for two or three?
2. Can the activity be performed in a less strenuous way, such as by sitting or using a rolling basket?
3. Are there easier ways to perform the activity with modern comforts and technology, including motorization and electronics?
4. Can the activity be broken up into parts with change of activity or rest?
5. Are there other people who can perform some of the physical aspects of the activity?

Weight reduction. Weight reduction is the single most effective way to decrease the muscle work load, but it is one of the most difficult. Weight loss is slow without exercise, but it can be accomplished. Weight control needs to be incorporated as a permanent modification of nutritional habits rather than achieved in a short-term diet. Dietetic counseling and support groups are important components of this difficult life-style modification.

Locomotion. Locomotion and related activities such as elevation and transfer of body weight or wheelchair loading require major modifications that are difficult for polio survivors to consider. They underwent extensive rehabilitation for months and years to achieve independence. Rehabilitation included long-term hospitalization with absence from families, extensive exercise, frequently painful stretching, wearing braces and corrective shoes, and often multiple surgical procedures. Many with only generalized weakness have a lifetime pattern of "passing" as normal by using shoe and clothing modifications, walking slowly, and avoiding activities that would reveal impairment. Those with noticeable signs of disability minimize impairments. They frequently describe their ability to compete with and often exceed the physical abilities of their siblings and peers. As walking or wheelchair activities become more difficult and painful, many permit their world to close in and become smaller rather than modify their methods of locomotion. They find more and more reasons to avoid activities. Many come to dread family outings and vacations, and some get into a cycle of going to work, going home to bed, and then going to work.

Prevention of this spiraling disability or restoration of lost function requires multiple interventions that include modifying the environment to decrease elevation activities of the body, avoiding stairs and floor sitting, using handicapped parking in those and assistive devices, and motorization for distance locomotion. Motorized off the road vehicles should be a consideration for almost all postpolio individuals, to decrease muscle work and preserve function. Light-weight wheelchairs at best only postpone problems. All-terrain vehicles (ATVs) permit continuing participation in farm, ranch, hunting, and country activities. Motorized carts for distance locomotion should be used at airports, in stores and malls (where available), for golf, at convention centers, and at large recreational or sports facilities. Persons currently using or considering manual wheelchairs should be directed to investigate the advantages and limitations of the many types of off-the-road vehicles and electric wheelchairs on the market. Some people may need motorization only at work, only at home, or only in the community. Others may need motorization as their primary form of locomotion.

Correction of posture and gait deviations. In addition to sitting in poorly supporting chairs, sofas, auto seats, and wheelchairs, the postpolio individual may have trunk muscle paresis or asymmetries of the pelvic base and may spend up to 16 hours per day in the seated position. The typical posture is slumped hanging on posterior vertebral ligaments with loss of lumbar and cervical curves. Neck, shoulder, and back pain are common. Mechanical restoration of the lumbar curve in all seating at home, during meals, at work, in automobiles, in wheelchairs, at church, in meetings, and at social events can correct the problem. This can be accomplished by use of properly fitted clerical chairs, ergonometric chairs, anterior tilt seats, gluteal pads, and the many types of lumbar rolls, back supports, and seating systems.

Persons with abdominal muscle paralysis benefit from custom-made thoracolumbar corsets with the posterior rigid stays bent to produce a normal standing lumbar curve. Paretic or paralyzed neck muscles can be rested and supported by soft foam collars or the more supportive microcellular neck collars.

People with severe trunk muscle paralysis or scoliosis with or without spinal fusion often support their trunk or relieve pain by pushing down with their hands or elbows on chairs, tables, and on their hips (Fig. 17-4). In time such self-traction results in pain and weakness in their arms. Chair inserts and fixed supports as well as custom-made corsets, back braces, and molded body jackets should be considered. The rigid trunk supports, however, take away mobility used for function. Usually they can be worn for part of the day in activities where trunk mobility is not essential.

Most postpolio individuals long ago discarded orthotic assistance and have relied on body compensations. The abnormal deviations in standing and walking cause increased energy expenditure and in time lead to pain, fatigue, or loss of safety. Orthotic applications are necessary for prevention and correction of these problems. Attempts at gait training only place more stress on the person and may be dangerous. Biomechanical objectives for application of orthotics are to (1) minimize leg length differences, (2) restore weight bearing on the weaker leg, (3) control unstable or painful joints, (4) gain an erect posture, (5) minimize gait deviations, (6) increase shock absorption, and (7) decrease energy expenditure. Achievement of these ob-

jectives requires attention to cosmesis, provision of alternatives for different activities, and simulation or trial use of the orthosis as possible.

Heel lifts, shoe inserts, molded foot orthoses, and some normal footwear can provide a number of unobtrusive corrections. Positive heel shoes with a broad base, such as cowboy boots, stacked or Cuban heels, or the Swedish clog,[32] decrease the amount of dorsiflexion and plantar flexion motion and work needed in the gait cycle. Rocker bottom soles provide mechanical heel rise to assist the calf muscles and are available commercially or can be added to shoes. Work boots, dress boots, or basketball shoes may provide needed ankle stability.

People with unilateral lower-extremity paralysis or pain stand with weight on the stronger limb, which must perform continuous, high-level isometric contractions (Fig. 17-5). Unloading the stronger leg requires restoration of weight bearing on the more involved leg using a knee-ankle-foot orthosis (KAFO) or, in some instances, an ankle-foot orthosis (AFO), which prevents advance of the tibia in the stance phase.[26,37,42,50]

Fifty percent of ambulatory postpolio individuals were found to walk with an obvious forward lean (see Fig. 17-4). This posture requires continuous contraction of the erector spinae muscles and leads to back pain, often radiating to the hip and leg. The forward lean posture is found in people with quadriceps muscle paresis and in persons

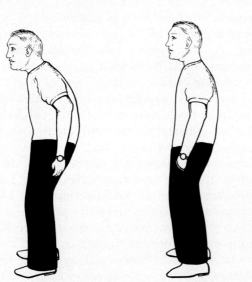

Fig. 17-4. Polio paralysis of the erector spinae (and abdominal) muscles with inability to sit or stand erect. Erect posture is frequently achieved by casual appearing activities such as pushing down on the body and chairs.

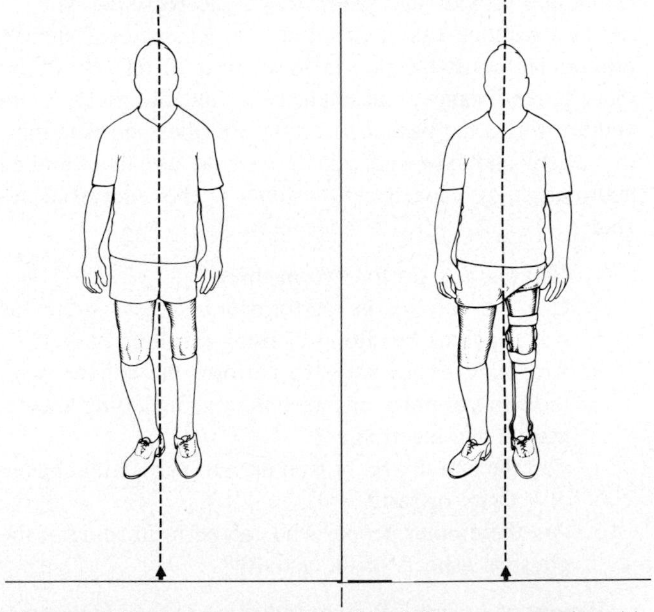

Fig. 17-5. This man has paralysis of the left lower extremity with severe fatigue, low-back pain, pain and weakness in the right lower extremity, and decreased function. He can be seen to bear weight and stand on the right leg. Application of a left KAFO with a free knee joint (with a drop lock for use in prolonged standing and walking on rough terrain) and a limited motion ankle joint unloaded his right leg and permitted him to walk in an erect posture. His pain disappeared and he has regained function at work and in social activities.

with ankle weakness. Those with quadriceps weakness must move the center of gravity of the body anterior to the knee axis to lock the knee and prevent knee flexion in stance. This posterior force also produces ligamentous instability and genu recurvatum (see Fig. 17-3). In some instances light-weight athletic knee braces allowing 10 to 15 degrees of hyperextension provide adequate control. More often a KAFO with an offset knee joint allowing necessary hyperextension is required.[4,31,33] People with dorsiflexor muscle paralysis or ankle instabilities walk in the forward lean posture to watch the floor and foot placement to avoid tripping and falling. Athletic ankle supports or boots may be sufficient to control some ankle instabilities. Molded and posted plastic AFOs with or without ankle joints are needed for more control. Flexible plastic AFOs and the dynamic spring dorsiflexion assists correct simple drop foot.[42] Once the need to walk in a forward leaning posture is removed, the person can walk upright, and back pain may disappear in a few days.

Walking with lateral trunk shift in the stance phase (gluteus medius gait) produces abnormal forces and joint dysfunction from the spine to the foot (Fig. 17-6). These forces can be reduced by use of a forearm crutch or cane.

People who are long-term crutch walkers with or without orthoses and those whose walking is slow, precarious, or labored should be guided to consider use of motorized vehicles as their primary form of locomotion. Orthotic corrections or applications may be indicated to improve transfers and short-distance walking.

Exercise. Strengthening, aerobic, and sports exercise

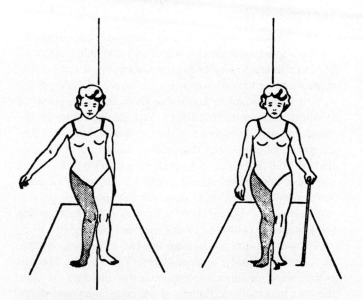

Fig. 17-6. Lateral trunk shift in a postpolio individual to illustrate abnormal forces occurring in the back, knee, and ankle with resulting joint dysfunction and pain. Prevention of these abnormal forces and some correction can be provided by use of a cane or forearm crutch. (Adapted from Ducroquet and others: Walking and limping—a study of normal and pathological walking, Philadelphia, 1968, JB Lippincott Co.)

programs add to the work load of the already overloaded motor units with further depletion of reserve capacity. Most postpolio individuals have been directed or self-directed to engage in or increase exercise activities. Instead of correction of problems, they have found an increase in pain, fatigue, and weakness in function as well as increase in fasciculations, muscle cramps, tremor, and sometimes sudden muscle atrophy. Unless there is EMG evidence to prove absence of polio involvement in extremities, the postpolio individual should be advised to forego exercise or heavy activity. Because of the neuromuscular deficit, use of exercise for weight reduction, diabetic control, or cardiovascular rehabilitation should not be considered unless the exercise can be limited to extremities without EMG evidence of prior polio. Those without such evidence in the upper extremities can be directed toward swimming with the legs trailing, supine weight programs, or arm ergometry.

Beneficial exercises include relaxation exercises and imagery to maximize rest periods, passive stretching (particularly of the neck and trunk), body awareness techniques, beginning yoga within abilities, nonresistive underwater exercise, or easy, noncompetitive recreational swimming.

Carefully supervised exercise programs have been advocated to determine if the new weakness is a result of overuse or disuse.[14] Weakness from disuse is rare. Usually the cause of the new weakness can be determined by the physical therapy evaluation with careful attention to the activity and exercise history and the physical examination. Weakness from disuse and deconditioning may occur with illness, injury, or surgery and treatment. In addition, new peripheral nerve lesions and aggravation of the postpolio syndrome may occur. Again, a careful evaluation plus the creation of a preillness gross muscle test is helpful to sort out causes of the weakness. Postpolio individuals know what they could move previously and how much if the right questions are asked. Exercise programs should be directed to previously functional muscles using low-resistance, low-repetition interval training. Careful monitoring is essential to determine increases, decreases, or plateaus of strength to avoid overload.

PSYCHOSOCIAL CONSIDERATIONS

The psychosocial problems of facing a second disability equal or exceed the physical problems.* Polio survivors worked long and hard to achieve a high level of function, and most have not considered themselves handicapped. Many are in a prime period of their lives with extensive work, family, and community responsibilities. These people are willing to work even harder, but efforts to preserve muscles and build a reserve capacity through life-style modifications or use of orthotics are difficult. Compliance

*References 13, 16, 21, 24, 25, 47.

is improved by the physical therapist's ability to provoke and allieviate pain during the initial evaluation, to begin with nonthreatening suggestions, such as seating corrections, and to provide options and alternatives. Most of all, postpolio individuals need support, patience, and time for processing and decision making.

Part II Human immunodeficiency virus (HIV) illness*

Johnny Bonck and Anne MacRae

IDENTIFICATION OF THE CLINICAL PROBLEM

Acquired immunodeficiency syndrome (AIDS) has been considered an epidemic since 1985.[51] The vast array of physical and psychological dysfunctions associated with AIDS, as well as the social and political implications of the disease, will continue to have a profound impact on all rehabilitation professionals.

The nomenclature and acronyms developed for the study of AIDS can be confusing. Furthermore, the clinical and pathological information about the disease is increasing weekly. Certainly our understanding of the disease process will be different at the time of publication of this textbook from what it was at the time of writing. Changes in terminology will reflect this. Let us attempt to define the terms in current use.

The virus thought to be responsible for the transmission of AIDS was named HIV (human immunodeficiency virus) in July, 1986 at the International Conference on AIDS in Paris.[54] However, some literature continues to refer to the etiological virus by an earlier term known as HTLV-III (Human T cell lymphotropic retrovirus type III).[62] A second AIDS virus, HIV-2, has been identified and is now being tracked epidemiologically.[71] It is possible to test seropositive for the HIV antibody while displaying no symptoms of AIDS. Estimates of the incubation period of the AIDS virus are constantly changing and will probably continue to do so as the AIDS epidemic progresses. Several studies have suggested that the mean period between infection by the HIV and the development of symptoms is 1 to 2 years in infants and 5 to 10 years in adults.

During the early attempts to understand the natural history of HIV infection, the term AIDS related condition (ARC) was used to describe a host of immunodeficiency-related illnesses that did not fit the formal diagnostic categories for AIDS. It was speculated that, as in hepatitis-B infection, there might be milder forms of the illness that are self-limiting or chronic but nonprogressive. However, the evidence does not support this theoretical model, and therefore the Center for Disease Control (CDC) of the

*Acknowledgments: A. Boccellari, Ph.D., Department of Psychiatry; and Kate Zimmerman, R.P.T., Department of Rehabilitation, San Francisco General Hospital.

United States has broadened its criteria for AIDS diagnosis.[52] The entire spectrum of the illness from asymptomatic seroconversion to full-blown AIDS can be covered by the term *HIV illness*, but it is important for the practitioner to be precise in the use of these terms for epidemiological, clinical, and psychosocial reasons.

Epidemiology

The estimates of the numbers of people worldwide who are infected with HIV range as high as 5 million.[66] Diagnosed cases of AIDS have been reported from all over the world. The World Health Organization, taking into account the inaccuracy of the reports from the developing nations, has estimated that the numbers of people with AIDS had reached 150,000 as of the end of 1987. The United States has the highest reported incidence of AIDS as of July 1988, with 66,464 cases reported and 37,535 dead of the disease;[63] the best-case scenarios estimate that 200,000 to 1,000,000 Americans are infected (many of them since before the disease was identified) and will presumedly require some kind of medical intervention by the end of the century.[57] It is speculated that the epidemic is far more widespread in Africa than it is in the developed nations.

It has been theorized that HIV was present in Africa as early as 1959 as supported by evidence of HIV antibody in frozen blood from Zaire. However, at the time of this writing, clinical samples from Europe and North America from that period are not available; therefore it is premature to conclude that the virus originated in Africa.[71]

The immune system

The immune system is very complex and dynamic, comprising a multitude of components and subsystems, all of which interact more or less continuously. It can be conceptualized in various ways; for the study of HIV pathology, it is important to know that there are many kinds of leukocytes, or white blood cells, that are central to the immune function. Lymphocytes and phagocytes are two subcategories of leukocytes that will be discussed in the context of HIV infection. Researchers are discovering more and more specialized subcategories of this group of cells. Furthermore, the effort to discover treatment and prevention techniques against HIV illness is rapidly expanding the knowledge of these cellular mechanisms.

The normal immune system has two main components, or "lines of defense," against illness (Table 17-3). The first is the innate, or inborn, component that includes the skin, the cilia and mucosal linings of the respiratory and digestive systems, the gastric fluids and enzymes of the stomach, and the phagocytes, or "cell eating" cells, that are found in specific organs such as the lungs and liver. This innate component of the immune system keeps pathogens out of the body by creating barriers against them, by ejecting them, or by enveloping and eliminating them.

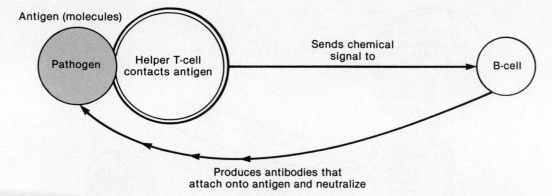

Fig. 17-7. Interaction of helper T-cells and B-cells in the acquired immune system. This simplified diagram eliminates several major processes including the role of the suppressor T-cell and the production of "memory" cells by which the acquired immune system is prepared to more effectively eliminate certain pathogens that are reintroduced into the body.

Table 17-3. Components of the immune system

Innate	Skin
	Cilia and mucosal linings of respiratory and digestive systems
	Gastric fluids and enzymes of the stomach
	Phagocytes: a form of white blood cell of leukocyte
Acquired	Humoral: substances produced by specialized cells and tissue (e.g. interferon, interleukon, and specific antibodies produced by B-cells which are also leukocytes)
	Cell-mediated: various cells, including at least eight kinds of T-cells, also a subcategory of leukocytes

The second, or acquired, component of the immune system, which develops defenses against specific pathogens, starts in utero and continues throughout life. In the context of the acquired immune system, pathogens are also known as antigens. Miller and Keane[68] define an antigen as "any substance which is capable, under appropriate conditions, of inducing a specific immune response and of reacting with the products of that response." Antigens are specific substances that the body identifies as destructive to itself. The acquired immune system destroys these antigens by the interaction of two basic processes, the humoral system and the cell-mediated system, both of which operate at the cellular level.

In the process of identifying and destroying these antigens, the acquired immune system also retains a "memory" of the antigen, which allows it to respond more rapidly and more effectively to the pathogen if it is reintroduced into the body. Thus the phenomenon of "being immune to" an illness.

The cells of the acquired immune system are lymphocytes, which are a subcategory of leukocytes. The B-lymphocytes, or B-cells, which are produced in the bone marrow, produce antibodies effective against antigens. These antibodies are part of the humoral system. The humoral system is also responsible for the substances, such as interferon and interleukon, that have shown promise in the elimination of certain kinds of neoplasms (cancers). Another important lymphocyte is the T-cell. There are at least eight kinds of T-cells that have various functions. Some T-cells function as monitors and activators of B-cells, signalling the B-cells to produce antibodies to attack an antigen; these are the helper T-cells. Other T cells send the signal to stop the attack; these are the suppressor T-cells. It is at this cell-mediated level that the HIV does the most damage to the immune system (Fig. 17-7).

Pathogenesis of AIDS

The HIV is a retrovirus, a class of virus that survives and multiplies by injecting genetic material into a host cell, thereby causing it to produce more of the virus—to become a "virus factory"—and to destroy itself. There is evidence that the HIV can do this to at least two kinds of cells of the immune system—the macrophages, which are a form of phagocytes, and the helper T-cells. Using its special destructive talent, the HIV eventually reduces the number of available healthy helper T-cells. This alters the critical ratio of helper to supressor T-cells; the B-cells do not receive the proper signals and are therefore less effective in producing the antibodies that are the body's response to the attack of the HIV as well as other opportunistic infections and neoplasms (Fig. 17-8). Metaphorically, the HIV is a guerilla warrior who sneak-attacks the lieutenants' and sergeants' barracks and leaves the rest of the soldiers without guidance or communication. The retrovirus is also protected from antibodies that cannot eliminate it as an antigen while it is "disguised" and replicating inside the cells of the immune system. This simplified de-

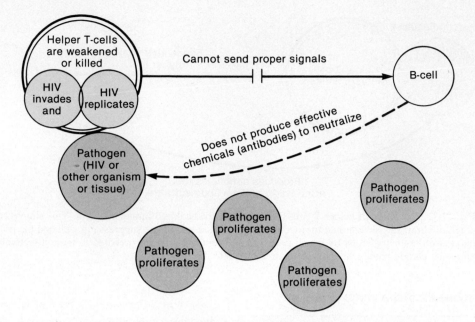

Fig. 17-8. The process by which HIV weakens the acquired immune response.

scription accounts for what may prove to be only one of many processes by which the HIV attacks the body at the cellular level. Several additional and alternate models are currently being researched;[73] among them are an autoimmune process, in which otherwise functioning cells, slightly altered by viral material, are identified as foreign and attacked by the immune system.[60] This is an alternative to the theory that the virus "hides" in T-cells and macrophages to foil the normal immune response. Gallo and Montagnier[60] also discuss a process by which "infection by HIV can cause infected and uninfected cells to fuse into giant cells called syncytia, which are not functional." A great deal needs to be learned about how these indirect mechanisms contribute to the depletion of healthy cells seen in HIV illness.

Systemic manifestations

Although the clinical course of HIV disease can vary greatly in individuals, researchers and practitioners have begun to track the overall course of the disease, and a frustratingly progressive pattern of clinical manifestations of the pathological process has emerged. Fig. 17-9 very broadly depicts a time line for the progression of HIV illness. The relative time values of the various stages will fluctuate for individuals. The 5- to 8-year period between infection with HIV and death from AIDS mentioned earlier in the text is an estimate and an average. There are individuals who remain asymptomatic or relatively free of symptoms longer than this estimated period, even with some evidence of changes in the immune process. This is understandably of great interest to all concerned.

Most people are able to live full lives during the early stages of HIV illness. Before the disease process was

tracked, many were unaware of their condition until they developed the secondary diseases that are the hallmarks of an AIDS diagnosis. The interim stages of HIV illness are marked by generalized swelling of the lymph nodes followed by an extended period when the infected person will not necessarily develop further symptoms but laboratory tests will reveal immune dysfunction, particularly a decline in the number of helper T-cells. When the immune system can no longer protect the body from recrudescent (already existing in the body) or ubiquitous (commonly found in the environment) pathogens, a variety of systemic diseases develop. The most common of these diseases has been a pneumonia known as PCP (*Pneumocystis carinii* pneumonia). Other serious conditions of the syndrome include a yeast infection of the mouth and throat called esophageal candidiasis, which has implications for nutritional intake; cryptosporidiosis, a cause of chronic diarrhea; a form of blindness caused by cytomegalovirus (CMV); and other CNS infections that can affect sensation and perception. Lymphomas are tumors of the lymph glands, a part of the immune system. Kaposi's sarcoma (KS) is a form of lesion in the blood vessel wall that can also appear in the earlier stages of the disease (for reasons that are not clear) but can be relatively stable and benign for years before spreading systemically, causing major organ dysfunction or death in the later stages of HIV illness.[73] Infants with HIV illness exhibit "failure to thrive" syndrome and adults may also experience serious weight loss. The incidence of certain secondary illnesses can vary regionally and seems to be changing over time as well, possibly because of changes in survival time or viral neurotropism.[62,71] The functional level of any person with HIV illness will fluctuate with the overall energy level and in re-

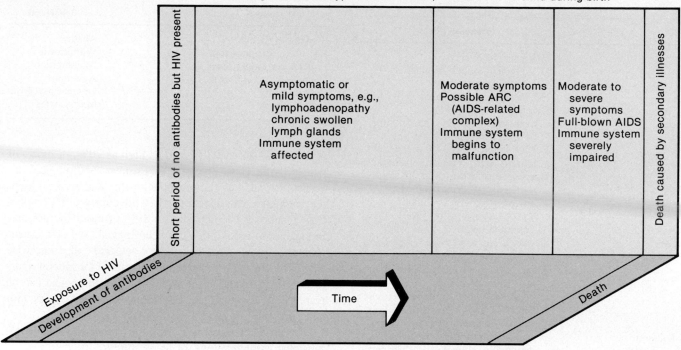

Fig. 17-9 HIV present and possibly transmissable through unprotected sexual intercourse, sharing infected hypodermic needles, and from mother to child during birth.

sponse to such specific symptoms as have been previously mentioned.

Treatments are being developed for some of these illnesses and are enhancing the quality and length of the lives of the person with AIDS (PWA). Antibiotics can now control or even prevent attacks of pneumonia (PCP). Antiviral drugs are being used against cytomegalovirus and herpes simplex virus. Chemotherapy and radiation are used against neoplasms and Kaposi's sarcoma. Some of these treatments have serious side effects, such as thrombocytopenia and anemia (which are conditions of the blood). Some can confound the diagnosis of other CNS illnesses by causing neurogenic pain and neuropathy.[64] This adds to the complication of medical management of the disease and challenges the rehabilitation therapist to provide significant input to the diagnostic process and to plan realistic and meaningful intervention.

Neuropathology

Table 17-4 lists a wide variety of organisms and/or conditions responsible for the neurological manifestations associated with HIV illness. These include primary and secondary viral, protozoan, fungal, and mycobacterium infection, as well as neoplasms and iatrogenic conditions (caused by the treatment for an illness).

It has been evident from early in the investigation of this disease that there was a potential for a devastating effect on the central nervous system (CNS). However, it was initially assumed that opportunistic infections were responsible. It is now known that the HIV, either through direct infection or through indirect mechanisms, is responsible for signs and symptoms of encephalopathy and neuropathy in the absence of opportunistic illness. Laboratory and pathological evidence of the virus in CNS tissue has led researchers to the conclusion that one or more neurotrophic processes can occur. It is theorized that the inflammatory process in the glial cells, a supporting structure of the CNS, leads to demyelination and cell death of neurons of the brain and spinal cord. It has now been demonstrated that the CD4 molecule, the receptor for the virus, is located on neurons as well as glial cells in cerebellum, pons, and thalamus.[58] Gray, Gherardi and Scaravilli[62] describe involvement of the hemisphere white matter associated with subacute (HIV) and nonspecific encephalopathy. They refer to several reports of HIV-related vascuolar myelopathy in the lateral and posterior columns of the thoracic area of the spinal cord that are similar to that caused by vitamin B12 deficiency. Peripheral neuropathy may be the result of nutritional and toxic factors, the result of an HIV-mediated auto-immune process, or may be the result of direct HIV infection of the sensory ganglia.[62,69]

It is not possible in this context to discuss the neuropathology of each of the many secondary infections and neoplasms of HIV illness. However, it is important to realize that the clinical manifestations of these pathological processes overlap with one another as well as with the signs

Table 17-4. Neurological diseases associated with AIDS*

	Organism/disease
Primary viral	HIV/encephalopathy
	HIV/atypical aseptic meningitis
	HIV/vacuolar myopathy
	HIV/peripheral neuropathy
Secondary viral	Cytomegalovirus (CMV)/ meningoencephalitis, retinitis, peripheral neuropathies
	Herpes simplex I and II/encephalitis, retinitis, peripheral neuropathies
	Herpes varicella zoster/encephalitis, retinitis, peripheral neuropathies
	Papovavirus/progressive multifocal leukoencephalopathy (PML)
Protozoan	Toxoplasma gondii/toxoplasmosis
Fungal	*Cryptococcus neoformans*/cryptococcal meningitis
	Candida albicans/intracerebral candidiasis (rare abscess)
	Aspergillus fumigatus/meningitis, encephalitis and/or abscess (rare)
	Coccidioides immitis/meningitis
Bacterial	*M. avium*-intracellulare/encephalitis, meningitis, cranial and/or peripheral neuropathy
	M. tuberculosis hominis/meningitis and/or CNS mass lesion
Neoplastic	Primary CNS lymphomas
	Metastatic systemic lymphoma
	Metastatic Kaposi's sarcoma
Iatrogenic	Extrapyramidal motor symptoms (EPS)
	Acute myelopathies
	Neuropathy

*Many of these organisms are responsible for profound nonneurological disease.

and symptoms of primary HIV infection of the CNS; lesions of the CNS can be the site of more than one opportunistic disease process simultaneously. The following list, adapted from Levy and Bredesen,[64] includes signs and symptoms of CNS illness in persons with AIDS (PWAs):

- Altered consciousness
- Aphasia
- Cranial neuropathies
- Decreased cognition
- Disordered gait
- Dizziness
- Headache
- Hemiparesis
- Incontinence
- Incoordination
- Pain
- Paresthesia
- Perceptual disturbances
- Seizures
- Sensory loss
- Visual disturbances
- Weakness

Neurological manifestations

Studies estimate that the prevalence of neurological involvement from some combination of primary or second-

Table 17-5. Symptoms of AIDS dementia complex

Cognitive	Behavioral
Slowing of mentation	Apathy
Short-term memory loss	Withdrawal
Projective memory loss	Disinhibition
Decreased concentration	Agitation
Distractability	Organic psychosis
Confusion	Manic states

ary illness is at least 30% and as high as 70%, or more, of people with HIV illness.[62,64] Primary neurological involvement, such as HIV encephalopathy and atypical aseptic meningitis, can appear early in the course of HIV infection. One study[64] found that in 10% of cases the presenting symptoms of AIDS were neurological, and subtle neuropsychological deficits were detected in otherwise asymptomatic HIV-positive individuals.[61] Peripheral neuropathies can appear at all stages of HIV illness and can be responsible for the gait disturbances caused by painful soles and paresthesias of the feet.[53]

The array of signs and symptoms related to the neuromuscular complications of HIV illness, listed above, is somewhat daunting. The number and/or severity of symptoms a person will develop is idiosyncratic. These signs and symptoms will be the sequelae of one or more of the illnesses listed in Table 17-4. In addition, neurological disorders can result from the breakdown of tissue seen with neoplasia and resulting cerebrovascular infarction, hemorrhage, or vasculitis.

AIDS dementia complex is considered the most common nervous system complication of HIV illness.[59] This disorder is characterized by changes in both cognition and behavior as described in Table 17-5. In addition to the symptoms of AIDS dementia, HIV encephalopathy can produce a variety of physical symptoms including lethargy, malaise, decreased motor control, paraparesis, seizures, incontinence, blindness, and mutism. It is estimated that at the time the AIDS diagnosis is made, one third of all patients have overt dementia complex and an additional one fourth have a subclinical case.[72] As the disease progresses to the preterminal stage, two thirds of all patients have overt dementia and an additional one fourth have subclinical dementia.

MEDICAL MANAGEMENT

In the earliest days of the epidemic, medical management focused exclusively on palliative care and the treatment of the symptoms of the secondary illnesses of AIDS, while researchers searched for the etiology of the mysterious malady. An array of diagnostic techniques such as surgical biopsy, bronchoscopy, extensive blood work, and radiology are used to identify the various possible infections, neoplasms, and related conditions of the syndrome. Antibiotics, chemotherapy, analgesics, and antiinflammatory agents are still important tools in the task of controlling or curing these related diseases. Neuroleptics and antianxiety medications are used with some success to alleviate the psychiatric manifestations of HIV dementia.[70]

Now that a viral etiology has been established with some certainty, the emphasis of researchers is on developing effective antiviral agents and a safe vaccine. At least a dozen known antiviral agents are being studied in clinical trials, the most successful so far being azidothymidine (AZT), which is effective at the genetic level of the viral life cycle. AZT attaches its own genetic material to the DNA chain and blocks the process by which the HIV replicates in the living cell. This substance has also proven to be toxic and can cause side effects as mild as a general feeling of discomfort or as severe as the complete suppression of bone marrow production of red blood cells. The effectiveness of the drug has apparently diminished over time in some cases, for reasons that are not clear. A possible explanation is that the virus mutates so that its replication is not affected by the very specific alteration of genetic material accomplished by the AZT.[74]

In the few years since the HIV was isolated in infected tissue, the amount of information generated about the life cycle of the retrovirus has been considerable. Theoretically, the complexity of the life cycle of the virus should provide researchers with many "points of entry" at which a treatment or vaccine might effectively interfere with its deadly progress. But just as the HIV confounds the body's immune system, so has it confounded medical science in its attempts to formulate antiviral drug treatments or a vaccine. Other impediments to the research are the ethical and practical concerns of human subject research with a vaccine that might potentially be harmful or a promising treatment that needs to be withheld from a control group of patients in a clinical trial. Dr. Koop, the former United States Surgeon General, has warned that a vaccine is not expected until the end of the century.[67]

EVALUATION PROCESS

The evaluation procedures for HIV illness are broadly outlined below. Of course, each case varies and the evaluation process is individualized according to the specific needs of the client.

A. Baseline data (premorbid functional level)
   1. Accustomed life roles
B. Stage in disease process
C. Psychosocial issues
   1. Coping mechanisms
   2. Social support system
D. Cognitive/perceptual status
   1. Reality orientation
   2. Memory
   3. Organizational skills
   4. Visual perception
   5. Motor planning

6. Safety awareness
   7. Judgment
E. Communication
   1. Oral language
   2. Written language
F. Sensory/motor status
   1. Balance
   2. Gait
   3. Coordination
   4. Sensation/pain
   5. Muscle tone
   6. Strength
G. Activities of daily living (ADL)
   1. Grooming/hygiene
   2. Feeding
   3. Bathing
   4. Dressing
   5. Housework
   6. Community management
   7. Other self-care regimens (i.e., medications)
   8. Avocational interests
   9. Activity tolerance

What is the relationship of the person with HIV illness to the environment, both at present and in the future? The rehabilitation therapist should keep this important question in mind throughout the evaluation process, using the term "environment" broadly to include not only the physical aspects of the environment, but also the psychological and emotional climate in which the client functions.

The evaluation process will have a different focus, depending on the stage of the disease. If the client is in the early stages of the disease, the therapist should determine if he or she is still managing in accustomed life roles. Important issues might include new or adapted vocational and avocational skills. At a later stage, the focus may change to more basic daily functional concerns. It is especially crucial to determine if the hospitalized client is going to be discharged to some other supervised setting or to home.

Evaluative questions about the psychosocial status of the client include the following:

1. Does the client's perception of his or her current status and prognosis agree with that of the treatment team?
2. What is the client's predominant coping style?
3. Who is the client's social support system?

The support system can be a critical issue for many people with HIV illness who are part of the high-risk groups of homosexual and bisexual men and intravenous (IV) drug users. Many of these men and women have traditional networks of family, spouse, and friends; a significant number have equally strong nontraditional support systems. Some will be lacking in the kinds of support needed to cope with the devastating effects of the disease.

It is possible to use models developed for oncology and

progressive neurological disorders, such as amyotrophic lateral sclerosis for HIV neurological rehabilitation. However, the sometimes dramatic fluctuations in signs and symptoms of dysfunction that characterize HIV, especially in response to treatment of secondary illnesses or the temporary efficacy of antiviral medications, must be taken into consideration.

The neurorehabilitation evaluation for HIV illness will, of course, include a standard evaluation of cognitive, perceptual, and motor systems, all of which are at risk as a result of the neuropathology of the disease. However, because of the idiosyncratic nature of the disease, a detailed evaluation of one or more specific areas of cognition, perception, and/or motor skills may be indicated. In addition to the neuromuscular sequelae of CNS disease, a thorough evaluation considers the systemic, nonneurological symptoms of HIV illness. The results of the total evaluation are of use not only in the development of an appropriate rehabilitation plan, but also in assisting medical personnel in the differential diagnosis of the many potentially related conditions of HIV illness.

Particular attention to the evaluation of cognitive/perceptual dysfunction, prevalent in HIV illness, is essential. The cognitive/perceptual evaluation should be both formal and observational. The initial screening includes a check of reality orientation and an investigation into the maximal premorbid functional level.

The clinical picture that emerges in AIDS dementia complex includes a general slowing of mental processes, but deficits will not necessarily show up in a bedside minimental status examination. Clients often have a subjective experience of more severe memory loss than is demonstrated by formal testing.[72] In addition, symptoms of AIDS dementia complex can include behavioral and affective changes such as agitation or euphoria. Social skills and general fund of knowledge can remain largely intact in the face of significant loss of organizational abilities.

Safety and judgment need to be assessed at the gross level, such as potential for falls and fire safety awareness, as well as at a more subtle level. Deficits in money management and/or decreased ability to engage in business or professional activity are commonly seen with subtle cognitive changes. Formal evidence of deficits is often helpful to the client's support system in determining how to protect the client's best interests.

A check of language skills may reveal some word-finding problems, which are associated with AIDS dementia complex. A more serious aphasia or agnosia could be symptomatic of a focal lesion. Neglect, hemianopsia, and apraxias are all possible symptoms of the opportunistic-infectious and neoplastic illnesses associated with the syndrome, and any sudden change in the cognitive/perceptual status of a client could be indicative of a developing lesion in the brain.

Sensory loss and pain are a part of the neurological picture of HIV illness. Because of the prevalence of CMV retinitis, any changes in vision should be a focus of the neurological evaluation, especially now that there are promising pharmacological treatments for it. The paresthesias associated with peripheral neuropathy are evaluated for pain management.

The motor component of the neurorehabilitation evaluation assesses for abnormal tone, balance, and gait as well as fine and gross motor planning and performance. Impaired ambulation can be the result of decreased strength and endurance and/or gait disturbances. A careful evaluation can determine the underlying cause. For example, concurrent urinary incontinence could be indicative of spinal cord involvement; concurrent dementia and motor planning deficits may indicate a supraspinal origin; incoordination and speech articulation problems may indicate cerebellar involvement; and specific weakness could be the result of a myopathy.[58]

The activities of daily living (ADL) evaluation is done in the context of the immediate and projected life roles of the client. The maximal level of independent function is the goal of rehabilitation at whatever the stage of the illness. Some clients will insist on participating in their own daily care even when they are critically ill; others will demand total assistance and may need structured redirection toward basic self-care as an appropriate means of remaining in touch with their environment and their bodies. Again, the critical factor is the therapist's assessment of the psychosocial status of the client.

If the client is at home or being discharged to home, a crucial part of the ADL evaluation is the assessment of community management skills. These include access to transportation, socialization opportunities, and community involvement. Many clients with HIV illness and their support systems have little or no experience with disability because of their age and social status. This, combined with the mental status changes of AIDS dementia complex, can create very unrealistic expectations for home and community management.

TREATMENT PROCESS

The neuromuscular rehabilitation treatment procedures for HIV illness are outlined below.

A. Psychosocial intervention
   1. Facilitation of the expression of grief
   2. Validation and education of the support system
B. Cognitive/perceptual intervention
   1. Rehabilitation
   2. Maintenance
   3. Compensation (includes communication)
C. Sensory/motor intervention
   1. Sensory stimulation
   2. Maintenance of strength, range of motion, and endurance

3. Tone normalization
4. Gait training (includes ambulation aids)
D. Pain control
   1. Psychological modalities
   2. Physical modalities
E. ADL training
   1. Leisure time or avocational skills development
   2. Community management skills
   3. Transfer training
   4. Recommendations for adaptive equipment and assistive devices
   5. Self-care retraining
   6. Energy conservation
   7. Work simplification

Many rehabilitation techniques and modalities have beneficial effects on the overall psychosocial status of the client with HIV illness. Active listening, empathy, and unconditional positive regard are effective aspects of the therapeutic persona. The use of expressive modalities can facilitate the development of coping skills and provide a focus for the appropriate exploration and release of powerful emotions. The emotional climate of the client's environment can be affected by optimizing pleasant sensory stimulation, especially tactile. Human touch can counter the powerful isolating effect of fear of contagion. Several grieving processes might overlap for different kinds of losses, and the stages can occur in patterns specific to the individual. Grieving, mistakenly associated only with the death of a loved one, is a natural and normal reaction to loss. Typical losses seen include the loss of the use of limbs or senses, poor endurance, and potential loss of life. However, one may also grieve over the loss of abstract human qualities such as perceived attractiveness, productivity, independence, and a general sense of well-being. These feelings are often difficult for a client to articulate; therefore it is the therapist's responsibility to be sensitive to the individual client's pattern of grieving.

An additional role of the therapist is to address the needs of the members of client's support system. This includes education on treatment issues and validation of their concerns in the unfamiliar role of caregiver. This is especially true when the client is a young and recently vital person.

Although specific cognitive/perceptual retraining techniques are sometimes used in the treatment of HIV illness, maintenance and compensatory techniques are used more often, especially because of the prevalence of AIDS dementia complex and the resulting organicity of the deficits. Once again, the most effective intervention focuses on environmental modification, incorporating the training of staff and the social support system in optimizing communication style and interactive approach.

When cognitive deficits are present, communication with the client should be repetitive and carefully paced.

Also, information needs to be broken down into components. Consistency of personnel, location, and schedule can reduce confusion and resulting anxiety. The overall level of stimulation, and specifically the number and timing of visitors and treatments, should be monitored to maximize their effectiveness. This is an area over which the client ideally should be given as much control as possible to increase empowerment and maximize comfort.

The evaluation process will already have determined if the client has begun to use compensatory techniques in the self-treatment of memory dysfunction by "writing everything down." Obviously some clients will be too disorganized to benefit from lists of information. At this level of dysfunction, large signs identifying hospital rooms or the location of needed personal items can be effective. For the client who is disoriented in time and/or has short-term memory deficits, calendars and daily journals or records of visitors can be very reassuring. Because he or she may not remember the visits, the client can feel abandoned when alone.

If the evaluation reveals that the client's judgment has been affected by cognitive and behavioral changes, then adaptation may be the optimal treatment approach to ensure environmental safety. Toxic substances, sharp items, electrical appliances, and dangerously hot or cold objects need to be put behind barriers. Stairwells need to be blocked off, and obstructive or unsteady furnishings need to be removed from the client's access. At this point, the support system may need validation from the rehabilitation team to take a proactive stance in assuming responsibility for the financial and business matters of a loved one who does not appreciate the extent of his or her disability. Social services consultation, backed by the results of a neurological rehabilitation evaluation, can be of value in this delicate area.

One of the reasons that sensory stimulation is so beneficial to the psychosocial well-being of the client is that it is a primitive and basic arousal mechanism of the nervous system and, as such, can be used effectively to increase the response level of the unmotivated, drowsy, or obtunded patient. Olfactory receptors are part of the reticular activating system and are closely connected physiologically to the brain centers for memory and emotion.[56]

Neuromuscular facilitation and inhibition, positioning, and splinting are all possible modalities for the treatment of abnormal tone associated with HIV-related or secondary hemiparesis and paraparesis. Depending on the results of the evaluation, gait training, including the use of ambulation aids, focuses on motor planning, balance, endurance, and/or muscle tone with an overall concern for safety awareness. In addition, the maintenance of strength and endurance as well as passive and active range of motion are important components of any motor function treatment plan.

Pain control, especially pain associated with peripheral

neuropathies, can be approached psychologically as well as physically. Stress reduction through education and training in deep breathing, progressive relaxation, autogenic training, music meditation, guided imagery, and visualization are all effective modalities. In addition, transcutaneous electric nerve stimulation (TENS), ultrasound, and massage may be utilized.

The specific treatment modalities in the area of activities of daily living will depend on the information gathered in the evaluation regarding the client's life roles, status at home and in the community, and activity tolerance. If the client is no longer able to work at his or her job, then suitable and meaningful avocational and leisure skills will be the focus of ADL training. These are particularly difficult issues for clients who are considered to be in "high-risk groups" because accustomed life roles may involve behaviors that jeopardize their own health or that of others. If the client is in need of assistance with community management, then equipment and community reorientation are appropriate modalities. Some clients will be reluctant to accept the use of ambulatory aids out in the community, saying that they are "too independent." It requires a great deal of skill on the part of the rehabilitation therapist to recognize and deal effectively with psychosocial issues of self-image and need for autonomy that complicate the process of providing for maximum independence. If the client is in need of assistance with daily self-care, then compensatory techniques, assistive devices, and equipment to maximize safety and increase or maintain function are appropriate, along with retraining in feeding, transfers, bathing, dressing, grooming, and hygiene. Incorporated into all of these ADL modalities is training in energy conservation and work simplification. An understanding of how to apply the principles of energy conservation is of great benefit to the person with HIV illness because of the sometimes erratic fluctuations in available energy that are a symptom of the disease.

IMPLICATIONS FOR THE HEALTH CARE WORKER

Any discussion of the clinical manifestations of HIV infection must include important emotional-affective considerations regarding the high morbidity of the disease. The attitude of persons with the disease and of health professionals is changing as research promises hope of effective treatment and as infected people learn how to cope with the illness and its disabling conditions. The presence of HIV is no longer considered an automatic death sentence. Reluctance to invest rehabilitation resources in a person with a "terminal" illness has given way to an awareness that appropriate intervention can prolong function and maintain quality of life for people whose long-term prognosis may be no worse than that of others with more familiar progressive diseases.[54,58]

Fear of infection is a valid concern for the health care worker. It should be addressed with accurate information about the risk factors as well as the methods of transmission. Although HIV has been isolated from nearly all body fluids, the only documented mechanisms of transmission as of this writing are (1) sexual contact, (2) parenteral contact with blood or blood products, and (3) perinatal infection from an infected mother to her offspring.[65]

The actual danger of infection by HIV to a health care worker is very low. However, the association of the illness it causes with the highest-risk groups of homosexual men and IV drug users, as well as the high mortality rate of the disease, caused an inordinate fear response in many health care workers in the early years of the epidemic. Partly in response to this, the health care industry and governmental regulating agencies have recommended new standards of infection control. Universal precautions and body substance isolation remove from the health care worker the need to determine which clients or which body substance is dangerous. Precautions are to be taken with all clients whenever there is any possibility of exposure to body fluids. For rehabilitation therapists this means gloves and gowns are used in handling clients who are incontinent or who have open lesions or wounds with which the therapist will come into contact. Gloves are necessary for feeding training or oral-bulbar facilitation if the therapist puts a hand in the client's mouth. Handwashing is still indicated even with gloves. Gloves are especially important if there is a lesion or dermatitis on the therapist's hands. These precautions are for the protection of all clients as well as health care workers. Finally, there is no reason for pregnant therapists to avoid or be prevented from working with HIV-infected clients as long as infection control procedures are followed.[65]

Another concern is that the sociocultural background of many clients with HIV illness may be foreign to the therapist. This is usually an issue in theory more than in practice. The competent and caring health care worker tends to respond to the client as an individual, putting aside personal moral and political points of view and focusing on the needs that result from the illness.

SYNOPSIS

AIDS is the end-stage syndrome of an epidemic of alarming proportions that will have disabled or killed hundreds of thousands of men and women worldwide before effective medical interventions are developed. As treatments are developed, more and more people will be in need of rehabilitation to maximize function and quality of life in the face of the many secondary and opportunistic diseases that are associated with this illness.

HIV illness is caused by a retrovirus that attacks the humoral and cellular immune system, the CNS, and possibly other tissue at the cellular level, leaving the body open to attack by other organisms and neoplasms and causing a wide range of symptoms including dementia, peripheral neuropathies, and vacuolar myelopathies. The disease progresses in stages. Initial "flulike" symptoms at the time of seroconversion of the blood to antibody positive (when the immune system first responds to the organism) are followed by an asymptomatic period during which disruption of the immune function or of the CNS will be demonstrated only in laboratory tests or pathological studies. The latter stages of the disease are marked by the development of a complex of signs, symptoms, and illnesses.

HIV illness produces many neurological sequelae, caused by both the primary HIV disease process and the many secondary diseases that can attack the CNS. Medical management has focused on the treatment of the secondary illnesses and conditions and on palliative care because of the lack of effective antiviral therapies. Research developments are occurring rapidly as the world community gears up to cope with the epidemic. There is promise of the availability of effective antiviral therapies soon, but the development of an effective vaccine against HIV is not expected until the turn of the century.

Neuromuscular rehabilitation evaluation procedures for HIV illness are similar to those of other progressive neuromuscular illnesses; the later stage of the disease, known as AIDS, can be evaluated according to models for wasting diseases such as cancer, with special focus on cognitive/perceptual deficits because of the neurotrophic quality of the virus and the prevalence of AIDS dementia complex.

Treatment focuses on the specific deficits of the illnesses of the syndrome, with special attention to the psychosocial sequelae of the disease. Compensatory techniques for cognitive deficits, education of the client's support system, gait training, and pain control are further treatments used to maximize function and quality of life.

The epidemic is a major challenge on a personal as well as a cultural level because of the natural fear of contagion, because the illness initially has stricken subpopulations that are disenfranchised as a result of social, racial, and economic status, and because of the controversial nature of the behaviors associated with the transmission vectors of the organism, mainly sexual intercourse and intravenous injection of illegal addictive drugs. Rehabilitation professionals have responded significantly to this challenge. This response must continue throughout the course of the epidemic to minimize its devastating effect.

Summary

This chapter has presented ideas regarding pathology, evaluation, and treatment of two relatively new clinical problems: postpolio syndrome and HIV infection, which is the precursor to AIDS. In the first clinical problem, the virus was contracted many years ago and the residual problems are the result of initial damage, not of a reinfection of the virus. The second problem is directly related to the invading virus and its potentially disastrous effect on the CNS. The progressions, treatment procedures, and social attitudes toward these two disease processes do vary. Yet the generalities of treatment in both cases focus on client function, self-management, and psychosocial considerations. Both were feared by society when they first reached epidemic form. The newness of the problems, whether acute or chronic, creates many unknowns regarding the progression to overall outcome of the disease process. New diseases in the future may be added to this chapter and the diseases presented here may become less important, or these diseases may become so important that larger sections will need to be added.

Both clinical problems presented have tremendous social significance not only to the clients and their families, but also to society as a whole. Acute polio is a forgotten issue within industrialized countries, yet past victims are now facing new problems that drastically affect their lives and future. HIV infections have created a new challenge to the health care fields. It, like acute polio, may be eradicated as a health risk in the future, but clients who have already contracted the virus will still face unknown problems that a therapist my be asked to help solve. It is hoped that the reader will find this chapter not only intellectually challenging, but also emotionally stimulating.

REFERENCES
Poliomyelitis and the postpolio syndrome

1. Bach J and others: Mouth intermittent positive pressure ventilation in the management of postpolio respiratory insufficiency, Chest 91,859, 1987

2. Bodian D: The virus, the nerve cell, and paralysis, Bull Johns Hopkins Hosp 83:1, 1948.

3. Bennett RL and Knowlton GC: Overwork weakness in partially denervated skeletal muscle, Clin Orthop 12:22, 1958.

4. Clark D, Perry J, and Lunsford T: Case studies—orthotic management of the adult post polio patient, Orthop Prosthet 40:43, 1986.

5. Cornill L: Sur un cas de paralysie generale spinale anterieure subaipue, suivi d'autopsie, Gaz Med (Paris) 4:127, 1875.

6. Dail C: Clinical aspects of glossopharyngeal breathing: report of its use by 100 post-polio patients, JAMA 158:445, 1955.

7. Dalakas MC and others: Late effects of poliomyelitis muscular atrophy: clinical, virologic and immunologic studies, Rev Inf Dis 6(suppl):S562, 1984.

8. Dalakas M and others: A long term follow-up study of patients with post-poliomyelitis neuromuscular symptoms, N Eng J Med 314:959, 1986.

9. Ducroquet R, Ducroquet J, and Ducroquet P: Walking and limping—a study of normal and pathological walking, Philadelphia, 1968, JB Lippincott Co.

10. Fergelson C: Glossopharyngeal breathing as an aid to the coughing mechanism in patients with chronic poliomyelitis in a respirator, N Eng J Med 254:611, 1956.

11. Fetell MR and others: A benign motor neuron disorder: delayed cramps and fasciculations after poliomyelitis or myelitis, Ann Neurol 11:423, 1982.

12. Fisher A: Sleep-disordered breathing as a late effect of poliomyelitis. In Halstead L and Wiechers D, editors: Research and clinical aspects of the late effects of poliomyelitis, White Plains, NY, 1987, March of Dimes Birth Defects Series 23:4.

13. Frick N: Post-polio sequelae and the psychology of second disability, Orthopedics 8:851, 1985.

14. Halstead L: The residual of polio in the aged, Top Geriatr Rehab 3:9, 1988.
15. Halstead L and Wiechers D, editors: Late effects of poliomyelitis, Miami, 1985, Symposia Foundation.
16. Halstead L and Wiechers D, editors: Research and clinical aspects of the late effects of poliomyelitis, White Plains NY, 1987, March of Dimes Birth Defects Series 23:4.
17. Hamilton EA, Nichols PIR, and Tair GBW.: Late onset of respiratory insufficiency after poliomyelitis: a preliminary communication, Ann Physiol Med 10:223, 1970.
18. Hill R and others: Sleep apnea syndrome after poliomyelitis, Am Rev Resp Dis 127:129, 1983.
19. Huckstep RL: Poliomyelitis: a guide for developing countries including appliances and rehabilitation of the disabled, New York, 1975, Churchill Livingstone.
20. Jubelt B and Cashman N: Neurological manifestation of the post-polio syndrome, Crit Rev Neurobiol 3:199, 1987.
21. Kaufert J and Kaufert PA: Aging and respiratory polio, Rehab Digest 13:15, 1982.
22. Kayser-Gatchalian MC: Late muscular atrophy after poliomyelitis, Eur Neuro 10:371, 1973.
23. Kendall H and Kendall F: Orthopedic and physical therapy objectives in poliomyelitis treatment, Physiotherapy Rev 27:2, 1947.
24. Laurie G and Raymond J, editors: Proceedings of Rehabilitation Gazette's Second Internation Post-Polio Conference and Symposium on Living Independently with a Severe Disability, St Louis, 1984, Gazette International Networking Institute.
25. Laurie G and Raymond J, editors: Proceedings of Gazette International Networking Institute's Third Internation Polio and Independent Living Conference, St Louis, 1986, Gazette International Networking Institute.
26. Lehmann J and others: Ankle-foot orthoses: effect on abnormalities in tibial nerve paralysis, Arch Phys Med Rehabil 66:212, 1985.
27. McComas A, Upton A, and Sica R: Motor neuron disease and aging, Lancet 2:1474, 1973.
28. Martinez A, Ferrer M, and Conde M: Electrophysiological features in patients with non-progressive and late progressive weakness after paralytic poliomyelitis: conventional EMG automatic analysis of the electromyogram and single fiber electromyography study, EMG Clin Neurophysical 24:469, 1984.
29. Martinez A, Perez M, and Ferrer M: Chronic partial denervation is more widespread than is suspected clinically in paralytic poliomyelitis—an electrophysiological study, Eur Neurol 22:314, 1983.
30. Maynard F: Post-polio sequelae—differential diagnosis and management, Orthopedics 8:857, 1985.
31. Perry J and Fleming C: Polio: long-term problems, Orthopedics 8:877, 1985.
32. Perry J, Gromley J, and Lunsford T: Rocker shoe as a walking aid in multiple sclerosis, Arch Phys Med Rehabil 62:59, 1981.
33. Perry J and Hislop H, editors: Principles of lower extremity bracing, Washington, DC, 1967, American Physical Therapy Association.
34. Potts CS: A case of progressive muscular atrophy occuring in a man who had acute poliomyelitis nineteen years previously, University of Pennsylvania Medical Bulletin 16:31, 1903.
35. Rosenheimer J: Effects of chronic stress and exercise on age-related changes in end-plate architecture, J Neurophysiol 53:1582, 1985.
36. Rosenheimer J and Smith D: Differential changes in the end-plate architecture of functionally diverse muscles during aging, J Neurophysiol 53:1567, 1985.
37. Saltiel J: A one piece laminated knee locking short leg brace, Orthop Prosthet 23:68, 1969.
38. Schenck J and Forward E: Quantitative strength changes with test repetitions, Phys Ther 45:562, 1965.
39. Sharrard WJW: The distribution of permanent paralysis in the lower limb in poliomyelitis, J Bone Joint Surg 37(B):540, 1955.
40. Sleeper G, Kignman P, and Armeni M: Nasal continuous positive pressure for at-home treatment of sleep apnea, Respir Care 30:90, 1985.
41. Smith E, Rosenblatt P, and Limauro A: The role of the sympathetic nervous system in acute poliomyelitis, J Pediatr 34:1, 1949.
42. Smith L and McDermott K: Pain in post-poliomelitis: addressing causes versus effects. In Halstead L and Wiechers D, editors: Research and clinical aspects of the late effects of poliomyelitis, White Plains, NY, 1987, March of Dimes Birth Defect Series 23:4.
43. Spencer GT: Respiratory insufficiency in scoliosis: clinical management and home care. In Zorab PA, editor: Scoliosis, London, 1977, Academic Press.
44. Spencer WA: Treatment of acute poliomyelitis, Springfield, Ill, 1956, Charles C Thomas, Publisher.
45. Thompson W and Jansen JKS: The extent of sprouting of remaining motor units in partly denervated immature and adult rat soleus muscle, Neuroscience 2:523, 1977.
46. Tomlinson BE and Irving D: The numbers of limb motor neurons in the human lumbosacral cord throughout life, J Neurol Sci 34:213, 1977.
47. Trieschmann R: Aging with a disability, New York, 1987, Demos Publications.
48. Wiechers D and Hubbel S: Late changes in the motor unit after acute poliomyelitis, Muscle Nerve 4:524, 1981.
49. World Health Organization: Poliomyelitis in 1985. Part I, Weekly Epidemiological Record 62:273, 1987.
50. Yang C and others: Floor reaction orthosis: clinical experience, Orthop Prosthet 40:33, 1986.

Human immunodeficiency virus illness

51. Beckham M and Rudy E: Acquired immunodeficiency syndrome: impact and implication for the neurological system, J Neurosci Nurs 18(1):5, 1986.
52. Center for Disease Control: Revision of the CDC surveillance case definition for acquired immunodeficiency syndrome, Atlanta, 1987, Center for Disease Control.
53. Cornblath D and McArthur J: Predominantly sensory neuropathy in patients with AIDS and AIDS-related complex, Neurol 38(5):794, 1988.
54. Curran J and others: Epidemiology of HIV infection and AIDS in the United States, Science 239:610, 1988.
55. Denton R: AIDS: guidelines for occupational therapy intervention, Am J Occup Ther 41(7):427, 1987.
56. Farber S: Neurorehabilitation: a multisensory approach, Philadelphia, 1982, WB Saunders Co.
57. Fauci A: The human immunodeficiency virus: infectivity and mechanisms of pathogenesis. Science 239:617, 1988.
58. Galantino M and Levy J: Neurological implications for rehabilitation, Clin Man 8(1):6, 1988.
59. Gallo P and others: Central nervous system involvement in HIV infection, AIDS Res Hum Retroviruses 4(3):211, 1988.
60. Gallo R and Montagnier L: AIDS in 1988, Sci Am 259(4):40, 1988.
61. Grant G and others: Evidence for early central nervous system involvement in the acquired immunodeficiency syndrome (AIDS) and other human immunodeficiency virus (HIV) infections, Ann Intern Med 107:828, 1987.
62. Gray R, Gherardi R, and Scaravelli F: The neuropathology of the acquired immune deficiency syndrome (AIDS), Brain 111:245, 1988.
63. Heyward W and Curran J: The epidemiology of AIDS in the U.S., Sci Am 259(4):72, 1988.
64. Levy R and Bredesen D: Central nervous system dysfunction in acquired immunodeficiency syndrome, Journal of Acquired Immune Deficiency Syndromes 1 (1):41, 1988.
65. Loschen D: Protecting against HIV exposure in family practice, Am Fam Physician 37(1):213, 1988.

66. Mann J and others: The international epidemiology of AIDS, Sci Am 259(4):82, 1988.
67. Matthews T and Bolognesi D: AIDS vaccines, Sci Am 259(4):120, 1988.
68. Miller B and Keane C, editors: Encyclopedia and dictionary of medicine, nursing and allied health, Philadelphia, 1987, WB Saunders Co.
69. Parry G: Peripheral neuropathies associated with human immunodeficiency virus infection, Ann Neurol 23(suppl):49, 1988.
70. Perry S and Jacobsen P: Neuropsychiatric manifestations of AIDS-spectrum disorders, Hosp Community Psychiatry 37(2):135, 1986.
71. Piot P and others: AIDS: an international perspective, Science 239:573, 1988.
72. Price R and others: The brain in AIDS: central nervous system HIV-1 infection and AIDS dementia complex, Science 239:586, 1988.
73. Redfield R and Burke D: HIV infection: the clinical picture, Sci Am 259(4):90, 1988.
74. Yarchoan R, Mitsuya H, and Broder S: AIDS therapies, Sci Am 259(4):110, 1988.

Chapter 18

MULTIPLE SCLEROSIS

Debra I. Frankel

BACKGROUND

Multiple sclerosis (MS) is one of the most common neurological diseases of young adults. It was first recorded in 1822 by an English nobelman, Sir Augustus D'Este, who apparently had the disease and documented in his diary a 25-year search for a cure.[5]

In 1838, Robert Carswell, a British medical illustrator, made drawings of a brainstem and spinal cord, showing patchy, hardened, and discolored tissue he had seen during an autopsy, and in 1842, Jean Cruveilhier, a French physician, observed similar patchy areas that he called "islands of sclerosis" on an autopsy of a paralyzed woman.[5]

It was not, however, until 1868 that Jean Martin Charcot formally identified and described MS. He called the disease "sclerose en plaques," describing the hardened

patch-like areas found (on autopsy) disseminated throughout the central nervous system (CNS) of individuals with the disease.[5]

In the normal human nervous system, impulses in many nerve fibers travel in excess of 200 mph. This remarkable velocity is achieved, to a large extent, by the insulation property of myelin, a complex of lipoprotein layers formed early in development by oligodendroglia in the CNS, which sheaths the axons.

MS is characterized by lesions (plaques)—distinct areas of myelin loss scattered throughout the CNS, primarily in the white matter (Fig. 18-1). These plaques of demyelination are accompanied by destruction of oligodendroglia and by inflammation (or the accumulation of white blood cells and fluid around blood vessels that lie within the CNS). Cell bodies and axons are, for the most part, spared; however, axons may be destroyed when fibrous gliosis (scarring) occurs—thus the observation of sclerotic plaques by medical historians. Because of destruction of myelin, neurotransmission is disrupted.

MS involves demyelination in the CNS only. CNS demyelination also occurs as a predominant finding in several other less common disorders, including acute, disseminated encephalomyelitis, optic neuromyelitis, and diffuse cerebral sclerosis.

AN OVERVIEW OF MULTIPLE SCLEROSIS
Epidemiology

In general, MS is diagnosed in individuals between the ages of 15 and 50. Although childhood MS has been reported, it is fairly uncommon. A clear geographical distribution has been supported by epidemiological studies over the last 50 years. An initial study by Kurland,[15] for example, compared cases of MS in Halifax, Nova Scotia, with cases in Charleston, South Carolina, and found that the

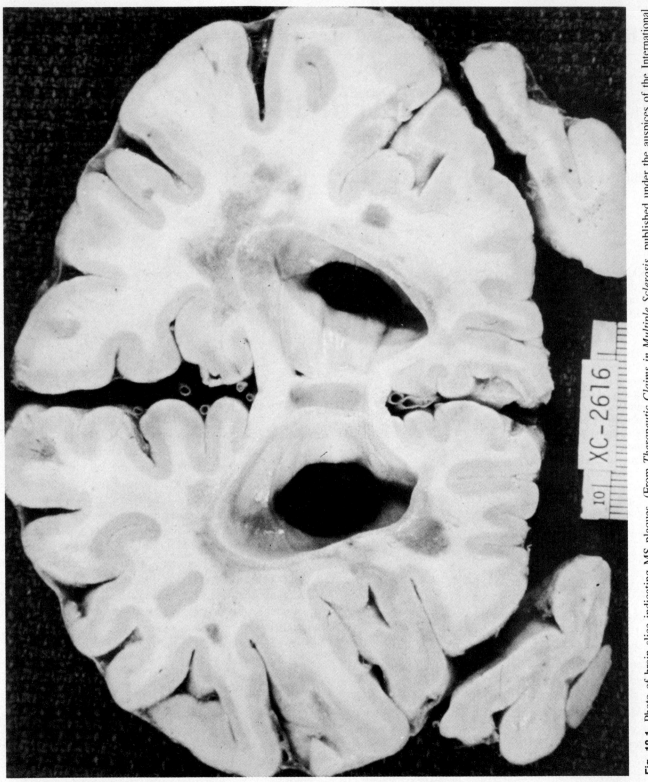

Fig. 18-1. Photo of brain slice indicating MS plaques. (From *Therapeutic Claims in Multiple Sclerosis*, published under the auspices of the International Federation of Multiple Sclerosis Societies, 1982; photo, courtesy Cedric Raine M.D., Albert Einstein College of Medicine, Yeshiva University, New York.)

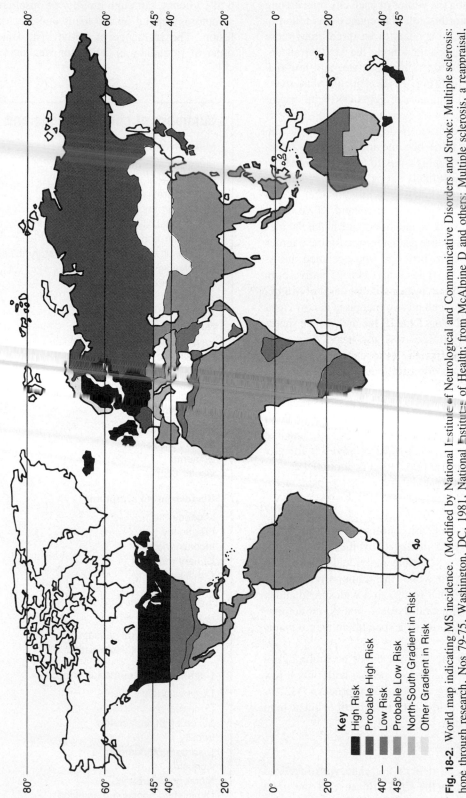

Fig. 18-2. World map indicating MS incidence. (Modified by National Institute of Neurological and Communicative Disorders and Stroke: Multiple sclerosis: hope through research, Nos 79-75, Washington, DC, 1981, National Institutes of Health; from McAlpine D and others: Multiple sclerosis, a reappraisal, 1965, Edinburgh, E & S Livingstone, Ltd.)

Key
High Risk
Probable High Risk
Low Risk
Probable Low Risk
North-South Gradient in Risk
Other Gradient in Risk

disease was three times more prevalent in the northern city than in the southern one. Kurland also found the disease to be more prevalent among the whites of each city than among the blacks. A similar north/south discrepancy was found in Europe, where the disease appears to be three times more common in northern Europe than along the Mediterranean. In other areas of the world, high, moderate, and low-risk zones have been identified (Fig. 18-2). This distribution reflects the probable dual influence of genetics (racial origin) and an environmental factor (such as a virus).

Another factor with regard to epidemiology has to do with the risk to immigrants. It has become apparent that an individual who migrates from a high-risk to a low-risk zone before the age of 15 will most likely adopt the risk factor of the new home. However, individuals who migrate after age 15 carry with them the risk rate of their native land.[1] Two seeming epidemics of MS have been identified: one in the Faeroes and one in Iceland.[17] Evidence as to a source for the Faeroes epidemic points to the British troops who occupied the islands in great numbers from 1940 to 1945; 25 native-born Faeroeses were discovered to have a clinical onset of MS between 1943 and 1960. In Iceland two increases in new cases of MS came after World Wars I and II. Iceland, which shares ethnic origin with the Faeroese, was also heavily occupied during World War II by British, American, and Canadian troops. These findings provide additional support to the acquired viral theory of the disease in a genetically susceptible population. Family studies have supported the importance of genetic factors in MS. The clinical concordance rate in monozygotic twins, for example, is as high as 30%, and that of dizygotic twins of other first-order relatives is roughly 3%. The risk for the general population is about 0.1%.[13,31] The overall sex ratio appears to be about 3:2 (women:men).

Etiology

MS may be a disease of viral etiology, and it is probable that myelin damage is mediated by the immune system. It appears that in susceptible individuals there is an abnormality in the way in which the immune response is regulated and controlled that results in a widespread attack on the individual's own neural tissue—that is, an autoimmune response. Identification of a specific antigen remains to be accomplished.

If a virus is responsible, it must either be a ubiquitous virus that infects a large number of people with only a few of the infected developing the secondary process (MS) or an unusual virus with a low rate of infection but a high rate of clinical expression.[13]

Signs and symptoms

Functional and clinical deficits correlate with localized areas of demyelination in the CNS. Because of the great variability of the anatomical location and time sequence of lesions in clients with MS, the clinical manifestations of the disease vary from one individual to another. Symptoms may develop quickly, within hours, or slowly over several days or weeks. Most commonly, symptoms develop within 6 to 15 hours, although rapidity of onset and appearance of symptoms depend on the locus and size of the underlying lesion. The incidence of initial symptoms in descending order of frequency is (1) motor weakness, (2) retrobulbar

---

Summary of common signs and symptoms

Motor symptoms

Spasticity and reflex spasms
Weakness
Contractures
Gait disturbance
Easy fatigability
Cerebellar and bulbar symptoms
- Resultant swallowing/respiratory difficulties
- Nystagmus
- Intention tremor

Sensory symptoms

Numbness
Pain (most often of musculoskeletal origin)
Paresthesia
Dysesthesia
Distortion of superficial sensation

Visual symptoms

Diminished acuity
Double vision
Scotoma
Ocular pain

Bladder/bowel symptoms

Urgency
Frequency
Incontinence
Urinary retention
Constipation

Sexual symptoms

Impotence
Diminished genital sensation
Diminished genital lubrication

Cognitive and emotional symptoms

Depression
Euphoria
Mixed emotional states
Lability
Disorders of judgment
Agnosia
Memory disturbance
Diminished conceptual thinking
Decreased attention and concentration
Dysphasia

neuritis, (3) paresthesia, (4) unsteady gait, (5) double vision, (6) vertigo/vomiting, and (7) micturition disorder. Other types of onset, such as hemiplegia, trigeminal neuralgia, and facial palsy, are seen in fewer than 3% of the cases.[19] In many individuals a history of vague functional impairment precedes definite symptoms, and there are some in whom definite neurological signs do not confirm initial complaints.

A wide variety of symptoms are associated with the disease and should be understood by a therapist dealing with these problems (see the box on p. 534 for a summary of the most common signs and symptoms of MS).

Course and prognosis

The clinical course of MS can be roughly divided into three patterns. One is the classic pattern, characterized by exacerbations and remissions. It features sudden onset or reappearance of symptoms that indicate the development of a fresh lesion or extension of an old one. This is followed by partial or total disappearance of the symptom or symptoms. In benign cases (which may account for 20% of the total MS population) this pattern may recur throughout life with little or no residual disability. Mild cases may be evidenced by deficits that accumulate over the series of exacerbations but are not severe enough to interfere with near-normal functioning. Moderate cases carry a more severe degree of residual deficit, which subsequently may become progressive, resulting in significant disability.

The second pattern, progressive MS, is characterized by slow or rapid worsening of disability from the onset, without delineated periods of relapse and remission. Existing deficits may increase in severity, and new symptoms occur as the disease progresses. For the most part, progression is slow; however, in a small number of cases the disease fulminates, progressing rapidly over a few years, leading to severe disability or death.

The third pattern consists of a combination of the first two. It starts with a classic relapsing/remitting course but becomes progressive, with limited remissions.

Overall prognosis is variable and the course of the disease quite unpredictable (Fig. 18-3). Although there have

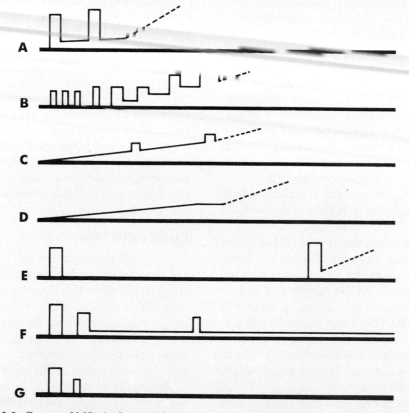

Fig. 18-3. Course of MS. **A,** Severe relapses, increasing disability and early death. **B,** Many short attacks, tending to increase in duration and severity. **C,** Slow progression from onset, superimposed relapses, and increasing disability. **D,** Slow progression from onset without relapses. **E,** Abrupt onset with good remission followed by long latent phase. **F,** Relapses of diminishing frequency and severity; slight residual disability only. **G,** Abrupt onset; few if any relapses after first year; no residual disability. (From McAlpine D and others: Multiple sclerosis: a reappraisal, 1965, Edinburgh, E & S Livingstone, Ltd.)

been efforts to identify prognostic guidelines, these guidelines have not proved to be reliable.

Various factors have been associated with exacerbations or temporary worsening. These include excessive fatigue, trauma, rise in body temperature because of fever, hot bath or shower, hot weather conditions, and pregnancy. However, no specific cause-effect relationship has been identified. For the most part, the exacerbating/remitting pattern remains unpredictable.

Problems of diagnosis

The diagnosis of MS rests on clinical criteria because there are no specific laboratory aids that are conclusive. The basic criteria that support a diagnosis are (1) evidence of multiple lesions in the CNS, (2) evidence of discrete episodes of neurological disturbance, (3) evidence that the clinical signs and symptoms are compatible with a diagnosis of MS, and (4) lack of a better neurological explanation for the disturbance.

Differential diagnosis and the exclusion of other disease states are mandatory because of the extreme variation in the sites of CNS involvement and in the temporal sequence of symptoms and signs. Disease states to be ruled out include orthopaedic pathology, tumor, metabolic or toxic disorders, transverse myelitis, and motor neuron disease.

Although no specific diagnostic laboratory test for MS exists, laboratory studies, helpful in establishing a broad clinical picture, have aided the identification of clinically silent lesions in some individuals. Lumbar puncture and analysis of the cerebrospinal fluid (CSF) can provide significant information. Approximately one quarter of all persons with active disease show an increase in the number of white blood cells in the CSF. Total CSF protein is elevated in approximately 30% of those with active disease, and the gamma-globulin fraction[14] is found increased 70% to 90%, especially when electrophoretic analysis is applied. Analysis of CSF may show fragments of myelin or myelin-basic protein in individuals with acute episodes.

Visual, auditory, and somatosensory evoked response evaluation provide objective measures of impulse conduction in CNS white-matter tracts. An evoked response is the electrical manifestation of the brain's reception of and response to an external stimulus; it is a way of measuring conduction efficiency in the CNS (see Chapter 26). In persons with MS, evoked response abnormalities are quite common, and they may enable otherwise clinically "silent" lesions (where the individual may not be aware of any symptom) to be discovered.

A number of disorders of immunological function have recently been found in MS, but these research studies have not yet proved helpful in diagnosis. Neuroradiological studies such as isotope scanning, angiography, computed axial tomography (CT) scan, myelography, and pneumoencephalography are sometimes performed to rule out other pathologies. In addition, the CT scan can

---

Diagnostic guidelines for multiple sclerosis

Clinically definite multiple sclerosis

1. Relapsing and remitting course with at least two bouts separated by no less than 1 month
2. Slow or step-by-step progressive course over at least 6 months
3. Documented neurological signs attributable to more than one site of predominantly white-matter CNS pathology
4. Onset of symptoms between ages 10 and 50
5. No better neurological explanation

Probable multiple sclerosis

1. History of relapsing and remitting symptoms without documentation of signs and with only one neurological sign commonly associated with MS
2. A documented single bout of symptoms with signs of multifocal white-matter disease, with good recovery and followed by variable symptoms and signs
3. No better neurological explanation

Possible multiple sclerosis

1. History of relapsing and remitting symptoms, without documentation of signs
2. Objective neurological signs insufficient to establish more than one site of CNS white-matter pathology
3. No better neurological explanation

---

sometimes demonstrate the MS plaques directly. Magnetic resonance imaging (MRI) has recently been used to evaluate MS, and in one study it was used to identify very small lesions.[32] MRI will probably supplant CT as the diagnostic scanning procedure of choice. It is about 10 times more sensitive than unenhanced CT for detection of MS lesions.[13]

Psychosocial considerations

The total personality of the individual and the family and community environment before the development of any physical disability crucially affect the response to illness. The nature of the disability itself will also, obviously, help to determine the response. MS is a tremendously demanding disease from a psychological point of view. Several clinical characteristics of the disease are of particular importance in this regard.

Ambiguity of diagnosis. Because a specific laboratory test for MS is lacking, many individuals are initially given a vague or an indefinite diagnosis or perhaps even none at all. They may therefore seek numerous medical opinions and undergo extensive and exhaustive neurological, medical, and psychiatric evaluations. Fantasies of what may be wrong abound during this period of not knowing. Most people feel that they can handle most things if they know where they stand, but unfortunately MS does not always afford this privilege.

Unpredictability of course. Adjustment to a stable and clearly defined loss is not usually possible with MS. The uncertainty of the future—and even the changes from week to week, month to month, year to year—demand an ongoing adjustment and readjustment process. Additionally, an individual diagnosed with MS cannot be sure of the subsequent pattern or level of severity of the disease. At one extreme are individuals with relatively benign disease; at the other are those with quickly progressive, debilitating MS. A study carried out in 1971,[24] however, did indicate a more optimistic outlook than previously believed for most persons with MS. Investigators in this study followed persons with MS for 25 years after diagnosis. Their study showed that 74% were still living at the end of 25 years compared with an expected figure of 86% for the general population. Even more impressive, however, is the fact that two thirds of the 25-year survivors were still ambulatory. It is therefore the minority of persons with MS who experience severe levels of disability. It is easy for clinicians to lose sight of this reality because they are less likely to come in contact with clients with MS who have benign or mild disease and who are conducting their everyday activities with minimal or no limitations.

"Borderline" factor. Many individuals with an exacerbating/remitting pattern of the disease are sometimes disabled, sometimes ablebodied. They walk a borderline, in a sense, between two worlds. Additionally, many persons with MS experience covert or invisible symptoms that may limit their activities but that are not apparent to others. Because they look so well, unreasonable expectations and confusion may result on the part of employers, family, and friends.

• • •

Certainly, the stress of MS is in many ways like the stress of any kind of serious illness. A profound sense of fear, vulnerability, and exhausting self-concern underlies the coping process. The loss of a sense of control over one's body and life-style may precipitate an ongoing grieving process and a search to make some sense and give meaning to an otherwise confusing and purposeless event.

MEDICAL MANAGEMENT

There are no specific treatments available that can prevent or reverse the demyelination process. Therefore major treatment measures focus on easing of symptoms and attempting to maximize health, minimize associated complications, and lessen the severity or length of an exacerbation. Overall nursing and medical management calls for principles that will effect maximal health in general. These include ensuring adequate nutrition, encouraging balanced

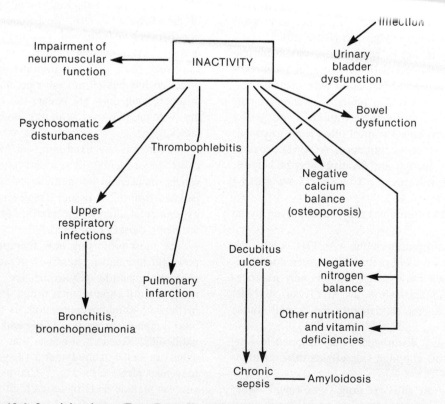

Fig. 18-4. Inactivity chart. (From Bauer H: A Manual on Multiple Sclerosis, published under the auspices of the International Federation of Multiple Sclerosis Societies, 1977.)

rest and exercise, avoiding exposure to infections, and—certainly of importance—preventing complications secondary to reduced activity (Fig. 18-4). Psychosocially, it is also important to facilitate coping resources and to avoid psychiatric disturbance or severe family problems. Specifically, the following medical treatments can be beneficial.

1. Spasticity of skeletal musculature and external urethral sphincter may be reduced by baclofen (Lioresal), diazepam (Valium), and dantrolene (Dantrium). Attention needs to be paid to side effects of these medications—such as increased weakness, fatigue, lethargy, and problems with mentation—and the dosage regulated accordingly. Phenol blocks or tendon-release procedures may be required where severe spasticity interferes with personal hygiene, mobility, and activities of daily living (ADL).[6]

2. Therapy of incoordination related to cerebellar dysfunction is not reliably effective. Isoniazid (INH) may have inhibitior properties in the cerebellum. Propanolol (Inderal) may be moderately useful in controlling tremor. For severe and uncontrollable tremor, some individuals may benefit from thaomotomy (the surgical destruction of part of the thalamus) or by electrical stimulation of the thalamus by implanted electrodes.[30]

3. Substantial improvement in vision, strength, and coordination has been obtained in clinical trials of 4-aminopyridine, which enhances conduction in demyelinated axons. Its effects only last a few hours, however, and this drug in under further investigation.[30]

4. Urinary frequency and urgency may be reduced by smooth muscle relaxants or nerve blockers such as propantheline (Pro-Banthine) and oxybutynin (Ditropan).[4]

5. Urinary retention can be reduced by smooth muscle stimulants such as bethanechol (Urecholine) or phenoxybhenzamine (Dibenzyline) in association with manual pressure over the bladder (Credé's method). Some patients may require intermittent self-catheterization.[4]

6. Absence of good bowel control often leads to constipation and at times fecal incontinence. A bowel program or appropriate use of enemas and laxatives may be helpful. (For additional information, see Chapter 25 on nursing procedures.)

7. Visual distortion (diplopia) may be improved by an eye patch.

8. Adrenocorticotropic hormone (ACTH), cortisone, prednisone, and other steroid preparations given during exacerbation sometimes may be associated with improvement. Long-term administration of ACTH or steroids, however, does not appreciably modify the overall course of the disease.[8]

9. Pain and sensory disturbances may respond to Carbamazepine (Tegretol) although side effects may contraindicate its use.

10. Amantadine, an antiviral drug, was found somewhat by chance to be effective in relieving fatigue in a significant number of persons with MS.[30]

11. Speech therapy, occupational therapy, and physical therapy should be prescribed (these are discussed in greater detail in the section on treatment of sensorimotor dysfunction).

12. Emotional or psychological symptoms may warrant drug (e.g., tricyclic antidepressants) therapy in addition to counseling or adjustment programs.

In considering any therapy or treatment, one must keep in mind that a large percentage of persons with MS show improvement at various times during their illness regardless of what is done. Recent research regarding the placebo effect and the "mind-body" effect are further evidence that improvement is not always a direct result of treatment procedures themselves.

THERAPEUTIC CLAIMS AND RESEARCH CONSIDERATIONS

Epidemiological evidence provides strong support for the hypothesis that MS is initiated by a virus infection. Attempts to isolate a specific MS virus, however, have to date failed, and various common viruses continue to be studied. Antibodies to measles, for example, appear to be elevated in persons with MS as compared to individuals in control groups. Antibodies to components of myelin basic protein and to oligodendrocytes are also found in significant quantity in persons with MS. In addition, there is a striking abnormality of one kind of T lymphocyte, specifically the T-suppressor cell in persons with MS. Normally, T cells help maintain the delicate balance of the immune system. Researchers postulate a correlation between a failure of T-suppressor cells and autoimmunity. Investigators hypothesize that the suppressor cells that "turn off" the immune response when a viral infection has passed are not operating, and if this immunosuppression does not occur, the immune attack continues without purpose, with the body's own tissue under attack.[18]

Researchers are examining an MS-like animal disease called experimental allergic encephalomyelitis (EAE) that can be induced in lab animals using myelin basic protein isolated from CNS tissue. Treatment procedures that alter experimental allergic encephalitis or initiate remyelination are being closely examined.

The most promising new therapies involve the use of powerful immunosuppressives. Azathioprine (Imuran) and cyclophosphamide (Cytoxan) are the most commonly used, yet still experimental drugs. Plasmapheresis, another method of immunosuppression, is also under study as is total lymphoid irradiation (TLI) and the use of monoclonal antibodies. Research suggests that interferon (an antiviral agent) as well as Copolymer 1 (a synthetic myelin protein) may also prove effective.[30] Claims regarding therapeutic success include diets of foods high in polyunsaturated fat; gluten-free, raw food; and megavitamin supplements. Hyperbaric oxygen, snake venom (Pro-ven), acupuncture, vertebral and carotid artery manipulation to increase blood flow, and a variety of other relief measures have failed to show effectiveness. Until a specific preventive or curative treatment is developed, undocumented claims of therapeutic success will undoubtedly remain prominent. Given the circumstances and the still unanswered questions about MS, a guarded and careful approach to speculative treatments should be taken.

EVALUATION PROCEDURES

The clinician must take into consideration various factors in evaluating the individual with MS. Subjective perceptions of problems by the individual and family members are of great importance. Functional assessment at times may not correlate with clinical measure—that is, MS lesions may be functionally silent in some cases; yet in others, significant functional impairment may result from apparently minimal clinical disease activity. Evaluation of the individual with MS must be done at intervals during the fluctuating course of the disease. Additionally, factors that influence performance such as heat and time of day (fatigue factor) must be considered when the client is evaluated.

Disability profiles and indexes

A number of assessment profiles have been designed to gauge the abilities and rehabilitation needs of disabled individuals. These measures have been useful in planning a rehabilitation program.

Pulses Profile is a scale developed in 1957 by Moskowitz and McCann.[20] It consists of six components indicated by the acronym PULSES (see boxed material below).

The Barthel Index (BI) is another profile scale (see box on p. 541); it includes 10 self-care, sphincter control, and mobility factors (Table 18-1).[18] The specific details used in scoring this index are presented in the boxed material. The advantage of the Barthel Index is its simplicity and usefulness in evaluating patients before, during, and after

---

PULSES Profile

P. *Physical condition* including diseases of the viscera (cardiovascular, pulmonary, gastrointestinal, urologic, and endocrine) and cerebral disorders which are not enumerated in the lettered categories below
   1. No gross abnormalities considering the age of the individual
   2. Minor abnormalities not requiring frequent medical or nursing supervision
   3. Moderately severe abnormalities requiring frequent medical or nursing supervision yet still permitting ambulation
   4. Severe abnormalities requiring constant medical or nursing supervision confining individual to bed or wheelchair

U. *Upper* extremities including shoulder girdle, cervical, and upper dorsal spine
   1. No gross abnormalities considering the age of the individual
   2. Minor abnormalities with fairly good range of motion and function
   3. Moderately severe abnormalities but permitting the performance of daily needs to a limited extent
   4. Severe abnormalities requiring constant nursing care

L. *Lower* extremeties including the pelvis, lower dorsal, and lumbosacral spine.
   1. No gross abnormalities considering the age of the individual
   2. Minor abnormalities with fairly good range of motion and function

   3. Moderately severe abnormalities permitting limited ambulation
   4. Severe abnormalities confining the individual to bed or wheelchair

S. *Sensory* components relating to speech, vision and hearing
   1. No gross abnormalities considering the age of the individual
   2. Minor deviations insufficient to cause any appreciable functional impairment
   3. Moderate deviations sufficient to cause appreciable functional impairment
   4. Severe deviations causing complete loss of hearing, vision or speech

E. *Excretory* function, i.e., bowel and bladder control
   1. Complete control
   2. Occasional stress incontinence or nocturia
   3. Periodic bowel and bladder incontinence or retention alternating with control
   4. Total incontenence, either bowel or bladder

S. *Mental* and *emotional status*
   1. No deviations considering the age of the individual
   2. Minor deviations in mood, temperament and personality not impairing environmental adjustment
   3. Moderately severe variations requiring some supervision
   4. Severe variations requiring complete supervision

Each component is rated on a 1 to 4 scale with no. 1 being most stable, independent, and close to normal function and no. 4 indicating total dependence in mobility and ADL, with medical problems requiring intensive attention and significant impairment. Thus the "best" score is 6 and the score 24 indicates the greatest involvement.

Table 18-1. Barthel Index*

	With help	Independent
1. Feeding (if food needs to be cut = help)	5	10
2. Moving from wheelchair to bed and return (includes sitting up in bed)	5-10	15
3. Personal toilet (wash face, comb hair, shave, clean teeth)	0	5
4. Getting on and off toilet (handling clothes, wipe, flush)	5	10
5. Bathing self	0	5
6. Walking on level surface	10	15
(or if unable to walk, propel wheelchair)	0†	5
7. Ascend and descend stairs	5	10
8. Dressing (include tying shoes, fastening fasteners)	5	10
9. Controlling bowels	5	10
10. Controlling bladder	5	10

From Mahoney FI and Barthel DW: Md State Med J 14:61, 1965.
*A patient scoring 100 BI is continent, feeds himself, dresses himself, gets up and out of bed and chairs, bathes himself, walks at least a block, and can ascend and descend stairs. This does not mean that he is able to live alone. He may not be able to cook, keep house, and meet the public, but he is able to get along without attendant care.
†Score only if unable to walk.

treatment. It is functionally oriented and may be best used accompanied by a clinical evaluation.[12]

A third assessment, designed by Kurtzke,[16] is a two-part scale measuring disability specifically related to MS. The first part documents neurological functions scored on a scale of 0 to 6. Specific functions to be rated are outlined in the box on p. 542. The scoring instructions are presented in the box at the top of p. 543.

One difficulty in utilizing these three scales is that there is no satisfactory system for measuring fatigue, an issue that plays a significant part in the performance capacity of individual clients. Second, capacity may depend on such factors as time of day, domestic situation, and the person's mood, which are not measured fully in these scales. Third, as previously mentioned, physical signs in themselves often have little relevance in measuring capacity. For example, many individuals with grade 1 on pyramidal function (Kurtzke, Part 1) may be homebound while others with a grade 5 on pyramidal function may work full time.

A minimal record of disability (MRD) for multiple sclerosis was developed in 1985 under the aegis of the International Federation of MS Societies.[25] The format combines neurological assessment and status of daily living circumstances in a single page that can be completed in a short time. The MS Society is encouraging its use. The MRD was designed to adhere to the following three-tier classification developed by the World Health Organization:

1. *Impairment:* caused by underlying organic disorders resulting in clinical signs and symptoms
2. *Disability:* reflecting the personal limitations imposed upon activities of daily living
3. *Handicap:* reflecting the environmental situation that limits the disabled person from achieving an optimal role

The scale was constructed to correlate with the Kurtzke, PULSES, and Barthel systems. The scale consists of five parts: Demographic Information, Neurological Functional Systems of Kurtzke, Disability Status Scale of Kurtzke, Incapacity Status Scale, and Environmental Status Scale. The MRD can be obtained directly from the National MS Society (205 E. 42 St., New York, NY 10017). Because it is specifically designed for the person with MS, this useful tool provides a simple, comprehensive, and standardized profile that can assist the health care team in planning and coordinating the management of these individuals.

Standardized scales are necessary in comparing standardized work of one center with the work of other centers, and they can be useful in monitoring treatment results and providing clients with goals.

Rehabilitative data base

A more flexible and comprehensive physical occupational therapy evaluation for an individual with MS is also used by therapists. These evaluations include sensorimotor control, functional status, developmental activities, respiratory status, and psychosocial behaviors (i.e., cognitive, affective, and perceptual). (See p. 543 for the box on formulating a rehabilitative data base.)

SETTING GOALS

A statement from *A Manual on Multiple Sclerosis*[2] summarizes important guidelines in setting goals:

In every rehabilitation program, the patient must be treated as a whole, the best physical and psychological condition under the circumstances must be achieved, complications eliminated as far as possible and realistic motivations exploited. This can only be accomplished by the well-coordinated teamwork of doctors, nurses, physiotherapists, occupational therapists, clinical psy-

Text continued on p. 544.

Rating guidelines for Barthel Index*

1. Feeding
   10 = Independent. The patient can feed himself a meal when someone puts the food within his reach. He must put on an assistive device if this is needed, cut up the food alone. He must accomplish this in a reasonable time.
   5 = Some help is necessary (with cutting up food, etc., as listed above).

2. Moving from wheelchair to bed and return
   15 = Independent in all phases of this activity. Patient can safely approach the bed in his wheelchair, lock brakes, lift footrests, move safely to bed, lie down, come to a sitting position on the wheelchair, if necessary, to transfer back into it safely, and return to the wheelchair.
   10 = Either some minimal help is needed in some step of this activity or the patient needs to be reminded or supervised for safety of one or more parts of this activity.
   5 = Patient can come to a sitting position without the help of a second person but needs to be lifted out of bed, or if he transfers with a great deal of help.

3. Doing personal toilet
   5 = Patient can wash hands and face, comb hair, clean teeth, and shave. He may use any kind of razor but must put in blade or plug in razor without help as well as get it from drawer or cabinet. Female patients must put on own makeup.

4. Getting on and off toilet
   10 = Patient is able to get on and off toilet, fasten and unfasten clothes, prevent soiling of clothes, and use toilet paper without help. If it is necessary to use a bedpan instead of a toilet, he must be able to place it on a chair, empty it, and clean it.
   5 = Patient needs help because of imbalance or in handling clothes or in using toilet paper.

5. Bathing self
   5 = Patient may use a bathtub, a shower, or take a complete sponge bath. He must be able to do all the steps involved in whichever method is employed without another person being present.

6. Walking on a level surface
   15 = Patient can walk at least 50 yards without help or supervision. He may wear braces or protheses and use crutches, canes, or a walkerette but not a rolling walker. He must be able to lock and unlock braces, if used, assume the standing position and sit down, get the necessary mechanical aids into position for use, and dispose of them when he sits. (Putting on and taking off braces is scored under dressing.)
   10 = Patient needs help or supervision in any of the above but can walk at least 50 yards with a little help.

6a. Propelling a wheelchair
   5 = If a patient cannot ambulate but can propel a wheelchair independently. He must be able to go around corners, turn around, maneuver the chair to a table, bed, toilet, etc. He must be able to push a chair at least 50 yards. Do not score this item if the patient gets score for walking.

7. Ascending and descending stairs
   10 = Patient is able to go up and down a flight of stairs safely without help or supervision. He may and should use handrails, canes, or crutches when needed. He must be able to carry canes or crutches as he ascends or descends stairs.
   5 = Patient needs help with or supervision of any one of the above items.

8. Dressing and undressing
   10 = Patient is able to put on and remove and fasten all clothing, as well as tie shoe laces (unless it is necessary to use adaptions for this). The activity includes putting on and removing and fastening corset or braces when these are prescribed.
   5 = Patient needs help in putting on and removing or fastening any clothing. He must do at least half the work himself. He must accomplish this in a reasonable time. Women need not be scored on use of a brassiere or girdle unless these are prescribed garments.

9. Continence of bowels
   10 = Patient is able to control his bowels and have no accidents. He can use a suppository or take an enema when necessary.
   5 = Patient needs help in using a suppository or taking an enema or has occasional accidents.

10. Controlling bladder
   10 = Patient is able to control his bladder day and night. Patients who wear an external device and leg bag must put them on independently, clean and empty bag, and stay dry day and night.
   5 = Patient has occasional accidents or cannot wait for the bedpan or get to the toilet in time or needs help with an external device.

Mahoney FI and Barthel DW: Md State Med J 14:63, 1965.
*A score of 0 is given in the activity when the patient cannot meet the criteria as defined.

Kurtzke Disability Scale

1. Pyramidal functions
   0 = Normal
   1 = Abnormal signs without disability
   2 = Minimal disability
   3 = Mild or moderate paraparesis or hemiparesis; severe monoparesis
   4 = Marked paraparesis or hemiparesis; moderate quadriparesis; or monoplegia
   5 = Paraplegia, hemiplegia, or marked quadriparesis
   6 = Quadriplegia
   V = Unknown

2. Cerebeller functions
   0 = Normal
   1 = Abnormal signs without disability
   2 = Mild ataxia
   3 = Moderate truncal or limb ataxia
   4 = Severe ataxia all limbs
   5 = Unable to perform coordinated movements due to ataxia
   V = Unknown
   X is used after 0-3 when weakness of grade 3 or more interferes with testing.

3. Brainstem functions
   0 = Normal
   1 = Signs only
   2 = Moderate nystagmus or other mild disability
   3 = Severe nystagmus, marked extraocular weakness or moderate disability of other cranial nerves
   4 = Marked dysarthria or other marked disability
   5 = Inability to swallow or speak
   V = Unknown

4. Sensory functions
   0 = Normal
   1 = Vibration or figure-writing decrease only
   2 = Mild decrease in touch or pain; moderate decrease in position, vibration, or discrimination
   3 = Marked hyposensitivity (not complete)
   4 = Analgesia or anesthesia to groin; hemianesthesia or hemianalgesia
   5 = Analgesia and anesthesia to neck
   V = Unknown

5. Bowel and bladder functions
   0 = Normal
   1 = Mild hesitancy, urgency or retention
   2 = Moderate hesitancy, urgency, retention, or rate urinary incontinence
   3 = Frequent incontinence
   4 = In need of almost constant catheterization but with intact bladder sensation; severe bowel retention and/or incontinence
   5 = Lack of sensation and control of bowel and bladder function
   V = Unknown

6. Visual functions
   0 = Normal
   1 = Scotoma with visual acuity (corrected) better than 20/30
   2 = Worse eye with scotoma with maximal visual acuity (corrected) of 20/30 to 20/59
   3 = Worse eye with large scotoma, or moderate decrease in fields, but with maximal visual acuity (corrected) of 20/60 to 20/99
   4 = Worse eye with marked decrease of fields and maximal visual acuity (corrected) of 20/100 to 20/200; grade 3 plus maximal acuity of better eye 20/60 or less
   6 = Grade 5 plus maximal visual acuity of better eye 20/60 or less
   V = Unknown
   X is added to grade 0-6 for presence of temporal pallor.

7. Mental functions
   0 = Normal
   1 = Mood alteration only
   2 = Mild decrease mentation
   3 = Moderate decrease mentation
   4 = Marked decrease in mentation (chronic brain syndrome, moderate)
   5 = Dementia; or chronic brain syndrome, severe, incompetent
   V = Unknown

8. Other functions
   0 = None
   1 = Any other findings (specify)
   V = Unknown

Kurtzke JF: Neurology 11(8):688, 1961.

Specific scoring of the disability scale: Kurtzke Scale

0 = Normal neurologic examination (all grade 0 in functional groups)

1 = No disability, minimal signs (Babinski, minimal finger-to-nose ataxia, diminished vibration sense) (grade 1 in functional groups)

2 = Minimal disability—slight weakness or stiffness, mild disturbance of gait, or mild visuomotor disturbance (1 or 2 functional grade 2)

3 = Moderate disability—monoparesis, mild hemiparesis, moderate ataxia, disturbing sensory loss, or prominent urinary or eye symptoms, or combinations of lesser dysfunctions (1 or 2 functional grade 3 or several grade 2)

4 = Relatively severe disability not preventing ability to work or carry on normal activities of living, excluding sexual function. This includes the ability to be up and about 12 hours a day (1 functional grade 4 or several grade 3 or less)

5 = Disability severe enough to preclude working, with maximal motor function walking unaided up to several blocks (1 functional grade 5 alone, or combination of lesser)

6 = Assistance (canes, crutches, braces) required for walking (1 functional grade 6 alone or combination of lesser)

7 = Restricted to wheelchair—able to wheel self and enter and leave chair alone (combinations with at least 1 above functional grade 4)

8 = Restricted to bed but with effective use of arms (combinations usually junctional grade 4 or above in several functional groups)

9 = Totally helpless bed patient (combinations usually functional grade 4 or above in most functional groups)

10 = Death due to multiple sclerosis

Kurtzke JF: Neurology 11(8):688, 1961

Rehabilitative data base

Sensorimotor control

1. Patterns of muscle weakness
2. Tonal dominance of postures, spasticity, reflexes
3. Hyperactive/hypoactive reflexes
4. Cerebellar dysfunction (such as tremor, dysmentria, coordination: upper and lower extremities)
5. Sensation
6. Range of motion, contractures

Functional status

1. Ambulation patterns (walking, braiding, tandem walking, hopping, skipping, running, stair climbing), speed, endurance, stability, safety
2. Wheelchair activities (propulsion, retropulsion, ramps, handling of brakes, footrests, armrests, wheelchair maintenance)
3. Transfers (car, bed, toilet, tub)
4. Activities of daily living (personal hygiene, toileting, bathing, dressing, bed mobility, feeding, writing and communication, driving, homemaking, child care, prevocational and vocational skills)

Developmental activities

1. Rolling side to side
2. Prone on elbows, creeping
3. Lower trunk rotation
4. Bridging, sitting, quadruped
5. Kneeling, half kneeling
6. Standing

Respiratory evaluation

1. Breathing patterns (relative movement of abdomen and chest and use of abdominal, diaphragmatic, intercostal, and accessory muscles)
2. Cough and breath control
3. Voice volume

Cognitive, affective, and perceptual evaluation

1. Motivation
2. Judgment and understanding of illness
3. Cognition (memory, language, attention span, conceptual thinking)
4. Affective assessment (such as depression, euphoria, and lability)
5. Perception (such as visual-spatial skill, sequencing, and apraxia)

chologists, social workers, the patient and his family and friends, and organizations with a genuine interest and sense of responsibility for him (p. 34).

The ideal rehabilitation model acknowledges the client's responsibility and resources. It recognizes both the client's and family members' priorities and values; it considers not only the home environment but community resources, medical issues, history of the disease, and the cognitive and affective status of the individual.

To date there is no evidence that rehabilitation efforts have an influence on the principal pathological process in MS. Therefore the overriding principle in setting rehabilitation goals is to maximize independence, self-determination and quality of life within the context of the individual's life-style and abilities, (see box at right).

Often, for more stable or clear-cut disabilities, goals are set according to a functional skill such as ambulatory or wheelchair level. This may not be appropriate for clients with MS. A large number may be ambulatory for short distances but require a wheelchair for more demanding tasks. Additionally, for periods of exacerbation, training in wheelchair mobility may be a temporary yet important necessity. The variations in MS confirm the need for ongoing reestablishment of goals in response to therapy and to changes in the client's condition, home environment, and the family situation.

TREATMENT CONSIDERATIONS

Involvement in a rehabilitation program may take several forms. From a practical point of view, fiscal considerations may dictate the frequency and duration of therapy visits as well as location, that is, whether the care is administered at home or on an inpatient or outpatient basis. Unfortunately, the availability of third-party payment for therapy is often conditional, with many individuals ineligible for reimbursement, particularly for maintenance and preventotive therapies.

The place at which treatment is provided can often dictate the form it takes. An inpatient setting, for example, provides an opportunity for intensive therapies, a therapeutic community, multidisciplinary support, a comprehensive treatment environment, and easy availability of equipment and modalities. It is also important to realize that such a setting requires learning skills outside of the home environment, transferring those skills after discharge, and adjusting psychologically to the home setting, where the client has the opportunity and responsibility to carry out his or her program.

Home-based treatment, as an alternative, provides a familiar environment; however, availability of equipment or modalities may be limited. The treatment environment selected needs to be based on the client's needs, the availability of resources, and cost.

Aspects of quality of life

Psychophysiological equilibrium

Understanding of the disease, the symptoms, and how to manage them

Understanding of limitations and strengths; functioning up to but respecting limits

Maintenance of function with minimum effort and maximum safety (balancing rest and activity appropriately)

Functional improvement in spite of persistent neurological signs

Return to preexacerbation physical status

Altering environment to support independence, diminish disability

Wellness lifestyle

Mastery over potential uncertainty and loss of control

Interrelatedness

Realistic expectations for patient and family

Preservation of family unit

Learning new ways to fulfill family/friendship roles

Knowing and practicing how to be realistically independent—not being a burden—but also being able to communicate when and how help is needed

Avoiding social isolation

Knowing and appropriately using community resources

Productivity

Developing alternative plans to already established vocational goals (job, education, other training)

Establishing a productive life (paid or volunteer)

Creativity

Developing problem-solving skills

Developing avocational interests

Reaching important life goals; focusing on remaining possibilities

Developing an enjoyable, personally meaningful life (MS not being the focus of one's life)

Adapted from Maloney FP and others: Interdisciplinary rehabilitation of multiple sclerosis and neuromuscular disorders, Philadelphia, 1985, JB Lippincott Co.

Treatment of sensorimotor dysfunction

A primary area of difficulty for persons with MS arises from poor sensorimotor integration. Several important general areas to consider in treatment planning include spasticity, weakness, cerebellar dysfunction, sensory loss, impaired range of motion (ROM), pain, and speech problems.

To manage spasticity and maintain joint mobility the therapist should consider reflex dominance, hypertonicity, and abnormal movement. Daily passive and active stretching and active range of motion should be performed. Prolonged icing (ice packs or ice massage) has been useful in some cases to reduce spasticity—as have relaxation (inhibitory) techniques, which include joint approximation, slow rolling of the client from supine to side, slow rocking, slow stroking of the posterior rami, and pressure on the tendinous insertion of the spastic muscle. Proper bed and wheelchair positioning to maximize normal tone, inhibit primitive reflex patterns, and normalize posture is also important. Strengthening exercises for the relatively weaker agonistic muscles while relaxing the antagonistic may lead to improved functional mobility. Pharmaceutical intervention, as discussed earlier, may augment therapy. In severe cases, where joint range is compromised and where spasticity interferes with hygiene or nursing care, phenol injection may be indicated. (See Chapter 6 on neurophysiological classification of treatment procedures for the neurophysiological explanation.)

Decreased muscle function results from a variety of causes, including the disease process, disuse, or overriding spasticity by the antagonistic muscle. To increase or maintain strength, progressive resistive exercises and flexibility programs should be performed daily. Equipment needs will vary depending on the individual situation. Active or active-assistive exercises, perhaps done in proprioceptive neuromuscular facilitation (PNF) diagonals, require no equipment. Resistive exercise programs may require pulley systems, wall weights, wrist cuffs, barbells, or sandbags. Although strengthening exercises will not reverse the disease process, compensatory strengthening of nonaffected muscle groups, strengthening of agonistic muscles to overcome spastic antagonistic muscles, and prevention of weakness secondary to disuse can be achieved. For a home program it is important to prescribe a specific strengthening program without sacrificing ability to perform daily functional activities. Energy-conserving techniques must become habitual to maximize and prolong strength and endurance. To maximize the conservation of energy, the time of day when exercises are performed should be considered. If compensatory strengthening proves to be limited in improving mobility, bracing may be used to diminish gait abnormalities and improve the individual's ability to function with less effort. Ankle-foot orthoses (AFOs) are used to stabilize the ankle and compensate for foot drop. Rocker shoes (a clog-type shoe) may be helpful in improving ambulation in individuals with specific patterns of lower-extremity weakness and spasticity.[25] Other orthotics to compensate for weakness may also be prescribed. Static upper-extremity splints, such as a resting-pan or wrist extension splints, may be useful in some cases.

MS patients with cerebellar dysfunction may exhibit signs of ataxia, tremor, and dysmetria (see Chapter 21). These types of symptoms are seen not only in the extremities but in the trunk as well. They are often the most difficult to manage of all MS problems and, for the most part, treatment is compensatory. Strengthening of fixation musculature by way of rhythmic stabilization, adapting techniques for proximal stabilization, and facilitating co-contraction at proximal joints may improve stability and coordination. In addition, providing general coordination activities progressing from gross to fine control may be helpful. Adapted games and upper-extremity exercises with increasing demands for speed and accuracy may yield improvement; however, this is inconclusive and may often be frustrating for the patient. Where ataxia is related to decreased proprioception, Frenkel's coordination exercises[9] may be useful (see Appendix). Further, utilizing visual feedback and engaging in coordination activities to decrease velocity of tremor, promote increased feedback, and improve stability may also be useful. Effects of weighted cuffs or weighted belt devices must be monitored; increased fatigue is an indicator that weights need to be altered or removed. If head and neck ataxia interferes with the ability to eat, drink, and swallow, an adapted cervical collar may help to improve these functions. In extreme cases, where tremor significantly interferes with functional tasks, cryosurgery of the thalamus may be indicated.

Impaired sensation is frequently a problem with this client population. Treatment in this area is aimed at compensating for the loss, maximizing safety utilizing visual feedback, and increasing awareness of the distribution of sensory impairment. Coordination exercises in combination with sensory stimulation may enhance sensory awareness. Inability to perceive temperature or pain must be particularly attended to by training in safety techniques. Skin breakdown or pressure areas must be prevented in cases in which sensory loss or immobility is present. Routine pressure relief and use of cushions and air or water mattresses may be indicated; skin inspection and care should be accomplished regularly.

Daily active and passive stretching and passive, active, and active-assisted ROM exercises repeated several times a day will help maintain joint range. Training in self-ROM and encouragement of participation in functional tasks will aid in the prevention of contractures. Severe ROM limitations may require myotenotomy or other surgical procedures.

Pain from MS may result from several sources. Pain related to spasticity, particularly in the lower extremities, may be relieved by spasticity-reducing measures along with pain-relief medication. Painful paresthesias, such as burning and tight banding sensations, may be experienced by some individuals. Treatment with pain medication is unpredictably effective, however. Transcutaneous nerve stimulation (TENS) may be tried for pain control.

A significant number of persons with MS have symptoms of dysarthria and dysphagia. These individuals may derive benefit from an evaluation by a speech and language specialist. Assessment of oral-facial structures with regard to such factors as strength, coordination, spasticity, tremor, and range of motion as well as of the speech, vocal, temporal, and respiratory aspects of communication can reveal the important clinical and functional problems. Treatment of spasticity, ataxia, and fatigue as it relates to speech and swallowing as well as therapy to improve articulation may be beneficial for some individuals (see Chapter 24).

Other treatment procedures

Specific rehabilitation techniques to improve mobility include gait training, developmental activities, wheelchair mobility training, ADL training, driver training, and vocational counseling.

The goals of gait training are to provide encouragement, the opportunity to prevent development of symptoms secondary to disuse, and the possibility of learning or relearning to walk. The client with MS may require a graduated sitting tolerance program, tilt-table routine, graduated standing tolerance schedule, balancing exercises, progressive resistive exercise for certain lower-extremity muscle groups, upper-extremity exercises for good control of crutches and other assistive devices, stretching and relaxation exercises to reduce spasticity, visual training to reinforce proprioception, and specific gait training.

Developmental activities are useful in several ways both from functional and neurotherapeutic points of view. Developmental mat exercises are necessary prerequisites to bed mobility, self-care training, and general mobility. On-elbows and quadruped tasks facilitate cocontraction at proximal joints and may improve coordination and stability. Advanced developmental tasks (i.e., kneeling, half-kneeling, and standing) are prerequisite to ambulation and general mobility training. Holding a position, assuming the position, and withstanding challenge in the position can improve strength, help to normalize tone, and facilitate independence in ADL tasks.

Proper wheelchair prescription will precede mobility training. Functional training should include propulsion, retropulsion, and maneuvering in narrow areas and on various terrains. Manipulation of arm rests, leg rests, foot rests, brakes, and other wheelchair parts must be included in the wheelchair mobility program. Use of power wheelchairs with adapted control devices may be required. In addition, use of three wheeled, scooter-type vehicles such as the Amigo* or Portascoot† may compensate for poor endurance or weakness for some clients with good sitting balance and some upper extremity control.

Functional improvement or maintenance of functional independence is the overall goal of the rehabilitation program. Carry-over of therapeutic exercise, mat exercises, and ambulation training to ADL tasks is vital. In addition,

*Amigo Sales, Inc, 6693 Dixie Highway, Bridgeport, MI 48722.
†EF Brewer Co, PO Box 159, Menomonee Falls, WI 53051.

specific training in techniques of dressing, bathing, toileting, personal hygiene, feeding, and bed mobility can improve or maintain independence in ADL. Adaptive equipment can be used to conserve energy and compensate for weakness and incoordination. For example, weighted silverware and plate guards can compensate for tremor and incoordination in self-feeding. Button hooks, reachers, stocking aids, and Velcro may improve independence in dressing. Transfer training should be incorporated into functional activities. The use of sliding board, hydraulic lift, or assistance from another individual must be geared to the client's ability and priorities regarding expenditure of energy.

Adapted tools for communication skills (i.e., writing or typing), such as built-up pencils, typing shield, or universal cuffs, may assist written communication. Severe dysarthria combined with mobility impairment may necessitate the use of electronic communication boards with scanners or mouth/head stick pointers, page turners, tape recorders, speaker phones, or other adapted telephones. Homemaking tasks and child care from a wheelchair level, ambulatory-assisted level, or ambulatory level can be practiced with the aid of assistive devices and energy conservation techniques. Several cookbooks and guides for the handicapped homemaker and parent have been included in the references for specific ideas in this area.[10,11]

Driving often presents multiple problems for the individual with MS. Diplopia or blurred vision, decreased coordination, weakness, and spasticity may interfere with safe driving or require the use of hand controls or adapted van. Perceptual and cognitive considerations must be made in a predriving evaluation or in driver training.

Persons with MS, whether they are experiencing mild or severe symptoms, may have job and career concerns. Individuals engaged in heavy physical labor may not be able to continue. Persons who are unable to stand for long periods or walk long distances and those who fatigue easily or have visual or coordination problems may need to make adjustments at the work site or build flexibility into their career plan. Although some persons with MS may be severely disabled, there are often significant areas of good functioning remaining as well as periods of disease stability. Attention to these in prevocational and vocational counseling is, of course, important. Psychological adjustment, as well as cognitive and perceptual status, will also influence career planning and vocational goal setting.

Cognitive, perceptual, and affective issues

Recent studies in the neuropsychology of MS suggest that 30% or more of diagnosed individuals experience cognitive impairment to some degree.[26,27] Short-term memory and conceptual reasoning (ability to solve complex and abstract problems that require planning, judgment, concentration, and organizational abilities) appear to be the most often affected functions. Also, while not entirely in agreement, some longitudinal studies of people with MS suggest slight deterioration of overall intelligence over time.[26,29]

Although the number of studies devoted to language function is limited, it is generally believed that language function is not commonly affected.

Several investigators have noted changes in affect as an accompaniment to cognitive decline in MS. Euphoria, apathy, lack of interest, and irritability are noted to occur in some individuals with widespread cerebral dysfunction.[26] Several studies have also shown a high rate of depression among those with MS and noted that reactive depression is not always sufficient to explain the high rate.[21] This is a complicated issue, as making a distinction between a reactive and endogenous depression may be difficult. Doing so, however, may have significant implications for treatment.

It is important to remember that people with MS do not make up a uniform group of individuals, nor is there an "MS personality." Also, the relationships among age, severity of disability, and duration of illness are not good predictors of cognitive or affective changes.

Given this information, many persons with MS would derive benefit from a neuropsychological evaluation. Such an evaluation could be helpful in several ways: the person with MS as well as family members can gain a better understanding of the nature and extent of the illness; the evaluation can identify impaired functions as well as intact functions; the evaluation may assist the person in developing realistic vocational and other life goals; the results can clarify misconceptions on the part of others who may incorrectly attribute cognitive problems to uncooperative or oppositional behavior; and, finally, the results can suggest compensatory techniques.

In regard to psychosocial functioning, many families cope well with MS and find that, along with the problems, MS has brought about useful changes. Yet it is important to recognize that the family feels the pain of this disease too. Family members may wonder how much to help the person with MS, they may feel burdened with his or her dependence, and they may be worried about the future, concerned about financial pressures, and exhausted by the care requirements of their family member. Sexual dysfunction, which is often not addressed by care givers, may also have a significant impact on family functioning. This aspect of daily living merits attention, counseling, and practical information, and these should be made available to families.

The meaning of illness or disability in a family relates to culture, religion, and personal values and beliefs. For some, illness means weakness, imperfection, asexuality, and a result of sin or wrongdoing. For others, illness may be seen as a learning opportunity or an enriching experience—a challenge to confront or a catalyst to making one more compassionate and aware of what is really important

in life. We are also influenced strongly by the viewpoints of our friends, family, medical care givers, and rehabilitation team members. Personal awareness of attitudes and beliefs about disability are important to examine because therapists sometimes communicate these beliefs in subtle ways to their clients.

Helping families cope with MS may also involve an examination of their premorbid patterns of dealing with stress, conflict, and tragedy. Often, MS magnifies preexisting problems and tensions so that families who present "MS-generated" problems may be found to have had these problems before the diagnosis.

The relationship among attitude, psyche, and physical wellness or disease is well documented.[3,23] Although stress cannot be implicated in causing exacerbations per se, the ability to manage stress can positively influence overall health and well-being. To treat the body without adequate consideration of the accompanying psychological and emotional issues would be a great injustice.

SUMMARY

MS is a chronic and usually progressive disease of the CNS, characterized by disseminated patches of demyelination in the brain and spinal cord, resulting in multiple and varied neurological symptoms and signs. Destruction of myelin, accompanied by edema and inflammation and followed by tissue scarring, appears to be the underlying cause that impedes or prevents neurotransmission.

The clinical diagnosis of MS is dependent on evidence of two or more distinct CNS lesions, of symptoms and signs that have appeared in distinct episodes or have progressed over time, and the exclusion of other neurological explanations. Laboratory and electrophysiological tests provide support of a clinical diagnosis; however, at the present time no test is pathognomonic for MS.

The course of the disease is characterized by an unpredictable series of exacerbations and remissions in some cases, progressive disability over time in other cases, or a combination of the two, often accompanied by periods of disease stability.

The etiology of MS appears to be an autoimmune process in which myelin is destroyed. The trigger of this abnormal immune response is unknown although a viral cause is under examination.

Treatment of MS is primarily symptomatic. Therapeutic trials of immunosuppressive, antiviral, and antiinflammatory agents remain inconclusive to date. Rehabilitative measures, including physical, occupational, and speech therapy, do not appear to alter the underlying pathology of the disease. Therefore the overriding principle in setting rehabilitation goals for a person with MS is to maximize functional independence, minimize complications and problems secondary to decreased mobility, and compensate for loss of function. Psychosocial adjustment, vocational disposition, and family issues merit significant attention by the treatment team, since MS generates tremendous need in these areas.

REFERENCES

1. Alter M and others: Migration and risk of multiple sclerosis, Neurology 28:1089, 1978.
2. Bauer H: A manual on multiple sclerosis, Vienna, 1977, International Federation of Multiple Sclerosis Societies.
3. Benson H: The mind/body effect, New York, 1979, Simon & Schuster.
4. Catanzaro M: Nursing care of the person with MS, Am J Nurs 80(2):286, 1980.
5. Dean G: The multiple sclerosis problem, Sci Am 223(1):40, 1970.
6. Dimitrijevic MR and Sherwood AM: Spasticity: medical and surgical treatment, Neurology 30(7, pt 2):19, 1980.
7. Eggert GM and others: Caring for the patient with long term disability, Geriatrics 32(10):102, 1977.
8. Ellison GW and Myers LW: Immunosuppressive drugs in multiple sclerosis: pro and con, Neurology 30(7, pt 2):28, 1980.
9. Frenkel HS: In Granger FB, editor: Physical therapeutic technique, Philadelphia, 1929, WB Saunders Co.
10. Gifford L: If you can't stand to cook, Grand Rapids, Mich, 1973, The Zondervan Corp.
11. Gilbert A: You can do it from a wheelchair, Westport, Conn, 1973, Arlington House Publishers.
12. Granger CV and others: Outcome of comprehensive rehabilitation: measurement by Pulses Profile and the Barthel Index, Arch Phys Rehabil 60:145, April 1979.
13. Hashimoto SA and Paty DW: Multiple sclerosis, Disease-A-Month 32(9):518, 1986.
14. Johnson KP: Cerebrospinal fluid and blood assays of diagnostic usefulness in multiple sclerosis, Neurology 30(2):107, 1980.
15. Kurland LT: The frequency and geographic distribution of multiple sclerosis as indicated by mortality statistics and morbility surveys in the U.S. and Canada, Am J Hyg 55:457, 1952.
16. Kurtzke JF: On the evaluation of disability in multiple sclerosis, Neurology 11(8):686, 1961.
17. Kurtzke JF and Hyllested K: Multiple sclerosis in the Faroe Islands. I. Clinical and epidemiological features, Ann Neurol 5:6, 1979.
18. Lisak RP: Multiple sclerosis: evidence for immunopathogenesis, Neurology 30(2):99, 1980.
19. Mahoney FI and Barthel DW: Functional evaluation: Barthel Index, Md State Med J 14:61, 1965.
20. McAlpine D and others: Multiple sclerosis: a reappraisal, Edinburgh, 1965, E & S Livingstone, Ltd.
21. Minden SL and others: Depression in multiple sclerosis, Gen Hosp Psychiatry 9:426, 1987.
22. Moskowitz E and McCann CB: Classification of disability in the chronically ill and aging, J Chronic Dis 5(3):342, 1957.
23. Pelettier K: Mind as healer, mind as slayer, New York, 1977, Dell Publishing Co.
24. Percy AK and others: MS in Rochester, Minn.: a 60-year appraisal, Arch Neurol 25:105, 1971.
25. Perry J and others: Rocker shoe as walking aid in multiple sclerosis, Arch Phys Med Rehab 62:59, 1981.
26. Rao SM: Neuropsychology of multiple sclerosis: a critical review, J Clin Exper Neuropsychol 8(5):503, 1986.
27. Schiffer RB and Slater RJ: Neuropsychiatric features of multiple sclerosis: recognition and management, Semin Neurol 5(2):127, 1985.
28. Slater RJ and others: Minimal record of disability for multiple sclerosis, New York, 1985, National Multiple Sclerosis Society.
29. Surridge D: Psychiatric aspects of multiple sclerosis, Br J Psych 115:524, July 1969.
30. Waksman BH and others: Research on multiple sclerosis, ed 3, New York, 1987, Demos Publications.
31. Williams A and others: An investigation of multiple sclerosis in twins, Neurology 30:1139, 1980.
32. Young IR and others: Nuclear magnetic resonance imaging of the brain in multiple sclerosis, Lancet 2:1063, 1981.

ADDITIONAL READINGS

Broman T: Management of patients with multiple sclerosis. In Vinken PT and Bruyn GW, editors: Handbook of clinical neurology, vol 9, New York, 1970, Elsevier North-Holland, Inc.

Brown JR: Therapeutic claims in multiple sclerosis, New York, 1982, International Federation of Multiple Sclerosis Societies.

Hartings MF and others: Group counseling of MS patients, J Chronic Dis 29:65, 1976.

Maloney FP and others: Interdisciplinary rehabilitation of multiple sclerosis and neuromuscular disorders, Philadelphia, 1985, JB Lippincott Co.

Marinelli RP and Demorto AE: The psychological and social impact of physical disability, New York, 1977, Springer Publishing Co, Inc.

McFarlin DE and McFarland HF: Multiple sclerosis. I. N Engl J Med 307(19):1183, 1982.

McFarlin DE and McFarland HF: Multiple sclerosis. II. N Engl J Med 307(20):1246, 1982.

Pavlou M, editor: Variety and possibility in multiple sclerosis, Chicago, 1979, Bio Service Corp.

Tourtellotte WW: Therapeutics of multiple sclerosis. In Klawans HL, editor: Clinical neuropharmacology, vol 2, New York, 1977, Raven Press.

Waksman BH: Current trends in multiple sclerosis research, Immunol Today 2:87, 1981.

Weinstein EA: Behavioral aspects of multiple sclerosis, Mod Treatment 7(5):961, 1970.

APPENDIX
Frenkel exercises

Frenkel exercises are begun from one of four positions: lying, sitting, standing, or walking. Concentration of attention on each movement is mandatory. Each movement is done slowly and with repetition. The exercises are as follows*:

1. Lying position: Flexion and extension of each leg at the knee and hip joints. Abduction and adduction with the knee bent; later, abduction and adduction with the knee extended
2. Flexion and extension of one knee at a time with the heel raised from the bed
3. Knee flexed and heel placed on some definite part of the other leg; for example, on the patella, the middle of the leg, ankle, and toes. These exercises may be adapted by changing the heel from one position to another or else by calling for extension between different placings (the neurological heel-to-knee test)
4. Knee flexed, heel placed on knee of other leg, heel of flexed leg gliding down the tibia to the ankle joint and back to knee
5. Flexion and extension of both legs, together with knees and ankles held close together

*When the performance of exercises *1* through *7* becomes easy, the client should repeat them with the eyes closed.

6. Flexion of one leg during extension of the other (reciprocal movement)
7. Flexion or extension of one leg during adduction and abduction of the other
8. From the sitting position the client tries to place a foot with precision in the hand of the therapist who constantly changes the position of the hand. Exercises may be performed by means of special apparatus, consisting of a board with holes in which to place the heels and a bar that may be placed across the bottom of the bed at different heights and varying distances. The client is encouraged to place the heels in the holes. The position of the board is changed after each attempt

9. Maintaining the fundamental sitting position for a few minutes at a time
10. Raising each knee alternately and placing the foot firmly on the ground on a traced footprint
11. Learning to rise from a chair and sit again with knees held together
12. Placing foot forward and backward on a straight line. These exercises should be followed by walking maneuvers (e.g., walking along a zigzag strip following markings)
13. Walking between two parallel lines
14. Walking, placing each foot on tracing on floor that should be marked in fairly close adduction position, straight line walking (not toe out)

Chapter 19

BASAL GANGLIA DISORDERS
Metabolic, hereditary and genetic disorders in adults

Marsha E. Melnick

This chapter considers the metabolic, hereditary, and genetic disorders that typically have their onset in adulthood, including Huntington's chorea, Wilson's disease, alcoholism, heavy metal poisoning, and drug intoxication. Because of the wide variety of diseases with a wide variety of causes, the concentration here is on understanding the clinical problems and commonalities that exist within this grouping. The predominant area of the brain affected by these disorders is the basal ganglia. For this reason Parkinson's disease, a degenerative disease of the basal ganglia, is also included. Therefore the first part of this chapter is devoted to the diseases of these structures, and the second part incorporates diseases of other areas of the brain. The reader should also review other chapters of the book that discuss in particular cerebellar dysfunction and hemiplegia.

THE BASAL GANGLIA

The most commonly seen disorders affecting the basal ganglia include Parkinson's disease, Huntington's chorea, Wilson's disease, and the drug-induced dyskinesias. All involve changes in muscle tone, a decrease in movement coordination, and the presence of extraneous movement. Taken together, these disorders affect approximately 450,000 people.[3]

To understand how one interrelated area of the brain can account for such a wide variety of symptoms, it is first necessary to understand the anatomy, physiology, and pharmacology of these structures.

Anatomy

The basal ganglia are comprised of three nuclei located at the base of the cerebral cortex—hence their name. These nuclei are the caudate nucleus, the putamen, and the globus pallidus. Two brainstem nuclei, the substantia nigra and the subthalamic nucleus, are included here as part of the basal ganglia because they have a close functional relationship to the forebrain nuclei. Some authors include the amygdala, the claustrum, and the red nucleus as part of the basal ganglia. Functionally, the amygdala and claustrum are not part of this system despite their anatomical location, and the red nucleus has not been shown to be anatomically connected with the other nuclei of the basal ganglia. Therefore these structures will not be included in this portion of the chapter. (The anatomical location of the various parts of the basal ganglia is shown in Fig. 19-1.)

The varying terminology associated with this brain region can be confusing. Based on their location and shape, the putamen and globus pallidus together have been referred to as the lentiform (lens-shaped) nucleus. However, embryologically, anatomically, and functionally the caudate nucleus and the putamen are similar, and many recent texts and articles refer to the caudate and putamen together as the neostriatum—a term derived from *striate* and used to denote pathways from and to the caudate and putamen. Further, the term *corpus striatum* refers to the caudate, putamen, and globus pallidus. The various connections and interconnections of this system will be discussed on the basis of these definitions.

The basal ganglia may contain two functional but interacting units. The dorsal portion of the system, or dorsal striatum, is the functional unit related to movement. The ventral portion, or ventral striatum, is related to motivation and therefore is closely related to the limbic system.[54] This chapter will concentrate on the dorsal striatum, but the reader should examine Chapter 4 for a full appreciation and understanding of the limbic system.

Afferent pathways. Functionally, the basal ganglia can be divided into an afferent portion and an efferent portion (Fig. 19-2). The afferent structures are the caudate and putamen. They receive input from the entire cerebral cortex, the intralaminar thalamic nuclei, and the centromedian-parafascicular complex of the thalamus, as well as from the substantia nigra and the dorsal raphe nucleus. The projections from the cortex are systematically arranged so that the frontal cortex projects to the head of the caudate and putamen and the visual cortex projects to the tail (Fig. 19-3). In addition, the prefrontal cortex projects mainly to the caudate, while the sensorimotor cortex projects mainly to the putamen.[78] Those projections from the cortical regions, which represent the proximal muscu-

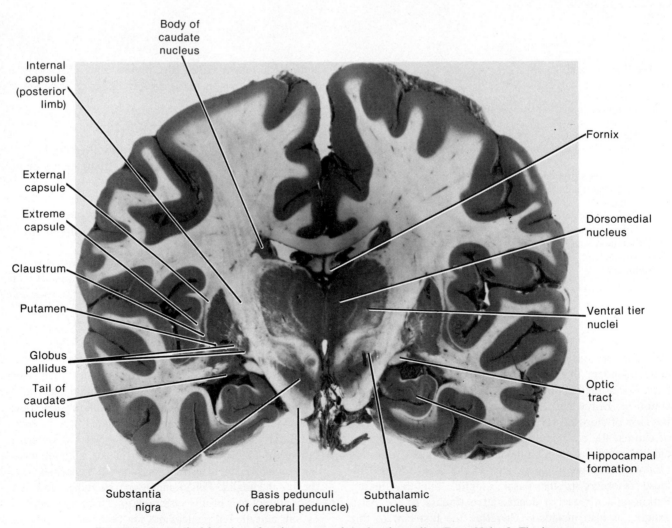

Fig. 19-1. Anatomical location of various parts of the basal ganglia. (From Nolte J: The human brain: an introduction to its functional anatomy, St Louis, 1981, The CV Mosby Co.)

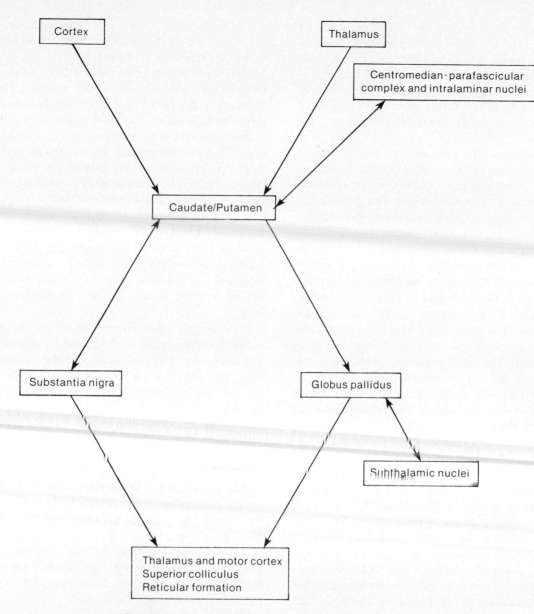

Fig. 19-2. Afferent and efferent portions of the basal ganglia.

lature, and those from the premotor regions may be bilateral.[64,77] Further, if two areas of the cortex are closely interconnected, their projections to the caudate-putamen will overlap.[150] These very close and very profuse connections between the cortex and the basal ganglia are suggestive of a close interfunctional relationship between the cortex and the neostriatum. The projections from the thalamus to the caudate-putamen are also somatotopically arranged. The heaviest projections are from the centromedian nucleus, which also receives massive input from the motor cortex.[64,78]

The internal (microscopic) structure of the caudate-putamen is such that the neurons are heavily interconnected; thus before a message is sent out of this afferent

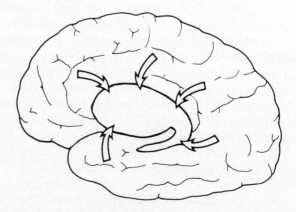

Fig. 19-3. Somatotopic projections from cortex to caudate nucleus.

portion a great deal of processing has already occurred. Of these neurons 95% are small with numerous dendritic spines.[64] At one time it was thought that all of these small neurons were intrinsic to the neostriatum. However, because anatomical techniques for visualizing neurons have improved, it is now believed that approximately 40% of caudate neurons do project to structures located outside the caudate.

Efferent pathways. The input that has been processed in the caudate-putamen is then sent to the globus pallidus (pallidum) and substantia nigra (nigra), which comprise the efferent portion of the basal ganglia. The globus pallidus and substantia nigra are each divided into two regions. The globus pallidus has an external and an internal region; the substantia nigra consists of the dorsal pars compacta and the ventral pars reticulata. Embryologically and microscopically the internal segment of the globus pallidus and the pars reticulata of the substantia nigra are very similar. These two regions are the primary efferent structures for the basal ganglia. The projections from the caudate and putamen to the pallidum and nigra maintain the somatotopic arrangement. The caudate projects primarily to the rostral and dorsal third of the pallidum and the anterior portion of the substantia nigra. The putamen projects to the caudal and ventral portions of the pallidum and the caudal nigra.[22,38] Recent evidence suggests that the projection from the caudate and putamen are separate in the pallidum and nigra.[64] From these structures the information is transmitted to the thalamus and then to the cortex. The pallidum projects to the lateral portions of the ventrolateral and ventroanterior nuclei of the thalamus. The nigra projects to the medial portions of these nuclei. The superior colliculus and other less defined brainstem structures (perhaps the reticular formation) also receive pallidal and nigral output. All output of the basal ganglia has then been processed through the globus pallidus and/or the substantia nigra before proceeding to other areas of the brain (see Fig. 19-2).

Pathways to the motor system. Information processed in the basal ganglia can influence the motor system in several ways, but no direct pathway to the alpha or gamma motor neurons exists. This first route is the projection to the ventroanterior and ventrolateral nuclei of the thalamus, which then projects to the motor and premotor cortex. Another pathway is through the superior colliculus and then to the tectospinal tract. There are also pathways from the globus pallidus and substantia nigra that terminate in areas of the reticular formation (e.g., the pedunculopontine nucleus) and then through the reticulospinal pathways. Anatomically therefore the basal ganglia are in good position to affect the motor system.

In addition to these external connections, there are several important internal basal ganglionic loops. The loop that receives the most attention, perhaps because of its involvement in Parkinson's disease, is the caudate-substantia nigra-caudate loop. The pars compacta of the nigra projects to the caudate nucleus, which then projects back to the pars reticulata of the nigra.

Additionally there is an internal loop between the globus pallidus and the subthalamic nucleus. The external segment of the pallidum projects somatotopically to the subthalamic nucleus. The subthalamus then projects back to both segments of the pallidum and also to the substantia nigra.[107] Ballismus results when a lesion occurs in this loop. It is believed that this loop acts to affect the gain of the system, that is, it can amplify a small signal or diminish a large signal. The subthalamic nuclei receive information from the premotor and motor cortex as well as from the pallidum.[51] Another important loop exists between the basal ganglia and the thalamus (see Fig. 19-2). The reciprocal interaction between these two structures may adjust the activity of the basal ganglia to ensure smooth, sequential movements; it also provides an important feedback loop.

In summary, input from the motor cortex, all other areas of the cortex, parts of the thalamus, and the substantia nigra enter the basal ganglia through the caudate and putamen. Here they are processed and sent on to the globus pallidus and substantia nigra. The appropriate "gain" of the system is adjusted, and the information is sent to the muscles by way of the thalamus and motor cortex, the superior colliculus, or the reticular formation.

Physiology

The understanding of the physiology of the interactions among areas of the basal ganglia has greatly increased in the last decade. Initially the prevalent view was that the basal ganglia exerted an inhibitory influence on the motor system. An early study by Mettler and others[104] demonstrated an inhibition of cortically evoked movements following caudate stimulation. More recent studies show both excitatory and inhibitory influences.

The caudate and putamen are composed of neurons that fire very slowly, whereas the neurons in the globus pallidus fire tonically at fairly high rates. (The spontaneous activity of the caudate and putamen is therefore low while that of the globus pallidus is high.) The low firing rates of neostriatal neurons are partially a result of the nature of thalamic synaptic inputs.[19]

Stimulation of the cortex, thalamus, and substantia nigra almost always produces excitatory postsynaptic potentials (EPSP) followed by longer inhibitory postsynaptic potentials (IPSP)—EPSP-IPSP sequence. Further, input from the cortex seems to have priority over input from the thalamus and substantia nigra.[61] The data provide evidence that the cortex is instrumental in regulating the responsiveness of caudate neurons.[19]

The concept that the neostriatum is not totally inhibitory also receives support from intracellular studies. Stimulation of caudate neurons evokes a mixture of excitatory and inhibitory responses in the globus pallidus.[82] Further, cortical recruiting responses have been demonstrated following caudate, putamen, and pallidal stimulation.[17,18,29] especially over the area of the motor cortex. This led Dieckmann and Sasaki[29] to conclude that the neostriatum and pallidum have an important functional role in controlling the activity level of the cerebral cortex. The cortical response from caudate stimulation is a long-term hyperpolarization. Hull and co-workers[59] hypothesized that this hyperpolarization served to "enhance the magnitude of subsequent excitatory inputs" (p. 97), that is, the caudate would affect the bias of cortical neurons. They also suggested that a long-lasting hyperpolarization might be a useful model for the "timing and sequencing of behavioral responses in the presence of relatively constant stimulus inputs as for example, in a delayed response situation" (p. 175).[60]

Thus the behavior of basal ganglia neurons and the synaptic interactions provide some hints regarding the function of the basal ganglia. The afferent portion, the neostriatum, receives excitatory information from other brain structures. It then processes this information and produces a modulated output that is a mixture of excitation and inhibition to the efferent portion, the pallidum and nigra. The efferent portion can then amplify the message it receives: "small changes in slowly firing neostriatal neurons are translated into much larger changes in faster firing pallidal cells" (p. 171).[19]

Relationship of the basal ganglia to movement and posture

Functionally, what might be happening in these anatomical and physiological connections? Researchers and clinicians have been attempting to answer this question for several centuries. Lesion experiments, single unit recording in awake, behaving animals, and careful observations of the sequelae of human disease processes have provided some answers.

Automatic movement. Based on the anatomical knowledge of his time, Willis in 1664 wrote that "the corpus striatum represents an exchange between brain stem and cortex" (p. 7).[146] He therefore suggested that this structure "receives the notion of spontaneous localized movements in ascending tracts. . . . Conversely, from here tendencies are dispatched to enact notions without reflection [automatic movements] over descending pathways" (p. 7).[146] Magendie in 1841 demonstrated that removal of the striatum bilaterally produced compulsive movements. He described the response of acaudate rabbits as follows: "The animal runs forward as if under an irresistible impulse. . . . One may say that the animal believes it is hunted and hears the barking of the dogs running in its footsteps" (p. 8).[94] Removal of only one striatum produced no visible effect. Studies by Nothnagel[110] demonstrated that destruction of the globus pallidus produced a

twisting of the spine with the convexity toward the side of the lesion. Lesions of the nigra tended to produce immobility. With the advent of the use of electrical stimulation in the late nineteenth century, further information on the function of the basal ganglia was gathered. Stimulation of the caudate nucleus did not (and does not) produce movement of muscles or limbs as did stimulation of the motor cortex. However, total body patterns and postures were usually evoked.

Ferrier[40] was the first to describe the results of stimulation of the caudate nucleus. He noted that there was an increase of flexion of the head and trunk, that the limbs remained in a flexed position, and that the facial muscles also went into tonic contraction. Ferrier concluded that "in the corpus striatum there would thus appear to be an integration of the various centers which are differentiated in the cortex."[40] From these early experiments came the idea that the basal ganglia are involved not only in sensorimotor integration but in initiation of movements and postural and movement programming. (Recent experimental evidence continues to support the concept that the basal ganglia are involved in the preparatory stages but not in the excitation of movement.)

Motor problems in animals. Contemporary experiments concerning lesions show a wide variety of motor problems in a variety of animals. Hypokinesia following the occurrence of lesions in the basal ganglia is one frequent result. Stern[132] observed that bilateral lesions of the substantia nigra produced poverty of movement and a tendency to assume fixed postures. Monkeys with large lesions in the basal ganglia have been shown to assume a "somersault" position; that is, the animal is flexed so that the head rests on the floor while the animal is standing.[32] Cooling of the putamen and the pallidum in the monkey has been shown to produce a slowing of movements as well as the tendency toward flexed postures.[52] In one experiment electromyogram (EMG) recordings of the biceps and triceps of monkeys demonstrated an increase in cocontraction of these muscles.[56] Although movement is still possible, it must be made with an abnormal starting position and a delay in appropriate activation of the prime movers.

Movement initiation and preparation. The hypothesis that the basal ganglia are involved in movement initiation and preparation also receives support from human experiments. Kornhuber[73] observed, while recording from the scalp in humans, a slow negative potential bilaterally just before movement. This "Bereitschafts-potential" or "readiness potential" was not present in individuals with Parkinson's disease. Kornhuber hypothesized that the generator for this readiness potential was not in the motor cortex but rather in subcortical structures and, further, that there were two types of movement generators: one for ramp function, or "voluntary speed smooth movement," and another for ballistic, or fast, movement. Ramp movements require integration among the parts of the body for control of constant speed and fluidity of movement. Based on his observations that the signs of lesions in the basal ganglia produced a deficiency in the voluntary production of smooth movements and that lesions of the motor cortex did not, Kornhuber concluded that the generator for ramp movements in the extremities, trunk, and head was the basal ganglia.

A more precise investigation into how movements were programmed and initiated used the technique of single unit recording in awake, performing animals: Evarts[39] in the motor cortex, Delong[30] in the basal ganglia, Thach[137,138] in the cerebellum, and Massion and Smith[98] and Strick[133] in the ventroanterior-ventrolateral nuclei of the thalamus. All these researchers found that units in these areas alter their activity before changes in the EMG activity of the muscles performing the task; that is, before arrival of sensory feedback information from the muscles, joints, and skin could modify the centrally generated movement program. These changes in neuronal activity occurred 50 to 200 msec before the EMG activity changes, and there was enough overlap of the onset of these changes so that no clear answer established which of these areas gave the command to move. However, these results do indicate that all of these brain sites are involved in movement generation. Delong's experiments showed that some units in the basal ganglia changed their activity preferentially with performance of slow (ramp) movements and that units in the cortex, cerebellum, and some pallidal units showed activity changes in both ramp and ballistic movements,[30] in partial agreement with Kornhuber's hypothesis. Experiments using cooling procedures demonstrated that cooling the ventrolateral nucleus,[11] the cerebellum, or basal ganglia[16,57] produced a delay in the onset of the movement but also a slowing in the velocity of the movement itself, again indicating that these structures are involved in the initiation phase of the movement.

Neafsey and others[108,109] and Melnick and co-workers[102] presented further evidence for the involvement of the globus pallidus, ventroanterior-ventrolateral nuclei, and motor cortex in the preparation of movement. Of the units recorded in the globus pallidus, ventroanterior-ventrolateral nuclei, and medial precruciate cortex of the cat, 30% to 70% changed their firing pattern more than 250 msec before changes in EMG activity. Neafsey hypothesized that these early unit activity changes were the "neural correlate of the state of set" (p. 712), or readiness that exists as a preparatory adjustment for performing a task, as proposed by Woodworth and Schlosberg.[149] Buchwald and others[18] have defined this preparatory activity as "response set," which entails "the ability to initiate and carry out smoothly and in proper sequence a set of movements that comprise a defined response" (p. 175).[19] Denny-Brown,[32] in studying the effects of lesions of the basal ganglia on movement, has also suggested that the basal ganglia participate in the "activating set." He defined this "set" as the "preparation of the mechanism preparatory to a motor performance oriented to the environment."[33] The difficulty in parkinsonism of initiating movements or in changing from one movement to another is an example of a disruption in this "response set" process.

Postural adjustments. The involvement of the basal ganglia in the initiation of movement may include a role in directing the postural adjustments necessary before distal movement can take place. In fact, in addition to the assumption of flexed, fixed postures, other postural abnormalities have been observed following lesions of the basal ganglia. In an experiment by Winkelmuller and Nitsch,[148] rats with bilateral lesions of the substantia nigra were unable to balance skillfully or correct imbalance by quick movements or by shifting their weight. Cats with lesions of one caudate nucleus who had been trained to alternate bar presses have been shown to have similar deficits in postural adjustments. The normal animal keeps the body in a central position and moves only its paws in these alternating movements. The animals with lesions had to move the entire body back and forth between the bars in order to perform the task.[115] Similar postural deficiencies have been observed in monkeys with lesions of various parts of the basal ganglia. These deficiencies led Denny-Brown and Yanagesawa to conclude that the basal ganglia "must be concerned in the elaboration of specialized motor reactions to the environment by modification of the labyrinthine and body-contact righting reactions."[33] Similarly, Potegal[121] observed that animals with lesions in the anterior caudate were unable to guide their behavior by taking their own body position into account. He referred to this deficit as a breakdown in "egocentric localization." Similarly studies of human disease processes support the hypothesis that the basal ganglia have a role in the postural mechanisms active before movement. Martin,[97] in his extensive studies of individuals with Parkinson's disease, found that these patients, in addition to their akinesia, demonstrated severe disturbances in posture. He noted that especially when vision was occluded these persons were unable to make the normal postural shifts involved in equilibrium reactions.

Despite the preceding discussion regarding the role of the basal ganglia in postural mechanisms, the data are inconclusive. The early unit activity changes seen in the basal ganglia are not related in a simple fashion to early EMG activity in the proximal and axial muscles. Neither Melnick and others[102] nor Neafsey and co-workers[108,109] found early EMG changes in the proximal muscles that correlated with changes in basal ganglia neuronal activity changes. It is possible that the basal ganglia are involved in biasing and setting the gamma motorneuron system in preparation for extrafusal muscle contraction. The lack of early EMG activity is not inconsistent with a theory of biasing spinal reflex mechanisms to enhance or inhibit the eventual firing of alpha motor neurons of specific muscles.[45] Perhaps the central nervous system (CNS) prepares the muscles for a certain amount of postural tone; if this tone is already present, then no activity changes occur in the muscles. Changes in neuronal activity in preparation for movement would therefore occur with no corresponding change in the EMG activity. Kubota and Hamada[75] reported gradual changes in pyramidal tract neuronal activity up to 1 second before movement without any visible changes in the posture of the monkey or any changes in EMG activity. They interpreted their finding as also indicating a preparatory state for voluntary movement. This early neuronal activity might also be preparing neurons in the reticulospinal, tectospinal, and corticospinal pathways so that when movement is required, the alpha motor neuron will be more ready or less ready to fire and therefore the movement will occur with the appropriate speed and coordination. This would be similar to the theory of long-term biasing of the cortex discussed earlier. Stimulation of the caudate nucleus or globus pallidus can modify alpha and gamma motor responses evoked by motor cortex or pyramidal tract stimulation.[47,110] Delong and Strick[31] interpreted the changes in basal ganglionic activity preceding movement to be a facilitory discharge to "establish the climate for the performance rather than the detailed pattern of the movement" (p. 334).

Perceptual and cognitive functions. The basal ganglia's function is not solely in the initiation and control of movement and posture. There is also evidence to show that they are involved in perceptual and cognitive functions. Following lesions of the basal ganglia, deficits appear in the performance of a variety of alternation tasks in rodents, carnivores, primates, and humans (see Teuber[136] for a review). One reason for these deficits is the animal's tendency toward perseveration of a previously reinforced cue. In learning a delayed spatial alternation task, the animal must learn the temporal sequence (i.e., the alternation of position) and must be able to remember the location and consequences of its last response.[90] Stimulation of the caudate nucleus immediately following movement to the goal prevents the acquisition of this task and also disrupts performance of the task once it is learned, but it does not affect motor ability. Livesey and Rankine-Wilson[90] therefore concluded that interference in caudate functioning at this time selectively disrupted the registration of information generated internally. Frontal cortical lesions also produce deficits in delayed spatial response tasks, but the cortex and the neostriatum appear to mediate separate aspects of delayed response behavior.[34,90,141]

Further support for differences between the cortex and caudate in these tasks comes from experiments involving lesions of these areas in neonatal primates and cats. Kling and Tucker[70] found that early combined lesions of the frontal cortex and caudate nucleus had "devastating" effects on early survival, on somatomotor function, and on

the ability to perform delayed-response tasks. Lesions of the frontal cortex alone, occurring at the same period in development, did not show these effects.[140] Kling and Tucker concluded that subcortical structures were more important in control of movement in the neonate and also for the retention of certain cognitive functions if the animal had sustained early brain injury. Goldman[46] obtained similar results in early lesions of the cortex or caudate nucleus. She suggested that the caudate nucleus might be responsible for mediating delayed-response performance in both normal monkeys and those with cortical lesions at early ages. She also hypothesized that the caudate "does not take over functions of the dorsolateral cortex in a compensatory sense, by assuming functions it would not normally have, but is simply the structure primarily responsible for mediating spatial-mnemonic abilities in monkeys under 2 years of age" (p. 409). Olmstead and Villablanca,[115] however, found that cats with lesions of the caudate nucleus made early in life were not as impaired on tasks such as alternating bar pressing and reversal of a spatial discrimination task as cats who sustained this lesion later in life. The kittens used in the experiment showed fewer perseveration tendencies than the adult animals. Deficits have been found in tasks other than delayed-response tasks in animals with basal ganglia lesions. Animals show difficulties in performance of *go-no go* tasks because of a difficulty in suppressing a response to the *no-go* cue.[10]

Humans with basal ganglia disease also show problems in perceptual abilities. Bowen[15] found that these individuals exhibited deficits in a variety of tasks involving perception of interpersonal and intrapersonal space. In pursuit-tracking tests individuals with Parkinson's disease had particular difficulties in correcting errors, which is consistent with Teuber's view that "the basal ganglia may play a role in the regulation of 'corollary' discharges, that is, in presetting of the motor system by sensory stimuli" (p. 164).[136] If the motor system is infexibly set, corrections can be made only by a complete reprogramming. Further, Bowen noted differential responses when individuals with Parkinson's disease were categorized according to the side of their major neurological symptoms. She suggested that hemispheric specialization in humans may be affected by basal ganglia lesions.[15] It is interesting to note that children with learning disabilities frequently display deficits in the postural mechanisms thought to be mediated by the basal ganglia.[3]

Further evidence that the basal ganglia participate in the performance of delayed-response tasks is found in the results of single unit recording studies. Units in the frontal cortex change their activity during the delay period in these types of tasks.[42,76] Soltysik and others[131] found neuronal activity changes related to at least one epoch of the delayed-response paradigm in 60% of the units recorded from the globus pallidus, putamen, and caudate. In particular, they found a high percentage of these units responded during the delay period, which would be expected if these structures play a role in the regulation of this task. They stated: "If we consider the delay period to represent a maintaining of a response set, and the pre-response epoch to be a preparatory period enabling the specific response, then neurons of both the pallidum and caudate appear to be associated in significant numbers with this behavior" (p. 75).[131]

Based on the literature indicating involvement of the basal ganglia in these complex behaviors, Buchwald and others[19] have hypothesized that the basal ganglia are involved in "cognitive set" as well as "response set." They defined "cognitive set" as "the ability to discriminate a situational context and make an appropriate response to a given signal" (p. 175). The term *cognitive* was used for "situations where information has to be transferred across some period of time before a response is initiated" (p. 177). They further suggested that the basal ganglia were more involved in complex tasks than in simpler behaviors. Animal experiments seem to indicate that complex learned responses are the ones most affected by basal ganglia lesions.[31,97]

The ability to perform cognitive activities involves integrating sensory information and, based on this information, making an appropriate response. The basal ganglia seem to have a sensory integrative function as evidenced by experiments that show a multisensory and heterotopic convergence of somatic, visual, auditory, and vestibular stimuli.[74,99,106,125] Segundo and Machne[125] observed unitary discharges of the basal ganglia to both somatic and vestibular stimuli. They hypothesized that the function of the basal ganglia was not in a subjective recognition of the stimuli but rather in the regulation of posture and movements of the body in space and in the production of complex motor acts (see Potegal[122] for a similar hypothesis).

For movements to be properly controlled and properly sequenced, the two sides of the body need to be well integrated. Some anatomical evidence exists that suggests some means of bilateral control for the basal ganglia. A lesion of one caudate nucleus or nigrostriatal pathway produces a change in the unit activity of the remaining caudate.[82,84] Studies of the dopaminergic pathway also indicate interactions between the two sides of the body.[88] For this reason one may find deficits in function even on the "uninvolved" side of an individual with disease of the basal ganglia. It is also possible that diseases of the basal ganglia may go unnoticed until damage is found bilaterally.

It is hoped that this summary of experimental results on the function of the basal ganglia illustrates several points. Despite many years of research an exact and precise role for these structures remains to be discovered. However, it does appear that at least in some general way the basal ganglia are involved in the processes of movement related to preparing the organism for future motion. This may in-

clude preparing the cortex for approximate time activation, "setting" the postural reflexes or the gamma motor neuron system, and perhaps organizing sensory input to produce a motor response in an appropriate environmental context. The various parts of the basal ganglia may subserve different aspects of movement, which might account for the differences between an individual with Parkinson's disease and one with Huntington's disease. In a clinical assessment one must carefully examine the loss of automatic postural adaptations appropriate for the task at hand. One, hopefully, approaches the day when it will no longer be necessary to say, "The exact nature and function of the large mass of basal grey matter known as the corpus striatum have hitherto constituted, it is no exaggeration to say, one of the unsolved problems of neurology" (p. 428).[147] The therapist's job will certainly be easier. Until then it is crucial that clinicians carefully observe all aspects of movement and postural tone during treatment. For additional information refer to the chapter on motor control.

Neurotransmitters

Before a detailed analysis of the diseases of the basal ganglia can be considered, a brief description of the neurotransmitters of this region is necessary. The primary diseases discussed in this chapter indicate a deficit in specific neurotransmitters. The pharmacological treatment of Parkinson's disease and, in the future, perhaps of Huntington's disease is based on these neurochemical deficits. The basal ganglia possess high concentrations of many of the suspected neurotransmitters: dopamine (DA), acetylcholine (ACh), gamma-aminobutyric acid (GABA), substance P, and the enkephalins and endorphins. This discussion, however, includes only the first three neurotransmitters.

DA is the major neurotransmitter of the nigrostriatal pathway. It is produced in the pars compacta of the substantia nigra. The axon terminals of these dopaminergic neurons are located in the caudate nucleus. For years a battle raged as to whether DA was excitatory or inhibitory. At present there is evidence that DA is both excitatory and inhibitory.[22] It is also hypothesized that DA has a modulatory influence on the caudate neurons.[22] In essence this means that DA in the caudate nucleus may not satisfy all the criteria of a neurotransmitter but will make a cell more excitatory or less excitatory to other input. It has also been speculated that DA may play a role in maintaining metabolic competency of the caudate neurons it innervates.[44]

It is also known that there are at least two types of DA receptors, D_1 and D_2. Many new drugs will influence only one of these receptors. Recent experiments have been trying to determine which behaviors are mediated by which DA receptor in the hope that this research may lead to more effective drug treatment with fewer side effects. All dopamine receptor agonists useful in treating Parkinson's disease are D_2 receptor agonists. The exact role of D_1 receptors is still under investigation.

Because various drugs and chemicals can act as agonists (similar to) and antagonists (block the action of) of DA, they are used in treating disease involving the basal ganglia. Agonists include amantadine, apomorphine, and a class of drugs called the ergot alkaloids (e.g., bromocriptine). Amphetamine, which prevents the reuptake of DA, can enhance the effect of any DA present in the system. Antagonists include haloperidol and other antipsychotic drugs of the phenothiazine class. With time these drugs may deplete the basal ganglia of DA and thus cause Parkinson's disease or tardive dyskinesia. The DA agonists and antagonists will be discussed further in the treatment of Parkinson's disease and the occurrence of drug-induced dyskinesia.

ACh is believed to be the neurotransmitter of the small interneurons of the caudate and putamen. It is presumed to inhibit the action of DA in this region and classically must be "in balance" with DA (and GABA). Dopaminergic axon terminals are found on cholinergic neurons. Substances that increase dopaminergic activity decrease release of ACh and vice versa.[111] The antagonists of ACh, such as belladonna alkaloids and atropine-like drugs, were one of the first class of drugs used in the treatment of Parkinson's disease.

GABA is an inhibitory neurotransmitter that is found throughout the brain. In the basal ganglia it is synthesized in the caudate nucleus and transmitted to the globus pallidus and substantia nigra.[122] GABA in the basal ganglia may permit movement to occur by allowing a distribution of neuronal firing. It also may provide a means of feedback inhibition in the efferent parts of the basal ganglia so that the program of activity is not repeated unless needed (see reference 123 for a summation of the role of GABA). Individuals with Huntington's disease have a deficiency of this chemical. Although agonists of GABA exist (e.g., muscimol and imidazole-acetic acid), a successful drug for the treatment of Huntington's disease has not yet been found. This may be a result of either the ubiquitous nature of GABA or the very complex circuitry and interrelationships that exist among GABA, ACh, and DA.

In addition to the transmitters discussed, there may be cotransmitters in the basal ganglia. Two such cotransmitters are cholecystokinin and neurotensin. The interactions of these cotransmitters may alter the sensitivity of DA receptors. Fuxe and others[43] suggest that the interactions of cotransmitters may alter the "set point" of transmission in synapses. They may therefore be important in one of the side effects of DA therapy, supersensitivity.

SPECIFIC CLINICAL PROBLEMS ARISING FROM BASAL GANGLIA DYSFUNCTION
Parkinson's disease

Parkinson's disease is so named because it was first described by Parkinson in 1868. It is a disease characterized by rigidity, bradykinesia (slow movement), micrography,

masked facies, postural abnormalities, and a resting tremor. As might be suspected from the review of functional physiology of the basal ganglia, the postural abnormalities include an assumption of a flexed posture, a lack of equilibrium reactions, especially of the labyrinthine equilibrium reactions, and a decrease in trunk rotation.

The pathology of Parkinson's disease consists of a decrease in the DA stores of the substantia nigra with a consequent depigmentation of this structure and the presence of Lewy bodies (intracellular inclusions). It is DA that gives the substantia nigra its coloration (and hence its name); therefore the lighter the nigra the greater the DA loss. It has been proposed that Parkinson's disease is an abnormal acceleration of the aging process.[100] DA shows an increase in concentration very early in life, followed by a rapid decrease from 5 to 20 years of age and a slow continuous loss between ages 20 to 80. Carlsson proposed that while a loss of or damage to the DA neurons early in life (because of, for example, infection or toxicity) may be insufficient to precipitate Parkinson's disease, the additional loss of neurons with the natural physiological aging process may add cumulatively to that early loss and the signs of Parkinson's disease are seen when some critical level is reached.[22] Indeed the average age of onset for Parkinson's disease is 35 to 60 years. The disease is equally distributed between men and women.

The etiology of most cases of Parkinson's disease is idiopathic (i.e., no cause can be found). A slow viral process or long term effects of early infection have been implicated. There was a large increase in the number of individuals with Parkinson's disease following the worldwide epidemic of influenza in 1917 to 1926. Other possible causes of Parkinson's disease include arteriosclerosis, intoxication, tumor, metabolic deficits, environmental toxins, and drug intoxication. An inherited disorder may be responsible for a very rare form of the disease with an early onset (below age 30).

What are the mechanisms by which a decrease in DA and a loss of dopaminergic cells lead to the development of the clinical signs and symptoms of Parkinson's disease? As explained earlier in the chapter, the exact role of the basal ganglia in movement is still under investigation. This is even more true of the nigrostriatal dopamine pathway. The nigra fires at a slow, fairly regular rhythm without varying its unit activity even with movement. Without this low, steady firing, however, the caudate loses some of its source of excitation, the disinhibition that enables movement to occur. There are several theories as to what may be happening "downstream" in the motor system following a loss of the dopaminergic nigral cells. A discussion of each symptom follows.
Symptoms
Bradykinesia and akinesia. Bradykinesia (a decrease in motion) and akinesia (a lack of motion) are characterized by an inability to initiate and perform purposeful

movements. They are also associated with a tendency to assume and maintain fixed postures. All aspects of movement are affected, including initiation, alteration in direction, and the ability to stop a movement once it is begun. Spontaneous or associated movements, such as swinging of the arms in gait or smiling at a funny story, are also affected. The decreased nigral activity transmitted through the basal ganglia pathways could lead to an imbalance in the information transmitted to the motor and premotor cortices.[117] The resting level of activity in these areas of the cortex may be decreased so that a greater amount of excitatory input from other areas of the brain would be necessary before movement patterns could be activated. In the individual with Parkinson's disease, an increase in cortically initiated movement even for such "subcortical" activities as walking supports this hypothesis. These automatic activities are now cortically controlled, and each individual aspect seems to be separately programmed. Associated movements in the trunk and other extremities are not automatic activity. This means that great energy must be expended whenever movement is begun.

It is important to remember that bradykinesia is *not* caused by rigidity or an inability to relax. This was demonstrated in an EMG analysis of voluntary movements of persons with Parkinson's disease.[49] On both fast and slow flexion of the elbow, EMG activity was abnormal, but the duration of the EMG bursts in agonistic and antagonistic muscles was normal. Even in slow, smooth movements, however, these individuals demonstrated alternating bursts in the flexor and extensor muscle groups. This type of pattern is expected in rapid movements that require the immediate activation of the antagonist to halt the motion, but it would interfere with slow, smooth, continuous motion. Other experimenters[48,105] found an alteration in the recruitment order of single motor units. Milner-Brown and others[105] hypothesized that recruitment of the first motor units participating in the initiation of movement involved a pathway from the substantia nigra to the caudate, then through loops to the thalamus and motor cortex, and on down by way of the pyramidal system. Once initiated, smooth movement can continue only with a continuous firing of agonist motor units, along with recruitment of more motor units or the ability to increase firing rates. In individuals with Parkinson's disease, there was a delay in recruitment, pauses in the motor unit once it was recruited, and inability to increase firing rates. These persons therefore would have a delay in activation of muscles and an inability to properly sustain muscle contraction for movement.

Rigidity. The rigidity of Parkinson's disease may be characterized as either "lead pipe" or "cogwheel." The cogwheel type of rigidity is a combination of lead-pipe rigidity with tremor. In rigidity there is an increased resistance to movement throughout the entire range in both directions without the classic clasp-knife reflex so characteristic of spasticity. Rigidity does involve a hyperactivity of the tonic stretch reflex.[111] And again it must be reemphasized that rigidity is a symptom separate from bradykinesia. Procaine injections can decrease the rigidity without affecting the decrease of spontaneous movements.[120,144]

It was originally believed that rigidity resulted from an increase in alpha motor neuron activity. Gamma motor neuron activity also seems to be implicated. Yet neither altered gamma nor alpha activity can account for both the tone alterations and the seemingly selective disruption of reflex activity. The tendon jerk, for example, is usually a normal occurrence with Parkinson's disease whereas slow-stretch responses are hyperactive. In other words, although the phasic, monosynaptic stretch reflex is normal, static stretch reflexes are impaired. One proposed mechanism to account for these phenomena is that there is an alteration in the convergent synaptic input to the interneurons of the spinal cord. An increase in alpha motor neuron input could then be limited to the activation of selected reflex pathways without a generalized increase in alpha motor neuron activity.[135] Tatton[135] found differences in certain cortical long-loop reflexes in normal and drug-induced parkinsonian monkeys, which led him to speculate that the "reflex gain" of the CNS may lose its ability to adjust to changing environmental situations. That is, in normal persons the descending input that would establish the appropriate level of excitability of the alpha and gamma motor neurons for writing is different from that necessary to lift a heavy object; in individuals with Parkinson's disease it would be at the same level. (The descending input for excitability of the motor neurons to the commands "push" or "pull" would also be the same in the parkinsonian person.) In other words, for the normal person the command to "push" in response to an external perturbation would increase the excitability of the triceps motor neuronal pool; the command to "pull" would decrease triceps excitability. In the individual with Parkinson's disease, the excitability of the triceps motor neuronal pool would be the same to both commands, and therefore the response to either would be delayed. It is possible that the basal ganglia help to modulate the gain of proprioceptive feedback occurring through the motor cortex. Disease in these structures might then limit the range of this modulation so that all inputs are treated the same and the whole system is adjusted at a higher level of activity.

Another—though perhaps not competing—theory is that reciprocal Ia (muscle spindle afferent) inhibition is increased in the parkinsonian person. Studies of this phenomenon have used the H reflex. A study by Bathien and Rondot[9] demonstrated an increase in H-reflex amplitude of individuals with Parkinson's disease following lidocaine block to the peroneal nerve. This led the researchers to conclude that reciprocal Ia inhibition of ankle dorsiflexors on plantar flexors was strong and continuous in the parkinsonian person at rest; that is, the lidocaine block removed a continuous source of inhibition from the anterior tibial muscle via the Ia inhibitory pathway. Reciprocal Ia inhibition of the dorsiflexors onto the plantar flexors is not present at rest in the normal person. These findings, however, could be compatible with the viewpoint that the descending input which "biases" the alpha and gamma motor neurons is always at a constant level. It is interesting that a preliminary study by Ahrens[1] did demonstrate Ia inhibition in elderly as well as parkinsonian persons at rest.

Tremor. The tremor observed in Parkinson's disease is present at rest, it usually disappears or decreases with movement, and it has a regular rhythm of about 4 to 7 beats per second. The EMG tracing of a person with such a tremor shows rhythmic, alternating bursting of antagonistic muscles. Tremor can be produced as an isolated finding in experimental animals that have lesions in various parts of the brainstem or that have been treated with drugs, especially DA antagonists. DA depletion, however, is not the sole cause of tremor. It appears that efferent pathways, especially from the basal ganglia to the thalamus, must be intact because lesions of these fibers decrease or abolish the tremor.[119] Poirier[119] proposed that tremor results from a combined lesion of the basal ganglia and cerebellar-red nucleus pathways. Because both the basal ganglia and the cerebellum project to the thalamus, a lesion of the thalamus can abolish the tremor regardless of the specific pathway(s).

Postural alterations. The pathophysiology of the postural alterations is far more difficult to pinpoint. One hypothesis is that these are simply manifestations of bradykinesia. Another is that perhaps there is an alteration in the processing of sensory stimuli, especially of the vestibular and proprioceptive systems. In fact, parkinsonian individuals do have difficulty in assessing the feeling of "upright." They cannot pick out a vertical line when their own body is not vertical, they cannot tell when they are aligned vertically with their eyes closed, and they have diminished or absent equilibrium responses with the eyes closed.[15,97] To date, however, results of tests specifically assessing either proprioception or vestibular function have been normal in these persons.[96] One should bear in mind that the means of assessing proprioception can test only peripheral function, for example, the shoulder, hip, elbow, or knee. There is no test for lack of trunkal proprioception.[95]

More recent clinical evaluations indicate that postural instability is a separate symptom of Parkinson's disease that is distinct from *bradykinesia or rigidity.* Drug treatment using L-dopa may reduce the number of falls in some individuals as rigidity decreases; in other patients, falling continues. In the first group, the lack of or the delay in equilibrium reactions may be the result of an inability to initiate the appropriate postural response and not a defect in proprioception per se. In the other group, further investigation is needed to determine the function of the basal ganglia in postural reactions.

Gait. Another characteristic of Parkinson's disease is the presence of a festinating gait. This is a gait characterized by a progressive increase in speed and shortening of stride as if the individual is trying to catch up with his or her center of gravity. Forward festination is called propulsion; backward festination is known as retropulsion. The festinating gait may be caused by the decreased equilibrium responses. If walking is a series of controlled falls and if normal responses to falling are delayed or not strong enough, then the individual will either fall completely or continue to take short, runninglike steps. The abnormal motor unit firing seen with bradykinesia may also be the cause of ever-shortening steps. If the motor unit cannot build up a high enough frequency or if it pauses in the middle of the movement, then the full range of the movement would decrease; in walking this would lead to shorter steps. Festination may be similar to the description of a rabbit running as if chased by dogs. In this regard then it could be similar to what Villablanca and Marcus call "obstinate progression."[141] Cats with lesions of the basal ganglia will fixate on a singular sensory object and follow it continuously even if they bump into the wall. If a new, more potent stimulus is presented, the animal will refocus its attention or at least halt the activity. A client walking with a festinating gait can be made to alter this gait pattern by introduction of a potent new stimulus (e.g., a loud clap) which is similar to the cat displaying "obstinate progression."

The gait of a person with Parkinson's disease shows other abnormalities besides festination. Typically, there is a loss in the heel-toe progression of the normal gait cycle. Instead there is a flat-footed or, with progression, a toe-heel sequence. It is as if the Parkinsonian patient has lost the adult gait pattern and is using a more primitive pattern. The flat-footed gait decreases the ability to step over obstacles or to walk on carpeted surfaces.

Stages of the disease. Parkinson's disease is a progressive disorder. Usually the initial symptom is a resting tremor or micrography (bradykinesia of the upper extremity). With time rigidity and bradykinesia are seen and postural alterations begin to occur. This commonly starts with an increase in neck, trunk, and hip flexion, which, accompanied by a decrease in righting and equilibrium responses, leads to a decreasing ability to balance.

While these postural changes are occurring, there is also an increase in rigidity, which is most apparent in the trunk and proximal musculature. Trunk rotation is severely decreased. As the rigidity progresses, the bradykinesia becomes akinesia. There is no arm swing in gait, no spontaneous facial expression, and movement becomes more and more difficult to initiate. What movement occurs is usually produced with great concentration and is perhaps cortically generated, therefore bypassing the damaged basal ganglia pathways. This great concentration then makes movement tiring, which also heightens the debilitating effects of the disease.

Eventually the individual becomes wheelchair bound and dependent. In the late and severe stages of the disease, especially without therapeutic attention to movement, the client may become bedridden and may demonstrate a fixed trunk-flexion contracture no matter what position the person is placed in. This posture has been called the "phantom pillow" syndrome because, even when lying supine, the person's head is flexed as if on a pillow.

Throughout this progressive deterioration of movement, there is also a decrease in higher-level sensory processing. This is especially evident in the performance of spatial tasks,[7,15] for example, following a map. The difficulty occurs because these individuals cannot orient their own body in space with reference to the map; they display a loss of egocentric localization. In addition, they can perform only one task at a time. They also lose the ability to walk and chew gum at the same time. Despite these changes there is no conclusive evidence of a loss in cognitive abilities.[15] Reports of dementia do exist and, depending on the article read, range from 30% to 93% of Parkinson's disease patients.[62] It is generally thought that the appearance of dementia in Parkinsonian patients is a result of the presence of extranigral and/or cortical changes similar to those seen in Alzheimer's disease. Frequently the amount of dementia is related to the age of the patient, and these patients may represent a subset of Parkinson's disease. The presence of dementia with Parkinson's disease may indicate involvement of acetylcholine and/or the noradrenergic mesolimbic system. In this case, treatment with anticholinergic drugs may increase a tendency toward dementia, especially in older patients. Sometimes cognitive deficits are inferred because of spatial problems, sensory processing problems, and a masked face.

The most serious complication of Parkinson's disease is bronchopneumonia. Decreased activity in general, along with decreased chest expansion, may be contributing factors. The mortality rate is greater than in the general population, and death is usually from pneumonia.

Pharmacological considerations and medical management. The knowledge that the symptoms of Parkinson's disease are caused by a decrease in DA led to the pharmacological management of this disease. DA itself does not cross the blood-brain barrier, but levo-dihydroxyphenylalanine (L-dopa), a precursor of DA, does. This led to the use of L-dopa in treatment in the late 1960s.[26,58,91] Because L-dopa can be changed to DA in the body before ever reaching the brain, it is now usually given with an inhibitor of aromatic amino acid decarboxylation (carbidopa). These inhibitors do not enter the brain readily; thus at the dosages used, their actions are limited to peripheral tissue. This then allows more of the L-dopa to enter the brain and undergo decarboxylation where it will do the most good. Further, the decarboxylase inhibitor allows a reduction in dosage of L-dopa itself, which helps decrease the cardiac and gastrointestinal side effects it causes through the increase in DA in the peripheral organs.

Amantadine is another drug that has been effective in treatment of Parkinson's disease. Although the mechanism of action of this antiviral medication is unknown, it is thought to include a facilitation of release of catecholamine (of which DA is one) from stores in the neuron that are readily releasable. It is often administered in combination with L-dopa.

Treatment of Parkinson's disease with L-dopa in these various combinations has been shown to be extremely helpful in reducing bradykinesia and rigidity. It is less effective in reducing tremor. Because Parkinson's disease involves the nigral neurons, the receptors and the neurons in the striatum (which are postsynaptic to DA neurons) remain intact and initially are somewhat responsive to DA.[58] With time, however, the receptors appear to lose their sensitivity, and the prolonged effectiveness (10 years or more) of L-dopa therapy is questionable.[63,101] A further complication of L-dopa therapy is the development of involuntary movements (dyskinesias) and the "on-off" phenomenon—a short-duration response resulting in sudden improvement of symptoms followed by a rapid decline in symptomatic relief and perhaps the appearance of dyskinesias. With time the "on" effect becomes of shorter and shorter duration.[63] The effectiveness of L-dopa does not appear to be closely correlated with the stage of the disease.

The use of L-dopa alone or in combination with carbidopa has not provided a cure or even prevented the degeneration of Parkinson's disease. Therefore many new drugs are being tested and tried. As scientists learn more about the dopamine receptors and their role in motor control, more effective medications may be found. Some of these "newer" drugs that are being clinically tested include Bromocriptine and Pergolide, both D_2 receptor agonists. Low doses of bromocriptine seem to decrease the wearing off phenomenon of L-dopa and may also decrease the dyskinesia.[21] However, the side effects include hallucinations, nausea, and vomiting. Pergolide also appears to be effective in treatment; however, double-blind studies seem to indicate recovery in placebo as well.[28] Testing on both these drugs is now aimed at new Parkinson's patients and not exclusively at those with long-term disease.

Another approach to pharmacologic treatment of Parkinson's disease came out of research on a designer drug that contained the neurotoxin 1-methyl-4-phenyl-1,2,3,6-tetrahydropyridine (MPTP) (see p. 747 for additional information on drug consideration). It was found that the conversion of MPTP to the active neurotoxin MPP+ could be prevented by monamine oxidase inhibitors such as deprenyl and pargyline.[53] Deprenyl is now undergoing multiple-site testing to determine its effectiveness in retarding progression of the disease. MPTP research has also indicated the involvement of free radicals as a cause of cell damage.[24,72] Alpha-tocopheral is a protective, fat-soluble antioxidant, and therefore this drug is being tested by itself and with Deprenyl.

In addition to drug management, stereotaxic surgery has also been attempted to relieve the symptoms of Parkinson's disease. Discrete lesions are made in the brain, usually in the thalamus or pallidothalamic pathway. As might be expected this technique has been highly effective in reducing tremor and somewhat effective in reduction of rigidity. The relief of symptoms following the surgery is also reported to be of short duration, that is, less than 10 years.[63]

The newest therapeutic intervention for treatment of Parkinson's disease is the use of adrenal medulla transplants.[93] In this procedure the person's own adrenal medulla is transplanted to the ventricle overlying the caudate nucleus. The cells of the adrenal medulla have all the enzymatic machinery to produce DA (which is a precusor of epinephrine).[41] Trophic factors in the brain halt the adrenal medulla's production of epinephrine at DA.[41] It is hypothesized that this is a more natural method of DA replacement therapy. The initial reports appeared very promising; however, the true effectiveness of this treatment must be proven over time. For some patients there is dramatic improvement, but for others improvement is difficult to see.

Evaluation of the client with Parkinson's disease. Evaluation of the client with Parkinson's disease should focus on the degree of rigidity and bradykinesia and how much these symptoms interfere with activities of daily living. These evaluations should of course be as objective as possible, and one method is the rating scale developed by Webster (1968) and shown in Fig. 19-4.[55] This type of scale also allows assessing the progression of the disease. Additionally, active and passive range of movement should be measured.

In assessing function of the client with Parkinson's disease, the therapist must note not only that an activity can be accomplished but also how long it takes to perform a task. Gait can be assessed by general pattern and also by speed and distance. Forward and backward walking as well as braiding should be evaluated. (Similarly, the time it takes to go from sitting to standing, standing to sitting, and supine-lying to sitting and back again should be recorded.) Handwriting should be periodically sampled.

A careful analysis of equilibrium is imperative for the parkinsonian client. This must include assessment with and *without* vision and the differences in the two recorded. The author's own investigation also highlights the importance of assessing tandem walking, especially in the early stages of the disease. This may be the first sign of equilibrium impairment.

An assessment of chest expansion and vital capacity should also be included in the evaluation. This is important because of the complication of pneumonia.

General treatment goals and rationale. As with all treatment, the general goals will be related to the findings on evaluation of each client. In general, goals include increasing movement as well as range of motion, maintaining or improving chest expansion, improving equilibrium reactions, and maintaining functional abilities. Increased movement may in fact modify the progression of the disease and prevent contractures.[36] It may further help to retard dementia. Although L-dopa decreases the bradykinesia, it alone will not be effective in increasing movement, and therefore aggressive intervention in the early stages is necessary. Increasing trunk rotation goes hand in hand with increasing range of movement and motion in general. The longer clients are kept mobile the less likely they are to develop pneumonia.

Treatment procedures. To increase movement there must be a decrease in rigidity. Many relaxation techniques appear to be effective, including gentle, slow rocking, rotation of the extremities and trunk, and even the use of yoga. With the parkinsonian client success in relaxation may be better achieved in the sitting position because rigidity may increase in the supine position.[6] Further, because the proximal muscles are often more involved than the distal muscles, relaxation may be easier to achieve by following a distal to proximal progression. The inverted position may be used with care. Initially this position facilitates total relaxation (increase in parasympathetic tone) and then increases trunk extension, which is important for the parkinsonian client.

Once a decrease in rigidity is achieved through relaxation, movement must be initiated. For the client with Parkinson's disease, this movement should be large and through the entire range. As with relaxation techniques it may be easier to start with distal motions first and gradually increase the movement, bringing in proximal and trunk muscles. Sitting is a good position from which to begin, starting perhaps with swinging of the arms in ever-increasing amplitude. Because bilateral symmetrical patterns are easier than reciprocal patterns, they should be used first. To add trunk rotation (which will also help decrease the proximal rigidity)[13] proprioceptive neuomuscular facilitation (PNF) patterns and rhythmic initiation might be used.[71] Additionally, neurodevelopmental treatment (NDT) and mobilization techniques may be useful to increase scapular and pelvic mobility.

The use of rhythm and auditory cues facilitates movement. Rhythm, especially as in a march, seems to enable the client to move continuously with alternating flexion and extension without becoming fixated. Clapping or music enhances this effect. At present no explanation can be given for this phenomenon, but perhaps it diminishes cortical initiation and abnormal EMG activity (which was discussed earlier). Movement is thus accomplished in a more automatic, nonfragmented manner.

As the client's movement increases, bilateral activities

PARKINSON'S DISEASE PATIENT EVALUATION

Select the appropriate rating for each symptom and mark it in the space provided
in the right-hand column.

BRADYKINESIA
OF HANDS—
INCLUDING
HANDWRITING
- 0　No involvement
- 1　Detectable slowing of the supination-pronation rate evidenced by beginning difficulty in handling tools, buttoning clothes, and with handwriting
- 2　Moderate slowing of supination-pronation rate, one or both sides, evidenced by moderate impairment of hand function. Handwriting is greatly impaired, micrographia present
- 3　Severe slowing of supination-pronation rate. Unable to write or button clothes. Marked difficulty in handling utensils

RIGIDITY
- 0　Nondetectable
- 1　Detectable rigidity in neck and shoulders. Activation phenomenon is present. One or both arms show mild, negative, resting rigidity
- 2　Moderate rigidity in neck and shoulders. Resting rigidity is positive when patient not on medication
- 3　Severe rigidity in neck and shoulders. Resting rigidity cannot be reversed by medication

POSTURE
- 0　Normal posture. Head flexed forward less than 4 inches
- 1　Beginning poker spine. Head flexed forward up to 5 inches
- 2　Beginning arm flexion. Head flexed forward up to 6 inches. One or both arms raised but still below waist
- 3　Onset of simian posture. Head flexed forward more than 6 inches. One or both hands elevated above the waist. Sharp flexion of hand, beginning interphalangeal extension. Beginning flexion of knees

UPPER
EXTREMITY
SWING
- 0　Swings both arms well
- 1　One arm definitely decreased in amount of swing
- 2　One arm fails to swing
- 3　Both arms fail to swing

GAIT
- 0　Steps out well with 18-30 inch stride. Turns about effortlessly
- 1　Gait shortened to 12-18 inch stride. Beginning to strike one heel. Turn around time slowing. Requires several steps
- 2　Stride moderately shortened now 6-12 inches. Both heels beginning to strike floor forcefully
- 3　Onset of shuffling gait, steps less than 3 inches. Occasional stuttering-type of blocking gait. Walks on toes turns around very slowly

TREMOR
- 0　No detectable tremor found
- 1　Less than 1 inch of peak-to-peak tremor movement observed in limbs or head at rest or in either hand while walking or during finger to nose testing
- 2　Maximum tremor envelope fails to exceed 4 inches. Tremor is severe but not constant and patient retains some control of hands
- 3　Tremor envelope exceeds 4 inches. Tremor is constant and severe. Patient cannot get free of tremor while awake unless it is a pure cerebellar type. Writing and feeding self are impossible

FACIES
- 0　Normal. Full animation. No stare
- 1　Detectable immobility. Mouth remains closed. Beginning features of anxiety or depression
- 2　Moderate immobility. Emotion breaks through at markedly increased threshold. Lips parted some of the time. Moderate appearance of anxiety or depression. Drooling may be present
- 3　Frozen facies. Mouth open ¼ inch or more. Drooling may be severe

SEBORRHEA
- 0　None
- 1　Increased perspiration, secretion remaining thin
- 2　Obvious oiliness present. Secretion much thicker
- 3　Marked seborrhea, entire face and head covered by thick secretion

SPEECH
- 0　Clear, loud, resonant, easily understood
- 1　Beginning of hoarseness with loss of inflection and resonance. Good volume and still easily understood
- 2　Moderate hoarseness and weakness. Constant monotone, unvaried pitch. Beginning of dysarthria, hesitancy, stuttering; difficult to understand
- 3　Marked harshness and weakness. Very difficult to hear and to understand

SELF-CARE
- 0　No impairment
- 1　Still provides full self-care but rate of dressing definitely impeded. Able to live alone and often still employable
- 2　Requires help in certain critical areas, such as turning in bed, rising from chairs, etc. Very slow in performing most activities but manages by taking much time
- 3　Continuously disabled. Unable to dress, feed self, or walk alone

TOTAL _____

OVERALL DISABILITY (total value of):
1-10, Early illness; 11-20, moderate disability; 21-30, severe or advanced disease.

Fig. 19-4. Parkinson's disease patient evaluation form. (From Endo Laboratories, Inc, Garden City, NY, Copyright 1979.)

can be replaced with reciprocal patterns. Use of functional types of activities is likewise important. In gait activities large steps with large arm swings should be encouraged. Additionally, changes in direction, changes in movement patterns, and stopping and starting activities should be stressed.

Equilibrium reactions in the developmental sequence should be encouraged. These should be kept at an automatic level. Rhythmic stabilization may be used *if* the use of resistance does not lead to an increase in truncal rigidity. The timing of the resistance must be very gradual, allowing the client time to develop force in one set of muscles before increasing resistance and then switching directions. If proper time is not allowed, the therapist will be reinforcing the already abnormal patterns of motor neuron activity. (See Chapters 6, 9, 13, 16, 21, and 22 for other procedures.)

While working on upper-extremity activities, chest expansion may be increased as arm swings increase. The clinician may also have the client shout—again, especially with some kind of rhythmic chant, even a simple "left, right" while walking. If needed, specific breathing exercises can be incorporated.

In addition to treatment in the therapy department, the parkinsonian client should also be given a home program, which is necessary to encourage making moderate, consistent exercise a part of the normal day. Fatigue should be avoided and the exercise graded to the individual's capability. The therapist should keep in mind that learned skills such as various sports are sometimes less affected than automatic movements,[38] perhaps because these skills may rely on cortical involvement.

Physical or occupational therapy in the treatment of Parkinson's disease can be quite effective whether or not the client is taking medication. Physical therapy is suggested in most brochures and books[36] for parkinsonian individuals and their families. However, little has been published on effective therapeutic procedures for the individual with Parkinson's disease.[5] One recent report by Palmer and others[116] utilized precise, quantitative measures to assess motor signs, grip strength, coordination, and speed as well as measurements of the long latency stretch reflex following two exercise programs in Parkinson's patients. These two programs were the United Parkinson Foundation program and karate training. Their results indicated improvement over 12 weeks in gait, grip strength, and coordination of fine motor control tasks but no change in a decline in movements requiring speed. The patients all felt an increase in general well-being. The results of this careful study indicate that more research and careful documentation of exercise programs are needed.

Physical activity and movement appear to increase quality of life by decreasing the depression and lack of initiative that occur in Parkinson's disease. Group classes can serve as an extra support system for Parkinson's patients and their spouses. A carefully structured low-impact aerobics program appears to be a benefit to patients even with long-standing disease (Melnick and others, unpublished results). One program begins with seated activities for upper extremities (Fig. 19-5, *A*) and then combination movements for warm-up (Fig. 19-5, *B*). The participants then progress to standing and marching activities that incorporate coordinated movements of arms and legs as well as balance and trunk rotation (Fig. 19-6). All movements are performed to music similar to that used in aerobics classes in any gym or health spa. Heart rate should be monitored periodically. Many Parkinson's disease associations also have audio tapes for exercises (e.g., United Parkinson's Foundation). Ballroom dancing is also an excellent form of therapy for Parkinson's patients as it promotes rhythmic movement, rotation, balance, and coordination. The waltz or fox trot is a good beginning dance as it is easy and somewhat slow (Fig. 19-7). The mambo promotes separation of the pelvis from the trunk and increases coordination. A modified Charleston can be used to increase one-legged balance, as can modified tap dancing. The use of dance also facilitates changing direction.

Some of the group activities and possible exercises are depicted in Figures 19-5 to 19-8. Data are presently being gathered on functional changes and range of motion changes in patients participating in a weekly program of aerobics.

The use of assistive devices in gait for the Parkinson's patients is an area with no clear-cut guidelines. Because coordination of upper and lower extremities is often difficult, the ability to utilize a cane or walker is often impossible. The patient may drag the cane or carry the walker. Walkers with wheels seem to increase the festinating gait, and the patient may just fall over the walker. For those patients with a tendency to fall backwards, an assistive device may simply be something to carry backwards with them. Therefore the reason for utilizing the assistive device must be carefully assessed. Walkers or canes can be helpful for the person with postural instability and the ability to walk with a heel-toe gait. The height of walker or cane should be adjusted carefully to promote extension and avoid an increase in trunk flexion. Parkinson's patients may also benefit from assistive devices for eating and/or writing. For a few patients small cuff weights may decrease tremor when walking; however, for many patients cuff weights only exacerbate the tremor.

Bed mobility is another important consideration for Parkinson's patients. A firm bed may make getting in and out of bed easier. Most patients report that satin sheets with silk or satin pajamas make moving in bed far easier. This is true in both the early and later stages of the disease. Beds with a head that can be raised electrically may be helpful as the disease progresses, but while sleeping the patient should lower the head as close to horizontal as pos-

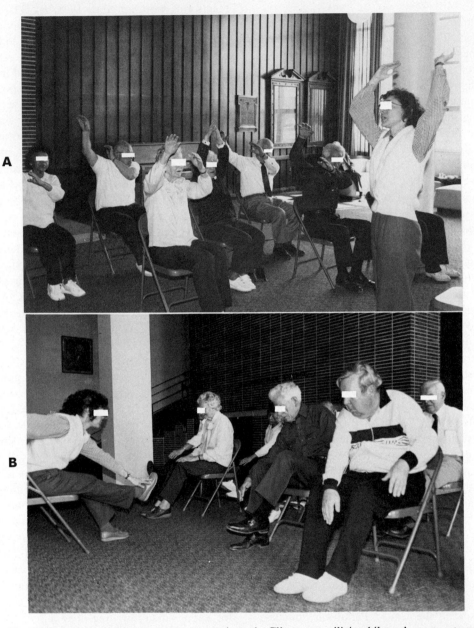

Fig. 19-5. Seated aerobics or warm-up exercises. **A,** Clients are utilizing bilateral upper-extremity patterns to facilitate trunk rotation. Instruction was to let the head follow the hands. **B,** This exercise encourages trunk rotation, large movements, and coordination of the upper and lower extremities. Clients are to reach with the arms and touch the opposite foot. This coordination is very difficult in Parkinson's disease, and initially many clients could not move the arms and legs at the same time.

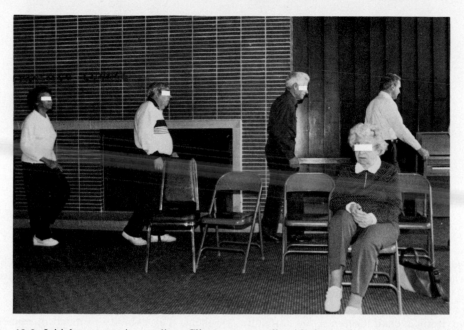

Fig. 19-6. Initial warm-up in standing. Clients are to walk with the head up, back as straight as possible, and take large steps. When the group began, walking was the major aerobic activity and used to influence flexibilities and encourage movement. Nonambulatory patients march in place in the chair.

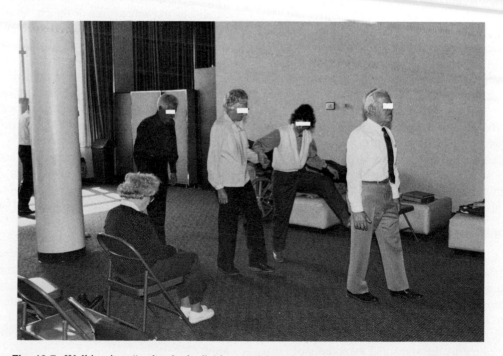

Fig. 19-7. Walking in a "waltz rhythm" (slow, quick, quick) emphasizing a big step for the slow step. Notice lack of automatic arm swing. Also notice flexed posture of seated patient during rest period.

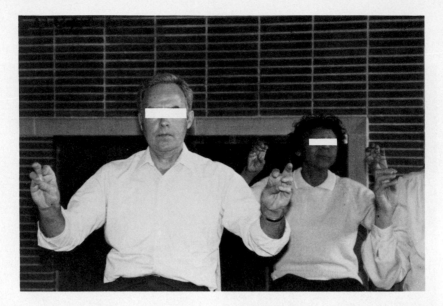

Fig. 19-8. Cool-down period allows time to work on fine finger movements. Thumb abduction with rounded fingers and various rhythms is used to increase coordination. Notice "masked face."

sible. If getting up from a chair becomes too difficult, chairs with seats that lift up have been used effectively.

As Parkinson's disease progresses the patient may experience difficulty in swallowing and even in chewing. Therapy for oral-motor control should be initiated, and a dietician consult may be necessary to ensure adequate nutrition.

A dietician may also be beneficial in guiding the patient's protein intake. High protein may reduce the responsiveness of the patient to dopamine replacement therapy.[114] Regulating the amount and timing of protein ingestion can improve the efficacy of drug treatment in some patients.

Finally, Parkinson's disease is a progressive, degenerative disease. Therapy and exercise may modify the progression but cannot halt or reverse it. Quality of life throughout the course of the disease may be enhanced, however, and the therapist can assist the client and family in coping with the constraints of this disease.

Huntington's disease

Huntington's disease (formerly Huntington's chorea) is another degenerative disease of the basal ganglia. This disease gets its name from the family of physicians who described its patterns of inheritance. Huntington's disease is inherited as an autosomal dominant trait and affects approximately 6.5/100,000 people.[38]

Symptoms. Some of the signs and symptoms of Huntington's disease are similar to Parkinson's disease: abnormalities in postural reactions, trunk rotation, distribution of tone, and extraneous movements. However, individuals with Huntington's disease may be considered to be at the other end of the spectrum; rather than a paucity of move-

ment, they exhibit too much movement, which is evident in the trunk and face in addition to the extremities. The gait takes on an ataxic, dancing appearance (in fact, chorea means *to dance*), and fine movements become clumsy and slowed. As with the parkinsonian individual there is a decrease in associated movements (e.g., arm swing). The extraneous movements are of the choreoathetoid type, consisting of "single, isolated muscle action, producing a short, rapid uncoordinated jerk of the trunk, limb or face" (p. 312).[59] Usually, however, these occur in successive movements so that the entire picture is one of complex movement patterns. It is as if the "movement generator" aspects of the basal ganglia are continuously active. As the disease progresses, the choreic movements may give way to akinesia and rigidity.

In addition to the involvement of the motor systems, the individual with Huntington's also shows signs of dementia and emotional disorders that become worse as the disease progresses. The client may show lack of judgment and loss of memory, a deterioration in speech and writing (i.e., severe decrease in ability to communicate), depression, hostility, and feelings of incompetence. There is a decrease in IQ with performance measures decreasing more rapidly than verbal levels. Suicide is fairly common.

Huntington's disease is usually manifested after the age of 30 although childhood forms appear rarely. Death from this disease occurs about 15 years after the onset of symptoms.

The movement disorders of Huntington's disease are presumed to be related to degeneration of the striatal neurons; the dementia is associated with cortical destruction. Recently, the locus of the gene for Huntington's disease has been found. It is located on the short arm of chromosone 4. Although neither the abnormal gene product nor the gene itself has been identified, a marker close to the gene has been detected.[50] If the family pedigree is known and the chromosomes of the parents can be obtained, it is now possible to detect which offspring have the faulty chromosome presymptomatically.

Although this may be a great step forward, genetic testing is still fraught with ethical considerations. At present, although testing is available it is not widely utilized. Further, testing for Huntington's disease is typically only available to those over the age of 18. Despite these problems, localizing the portion of the chromosome involved means that ultimately the gene product will be identified, and this will perhaps lead to improved means of treatment.

In contrast to Parkinson's disease (in which there is involvement of the dopaminergic nigrostriatal pathway) Huntington's disease is characterized by a loss of the intrinsic neurons of the striatum that receive DA. Thus the earliest theories involved striatal dysfunction in response to normal DA concentrations. This abnormal response would in turn prevent the normal *modulation* of movement. Again, it is important to remember that, although the choreiform movements involve contraction of single muscles, they are usually linked together. That is, they are not random jerks but a series of contractions that resemble normal movements or parts of movements. These movements are fairly stereotypical, especially for each individual. The administration of DA agonists can produce these movements in experimental animals and can also make the individual with Huntington's disease worse. In other words, these persons appear to have too much DA whereas those with Parkinson's disease have too little.

The exact mechanisms for the production of choreoathetoid movements are unknown. Because these extraneous movements are part of a person's normal repertoire of movement patterns, it is possible that they are "released" at inappropriate times and without any modulation. A postmortem examination shows a decrease in GABA that could be associated with a decrease in inhibitory feedback. Recent use of positron emission tomography (PET) scans demonstrates loss of ACh and GABA neurons. A pattern may therefore be released before it is necessary, and inappropriate portions of pattern cannot be inhibited. Petajan and others also found motor unit activity indicative of bradykinesia.[118] Recordings of single motor units in the muscles indicates that persons with Huntington's disease have a loss of control evidenced by an inability to recruit single motor units.[118] As the efforts at control increased, these individuals demonstrated an overflow of motor unit activity that resulted in full choreiform movements. Those in the earlier stages of the disease demonstrated what the experimenters termed "microchorea," small ballistic activations of motor units.[118] As in Parkinson's disease, difficulty occurs in modulating motor neuron excitability. An-

other finding in this experiment revealed motor unit activity indicative of bradykinesia.

The abnormal postural reactions of the person with Huntington's disease may occur from a misinterpretation of sensory input, especially vestibular and proprioceptive (similar to the parkinsonian syndrome). However, the dementia of Huntington's disease precludes further testing. Although it appears as if the thalamus also plays a role in the movement disorders of Huntington's disease, the specifics are unknown at present.[33,117]

Stages of the disease. Huntington's disease is a progressive disorder. The initial symptoms are most often complaints of incoordination, clumsiness, or jerkiness. A classic test for eliciting choreiform movements in this early stage is a simple grip test. The client grips the examiner's hand and maintains that grip for a few seconds. The person with Huntington's disease will display what is descriptively called the "milkmaid's sign"; there will be alternate increases and decreases in the grip. Facial grimacing or the inability to perform complex facial movements may also be present very early.

In many cases the dementia and psychological symptoms of Huntington's disease occur after the onset of the neurological signs. In those cases where very subtle personality changes occur first, the diagnosis may be more difficult. Such persons may appear forgetful or unable to manage appointments and financial affairs. They may be thought to have early senility, or they may show signs of severe depression or schizophrenia.

With time, the combination of the psychological and neurological problems causes the individual to lose all ability to work and perform activities of daily living (ADL). This person eventually can be cared for only in an extended care facility. By this time the choreiform movements have given way to rigidity, and the patient is bedridden. Fig. 19-9 shows the stages of Huntington's disease according to Shouldon and Fahn.[127]

Pharmacological considerations and medical management. The great advances in pharmacological management of Parkinson's disease have led to a great deal of research to find appropriate drugs for the management of Huntington's disease. At present, however, there is no fully effective medication for this disease.

The symptoms of Huntington's disease indicate an increase in dopaminergic effect. At autopsy there is a decrease in the number of intrinsic neurons of the striatum that contain the neurotransmitter GABA or ACh. Biochemical studies reveal a definite decrease in GABA concentration in addition to a decrease in ACh concentration in the basal ganglia. Therefore drug therapy depends on those drugs that are cholinergic or GABA-containing agonists and those that act as DA antagonists. To date the DA antagonists have been more effective in ameliorating neurological symptoms.

In general, pharmacological treatment is not started un-

	Engagement in occupation	Score	Capacity to handle financial affairs	Score	Capacity to manage domestic responsibility	Score	Capacity to perform activities of daily living	Score	Care can be provided at	Score
Stage 1	Usual level	3	Full	3	Full	2	Full	3	Home	2
Stage 2	Lower level	2	Requires slight help	2	Full	2	Full	3	Home	2
Stage 3	Marginal	1	Requires major help	1	Impaired	1	Mildly impaired	2	Home	2
Stage 4	Unable	0	Unable	0	Unable	0	Moderately impaired	1	Home or extended care facility	1
Stage 5	Unable	0	Unable	0	Unable	0	Severely impaired	0	Total care facility only	0

Fig. 19-9. Functional stages of Huntington's disease. (From Shoulson I and Fahn S: Neurology 29:2, 1979.)

From Shoulson and Fahn (1979).

til the choreiform movements interfere with function[50] because these drugs have side effects that may be worse than the chorea (see the section on tardive dyskinesia). According to the report of the Committee to Combat Huntington's Disease,[128] the following drugs are listed as preferred medication: perphenazine, haloperidol (Haldol), and reserpine. The first two block the DA receptors themselves; reserpine depletes DA stores in the brain. Side effects include depression, drowsiness, a parkinsonian type of syndrome, or sometimes dyskinesia. Drugs such as choline, which would increase ACh concentrations, have produced only transient improvement.[134] There have been many efforts to find a GABA agonist that would reduce the symptoms of Huntington's disease, but these have so far been unsuccessful.[12,129] The problem with finding a medication to increase GABA is that such a drug will probably cause inhibition throughout the brain, not just in the basal ganglia. Thus the individual's level of alertness and ability to function might be reduced—something the person with Huntington's disease can ill afford.[12]

Because management of the dementia and personality problems is not satisfactory with any present drug therapy, it becomes more difficult than the choreiform problem. Cortical degeneration is most certainly involved, but disruption of the heavy corticostriate projections may also be a factor in the progression of this disease. Although alterations in DA have been implicated in psychotic problems such as schizophrenia, the role of the basal ganglia in thought processes is, at best, little understood. In the words of Woody Guthrie:

> There's just not no hope
> Nor not no treatment known
> to cure me of my dizzy
> called Chorea.[52]

At present the best hope for the person with Huntington's disease lies in a better understanding of the genetic mechanisms causing destruction of the GABA-containing cells in the striatum and cortical destruction. In the meantime correct and early diagnosis is important in providing the proper early intervention, which must include counseling.[68] The Committee for the Control of Huntington's Disease has set up several research centers, including a brain and tissue bank, in an effort to facilitate research into the causes of the disease.

Evaluation of the client with Huntington's disease. In evaluating a person with Huntington's disease, one must assess the degree of functional ability and how the chorea interferes with function. Which extremities, including the face, are involved? Does the client have any cortical control of the chorea or any means of allaying these extraneous movements? What exacerbates the symptoms? What lessens them? At present no rating scale exists other than the capacity to perform ADL (see Fig 19-9). A standard ADL form with space to write in how the client performs these activities or why she or he cannot perform them would be helpful.

In addition, posture and equilibrium reactions should be tested. What associated reactions, if any, are present? In assessing posture, care should be taken to observe the posture of the extremities in addition to the trunk, head, and neck. Dystonic posturing should be carefully noted, especially if the client is taking medication. Any changes should be reported to the physician.

A gross assessment of strength should be made with particular attention paid to the ability to stabilize the trunk and proximal joints. To reduce the effects of rigidity, range of motion becomes important as the disease progresses.

In the assessment of the client with Huntington's disease, the stage of psychological involvement and mental state must be reliably assessed both during evaluation and treatment. Computerized axial tomography data will give some clues to the amount of cortical and basal ganglia degeneration, which can assist in determining possible cortical functioning.

General treatment goals and rationale. Maintaining the optimal quality of life is the most important goal for treatment of persons with Huntington's disease and their families. This will include maintenance of functional skills and advice to the family on adaptive equipment. Techniques that reduce tone may also reduce choreiform movements. Increasing stability about the shoulders, trunk, neck, and hips will help maintain function. Again, it must be reiterated that the evaluation results will dictate treatment procedures.

Treatment procedures. The Commission on the Control of Huntington's Disease[68] stated that these individuals are underserved by physical and occupational therapy. Hayden[52] mentions that therapy can improve the quality of life. Yet there are no articles on treatment procedures. Theories as to which techniques may prove most beneficial are offered here with the warning that to date none have been documented. (See also Chapter 6 for specific techniques of facilitation and inhibition.)

The treatment of the person with Huntington's disease has some parallels with the treatment of cerebral palsy athetosis. These techniques, however, must be adapted to the adult. Of critical importance are the techniques for improving cocontraction and trunk stability. The use of the pivot-prone and withdrawal patterns of Rood are helpful, and their benefit may be increased with the use of theraband. Neck cocontraction and trunk stability may improve or at least maintain oral functions. Additionally, the techniques of rhythmic stabilization in all positions as well as heavy work patterns of Rood should be helpful.[71]

Relaxation aids reduction of extraneous movements. In the early stages methods that require active participation of the client, such as biofeedback and traditional relaxation exercises, may be included. As dementia becomes more apparent, more passive techniques such as slow rocking and neutral warmth must be employed. These techniques are also helpful in reducing the choreiform movements of the mouth and tongue, which may prove useful for the dentist and those responsible for proper nutrition of the client. In most cases of Huntington's disease, the individual is quite thin (almost emaciated) and begins to age rapidly as the disease progresses. The extraneous movements, especially as they become more severe, increase metabolic demands, and nutrition therefore becomes increasingly important. Attention, therefore must be paid to head, neck, and oral-motor control. Increased pressure on the lips may aid in lip closure and facilitate swallowing. Special straws with a mouthpiece similar to a pacifier may therefore be useful. A dietitian should be consulted for assistance in teaching the family how to prepare balanced and appetizing meals and snacks that are still easy to swallow.

The degree of dementia influences the treatment. Conscious efforts to control extraneous movements will be more difficult as cognitive function decreases. Further, new memories and new patterns of movements will be difficult to establish. The therapist therefore must use techniques that require subcortical control and must keep in mind that the client can sometimes remember old, normal patterns of movement.

No amount of physical therapy can prevent neuronal cell loss. Because Huntington's disease is a progressive, degenerative disease, the client will get worse. Eventually, goals must be aimed at preventing total immobility and assisting caretakers in transfer techniques and advising them in the use of adaptive equipment. One aspect of treatment that cannot be measured but is important in the author's view is the degree of hope offered just by the fact that a health professional is providing ongoing care. This may lessen the client's degree of despair and depression and may help maintain quality of life.

Wilson's disease

Wilson's disease, or hepatolenticular degeneration, is a disease caused by faulty copper metabolism. The toxic effects of copper lead to degeneration of the liver and the basal ganglia, hence the name. Wilson's disease, inherited as an autosomal recessive trait, affects a very small percentage of the population.

In Wilson's disease there is an increase in the amount of copper absorbed from the intestinal tract, a subsequent elevation in the amount of copper in the blood serum, and an increase in the amount of copper deposited in tissue.[145] There is a concomitant reduction in ceruloplasmin. The increase in tissue copper may interfere with various enzyme systems of particular cells. The connection of copper with DA metabolism may account for the basal ganglia involvement.

Neuronal degeneration is present in the globus pallidus and putamen and to a lesser extent in the caudate nucleus. There may also be atrophy in the gray matter of the cortex and the dentate nucleus of the cerebellum.

Symptoms. The deposition of the excess copper in the cornea results in the classic diagnostic sign of Wilson's disease, the Kayser-Fleischer ring—a brownish-green or brownish-red colored ring found in the sclerocorneal junction.

Based on constellations of the signs and symptoms, there are several forms of Wilson's disease. One type entails only liver involvement and no neurological signs. A dystonic form is most common in those with an onset of the disease after the age of 20. The individual shows the same abnormal positioning of the limbs and trunk that characterizes the dystonia, rigidity, and bradykinesia seen in Parkinson's disease. Associated reactions and facial expressions are absent. There is a festinating gait and flexed posture. There may be a tremor of the hand, head, and body.

If the onset of the disease occurs before age 20, the appearance of choreoathetoid movements of the face and upper extremities is usually present. The gait resembles that of the individual with Huntington's disease. This early onset form is accompanied by a very rapid deterioration.

Common to all forms of Wilson's disease that involve brain structures is difficulty in speaking and swallowing, incoordination, and personality changes. The personality changes are the first signs of the disease, especially emotional lability and impaired judgment. If the disease progresses, there is increased dementia, increased cirrhosis of the liver, and progressive decrease in motor function.

The term *dystonia* is used for involuntary movements with a sustained contraction at the end of the movement.[38] Usually these movements involve a twisting of the extremity. If the contraction at the end of the movement is prolonged, the term *dystonic posture* is used. A very peculiar aspect of dystonia is that it can be decreased with proprioceptive or tactile input.[38] Dystonia is usually seen with widespread involvement of the basal ganglia and intralaminar nuclei of the thalamus.[117] The cerebellum may also be involved.[25]

Dystonia, like bradykinesia and choreoathetosis, belongs on a continuum of the extraneous movements present with basal ganglia involvement. The movement patterns are total and involve rotation of the limb. As in the other diseases of the basal ganglia discussed so far, there is also a decrease in the normal associated movements. As Wilson's disease progresses, the classic abnormal posture of increased flexion occurs, along with rigidity and, if severe enough, the total inability to move. As with other diseases of the basal ganglia, there appears to be an imbalance or abnormal response in the neurotransmitters; however, the precise imbalance is not yet known.

Stages of the disease. The first symptom of Wilson's disease is usually a change in the individual's personality. Either when this becomes severe enough or when the movement disorder appears, a diagnosis can be made by the presence of the Kayser-Fleischer ring or by an analysis of copper metabolism. Because Wilson's disease is now treatable by chemical means, the full progression of this disease is usually not seen. If left untreated, the dystonia becomes worse and the person becomes more rigid. Additionally, muscle weakness can occur and progress, seizures may develop, and the dementia and personality disorder also become worse.

Medical management. Because the signs and symptoms of Wilson's disease are caused by an increased absorption of copper, treatment consists of drugs that will inhibit this absorption. Concomitantly, copper intake in the diet should be restricted. Penicillamine is the drug of choice, usually in combination with vitamin B_6.[38] There are some side effects of penicillamine, but these appear to be infrequent. If the copper imbalance is treated, the neurological signs do not progress.

Evaluation and treatment intervention. Because Wilson's disease is fully treatable and can be diagnosed early, it is possible that it will not concern the physical therapist. If the client is referred for physical therapy, treatment techniques should be wholly based on symptomatology. Evaluation is similar to that of the parkinsonian or Huntington's person. It consists of describing the type of extraneous movement present, when it is present, and factors that influence the degree of dystonia. Ease of movement should also be assessed, and it may be timed as for the parkinsonian client. Additionally, range of movement and strength should be evaluated, especially if the disease is progressing.

Treatment will then be designed to alleviate the problems. Extraneous movements may be reduced by any technique that will reduce tone. Positioning is important. If bradykinesia is the major sign, then treatment would be similar to that used in Parkinson's disease; if trunk stability is poor, the therapist proceeds as in Huntington's disease. The client with Wilson's disease has knowledge of what normal movement feels like and usually has good cognitive abilities at the time treatment is started. Because of the emotional lability, which is one of the first symptoms in this disease, the treatment session should be well planned and quite structured.

Tardive dyskinesia

Tardive dyskinesia is a drug-induced disorder and thus will be used to indicate the problems that can arise from drug intoxication. In particular this section concentrates on the problems associated with drugs that affect DA metabolism, including amphetamine, haloperidol, and classes of drugs used in treatment of psychotic disorders: the phenothiazines, butyrophenones, and thioxanthenes. As the use and misuse of drugs becomes more common, these types of disorders may become more frequent.

The use of phenothiazines (one of the neuroleptics) has become a very effective and common treatment for schizophrenia. This treatment protocol has enabled many schizophrenics to leave the mental institution. These drugs are DA antagonists and thus decrease the amount of DA in the brain. The exact site of the brain involved in schizophrenia itself is not within the scope of this chapter, but the neurological signs that occur will be discussed. These, as might be expected, involve structures within the basal ganglia. Tardive dyskinesia is a gradual disease that occurs after long-term drug treatment. The most typical involvement is of the mouth, tongue, and muscles of mastication; therefore tardive dyskinesia may be called orofacial or buccolingual-masticatory (BLM) dyskinesia.

Symptoms. Dyskinesia is defined as an inability to perform voluntary movement.[67] However, in practical terms dyskinesia is usually a series of rhythmic extraneous movements. In tardive dyskinesia this typically begins with, or may be confined to, the region of the face. These extraneous movements may include choreoathetoid or dystonic movements. Because of abnormality in basal ganglia function, there are also accompanying abnormalities in postural tone and postural adjustments. Instead of the typical flexed posture of Parkinson's disease, clients with tardive dyskinesia show extension of the trunk with increased lordosis and neck flexion.[92] This description of the disease is rather broad, but the problems of drug-induced movement disorders are varied. They may take the form of drug-induced Parkinson's disease or dystonia. In tardive dyskinesia, akinesia and rigidity similar to that seen in parkinsonism may exist simultaneously with the choreoathetoid-like movements. The key factor in tardive dyskinesia is its slow onset after the ingestion of neuroleptic medications.

Etiology. Although many people take neuroleptic medication, only a small percentage acquire tardive dyskinesia. Many factors may predispose an individual to movement disorders. One of these is age.[130] This might be expected because of the influence of aging processes on the concentration of DA. Sex may also be a factor. Women are more at risk for tardive dyskinesia.[92] The fact that sex can affect DA levels is supported in studies of animals with brain lesions. In one study, female rats had a lower concentration of DA following early brain lesion than did their male litter mates.[126] The absolute amount of neuroleptic ingested may also be a factor, but to date definitive studies have not been completed. So far it appears that the length of time the individual takes medication is not a strong predisposing factor. As the biological abnormalities of schizophrenia become better understood, further understanding of the causes of tardive dyskinesia may also be elucidated. It is hypothesized that the development of tardive dyskinesia is caused by supersensitivity.[4,67] With the use of drugs that deplete the brain of DA, the brain becomes more sensitive to it. And, in fact, in humans the withdrawal of neuroleptics tends to heighten the disease;

essentially, withdrawal of the DA antagonist means that far more DA is able to act on these already sensitive terminals.[4,20,67]

Because of the effectiveness of long-term treatment for schizophrenia provided by neuropletics, research into the underlying cause and therefore treatment of the major side effect, the motor disorders, has greatly increased. But as with Parkinson's disease and Huntington's disease, animal models are difficult to produce. For one thing, the normal function of the basal ganglia in movement is obscure. However, experimental evidence indicates that the basal ganglia are involved in movements about the face, especially the mouth, and buccolingual dyskinesia is the most frequently encountered symptom in tardive dyskinesia.[88,89,90] Lidsky and others[87] hypothesized that sensory input about the face was involved in the high number of globus pallidus units responsive to licking. Further experiments showed that basal ganglia stimulation could alter the threshold of mouth reflexes.[79] The response of basal ganglia neurons to sensory input shows increasing localization of response with age; the region about the mouth becomes increasingly sensitive.[124] Further research along these lines, both in normal animals and those with lesions, may answer the question of what is happening at a neuronal level. This would facilitate drug and physical therapy intervention.

Pharmacological and medical management. One serious problem of tardive dyskinesia is that it is often irreversible. The withdrawal of medication, in fact, may increase the movement disorders. Or it may be that recovery takes even more time than the time required for the onset of the disease. It is a strange fact that sometimes the drug that caused the disease may be the drug that reduces the symptoms; that is, increasing the dose may lessen the movement disorder. This might be expected if supersensitivity to DA is involved. But again, with time the increased dose will also cause a reappearance of the symptoms.

The use of other drugs in conjunction with the neuroleptics has been tried in various animal models of the disease. As might be expected, anticholinergic drugs (which would worsen an imbalance between DA and ACh) worsen the dyskinesia. Lithium has been successful in one animal model of dyskinesia.[67] Some neuroleptic drugs seem to have less effect on movement than others; however, the side effects of one such drug, chlorpromazine, are life threatening. More research is needed into both the mechanisms of schizophrenia and the mechanisms for the production of the abnormal movements.

Evaluation and treatment intervention. The effectiveness of physical therapy intervention in drug-induced dyskinesia is, as yet, not completely known. However, since the neuroleptics do provide an effective long-term treatment of schizophrenia, it is the author's opinion that therapists need to become aware of the problem and offer some assistance. Early drug holidays (time without use of drugs) may be of value in treatment of tardive dyskinesia, and therefore early awareness of incipient changes in motor function may be of value. Assessment of patients receiving drug therapy could perhaps begin before treatment and then at prescribed intervals. The knowledge that postural adjustments are abnormal in most basal ganglia diseases means that analysis of posture statically and in motion might provide early clues of development of movement disorders. The same would be true for equilibrium reactions and changes in tone with changes in position. Once movement disorders appear, an assessment of when and where the extraneous movements occur is important.

General treatment is similar to that used in Huntington's disease; oral treatment corresponds to that for the athetotic child with cerebral palsy. If a hyperreactivity to sensory stimulus exists, then oral desensitization may be of value.

Ameliorating the oral grimacing would, of course, be helpful for the schizophrenic person who is trying to return to society. The effectiveness of physical and occupational therapy treatment cannot be assessed until therapists become involved with these clients and record their results. In cases in which the parkinsonian-like symptoms are stronger than the dyskinetic movements, treatment would follow the plan for the individual with Parkinson's disease.

Other considerations

Other drugs besides neuroleptics may also produce movement disorders. Amphetamine, for example, has been shown to cause long-term changes in brain function even from very small doses.[85,86,142] Adults who were hyperactive children sometimes show a decrease in the readiness potential.[14] Further research is under way to determine the role that medications, such as methylphenidate (Ritalin), used in treating hyperactive children might play in causing movement disorders. The problem of drug-induced movement disorders may become an ever-increasing one for the therapist.

In 1982 several young people were treated for rigidity and "catatonia" after the use of what they thought was heroin. Careful examination of these patients revealed that they had parkinsonian-like symptoms.[27,80] The chemical responsible for the symptomatology was 1-methyl-4-phenyl-1,2,3,6-tetrahydropyridine (MPTP), a meperidine analogue that was an impurity in the designer heroin. This discovery has enabled research in animals and clinical studies in humans. Although there are some differences among idiopathic Parkinson's disease, MPTP-induced Parkinson's disease, and MPTP-induced parkinsonism, there are important similarities: MPTP selectively damages DA cells in the substantia nigra; L-dopa is effective in alleviating the symptoms; and the symptoms seen are irreversible and progressive. In animal studies, age does affect the degree of damage,[103,143] and in humans, some of those who utilized the drug MPTP are now beginning to show symptoms of parkinsonism.[81] This delay in appearance of symptoms fits a model of Parkinson's disease that suggests that an initial insult to the DA system may not result in disease until a critical level is reached. The critical level of DA depletion may occur with age because of a gradual loss of DA in the aging process. The real importance of the discovery of MPTP-induced parkinsonism is that it may enable better understanding of the pathogenesis and, in turn, of the treatment of the disease. One hypothesized cause of Parkinson's disease implicated environmental toxins (because some herbicides such as paraquot resemble the chemical structure of MPTP) and the involvement of superoxide free radical.[8,24,72] Epidemiology studies are now underway to investigate Parkinson's disease in areas known for high herbicide usage, and alpha tocopheral is under investigation as a protective agent.

It will be interesting to follow the MPTP story to see how many questions will be answered in the future.

METABOLIC DISEASES AFFECTING OTHER REGIONS OF THE BRAIN

All alterations of metabolism, if allowed to continue, will affect nervous system function. This includes alterations in sodium, water, sugar, and hormonal balance. Table 19-1 lists metabolic diseases that often have neurolog-

ical sequelae. Proper treatment is usually medical management of the imbalance. Physical therapeutic intervention, if necessary, should address specific neurological symptoms. (See other chapters that discuss these individual problems.)

Ingestion of or exposure to heavy metals may also lead to CNS disease. Table 19-2 describes the sequelae of these problems.

One metabolic problem, however, warrants in-depth consideration: drug-induced neurological disorders that arise from over ingesting alcohol. Movement disorders involve the effects of alcohol on the CNS and the effects of nutritional deficiency that are part of the alcoholic syndrome.

Alcoholism

Alcohol, as a drug, has a direct effect on the nervous system. Additionally, the chronic effects of alcohol include vitamin and general nutritional deficiency. Alcohol has a high caloric value and therefore the chronic alcoholic tends to decrease food intake: the classic "drinking lunch or dinner." Thus acute intoxication, while not producing nutritional deficiency, contributes to it.

Signs and symptoms of acute alcohol intoxication. Most people are well aware of the symptoms of acute al-

Table 19-1. Neurological complications of metabolic disorders

Metabolic problem	Treatment	Neurological complication
Decreased sodium (too much H₂O)	Restricted water intake	Muscle twitching, seizures, coma
Increased sodium	Rehydration, *slowly*	Cerebral edema, muscle rigidity, decerebrate rigidity
Decreased potassium (hypokalemia) often caused by aldosteronism	Restoration of calcium levels after assessing primary cause	Changes in resting potential of neuron; hyperpolarization; muscle weakness and fatigue with eventual total paralysis
Magnesium imbalance	Improved diet, intravenous magnesium	Mental confusion, muscle twitching, myoclonus, tachycardia, hyperreflexia, extraneous movements, seizures
Diabetes mellitus	Proper control of diabetes	Peripheral neuropathy, pseudotabes, possible seizures and coma
Hypoglycemia	Treatment of primary cause; diet adjustment	Anoxia of the brain, seizures, mental confusion
Hyperthyroidism	Thyroid-blocking agents; intravenous fluids, hydrocortisone and propranolol if patient in thyroid crisis	Hyperkinesia, irritability, nervousness, emotional lability, symmetrical peripheral neuropathy
Hypothyroidism	Thyroid supplement	Sluggishness, mental and motor retardation, muscle weakness, sometimes muscle pain
Hypercalcemia	Treatment of primary cause, which is often hyperparathyroidism, vitamin D malignancy (therefore surgical removal)	Headache, weakness, fatigue, proximal neuropathy, rigidity, tremor, disorientation
Hypocalcemia	Intravenous administration of calcium (possible medical emergency)	Hyperexcitability of the peripheral and central nervous systems, which can lead to tetany and convulsions

Table 19-2. Neurological complications of heavy metal poisoning

Type of metal	Treatment	Neurological complication
Lead		
Source: lead paint, industrial (fumes of molten lead)	Elimination of source, reduction of fluids, intravenous urea or mannitol, use of chelating agents	Interstitial edema and hemorrhage (especially in cerebellum) in acute poisoning; all levels of CNS affected in chronic poisoning
		In children: seizures, mental retardation, behavior problems, and hyperactivity
		In adults: spasticity, rigidity, dementia, personality changes
		Peripheral neuropathy may occur in adults and children
Arsenic		
Source: paint and insecticides	Removal of source, gastric lavage, intravenous fluids, and maintenance of electrolyte balance; penicillamine used in acute poisoning	Demyelinization of peripheral nerves in all extremities
Manganese		
Source: industrial if manganese dust is not removed; symptoms appear 2 to 25 years after exposure	L-dopa	Neuronal loss in basal ganglia, substantia nigra, and cerebellum
		Initially psychiatric disturbances, including nervousness, irritability, and a tendency toward compulsive acts
		Later, muscular weakness and parkinsonian-like symptoms
Mercury		
Rare but may affect farmers and dental office workers	Penicillamine; function returns only with physical, occupational, and speech therapy	Loss of neurons, especially in cerebellum; also in cortex near calcarine fissure
		Alternating periods of confusion, drowsiness, and stupor with restlessness and excitability
		Ataxia, dysarthria, visual deterioration

cohol intoxication, perhaps through personal experience. Initially, alcohol produces relaxation and a loss of inhibitions. This is followed by a loss of judgment and coordination. If alcohol ingestion continues, a stuporous stage may be reached: the person "passes out" and awakens the next morning with a hangover. Drinking water and eating tend to alleviate the sick feeling, and the neurological signs are reversible at this stage. However, overly large volumes of alcohol can lead to coma and death. The symptoms of acute intoxication result from the direct effect of alcohol on the excitability of neurons, that is, inhibitory neurons become less excitable. Alcohol causes a decrease in membrane excitability. The cortex is usually affected first, and this effect descends the neuraxis. Coma is an indication of medullary involvement.

The individual with signs of acute intoxication will rarely, if ever, be seen in the clinic. However, the person with chronic alcohol intoxication will often show neurological complications. The most prevalent problems involve cortical function, cerebellar function, and peripheral neuropathies. The cortical and cerebellar problems involve the combination of alcohol effects and nutritional deficiency; peripheral neuropathies are believed to be a result of nutritional deficiencies.[66] Because large neurons are more difficult to excite, it is possible that the large neurons of the cortex and cerebellum are more easily affected by decreases in excitability. The cerebellum and frontal lobes of the cerebral cortex are more sensitive to the deleterious effects of alcohol. The nutritional deficits further exacerbate these problems as the lack of food causes a decrease in glucose available for brain metabolism. Vitamin deficiency, especially of the B vitamins, is a further cause of the symptomatology seen.

In addition to the effects of chronic alcohol on the

adult, alcohol can also be devastating to an unborn child. Because alcohol crosses the placenta, the developing brain with its high metabolic rate may be affected even in the absence of symptoms in the mother. Binge drinking by the mother can be as detrimental as abuse. This has become a great enough problem with enough similarities among affected infants that fetal alcohol syndrome is a recognizable disease at birth. In addition to a low birth weight and irritability, there are also distinct facial anomalies associated with this disease. A long-term evaluation of these children will provide information on other neurological problems that may become more evident as the child ages. Animal research indicates that brain maldevelopment and delays in reflex and motor development are not reversible.[112] One of the areas showing a decrease in size is the frontal cortex.[112] (See Chapters 8, 9, and 10 for further information on pediatric problems.)

Signs and symptoms of chronic alcoholism. The individual suffering from chronic alcoholism can have neurological and psychological impairment. Neurological symptoms include ataxia (especially in the trunk and lower limbs), incoordination, and peripheral neuropathy. Seizures may also be a complication. The ataxia that occurs is the classic staggering, wide-based gait depicted on every television program showing an alcoholic. The person cannot perform a tandem gait (walking forward in heel-to-toe fashion on a straight line) and has difficulty maintaining an upright posture with the feet together. If weakness because of neuropathy is present, the ataxia, of course, is worsened.

The psychological problems are also probably fairly well-known. These include delirium tremens (DTs), dementia, and the Wernicke-Korsakoff syndrome. DTs are most frequently seen in any withdrawal from alcohol. This is when the alcoholic sees the "pink elephants." The individual is restless, irritable, disoriented, and often hallucinates when awake; speech may be unintelligible. Temperature is elevated, and the person is dehydrated. DTs are probably caused by a type of rebound phenomenon: the depressed neuronal firing is freed from the alcohol and neurons are overly irritable. Deep tendon reflexes are also hyperactive.

Wernicke-Korsakoff syndrome (hyphenated because the two syndromes are usually seen together) is caused by frontal lobe involvement complicated by vitamin B_1 deficiency. In Korsakoff's syndrome there is a loss of memory, especially short-term and recent memory. The individual then tends to make up answers and may "remember" the physician or even the therapist as someone she or he met in a bar; a simple breakfast just completed may become a banquet feast. These confabulations are a classic sign of the chronic alcoholic. They are probably an attempt to function without recent memory. Wernicke's syndrome includes ataxia (already described), disorientation, dementia, and ophthalmoplegia. The eye problems

include nystagmus followed by lateral rectus weakness and double vision.

The peripheral neuropathies exacerbate all of these problems. The muscles are tender to touch and there may be a burning sensation in the hands and feet, which intensifies the irritability of DTs. Muscle weakness will increase the apparent ataxia, and decreased sensation causes a further loss of proprioceptive cues the individual might otherwise use.

Pharmacological considerations and medical management. The biggest factor in treatment is, of course, withdrawal from alcohol. Librium, which is synonymous with chlorpromazine and chlordiazepoxide, is used to keep the individual sedated and to reduce DTs. At the same time, the electrolyte and water balance of the body must be restored. Because alcohol usually causes dehydration, the body's fluids must be replaced, but refurnishing necessary electrolytes also requires attention. In addition, nutrition is important because the nutritional deficiencies are as harmful as the effects of alcohol itself. Large supplements of B complex vitamins should be added to the diet.

If the individual has been hospitalized fairly early, abstains from alcohol, and controls the diet, some of the symptoms of the disease can be reversed. This is especially true of the eye involvement and of much of the ataxia. Permanent memory deficits, however, often occur; the longer the alcoholism, the worse the memory. The neuropathies, if they recover, recover very slowly. Both the myelin sheath and the axon have been damaged. In long-standing alcoholism the nerve roots also become involved, lessening the chances for regeneration and recovery. The best cure therefore is prevention.

Evaluation. Before proceeding with a neurological evaluation, the therapist needs to assess the client's mental status. Is there any short-term retention? Can the individual's perception of sensation be trusted as accurate? If the client cannot perform a task, is it because he or she did not understand the instructions or has forgotten them? All commands should be single commands and kept as short as possible. Because weakness and loss of sensation, especially proprioception, can produce signs similar to ataxia, it is a good idea to evaluate peripheral nerve function first. Nerve conduction tests are useful evaluation tools for the alcoholic patient.

In assessing the degree of cerebellar involvement, static posture and movement need to be evaluated. This includes the ability to stand upright with the feet together, the width between the legs in standing or walking, and the presence or absence of equilibrium reactions. Sometimes there is a delay in equilibrium reactions that needs to be recorded.

Treatment considerations. Chapter 21 on cerebellar disease deals with actual treatment methodologies; however, treatment of the alcoholic adds a few problems that may not be encountered in these other disease entities. The first problem encountered is one of setting goals because the client may not be sufficiently mentally alert to participate in goal setting. Second, the degree of recovery is impossible to know; the therapist should strive for as much recovery as possible. Of course, the achievement of whatever goals are established depends on abstinence from alcohol.

In treatment of alcoholism, the mental status is a crucial problem. If dementia is present, the client will not be able to use higher-level thought processes or achieve cortical control over movement. Therefore techniques that require attention or learning may have very limited success. In addition, carry-over from one session to the next will be hampered because the client may have no recollection of the previous treatment or even of the therapist. The lack of attention and memory also means that, just as in evaluation, all commands must be brief and simple. The treatment session should be well-structured so that the client's thoughts are not allowed to wander. Sometimes it may also be advisable to adjust the length of treatment to the individual's tolerance.

There is another consideration in the treatment of the alcoholic, and this is the effect of exercise on physical well-being in general. Even without neurological signs, alcoholic individuals may benefit from a carefully monitored program of physical activity—carefully monitored because this client may be in a debilitated condition with generalized weakness and even respiratory problems. A study in Japan has shown that physical exercise can help the alcoholic's general rehabilitation progress.[139] As in all diseases discussed so far, the exact treatment procedures will depend on the results of the evaluation. Documentation of the effects of therapy should be clear and, whenever possible, quantifiable.

SUMMARY

This chapter has focused on the pathophysiology, evaluation, and treatment of genetic, hereditary, and metabolic diseases affecting adults. In all of these diseases the therapist is an important (though sometimes underused) part of the rehabilitation team. A knowledge of the possible mechanisms involved in the production of the varying movement disorders may make the appropriate evaluation and subsequent treatment more meaningful. Even with degenerative, progressive disorders the therapist plays an important role in maintaining quality of life and assists the client and family in coping with the disease. Throughout this chapter the importance of documentation and publication has been stressed. This will assist in the development of improved therapeutic techniques and may also be of help to researchers in planning and interpreting appropriate experimental studies.

REFERENCES

1. Ahrens J: Reciprocal Ia inhibition in the Parkinson patient at rest, master's thesis, University of Iowa, Iowa City, 1980.
2. Amato G and others: The role of internal pallidal segment on the initiation of a goal directed movement, Neurosci Lett 9:159, 1978.
3. Ayres AJ: Sensory integration and learning disorders, Los Angeles, 1972, Western Psychological Services.
4. Baldessarini RJ and Tarsy D: Dopamine and the pathophysiology of dyskinesias induced by antipsychotic drugs, Annu Rev Neurosci 3:23, 1980.
5. Ball J: Demonstration of the traditional approach in the treatment of a patient with parkinsonism, Am J Phys Med 46:1034, 1967.
6. Ball J: Personal communication, 1983.
7. Barbeau A: Parkinson's disease: etiologic considerations. In Yahr, MD, editor: The basal ganglia, New York, 1976, Raven Press.
8. Barbeau A and others: Ecogenetics of Parkinson's disease: prevalence and environmental aspects in rural areas, Can J Neurol Sci 14:36, 1987.
9. Bathien N and Rondot P: Reciprocal continuous inhibition in rigidity of parkinsonism, J Neurol Neurosurg Psychiatry 40:20, 1977.
10. Battig K and others: Comparison of the effects of frontal and caudate lesions on discrimination learning in monkeys, J Comp Physiol Psychol 55:458, 1962.
11. Benita M and others: Effects of ventrolateral thalamic nucleus cooling on initiation of forelimb ballistic flexion movements by conditioned cats, Exp Brain Res 34:435, 1979.
12. Bird ED: Biochemical studies on γ-aminobutyric acid metabolism in Huntington's chorea. In Bradford HF and Marsden CD, editors: Biochemistry and neurology, London, 1976, Academic Press, Ltd, pp 83-90.
13. Bobath B: Adult hemiplegia: evaluation and treatment, London, 1976, William Heinemann Medical Books, Ltd.
14. Boop R and others: Methylphenidate (MPH): absence of readiness potential in patients with Parkinson's disease and in patients following long-term MPH treatment, Neurosci Abst 7:779, 1981.
15. Bowen FP: Behavioral alterations in patients with basal ganglia lesions. In Yahr MD, editor: The basal ganglia, New York, 1976, Raven Press, pp 169-180.
16. Brooks VB: Roles of cerebellum and basal ganglia in initiation and control of movements, Can J Neurol Sci 2:265, 1975.
17. Buchwald NA and others: The "caudate-spindle." III. Inhibition by high frequency stimulation of subcortical structures, Electroencephalogr Clin Neurophysiol 13:525, 1961.
18. Buchwald NA and others: The "caudate-spindle." IV. A behavioral index of caudate-induced inhibition, Electroencephalogr Clin Neurophysiol 13:536, 1961.
19. Buchwald NA and others: The basal ganglia and the regulation of response and cognitive sets. In Brazier, MAB, editor: Growth and development of the brain, New York, 1975, Raven Press.
20. Burt DR and others: Antischizophrenic drugs: chronic treatment elevates dopamine receptor binding in brain, Science 196:326, 1977.
21. Calne DB and others: Bromocriptine in parkinsonism, Br Med J 4:442, 1974.
22. Carlsson A: Some aspects of dopamine in the basal ganglia. In Yarh MD, editor: The basal ganglia, New York, 1976, Raven Press.
23. Carpenter MB: Anatomy of the basal ganglia and related nuclei: a review. In Yahr MD, editor: The basal ganglia, New York, 1976, Raven Press.
24. Cohen G and Heikkila RE: The generation of hydrogen peroxide, superoxide radical and the hydroxyl radical by 6-hydroxy dopamine, dialuric acid and related aytotoxic agents, J Biol Chem 249:2447, 1974.
25. Cooper IS: Involuntary movement disorders, New York, 1969, Paul B Hoeber, Inc.
26. Cotzias GC and others: Modification of parkinsonism: chronic treatment with L-dopa, N Eng J Med 280:337, 1969.

27. Davis CG and others: Chronic parkinsonism secondary to intravenous injection of meperidine, Psychiat Res 1:249, 1979.
28. Diamond SG and Markham CH: One year trial of pergolide as an adjunct to sinemet in the treatment of Parkinson's disease, Adv Neurol 40:537, 1984.
29. Dieckmann G and Sasaki K: Recruiting responses in the cerebral cortex produced by putamen and pallidum stimulation, Exp Brain Res 10:236, 1970.
30. DeLong MR: Activity of basal ganglia neurons during movement, Brain Res 40:127, 1972.
31. DeLong MR and Strick P: Relation of basal ganglia, cerebellum and motor cortex units to ramp and ballistic limb movements, Brain Res 71:327, 1974.
32. Denny-Brown D: The basal ganglia and their relation to disorders of movement, Liverpool, UK, 1962, Liverpool University Press.
33. Denny-Brown D and Yanagesawa N: The role of the basal ganglia in the initiation of movement. In Yahr MD, editor: The basal ganglia, New York, 1976, Raven Press, pp 115-150.
34. Divac I: Neostriatum and functions of perfrontal cortex, Acta Neurobiol Exp 32:461, 1972.
35. Dom R and others: Neuropathology of Huntington's chorea, Neurology 26:64, 1976.
36. Duvoisin RC: Parkinson's disease: a guide for patient and family, New York, 1978, Raven Press.
37. Evarts EV: Pyramidal tract activity associated with a conditioned hand movement in the monkey, J Neurophysiol 29:1011, 1966.
38. Fahn S: The extrapyramidal disorders. In Wyngaarden JB and Smith LH, editors: Cecil's textbook of medicine, ed 16, Philadelphia, 1982, WB Saunders Co.
39. Feltz P: γ-Aminobutyric acid and a caudate nigral inhibition, Can J Physiol Pharmacol 49:1113, 1971.
40. Ferrier D: The functions of the brain, London, 1876, Smith, Elder.
41. Freed WJ and others: Transplanted adrenal chromaffin cells in rat brain reduce lesion-induced rotational behavior, Nature 292:351, 1981.
42. Fuster JM and Alexander GE: Neuron activity related to short-term memory, Science 173:652, 1971.
43. Fuxe K and others: Heterogeneities in the dopamine neuron systems and dopamine cotransmission in the basal ganglia and the relevance of receptor-receptor interactions. In Fahn S and others, editors: Recent developments in Parkinson's disease, New York, 1986, Raven Press.
44. Garcia-Rill E and Anchors JM: Effects of nigral and cortical stimulation on caudate carbohydrate metabolism, Brain Res 156:407, 1978.
45. Gelfand IM and others: Some problems in the analysis of movements. In Gelfand VS and others, editors: Models of the structural-functional organization of certain biological systems, Cambridge, 1971, The MIT Press.
46. Goldman PS: The role of experience in recovery of function following orbital prefrontal lesions in infant monkeys, Neuropsychologia 14:401, 1976.
47. Granit R and Kaada BR: Influence of stimulation of central nervous structures on muscle spindles in cat, Acta Physiol Scand 27:130, 1952.
48. Grimby L and Hannerz J: Disturbances in the voluntary recruitment order of anterior tibial motor units in bradykinesia of parkinsonism, J Neurol Neurosurg Psychiatry 37:47, 1974.
49. Hallett M and others: Analysis of stereotyped voluntary movements at the elbow in patients with Parkinson's disease, J Neurol Neurosurg Psychiatry 40:1129, 1977.
50. Harper PS: Localization of the gene for Huntington's Chorea, Trends Neurosci 7:1, 1984.
51. Hartmann-von Monakow K and others: Projections of the precentral

52. motor cortex and other cortical areas of the frontal lobe to the subthalamic nucleus in the monkey, Exp Brain Res 33:395, 1978.
52. Hayden MR: Huntington's chorea, Berlin, 1981, Springer-Verlag.
53. Heikkila RE and others: Protection against the dopaminergic neurotoxicity of MPTP by monoamine oxidase inhibitors, Nature 311:467, 1984.
54. Heimer L: The human brain and spinal cord: functional neuroanatomy and dissection guide, New York, 1983, Springer-Verlag.
55. Hoehn MM and Yahr MD: Parkinsonism: onset, progression and mortality, Neurology 17:427, 1967.
56. Hore J and Vilis T: Arm movement performance during reversible basal ganglia lesions in the monkey, Exp Brain Res 39:217, 1980.
57. Hore J and others: Basal ganglia cooling disables learned arm movements of monkeys in the absence of visual guidance, Science 195:584, 1977.
58. Hornykiewicz O: The mechanisms of action of L-dopa in Parkinson's disease, Life Sci 15:1249, 1974.
59. Hull CD and others: Intracellular responses in caudate and cortical neurons. In Crane G and Gardener R, editors: Psychotropic drugs and dysfunctions of the basal ganglia, Washington, DC, 1969, US Public Health Service.
60. Hull CD and others: Intracellular responses of caudate neurons to brainstem stimulation, Brain Res 22:163, 1970.
61. Hull CD and others: Intracellular responses of caudate neurons to temporally and spatially combined stimuli, Exp Neurol 38:324, 1973.
62. Jellinger K: Pathology of parkinsonism. In Fahr S and others, editors: Recent developments in Parkinson's disease, New York, 1986, Raven Press.
63. Kelly PJ and Gillingham FJ: The long-term results of stereotaxic surgery and L-dopa therapy in patients with Parkinson's disease: a ten-year follow up study, J Neurosurg 53:332, 1980.
64. Kemp JM and Powell TPS: The connexions of the striatum and globus pallidus: synthesis and speculation, Philos Trans R Soc Lond (Biol) 262:441, 1971.
65. Kim R and others: Projections of globus pallidus and adjacent structures: an autoradiographic study in the monkey, J Comp Neurol 169:263, 1976.
66. Kissin B and Begleiter H, editors: The biology of alcoholism, vol 5, New York, 1977, Plenum Publishing Corp.
67. Klawans HL: Therapeutic approaches to neuroleptic induced tardive dyskinesia, Res Publ Assoc Res Nerv Ment Dis 55:447, 1976.
68. Klawans HL and others: Presymptomatic and early detection in Huntington's disease, Ann Neurol 8:343, 1980.
69. Klawans HL Jr and Weiner W: The effect of δ-amphetamine of choreiform disorders, Neurology 24:312, 1974.
70. Kling A and Tucker TJ: Effects of combined lesions of frontal granular cortex and caudate nucleus in the neonatal monkey, Brain Res 6:428, 1967.
71. Knott M and Voss D: Proprioceptive neuromuscular facilitation patterns and techniques, ed 2, New York, 1968, Harper & Row, Publisher, Inc.
72. Kopin IJ and others: Mechanisms of neurotoxicity of MPTP. In Fahr S and others, editors: Recent developments in Parkinson's disease, New York, 1986, Raven Press.
73. Kornhuber HH: Motor functions of cerebellum and basal ganglia: the cerebellocortical saccadic (ballistic) clock, the cerebellonuclear hold regulator, and the basal ganglia ramp (voluntary speed smooth movement) generator, Kybernetik 8:157, 1971.
74. Krauthamer GM and Albe-Fessard D: Electrophysiological studies of the basal ganglia and striopallidal inhibition of non-specific afferent activity, Neuropsychologia 2:73, 1964.
75. Kubota K and Hamada I: Preparatory activity of monkey pyramidal tract neurons related to quick movement onset during visual tracking performance, Brain Res 168:435, 1979.

76. Kubota K and Niki H: Prefrontal cortical unit activity and delayed alteration performance in monkeys, J Neurophysiol 34:337, 1971.

77. Kunzle H: Bilateral projections from precentral motor cortex to the putamen and other parts of the basal ganglia: an autoradiographic study in Macaca fascicularis, Brain Res 88:195, 1976.

78. Kunzle H: Projections from the primary somatosensory cortex to basal ganglia and thalamus in the monkey, Exp Brain Res 30:481, 1977.

79. Labuszewski T and Lidsky TI: Basal ganglia influences on brain stem trigeminal neurons, Exp Neurol 65:471, 1979.

80. Langston JW and others: Chronic parkinsonism in humans due to a product of meperidine analog synthesis, Science 219:979, 1983.

81. Langston JW: MPTP neurotoxicity: an overview and characterization of phrases of toxicity, Life Sci 36:201, 1985.

82. Levine MS and others: Pallidal and entopeduncular intracellular responses to striatal, cortical, thalamic and sensory inputs, Exp Neurol 44:448, 1974.

83. Levine MS and others: The spontaneous firing patterns of forebrain neurons. II. Effects of unilateral caudate nuclear ablation, Brain Res 78:411, 1974.

84. Levine MS and others: The spontaneous firing pattern of forebrain neurons. III. Prevention of induced asymmetries in caudate neuronal firing rates by unilateral thalamic lesions, Brain Res 131:215, 1977.

85. Levine MS and others: Long-term decreases in spontaneous firing of caudate neurons induced by amphetamine in cats, Brain Res 194:263, 1980.

86. Levine MS and others: Long-term behavioral and neurophysiological effects of neonatal δ-amphetamine administration in kittens, Neurosci Abst 8:965, 1982.

87. Lidsky TI and others: Pallidal and entropeduncular single unit activity in cats during drinking, Electroencephalogr Clin Neurophysiol 39(1):79, 1975.

88. Lidsky TI and others: The effects of stimulation of trigeminal sensory afferents upon caudate units in cats, Brain Res Bull 4:9, 1979.

89. Lidsky TI and others: Trigeminal influences on entopeduncular units, Brain Res 141:227, 1978.

90. Livesey PJ and Rankine-Wilson J: Delayed alternation learning under electrical (blocking) stimulation of the caudate nucleus in the cat, J Comp Physiol Psychol 88:342, 1975.

91. Lloyd KG and others: The neurochemistry of Parkinson's disease: effect of L-dopa therapy, J Pharmacol Exp Ther 195:453, 1975.

92. MacKay AVP: Clinical controversies in tardive dyskinesia. In Marsden CD and Fahn S, editors: Movement disorders, Boston, 1981, Butterworth Publishers, Inc.

93. Madrazo I and others: Open neurosurgical autograft of adrenal medulla to the right caudate nucleus in two patients with intractable Parkinson's disease, N Engl J Med 316:831, 1987.

94. Magendie M: Fonctions et maladies du système nerveux, Paris, 1841, Lecapalin. (Translated in Assoc Res Nerv Ment Dis 21:8, 1940.)

95. Markham CH: Personal communication, 1983.

96. Markham CH and Diamond SG: Evidence to support early levodopa therapy in Parkinson disease, Neurology 31:125, 1981.

97. Martin JP: The basal ganglia and posture, London, 1967, Pitman Books, Ltd.

98. Massion J and Smith AM: Activity of ventrolateral thalamic neurons related to posture and movement during contact placing responses in the cat, Brain Res 61:400, 1973.

99. Matsunami K and Cohen B: Afferent modulation of unit activity in globus pallidus and caudate neurons and changes induced by vestibular nucleus and pyramidal tract stimulation, Brain Res 91:140, 1975.

100. McGeer PL and others: Aging and extrapyramidal function, Arch Neurol 34:33, 1977.

101. Melmon KL and Morrelli HF: Clinical pharmacology: basic principles in therapeutics, ed 2, New York, 1978, Macmillan, Inc, pp 893-900.

102. Melnick M and others: Activity of forebrain neurons during alternating movement in cats, Electroencephalogr Clin Neurophysiol 57:57, 1984.

103. Melnick ME and others: Comparison of behavioral effects of MPTP in young adult and year-old rats. In Markey SP and others, editors: MPTP: a neurotoxin producing a Parkinsonian syndrome, Orlando, Fla, 1986, Academic Press.

104. Mettler FA and others: The extrapyramidal system, Arch Neurol Psychiatry 41:984, 1939.

105. Milner-Brown HS and others: Electrical properties of motor units in Parkinsonism and a possible relationship with bradykinesia, J Neurol Neurosurg Psychiatry 42:35, 1979.

106. Muskens L: The central connection of the vestibular nuclei with the corpus striatum and their significance for ocular movements and for locomotion, Brain 45:452, 1922.

107. Nauta HJW and Cole M: Efferent projections of the subthalamic nucleus: an autoradiographic study in monkey and cat, J Comp Neurol 180:1, 1978.

108. Neafsey EJ and others: Preparation for movement in the cat. I. Unit activity in the cerebral cortex, Electroenchephalogr Clin Neurophysiol 44:706, 1978.

109. Neafsey EJ and others: Preparation for movement in the cat. II. Unit activity in the basal ganglia and thalamus, Electroencephalogr Clin Neurophysiol 44:714, 1978.

110. Newton RA and Price DD: Modulation of cortical and pyramidal tract induced motor responses by electrical stimulation of the basal ganglia, Brain Res 85:403, 1975.

111. Nieoullon A and others: Interdependence of the nigrostriatal dopaminergic systems on the two sides of the brain in the cat, Science 198:416, 1977.

112. Norton S and others: Early motor development and cerebral cortical morphology in rats exposed prenatally to alcohol, Alcoholism 12:130, 1988.

113. Nothnagel H: Experimentalle Untersuchungen uber die Funktion des Geherns, Virchows Arch 57:184, 1873. (Translated in Assoc Res Nev Ment Dis 21:8, 1940.)

114. Nutt JG and others: The "on-off" phenomenon in Parkinson's disease: relation to levadopa absorption and transport, N Engl J Med 310:483, 1984.

115. Olmstead CE and Villablanca JR: Effects of caudate nuclei or frontal cortical ablations in kittens: bar pressing performance, Exp Neurol 63:244, 1979.

116. Palmer SS and others: Exercise therapy for Parkinson's disease, Arch Phys Med Rehab 67:741, 1986.

117. Pechadre JC and others: Parkinsonian akinesia, rigidity and tremor in the monkey, J Neurol Sci 28:147, 1976.

118. Petajan JH and others: Motor unit control in Huntington's disease: a possible presymptomatic test. In Chase TN and others, editors: Advances in neurology, vol 23, New York, 1979, Raven Press, pp 163-175.

119. Poirier LJ and others: Stereotaxic lesions and movement disorders in monkeys, Adv Neurol 10:5, 1975.

120. Pollock LJ and Davis L: Muscle tone in parkinsonian states, Arch Neurol Psychiat 23:303, 1930.

121. Potegal M: The caudate nucleus egocentric localization system, Acta Neurobiol Exp 32:479, 1972.

122. Potegal M and others: Vestibular input to the caudate nucleus, Exp Neurol 32:448, 1971.

123. Roberts E: Some thoughts about GABA and the basal ganglia. In Yahr MD, editor: The basal ganglia, New York, 1976, Raven Press.

124. Schneider JS and Lidsky TI: Processing of somatosensory information in striatum of behaving cats, J Neurophysiol 45:841, 1981.

125. Segundo JP and Machne X: Unitary responses to afferent volleys in lenticular nucleus and claustrum, J Neurophysiol 19:325, 1956.

126. Shellenberger MK: Persistent alteration of rat brain monoamine levels by carbon monoxide exposure: sex differences and behavioral correlation, Neurotoxicology 2:431, 1981.

127. Shoulson I and Fahn S: Huntington's disease: clinical care and evaluation, Neurology 29:1, 1979.

128. Shoulson I and others: Clinical care of the patient and family with Huntington's disease. In Commission for the Control of Huntington's Disease and its Consequences, vol 2, National Institutes of Health, Washington, DC, 1977, pp 421-451.

129. Shoulson I and others: Huntington's disease; treatment with muscimol, a GABA- mimetic drug, Trans Am Neurol Assoc 102:124, 1977.

130. Smith JM and Baldessarini RJ: Changes in prevalence, severity and recovery in tardive dyskinesia with age, Arch Gen Psychiatry 37:1368, 1980.

131. Soltysik S and others: Single unit activity in basal ganglia of monkeys during performance of a delayed response task, Electroencephalogr Clin Neurophysiol 39:65, 1975.

132. Stern G: The effect of lesions in the substantia nigra, Brain 89:449, 1966.

133. Strick PL: Anatomical analysis of ventrolateral thalamic input to primate motor cortex, J Neurophysiol 39:1020, 1976.

134. Tarsy D and others: Physostigmine in choreiform movement disorders, Neurology 24:28, 1974.

135. Tatton WG and others: Altered motor cortical activity in extrapyramidal rigidity. In Poirier LJ and others, editors: Advances in neurology, vol 24, New York, 1979, Raven Press.

136. Teuber HL: Complex functions of basal ganglia. In Yahr MD, editor: The basal ganglia, New York, 1976, Raven Press.

137. Thach WT: Discharge of cerebellar neurons related to two maintained postures and two prompt movements. I. Nuclear cell output, J Neurophysiol 33:527, 1970.

138. Thach WT: Discharge of cerebellar neurons related to two maintained postures and two prompt movements. II. Purkinje cell output and input, J Neurophysiol 33:537, 1970.

139. Tsukue I and Shohoji T: Movement therapy for alcoholic patients, J Stud Alcohol 42:144, 1981.

140. Tucker TJ and Kling A: Differential effects of early and late lesions of frontal granular cortex in the monkey, Brain Res 5:377, 1967.

141. Villablanca JR and Marcus R: Effects of caudate nuclei removal in cats: comparison with effects of frontal cortex ablation. In Buchwald NA and Brazier MAM, editors: Brain mechanisms in mental retardation, New York, 1975, Academic Press, Inc.

142. Wagner GC and others: Long-lasting depletions of striatal dopamine and loss of dopamine uptake sites following repeated administration of methamphetamine, Brain Res 181:151, 1980.

143. Wagner GC and Jarvis MF: Age-dependent effects of MPTP. In Markey SP and others, editors: MPTP: a neurotoxin producing a Parkinsonian syndrome, Orlando, Fla, 1986, Academic Press.

144. Walshe FMR: Nature of musculature rigidity of paralysis agitans and its relationship to tremor, Brain 47:159, 1924.

145. Walshe JM: Wilson's disease: the presenting symptoms, Arch Dis Child 37:253, 1962.

146. Willis T: Cerebri anatomie cui accessit nervorum descriptio et usus, 1664. (Translated in Assoc Res Nerv Ment Dis 21:8, 1940.

147. Wilson SAK: An experimental research into the anatomy and physiology of the corpus striatum, Brain 36:427, 1914.

148. Winkelmuller W and Nitsch FM: Quantitative registration of motor disorders following bilateral lesions of S.N. in the rat, Appl Neurophysiol 38:291, 1975.

149. Woodworth RS and Schlosberg H: Experimental psychology, New York, 1961, Holt, Rinehart & Winston.

150. Yeterian EH and Van Hosesen GW: Cortico-striate projections in the rhesus monkey: the organization of certain cortico-caudate connections, Brain Res 139:43, 1978.

Chapter 20

BRAIN TUMORS

Gertrude Freeman

Rehabilitation is the restoration or improvement of the physical function of a patient, which has been impaired by accidents, disease, or its treatment. Among the patients who may benefit from the rehabilitative services of the physical therapist are those with a brain tumor.[10] Until recently, most people could not see any rationale for applying the benefits of rehabilitation to a group of patients who, if not cured, were likely to die within a relatively short time, but today many people are cured of tumors, whereas others live with chronic illness that is interspersed by remissions. Unfortunately, these patients are often left with severe functional problems. The physical therapist can make a significant contribution towards improving the quality of life remaining to such patients.[4,10,11,25]

The management of a patient with a tumor is much like that of any patient with a chronic neurological condition (i.e., patients with problems resulting from vascular insult or trauma).[10,15] In patients with other conditions, however, the disease process usually has been arrested before rehabilitative measures are employed, enabling the therapist to make certain assumptions about the patient's future and to plan a rehabilitative strategy; absolute goals can be formulated in the secure knowledge that the rehabilitative program will not be complicated by a deteriorating physical condition. This may not be true of the patient with a brain tumor, although the rehabilitative plan may have essentially the same goals. As with any patient, the therapist must be flexible, adjusting his or her expectations as the patient's physical status changes in the course of the disease.[15]

The multifaceted team approach, using the combined skills of all its members, has been successful in the rehabilitation of chronic neuromuscular disability and can be profitably applied to managing the patient with a brain tumor. Rehabilitation results can be predicted with greater certainty when the natural history of the primary tumor, the therapeutic medical-surgical approach and its complications, and the patient's current clinical status are taken into consideration. It is essential for the physical therapist to work closely with the entire medical team to determine appropriate care.[26] Therapists must be sensitive to the patient's physical and psychological needs and adjust rehabilitation goals and methods accordingly. To be a respected member of the oncology team, a physical therapist needs to have a knowledge of tumor management, as well as management of the particular neurological deficit.[28]

AN OVERVIEW OF BRAIN TUMORS
History

The microscopic characteristics of brain tumors were first recognized during the latter half of the nineteenth century. However, an orderly scheme of classification based

□ Sincere appreciation is expressed to Bonnie Blossom, MA, PT and Lois Barnhart, PT for their contribution to the chapter on brain tumors in the first edition of this book.

on cell morphology was not established until 1926, when Bailey and Cushing published a monograph in which tumors were named according to the histological resemblance between their cells and cells of normal development. In more recent years, there has been a trend toward simplification so that a diagnosis with prognostic implication can be made. One of the easiest systems to understand is the classification of Kernahan and Sayre, in which the name of the tumor is based on the cells present in the adult brain combined with a malignancy grading of I to IV (IV being the most malignant).[1,22,23] In 1970 the World Health Organization (WHO), realizing the need for a universal classification of CNS tumors, established a center for this purpose. The resulting publication, in which tumors were named according to microscopic characteristics, appeared in 1979. The WHO classification has proven to be useful to many neuropathologists. The present classification will continue to evolve as our understanding of tumor cells increases.[36]

Etiology and incidence

The American Cancer Society estimates that 10,900 cases of primary brain and central nervous system tumors occur yearly, with a slightly greater incidence projected for males than females (5900 and 5000 respectively). Other statistics indicate that about 8500 deaths occur annually as a result of brain tumors.[18] Another 67,000 cases, or 18% of cancer patients, develop metastasis to the brain from other sites.[18] Metastatic tumors are currently more frequent in males, but this trend appears to be changing in tandem with the changing statistics for lung cancer.[36]

The majority of brain tumors occur in two age ranges: childhood (3 to 12 years) and later life (50 to 70 years). Pediatric tumors are quite different in histology and behavior than those of adults. Nearly two thirds of pediatric CNS lesions are infratentorial in location, whereas an equivalent proportion of adult tumors are supratentorial. Most pediatric tumors arise in the cerebellum, brainstem, or midbrain/thalamus region. Cortical or hemispheric lesions are seen with much greater frequency in the adult population.

The cause of brain tumors is unknown. Certain tumors appear to be congenital; others may be related to hereditary factors. It has been suggested that intracranial tumors may be secondary to craniocerebral trauma or inflammatory disease. Some interesting work suggests that living near or under high-voltage electrical transmission lines may have etiological significance. No conclusive evidence is currently available to support any of the hypotheses.[18,23]

Classification of tumors

It is important that physical therapists who find themselves treating patients with brain tumors have a knowledge of their classification. The understanding of the clinical behavior of a brain tumor depends on an accurate classification of the cell of origin and on the degree of aggressiveness of the cells. The brain tumor classification of Kernhan and Sayre, along with the percentage of occurrence, is presented in Table 20-1. Characteristics of the most common brain tumors are described in the following paragraphs, and biological as well as histological malignancy is discussed.

Tumors may be classed as primary or secondary (metastatic). As seen in Table 20-1, the common primary tumors include the glial series, meningiomas, pituitary tumors, and neurilemmomas. The glial series makes up the majority of primary tumors (40% to 50%). These tumors arise from neuroglial cells, which form the supporting substance of the central nervous system. Gliomas vary in their biological and growth characteristics; some are benign and slow growing whereas others are highly malignant. Gliomas produce symptoms that are focal in nature as a result of local infiltration, destruction, or pressure on the brain; they rarely metastasize.[5,23]

Table 20-1. Histological classification of tumors

Tumor	Percent
Gliomas	40-50
Astrocytoma grade I	5-10
Astrocytoma grade II	2-5
Astrocytoma grades III and IV (glioblastoma multiform)	20-30
Medulloblastoma	3-5
Oligodendroglioma	1-4
Ependymoma grades I-IV	1-3
Meningioma	12-20
Pituitary tumors	5-15
Neurilemmomas (mainly cranial nerve VIII)	3-10
Metastatic tumors	5-10
Blood vessel tumors	0.5-1
Arteriovenous malformations	
Hemangioblastomas	
Endotheliomas	0.5-1
Tumors of developmental defects	2-3
Dermoids, epidermoids, teratomas, chordomas, paraphyseal cysts, craniopharyngiomas	3-8
Pinealomas	0.5-0.8
Miscellaneous	
Sarcomas, papillomas of the choroid plexus, lipomas, unclassified, etc.	1-3

From Schwartz SI, editor: Principles of surgery, ed 2, New York, 1974, McGraw-Hill, Book Co.

Astrocytomas, the most commonly occurring gliomas, may develop in the cerebral hemispheres, the brainstem, or the cerebellum. They range from the benign, slow-growing variety to the highly malignant glioblastoma multiform. The peak incidence of cerebral astrocytomas occurs during the third and fourth decades of life with the frontal lobes the most common site of origin. The cerebellar astrocytoma is the most common infratentorial tumor of children.[13]

Glioblastoma multiform-astrocytoma (GM-A) grade III and IV, the most common intercranial neoplasm of the adult, occurs most often in the fifth and sixth decades. It may be found in any area of the brain, but occurs most frequently in one frontal lobe and may spread via the corpus callosum to the opposite side. It is somewhat more prevalent in males. Life expectancy after diagnosis of GM-A Grade III or IV is usually about 6 to 12 months.[23]

Medulloblastoma is the second most common posterior fossa tumor found in children. This highly malignant tumor usually develops in the vermis of the cerebellum, advancing upward into the ventricular system and down into the spinal cord. The presence of a tumor close to the fourth ventricle results in the early development of hydrocephalus.[30]

Oligodendrogliomas constitute approximately 5% of all gliomas. They are found in proximity to neurons and are made up of cells that are involved in the process of myelination. These tumors occur in adults, most often during the third and fourth decades, and are located predominately in the frontal lobes of the cerebral hemispheres. Oligodendrogliomas are usually benign and have a tendency to calcify. Patients often survive with this type of tumor for 15 to 20 years.

Ependymoma, a type of glioma that occurs most commonly in children, is derived from the lining of the walls of the ventricular system and spinal canal. Those found in the parietal occipital region show a tendency to malignancy whereas those in the spinal cord are relatively benign.[23]

The *meningioma* is the most important tumor of the meningeal group. The majority of these tumors are benign, encapsulated, and slow growing. They are common in later years of life, and are more frequent in women. Because meningiomas are slow-growing tumors that compress the underlying structures rather than infiltrate adjacent tissue, abnormal signs and symptoms may be overlooked and the diagnosis missed completely.

Pituitary adenomas are tumors derived from cells of the anterior portion of the pituitary gland. They are usually found in middle-aged or older individuals. The clinical signs and symptoms are caused by the secretion of hormones through compression of the normally functioning pituitary.

Neurilemmomas are slow-growing benign tumors that originate from Schwann cells; the most common is an acoustic neuroma beginning from sheath cells of the vestibular portion of the eighth nerve. Treatment consists of surgical removal, which usually results in facial paralysis and deafness.[13,22,30]

Metastases to the brain constitute a major problem in the management of patients with malignancies. The literature varies, reporting from 5% to 20% as the percentage of intracranial neoplasms that arise from metastatic lesions. Metastatic brain tumors are most frequently reported between the fourth and seventh decades. The lesions that most commonly give rise to metastases to the brain are carcinomas of the lung and breast. The incidence of lung metastases varies from 28% to 60%, paralleling the increase in the frequency of the primary tumor. Improved management of patients with generalized metastases has recently led to longer survival with a greater incidence of brain metastases. The use of multiagent chemotherapy, in particular, because of its ability to retard metastases in other sites, has contributed to this trend. Multiagent chemotherapy may fail to cross the blood-brain barrier, which affects the management of cerebral metastases. Thus, the combination of an increasing incidence of lung cancer, with its predilection for brain metastases, and of the development of metastases by patients on systemic chemotherapy has led to a large increase in this disease.

The metastatic lesion may be singular or multiple; unfortunately, a single metastasis is rare. The occurrence may be at a late stage in the metastatic process or may be the first sign of a previously unrecognized primary tumor. The great majority of metastases reach the CNS through the arterial system. The frontal lobe of the cerebrum is the most common site for metastatic disease with other frequent sites being the temporal, parietal, and occipital lobes. Cerebellar metastases are infrequent and those to the brainstem are rarest of all.[22,23]

The use of the word "benign" in the classification of brain tumors can be misleading. When a neoplasm is designated as benign, one assumes that a complete cure is possible; conversely, a malignant tumor indicates a poor prognosis. This distinction is made on the basis of histological examination and is termed cytological malignancy. In assessing the malignant potential of a brain tumor, we must also consider biological malignancy, which is the likelihood that a tumor will kill the patient. Most cytologically malignant brain tumors are also biologically malignant. Irrespective of the histological malignancy of the tumor, its unimpeded growth as a space-occupying and expanding lesion within the confines of the skull inevitably leads to death, which, by definition, is equated to clinical malignancy. Various other factors, including the brain's exquisite sensitivity to increased internal pressure, tumor volume, surrounding brain edema, or ventricular obstruction dictate that certain cytologically benign tumors are biologically malignant and inevitably fatal.[5,22,29,36] Many current difficulties in the classification of tumors arise from our incomplete knowledge of their nature and should dissipate as our understanding of the embryology of tumor cells increases.

Signs and symptoms

The progression and type of neurological symptoms depend on the site, growth rate, and type of brain tumor. Neurological deficits are generally thought to be the result of two factors: focal disturbances caused by a tumor and increased intercranial pressure. Focal disturbances are a result of direct invasion or infiltration, causing destruction of neural tissue, and of compression of the brain. Compression may also result in necrosis as a result of alteration in circulation.[18,23,30] The increased intracranial pressure may be a result of several factors: an increase in the mass within the skull, edema formation around the tumor, and alteration in cerebrospinal fluid circulation. By the time increased pressure appears, a significant tumor mass or corresponding amount of cerebral edema is present. The symptoms of increased pressure include lethargy, drowsiness, irritability, and difficulty with ambulation. It is not surprising therefore that these symptoms reflect an unfavorable prognostic value.[1,13,23,30]

The most frequent signs and symptoms of tumors are headache, vomiting, and papilledema, which are seen during the course of illness in approximately 70% of brain tumor patients. Headache is the most common presenting symptom. It may be in a generalized area, or there may be regional correlation, in which case it has a localizing value. The headache associated with brain tumor is caused by irritation, traction, or compression on pain-sensitive structures including blood vessels, venous sinuses, and cranial nerves. The pain may be described as deep, aching, steady, dull, or severe. It is most severe in the morning, gradually decreasing during the day because of the increased CSF drainage in the erect versus the recumbent position. Vomiting that is related to increased intracranial pressure and brainstem compression occurs as a result of stimulation of the emetic center in the medulla. It occurs most frequently in children, is most likely to occur in the morning, is unrelated to meals, may be unaccompanied by other symptoms, and may be projectile in nature. Papilledema is caused by venous stasis, which leads to engorgement and swelling of the optic disc. In association with the papilledema, disturbances in vision—such as decreased visual acuity, diplopia, and deficits in the visual fields—may occur.[18,23]

Other symptoms common in adults with brain tumors are seizure activity and personality changes. Seizures, as a manifestation of altered neuronal excitability, are related to compression invasion or alteration in blood supply. They may take the form of a generalized grand mal type or a focal Jacksonian seizure (which can be helpful in localization). Often the first seizure is a momentary loss of alertness or concentration and may be ignored by the patient. It is of interest that the presence of a seizure as an early presenting symptom has a positive correlation in prognosis.[13,18,23]

Encroachment on highly specialized cerebral tissue will produce specific neurological deficits, depending on the area and extent of involvement (Table 20-2). The most common frontal lobe symptoms involve higher-level reasoning and judgment skills and may manifest themselves as inappropriate behavior, inability to concentrate, or indifference. (See Chapter 4, limbic system.) Other frontal lobe symptoms involve hemiparesis, caused by pressure on the neighboring precentral cortex and pathways and unsteadiness in gait, often imitating cerebellar ataxia (patients with frontal ataxia tend to fall backward). When the dominant frontal lobe is affected, aphasia and apraxia may be evident.

Lesions in the parietal lobe pose particular problems. Removal of significant portions of this area produce major, and often disabling, deficits. The left parietal lobe controls speech as well as sensory and motor functions in patients who are right-handed. The right parietal lobe, which has control of the left side of the body, is concerned with complex cognitive functions (concepts of space, music, and other abstractions) and sensory-motor control.

Visual loss in the upper quadrant of the eye opposite the lesion, which may progress to a complete hemianopsia and psychomotor seizures (which are described as visual, auditory, or olfactory hallucinations), are two common symptoms that occur with temporal lobe involvement. Varying degrees of receptive aphasia, beginning with difficulty in naming objects, occur when the involvement is in the dominant hemisphere. Facial weakness may result from pressure in the frontal cortex, and total destruction of the temporal lobe will result in such mental changes as irritability, depression, poor judgment, and childish behavior.

Tumors of the occipital lobe occur less frequently than do tumors of the previously mentioned lobes. Symptoms include convulsive seizures preceded by an aura. When the occipital cortex is involved, contralateral homonymous hemianopsia, visual agnosia, difficulty in judging distances, and the tendency to get lost in familiar surroundings may occur.

Cerebellar tumors cause early papilledema and may produce a headache at the base of the skull. Lesions of the cerebellum produce a variety of movement disorders, depending on the location of the tumor. Ataxia often suggests a midline cerebellar lesion. Dysmetria and dysdiadochokinesia reflect cerebellar hemisphere deficits, usually of ipsilateral representation. Symptoms that are less obvious than movement disorders, but equally characteristic of a cerebellar tumor, are hypotonia and scanning speech—a tendency to speak with a staccato rhythm, pronouncing each syllable rather than the word. (Refer to Chapter 21, cerebellar dysfunction).

Cerebral tumors can manifest their effects through in-

Table 20-2. Correlation between clinical symptoms and common neuroantomical location of tumor sites

Symptoms	Frontal lobe	Parietal lobe	Temporal lobe	Occipital lobe	Lateral and third ventricle	Fourth ventricle	Cerebellum	Midbrain	Brainstem	Cerebellopontine angle	Pineal	Pituitary	Pons	Posterior fossa
Headache				X	X	X	X				X	X		X
Nausea and vomiting				X	X	X	X				X	X		X
Vertigo				X				X		X				X
Light-headedness														
Convulsions														
Personality changes	X													
Papilledema	X		X											
Cranial nerve palsies									X					
Loss of social and sexual inhibitions or apathy/lethargy	X													
Astereognosis		X												
Nystagmus		X					X	X					X	
Contralateral hemiparesis														
Interruptions of consciousness				X										
Visual and auditory hallucination														
Contralateral hemianopsia		X	X	X										
Aphasia		X	X											
Sensory loss		X				X								
Motor loss						X	X	X	X					
Ataxia							X	X		X				
Hearing loss	X													
Alexia				X										
Homonymous hemianopsia			X	X										

creased intracranial pressure, causing specific cranial nerve compression, such as optic nerve compression resulting in blindness or ocular motor nerve damage resulting in ocular motility defects. Increased pressure also can cause clinical symptoms indirectly with ventricular compression or blockage resulting in hydrocephalus. Another major area is pituitary dysfunction with all of its ramifications of changes in body function, hypopituitarism, giantism, acromegaly, and Cushing's syndrome, depending on the type of tumor and its location.[18,22,23,30]

Diagnosis

Evaluation. The history of a patient suspected of having a brain tumor is a crucial part of the evaluation, because a presumptive diagnosis can be made from the symptoms of headache, evidence of seizure, or indications of a progressive loss of function. The neurological examination enables one to determine the current overall neurological status of the patient and can be helpful in localizing the lesion and predicting outcome. Patients with the poorest level of neurological function have the worst prognosis, regardless of therapy.

The neurological evaluation of a patient suspected of having a brain tumor must encompass the following areas: intellectual, cranial nerve, motor, sensory, reflex, and coordination functions. The most crucial of these areas is intellectual orientation to person, place, and time. The more subtle evaluation of intellectual function involves speech, memory, arithmetic, verbal skills, and association. In general, intellectual functions can be associated with anatomic areas; for example, speech is involved with temporal and parietal areas, especially left parietotemporal (in right-handed patients), memory is frontal and temporal, and mathematical skills are parietal. Association functions are primarily frontal and temporal in location.

Visual field and cranial nerve deficiencies can be very important in diagnosis. Expanding tumors frequently affect cranial nerves III, IV, and VI, and similar dysfunction may be produced by the compression and stretching of the cranial nerves. Visual deficits involve the entire visual pathway from occipital lobe to optic nerve. Motor functions involve pathways from the contralateral parietal motor area through the midbrain and brainstem; lesions at any point in the course of these tracts can result in weakness.

Cerebral lesions affecting motor function tend to produce a spastic paralysis with distal parts and fine motor functions first to be affected.

Sensory functions follow a complex pathway from the sensory areas of the contralateral parietal lobes by way of the midbrain, thalamus, and medulla to the cord. Brain tumors of the parietal lobes often produce sensory loss in distal parts earlier than motor loss, and testing for reactions to a pin, temperature, or vibration, as well as for tactile discrimination are all effective. Reflexes are hyperactive with intracranial mass lesions, becoming hypoactive in the terminal phases. Careful determination of the amplitude of the reflex responses on a numerical scale is helpful. Tumors in the cerebellar area result in transient symptoms of incoordination that are frequently observable only for short intervals.[22,23]

Diagnostic studies. Definitive diagnostic studies are of value to further substantiate a suspected diagnosis of brain tumor. When the history and neurological examination are suggestive of a brain tumor, the performance of a CT scan is often the next step. The CT (computed tomography) scan has markedly changed the diagnostic approach to the patient with a possible tumor, allowing precise, detailed analysis of density changes with minimal risk to the patient. It distinguishes CSF, blood, edema, tumor, and normal brain tissue in specific areas in three dimensions illuminating differences in quantitative density.[22]

Positron emission tomography (PET scanning) has become a major clinical research tool for imaging of cerebral blood flow, brain metabolism, and other chemical processes. It does have some disadvantages, such as a lack of detailed resolution and the fact that most positron emitting nucleoids decay so rapidly that their transportation from the cyclotron becomes a problem. A few isotopes, such as ruthenium derivatives, can be made at the site of examination.[6]

Although brain scanning with intravenously injected radio-labeled isotopes was once very important in tumor diagnosis, presently its primary value lies in the detection of meningiomas and certain well-vascularized astrocytomas or in the three-dimensional visualization of a tumor prior to surgery. Its use, in combination with a CT scan, increases the accuracy of diagnosis.

Skull films are usually ordered, and an electroencephalogram is helpful in tumor localization in patients who present with seizures. Careful examination of the visual field provides information that is helpful in localizing the lesion, and funduscopic examination determines the presence of papilledema.[22,23]

Magnetic resonance imaging (MRI) appears to be highly sensitive to the presence and characteristics of brain tumors. In tumors of the midbrain and brainstem, where overlying bone can impair CT scan visualization, the use of MRI is particularly helpful. The increasing sophistication of MRI techniques is expected to broaden its clinical usefulness, and it is likely that further improvements will make the procedure faster and cheaper and therefore more frequently used. Like CT scanning, MR imaging requires correlation of results with the clinical history and physical examination for accurate diagnosis of an abnormality.[6,22,23]

From 1955 to 1975, angiography was crucial to cerebral-tumor diagnosis. The availability and success of the CT scan has altered the use of angiography, and currently its major role is in outlining the detailed vascular supply of a tumor. In certain instances, tumors are seen on angiography but not on CT scan.

The air contrast studies of pneumoencephalogram and ventriculography revolutionized the diagnostic approach to the brain tumor patient. Before their introduction in 1918, only the neurological examination and the occasional finding on the skull film were available for either tumor screening or localization. The pneumoencephalogram (PEG) is now of limited value and is used only in diagnosis of specific types of tumors (i.e., brainstem or suprasellar neoplasms). Other diagnostic tests include Tangent Screen and Perimetry, a test used to evaluate visual fields, and caloric testing, which is most useful with a comatose patient.[22,23]

Medical and surgical management

Once the presence of a brain tumor has been positively established, an appropriate therapeutic plan must be selected. The three general methods for the treatment of brain tumors are surgery, radiation, and chemotherapy. These modalities can be used alone or in any combination.[18] In most instances, surgery is the last step in a positive diagnosis of a brain tumor. The surgical procedure can be one of four types: biopsy, decompression, removal of the tumor, or lobectomy. In addition, a shunting procedure may be required to relieve the pressure from cerebrospinal fluid. Biopsy is the removal of sufficient tissue to establish the diagnosis without removing a significant portion of the tumor. Open biopsy is preferable because it allows the gross appearance of the tissue and location of major blood vessels to be seen. The general procedures for the three major operative approaches—decompression, tumor removal, and lobectomy—are similar; the major differences occur during surgery and vary according to the specific situation.[22] A major new development of brain tumor surgery involves microsurgical techniques. These techniques offer particular promise for tumors that are inaccessible to open surgical approaches. Many brain tumors cannot be completely removed; a tumor may not have a clear demarcation, or it may be in a strategic location or involved with vital areas of brain function. However, a partial resection will provide decompression and relieve the symptoms temporarily.[22]

Ventilation and blood pressure status are carefully monitored following surgery, and cerebral edema is controlled by continued fluid restriction, anticonvulsants, and corticosteroids. Changes in neurological status can be anticipated on the second to fourth day after the operation because of evolving cerebral edema. Because these patients are dehydrated and are usually in one position for a long interval, they are prime candidates for thrombophlebitis and pulmonary emboli. The use of anticoagulants is contraindicated postoperatively because of risk of intracranial bleeding; therefore elevation, bed rest, and elastic stockings are extremely important during the immediate postoperative period.[23]

Surgery, followed by radiation and/or chemotherapy, may be the most common approach to primary brain tumors. Radiation is planned for tumors that are surgically inaccessible or for remnants of a tumor that could not be completely removed. Tumor cells are more radio-sensitive than nontumor cells; therefore the objective is to destroy tumor cells without injury to the normal cells. Radiation has the advantage of treating locally a small, defined, and nonmetastasizing tumor. The toxicity affects only adjacent and potentially involved brain tissue, its vasculature, and supporting structures. Radiotherapy has as its limitations the maximally tolerated dose that normal brain tissue can accept without the development of radiation necrosis.[18]

The treatment dose for the tumor depends upon several variables, including histological type, radio responsiveness, location, and level of tolerance. Many patients improve remarkably after surgical decompression and radiation. If radiation is not preceded by surgery, radiation accompanied by large doses of corticosteroids can temporarily reverse and control symptoms of increased intracranial pressure. A number of experimental approaches have been tested and are currently undergoing investigation in an attempt to improve the efficacy and local control of irradiation for patients with malignant tumors.[18]

Chemotherapy as a treatment for brain tumors is in the developmental stages, but evidence of its effectiveness is encouraging. Drugs, such as nitrosoureas and procarbazine, do possess the appropriate pharmacological characteristics for passing the blood-brain barrier and have application in a wide variety of tumors. Chemotherapy cannot be considered independent of surgery and radiation, but as a part of the overall therapeutic plan. Chemotherapy may be applied regionally or systemically. This type of therapy almost always exhibits its primary toxicity in organs other than the brain; therefore the systemic side effects limit the application.[22] The drug choice and its dosage depend on the particular tumor, location, and body tolerance.[18]

Future advances in the chemotherapy of CNS tumors are likely to include the development of drugs with greater specificity, with a greater ability to penetrate the blood-brain barrier, a better tumoricidal effect, and a diminished toxicity for normal organs. In addition to new agents, the use of a combination of existing agents may prove valuable. There have been two developments in the area of drug delivery: a totally implantable system for maintaining constant CSF drug levels and the use of biological agents that modify the growth of tumor cells without killing them.

Hypothermia and immunotherapy are recent advances in the treatment of brain tumors. Hypoxia, poor blood flow, and acid pH make tumors more heat sensitive than normal tissue and therefore more vulnerable to cell death or tumor regression via hyperthermia. Although immunotherapy has been attempted in a variety of ways, researchers state that we must increase our knowledge of the immune response before it can be applied to the treatment of brain tumors.[22]

Management of a metastatic tumor differs from primary tumor management. In most cases, radiotherapy is the principal and often the sole treatment, although surgery may be considered for the young patient who has a solitary metastasis in a silent area, with the primary tumor a site other than the lung. The surgical techniques are essentially the same as those for primary tumors except that resection of surrounding normal brain, such as lobectomy, is rarely indicated. Certain medical approaches, such as the use of corticosteroids for management of the increased intracranial pressure, can often preclude the need for acute surgical intervention. Such surgery may be done on an elective basis later in the course of care. Recent research indicates that the recurrence of metastasis in the CNS is far lower following surgery combined with radiation than with radiation alone, suggesting that patients who might benefit from such prolonged suppression of symptoms should have surgery. The future of the treatment of human CNS neoplasms offers a tremendous challenge to all of those concerned with the treatment of these patients.[22]

REHABILITATION

Rehabilitation is an important component in the management of patients with brain tumors, and it is becoming more valuable as new technology lengthens the patient's life following diagnosis. The tumor makes its presence known through its symptoms—the functional limitations it imposes on the patient's activities and the pain it produces. The rehabilitation plan is essentially the same as that used in the management of other chronic CNS disabilities. The multifaceted team approach, successfully employed in the rehabilitation of patients with other disabilities, can be used with equal facility for patients with brain tumors. The patient must be a participant in the therapeutic plan. The physical therapist who interacts with the patient at the level of symptom management generally focuses his or her attention on the functional consequences of the disease. However, patients with brain tumors present problems and opportunities different from those of patients with other diagnoses. When developing a rehabilitation program for these patients, the therapist must consider the prognosis, the highly emotional impact of the disease, the consequences of immobilization, and the effect of therapeutic interventions on both the physical and emotional responses of the patient. In some patients, hemiparesis and aphasia can clear dramatically, whereas the resolution of symptoms following a vascular occlusion is slow. Unfortunately, the therapists' evaluations must frequently culminate in program changes to accommodate increasing disability; initial efforts directed at ambulatory self-care may be reoriented to wheelchair, then assisted self-care, and finally to supportive, total bed care.*

Evaluation

The patient with a brain tumor typically presents to physical therapy with problems of hemiplegia similar to those that occur as a result of CNS damage resulting from vascular or traumatic insult. For a detailed description of the definitive techniques employed in the evaluation of hemiplegia, refer to Chapter 22, Hemiplegia Resulting from Vascular Insult or Disease. The clinical label of hemiplegia may not be sufficient to explain all the problems encountered by these patients. Therefore the site and characteristics of the tumor dictate what other difficulties must be considered. The patient may exhibit deficits on the "uninvolved side" as well as greater changes in cognitive functioning and cranial nerve involvement than usually exhibited following a cerebrovascular accident (CVA). These areas should be carefully evaluated. Pain, fatigue associated with a limited cardiopulmonary reserve, and weakness as a side effect of tumor treatment are additional areas to assess before activity levels are established.[4,7,26]

The clinical picture for this type of patient is a changing one; we are dealing with a progressive disease that demands attentive, ongoing evaluation. Pain during assistive joint range of motion may be the first indicator of a metastasis or pathological fracture and progressive weakness the initial sign of increasing intracranial pressure.[26]

Functional assessment. The functional assessment is the most important evaluation to consider when developing a treatment plan. We must note the degree of functional difficulty, the factors that are preventing performance of the activity, and the level of energy expenditure involved. In addition to providing a system of analyzing the deficits and formulating a problem list, the assessment can assist in determining clinical care outcomes by comparing measures of function before and after treatment.[14]

Other evaluation scales. The physical therapist needs to be aware of the functional evaluation scales that are frequently employed by other oncology team members for monitoring treatment. The Karnofsky Scale of Performance Status (KPS)[20] is widely used in clinical research and treatment decisions. During early cancer therapy, radi-

ologists recognized the need to clinically evaluate the chemotherapeutic agents. Four general criteria were suggested: subjective improvement, objective improvement, performance status, and length of remission or prolongation of life. The KPS was the first evaluation scale in which performance status was included. An individual's performance status was rated on a numerical scale from 0 to 100, representing ability to perform normal activity and the patient's need for assistance (Table 20-3). The KPS has been employed in randomized trials of chemotherapeutic agents, in evaluating an individual's response to treatment, and in evaluating the impact of therapeutic agents on the patient's quality of life. Because of the relationship between KPS and prognosis, individual physicians also use the performance status as a guide to treatment plans.

A physician who routinely assesses the KPS may identify specific areas of difficulty indicating need to make referrals for rehabilitation services. These early referrals may lead to a better quality of life and care for patients with advancing tumors.[2,20,33]

Other measurements of functional ability that are employed in the field of oncology are the needs assessment of Lehman and others and the Long Range Evaluation System developed by Carl V. Granger. In 1978, Lehman and others[27] reported that a significant number of cancer patients they reviewed had functional disabilities that could be improved by rehabilitation techniques. Problems that contributed to the functional disabilities included pain, generalized weakness, and psychological problems. Primary barriers to rehabilitation were the failure to identify functional problems and unfamiliarity with the value of rehabilitation. As a result of the chart review, they defined a needs assessment system, followed by the development of a model of care.[4,16,27,32] The Long Range Evaluation System (LRES) is a functional assessment system designed, tested, and used in a variety of clinical settings. It is a measurement tool for describing areas of service need, severity of handicap, and change in individuals over a period of time. The data collection forms are descriptive checklists prepared for computer entry with allowance for descriptions. Scores are generated incorporating modified versions of the Barthel Index, a measure of independence in self-care and mobility, and the Pulses Profile, a measure of independence in personal care. For examples of the Barthel Index and the Pulses Profile, see Chapter 18. The level of social support is measured by the ESCROW scale profile. It is postulated that the physically disabled person with a marginal level of independence is more likely to have potential for independent living if social supports are high as represented by ESCROW scales.[24] The LRES was structured so that it measures change over time. Through periodic assessments the rehabilitation program can be adapted to the patient's needs in either a stable or progressive clinical situation. The utilization of this instrument for

---

*References 7, 11, 14, 15, 25, 26, 28.

Table 20-3. Karnofsky performance status scale

Condition	Performance status %	Comments
A. Able to carry on normal activity and to work. No special care is needed.	100	Normal. No complaints. No evidence of disease.
	90	Able to carry on normal activity. Minor signs or symptoms of disease.
	80	Normal activity with effort. Some signs or symptoms of disease.
B. Unable to work. Able to live at home, care for most personal needs. A varying degree of assistance is needed.	70	Care of self. Unable to carry on normal activity or to do active work.
	60	Requires occasional assistance, but is able to care for most of personal needs.
	50	Requires considerable assistance and frequent medical care.
C. Unable to care for self. Requires equivalent of institutional or hospital care. Disease may be progressing rapidly.	40	Disabled. Requires special care and assistance.
	30	Severely disabled. Hospitalization is indicated although death not imminent.
	20	Very sick hospitalization necessary. Active supportive treatment necessary.
	10	Moribund. Fatal processes progressing rapidly.
	0	Dead.

From Karnofsky DA and Burchenal JH: The clinical evaluation of chemotherapeutic agents in cancer. In Macleod CM, editor: Evaluation of chemotherapeutic agents, New York, 1949, Columbia University Press.

many years has permitted validation of interrater reliability, making it a well-established test.[4,14]

Rehabilitation plan

The problem list generated by the definitive evaluation dictates the rehabilitation plan. In carrying out this plan, physical therapists use their skills as they would with any similarly disabled patient. Realistic goals must be established. In addition, a program to achieve these goals, subject to adaptation to accommodate the patient's response to treatment and the course of the disease, must be initiated as early as possible.[26,28]

Dietz classification. At the Sloan-Kettering Cancer Center, the late J.H. Dietz, Jr. pioneered the establishment of standards of care based on which adaptation may be necessary to meet the patient's physical and personal needs. The Dietz classification, based on four phases of care (preventive, restorative, supportive, and palliative), is widely accepted. Through the use of this classification, the appropriate rehabilitation stage of the disease can be delineated and realistic goals set. Specific rehabilitation goals and a plan of care are established depending on individual need within each classification.

The majority of patients fall into the category of preventive rehabilitation, which seeks to apply appropriate interventions at an early stage to prevent or retard the development or reduce the impact of a potential disability. Patient education should be a significant facet of preventive rehabilitation. The patient in the restoration phase can be expected to return to his premorbid status without any significant handicap. The focus of physical therapy within this stage is defined as the process of evaluating the patient's condition and setting specific treatment goals to assist the restoration of function. Supportive rehabilitation seeks to provide the maximal level of independence. Patients in this phase may remain active with known residual tumor and the possibility of a slowly progressive disability. These patients require the most rehabilitation. Because they can easily be overlooked, reasonable and realistic goals may not be fully achieved. During the palliative phase increasing disability and decreasing functional capacity reflect the rapid progression of the tumor. Appropriate measures set in parameters of short-term goals can reduce complications, increase comfort or independence, and provide emotional support to patients during the terminal stage.[4,8,19,25,28]

Complications and side effects. Although the traditional goals of neurorehabilitation apply, the length of the immobilization period and the side effects of treatment are somewhat unique in tumor patients. For the patient with a brain tumor, there is often a prolonged period of inactivity. This period may actually precede the diagnosis of the tumor or be a consequence of the medical/surgical care. Although the control of the tumor usually causes a temporary improvement in activity, the complications of muscle weakness and the other effects of inactivity can deter this improvement. Because of its deconditioning effects, prolonged bed rest may shift the marginally independent patient to one requiring total care. The effects of immobilization may be more pronounced in patients whose systems have been subjected to chemotherapy.[4,7]

With bed rest, changes in blood volume and viscosity result in an increased risk of thrombophlebitis and pulmonary embolism. It has been determined that a reduction in plasma volume can be limited by exercise, with isotonic exercise being more effective than isometric. If a patient receives chemotherapy, the inability of the circulatory system to adapt to the upright position after a period of forced bed rest may occur sooner than with other types of patients. Early intervention in the form of exercise and carefully monitored patient activity helps to diminish the adverse effects of immobilization.[4,7]

Along with preventing the complications of immobilization, a stimulating and interesting environment including sound, color, and motion should be created for patients with a brain tumor. It is equally important to include a variety of individuals in the therapeutic environment; implementing a program for volunteers is an excellent means by which this can be accomplished. Evidence suggests that environmental enrichment is effective in enhancing recovery after brain damage. The environment may very well help to reduce inhibition to the suppressed system, prevent transneuronal degeneration, and stimulate sprouting, dendritic branching, and increased enzyme activity.[3]

Recent trends in treatment have resulted in intensive combinations of treatment modalities as well as patient multidrug chemotherapy protocols. As a result, more complications occur now than in the past, when treatment was simpler but less effective in reducing tumor mass. It has been observed that the patient and family usually benefit from knowing the potential psychological and neurological effects of chemotherapy and radiation. To hide the facts from the patient may cause unnecessary distress. Considering the relationship physical therapists build with their patients, they are often the ones the patients question. It is important that the therapist have a knowledge of the side effects of treatment and be aware of signs and symptoms that may develop.[4,7,10]

The ability of the patient to respond to rehabilitation measures may fluctuate during radiation and chemotherapy. Although the long-term effects of these therapies may be a "cure" or rapid improvement, during intensive treatment the patient may exhibit a transient decline in neurological or hematological conditions. Complications of tumor treatment, which should be anticipated in planning a rehabilitation program, include the toxic effect to the patient's gastrointestinal tract and hematopoietic system. In the case of the gastrointestinal tract, complications may include anorexia, difficulty in swallowing, nausea, and irritation of the gut lining. These problems may result in decreased caloric intake and markedly reduced tolerance for

activity. Tumor therapy may also result in decreases in platelet as well as white cell production. Decreased platelet counts may increase the potential for bleeding episodes (bruising) whereas decreased white counts herald the increased susceptibility to infections. These complications may require a reduction in activity for a limited period of time or may require a more complicated response, such as the use of reverse barrier precautions to reduce the risk of infection.[4,18]

Appropriate goal setting: adaptive or functional program. Use of the terms "adaptive" or "functional" discourages the misconceptions and unrealistic expectations by the patient of being restored to a former level of function. Their use creates an environment that permits the patient to adjust according to his or her needs or to develop better tolerance for a progressive disease. The long-term goal of rehabilitation for patients with brain tumors is to achieve an independent or maximal level of function in the patient's own environment despite the possibility of residual disability. Rehabilitation must be initiated soon after the presence of disability has been recognized or the likelihood of disability has been realized. The patient must not be made to wait until all therapeutic treatment for the tumor per se has been completed because readaptive measures first introduced at that point may well be too little and come too late.[4,7,8,9]

For patients in the restorative and supportive phases, efforts should be directed toward the expected functional recovery by providing early specific training in tasks in which the patient needs and wants to be engaged. Patients are helped to activate the required muscles in a goal-directed, task-oriented context. Principles of motor learning and currently accepted knowledge of the system control of movement must be taken into account for effective therapy (Refer to Chapter 3, motor control). Although therapy after brain damage has been shown to improve recovery, points to consider in providing optimal treatment are that treatment be initiated as early as possible and that the more specific the training, in some instances, the greater the improvement. The positive effects of postinjury training may depend on ensuring a functional level of excitability within the system and perhaps preventing transneuronal degeneration. Success may be the result of specific training preventing the use of compensation, thus stimulating the remaining intact nervous system to recover.[3]

Short-term goals include managing the problems and mastering the appropriate functional tasks. Approaches used to attain these goals include selection of exercise for muscle weakness, management of tone and reflexes, and maintenance of a functional range of motion. Adapting to sensory loss and cerebellar involvement and addressing the cranial nerve deficits that have occurred must also be a part of the treatment plan (see Appendix).

To assist a patient in gaining improvement, the functional task should be subdivided into its component skills. These components are practiced separately, and gradually added together into short sequences. Eventually, the sequences can be combined until the patient is performing the task as a whole. Once the patient understands the components and sequences on the intellectual and experiential levels, he or she may be able to recombine the components to solve additional functional problems as they occur. To attain the desired goals, principles of energy conservation, work simplification, and the use of adaptive equipment may be required.*

Obstacles to successful attainment of treatment goals may be lack of initiation and perceptual problems. Patients who lack the ability to initiate movement are often incorrectly described as obstinate, uncooperative, unmotivated, or depressed. Conversely, because some tumor patients have normal verbal skills, their impulsiveness and perceptual problems may be overlooked and their rehabilitation potential overestimated. They are at risk for accidents and need a fixed routine and predictable environment. Efforts should be made to involve the family in all levels of the patient's rehabilitation. Early efforts must be made to mobilize family and community resources for discharge planning.[7,26]

Hospice

A nontraditional role therapists might assume when treating patients with a brain tumor is that of a hospice team member. Referral to a hospice program is appropriate when the patient's tumor is unresponsive to therapy and therefore a "cure" or long-term remission is no longer possible. In medieval Europe, the word "hospice" was used to describe a place of shelter and comfort for travelers who were ill or suffering from wounds. Today hospice is the name given to a new health care movement in which the emphasis is placed on control of physical symptoms. These facilities assist both the patient and his or her family to live life fully before death. Because one person cannot fully meet the needs of the terminally ill, the hospice program is organized on the basis of the interdisciplinary team. The patient is the central figure in this team.

The physical therapist, like other members of the team, provides palliative care, including positioning for comfort, applying modalities to alleviate pain, and maintaining functional range of motion. An equally important area of involvement for the physical therapist is adapting the activities of daily living to accommodate the capabilities of the patient and family. It is important to employ techniques of energy conservation and to identify equipment that will enable the patient to maintain his or her independence or ease the family's burden of care. Although the physical therapist often will provide "hands-on" treatment

for the hospice patient, more prevalent roles are those of counselor, educator, and facilitator. With proper background in the psychological implications of terminal illness and the hospice philosophy of care, the physical therapist is well equipped to provide valuable assistance.[21,31,34]

PSYCHOSOCIAL PROBLEMS

Physical therapists develop a special supportive relationship with their patients. They are usually one of the few consistent providers of care in the acute setting and often continue to see the patient after discharge. This strong interpersonal relationship is a key to successful rehabilitation. When a therapist allows this bond to develop, he or she must be committed to continuing the relationship with a patient who potentially may die. The physical therapist can help the patient overcome the sense of helplessness that accompanies the diagnosis of a brain tumor by maintaining an active, positive approach and encouraging the patient to be an informed participant in treatment decisions.[10,12,17,26,35] In the palliative stage, when the purpose of treatment is limited to slowing the progression of the disease, physical therapy can continue to assist the patient by setting realistic short-term goals that focus on maintenance of comfort and reduction of pain. A patient's primary need at this time is to know he or she will not be abandoned.[10]

Another key role for the therapist is that of being an active listener: particularly important is the skill of listening without expressing pessimism or, conversely, not giving false hope. The physical therapist can also be a support to family and friends by encouraging active participation in the treatment plan.[10]

Physical therapy typically directs treatment toward the patient's recovery. It is thus natural for the therapist to experience a sense of frustration and depression when evidence of recurrent disease becomes apparent in the patient. Equally natural is the personal as well as professional challenge present in providing treatment for this patient. The therapist's success in meeting this challenge depends both on his or her personality and his or her professional support system. Success will require that the therapist develop insight into his or her own feelings or attitudes related to cancer, its disabling effects, dying, and death. When these issues have not been satisfactorily dealt with, the therapist may find himself or herself avoiding the patient by spending less time with the patient, avoiding eye contact, or limiting touch. These behaviors may reinforce the patient's feelings of loneliness and isolation. An excellent support system may be found within the oncology team, which encourages its members to express their feelings and helps them to strike an emotional balance between aloofness and over-involvement.[10,12,17,26,35] Both the patient and family members may experience a number of reactions when evidence of disease recurrence or progression is identified.

---

*Class notes based on NDT Seminars and information from the Rehabilitation Institute of Chicago.

The physical therapist who has not taken the opportunity to evaluate and address the psychosocial status of the patient and family will encounter obstacles to his or her attempts at treatment at this time.[10]

SUMMARY

Rehabilitation is a vital component of the treatment plan for patients with brain tumors. The first step in developing an appropriate plan is to identify what functional limitations will result from the tumor or the treatment procedures. These areas then become the focal point for rehabilitation. The ultimate goal is to improve the quality of survival so that patients will be able to lead lives as independent and productive as possible regardless of life expectancy. Even in instances where the patient's life expectancy is limited, efforts toward maintaining function at maximum potential may produce results that transcend economic return.[7,9]

REFERENCES

1. Barnard RO: Pathological classification of tumors of the central nervous system. In Walker MD and Thomas GT: Biology of brain tumor, Boston, 1986, Martinus Nijohff Publishers.
2. Cammack JM: Interdisciplinary care of the patient with cancer in a community hospital, Clin Man Phys Ther 2(4):7, 1982.
3. Carr JH and others: Movement science foundations for physical therapy in rehabilitation, Rockville, Md, 1987, Aspen Publishers.
4. Charrette EE and O'Toole DM: Cancer rehabilitation. In Higby DJ, editor: Issues in supportive cancer care, Boston, 1986, Martinus Nijhoff Publishers.
5. Clark RL and Howe CD: Cancer patient care at MD Anderson hospital and tumor institute, the University of Texas, Chicago, 1976, Year Book Medical Publishers.
6. De Groot J and Chusid JG: Correlative neuroanotomy, ed 20, San Mateo, 1988, Appleton & Lange.
7. De Lisa JA and others: Rehabilitation of the cancer patient. In De Vita VT and others, editors: Cancer: principles and practice of oncology, ed 2, vol 2, Philadelphia, 1985, JB Lippincott Co.
8. Dietz JH: Adaptive rehabilitation in cancer: a program to improve quality of survival, Post Grad Med 68(1):145, 1980.
9. Dietz JH: Rehabilitation oncology, New York, 1981, John Wiley & Sons.
10. Etherington ME: Physical therapy management of the cancer patient, Clin Man Phys Ther 7(3):12, 1987.
11. Fink DJ: Cancer rehabilitation the team approach. In McKenna RJ and Murphy GP, editors: Fundamentals of surgical oncology, New York, 1986, Macmillian Publishing Co Inc.
12. Flomenhoff D: Understanding and helping people who have cancer, Phys Ther 64(8):1232, 1984.
13. Gilroy J and Holliday PL: Basic neurology, New York, 1982, Macmillian Publishing Co Inc.
14. Granger CV and Seltzer GB: Primary care of the functionally disabled: assessment and management, Philidelphia, 1987, JB Lippincott Co.
15. Gunn AE and others: Physical rehabilitation. In Gunn AE, editor: Cancer rehabilitation, New York, 1984, Raven Press.
16. Harvey RF and others: Cancer rehabilitation an analysis of 36 program approaches, JAMA 247:2127, 1982.
17. Hersch SP: Psychological aspects of patients with cancer. In De Vita VT and others, editors: Cancer: principles and practice of oncology, ed 2, vol 2, Philadelphia, 1985, JB Lippincott Co.
18. Hickey JV: The clinical practice of neurological and neurosurgical nursing, ed 2, Philadelphia, 1986, JB Lippincott Co.
19. Hinterbuchner C: Rehabilitation of physical disability in cancer, NY State J Med 78(7):1066, 1978.
20. Karnofsky DA and Burchenal JH: The clinical evaluation of chemotherapeutic agents in cancer. In Macleod CM, editor. Evaluation of chemotherapeutic agents, New York, 1949, Columbia University Press.
21. Katterhagen JG: Specialized care of the terminally ill patient. In De Vita VT and others, editors: Cancer: principles and practice of oncology, ed 2, vol 2, Philadelphia, 1985, JB Lippincott Co.
22. Kornblith PL and others: Neurologic oncology, Philadelphia, 1987, JB Lippincott Co.
23. Kornblith PL and others: Neoplasms of the central nervous system. In De Vita VT and others, editors: Cancer: principles and practice of oncology, ed 2, vol 2, Philadelphia, 1985, JB Lippincott Co.
24. Kottke FJ, Stillwell K, and Lehman J: Krusen's handbook of physical medicine and rehabilitation, ed 3, Philadelphia, 1982, WB Saunders Co.
25. Kudsk EG and Hoffman GS: Rehabilitation of the cancer patient, Primary Care 14(2):381, 1987.
26. La Ban MM and Meerschaert JM: Cancer therapy: an emerging role for physical medicine and rehabilitation, Ariz Med 37(7):483, 1980.
27. Lehman JF and others: Cancer rehabilitation: assessment of need, development, and evaluation of model of care, Arch Phys Med Rehab 59:410, 1978.
28. McLaughlin WJ and Holz S: Cancer rehabilitation: an integrated support system, Clin Man Phys Ther 5(6):9, 1985.
29. Poulson S: Neurosurgical nursing care. In Tiffany R, editor: Cancer nursing: surgical, London, 1980, Farber & Farber.
30. Price SA and Wilson LM: Pathophysiology: clinical concepts of disease processes, ed 2, New York, 1982, McGraw-Hill Book Co.
31. Reuss R: Hospice: one physical therapist's personal account, Clin Man Phys Ther 4(6):28, 1984.
32. Romsaas EP and McCormick JM: Assessment and resource utilization for cancer patients, Arch Phys Med Rehab 67(7):459, 1986.
33. Schag CC and others: Karnofsky performance status revisited, J Clin Oncol 2(3):187, 1984.
34. Toot J: Physical therapy and hospice: concept and practice, Phys Ther 64(5):665, 1984.
35. Wellisch DK and Cohen RS: Psychosocial aspects of cancer. In Haskel CM, editor: Cancer treatment, ed 2, Philadelphia, 1985, WB Saunders Co.
36. Zulch KJ: Histological typing of tumors of the central nervous system, Geneva, 1979, World Health Organization.

APPENDIX

Cranial nerve evaluation

The cranial nerves should be addressed separately because they represent sensory and motor innervation, which is very specific. Cranial nerve deficits will be readily noted if one pays particular attention to the patient's face, eye movement, speech, and swallowing during the initial interview.

The facial nerve (cranial nerve VII) is primarily a motor nerve and innervates the superficial muscles of the face and scalp. The nucleus of the facial nerve lies in the pons. The visceral motor component of cranial nerve VII lies in the medulla and is responsible for tearing and some salivation. One clinical point of importance is that the oculomotor nerve (cranial nerve III) innervates the muscle that opens the eyes and the facial nerve innervates the muscle that closes them. Ptosis of the eyelids is often confused with or mistakenly associated with facial nerve involvement. Also, lower motor neuron damage to the facial nerve will render that entire side of the face paralyzed. The forehead on the same side will appear ironed out, the eye will not close, and there is flattening of the nasolabial fold. If the lesion is above the nucleus to the facial nerve (upper motor neuron lesion), only the area of the face below the eyes is paralyzed because of the bilateral innervation of the upper face by the two cerebral hemispheres.

The trochlear nerve (cranial nerve IV) is located in the midbrain as is the oculomotor nerve (cranial nerve III). These two cranial nerves and the abducens nerve (cranial nerve VI) are responsible for almost all eye movements. The abducens nerve is located in the pons, and it teams up with the trochlear nerve to allow the eyes to turn outward. Palsy of cranial nerve VI is common with increased intracranial pressure. This nerve has the longest intracranial course and is very subject to stretch. Isolated lesions of the trochlear nerve are rare, but damage to the abducens nerve would produce internal strabismus and diplopia. The oculomotor nerve provides inward movement of the eye and constriction of the pupil so that a lesion of this nerve would appear with external strabismus (outward deviation) and dilation of the pupil.

The optic nerve (cranial nerve II) is an outgrowth of the diencephalon and is responsible for vision. It is important to note visual deficits during a physical examination, primarily for the purpose of referring the client to an eye specialist. There are many disorders that affect vision, and only the proper diagnostic examination will pinpoint the problem. (For additional evaluation and treatment approaches for clients suffering from visual deficits refer to Chapter 25.) Generally, compression of the optic nerve causes central scotoma (loss of central vision), but macular cortex lesions present a similar visual defect in both eyes. This could lead to visual confusion and thus visual perceptual problems. Atrophy of the optic nerve affects some fibers but spares others, and there are usually areas of lost function in the peripheral part of the fields of vision of each eye. Complete lesion of the optic nerve blinds the eye. Temporal lobe lesions can block out the upper temporal visual quadrant on the lesion side and the upper nasal quadrant on the nonlesion side. Lesions of the superior peduncle, extensive parietotemporal gliomas, or complete middle cerebral artery occlusions cause a complete homonymous hemianopsia. Because there are so many causes of visual loss and several types of deficits, it is important to perform some gross visual field tests and take special effort to note eyeball appearance and eyeball movement.

The trigeminal nerve (cranial nerve V) arises from the pons and provides sensory branches to the mouth, nasal cavity, orbit, and skin of the face and scalp. Lesions in the lateral part of the medulla or lower pons, which damage the trigeminal lemniscus, are likely to include the lateral spinothalamic tract, which causes loss of pain and temperature sense on the same side of the face as the lesion and loss of pain and temperature sense on the opposite side of the body beginning at the neck.

The mandibular branch of the trigeminal nerve is motor and provides innervation to the temporalis, masseter, and pterygoid muscles. A lesion of this branch would leave jaw closure weak or paralyzed.

The vestibulocochlear nerve (cranial nerve VIII) exits the pontomedullary junction. The exteroceptive fibers (the cochlear division of this nerve) receive stimuli from the hair cells in the cochlear duct, projecting auditory input down cranial nerve VIII (hearing acuity). The proprioceptive fibers of the nerve, the vestibular division, have their peripheral endings on the hair cells in the ampullae of the semicircular canals and maculae of the sacculus and utriculus. The nerve provides proprioceptive afferent fibers for coordinated reflexes of the eyes, neck, and body for maintaining equilibrium consistent with the posture and movement of the head.

Clients with involvement of the eighth cranial nerve may complain of ringing, buzzing, or hissing noises in the ear, and various forms of deafness may occur. From the vestibular branch, vertigo, and nystagmus are common symptoms. These clients will also sometimes complain of nausea. Treatment that involves rapid movement may elicit vomiting. Thus therapy that emphasizes decrease of spasticity and movement through functional or developmental sequences should be done slowly.

The spinal root of the accessory nerve (cranial nerve XI) has its nucleus in the cervical cord levels 1 to 6 and supplies part of the trapezius and sternocleidomastoid muscles. The ability to shrug the shoulders and rotate the head may be diminished or lost, and muscle atrophy may be evident. The bulbar root of the accessory nerve arises out of the medulla, accompanies the spinal root for a short distance, and turns away to join the vagus nerve and is distributed with the terminal branches of the vagus.

Involvement of the glossopharyngeal nerve (cranial nerve IX) would present symptoms of slight dysphagia, diminished or lost gag reflex, deviation of the uvula to the uninvolved side, and loss of taste in the posterior third of the tongue. Complaints of choking while eating and less interest in eating may come out during conversations with these clients. The vagus nerve (cranial nerve X) also appears with difficulty swallowing and diminished gag reflex, but loss of voice (dysphonia) is also present.

The hypoglossal nerve (cranial nerve XII) is a motor nerve and innervates the muscles of the tongue. Depending on where a lesion may be, the symptoms will vary. For example, in tongue protrusion the tongue deviates toward the lesion side when there is a peripheral lesion. With a supranuclear lesion the tongue deviates away from the lesion. One should note the position of the tongue during protrusion and look for atrophy or tremors of the tongue.

Chapter 21

CEREBELLAR DYSFUNCTION

Nancy L. Urbscheit

Receipt of a referral of a client with cerebellar dysfunction can be a frustrating event for a physical therapist. The first problem facing the therapist is the proper recognition and evaluation of motor problems peculiar to cerebellar disease. Second, a treatment program with known beneficial effects for the improvement of the motor deficits must be implemented. In solving these two problems a therapist can run into difficulty for a number of reasons. Although physical therapists typically learn a list of signs and symptoms accompanying cerebellar disease, they are not taught precise methods of examination and quantification of these symptoms. In addition, the relative significance and progression of each symptom have not been clearly defined. Last, and perhaps the most serious of all, is the limited knowledge of the mechanisms underlying each motor symptom in cerebellar disease. This lack of awareness is the most serious limitation because it hampers development of effective treatment programs.

Therapists are not the only individuals struggling to understand the intricacies of cerebellar function. In this century scientists have generated tremendous volumes of literature on the anatomy and discharge characteristics of neurons of the cerebellum, yet much of this material does not readily explain normal or pathological motor control by the cerebellum. For example, the anatomy, synaptic interaction, and discharge behavior of neurons of the cerebellar cortex have been defined in detail. However, the link between the behavior of this complex sheath of neurons and normal coordination of movement remains obscure. In attempting to resolve the mystery of the cerebellum, scientists repeatedly have turned to the classic studies of cerebellar dysfunction by Holmes.[43-48] With relatively simple tools, Holmes carefully observed and evaluated the motor problems of soldiers who had sustained cerebellar wounds in World War I. From this data he offered definitions and proposed theories of cerebellar functions that have centralized the focus for both the inquisitive investigator and the clinician.

Although the observations of Holmes cannot be completely explained, new insight into cerebellar function has been developed since Holmes' work was done. Other studies on man and animals have revealed additional physical characteristics of the motor problems, the association of the lesion to the symptom, and the prognosis of the problem. Refer to Chapter 3 on motor control for additional information on cerebellar function.

IDENTIFICATION OF MOVEMENT DISORDERS ASSOCIATED WITH CEREBELLAR LESIONS
Hypotonicity

Hypotonicity is a typical symptom of a cerebellar lesion.* Hypotonicity occurs ipsilaterally to the lesions

*References 6, 7, 26, 30, 44, 48.

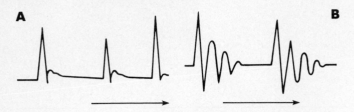

Fig. 21-1. Tracings of the excursion of the leg during a knee-jerk response in a normal person, **A,** and a person with cerebellar hypotonicity, **B.** Direction of arrows indicate progression of record in time. Note pendular response of a person with cerebellar damage. (From Holmes G: Lancet 1:1181, 1922.)

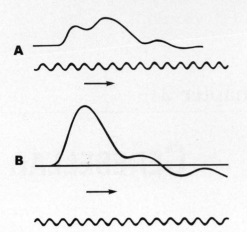

Fig. 21-2. Myogram of quadriceps muscle on normal knee-jerk response, **A,** and that evoked from a person with cerebellar lesion, **B.** Time indicated below each trace by vibrations of tuning fork at 25 Hz. Note absence of second peak of tension in response of person with cerebellar disease. (From Holmes G: Lancet 1:1181, 1922.)

that are restricted to the lateral cerebellum but may be bilateral or contralateral to lesions in the intermediate area of the cerebellum. If cerebellar hypotonicity is present bilaterally, the intensity is greater in the involved limbs than with unilateral hypotonicity. All muscles of the involved extremities are affected, but those muscles that move proximal joints are involved most significantly. In adult monkeys with acute cerebellar lesions, hypotonicity dissipates with time, resulting in minimal deficit after several months.[6]

Hypotonicity can be detected in a variety of ways.[3,36,44] The muscles of an involved limb have a reduced firmness or turgor to palpation. Upon passive shaking, the limb will move through a greater arc of motion than does a normal limb. In the case of unilateral lesions, hypotonicity may result in a wider, flatter barefoot print on the ipsilateral side. When the client attempts to maintain a hypotonic extremity against gravity, the extremity will tend to drop slowly. Also if a client is distracted while holding an object in his hand, the object may drop from his grasp. In addition, if an extremity is passively supported and the support withdrawn unexpectedly, the extremity will tend to fall heavily. The client's posture may also be poorly maintained or asymmetrical as a result of hypotonicity.

Although deep tendon reflexes may be subnormal, this symptom does not necessarily accompany hypotonicity.[3] Even though the amplitude of the deep tendon reflexes may be normal, the limb may briefly oscillate back and forth after tendon tap (Fig. 21-1). This phenomenon has been called a pendular deep tendon reflex. Pendular deep tendon reflexes are typically associated with hypotonicity.

Holmes compared the myogram of the knee jerk in hypotonic men with cerebellar damage to that of normal men.[44] The myogram of the normal knee jerk response displays two peaks of tension (Fig. 21-2, *A*). The initial peak is evoked by the tendon tap and is responsible for the brisk twitch of knee extension. The second contractile response is presumed to be caused by another stretch reflex of the quadriceps femoris muscle evoked by the descent of the leg. The descent of the leg is actually slowed by the second contractile response. In the myogram of the knee jerk of a client with a cerebellar lesion, only the early ten-

sion peak appears (Fig. 21-2, *B*). The second response, which would brake the return of the limb, is not present, and the limb falls heavily. Thus, during a knee jerk, the leg behaves as a pendulum that falls by its own weight and oscillates momentarily because of momentum.

A client with hypotonicity may be unable to fixate a limb posturally. This problem can lead to incoordination during voluntary movement. For example, flexion and extension of the elbow in an unsupported position can be very erratic in a hypotonic client, yet the same movement can become very smooth and controlled when the arm is supported on a table.[45] Also, a hypotonic client may be unable to flex one finger and hold the other in extension.[45] This may at first be considered incoordination but is really caused by lack of stability induced by hypotonicity.

Several mechanisms have been suggested for the appearance of cerebellar hypotonicity. Hypotonicity can occur in primates and humans who have isolated lesions in the lateral region of the hemispheres of the cerebellum.* Dow and Moruzzi[26] noted in primates that hypotonicity after cerebellectomy (total removal of the cerebellum) is very similar to that appearing after medullary pyramidotomy (section of the corticospinal tract at the pyramids), and they made the assumption that there is a common mechanism. The cortex of the lateral region of the cerebellar hemispheres or neocerebellum sends fibers to the dentate nucleus of the cerebellum, which in turn sends fibers to the ventral lateral nucleus of the thalamus via the superior cerebellar peduncle. The fibers from the ventral lateral nucleus of the thalamus terminate in the motor cortex. This pathway produces a facilitation of neurons of the motor cortex.[65,66,87,89] If this facilitation to the motor cortex

*References 3, 6, 7, 13, 39, 50.

is lost, the ability of the motor cortex to facilitate spinal motor neurons via the corticospinal tract will be reduced.

By recording the discharge of muscle spindle afferent fibers in response to stretch, gamma motor neuron discharge has been found to decrease after pyramidotomy, motor cortex ablation, and cerebellectomy in monkeys.[32-34] Following acute cerebellectomy in the monkey, Ia afferent fiber discharge decreases in response to both static and dynamic stretch (Fig. 21-3). Recovery of a relatively normal pattern of discharge is evident 56 days after the lesioning, which supports the observation that hypotonicity can improve after acute injury of the cerebellum. Interestingly, the discharge of secondary afferent fibers from the muscle spindles is not significantly influenced by cerebellectomy.[32]

The cerebellum can facilitate lower motor neurons not only through the corticospinal system but also via the vestibulospinal, rubrospinal, and reticulospinal pathways (refer to Chapter 3). The activity of these latter spinal pathways is influenced by the medial and intermediate regions of the cerebellum. In a study of clients with cerebellar tumors, Amici and others[3] noted a high incidence of hypotonicity with tumors located in the medial or intermediate regions of the cerebellum. Presumably, the facilitatory influence of the vestibulospinal, rubrospinal, and reticulospinal systems on alpha and gamma motor neurons is depressed by such tumors.

Asthenia

A lesion of the cerebellum can produce the condition of asthenia, or generalized weakness. Holmes noted that, in people with traumatic unilateral injury to the cerebellum, muscle strength on the involved side of the body may be reduced by 50% when compared to the normal limb.[43] Posture may also be poorly maintained in the client displaying asthenia. The clients complain of a sense of heaviness, excessive effort for simple tasks, and early onset of fatigue.[48] Asthenia is not as common a symptom as others accompanying cerebellar lesions. Amici and others[3] noted that the symptom occurred in only 10% of their clients with cerebellar tumors. Likewise, Gilman and others[36] noted it in only two of 162 clients with cerebellar lesions caused by a variety of problems.

The mechanism underlying asthenia is not clear. Hagbarth and others[40] performed an experiment that offered a possible model for cerebellar asthenia. They infiltrated lidocaine about the median nerve in normal subjects, producing weakness in the hand. Lidocaine blocks conduction in thin nerve fibers, including gamma motor neurons. During voluntary contraction both alpha and gamma motor neurons to a muscle are normally coactivated. If the gamma motor neurons are blocked by lidocaine, an excitatory input to alpha motor neurons from muscle spindles will be reduced. Without the excitatory input from muscle spindles, the supraspinal drive to alpha motor neurons may

have to increase to produce the voluntary movement. The normal perception of heaviness or force of effort is thought to be related to intensity of supraspinal signals required to produce the movement.[72] Thus any increase in the supraspinal drive to produce voluntary movement will be perceived as increased effort and fatigue, which is a common complaint in asthenic clients.

A decrease in fusimotor activity is known to occur in cerebellar lesions and has also been suggested as the mechanism for hypotonicity. Hypotonicity and asthenia, however, do not necessarily accompany one another. This suggests that although the conditions may share similar features, the mechanisms for them may not be identical.

Bremer[7] theorized that asthenia is caused by a loss of cerebellar facilitation to the motor cortex, which in turn could reduce the activity of spinal motor neurons during voluntary movement. A loss of facilitation of the cortex has also been suggested as a mechanism underlying hypotonicity. If loss of facilitation of the cerebral cortex is responsible for asthenia and hypotonicity, perhaps the areas of the cortex that are affected in asthenia and hypotonicity are not identical. Future research will need to be done to untangle the similarities and differences of these two symptoms of cerebellar dysfunction.

Ataxia

Ataxia is a general term used to describe the lack of coordination displayed by individuals with cerebellar lesions; however, the phenomenon of ataxia includes many distinctive traits, all of which need not be present in order for a person to be described as ataxic. Therefore, so that all the dimensions of ataxia may be covered, the phenomenon is described by body regions with the distinctions of ataxia associated with each.

Trunk and extremities

Disturbances of posture and balance. Acute or long-standing lesions of the cerebellum that affect one side of the body can result in lateral curvature of the spine.[46] Individuals with bilateral involvement of the cerebellum may assume extreme slouching and leaning positions when seated if support is not provided.[46] When standing, individuals have a tendency to spread their feet apart and use their arms for balance. Some clients fall to one side consistently. Opening or closing the eyes appears to have no significant effect on the ability to maintain standing balance.[43,48,79] Lateral deviation of the head can occur, but this is not a common symptom.[3,36]

Posture may be distorted by changes in proprioceptive control loops that operate via the cerebellum. There are several areas of the cerebellum in which these loops may exist. The dorsal spinocerebellar tract, the ventral spinocerebellar tract, and the spinoolivary tract carry proprioceptive information from the spinal cord to the midline cerebellum or vermis. The output of the vermis is to either the Deiter's nucleus (lateral vestibular nucleus) or to the

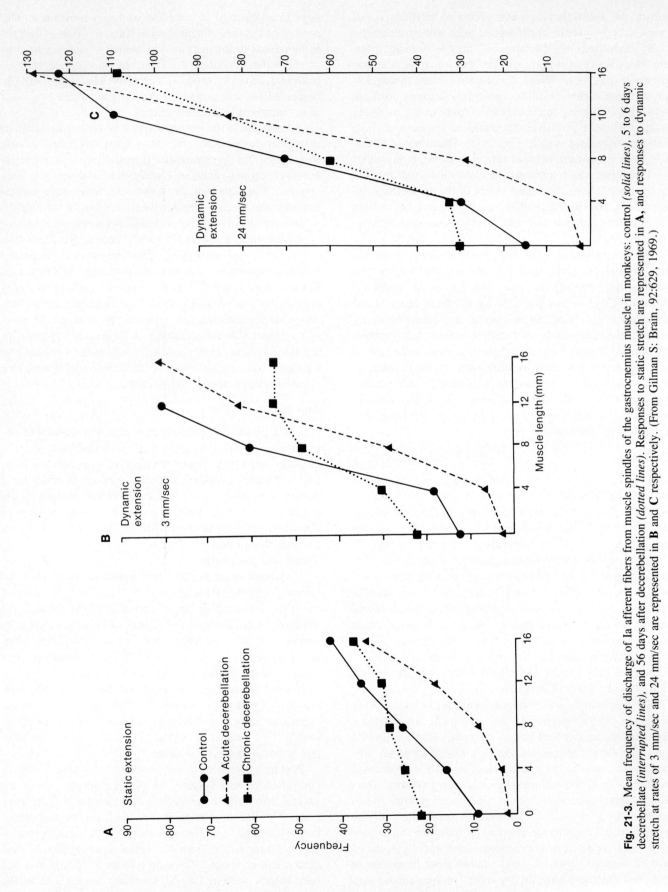

Fig. 21-3. Mean frequency of discharge of Ia afferent fibers from muscle spindles of the gastrocnemius muscle in monkeys: control (*solid lines*), 5 to 6 days decerebellate (*interrupted lines*), and 56 days after decerebellation (*dotted lines*). Responses to static stretch are represented in **A**, and responses to dynamic stretch at rates of 3 mm/sec and 24 mm/sec are represented in **B** and **C** respectively. (From Gilman S: Brain, 92:629, 1969.)

fastigial nucleus of the cerebellum. Both these nuclei can affect the excitability of the alpha and gamma motor neurons: the fastigial nucleus via the reticulospinal tract and Deiter's nucleus via the vestibulospinal tracts. Through these feedback loops the cerebellum can provide a corrective output for disruptions of body posture. Ablation or stimulation of the medial zone of the cerebellum in monkeys leads to disruption of equilibrium of the body.[14]

The intermediate region of the cerebellum also receives proprioceptive input from the spinal cord. The cortex of the intermediate region of the cerebellum has output to the interpositus nucleus in monkeys and cats and, in humans, to the globose and emboliform nuclei. These nuclei affect posture by connections with the motor cortex and red nucleus. Postural control exerted by such a feedback system appears to be associated with voluntary movements of the ipsilateral limb rather than with basic equilibrium of the entire body because electrical stimulation or ablation of the intermediate region of the cerebellum evokes postural changes only in the ipsilateral limbs.[5,14]

Lesions of the cerebellum might disrupt body posture by means other than loss of proprioceptive control loops operating via the cerebellum. The cerebellum normally has the ability to adjust the gain or sensitivity of proprioceptive reflexes that operate over segmental or suprasegmental paths. If this gain modulation is altered by cerebellar dis-

ease, the automatic postural adjustments may become distorted. An example of this has already been mentioned in relation to hypotonicity: decreased fusimotor activity (which decreases the sensitivity of the stretch reflexes) appears to be related to the inability of the person to support himself or herself adequately against gravity.

Nashner[79] noted that clients with cerebellar disease lacked the ability to adapt long-loop stretch reflexes in situations in which normal individuals could do so. A long-loop stretch reflex is evoked by stretch and has a latency of approximately 120 msec for the lower extremity. The pathway is presumably supraspinal, but the exact location is not clear. The reflex can be demonstrated in the medial gastrocnemius muscle of normal individuals when they stand on a platform that suddenly shifts backwards. The gastrocnemius muscle undergoes a long latency stretch reflex, which reduces the sway of the body in this situation (Fig. 21-4, *A*). After repeated trials, the long latency stretch reflex increases in amplitude. The reflex also occurs when the platform directly dorsiflexes the ankle; however, the reflex in this situation produces postural instability. After repeated trials the reflex disappears in normal individuals when the ankle is dorsiflexed by the platform (Fig. 21-4, *B*). Thus in normal people the long-loop stretch reflexes can be modified to fit the external circumstances. The medial gastrocnemius muscle of clients with

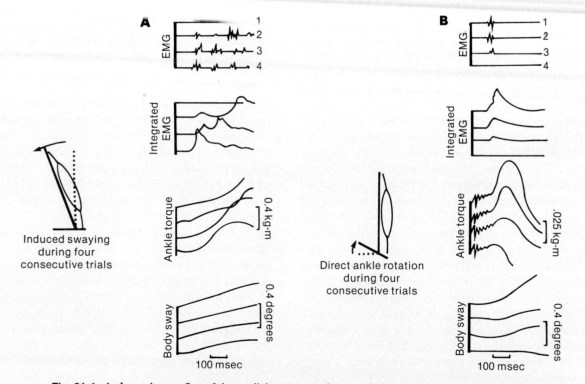

Fig. 21-4. A, Long-loop reflex of the medial gastrocnemius muscle in a normal subject induced by unexpected anterior sway of body. Note that the reflex increased in amplitude with each consecutive trial. **B,** Long-loop reflex of the medial gastrocnemius muscle in a normal subject induced by unexpected dorsiflexion of ankles. Note that amplitude of reflex decreases with each consecutive trial. (From Nashner LM: Exp Brain Res 26:65, 1976.)

cerebellar lesions also displays the long-loop stretch reflex under the above conditions. However, the amplitude of the reflex does not change with repeated trials with either type of stretch. These experiments suggest that the normal cerebellum is involved in the adaptation of postural reflexes to external conditions.

Another disturbance of posture that clients often display is postural or static tremor. The client's body may oscillate back and forth while standing, or a limb may oscillate up and down when the person attempts to hold it against the force of gravity. For example, a tremor may appear in an abducted arm but will disappear if support is provided at the axilla. The frequency of this oscillation is typically about 3 Hz, and both antagonistic muscles about a joint participate.[25,44,94] Although disturbances of balance and body position are common symptoms, postural tremor is an infrequent symptom occurring in 14 of 162 patients studied by Gilman and others[36] and in 13.1% of patients studied by Amici and others.[3]

The mechanisms underlying postural tremor are far from clear. Mechanisms for postural tremor and intention tremor (tremor during a movement) may not be identical. For example, administration of L-dopa will relieve postural tremor but not intention tremor.[37] Also, the two tremors are not always coincident, postural tremor being much less common than intention tremor.[3,81]

The postural tremor of cerebellar disease also displays differences from the typical resting tremor of parkinsonism. The tremor of parkinsonism has a higher frequency and can persist even when the subject is supine and relaxed.[61] The involvement of distal musculature is more prevalent in parkinsonian tremor than in cerebellar postural tremor. Although there are differences between the postural tremor of cerebellar disease and the resting tremor of parkinsonism (refer to Chapter 19), there are some similarities in that administration of L-dopa or stereotaxic lesions of the ventral lateral nucleus of the thalamus relieves both tremors.[21,37] In addition, the transection of the rubro-olivo-cerebello-rubral pathway in the monkey will lead to postural tremor if there is a concomitant depletion of dopamine in the animal's brain.[62]

The resting tremor of parkinsonism appears to be induced by a rhythmically discharging center in the brain. Neurons in the ventral lateral nucleus of the thalamus and the motor cortex have been found to discharge rhythmically with the tremor in parkinson clients. Although no one has recorded such activity in clients with postural tremor, a rhythmically discharging center in the thalamus might generate postural tremor, suggesting the importance of cerebellothalamocortical connections for normal posture and movement.[78]

Another possible mechanism for cerebellar postural tremor could be disruption of proprioceptive feedback loops. If the body shifts position, proprioceptors signal this change, and via a suprasegmental or long-loop pathway involving the cerebellum or another region in the brain, an automatic postural correction is made. When the limbs of a normal person shift because of gravity, sensory input will lead to a motor output that will return the limb automatically to the desired position. The motor output occurs in time to prevent a noticeable disruption of position. An oscillation can occur in this feedback system if there is a delay in the processing of sensory input or motor output because of a lesion. Thus clinically we see the limb tremor in a client with a cerebellar lesion when the client attempts to hold it steady against gravity.

Evidence for the actual delay of a long-loop reflex has been found in a variety of studies on clients with cerebellar disease. Marsden and others[70] noted that tonically contracting thumb flexors in normal individuals will undergo an initial segmental reflex with a latency of 25 msec in response to abrupt stretch, followed by two later reflexes with latencies of 42 msec and 55 msec, respectively. These latter two are considered to operate over a suprasegmental path. In these experiments clients with cerebellar disease display the early reflex at the same latency as normal people; however, only one late response occurs with a very long latency of 80 msec.

Rather than using the physical stimulus of stretch to activate muscle spindle afferents, Mauritz and others[71] electrically stimulated the tibial nerve to excite muscle spindle afferent fibers. Using this technique to evoke segmental and suprasegmental stretch reflexes, they found that persons with postural tremor had delayed long-loop reflexes. Postural tremor was also produced by this stimulation technique in persons with incipient degenerative cerebellar disease.

Postural tremor may also be explained by another hypothesis. Sensory feedback systems, which operate over supraspinal as well as spinal pathways, all oscillate even in a normal person. For example, the spinal stretch reflex pathway oscillates at 8 to 12 Hz, the corticospinal pathway has an oscillation of 3 to 5 Hz, and the transcerebellar pathway has an oscillation of 4 to 6 Hz. Yet in spite of these potentially oscillating circuits, a normal person displays no visually obvious tremor. The explanation lies in the fact that none of the feedback pathways operate in isolation from the others. By acting together these multiple pathways effectively dampen one another's oscillation so that little oscillation is actually expressed. However, if one of these multiple reflex pathways is absent or delayed, a noticeable oscillation of the body or limbs may occur. If the transcerebellar reflex path is absent, the spinal reflex path is ineffective in dampening the low frequency oscillation (3 to 5 Hz) induced by the corticospinal pathway.[96] Thus the body will tend to oscillate at the low frequency—that of postural tremor.

Clients with postural tremor display the tremor only when attempting to hold a fixed position, not necessarily all the time. Any limb displays a mechanical oscillation, similar to that of a metal spring or tuning fork when perturbed. When a limb or joint changes in stiffness, as from relaxation to an attempt at stabilization against gravity, its properties of mechanical oscillation also change. The mechanical oscillations of a stabilized limb may actually reinforce the low-frequency oscillation of the limb in a client with cerebellar disease and lead to a noticeable postural tremor, but not necessarily a movement tremor.

Dysmetria. People with cerebellar lesions often have difficulty placing their limbs correctly during voluntary motion. They typically overestimate or underestimate the range of movement needed. If normal individuals, with eyes closed, flex their shoulders to 90 degrees and then bring their arms quickly over their heads without hesitation, they can accurately reposition their arms to 90 degrees of flexion. People with cerebellar damage usually cannot return their arms to the original position without noticeable error. People with cerebellar damage may also display intention tremor, in which a hand oscillates back and forth as they try to touch their nose or the heel oscillates as they attempt to slide it down the opposite shin. The tremor has a frequency of 3 to 5 Hz and is typically enhanced during the termination of a goal-directed movement.[45]

Holmes[40] suggested that dysmetria results from errors in the level and rate of force production. He demonstrated this by having a client with a left cerebellar lesion press his right and left arms against springs of equal strength. Because of the ipsilateral cerebellar involvement, the tension developed by the left arm displayed a slow onset, reduced intensity, and a slow release compared to that of the right arm (Fig. 21-5). Holmes noted another error in the rate of force production, which he labeled as the rebound phenomenon.[44] If a restraining force is suddenly removed from an isometrically contracting limb in a normal person, the limb will not change position. In contrast, the limb of

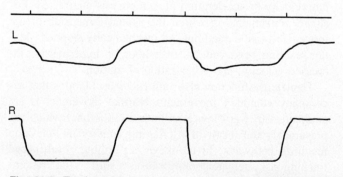

Fig. 21-5. Tracings on a slowly rotating drum of simultaneous depression of the right and left arms against springs of equal tension, from a man with a lesion of the left side of the cerebellum. The tracings show delay in starting and slowness in effecting the movements, reduced and irregular exertion of power, and slowness in relaxation on the affected side. Time in seconds. (From Holmes G: Brain 62:10, 1939.)

a person with a cerebellar lesion will move abruptly as if still opposing the resistance.

Recent studies have extended the observations of Holmes on the deficits of force production that accompany cerebellar lesions. If a normal subject performs a ballistic motion (high speed), the antagonist and agonist display a consistent triphasic pattern of activity (Fig. 21-6, *A*). The agonist undergoes an initial burst of activity, then the antagonist undergoes a burst, followed by a second burst from the agonist.[41,70] The first burst from the agonist has a consistent duration of 50 to 110 msec. The antagonist muscle burst displays a consistent duration of 40 to 100 msec. The duration of the second agonist muscle burst varies. The amplitude of the first agonist burst is related to the distance moved. The amplitude of the antagonistic muscle burst is not related to the amplitude of the movement or forces of deceleration but probably does assist in checking the movement. The amplitude of the second agonist burst varies with accuracy of movements and might serve as a means of correction.

Ballistic movements are assumed to be centrally programmed, the timing and amplitude of the activity being automatically signaled by the brain. A neural program does require sensory input to adjust for peripheral conditions, as evidenced by inaccurate ballistic movements in deafferented man.[9] The cerebellum may be an important part of this neural program because clients with cerebellar lesions lose the ability to perform normal ballistic motions. Although the triphasic pattern of antagonistic muscles still exists, the duration of the bursts is prolonged; thus the total motion has a longer duration and will obviously be dysmetric (see Fig. 21-6, *B*).[42] Clinical examples of this would be the overshoot when a client attempts to reach for something quickly or is unable to walk briskly and control the position of his or her feet.

Hallett and others[41,42] noted another abnormality in the activity of antagonist muscles of subjects with cerebellar lesions. If normal subjects isometrically extend their elbows against a resistance and then are unexpectedly told to flex their elbows very fast, the discharge of the triceps muscle will cease before the onset of the biceps activity. The triceps does not cease activity so abruptly in subjects with cerebellar lesions. In fact, the triceps may continuously discharge during the biceps activity. Such abnormal coactivation of the antagonists could contribute to dysmetria. This would lead to a delay in reversing any resistive movement, producing an overshoot and very imprecise alternating movement against resistance.

Other investigators utilizing normal and cerebellar-lesioned monkeys have examined aspects of cerebellar function related to the symptoms of dysmetria. In these studies the lateral and intermediate zones of the cerebellum and the associated deep cerebellar nuclei appear to control the onset, the rate, and the ultimate level of force produced by muscle contraction. Discharge of neurons of the

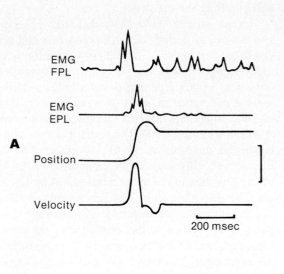

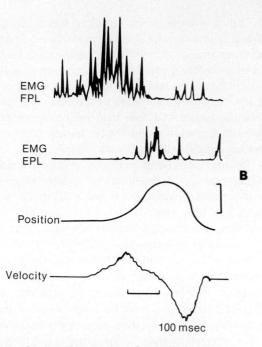

Fig. 21-6. A, Fast ballistic movements in normal man. Subject flexed distal joint of thumb through 20 degrees. Records are from top down, rectified EMG of flexor pollicis longus *(FPL),* rectified EMG of extensor pollicis longus *(EPL),* position, and velocity. Calibration is 200 msec and 20 μV, 27 degrees or 336 degrees/second. **B,** Fast thumb flexion from a 62-year-old man with unilateral cerebellar ataxia resulting from stroke. Records from top down are ordered as in **A.** Calibration is 100 msec and 100 μV, 25 degrees and 313 degrees/sec. Note the slower movement, inability to hold final position, and very prolonged bursts of activity in the agonist and antagonist muscle. (From Marsden CD and others: Physiological aspects of clinical neurology, Oxford, 1977, Blackwell Scientific Publications, Ltd. Edited by CF Rose.)

dentate nucleus has been observed to precede that of the motor cortex by 15 msec in monkeys trained to move in response to a light.[102] This suggests that the dentate nucleus acts as a trigger for the motor cortex during voluntary movement. Discharge of the dentate nucleus also appears to be tightly related to properties of intended movements as well as properties of ongoing movement.[8] Discharge of the interpositus nucleus is strongly related to properties of ongoing movement rather than those of intended movement.[8,98,102]

As might be expected, lesions of the dentate nucleus or interpositus nucleus in animals result in dysmetria. Specific, but temporary, lesions have been placed in the deep cerebellar nuclei in monkeys by use of a cooling probe. For example, during ipsilateral cooling of the dentate nucleus, the initiation of arm movements of two monkeys trained to respond immediately to a visual signal was delayed by 0.05 to 0.15 seconds.[74] Onset of movement-related discharge of neurons in the precentral motor cortex was also delayed by 0.05 to 0.15 seconds during dentate cooling. This suggests that disruption of the function of the dentate nucleus interferes with the trigger for the motor cortex during initiation of movement. Thus a client with a cerebellar lesion affecting the dentate nucleus might expe-

rience a delay in the initiation of movement and difficulty in movements that require bursts of speed.

Conrad and Brooks[18] also temporarily cooled the dentate nucleus in monkeys. The animals had been trained to perform fast alternating flexion and extension of the ipsilateral elbow. Range of movement was limited by mechanical stops at the end of flexion and extension. During the cooling, termination of the agonistic activity was delayed, but velocity or acceleration of motion was unaffected. For slower movements in which the spatial dimension of the movement was learned but not mechanically stopped, dentate cooling produced an overshoot or hypermetria, increased velocity, and acceleration of motion.[10]

Dentate dysfunction also influences oscillations that accompany voluntary movement. Normal movement is accompanied by very low amplitude oscillations, which are presumably the result of oscillating activity in long-loop feedback pathways. In monkeys performing a self-paced tracking task, dentate cooling causes a shift in the predominant peak of the power spectra of limb oscillation from 6 Hz to 3-5 Hz.[20] As mentioned before, intention tremor in clients with cerebellar disease also has a frequency of 3 to 5 Hz. Thus damage of the dentate nucleus could be involved in the generation of intention tremor. The slower oscillation of intention tremor might result from the time-consuming relay of sensory input to the motor cortex needed to modulate movement when the cerebellum no longer functions effectively.[2,73,106,107] Thus a client with intention tremor may have trouble performing tasks requiring precision of limb placement and steadiness, such as drinking from a cup, placing a key in the door, or putting on makeup.

Lesions of the interpositus nucleus in animals can also be responsible for dysmetria. Monkeys trained to perform a self-paced tracking task with the forearm displayed hypometria and decreased velocity of motion after local cooling of the interpositus nucleus. Thus very circumscribed lesions of the cerebellum may cause different characteristics of dysmetria.[103] Specific research on human subjects is not available, but the assumption is that lesions similar to those studied in the monkeys will cause similar symptoms in humans.

Disturbances of gait. Perhaps the most striking clinical feature of cerebellar dysfunction is the staggering gait, which resembles that of someone who is very intoxicated. Arm swing is typically gone. The individual cannot walk a straight line without lurching, step length is uneven, and the feet may be too close or too far apart or lifted without a regular rhythm or height. The gait pattern becomes even more distorted by walking heel to toe, walking in a small circle, or walking backward.

Gait disturbances are very common in cerebellar damage. Gilman and others[36] noted that 100 out of 162 clients with cerebellar lesions displayed the phenomenon. Amici and others[3] found ataxic gait the most frequent symptom in their clients with cerebellar tumors.

Although a disturbance of gait is considered a general manifestation of ataxia, gait can be the only feature of movement that is distorted. Gait is typically altered without changes in limb movement, muscle tone, or equilibrium with late atrophy of the cerebellum or chronic severe alcoholism.[68,105] Both of these conditions selectively involve the cortex of the anterior lobe of the cerebellum.

The cerebellum has been theorized to play a significant role in the generation of the pattern of locomotion. Activity of descending tracts during locomotion in cats is in phase with the gait cycle (Fig. 21-7). The rubrospinal pathway discharges in rhythm with the swing phase; the reticulospinal and vestibulospinal tracts discharge in rhythm with stance.[83] After cerebellectomy, rhythmic discharge disappears (see Fig. 21-7) in the descending tracts. Thus the cerebellum's control of gait extends beyond the integration of sensory input and correcting for errors in movement. In humans the clinical problem might be observed as a total disruption of the rhythm of gait: the stance and swing phase are totally irregular in duration, and the client cannot adjust for deviations in the surface on which he or she walks.

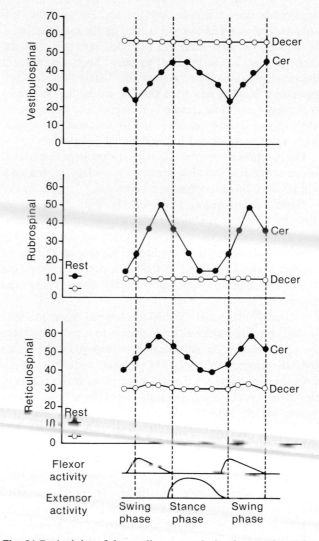

Fig. 21-7. Activity of descending tracts during locomotion. Mean values of the discharge rate of neurons of the vestibulospinal, rubrospinal, and reticulospinal tracts are plotted as a function of the hind limb position (ipsilateral for vestibulospinal and reticulospinal tracts; contralateral for rubrospinal tract). Curves obtained in cats with the cerebellum intact *(CER)* and those who have been decerebellated *(DECER)* are presented. A mean value of the resting discharge rate is also presented *(REST)*. Flexor and extensor activity is shown schematically. (From Orlovsky GN and Shik ML: Control of locomotion: a neurophysiological analysis of the cat locomotor system. In Porter R, editor: International review of physiology, neurophysiology II, vol 10, Baltimore, 1976, University Park Press.)

Gait disturbances can also occur in combination with other problems in cerebellar lesions. Gait disruption can be a result of errors in rate and absolute level of force of muscle contraction and can accompany dysmetria of isolated movement. Cerebellar lesions that affect posture will also influence the person's ability to walk.

Movement decomposition. A client with a cerebellar lesion may perform a movement in a distinct sequence of steps rather than in one smooth pattern. For example, if a supine client is asked to place a heel on the opposite knee, he or she may first raise the extended leg, then flex the knee, and last lower the heel to knee. Such a movement abnormality is called decomposition.[45] Based on such observations, Holmes theorized that the cerebellum functions to sequence and time simple movements into one smooth, complex act. In the absence of this function, the movement becomes separated into individual components.

Dysfunction of the dentate nucleus has been implicated in decomposition because temporary cooling of this area will produce this disturbance in monkeys.[18]

Dysdiadochokinesia. Many clients with cerebellar lesions are unable to perform rapidly alternating movements. This deficit can be demonstrated by having clients rapidly supinate and pronate their forearm or rapidly tap their hand on their knee. Compared to that of a normal person, the movement appears slow and quickly loses range and rhythm.

Holmes[43] attributed dysdiadochokinesia to an inability to stop ongoing movement rather than to a reduced velocity of motion. Use of electromyography has revealed discrete, nonoverlapping bursts of antagonistic muscle activity during rapid, alternating movements in normal people.[101] However, in people with cerebellar lesions, antagonistic muscle activity typically overlaps, resulting in a braking action for movement, such that activities like brushing one's teeth or stirring food will become ineffective.

Dysdiadochokinesia is related to dysmetria in that both result from the inappropriate timing of muscle activity. The inability to stop a goal-directed movement in one direction will be displayed as hypermetria, whereas the attempt to abruptly reverse the direction of movement will reveal dysdiadochokinesia.

In monkeys trained to perform rapid, rhythmic flexion and extension of the elbow, dentate cooling increased the duration of agonistic activity up to 0.1 to 0.2 seconds.[18] The onset of activity of the antagonist was delayed and often overlapped the activity of the agonist. No change in actual movement velocity was noted. Control of reciprocal motion by the cerebellum is also revealed by the observation that discharge of Purkinje cells in the intermediate zone of the cerebellum is related to reciprocal action of muscles. During cocontraction these same Purkinje cells become inhibited.[95] If the cerebellum is damaged, such neural discharge patterns may not occur.

Speech. Speech is a complex motor function that, as might be expected, is disturbed by cerebellar lesions. A client's grammar or word selection is not altered, but the melodic quality of speech is changed. The resultant disturbance is labeled dysarthria. Lechtenberg and Gilman[63] noted that 19% of 162 clients with various cerebellar lesions developed dysarthria, and Amici and colleagues[3] found dysarthria in 8.5% of a large population of clients with cerebellar tumors.

Scanning speech is a typical example of cerebellar dysarthria. Words or syllables are pronounced slowly, accents are misplaced, and pauses may be inappropriately short or long.[17] Clients may also display explosive speech or staccato speech.[116] The voice can become invariant in pitch and loudness, tremulous, nasal, or very soft.[11,44,46]

Attempts to localize areas of speech function in the cerebellum have revealed a relatively high incidence of dysarthria in clients with damage in the left cerebellar hemisphere.[63] The left cerebellar hemisphere is influenced by the right (nondominant) cerebral hemisphere, which has among its functions perception of melodies, tone, and rhythm.[84,91] If the left cerebellum plays a role in the melodic production of speech, input from the nondominant cerebral hemisphere seems appropriate in the context of this task.

Mechanisms responsible for dysarthria are most likely similar to those producing dysmetria of the limbs. For example, inability of muscles of the larynx to initiate or stop contractions quickly or hypotonicity of the larynx could produce a slurring in the pronunciation of consonants and vowels, slow speech, prolonged pauses, or uneven stress on syllables.[11,57] Hypotonicity of the larynx may also be responsible for the inability to increase loudness or vary pitch of the voice.

Eye movement. Although physical therapists are not expected to treat deviations of eye movement, they will see a relatively high frequency of such problems in clients with cerebellar lesions. An awareness of the variety of such problems and the underlying mechanisms should be helpful in interacting with a client who displays such phenomena.

Just like posture of the limbs, the *resting position of the eyes* is affected by cerebellar dysfunction. After an acute lesion of a cerebellar hemisphere, both eyes deviate toward the contralateral side.[29,80]

Voluntary movement of the eyes is also affected by cerebellar lesions. A relatively common disturbance in eye movement is gaze-evoked nystagmus.[4] As the eyes are voluntarily moved to gaze at an object in the periphery, they move quickly in the intended direction and then drift involuntarily to neutral. The sequence is repeated as long as the effort is sustained to keep the gaze deviated toward the periphery. Clients with cerebellar atrophy may display a permanent gaze-evoked nystagmus bilaterally, whereas those with an acute unilateral lesion may display nystagmus temporarily to the ipsilateral side.[54] A rebound nystagmus often appears if gaze deviation is maintained 20 seconds or longer. The nystagmus then occurs briefly in a direction opposite to the prior gaze when the eyes are voluntarily returned to neutral.[49]

The symptom in which the eyes cannot move accurately

toward an object in the periphery of vision is referred to as ocular dysmetria. When a normal person directs gaze toward an object in the periphery, the eyes move in a rapid step called a saccade. The amplitude of the saccade must be very accurate to place the intended image on the fovea of the retina. After cerebellar damage the saccadic movement of the eyes can become too large or too small, and corrective saccades will have to be made, resulting in ocular dysmetria.[59,86,90] Ocular dysmetria is related to the initial position of the eyes, such that hypermetria occurs when the eyes are eccentric to the target and hypometria occurs when the eyes move from neutral to a peripheral target.

Ocular dysmetria can also occur with pursuit movements of the eyes. When a normal person follows a slowly moving object, the eyes move in a smooth, continuous fashion but will stop abruptly if the object stops moving. However, if a client with cerebellar dysfunction visually pursues an object, the eyes may move only in saccades and will continue to move after the object stops.[15,16,108]

In the degenerative disease ataxia telangiectasia, clients are typically unable to initiate conjugate eye movement and accomplish lateral gaze by vigorous head movements.[4] Normal subjects can shift their eyes 30 degrees without accompanying head motion, but clients with cerebellar dysfunction typically move their heads within the first 30 degrees of eye movement.[93]

Reflex movements, as well as voluntary movements of the eyes, are also distorted by cerebellar lesions. The vestibular system influences the discharge of motor neurons of the extraocular muscles to appropriately regulate the velocity of eye movement with that of head movement. If such a reflex did not occur, the image on the retina would tend to shift with head movement and vision would be distorted. The effectiveness of the reflex can be demonstrated by watching a fixed object at arm's length while shaking the head. The visual image of the object remains clear because the eyes are held steady within the moving head. This response is called the vestibuloocular reflex. The sensitivity of the vestibuloocular reflex can be calculated by a ratio of eye velocity to head velocity. Although the sensitivity of the reflex is not universally altered in clients with cerebellar lesions, in such problems as the Arnold-Chiari syndrome and spinocerebellar degeneration, the ratio can exceed that of normal individuals.[113,114]

The amplitude of the vestibuloocular reflex will adapt to changes in internal or external conditions. For example, unilateral damage to the vestibular apparatus results in spontaneous nystagmus toward the damaged side, which typically disappears in a few weeks.[75] If normal subjects are asked to fix their eyes on a target attached to a rotating chair in which they are sitting, the vestibuloocular reflex nearly disappears.[113] These adaptations are possible only if the cerebellum is intact.

When a normal person watches stripes on a revolving drum moving horizontally or vertically, nystagmus develops in which the eyes snap quickly (fast phase) in the direction opposite to that of the revolving drum. The eyes then drift back slowly (slow phase) and the sequence is repeated. This phenomenon is called optokinetic nystagmus. In acute lesions of the cerebellum, the amplitude of the optokinetic nystagmus is often decreased, whereas in chronic problems, the amplitude of both phases or just one of the phases of optokinetic nystagmus is often increased.[36]

As might be expected, some clients with cerebellar lesions complain of visual defects. These defects include blurred vision, diplopia, loss of perspective, and difficulty seeing when their body is in motion.[112,113]

The *mechanisms* by which the cerebellum influences eye movement are not completely clear. Presumably lesions of different areas of the cerebellum affect different aspects of eye movement because a client may have distortion of one type of eye movement but not another. However, the diagnostic value of eye movements for cerebellar disease is limited because brainstem lesions can produce identical symptoms.

Gaze-evoked nystagmus has been explained by the loss of a holding function provided by the cerebellum. When the eyes are held steady at the end of a normal saccade, the discharge of motor neurons innervating the extraocular muscles is proportional to the position of the eyes in the head. However, the sensory systems that influence eye position transmit signals of velocity. For example, the semicircular canals detect velocity of head movement and the retina detects the velocity of the image moving across it. These signals must undergo a "mathematical" integration to code position rather than velocity. This process of neurointegration does not appear to occur in the cerebellum and is believed to occur in the brainstem.[12] However, the cerebellum is essential for the normal integration of the velocity signals. If the cerebellum is damaged, the integration undergoes a rapid decay, which is reflected in the poor maintenance of eye position. Thus the cerebellum is necessary to sustain or boost the output of the brainstem integrator of sensory signals influencing eye position.[115] The appearance of gaze-evoked nystagmus does not correlate with a specific cerebellar lesion in humans, although nystagmus occurring with downward gaze is particularly common in clients with the Arnold-Chiari malformation.[112] In addition, removal of the flocculus and paraflocculus in monkeys leads to a serious defect in the ability to sustain gaze in any direction.[115]

The ability of the eye to keep a smooth visual pursuit of a slowly moving target also appears to be related to the ability to keep gaze fixated on a still object. During normal smooth pursuit, the motor neurons to the extraocular muscles discharge at a rate proportional to eye movements. The sensory feedback from pursuit movement of the eyes codes target velocity rather than the position of the eyes. Thus velocity signals influencing smooth pursuit movements must be integrated to create a usable command for eye position. This neurointegration also presumably occurs in the brainstem. The control of the sensitivity of the integrator, however, is believed to be a function of the cerebellum. The flocculus and the paraflocculus are, again, presumed to be involved in this function because damage in these areas disrupts smooth pursuit movements.

Neurons that discharge before a saccade have been located in the thalamus, cerebellum, vestibular nuclei, superior colliculus, pontine reticular formation, and mesencephalic aqueductal grey matter. However, the area of the brain that appears primarily responsible for the generation of the saccades is the pontine paramedian reticular formation because specific lesions at this region will produce permanent loss of saccadic eye movement.[114] Damage to this region disrupts the rapid phases of both vestibular and optokinetic nystagmus. Although the cerebellum does not initiate saccades, it does influence their accuracy. To initiate saccades, the neurons in the pontine reticular formation send a burst of activity to the motor neurons of the extraocular muscles. This burst is believed to code the difference in the visual target position and the actual eye position at the start of the saccade. Thus, for this burst to move the eye to the exact location needed, the pontine reticular formation must have accurate estimates of the starting position of the eye as well as any other short-term or long-term changes in the eye and its muscles because of fatigue, injury, or aging. The cerebellum appears to provide this feedback to the saccadic pulse generator in the brainstem.[82]

Distortions of optokinetic nystagmus may be a result of disruption in the cerebellar systems, which control either smooth pursuit or saccadic movement of the eyes. For example, a client may display a loss of smooth pursuit movement and a disturbance of the slow phase of optokinetic nystagmus. Presumably, the cerebellar mechanisms responsible for these two features of eye movement are the same. Similarly, saccadic eye movement may be distorted as well as the fast phase of optokinetic nystagmus.

Theories of cerebellar function in coordination. Although studies of the normal function and consequences of lesions of the cerebellum strongly suggest that the cerebellum controls the onset, level, and rate of force production by muscles, there are only theories to explain how this is accomplished. One theory suggests that the cerebellum acts essentially as a comparator between sensory input and motor output.[27,28,88] The cerebellum is the recipient of a tremendous sensory input, including that from muscle spindles, Golgi tendon organs, cutaneous receptors, joint receptors, and the vestibular apparatus. The cerebellum also receives motor output from the motor cortex. Presumably, the cerebellum "compares" the voluntary command for movement with the sensory signals produced by the

evolving movement. If the motor commands and evolving sensory signals are not appropriately matched, the cerebellum will provide corrective feedback to motor pathways capable of influencing the movement.[28]

A second theory of function of the cerebellum suggests that it acts as a compensator, instead of a comparator. Rather than providing corrections to ongoing voluntary movement, the cerebellum is assumed to perform predictive compensatory modification of reflexes in preparation for movement.[67] The success of voluntary movement depends largely on the stability and adjustment of many different reflexes. For example, if the stretch reflexes of a limb are too sensitive, a high-speed movement may be impossible because of evoked stretch reflexes. Thus muscle spindle activity will have to be reduced before and during such movement. This reduction can be produced by inhibition of gamma motor neurons or interneurons in the stretch reflex pathway. In other circumstances the sensitivity of muscle spindles may have to be increased before movement. The cerebellum may be the initiator of such compensatory modification of the stretch reflex as well as many other reflexes.

The cerebellum has also been theorized to learn effective motor behavior. Ito[51] proposed that the cerebellum acts as an adaptive feed-forward control system, which programs or models voluntary movement skills based on a memory of previous sensory input and motor output. According to this theory, learned movement is controlled by an internal model stored in or triggered by the cerebellum. If the cerebellum is damaged, the learned motor programs cannot be utilized. Movement will then be guided by long delay sensory feedback loops through the cerebrum, just as in learning a new skill, and incoordination will result.

If the cerebellum learns or memorizes movements, are programs retained for complex movements, such as a serve in tennis, or for simple qualities of movements? Brooks[8] suggested that the lateral and intermediate cerebellum act to sequence simple movements that make up complex actions. The cerebellum may thus learn small, simple programs, which are then triggered in the order needed to produce the complex motion.

Although no one knows where and how learning in the cerebellum may take place, several ideas have been proposed that put heavy emphasis on the role of the inferior olivary nucleus.[1,69] The neurons of the inferior olive have a 1:1 relationship with Purkinje cells via the climbing fibers. Each olivary neuron is presumed to be activated by the cerebral cortex during a demand for an elemental or simple movement. The Purkinje cell activated by a particular inferior olivary neuron can then initiate this movement. The discharge of Purkinje cells is also affected by input from the mossy fibers, which reflects the sensory context in which the elemental movement is demanded. Possibly, the climbing fiber input potentiates the mossy fiber input so that mossy fiber input to the Purkinje cell may be able to evoke an elemental movement from the Purkinje cell in the absence of input from the cortex.

Currently, no one is certain whether the cerebellum functions in all three of these capacities or predominantly in just one. If the cerebellum does perform all three of the described functions, different lesions may disturb one function more than another. Recognition of these theories and the consequences of their disruption may help a therapist more carefully examine a client and plan a therapeutic program. For example, if the cerebellum no longer functions as a comparator, movement will obviously be dysmetric. This is the individual who will need time-consuming practice, but in selected activities that will be most useful for him or her and not in all movements. Even though the cerebellum may not automatically correct movement errors, the client may consciously be able to correct movement with practice or the remaining CNS may be able to assume a role of automatic correction.

If the cerebellar function of a reflex compensator is lost, the client may display abnormal muscle tone, inappropriate postural adjustment, and loss of associated limb movements, as well as being dysmetric. The therapist may need to evoke reflexes during an activity that would assist the postural stability and progression of movement. The presumption, again, is that the client can consciously learn to control the activity or that another part of the nervous system can begin to make the reflex adjustment automatically.

The concept of learning by the cerebellum is especially important for physical therapists to consider. If clients have lost "learned motor programs" controlled by the cerebellum, they will obviously be dysmetric. Physical therapy for any neurologically involved client is offered with the hope that a long-term modification of motor behavior will take place. However, if the cerebellum is the primary area where adaptive movement can be "learned," the client may never receive much benefit from therapy. Currently, there are no studies that quantify the ability of clients with cerebellar lesions to learn new motor skills or relearn lost skills with training. Obviously, such work would be a valuable guide to therapists in providing activities that can achieve better motor performance. Therapists, however, need to recognize that even though the best therapeutic program possible is offered, the motor learning capabilities of some clients with a cerebellar lesion may be very limited and gains achieved slowly at best.

RECOVERY FROM CEREBELLAR LESIONS

After a brain lesion there is always some level of spontaneous recovery or compensation; the level depends upon the severity of the lesion and its location. For cerebrovascular accidents and head trauma, therapists do have some published guidelines for recovery patterns to which they can refer; however, such information has not been well documented for cerebellar lesions. For this reason, this chapter cannot provide a complete description of recovery patterns following cerebellar damage. However, it is hoped that the information presented will provide therapists with some clarifying expectation for their clients.

Various investigators have attempted to study the recovery patterns following cerebellar damage with animal models. Poirier and others[85] observed the motor behavior of monkeys for up to 1 year after various surgical lesions had been placed in the cerebellum.[85] The most severe problems resulted from total cerebellectomy and included truncal ataxia, dysmetria of the limbs, hypotonicity, and postural tremor. These problems decreased in severity over the first 4 weeks after surgery but improvement then reached a plateau. The animal was still severely compromised, dysmetria and postural tremor being the least obvious of the above symptoms.

Goldberger and Growdon[38] bilaterally lesioned the dentate and interpositus nucleus in monkeys. The animals displayed gross oscillations of the limbs at a frequency of 2 per second, hypermetria of the limb, and primitive movement locomotion during the first 2 weeks. As the animals improved over the next 50 weeks, the limbs developed a smaller and faster amplitude tremor of 6 to 8 Hz and a marked improvement in gait and accuracy of movement of the extremities. In contrast, if only one cerebellar hemisphere is damaged with no nuclear involvement in a primate, the animal displays ipsilateral dysmetria, postural tremor, and awkward leaping gait for the first 1 to 2 weeks and becomes essentially normal over the next 2 months. If the midline structure of the cerebellum is involved, the animal's chief problem is truncal ataxia, which improves over the first 3 to 5 months but never disappears. Thus from animal work it appears that recovery is very poor from a total cerebellectomy; a bilateral lesion is more devastating than a unilateral lesion; damage to the deep cerebellar nuclei is more serious than that to the cortex; and spontaneous compensation will be complete within 6 months to a year.

Although one cannot assume that humans will respond to acute cerebellar injury exactly as primates do, the information provided by animal work does indeed provide a general framework for humans. A feature of cerebellar lesions that cannot be readily studied in animals is the effect of a degenerative disease or an expanding tumor. If a client develops a degenerative cerebellar disease or a tumor, the developing symptoms are generally milder than those produced by the same damage occurring acutely. Thus compensation appears to be concurrent with a steadily progressing lesion.

If compensation for a cerebellar lesion is possible, what other neurological structures are necessary for the compensation to take place? If the cerebellum is not totally destroyed, some available adaptation for the movement distortions may occur because of the remainder of the cerebellum. Evidence for this is displayed by the observation that compensation for a cerebellar lesion will be disrupted

---

Assessment of movement disorders

Hypotonicity

Specific tests
1. Muscle palpation
2. Deep tendon reflexes
3. Passive shaking of limbs

4. Wet foot print
5. Hold object while conversing
6. Voluntary flexion and extension of knee or elbow supported and unsupported
7. Flex one finger only

Observation
1. Resting posture

Positive
1. Reduced firmness
2. Pendular
3. Limbs move through greater arc of motion than does normal limb
4. Print broader on involved side
5. Drops object when distracted
6. Ataxic when unsupported; controlled when supported
7. All fingers flex

1. Slack, asymmetrical

Asthenia

Specific tests
1. Maintain arm(s) in 90-degree position of flexion or abduction
2. Maximal resisted muscle contraction for major muscle groups
3. Repeat submaximal muscle contractions, such as rising on toes, push-ups, squeezing tennis ball

Observation
1. Everyday activities

Positive
1. Arm(s) tire quickly

2. Weaker on involved side or unable to work against resistance, which is normal for size and age
3. Tires quickly

1. Tires easily, complains of heaviness

Balance and postural control

Specific test
1. Hold limb against pull of gravity
2. Nudge client unexpectedly when sitting or standing
3. Stand on one foot or walk backward

Observation
1. Standing posture

Positive
1. Postural tremor
2. Loses balance easily
3. Loses balance easily

1. Feet apart, trunk flexed slightly, needs to hold for stability, postural tremor of legs

---

by a second lesion in which deficits are more serious than those that have occurred if the second lesion had been produced alone.[3] The motor cortex is also considered to be an essential structure upon which compensation for a cerebellar lesion depends.[38]

EVALUATION AND GOALS

As for any neurologically involved client, the primary goal of physical therapy will be to make the client as functional as possible under conditions of maximum safety, reasonable energy cost to the client, and cosmesis. In deciding how to achieve this, a therapist will have to decide what basic functions the client cannot achieve and specific reasons why. Evaluation of a client with a cerebellar lesion should therefore include an initial determination of basic functional capabilities such as:

1. Bed mobility and posture
2. Ability to sit up from a reclining position
3. Maintenance of sitting posture
4. Ability to stand up from a sitting position
5. Maintenance of standing posture
6. Ambulation
7. Ability to dress, groom, and eat

No special tests are needed to isolate these abilities other than observing the client's attempts at each. Description of performance can include assistance needed, level of effort involved, time to complete the activity, potential hazards to the client, and unusual accompanying movements or noticeable features unique to that client.

Once an assessment of basic fundamental capabilities of clients has been completed, therapists should determine why their clients display the difficulties observed by looking carefully for the movement disorders associated with cerebellar lesions (described at the beginning of the chapter). A list of each movement disorder, a description of specific tests, and simple observations needed to determine the presence of each disturbance are presented in the boxed material. Both sides of the body need to be examined even if a unilateral cerebellar lesion has been diagnosed. Although therapists are not expected to provide de-

---

Assessment of movement disorders—cont'd

Dysmetria

Specific test

1. Flex arms to 90-degree position, quickly elevate overhead and then return to 90-degree position
2. Put peg in a hole, trace circle with pencil, trace circle on floor with big toe, slide heal down shin slowly, place feet on markers when walking
3. Therapist resists client's elbow flexion and releases unexpectedly
4. Voluntarily flex and extend knee or elbow in supported and unsupported position
5. Submaximal isometric effort against force transducer
6. Electromyogram of antagonistic pair of muscles during ballistic contraction

Posture

1. Not able to resume 90-degree position without initial error
2. Intention tremor, undershoots or overshoots target

3. Arm rebounds

4. Limb ataxic whether supported or not

5. Onset and release of force of involved limb delayed
6. Duration of triphasic pattern longer than 300 msec

Gait disturbance

Specific test

1. March to cadence
2. Walk on heels or toes
3. Walk clockwise and counterclockwise
4. Walk on uneven ground

Observation

1. Typical gait pattern

Positive

1. Unable to follow rhythm
2. Loses balance and rhythm
3. Stumbles in one direction
4. Cannot compensate and stumbles

1. Slow, stumbles easily, not rhythmic, step length and height irregular

Dysdiadochokinesia

Specific test

1. Tap hand on knee or toes on floor
2. Walk as fast as possible

Observation

1. Activities of daily living

Positive

1. Rapidly loses rhythm and range
2. Gait becomes very impaired only when fast

1. Unable to brush teeth, stir food, shake salt shaker

Movement decomposition

Specific test

1. Supine client touches heel to opposite knee

Observation

1. Typical movement

Positive

1. Movement broken up into separate phases, does not flow

1. Activity appears as if in slow motion, mechanical like a puppet

---

tailed evaluations of eye movement or speech, brief notations of obvious distortions may help clarify the total problem facing the client. If the client has multiple sites of brain involvement, the symptoms caused by cerebellar damage may be masked by spasticity or sensory loss, and tests for these features will need to be added.

The cerebellar movement disorders the client displays will help the therapist decide why any of the basic functions cannot be performed. The therapist can then select the therapeutic activities that would best correct the movement disorder and hence improve the client's functional behavior. For example, if an individual is hypotonic, his or her resting posture while reclining, sitting, and standing will be changed. The treatment for such a client would need to include activities that enhance tone of antigravity muscles. If asthenia exists, postural stability and ambulation will be affected. Resistive exercises to antigravity

muscles may improve such a client's posture and endurance in ambulation. If a client does not display hypotonicity or asthenia but still has poor postural stability, dysmetria may be the major problem. In this situation the client needs many sessions of practice in the precise posturing of the trunk, upper extremities, or legs in an attempt to make posture an automatic function or, second best, a consciously controlled function. If a client displays gait disturbances but does not have dysmetria, hypotonicity, or asthenia, the cerebellar motor program for gait may have been selectively disturbed and attention in therapy will need to be directed only toward gait. However, if dysmetria of isolated movements in the limbs is present as well as gait abnormalities, selected coordination exercises for the extremities as well as gait training should be implemented. Inability to dress, feed, or groom oneself effectively may be caused by hypotonicity, dysmetria, or asthe-

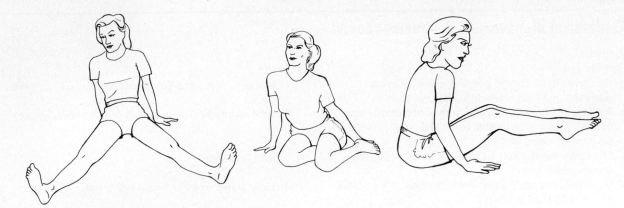

Fig. 21-8. Alternate positions in sitting to attempt with the client with a cerebellar lesion to promote control of posture and balance.

nia but may also be specifically caused by movement discomposition or dysdiadochokinesia. The predominant distortion will need to become the focus of treatment.

TREATMENT

The program described in this section is for the client with a relatively severe, but stabilized, lesion of the cerebellum, such as might be produced by trauma, cerebrovascular accident, or a tumor that has been surgically removed. Many parts of the program, however, could be used to help maintain function of the client with degenerative cerebellar disease. The reader should be aware that success of any of the following activities has not been well documented. Thus they are to be taken only as ideas for obtaining selective goals. Several goals toward which a physical therapist can work with a client having a cerebellar lesion are (1) postural stability, (2) functional gait, and (3) accuracy of limb movement.

Head and trunk control

A client with postural instability needs to be assisted sequentially to each level of independently maintained posture. Thus a client is a candidate for sitting only when there is sufficient head and trunk control and a candidate for standing only when sitting balance can be maintained. If clients have inadequate head control, they can be treated in the prone position while propped on elbows with pillow under chest or by being placed on a wedge bolster. If clients are not comfortable in the prone position, treatment can be performed with them seated with hips tucked back in a chair, feet flat on the floor, and elbows supported by a lap table or pillow. The goal is to have clients lift the head and hold it steady. This position is the same as that which a baby first learns in control of the head. It is called pivot prone and can be promoted by brushing of neck and upper back, 3 to 5 seconds of ice to the neck extensors, stretch to the neck extensors followed by heavy resistance to extensors to maintain extension in the shortened range, and downward compression on the shoulders.[97] To progres-

sively promote trunk control, less support to the elbows from the pillows and bolsters should be offered. The client in the prone position should attempt to prop on both elbows and progress to the use of just one elbow for support to promote weight shift at the shoulders (refer to Figs. 6-2 and 6-3 for additional information on head control treatment).

Biofeedback might be tried in an attempt to promote upright head position in the severely involved client. For example, the client could wear a helmet that provides a visual and auditory clue when the vertical position of the head is not maintained.[110]

Sitting balance

When clients can hold their heads up and have developed some trunk control, they need to be offered progressive challenges to sitting balance. This can be accomplished by treating the client in a chair without arms or a back, depending upon the individual's performance. If available, a safer and more versatile place to treat a client is on the edge of a mat table. To promote trunk stability the therapist applies joint approximation at the client's hips or shoulders. To help a client sustain contraction of the trunk muscles, rhythmic stabilization for trunk rotation may be utilized. In this situation rhythmic stabilization is provided not to increase strength but to give clients the sensation of stability, which they can then attempt alone. If clients cannot sustain an isometric contraction of the trunk muscles, a pattern of slow-reversal-hold over a steadily decreasing range of trunk rotation might be attempted instead.[58] Therapists can also help clients control balance by joining hands with them and having them meet a gentle resistance through their extended arms.

Clients next need to practice weight shift in all directions while sitting. This can first be practiced with clients using both hands for support, progressing to no support from their hands. Clients should also try to sustain balance with the arms overhead and the trunk rotated because this position will be used in activities of daily living. Although

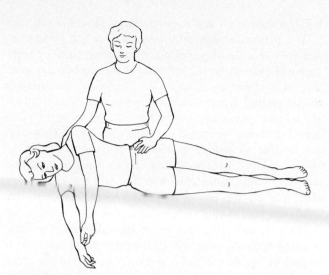

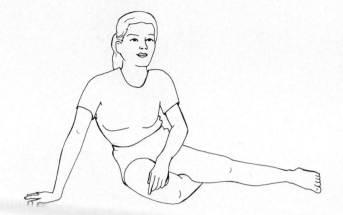

Fig. 21-10. Client pushing up from prone position and rotating back onto hips to sit up.

Fig. 21-9. Position in which to apply resistance to shoulder flexion, adduction, external rotation, and trunk rotation to promote rolling from supine to side-lying.

not essential, clients can be provided with practice in maintaining different sitting positions (Fig. 21-8). (Refer to Chapters 13 and 16 for additional information).

Rising from supine or prone position to sitting

At the same time the client is developing control of sitting balance, work on safe and efficient ways of moving from the supine or prone position to sitting will be necessary. Work toward this goal can also be done on a mat table. The procedure used will depend on the client's weight, side of involvement, and underlying muscle strength. A very heavy or weak individual may need first to roll to one side and push up from the sidelying posture. The client should first lie near the edge of the table with knees bent and feet flat on the table. As the knees drop passively to the side, the trunk should rotate as well. If clients still have difficulty getting to sidelying, their efforts can be strengthened by the therapist's providing gentle resistance in the sidelying position to flexion, adduction, external rotation of the shoulder, and trunk rotation (Fig. 21-9). As clients become stronger, the resistance can be applied when they are between the sidelying and supine positions. When clients can achieve a sidelying position alone, they can proceed to drop their legs off the edge of the table and push up with their arms to a sitting position. Ideally, clients should be taught to roll in both directions, but for practical purposes emphasis may need to be placed on one direction only. If clients have primary involvement on one side, they may find it easier to roll toward that side. However, this may create difficulty when they attempt to push up to sitting with the involved arm. Under these circumstances the therapist will have to decide the direction easiest for the client to roll and sit.

A more natural method of rising from the supine posi-

tion is to rely primarily on the action of the abdominal muscles. For stability, a client can drop one leg off the edge of the table, placing the foot on the floor if possible. The client can then rise to a sitting position using the abdominal and iliopsoas muscles. A weak or heavy client can use this method if a side rail is provided for a pull. The difficulty with external aids for clients with dysmetria is that the inaccuracy of reach may disrupt the ongoing flow of movement or actually be a hazard. If time allows, the client should practice assuming the sitting position from prone. Clients can push up on their arms and rotate their bodies backward onto their hips (Fig. 21-10). Clients can also push up on their hands and knees and drop onto a hip; however, this requires better control of balance.

Independent transfers

If clients develop adequate sitting balance but are not considered safe candidates for ambulation, they should be taught as many independent transfers as possible. A sliding transfer from a wheelchair to another chair or bed will be the safest. A trapeze over a bed or bars in the bath may increase the level of independence if the accuracy of limb movements allows such activity.

Preparing for ambulation

If the goal is to progress clients toward ambulation, a series of preliminary activities would be beneficial before they attempt to stand. The stability at the hip needed for standing can be developed by working initially in the crawling or kneeling position on a mat table. This allows the person to practice weight shifting through the hips without the harmful consequences of falling from standing. The client who is preparing to ambulate should be able to assume a quadriped position from sitting on the mat. If not, the therapist can help the client achieve this position from the prone position (Fig. 21-11). From hands and knees clients can, using the assistance of a therapist or stall bars, work their way up to a kneeling position or sit

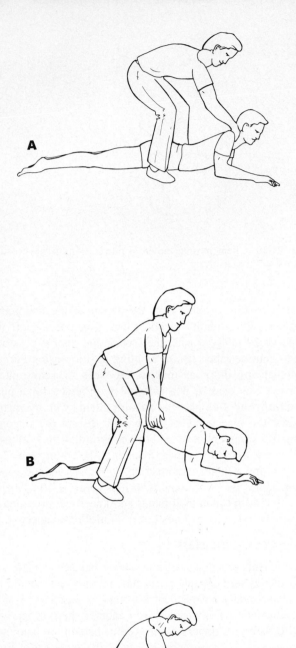

Fig. 21-11. Method to assist a client from prone to quadruped position. **A,** While lifting shoulders to prop client on forearms, therapist directs client to lift head. **B,** Therapist lifts client's pelvis to bring him up on knees. **C,** While lifting client's shoulders to place weight on hands, therapist directs client to lift head.

back on their heels and then straighten the trunk and legs.

If a person cannot easily practice crawling or kneeling activities because of age or other problems, standing activities will have to be started without this preliminary practice. If a client has been in a wheelchair, the therapist should prepare the person's cardiovascular system for being upright by placing him or her on a tilt table. Standing activities should be started in the parallel bars. Clients may not be able to assume a standing position without help. When standing up from sitting, clients need to remember to slide forward in the chair and flex their trunks considerably, placing the center of gravity over their feet. The trunk and legs should be extended only after gaining balance on the feet. This may be the most difficult step for an ataxic individual, who will either lean too far forward or extend the trunk too early and drop back into the chair. Another method a client may use to come to standing is to pull up on the stall bars from a kneeling position. However, this is less practical and will be useful only if the client should end up on the floor. Whatever the method used to come to standing, it will require much repetition by the client and verbal feedback from the therapist. In addition to verbal feedback, viewing a videotape may help a client recognize and correct mistakes.

Once upright, the person should practice balancing, which can be reinforced by approximation through the hips and shoulders. Tremor can be reduced by ankle weights or a weighted belt. Rhythmic stabilization applied to rotation of the trunk may also be valuable in gaining stability. Biofeedback from a force platform may also help the person control the center of gravity. Hopefully, the client can learn to come to standing and maintain standing without pulling on the bars; however, for some people this will be impossible. Those individuals who rely on the bars will not become independent ambulators but may, with the assistance of another person, be able to get up and walk. Once standing and stable, the client needs to practice alternate lifting of the feet. These activities can be practiced in rhythm with music to promote skill. A mirror will also be valuable at this time.

Ambulation

When the person begins to walk in the bars, he or she will need precise verbal feedback as to step length, body rotation, accessory movements, and trunk position. As in the initial learning of a sport, the therapist will need to isolate one problem at a time and provide practice. When the person is ready to walk outside of the bars, a decision will need to be made about an ambulatory aid. Aids may be necessary but also may be an obstacle because clients will now need to control position and movement of the device as well as themselves. Although a walker is typically the most stable, it can be so only when all legs are placed down together and at a correct distance from the body. Accuracy of placement may be facilitated by weighting the legs of the device. Also a piece of tape placed from side to side, midway across the walker, will help keep the client from walking too far into the walker and falling backwards. Crutches or canes may be used but require reciprocal movement of the arms and legs with appropriate timing and placement; this too can be very hard or impossible for some clients. The person may actually do better by using tall poles for support rather than the typical cane or crutches. Therapists can measure clients' progress in ambulation by the number of times they lose their balance in a treatment session, frequency of a specific error, the distance ambulated, or the level of assistance needed (refer to Chapter 13 for additional suggestions).

Activities for temporary reduction of dysmetria

Clients with cerebellar lesions will be frustrated in many activities by the presence of dysmetria. A therapist attempting to modify this impairment needs to recognize that no therapeutic procedure will totally eliminate dysmetria; however, before clients practice specific functional activities, the therapist can have them perform activities that will temporarily decrease dysmetria. For example, use of proprioceptive neuromuscular facilitation (PNF) patterns of rhythmic stabilization or slow-reversal-hold for the lower extremities will allow clients to ambulate with better control.[55,56] Similarly, functional tasks involving the arms can be preceded by PNF patterns for the arms.[77] Frenkel's exercises can also be used to modify dysmetria of the lower extremities.[60] These exercises can be performed in the supine, sitting, or standing positions. Each activity is to be performed slowly with the client watching the extremity very carefully. When the client has gained reasonable control of one activity, he or she should proceed to the next.

Although Frenkel's exercises are classically described for the leg (see the boxed material), they can be modified for the arm. For example, the client can first practice flexing and extending the elbow horizontally, supported on a sliding board, then move the arm without support to place the hand on the opposite elbow, next slide the hand down and up the forearm, and, finally, place the hand in the therapist's moving hand. Whether using Frenkel's exercises or PNF patterns to improve coordination, these activities should not comprise the entire therapy session but should be used to prime the client to practice a subsequent functional activity. Another procedure that can reduce dysmetria of an extremity is to place weights on the extremity.[76] The weights required vary from client to client. The greater the movement error, the heavier the weight needed; however, if the weight is too heavy, dysmetria will become worse.

The use of electromyographical or goniometrical biofeedback may also assist the client in receiving training in very specific acts. For example, brushing the teeth may be impossible because the toothbrush misses the mouth or hits

---

Frenkel exercises

Supine

1. Flex and extend one leg, heel sliding down a straight line on table.
2. Abduct and adduct hip smoothly with knee bent, heel on table.
3. Abduct and adduct leg with knee and hip extended, leg sliding on table.
4. Flex and extend hip and knee with heel off table.
5. Place one heel on knee of opposite leg and slide heel smoothly down shin toward ankle and back to knee.
6. Flex and extend both legs together, heels sliding on table.
7. Flex one leg while extending other leg.
8. Flex and extend one leg while abducting and adducting other leg.

Sitting

1. Place foot in therapist's hand, which will change position on each trial.
2. Raise leg and put foot on traced footprint on floor.
3. Sit steady for a few minutes.
4. Rise and sit with knees together.

Standing

1. Place foot forward and backward on a straight line.
2. Walk along a winding strip.
3. Walk between two parallel lines.
4. Walk, placing each foot in a tracing on floor.

---

the teeth and once inside the mouth does not effectively clean the teeth. Electromyographical feedback from the deltoids, biceps, wrist flexors, and extensors or goniometrical position of the shoulder and elbow may be relayed to clients as they try to learn a pattern that works for them or to duplicate the pattern of signals produced by normal individuals when brushing their teeth.

CEREBELLAR STIMULATION

Results of physiological studies of the function of the cerebellum have led to the use of electrical stimulation of the cerebellum in treatment of various neurological disorders. Electrical stimulation of the cerebellum in cats will disrupt seizure activity induced by electrical stimulation of the pericruciate cortex and the hippocampus.[19,52,53] Based on such observations, cerebellar stimulation has been tried for treatment of severe epilepsy uncontrolled by medication. The results of the treatment have been controversial. Cooper and others[22] reported substantial reduction of seizure frequency in 18 of 32 individuals receiving chronic cerebellar stimulation. Gilman and others[35] also reported favorable results in a study of seven clients with epilepsy. However, Van Buren and others,[104] who performed a double blind cross-over study in five people with epilepsy, were unable to demonstrate objective improvement in the character or frequency of the clients' seizures.

Spasticity in experimental animals can be reduced by electrical stimulation of the anterior lobe of the cerebellum.[64,92] Such findings led to the attempt to reduce involuntary movement disorders in humans by chronic cerebellar stimulation. The results of these efforts have also been controversial. Cooper and others[23] implanted stimulating electrodes over the anterior lobe of the cerebellum of 141 clients with cerebral palsy having severe spasticity and athetosis. In 124 of these individuals who were followed for 1 year after surgery, spasticity was considered improved in 41% and athetosis improved in 24%. Other studies using clients with a variety of movement disorders have also reported significant reduction in spasticity and improvement in the quality of voluntary movement.[99,111] However, double blind studies have not been positive for the effects of chronic cerebellar stimulation.[31,109] In these studies neither professional evaluators nor the clients themselves could tell when the stimulator was turned on.

Another problem with cerebellar stimulation has been to develop electrodes and methods of placement that do not induce damage yet provide adequate current on a long-term basis. Significant damage to the stimulating site and encapsulation of electrodes with connective tissue have been reported, but it is not known if this situation is a universal problem.[24,100] On the basis of the above uncertainties with chronic electrical stimulation of the cerebellum, the approach must still be considered experimental and a last resort for intractable epilepsy, severe spasticity, or other involuntary movement disorders.[52]

REFERENCES

1. Albus JS: A theory of cerebellar function, Math Biosci 10:25, 1971.
2. Allen GI and Tsukahara N: Cerebrocerebellar communications systems, Physiol Rev 54:957, 1974.
3. Amici R and others: Cerebellar tumors: clinical analysis and physiopathologic correlations, New York, 1976, S Karger.
4. Baloh RW and others: Vestibulo-ocular function in patients with cerebellar atrophy, Neurology 25:160, 1975.
5. Botterell EH and Fulton JF: Functional localization in the cerebellum of primates. II. Lesions of the midline structures (vermis) and deep nuclei, J Comp Neurol 69:47, 1938.
6. Botterell EH and Fulton JF: Functional localization in the cerebellum of primates. III. Lesions of the hemispheres (neocerebellum), J Comp Neurol 69:63, 1938.
7. Bremer F: Le cervelet. In Roger GH and Binet L: Traité de physiologie normale et pathologique, vol 10, Paris, 1935, Masson.
8. Brooks VB: Control of intended limb movement by the lateral and intermediate cerebellum. In Asanuma H and Wilson VJ: Integration in the human nervous system, New York, 1979, Igaku Shoin.
9. Brooks VB: Motor programs revisited. In Talbott RE and Humphrey DR: Posture and movement, New York, 1979, Raven Press.
10. Brooks VB and others: Effects of cooling dentate nucleus on tracking task performance in monkeys, J Neurophysiol 36:974, 1973.
11. Brown J and others: Ataxic dysarthria, Int J Neurol 7:302, 1970.
12. Carpenter RHS: Movement of the eyes, London, 1977, Pion, Ltd.
13. Carrea RME and Mettler FA: Physiologic consequences following extensive removals of the cerebellar cortex and deep cerebellar nuclei and effect of secondary cerebral ablations in the primate, J Comp Neurol 87:169, 1947.
14. Chambers WW and Sprague JM: Functional localization in the cerebellum. I. Organization in longitudinal corticonuclear zones and their contribution to the control of posture, both extrapyramidal and pyramidal, J Comp Neurol 103:105, 1955.
15. Chase RA and others: Modification of intention tremor in man, Nature 206:485, 1965.
16. Cogan DG: Ocular dysmetria: flutter like oscillations of the eyes and opsoclonus, Arch Ophthalmol 51:318, 1954.
17. Cole M: Dysprody due to posterior fossa lesions, Trans Am Neurol Assoc 96:151, 1971.
18. Conrad B and Brooks VB: Effects of dentate cooling on rapid alternating arm movements, J Neurophysiol 37:792, 1974.
19. Cooke PM and Snider RS: Some cerebellar influences on electrically induced cerebral seizures, Epilepsia 4:19, 1955.
20. Cooke JD and Thomas JS: Forearm oscillation during cooling of the dentate nucleus in the monkey, Can J Physiol Pharmacol 54:430, 1976.
21. Cooper IS: Involuntary movement disorders, New York, 1969, Harper & Row, Publishers, Inc.
22. Cooper IS and others: A long-term follow up study of cerebellar stimulation for the control of epilepsy. In Cooper IS: Cerebellar stimulation in man, New York, 1978, Raven Press.
23. Cooper IS and others: A long-term follow-up of chronic cerebellar stimulation for cerebral palsy. In Cooper IS: Cerebellar stimulation in man, New York, 1978, Raven Press.
24. Dauth GW and others: Long-term surface stimulation of the cerebellum in monkey. I. Light microscopic, electrophysiologic and clinical observation, Surg Neurol 7:377, 1977.
25. Dichgans J and others: Postural sway in normals and atactic patients, analysis of the stabilizing and destabilizing effects of vision, Agressologie 176:15, 1976.
26. Dow RS and Moruzzi G: The physiology and pathology of the cerebellum, Minneapolis, 1958, University of Minnesota Press.
27. Eccles JC: Long-loop reflexes from the spinal cord to the brain stem and cerebellum, Atti Accad Med Lomb 21:1, 1966.
28. Eccles JC: The dynamic loop hypothesis of movement control. In Leibovic KN, editor: Information processing in the nervous system, New York, 1969, Springer Publishing Co, Inc.
29. Fisher CN and others: Acute hypertensive cerebellar hemorrhage: diagnosis and surgical treatment, J Nerv Ment Dis 140:38, 1965.
30. Fulton JF and Dow RS: The cerebellum: a summary of functional localization, Yale J Biol Med 10:89, 1937.
31. Gahn NH and others: Chronic cerebellar stimulation for cerebral palsy: a double blind study, Neurology 31:87, 1981.
32. Gilman S: The mechanism of cerebellar hypotonia: an experimental study in the monkey, Brain 92:621, 1969.
33. Gilman S and others: Effects of medullary pyramidotomy in the monkey. II. Abnormalities of spindle afferent responses, Brain 94:515, 1971.
34. Gilman S and others: Spinal mechanisms underlying the effects of unilateral ablation of areas 4 and 6 in monkeys, Brain 97:49, 1974.
35. Gilman S and others: Clinical, morphological, biochemical, and physiological effects of cerebellar stimulation. In Hambrecht FT and Reswick FB: Functional electrical stimulation, New York, 1977, Marcel Dekker, Inc.
36. Gilman S and others: Disorders of the cerebellum, Philadelphia, 1981, FA Davis Co.
37. Goldberger ME and Growden JH: Tremor at rest following cerebellar lesions in monkeys: effect of L-dopa administration, Brain Res 27:183, 1971.

38. Goldberger ME and Growden JH: Pattern of recovery following cerebellar deep nuclear lesions in monkeys, Exp Neurol 39:307, 1973.

39. Growden JH and others: An experimental study of cerebellar dyskinesia in the rhesus monkey, Brain 90:603, 1967.

40. Hagbarth KE and others: The effect of gamma fiber block on afferent muscle nerve activity during voluntary contractions, Acta Physiol Scand 79:27A, 1970.

41. Hallett M and others: EMG analysis of stereotyped movements in man, J Neurol Neurosurg Psychiatry 38:1154, 1975.

42. Hallett M and others: EMG analysis of patients with cerebellar deficit, J Neurol Neurosurg Psychiatry 38:1163, 1975.

43. Holmes G: The symptoms of acute cerebellar injuries due to gunshot injuries, Brain 40:461, 1921.

44. Holmes G: The Croonian lectures on the clinical symptoms of cerebellar diseases and their interpretation, Lancet 1:1177, 1922.

45. Holmes G: The Croonian lectures on the clinical symptoms of cerebellar diseases and their interpretation, Lancet 1:1231, 1922.

46. Holmes G: The Croonian lectures on the clinical symptoms of cerebellar diseases and their interpretation, Lancet 2:59, 1922.

47. Holmes G: The Croonian lectures on the clinical symptoms of cerebellar diseases and their interpretation, Lancet 2:111, 1922.

48. Holmes G: The cerebellum of man, Brain 62:1, 1939.

49. Hood JD and others: Rebound nystagmus, Brain 96:507, 1973.

50. Horvath FE and others: Effects of cooling the dentate nucleus in alternating bar pressing performance in monkey, Int J Neurol 7:252, 1970.

51. Ito M: Neurophysiological aspects of the cerebellar motor control system, Int J Neurol 1:162, 1970.

52. Ivan LP and Ventureyra ECG: Chronic cerebellar stimulation in cerebral palsy, Appl Neurophysiol 45:51, 1982.

53. Iwata K and Snider RS: Cerebello-hippocampal influences on the electroencephalogram, Electroencephalogr Clin Neurophysiol 11:439, 1959.

54. Jung R and Kornhuber HH: Results of electronystagmography in man: the value of optokinetic vestibular, and spontaneous nystagmus for neurologic diagnosis and research. In Bender MB: The oculomotor system, New York, 1964, Harper & Row, Publishers, Inc.

55. Kabat H: Studies on neuromuscular dysfunction. XII. Rhythmic stabilization: a new and more effective technique for treatment of paralysis through a cerebellar mechanism, Permanente Found M Bull 8:9, 1950.

56. Kabat H: Analysis and therapy of cerebellar ataxia and asynergia, Arch Neurol Psychiatry 74:375, 1955.

57. Kent R and Netsell R: A case study of an ataxic dysarthric: cineradiography and spectrographic observations, J Speech Hear Disord 40:115, 1975.

58. Knott M and Voss DE: Preprioceptive neuro-muscular facilitation, ed 2, New York, 1968, Harper & Row, Publishers, Inc.

59. Kornhuber HH: Neurologie de kleinherns, Zbl ges Neurol Psychiat 191:13, 1968.

60. Krusen FH and others: Handbook of physical medicine and rehabilitation, ed 2, Philadelphia, 1971, WB Saunders Co.

61. Lamarre Y and others: Central mechanisms of tremor in some feline and primate models, J Can Neurol Sci 2:227, 1975.

62. Larochelle L and others: The rubro-olivo-cerebello nubral loop and postural tremor in the monkey, J Neurol Sci 11:53, 1970.

63. Lectenberg R and Gilman S: Speech disorders in cerebellar disease, Ann Neurol 3:285, 1978.

64. Lowenthal M and Horsley V: On the relations between the cerebellar and other centers (namely cerebral and spinal) with reference to the action of antagonistic muscles, Proc R Soc Lond 61:20, 1897.

65. Luciani L: Il cervelletto: nuovi studi di fisiologia normale e patologica, Florence, 1891, Le Monnier.

66. Luciani L: De l'influence qu'exercent les mutilations cérébelleuses sur l'excitabilité de l'écorce cérébrale et sur les réflexes spinaux, Arch Ital Biol 21:190, 1894.

67. MacKay WA and Murphy JT: Cerebellar modulation of reflex gain, Prog Neurobiol 13:361, 1979.

68. Marie P and others: De l'atrophie cerebelleuse tardive à predominance corticale, Rev Neurol (Paris) 38:849, 1082, 1922.

69. Marr D: A theory of the cerebellar cortex, J Physiol 202:437, 1969.

70. Marsden CD and others: Disorders of movement in cerebellar disease in man. In Rose CF, editor: Physiological aspects of clinical neurology, Oxford, 1977, Blackwell Scientific Publications, Ltd.

71. Mauritz KH and others: Delayed and enhanced long latency reflexes as the possible cause of postural tremor in late cerebellar atrophy, Brain 104:97, 1981.

72. McCloskey DI: Kinesthetic sensibility, Physiol Rev 58:763, 1978.

73. Meyer-Lohmann J and others: Effects of dentate cooling on precentral unit activity following torque pulse injections into elbow movements, Brain Res 94:237, 1975.

74. Meyer-Lohmann J and others: Cerebellar participation in generation of prompt arm movements, J Neurophysiol 38:871, 1977.

75. Miles FA and Fuller JH: Adaptive plasticity in the vestibulo-ocular responses of the rhesus monkey, Brain Res 8:512, 1974.

76. Morgan MH: Ataxia and weights, Physiotherapy 61:332, 1975.

77. Nakamura R and Taniguchi R: Kinesiological analysis and physical therapy of cerebellar ataxia. In Sobue I: Spinocerebellar degenerations, Baltimore, 1978, University Park Press.

78. Narabayashi H: Involuntary movements and cerebellar pathology. In Massion J and Sasaki K: Cerebro-cerebellar interactions, Amsterdam, 1979, Elsevier/North Holland Biomedical Press.

79. Nashner LM: Adapting reflexes controlling human posture, Exp Brain Res 26:59, 1976.

80. Nashold BS and others: Ocular reactions in man from deep cerebellar stimulation and lesions, Arch Ophthalmol 81:538, 1969.

81. Nyberg-Hansen R and Horn J: Functional aspects of cerebellar signs in clinical neurology, Acta Neurol Scand 48(suppl 51):219, 1972.

82. Optician LM and Robinson DA: Cerebellar-dependent adaptive control of primate saccadic system, J Neurophysiol 44:1058, 1980.

83. Orlovsky GN and Shik ML: Control of locomotion: a neurophysiological analysis of the cat locomotor system. In Porter R, editor: International review of physiology neurophysiology II, vol 10, Baltimore, 1976, University Park Press.

84. Oscar-Barman M and others: Dichotic ear-order effects with nonverbal stimuli, Cortex 10:270, 1974.

85. Poirier LJ and others: Physiopathology of the cerebellum in the monkey. II. Motor disturbances associated with partial and complete destruction of cerebellar structures, J Neurol Sci 22:491, 1974.

86. Ritchie L: Effect of cerebellar lesions on saccadic eye movements, J Neurophysiol 39:1246-1256, 1976.

87. Rossi G: Sugli effetti consequenti alla stimolazione contemporanea della corteccia cerebrale e di quella cerebellare, Arch Fisiol 10:389, 1912.

88. Ruch TC: Motor systems. In Stevens SS, editor: Handbook of experimental psychology, New York, 1951, John Wiley & Sons, Inc.

89. Russell JSR: Experimental research into the functions of the cerebellum, Philos Trans R Soc Lond 185:819, 1894.

90. Selhorst JB and others: Disorders in cerebellar ocular motor control. I. Saccadic overshoot dysmetria, Brain 99:497, 1976.

91. Shankweiler D: Effects of temporal lobe damage on perception of dichotically presented melodies, J Comp Physiol Psychol 62:115, 1966.

92. Sherrington CS: Double (antidrome) conduction in the central nervous system, Proc R Soc Lond 61:243, 1897.

93. Shimizu N and others: Eye-head co-ordination in patients with Par-

kinsonism and cerebellar ataxia, J Neurol Neurosurg Psychiatry 44:509, 1981.

94. Silfverskjold BP: A 3 sec leg tremor in a cerebellar syndrome, Acta Neurol Scand 55:385, 1977.

95. Smith AM and Bourbonnais D: Neuronal activity in cerebellar cortex related to control of prehensile force, J Neurophysiol 45:286, 1981.

96. Stein RB and Oguztoreli MN: Reflex involvement in the generation and control of tremor and clonus. In Desmedt JE, editor: Physiological tremor, pathological tremor and clonus, Prog Clin Neurophysiol (Basel) 5:28, 1978.

97. Stockmeyer S: An interpretation of the approach of Rood to the treatment of neuromuscular dysfunction, Am J Phys Med 46:900, 1967.

98. Strick PL: Cerebellar involvement in "volitional" muscle response to load changes, Prog Clin Neurophysiol 4:85, 1978.

99. Sukoff MH and Ragatz RE: Cerebellar stimulation for chronic extensor-flexor rigidity and opisthotonus secondary to hypoxia, J Neurosurg 53:391, 1980.

100. Tennyson VM and others: Long-term surface stimulation of the cerebellum in the monkey. II. Electron microscopic and biochemical observations, Surg Neurol 8:17, 1977.

101. Terzuolo TA and Viviani P: Parameters of motion and EMG activities during some simple motor tasks in normal subjects and cerebellar patients. In Cooper IS and others, editors: The cerebellum, epilepsy and behavior, New York, 1973, Plenum Press.

102. Thach WT: Correlation of neural discharge with pattern and force of muscular activity, joint position, and direction of the intended movement in motor cortex and cerebellum, J Neurophysiol 41:654, 1978.

103. Uno M and others: Effects of cooling the interposed nuclei on tracking-task performance in monkeys, J Neurophysiol 36:996, 1973.

104. Van Buren and others: Preliminary evaluation of cerebellar stimulation and other biologic criteria in the treatment of epilepsy, J Neurosurg 48:407, 1978.

105. Victor M and others: A restricted form of cerebellar cortical degeneration occurring in alcoholic patients, AMA Arch Neurol 1:579, 1959.

106. Vilas T and Hore J: Effects of changes in mechanical state of limb on cerebellar intention tremor, J Neurophysiol 40:1214, 1977.

107. Vilas T and others: Dual nature of the precentral responses to limb perturbations revealed by cerebellar cooling, Brain Res 117:336, 1976.

108. von Noorden GK and Preziosi TJ: Eye movement recordings in neurological disorders, Arch Ophthalmol 76:162, 1966.

109. Whittaker CK: Cerebellar stimulation for cerebral palsy, J Neurosurg 52:653, 1980.

110. Woolridge CP and Russell G: Head position training with the cerebral palsied child: an application of biofeedback techniques, Milbank Mem Fund Q 57:407, 1976.

111. Wong PKH and others: Cerebellar stimulation in the management of cerebral palsy: clinical and physiological studies, Neurosurgery 5:217, 1979.

112. Zee DS and others: The mechanism of downbeat nystagmus, Arch Neurol 30:227, 1974.

113. Zee DS and others: Ocular motor abnormalities in hereditary ataxia, Brain 99:207, 1976.

114. Zee DS and others: Slow saccades in spinocerebellar degeneration, Arch Neurol 33:243, 1976.

115. Zee DS and others: Effects of ablation of flocculus and paraflocculus on eye movements in primate, J Neurophysiol 46:878, 1981.

116. Zentay PJ: Motor disorders of the nervous system and their significance for speech. I. Cerebral and cerebellar dysarthrias, Laryngoscope 47:147, 1937.

Chapter 22

HEMIPLEGIA RESULTING FROM VASCULAR INSULT OR DISEASE

Susan D. Ryerson

OVERVIEW

The treatment of hemiplegia is controversial. Various treatment methods have been devised and advocated. This chapter reviews the problems and management of hemiplegia and will use normal movement as a base on which appropriate techniques of facilitation and inhibition can be chosen to allow the person with hemiplegia to return to life with the highest quality of function.

Definition

Hemiplegia, a paralysis of one side of the body, is the classic sign of neurovascular disease of the brain. It is one of many manifestations of neurovascular disease, and it occurs with strokes involving the cerebral hemisphere or brainstem. A stroke, or cerebrovascular accident (CVA), results in a sudden, specific neurological deficit. It is the suddenness of this neurological deficit—seconds, minutes, hours, or a few days—that characterizes the disorder as a vascular one. Although hemiplegia may be the most obvious sign of a cerebrovascular accident and a major concern of therapists, other symptoms are equally disabling, including sensory dysfunction, aphasia or dysarthria, visual field defects, and mental and intellectual impairment. The specific combination of these neurovascular deficits enables a physician to detect both the location and the size of the defect. Cerebrovascular accidents can be classified according to pathological type—thrombosis, embolus, or hemorrhage—or by temporal factors—completed, in-evolution, or transient ischemic attacks (TIA).

Epidemiology

Although the incidence of cerebrovascular disease has been decreasing for the past 25 years, stroke is still the third most common cause of death in the United States.[1] The incidence of stroke rises rapidly with increasing age; in the 80- to 90-year-old age group, the mortality rates approach the corresponding incidence rates. In the United States, the incidence of stroke is greater in males than in females, and it is greater in the black population than in the white population.[64] Cerebral infarction (thrombosis or embolism) is the most common form of stroke, accounting for 70%. Hemorrhages account for another 20%, and 11% remain unspecified. An idea of the prevalence of stroke can be gained by looking at the results of a study of three states: out of every 100 persons who survive a stroke, 10 return to work without impairment, 40 have mild residual disability, 40 are disabled and require special services, and 10 need institutional care.[63]

The three most commonly recognized risk factors for cerebrovascular disease include hypertension, diabetes mellitus, and heart disease. The most important of these factors is hypertension.[53] Systolic and/or diastolic blood pressure, pulse pressure, and variability of pressure are all good predictors of stroke for all age groups.

Clinically evident diabetes is also significantly related to stroke. Interestingly, the risk of stroke for a diabetic client is not related to the treatment or nontreatment of the disease.

Heart disease, especially electrocardiogram (ECG) abnormalities and heart enlargement, also increases the chance of a completed stroke. Cardiac and cerebrovascular disease are concomitant lesions. See Irwin and Tecklin: *Cardiopulmonary Physical Therapy* for more information.

Risk factors that have been correlated to stroke include increased blood fat levels, obesity, and cigarette smoking. Because high blood pressure is the greatest risk factor for stroke, human characteristics and behavior that increase one's blood pressure will increase the risk of stroke.

Ostfeld[53] has noted that mortality rates for stroke have declined, slowly at first (from 1900 to 1950), then more quickly (from 1950 to 1970), and with a sharp drop noted around 1974. Experts have speculated that the greater use of hypertensive drugs in the 1960s and 1970s started this decline, and the creation of screening and treatment referral centers for high blood pressure may account for the marked decline of the late 1970s. Although approximately 100,000 people die from cerebrovascular disease each year, an additional 1,000,000 people survive strokes but are left disabled.

Outcome

The long-term follow-up on the Framingham study revealed that long-term stroke survivors, especially those with only one episode, had a good chance for full functional recovery.[26] For those people left with severe neurological and functional deficits following a stroke, studies have demonstrated that rehabilitation is effective and that it can improve functional ability.[22,38,66] It has been dem-

onstrated that age is not a factor in determining the outcome of the rehabilitation process.[2] Presently, it is thought that all clients should be given an opportunity to participate in the rehabilitation process unless it is medically contraindicated.[38]

The prediction of ultimate functional outcome has been hampered by the inaccuracy of commonly used predictors (medical items, income level, intelligence, functional level). Computed tomography (CT) scanning and regional cerebral blood flow (rCBF) studies are presently being studied for their potential use as predictors of functional recovery following stroke.[43,59]

Pathoneurological and pathophysiological aspects

Classification

The pathological processes that result from a cerebrovascular accident can be divided into three groups—thrombotic changes, embolic changes, and hemorrhagic changes.

Thrombotic infarction. Atherosclerotic plaques and hypertension interact to produce cerebrovascular infarcts.[1] These plaques form at branchings and curves of the arteries. Plaques usually form in front of the first major branching of the cerebral arteries. These lesions can be present for 30 years or more and may never become symptomatic. Intermittent blockage may procede to permanent damage. The process by which a thrombus occludes an artery requires several hours and explains the division between stroke-in-evolution and completed stroke.

Transient ischemic attacks (TIAs) are an indication of the presence of thrombotic disease and are the result of transient ischemia. Although the cause of TIAs has not been definitively established, cerebral vasospasm or transient systemic arterial hypotension are thought to be responsible factors.

Embolic infarction. The embolus that causes the stroke may come from the heart, from an internal carotid artery thrombosis, or from an atheromatous plaque of the carotid sinus. It is usually a sign of cardiac disease. The infarction may be of pale, hemorrhagic, or mixed type. The branches of the middle cerebral artery are infarcted most commonly as a result of its direct continuation from the internal carotid artery. Collateral blood supply is not established with embolic infarctions as a result of the speed of obstruction formation, so there is less survival of tissue distal to the area of embolic infarct than with thrombotic infarct.[1]

Hemorrhage. The most common intracranial hemorrhages causing stroke are hypertensive, ruptured saccular aneurysm, and atrioventricular (AV) malformation. Massive hemorrhage frequently results from hypertensive cardiac-renal disease and causes bleeding into the brain tissue in an oval or round mass that displaces midline structures. The exact mechanism of hemorrhage is not known. This mass of extravasated blood decreases in size over 6 to 8 months.

Table 22-1. Clinical symptoms of vascular lesions

Vessel	Clinical symptoms	Structures involved
Middle cerebral artery	Contralateral paralysis and sensory deficit	Somatic motor area
	Motor speech impairment	Broca's area (dominant hemisphere)
	"Central" aphasia, anomia, jargon speech	Parietooccipital cortex (dominant hemisphere)
	Unilateral neglect, apraxia, impaired ability to judge distance	Parietal lobe (nondominant hemisphere)
	Homonomous hemianopsia	Optic radiation deep to second temporal convolution
	Loss of conjugate gaze to opposite side	Frontal controversive field
	Avoidance reaction of opposite limbs	Parietal lobe
	Pure motor hemiplegia	Upper portion of posterior limb of internal capsule
	Limb-kinetic apraxia	Premotor or parietal cortex
Anterior cerebral artery	Paralysis—lower extremity	Motor area—leg
	Paresis in opposite arm	Arm area of cortex
	Cortical sensory loss	Sensory area
	Urinary incontinence	Posteromedial aspect of superior frontal gyrus
	Contralateral grasp reflex, sucking reflex	Medial surface of posterior frontal lobe
	Lack of spontaniety motor inaction, echolalia	Uncertain
	Perseveration and amnesia	Uncertain
Posterior cerebral artery		
Peripheral area	Homonomous hemianopsia	Calcarine cortex or optic radiation
	Bilateral homonomous hemianopsia, cortical blindness, inability to perceive objects not centrally located, ocular apraxia	Bilateral occipital lobe
	Memory defect	Inferomedial portions of temporal lobe
	Topographic disorientation	Nondominant calcarine and lingual gyri
Central area	Thalamic syndrome	Posteroventral nucleus ophthalmus
	Weber's syndrome	Cranial nerve III and cerebral peduncle
	Contralateral hemiplegia	Cerebral peduncle
	Paresis of vertical eye movements, sluggish pupillary response to light	Supranuclear fibers to cranial nerve III
	Contralateral ataxia or postural tremor	
Internal carotid artery	Variable signs according to degree and site of occlusion—middle cerebral, anterior cerebral, posterior cerebral territory	Uncertain
Basilar artery		
Superior cerebellar artery	Ataxia	Middle and superior cerebellar peduncle
	Dizziness, nausea, vomiting, horizontal nystagmus	Vestibular nucleus
	Horner's syndrome on opposite side, decreased pain and thermal sensation	Descending sympathetic fibers / Spinal thalamic tract
	Decreased touch, vibration, position sense of lower extremity greater than upper extremity	Medial lemniscus
Anterior inferior cerebellar artery	Nystagmus, vertigo, nausea, vomiting	Vestibular nerve
	Facial paralysis on same side	Cranial nerve VII
	Tinnitus	Auditory nerve, lower cochlear nucleus
	Ataxia	Middle cerebral peduncle
	Impaired facial sensation on same side	Fifth cranial nerve nucleus
	Decreased pain and thermal sensation on opposite side	Spinal thalamic tract
Complete basilar syndrome	Bilateral long tract signs with cerebellar and cranial nerve abnormalities	—
	Coma	—
	Quadriplegia	—
	Pseudobulbar palsy	—
	Cranial nerve abnormalities	
Vertebral artery	Decreased pain and temperature on opposite side	Spinal thalamic tract
	Sensory loss from a tactile and proprioceptive	Medial lemniscus
	Hemiparesis of arm and leg	Pyramidal tract
	Facial pain and numbness on same side	Decending tract and fifth cranial nucleus
	Horner's syndrome, ptosis, decreased sweating	Decending sympathetic tract
	Ataxia	Spinal cerebellar tract
	Paralysis of tongue	Cranial nerve XII
	Weakness of vocal cord, decreased gag	Cranial nerves IX and X
	Hiccups	Uncertain

Adapted from Adams RD and Victor M: Principles of neurology, New York, 1981, McGraw-Hill Inc.

Saccular, or berry, aneurysms are thought to be the result of defects in the media and elastica that develop over the course of years. This muscular defect plus over stretching of the internal elastic membrane from blood pressure causes the aneurysm to develop. Saccular aneurysms are found at branchings of major cerebral arteries, especially the anterior portion of the Circle of Willis. Averaging 8 to 10 mm in diameter and variable in form, these aneurysms rupture at their dome. Saccular aneurysms are rare in childhood.

AV malformations are developmental abnormalities that result in a spaghetti-like mass of dilated arteriovenous fistulas varying in size from a few millimeters in diameter to huge masses located within the brain tissue. Some of these blood vessels have extremely thin, abnormally structured walls. Although the abnormality is present from birth, symptoms usually develop between the ages of 10 and 35. The hemorrhage of an AV malformation presents a pathological picture similar to the saccular aneurysm. The larger AV malformations frequently occur in the posterior half of the cerebral hemisphere.[1]

Clinical findings. The focal neurological deficit resulting from a stroke, whether embolis, thrombus, or hemorrhage, is a reflection of the size and location of the lesion and the amount of collateral blood flow. Unilateral neurological deficits result from interruption of the carotid vascular system, and bilateral neurological deficits result from interruption of the vascular supply to the basilar system. Clinical syndromes resulting from occlusion or hemorrhage in the cerebral circulation vary from partial to complete. Signs of hemorrhage may be more variable as a result of the effect of extension to surrounding brain tissue

and the possible rise in intracranial pressure. Table 22-1 summarizes the clinical symptoms and the anatomical structures involved according to specific arterial involvement.

The frequencies of the three types of cerebrovascular disease—thrombotic, embolism, and hemmorrhage—vary according to whether they were taken from a clinical study or from an autopsy study, but their frequency ranks in the order presented in this section (National Stroke Survey[72]). The clinical symptoms and laboratory findings for each type have been condensed in Table 22-2.

Movement disturbances. Hemiplegia, the motor dysfunction of stroke, is one of the most obvious clinical signs of the disease. Although the site and size of the cerebral vascular lesion initially determines the degree of motor function, the concomitant presence of sensory impairment adds to and compounds the problem of motor dysfunction. Although theories of generator control systems and efferent drive have explained how purposeful movements can occur without "input" from integrated sensory systems, movement is refined, coordinated, and adapted through the interaction of exteroceptive and kinesthetic messages.

Following the onset of a cerebrovascular accident with hemiplegia, a state of low tone or flaccidity exists. The length of this state of flaccidity varies from a short time to a period of weeks or months.

This state is followed by the development of patterns of returning muscle function and patterns of increased tone. The rate at which these patterns of muscle function return is dictated by the site and severity of the lesion and by the focus of the rehabilitation process. Early return of move-

Table 22-2. Clinical symptoms and laboratory findings for neurovascular disease

Disease type	Clinical picture	Laboratory findings
Thrombosis	*Extremely variable*	
	Proceeded by a prodromal episode	Cerebrospinal fluid pressure is normal
	Uneven progression	Cerebrospinal fluid is clear
	Onset develops within minutes, hours, or over days ("thrombus in evolution")	EEG: limited differential diagnostic value
		Skull radiographs are not helpful
	60% occur during sleep—awaken unaware of problem, rise, and fall to floor	Arteriography is the definative procedure, it demonstrates site of collateral flow
	Usually no headache, but may occur in mild form	CT scan is helpful in chronic state when cavitation has occurred
	Hypertension, diabetes, or vascular disease elsewhere in body	
TIAs	Linked to atherosclerotic thrombosis	Usually none
	Proceeded or accompanied by stroke	
	Occur by themselves	
	Last 2-30 minutes	
	Experience a few attacks or hundreds	
	Normal neurological examination between attacks	
	If transient symptoms are present on awakening, may indicate future stroke	

Adapted from Adams RD and Victor M: *Principles of neurology*, New York, 1981, McGraw-Hill Inc.

Table 22-2. Clinical symptoms and laboratory findings for neurovascular disease—cont'd

Disease type	Clinical picture	Laboratory findings
Embolism	*Extremely variable*	
Cardiac	Occurs extremely rapidly—seconds or minutes	Generally same as thrombosis except for following:
Non-cardiac	There are no warnings	If embolism causes a large hemorrhagic infarct, cerebrospinal fluid will be bloody
Atherosclerosis	Branches of middle cerebral artery are involved most frequently, large embolus will block internal carotid artery or stem of middle cerebral artery	30% of embolic strokes produce small hemorrhagic infarct without bloody cerebrospinal fluid
Pulmonary thrombosis		
Fat, tumor, air	If in basilar system, deep coma and total paralysis may result	
	Often a manifestation of heart disease, including atrial fibrillation and myocardial infarction	
	Headache	
	As embolus passes through artery, client may have neurological deficits that resolve as embolus breaks and passes into small artery supplying small or silent brain area	
Hemorrhage		
Hypertensive hemorrhage	Severe headache	CT scan can detect hemorrhages larger than 1.5 cm in cerebral and cerebellar hemispheres, they are diagnostically superior to arteriography; they are especially helpful in diagnosing small hemorrhages that do not spill blood into cerebrospinal fluid; with massive hemorrhage and increased pressure, cerebrospinal fluid is grossly bloody; lumbar puncture is necessary when CT scan is not available
	Vomiting at onset	
	Blood pressure > 170/90; usually "essential" hypertension but can be from other types	
	Abrupt onset, usually during day, not in sleep	
	Gradually evolves over hours or days according to speed of bleeding	Radiographs occasionally show midline shift (this is not true with infarction)
	No recurrence of bleeding	EEG shows no typical pattern, but high voltage and slow waves are most common with hemorrhage
	Frequency in blacks with hypertensive hemorrhage is greater than frequency in whites	
	Hemorrhaged blood absorbs slowly—rapid improvement of symptoms is not usual	Urinary changes may reflect renal disease
	If massive hemorrhage occurs, client may survive a few hours or days secondary to brainstem compression	CT scan detects localized blood in hydrocephalus if present
Ruptured saccular aneurysm	Asymptomatic before rupture	Cerebrospinal fluid is extremely bloody
	With rupture, blood spills under high pressure into subarachnoid space	Radiographs are usually negative
	Excrutiating headache with loss of consciousness	Carotid and vertebral arteriography are performed only if certain of diagnosis
	Headache without loss of consciousness	
	Sudden loss of consciousness	
	Decerebrate rigidity with coma	
	If severe—persistent deep coma with respiratory arrest, circulatory collapse leading to death; death can occur within 5 minutes	
	If mild—consciousness regained within hours then confusion, amnesia, headache, stiff neck, drowsiness	
	Hemiplegia, paresis, homonomous hemianopsia, or aphasia usually absent	

ment is seen in the spinal extensors and the shoulder and pelvic girdle elevators (upper trapezius, levator scapulae, quadratus lumborum, latissimus dorsi).[13,43] Often distal return is available early in recovery and is used by the client to reinforce weak proximal musculature. When these available motor components are used for function (without their corresponding flexor components), stereotypical movement patterns are seen:

1. Extension of the occiput on the first cervical vertebra without corresponding neck flexor activity results in a forward head position
2. Use of unilateral paracervical muscles of the neck results in ipsilateral flexion (the ear approximates the affected shoulder) and contralateral rotation (turning the face away from the affected side) (Fig. 22-1)
3. Use of shoulder elevators slowly changes the position of the scapula from one of depression on the thorax to elevation on the thorax
4. Use of pelvic hikers slowly changes the position of the pelvis from listing downwards on the affected side to listing upwards

The development of spasticity occurs not only in the arm and leg, but also in the musculature of the head, neck, and trunk. The trunk musculature, especially the shoulder and the pelvic girdle, is the initial site of the development of spasticity. This is the same phenomenon displayed in children with cerebral palsy (see Chapter 9). The development of spasticity in the girdle musculature results initially in downward rotation of the scapula and listing upwards of the pelvis, which may cause the trunk on the affected side to appear laterally flexed.

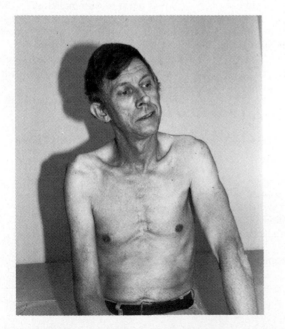

Fig. 22-1. Side bending of the head toward the affected side with the face directed away from the affected side.

The pattern of available spinal and girdle extension without the corresponding abdominal flexors allows the rib cage to rotate backwards on the affected spine. The thoracic vertebrae rotate in a compatible direction. This gives the body an appearance of being "retracted" as described by Bobath.[10]

The initial development of abnormal tone in the trunk and the downward pull of gravity are responsible for the development of the "typical synergistic" patterns seen in the extremities. These typical clinical signs have a neurological base according to established tracts within the CNS. The exact tracts released from higher control or the release of organized recruitment of motor units within the spinal cord is not known. (See Chapter 3 for additional information.)

Upper extremity. With a severe insult to the central nervous system, the upper extremity has no active movement and the scapula assumes a downwardly rotated position (the superolateral angle moves inferiorly and the inferior angle becomes adducted). With scapular downward rotation, the glenoid fossa orients downward, and the passive locking mechanism of the shoulder joint is lost. The loss of this mechanism, the loss of postural tone, and the loss of the shoulder capsule result in an inferior humeral subluxation of the hemiplegic shoulder. The humerus hangs by the side in internal rotation and the elbow is extended (Fig. 22-2).

A second pattern develops as the trunk gains more extension control than flexion control. An increase in cervical and lumbar extension becomes evident. The head and neck assume a position of ipsilateral flexion and contralateral rotation. The rib cage loses its abdominal "anchor" and rotates backward. The scapula and humerus are strongly influenced by this rib cage deviation. The downwardly rotated scapula begins to move superiorly on the thorax, and the humerus hyperextends with internal rotation. This combination of rib cage rotation, humeral hyperextension, and internal rotation allows the humeral head to sublux anteriorly (Fig. 22-3).

Because humans function in the upright position, the battle against gravity is often responsible for compensations. If a person with hemiplegia is in an unsupported sitting position and exhibits the previously described upper-extremity pattern of greater trunk extensor activity, the body will try to keep from falling backward into gravity by pulling the head forward (turtle-like) and rounding the shoulders. This forward compensation begins to accentuate the forward pull of the pectorals, and with the continued development of spasticity the humerus may be pulled forward across the thorax in horizontal adduction (Fig. 22-4).

The third movement pattern is characterized by abnormal coactivation of the limb muscles. This gives an appearance of "mass" flexion in the hemiplegic upper extremity. The head and neck control in clients with this upper-extremity pattern contains elements of both flexion and extension. The control patterns are not sufficiently inte-

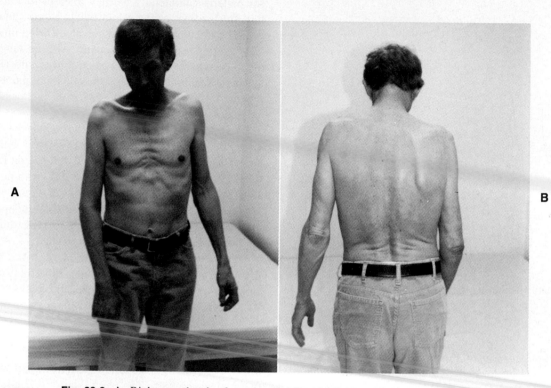

Fig. 22-2. A, Right arm dangles from the client's side. **B,** Scapula is rotated downward.

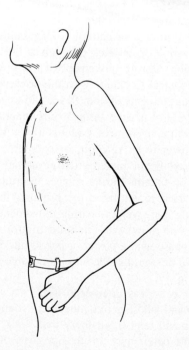

Fig. 22-3. Humerus hyperextends with internal rotation and subluxes anteriorly.

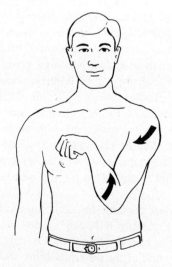

Fig. 22-4. Humeral adduction, internal rotation, elbow flexion, forearm pronation, and wrist and finger flexion.

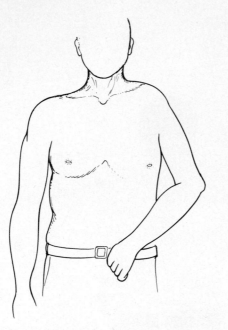

Fig. 22-5. Humerus abducts with internal rotation and subluxes superiorly.

grated to allow selective combinations of movement. The scapula is usually elevated and abducted on the thorax. The head of the humerus is held tightly beneath the acromial process. Although the deltoid and biceps attempt to initiate humeral motion, no disassociation occurs between the humerus and scapula. The upper-extremity pattern available as a result of the position of the scapula and humerus is shoulder elevation with humeral abduction, internal rotation, and elbow flexion[61] (Fig. 22-5).

Lower extremity. In the acute stage of recovery or following a severe stroke, when the client's motor control is one of low postural tone and little motor activity, the movement pattern is strongly influenced by gravity. As the client attempts to assume a standing position, the pelvis will either tilt anteriorly or posteriorly, and will list downwards on the affected side. As a result of this position and the loss of motor control, the hip and knee will flex. This hip and knee flexion combined with an inability to bear weight on the affected side places the ankle in plantarflexion. Because the calcaneus becomes non–weight bearing, any weight that is placed on the leg will be borne by the forefoot.

As functional training for activities such as transfers, standing, and walking is begun, clients are often encouraged to put the heel down on the ground. If this is done without correction of the proximal trunk and hip problems, the knee will move into recurvatum and the ankle will continue to move in the direction of plantarflexion.

During recovery or with a less severe stroke, a second pattern becomes evident. Motor return causes an imbalance of control between trunk flexor and extensor muscle

groups. Spinal extensor patterns are more available to the client than spinal flexor patterns. Clients use these extensor patterns unilaterally as they attempt functional activities. In standing, active use of pelvic hikers causes the pelvis to be tilted anteriorly and elevated (listed upward). The knee will extend unless the client has been taught to push the knee into flexion. If the knee moves into recurvatum, the ankle will plantarflex and the talus will move anteriorly relative to the calcaneus. If soft tissue tightness develops, ankle dorsiflexion range is lost.

These clients use this lower trunk extension and pelvic hiking to initiate the swing phase of gait. Pelvic hiking prevents any lower trunk rotational component from occurring. The hip and pelvis become a unit (with no disassociation present), the knee is extended stiffly, and the ankle is "pushed" into plantarflexion as the client attempts to swing the leg forward. As the client tries to clear the foot from the floor, the foot will begin to supinate.

At heel strike, the client's forefoot strikes the ground first. When body weight is placed on the foot, the midfoot collapses and weight is transferred back toward the heel. As weight shift during stance is attempted, the knee remains in recurvatum, hip extension is blocked, and the pelvis is not able to initiate a forward diagonal movement pattern. Therefore these clients compensate with either the upper trunk or the unaffected side to initiate weight shift over the stance limb. The pelvis stays elevated, tilted anteriorly, and rotated backwards. The hip is in relative flexion and varying degrees of internal rotation. There is a strong, rigid push of the leg into the ground.

The third movement pattern is characterized by abnormal coactivation of muscles. This gives the appearance of "mass flexion" during movement of the lower extremity. The trunk control in clients with this lower-extremity pattern contains elements of both flexor and extensor patterns, but the control of these patterns is not integrated enough to allow selective movement patterns (i.e., lateral flexion, upper or lower trunk rotation, or counter rotation). Such clients recruit flexor patterns during swing phase of gait and extensor patterns during stance. Recruitment of distal motion is used to reinforce the proximal motions, especially during non–weight-bearing movements.

Clients who move with this third control pattern initiate the swing phase with a posterior pelvic tilt. The hip moves into relative flexion, but the most noticeable hip movement is abduction.[60]

Another pattern is often seen in clients whose tone remains low and whose active movement control is minimal. This client will tend to sit more than walk. In the sitting position, the pelvis may roll to a position of posterior tilt. Because the activity level of these clients is low, the pelvis often becomes fixed in this position. When standing, these clients tend to hold the pelvis in this familiar posterior position and will lean the thoracic spine backward over the pelvis using the forward position of the head to counterbalance themselves. The posterior tilt of the pelvis tends to place the hip in a position of relative external rotation.

Although the main tonal movement problems of stroke are spasticity, flaccidity, or combinations thereof, other motor disturbances, such as ataxia, do occur. In ataxia, the main movement problem is one of low, fluctuating tone, which results in instability of the trunk, shoulder, and girdles. The compensation for this central instability is excessive movement of the extremities. Voluntary extremity movements are usually present but uncoordinated. The person with ataxia has low trunk and girdle tone. Occasionally, high tone is present in the extremities as a result of compensatory movements (see Chapter 21).

Sensory disturbances. A cerebrovascular accident with resultant hemiplegia and sensory loss is a devastating event. It is best appreciated by the client. Whereas some clients with hemiplegia experience a total loss of tactile and/or proprioceptive sensation, a majority experience partial impairment, which usually affects the higher discriminatory sensations. A client may feel touch but be unable to localize it, may interpret pressure as light touch, or may be unable to distinguish variations in temperature. Sensory deficit may be so complete as to lead to a loss of recognition of the affected side. The suddenness of the sensory loss leaves the two sides of the body with different sensory recognition, thus providing the brain with different forms of sensory feedback. With impaired sensation and sensory feedback, the client loses control and coordination of movements. This loss of control and disturbed sensory feedback results in disturbances of movement in the "good" side of the body also.[11] Perhaps there is no such thing as an "uninvolved" side.

Even if the client has suffered no loss of sensation but has experienced an abnormality of muscle tone, the abnormal sensations from the spastic muscles and the resultant abnormal feedback provided from the joints result in abnormal sensory feedback from the periphery to the CNS.

Sequential stages of recovery from acute to long-term care

Evolution of recovery process. The evolution of the recovery process from onset to the return to community life can be divided into three stages—acute, active (rehabilitation), and adaptation to personal environment.

The acute state involves the stroke-in-evolution, the completed stroke, or the TIA and the decision whether or not to hospitalize.

The stroke-in-evolution develops gradually with distinct demarcation of the events over a period of 6 to 24 hours. The thrombosis, the most common cause for stroke, results first in ischemia and finally in infarction. Its gradual onset has led researchers to believe that a "cure" may be found for this type of stroke. If ischemic tissue can be treated and saved before infarction occurs, the neurological damage may be reversible. Small hemorrhages may also become a stroke-in-evolution by effusing blood along nerve pathways and by attracting fluid.[42] A completed stroke has a sudden onset and produces distinct nonprogressive symptoms and damage within minutes or hours. In contrast, the TIA has a brief duration of neurological deficit and spontaneous resolution with no residual signs. TIAs vary in number and duration.

The need for hospitalization is decided on by the physician. The trend to hospitalize is more common today than years ago.[72] However, a mild stroke or TIA may produce minimal physical-mental symptoms and the person may not even seek medical help.

Once the stroke is completed the clinical symptoms begin to decrease in severity. Stroke caused by an embolic episode may have symptoms that reverse completely in a few days; more frequently however, improvement takes place very slowly with a marked deficit. The fatality rate is high within the first day but decreases substantially in the following months of recovery.[72]

The Framingham study population has revealed that long-term stroke survivors have a good chance of returning to independent living. The greatest deficit in those persons with hemiplegia who have recovered basic motor skills and who have returned home is in the psychosocial and environmental areas.[25]

Recovery of motor function. Recovery of motor function following a stroke was thought historically to be complete after 3 to 6 months of onset. Research has shown that functional recovery from a stroke can continue for months or years.[5,71]

The initial functional gains following the stroke are attributed to reduction of cerebral edema, absorption of damaged tissue, and improved local vascular flow. However, these factors do not play a role in long-term functional recovery.[5] The brain damage that results from a stroke is thought to be circumvented rather than "repaired" during the process of functional recovery. The CNS reacts to injury with a variety of potentially reparative morphological processes. Presently, the two mechanisms underlying functional recovery following stroke are collateral sprouting and the unmasking of neuropathways.[5,9] Research will continue to provide important insights into the fundamental capabilities of the brain to respond to damage. Therapeutic intervention and retraining of functional skills will also improve the functional ability of the person following a stroke.

Predictable traits. The CNS has some predictable traits in response to injury. Because the developing nervous system is more plastic than the adult nervous system, a stroke in an 8-year-old child is usually characterized by good recovery of function. However, a stroke at 80 years of age may be more devastating as a result of poorer functional recovery. Secondly, the less complete the lesion is, the more likely significant recovery will occur. Thirdly, damage to primary motor or sensory pathways is more likely to result in greater functional deficit than is damage to other areas.[45] Clinically, we have found some predictable events following a stroke. Twitchell, in his classic study, first documented the initial loss of voluntary function.[12] Although flaccidity initially exists, there is seldom if ever total flaccidity.[12] He reported both an increase in deep tendon reflexes after 48 hours and the emergence of synergistic patterns of movement. The synergistic movement patterns of the upper extremity and lower extremity have been described in detail by many, including Bobath,[10] Brunnstrom,[13] and Kabat and Knott.[33] Although the descriptions at first glance may seem at odds with each other, each is describing the same phenomenon. Semantics, differences in British and American terminology, and the degree of completeness of description cause the confusion. Verbal description of a visual phenomenon often leads to differences in written and spoken communication, yet the visual array or behavioral patterns may be exactly the same.[8]

The severity of the stroke, compensations, and deformity as well as the type of treatment may cause variations in or combinations of these described patterns of movement.

Synergistic patterns do not allow normal functions to occur. Synergistic patterns are not the same as the movement combinations necessary for function. Although it is said that the leg recovers more quickly or better than the arm, a leg that is bound by an extensor synergy and that is as "rigid as a pillar" during gait has not recovered quicker and/or better than an arm that is flexed and held across the chest and that can only grasp in a gross pattern with no ability to release.[46]

Although the relationship of voluntary movement to spasticity has not been clearly defined, clinical evidence demonstrates that as voluntary function increases, the dependence on synergistic movement decreases and spasticity decreases.[62] Twitchell concluded that at the point of complete motor recovery, the only remaining deficit may be an increased tendency to fatigue.[13]

With the knowledge that the CNS is capable of reacting to injury with a variety of morphological processes, we should no longer view the effect of a stroke as a negative event. The brain immediately institutes neuromechanisms that reconstitute normal function. Therapy should emphasize normality through long-term events and direct treatment goals and should attempt to achieve the highest level of function by concentrating on the quality, not the quantity, of recovery.

Medical management and pharmacological considerations

Acute medical care

Thrombosis and TIAs. Although infarcted tissue cannot be restored presently, medical management of the acute stroke from thrombosis or TIA is geared toward re-

storing the cerebral circulation as quickly as possible to prevent ischemic tissue from becoming infarcted tissue. Cerebral circulation is maintained by preventing upright posture for the first few days, avoiding dependency in the systemic circulation, maintaining blood pressure, and correcting anemia.

Anticoagulant drugs may prevent TIAs and may stop a stroke-in-evolution. Before anticoagulant drugs are used, an accurate differential diagnosis is necessary because of the danger of excessive bleeding if hemorrhage is present. Heparin is often used in the early stage of the stroke, and warfarin (Coumadin) is commonly used in the months following the stroke. Cerebral edema, if present, is managed pharmacologically during the first few days. Antiplatelet drugs such as aspirin, dipyridamole (Persantine), and sulphin pyrazone (Anturane) are being used, and their effects are being studied as a means to prevent clotting by decreasing platelet "stickiness."[1]

Surgical treatment, thromboendarterectomy, or grafting are used when TIAs are the result of arterial plaques. Areas accessible and suitable for surgery include the carotid sinus and the common carotid, innominant, and subclavian arteries. Although surgery and anticoagulant therapy is used in TIA, Adams[1] extensively reviews the wide divergence of opinions. For clients who have had a stroke yet recovered quickly and well, medical care focuses on prevention. Prevention usually includes maintaining blood pressure and blood flow, monitoring hypotensive agents (if given), and avoiding oversedation, especially for sleep, to prevent cerebral ischemia.

Embolic infarction. Management of embolic infarction is similar to that of thrombotic infarction. The primary emphasis is on prevention. Long-term anticoagulant therapy has been shown to be effective in preventing embolic infarction in clients with cardiac problems such as atrial fibrillation, myocardial infarction (MI), and valve prostheses. The diagnostic use of CT scans is important in anticoagulant therapy to rule out hemorrhage following the infarct.

Hypertensive hemorrhage. Medical procedures for hypertensive hemorrhage parallel those for thrombosis and embolis. Surgical removal of the clot and lowering of the systemic blood pressure to decrease hemorrhage have generally not been helpful. Again, the preventive use of antihypertensive drugs in clients with essential hypertension is the soundest medical management available.[1]

Ruptured aneurysm. Comatose clients are not good candidates for surgery. However, if the client survives the first few days and if the state of consciousness improves, surgical intervention whether extracranial or intracranial is the treatment of choice. Medical treatment consists of lowering arterial blood pressures. Bed rest for 4 to 6 weeks with all forms of exertion avoided is prescribed. Antiseizure medication may be used. Often a systemic antifibrinolysin is given to impede lysis of the clot at the site of rupture. Vasospasm, resulting in severe motor dysfunction, is present with the use of drugs such as reserpine (Serpasil) and kanamycin (Kantrex).

Regardless of the cause, comatose stroke clients are managed by (1) treatment of shock, (2) maintenance of clear airway and oxygen flow, (3) measurement of arterial blood gases, blood analysis, CT scan, and spinal tap, (4) control of seizures, and (5) gastric tube feeding (if coma is prolonged). Hypertensive hemorrhage is one of the most common vascular causes of coma.[69]

Medical management of associated problems with hemiplegia

Spasticity. Spasticity and its treatment present a major medical problem because there are several types of spasticity and because the relationship between spasticity and movement has not been universally accepted. Various pharmacological, surgical, and physical means have been used to decrease spasticity and therefore ameliorate the problems it causes. The pharmacological and surgical means are examined here, and the physical treatment is discussed later.

Three types of drugs are currently being used to counter the effects of spasticity. Centrally acting drugs (barbiturates and tranquilizers) have been used to depress the lateral reticular formation and thus its facilitory action on the gamma motor neurons. This form of drug is used widely to treat spasticity, even though the greatest disadvantage of centrally acting drugs is the fact they depress the entire CNS. Drowsiness and lethargy often result.

Peripherally acting drugs have also been used to block a specific link in the gamma group. Procaine blocks selectively inhibit the small gamma motor fibers, resulting in a relaxation of intrafusal fibers. The effect of procaine blocks is transient. Intramuscular neurolysis with the injection of 5% to 7% phenol has been used to destroy the small intramuscular mixed nerve branches.[16] Phenol blocks have been found to relieve spasticity and improve function, especially when followed by an intensive course of therapy.[55] They can provide relief from 2 to 12 months, and their effects have been documented to last as long as 3 years.[16,55] Disadvantages of phenol use include its toxicity to tissue and the complications of pain that occasionally result.

Dantrolene sodium has been used recently to interrupt the excitation-contraction mechanism of skeletal muscles. Trials have shown that it has reduced spasticity in 60% to 80% of clients while improving function in 40% of these clients. The side effects—drowsiness, weakness, and fatigue—can be decreased through gradation of dosage. Serious side effects, including hepatotoxicity, precipitation of seizures, and lymphocytic lymphoma, have been reported when the drug has been used in high dosages over long periods of time.[16]

The surgical treatment of spasticity through tenotomy or neurectomy has been considered when all other treatments fail, and it has been carried out for the purposes of correct-

ing deformity, especially of a hand or foot, and improving function. A peripheral nerve block is often used as a diagnostic tool to evaluate the effect of surgical treatment. If anatomical or functional gains are made through a temporary nerve block, considerations are given for surgical release. In the client with hemiplegia, the most common surgical sites include the hip adductors, ankle plantar flexors, and toe, wrist, and finger flexors.

Respiratory involvement. Fatigue is a major problem for the person with hemiplegia. This fatigability, which interferes with everyday life processes and active rehabilitation, is attributed to respiratory insufficiency resulting from paralysis of one side of the thorax. Haas[27] studied respiratory function and hemiplegia and found decreased lung volume and mechanical performance of the thorax to be significant factors, in addition to abnormal pulmonary diffusing capacity. Clients with hemiplegia consume 50% more oxygen while walking slowly (regardless of the presence or absence of orthotic devises) than nonhemiplegic subjects.[27] The decreased respiratory output and the increased oxygen demand that result from abnormal movement patterns are responsible for early fatigue in persons with hemiplegia. Treatment objectives and techniques must reflect the understanding of this respiratory problem. The use of standard respiratory functions as an objective measure of the efficacy of treatment techniques must not be overlooked.

EXAMPLE: Clients with left hemiplegia initially ambulate 5 to 20 feet with no ability to accept or bear weight on the left side.

Treatment objective: To facilitate weight acceptance onto left hip during standing and walking.

Results: Initial oxygen consumption 50% greater than normal; following treatment, oxygen consumption improved to 30% greater than normal.

Assessment: Gait deviations may not have changed dramatically, but the ability to shift weight onto the left hip did improve; the rate of oxygen consumption approached normal.

Conclusion: The functional ability of the client improved.

Common breathing pattern problems of the person with hemiplegia include clavicular breathing, a "breathy" quality of exhalation, inability to switch from oral to nasal breathing, and asymmetrical trunk control and tone.

Trauma. If the hemiplegic client is not trained in weight shifting and weight bearing to both sides, poor balance and resultant falls will occur.[49] Protective mechanisms may not be present, and the person often falls to the affected side. Frequent fractures include the humerus and femur. Treatment of femoral fractures is complicated by spasticity in the hip musculature. In addition to the loss of balance and protective mechanisms, the development of osteoporosis from disuse is a precipitating factor for fractures as a result of falls.[47]

Thrombophlebitis. Thrombophlebitis may occur in the early stages of rehabilitation. Vascular changes may have been present before the stroke, and they can be aggravated by the inactivity and dependent postures of the extremities.

Reflex sympathetic dystrophy. Medical treatment of reflex sympathetic dystrophy includes the use of chemical sympathetic blocks and oral or intramuscular steroids. The use of blocks and steroids often stops the burning pain. The length of time of the relief varies from client to client. Adverse reactions occur about 20% of the time.[14]

Pain. The pharmacological management of pain resulting from hemiplegia includes the use of corticosteroids. (For additional information regarding pain and its management see Chapter 27.)

EVALUATION PROCEDURES
General evaluation

Following or during the evolution of a stroke, a thorough medical examination is conducted; all systems are surveyed, with emphasis placed on the level of consciousness, mental, affective, and emotional states, cranial nerves, communication, perceptual ability, sensation, and motor function.

Scales of varying types are used to measure the client's level of consciousness, to assess the initial severity of brain damage, and to prognosticate recovery curves. The Glasgow Coma Scale, devised by Teasdale and Jennett[69] in collaboration with Plum, has been used for nontraumatic comas caused by stroke and cardiac disease. This scale records motor responses to pain, verbal responses to auditory and visual clues, and eye opening; it assigns numerical values according to graded scales.[72] Plum[56] and Levy[39] have also established criteria for correlating clinical signs of coma with prognosis.

The standard descriptions of level of consciousness—normal, semistupor, stupor, deep stupor, semicoma, coma, deep coma—are categorized by objective medical data but often leave a gap in the understanding of how the client functions in life.[69] This gap was closed by the creation of a scale, "Levels of Cognitive Functioning," devised at Rancho Los Amigos Hospital. This behavioral rating scale is not a test of cognitive skill but an observational rating of the client's ability to process information.[41]

The history portion of the neurological evaluation leads to an assessment of the mental, emotional, and affective state. The client's ability to describe the illness gives information on memory, orientation to time and place, the ability to express ideas, and judgment. If the examiner suspects a particular problem, a more thorough review is undertaken of the higher cortical function: serial subtraction, repetition of digits, and recall of objects or names. Emotional or behavioral traits are also documented. Clients with right hemiplegia may be cautious and disorganized in solving a given task, and clients with left hemiplegia tend to be fast and impulsive and seemingly unaware of the deficits present. These different response patterns stem from hemispheric involvement and prior hemispheric specialization. Loss of emotional control often exists following a stroke. Crying is a common problem. Although excessive, inappropriate, or uncontrollable crying is usually a result of brain damage and a sign of emotional lability, crying can also be an expression of sadness as a result of depression. This difference is distinguishable by the ease with which the crying can be stopped (see Chapter 7). Other signs of emotional lability in persons with hemiplegia from stroke include inappropriate laughter or anger.

A general evaluation of communication disorders is noted while taking the history. Cerebral disorder resulting from infarct or hemorrhage can produce a loss of production or comprehension of the spoken word, the written word, or both. Specific evaluation of aphasias and dysarthrias can be found in Chapter 24. The therapist should be familiar with all types of communication disorders and with alternate modes of communication in order to establish a good client interrelationship. The interrelationship between the therapist and client is critical for the retraining of the sensory, motor, and perceptual problems of hemiplegia.

Thorough cranial nerve evaluation is necessary in hemiplegia because a deficit of a particular cranial nerve helps to determine the exact size and location of the infarct or hemorrhage. In hemiplegia, it is imperative to check for visual field deficits, pupil signs, ocular movements, facial sensation and weakness, labyrinthine and auditory function, and laryngeal and pharyngeal function.

Standard areas of reflex testing include the triceps, biceps, supinator, quadriceps, and gastrocnemius muscles. According to Adams,[1] there are four plantar reflex responses: (1) avoidance—quick, (2) spinal flexion—slow, (3) Babinski—toe grasp, and (4) positive support.

Perceptual deficits in clients with hemiplegia are complex and are intimately linked to the sensorimotor deficit. Normal development has shown us that the acquisition of motor function is related to perceptual function.[4]

> **EXAMPLE:** In the sitting position, a 6- to 8-month-old child learns to hold midline with his or her trunk and then explores reaching up, reaching down, reaching from side to side, and reaching behind. As motor function allows exploration of the space around midline, the child's perception of midline up, down, side, front, and back is established.
>
> Sensory integration theory has begun to establish norms and objective data for testing and documenting perceptual deficits in children. Presently, norms and testing procedures for adults have not been standardized, but perceptual deficits have been identified in clients with hemiplegia. Common perceptual deficits found in left and right brain damage can be found in the box on p. 631

Perceptual retraining without standardized norms for the deficit is at best difficult. The soundest course presently available appears to be one that relates perceptual and motor learning rather than retraining perception in isolation (see Chapters 11 and 25).

Perceptual deficits in CNS dysfunction

Left hemiparesis: right hemisphere—general spatial-global deficits

Visual-perceptual deficits
  Hand-eye coordination
  Figure-ground discrimination
  Spatial relationships
  Position in space
  Form constancy
Behavioral and intellectual deficits
  Poor judgment, unrealistic behavior
  Denial of disability
  Inability to abstract
  Rigidity of thought
  Disturbances in body image and body scheme
  Impairment of ability to self-correct
  Difficulty retaining information
  Distortion of time concepts
  Tendency to see the whole and not individual steps
  Affect lability
  Feelings of persecution
  Irritability, confusion
  Distraction by verbalization
  Short attention span
  Appearance of lethargy
  Fluctuation in performance
  Disturbances in relative size and distance of objects

Right hemiparesis: left hemisphere—general language and temporal ordering deficits

Apraxia
  Motor
  Ideational
Behavioral and intellectual deficits
  Difficulty initiating tasks
  Sequencing deficits
  Processing delays
  Directionality deficits
  Low frustration levels
  Verbal and manual perseveration
  Rapid performance of movement or activity
  Compulsive behavior
  Extreme distractability

Traditional sensory testing is used to assess sensory deficits in the adult with hemiplegia, that is, light touch, deep pressure, kinesthesia, proprioception, pain, temperature, graph esthesia, two-point discrimination, appreciation of texture and size, and vibration. A comparison of the differences in the two sides of the body and qualitative as well as quantitative measurements are important features of sensory testing in clients with hemiplegia. Sensory testing is difficult because it relies on the client's interpretation of the sensation, the client's general awareness and suggestibility, as well as the client's ability to communicate a response to each test item.

The presence and quality of sensory loss is of greater importance during motor learning. Sherrington established the principle of interdependence of sensation and movement; current researchers have refined the concept and hypothesize that sensation modifies ongoing movement by providing feedforward, feedback, and corollary discharge, yet sensation is not an absolute prerequisite for movement.[12,68] Motor learning can occur in the absence of sensation through the learning of a "set," which is an equilibrium point between agonist and antagonist.[8] Although clinical investigations have correlated severe sensory loss with poor prognosis for motor function, the reason for this correlation may not be a cause and effect relationship but rather the state of the art of therapy. On the other hand, directing therapy only at movement will not give functional results if sensory preparation is not included. The ability to tolerate and appreciate light touch and pressure are related to the ability to tolerate weight bearing, and weight bearing is the beginning of functional muscle reeducation.[4]

Motor system evaluation

An evaluation of motor behavior can be broken down into three distinct but interrelated parts. The first part is an assessment of movement possibilities, postural mechanisms, and functional activities. The second part is an assessment of joint function, including pain. The third is an assessment of the sensory systems. This systematic evaluation of the client's motor capabilities must be conducted before beginning to plan a treatment program. Because human beings are motor driven creatures who achieve functional activity through movement, a motor system evaluation must be carried out with function in mind.

Assessment of movement possibilities

Active movement. When assessing active movement patterns, the therapist should be aware not only of whether or not the activity can be initiated or accomplished but of how the movement is done. The quality of the movement pattern will indicate which muscles are functioning and which muscles are not. Active movement patterns should be noted by joints and by position (supine, side-lying, sitting, and standing) because the effect of gravity and reflexes will influence the control of movement during changes of position.

EXAMPLE: Active movement patterns—sitting, shoulder flexion to 60 degrees, downward rotation of the scapula, and internal rotation of the humerus.

For the function of forward reach the missing components would be upward rotation and protraction of the scapula and external rotation of the humerus.

If the hemiplegic client is asked to perform a functional activity that requires use of components he or she does not have control of, a compensation will occur.

EXAMPLE: The client in the previous example cannot perform the function of forward reach. He or she will compensate for a lack of forward reach by recruiting shoulder elevators or by side bending away from the affected side, which gives the appearance of greater forward flexion and reach. If allowed to occur repeatedly, compensations for function will become habits, and habits will eventually lead to contractures. These contractures have the potential to become a fixed deformity. The presence of a fixed joint deformity rules out the possibility of facilitating new functional movement patterns.

The assessment of active movement in hemiplegia is commonly documented by therapists through the use of the synergistic stages as outlined by Brunnstrum[13] or by Bobath's long evaluation form, which relates postural abilities (righting, equilibrium, protection) to selective movement activities.[10] Each of these assessment methods lacks a numerical score to standardize the postural and motor performance of hemiplegic clients. Numerical rating scales for evaluating neuromotor performances are being devised.[21]

Postural mechanisms

Tone. The evaluation of postural mechanisms must always include an assessment of tone. Over the years, the great physiologists have split into two camps over the definition of tone. During the first half of the century, tone was thought of as postural reflexes. In the 1950s the concept of tone was thought of as a state of light excitation or a state of preparedness.[23] Granit[24] recently encouraged us to think of the relatedness of both these views. He felt that the same spinal organization is mobilized by the basal ganglia to produce *both* manifestations of tone, a state of preparedness and the postural reflexes.

It is heartening to hear such discussions occurring among the physiologists, because therapists are also questioned about their notations of and changes in tone, and they often have no objectively derived standard clinical system for quickly measuring tone. The debate over tone continues, but clients with CNS dysfunction clinically display changes of muscle tone that the therapist must identify.

The first noticeable change in tone is the change from the premorbid state. Clients in the acute phase of hemiplegia all exhibit, for varying periods of time, a lower than normal tonal state. Following the first 24 hours after injury, the client with hemiplegia begins to become more alert and more active. Because the client has moved before, he or she is motivated to move and will use whatever movement patterns are available. In the severe stroke, there is only one side to use for movement. Moving with half the body is hard, stressful work, and with that slow, laborious effort comes an increase in tone. The hemiplegic client's first automatic movement response is often one of primitive trunk extension on the affected side (a C curve, concavity to the affected side) and a weight shift to the unaffected side (Fig. 22-6).

A universally satisfactory definition of "tone" is hard to come by. For therapists retraining motor function in clients with CNS dysfunction, it is important to make a distinc-

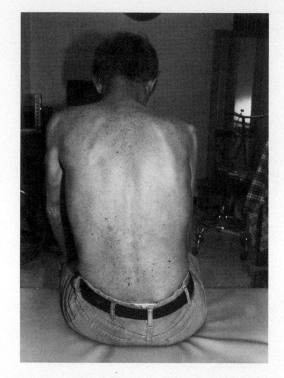

Fig. 22-6. This client with a right hemiplegia shows the tendency to shift weight to the unaffected side and the beginnings of a C curve of the spine with the concavity to the affected side.

tion between postural tone and muscle tone. Postural tone is tone that is "high" enough to keep the body from collapsing into gravity, but "low" enough to allow the body to move against gravity. It is influenced by the input from the corticospinal tracts, the vestibular system, the alpha and gamma systems, and peripheral-tactile and proprioceptive receptors.[18] Normal postural tone allows a constant interplay between the various muscle groups in the body and imparts a constant readiness to move and to react to changes in the environment (internal and external). It provides us with an ability to adjust automatically and continuously to movements. These adjustments provide the proximal fixation necessary to hold a given posture against gravity while allowing voluntary and selective movements to be superimposed without conscious or excessive effort. Fig. 22-7 illustrates this concept in diagrammatical form.

Muscle tone is defined as the passive resistance derived from the series and parallel elastic elements of a muscle. Although controversy now exists (see Chapter 2), spasticity (or increased muscle tone) is classically defined as increased resistance to passive stretch. Severe spasticity makes coordinated movements impossible because the balance between alpha and gamma firings seen in normal movement is lost.[57] Moderate spasticity can be defined clinically when movements are possible but characterized by great effort, slow velocity, and abnormal coordination. Slight spasticity allows gross movement patterns to occur with smooth coordination, but combined, selective move-

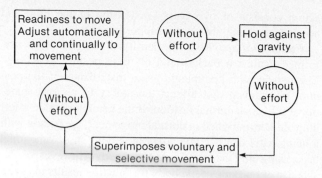

Fig. 22-7. Model for normal postural tone.

ment patterns will be incoordinated or not possible.[10]

Difference in tonal states lower than normal are also present in hemiplegia. The "floppy," or "almost zero," state is characterized by a feeling of total "dead weight" upon passive lifting. A limb with low tone feels heavy, but some "following" of passive movement patterns can be detected. When assessing and treating movement disorders, therapists should be aware of changes in both postural tone and muscle tone.

Righting and equilibrium reactions. Righting reactions enable a person to change position, such as rolling, rising from a lying position, and moving from a sitting to a standing position. The righting reactions are mediated by sensory receptors and begin to develop at birth. The five groups of righting reactions are:

1. Labyrinthine righting on the head
2. Body righting acting on the head
3. Neck righting
4. Body righting acting on the body
5. Optical righting

Equilibrium reactions develop as we become upright creatures, that is, as we are placed in a sitting or standing position. Equilibrium reactions help us to maintain or regain our balance by keeping the center of gravity within the base of support. Both the trunk and limbs are involved with equilibrium. Equilibrium reactions are often referred to as the body's first line of defense against falling. They occur when the body has a chance of winning the battle against gravity. If equilibrium reactions cannot preserve balance, the second line of defense emerges: protective reactions. One of the best known protective responses in the arm is the "parachute reaction." Protective responses in the leg include hopping or staggering.

The maintenance of balance or posture involves many postural reactions besides righting and equilibrium. In fact, it is most difficult to quantify where a righting reaction stops and where an equilibrium reaction begins. Antigravity control is an integral part of all skilled movement. The antigravity mechanism, first manifested as a supporting reaction, allows us to support the weight of our body

against gravity. Righting reactions and equilibrium reactions supplement this to allow us to move and stay upright. The postural fixation of varying parts of the body (the head on the trunk, the trunk on the pelvis, the shoulder girdle on the trunk) is maintained so that a movement can be made elsewhere while balance is maintained. This phenomenon has also been called "weight shift," "body sway," and "mobility superimposed on stability."

These baseline postural reactions must be evaluated following a stroke. For righting reactions to occur, rotation must be available and the ability to shift weight must be present. Rotation, a balance between flexors and extensors, occurs naturally at the extremes of pure lateral motion. The ability to shift weight in straight planes and in diagonal planes assumes the ability to accept and bear weight. Therefore to assess postural reactions, therapists must focus on available range, weight shift, and movement control.

For the person with a stroke, the presence of righting and equilibrium reaction varies according to the degree of abnormal tone and the amount of active movement present. As with head injury and cerebral palsy, a severe stroke will cause an absence of a righting reaction, but with a mild stroke, righting reactions are present but decreased in quality and timing and/or delayed. Although only one side of the body is impaired, the unaffected side of the body often loses the ability to normally right itself—in part because the inability of the affected side to accept and bear weight.

Hemiplegic clients with decreased or absent righting reactions move slowly and often stay in one position for uncomfortably long periods of time. When they do move, their movement is not automatic and smooth but willed, cautious, and jerky. Without righting reactions, the person with a hemiplegia thinks at a conscious level about how he or she will change position and has learned the one or two patterns of movement that are safe. If any unexpected change in the environment or learned patterns occurs, he or she will no longer be safe and may stumble or fall.

Righting reactions can be assessed in the person with hemiplegia. The following outline specifies positions and functional patterns:

1. Supine position
   a. rolling
2. Side-lying position (forearm and extended arm support)
   a. Moving into the sitting position from side-lying position*
   b. Moving into the side-lying position from a sitting position*

---

*Assessing righting reactions from both of these functional patterns is necessary because motor control of the upper body may be different from that of the lower body and thus affect the presence and/or quality of the reaction.

3. Sitting position
   a. Transferring to the left and right
   b. Sitting position to the standing position
      (1) Bilateral—moving from a chair to a standing position
      (2) Unilateral—moving from a kneeling position to a half kneel to a standing position
4. Standing position
   a. Right step to a stance
   b. Left step to a stance

Care should be taken to observe reactions of the head, neck, and trunk. When righting reactions are absent or diminished, the following questions should be addressed:

1. Is range of motion available?
2. Can the person accept some weight on each side?
3. Can the person bear full weight on each side?
4. Can the person shift weight to each side?
5. How does the person shift weight?

When assessing equilibrium reactions in the client with hemiplegia, the therapist must remember the distinction between equilibrium reactions and protective reactions. Equilibrium reactions should be assessed while slowly moving either the limb or trunk away from the base of support. The size of the base of support, the size of the supporting surface, and the range of joint movement of the joint supporting the body weight as well as the evaluator's handling skills will affect the quality and the timing of the reaction (Fig. 22-8).

Protective reactions can be tested in the prone position if the supporting surface is tilted and in the sitting, kneeling, half kneeling, and standing positions. Protective reactions are elicited by moving the person forward, backward, downward, and/or sideways quickly. Protective re-

action consists of two parts—extension of the limb and acceptance of weight on the supporting part.

Functional activities. Skilled functional activity is performed against a background of these postural reactions. The person with hemiplegia has a disturbance of the postural mechanism that affects the ability to perform functional skills in a normal fashion. If the hemiplegic side is left untreated or untrained in normal movement, the person with a hemiplegia can become adept at solving most functional tasks using only the sound side of the body. However, exclusive use of one side of the body for function results in asymmetry, poor balance, and an eventual deterioration of function of the unaffected side. This deterioration results from excessive stress and weight bearing and the marked exaggeration of movement patterns required to balance and simultaneously function with only one side of the body. Overcompensation is one reason for the abnormal movements seen on the unaffected side of hemiplegic clients.

Functional movement. To retrain motor function appropriately, it is necessary to evaluate motor function not only quantitatively but qualitatively. To assess how a functional activity is performed, it is important to measure the active movement components, the changes in tone, the available range, the ability to shift weight, and the need for adaptive devices.

Active movement components are identified descriptively at every joint involved. Limitation of degrees of movement and the movement's relations to gravity are documented. The movement components that are necessary for function to occur can then be assessed.

EXAMPLE: If in a sitting position, a person can move the humerus to 60 degrees of shoulder flexion only with abduction and internal rotation, the missing components of the *shoulder* for the function of finger feeding would be: shoulder external rotation, protraction, forward flexion, and neutral abduction/adduction.

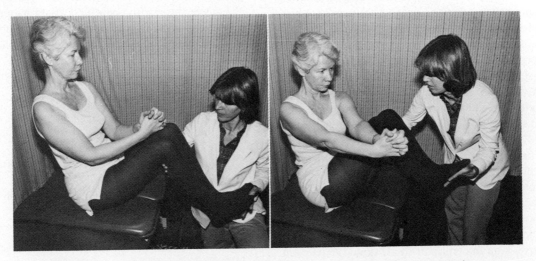

Fig. 22-8. Assessment of equilibrium reactions of a person with a right hemiplegia.

In CNS lesions, tonal changes occur with stress, effort, fear, or change of position. Documentation of the degree and type of tonal change at specific points in a functional activity will aid treatment planning.

EXAMPLE: Mrs. J. rises from a chair to a standing position; pushing down an armrest with the sound hand causes the involved leg to shoot out in an extensor pattern, which causes the pelvis and trunk to push back into the chair. Problem: The excessive effort and stress of trying to rise from the chair pushing with one hand increases the tone in the trunk and pelvic girdle, thus decreasing the chance of performing the function of rising from the chair independently.

The ability to shift and bear weight onto each side determines whether a functional activity can be performed and how it is performed.[37] To assess the ability to bear weight, the therapist can place a person with hemiplegia in the desired position, and the cocontraction pattern necessary to actively maintain the desired position can then be assessed.

EXAMPLE: To assess the ability of a client's hip to bear weight in the sitting position, the client's pelvis can be controlled and the trunk can be aligned over the hip. As the therapist's hands are removed, the question asked is, "Are the hip muscles working enough to maintain unilateral weight bearing?" Ability to shift weight can be noted both passively, with the therapist moving the client's body through the weight shift, and actively, with the client moving through the desired pattern.

If assistive devices are used, the following questions should be asked:

1. Is the device always used? If not, when is it used?
2. How is the device used?
3. Could the device be used in another fashion that would foster symmetry and weight bearing on the affected side?

When evaluating functional activities, three phases of the movement pattern can be assessed. The first phase is the initiation of the act, which includes the initial weight shift and the establishment of antigravity control. The transition phase, the second phase, represents the point in the functional activity at which there is a switch in the muscle groups that provide antigravity control. The third phase is the completion of the activity, involving a final weight shift and the ability to maintain postural control.

Passive range of motion. Passive range of motion is important in the assessment of hemiplegia because the knowledge of the degree of movement available at a joint will help the therapist decide if a normal movement pattern is at all possible. True, limited, passive range points to either a contracture or deformity. Treatment plans and goals for contracture and deformity are very different from treatment plans to correct compensatory movements. With normal range of motion, normal movement patterns can be experienced independently or with assistance. Preferred

posturing exhibited by the person with hemiplegia can be noted in the category of passive range. Some people with hemiplegia hold their head laterally flexed to the sound side and some hold their head laterally flexed to the involved side. Range of motion may be normal initially, but as a result of the preferred "hold" of a position, it may at a later date cause loss of joint motion and eventually result in a contracture.

The presence of pain is detrimental to safe movement patterns. A person with a hemiplegia should not be allowed to experience joint pain. Pain, if present, must be accurately assessed by answering the following questions:

1. Where is the pain? Pinpoint the location.
2. When does the pain occur?
3. What type of pain? Pins and needles, sharp, dull, stabbing?
4. How does pain relate to the joint or to the adjacent joints? Are there joint limitations?
5. How does active movement relate to pain?
6. What is the tone in the body part experiencing pain?

For an in-depth discussion of the topic of pain management, see Chapter 23.

Motor evaluation forms

The previous information, once gathered, can be placed on an evaluation form in many ways. Every medical institution seems to have its own evaluation form and its own system of recording data. At one hospital the documentation of pain may be descriptive, and at another it may be numerical. Active movement at the shoulder joint may be described in one institution in terms of percentages of synergistic stages and at another institution by a narrative of degrees and planes of movement. It is important to keep in mind the substance of the evaluative material, not the form in which it is described. A detailed motor evaluation form is necessary for the establishment of realistic goals and for subsequent treatment planning, but the specific form will depend on both the needs of the specific clinical setting and on the clinician's choice.

ESTABLISHMENT OF REALISTIC GOALS
Process

The process of establishing realistic goals for functional recovery for the person with hemiplegia is difficult because of the incomplete knowledge of underlying neurophysiological repair mechanisms in the CNS. The brain is incapable of myotatic regeneration, and it is probably incapable of axonal regrowth as occurs in peripheral nerves. Currently accepted "theories" that explain the reasons for long-term and short-term recovery in CNS deficits include renewed circulation, decreased edema, collateral sprouting, and unmasking. In spite of existing and changing reasons for neuroplasticity, we know from clinical experience

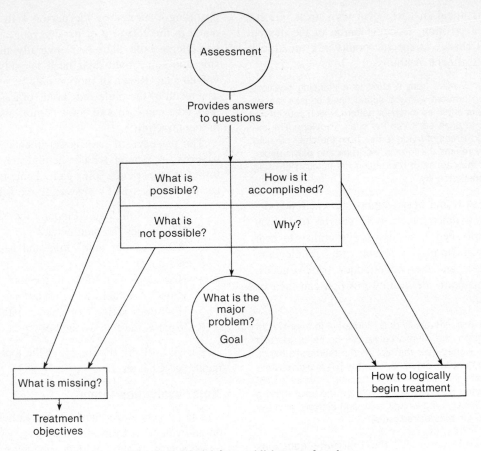

Fig. 22-9. Model for establishment of goals.

that functional recovery can occur for months or years following a stroke. Although some persons recover spontaneously from hemiplegia, in those persons with a residual deficit, rehabilitation offers the most effective means to re-establish a quality life.[3]

Although established means to restore functional movement deficits exist, cognitive and emotional barriers, such as the inability to learn or retain information, disoriented integrative skills, and disoriented emotional behavior, may interfere with the recovery process. With this in mind, we can begin to examine the needs of the person with hemiplegia. The key to the establishment of realistic goals lies in the accurate collection and interpretation of data from the assessment of the client. Fig. 22-9 presents a model that illustrates a framework for establishment of realistic goals.

Recognition of needs

The information obtained from the total evaluation provides the basis for answers to the questions: What movements and functions are possible? What movements and functions are not possible? By understanding the movement components a person with hemiplegia uses to move,

the therapist can answer the question: What movement components are missing? The answer to this question becomes the objective for treatment. *How* the *possible* is accomplished and *why* the *impossible* exists will provide logical suggestions for treatment procedures. *How* and *why* will give answers that ensure quality in treatment. A person with hemiplegia need not only know how to roll, stand, or walk but the safest and most efficient way to roll, stand, and walk. *Safest* ensures the closest to normal biomechanic and *efficient* means—the closest to symmetry and bilaterality.

The answer to the question: "What is the major problem?" provides the therapist with a *short-term goal*. The *major problem* of a person with a hemiplegia is related to what is possible and what is not possible. A realistic short-term goal should be the result of a change the therapist can produce in one or two treatment sessions that helps to eliminate or ameliorate the major problem. The *long-term goal* will be a functional skill that is directly linked through movement components to the short-term goal.

EXAMPLE: In the client with left hemiplegia, *What is possible?* The client sits unsupported and rises to a stand with assistance. *How?* With weight on the right side, he or she pushes up to a stand with the right hand, the left leg shoots out into extension, the trunk pushes back in the chair, and the head is in a forward position. *What is not possible?* Symmetrical sitting, symmetrical rise to a stand, and normal tonal situation in the left leg during rise to a stand is not possible. *Why?* Client cannot bear weight on left leg in sitting or standing position. *Why?* Because of lack of left hip control, lack of pelvic girdle control, lack of appropriate trunk reactions, and because spasticity rises dramatically with effort. *What is missing?* The ability to shift and bear weight on the left side.

Treatment objective: Facilitate weight shift and weight bearing to both sides, especially to the left.

Logically begin treatment
1. Weight on left side
   a. Side lying position—function rolling
   b. Sitting—assisted weight shift to both sides
2. Increase motor control of the left hip
   a. See 1 above.
   b. Lateral and diagonal weight shifts in sitting position with assistance
   c. Initiating the rise to a stand with assistance with weight equally distributed on both lower extremities

Major problem: The ability to bear weight and shift weight onto the left hip in the sitting position and in *coming to a stand.*

Short-term goal: Shift weight onto left and right hips with appropriate trunk elongation and shortening.

Long-term goal: Shift weight to both sides while standing, and bear weight on the left side in the left step stance and in the right step stance.

Goals for recovery phases

Two distinct types of goals may be established for a client with hemiplegia: compensatory goals and normalcy goals. The teaching of compensatory or splinter skills without regard for the symmetrical nature of the body will by design result in eventual contractures and possible deformity and pain.[15]

The establishment of compensatory goals may be necessary for a variety of reasons: e.g., for financial requirements, for the client's emotional needs, or the clinician's lack of experience/skill. It is important that the therapist accept the fact that teaching abnormal compensatory skills does not naturally lead to efficient, normal patterns of movement. Therefore when goals are set they should clearly state whether normality of motor function or compensatory strategies are the objectives. The client and family should also be aware of the direction of therapy. Using compensatory strategies while establishing goals of normal movement would falsely lead the client toward unattainable goals.

The teaching of normal movement may imply the attainment of an impossible level of function (100%) and with that the frustration of failure. Thus it is important that the clinician give the client a clear idea of the goals (along with their limits) of the treatment plan. The goals for the three recovery phases in hemiplegia are suggested and identified in Table 22-3.

Table 22-3. Goals for the three recovery phases

Acute	Completed	Long-term
Maintain mobility	Maintain mobility	$\longrightarrow$
	Teach client	
Give feeling of normal movement patterns	Begin to reproduce normal movement patterns	Move as normally as possible
Begin establishing symmetry in posture and movement	Allow symmetry to occur	Provide continued use of symmetry
Provide normal sensory input	$\longrightarrow$	$\longrightarrow$
Bedside care	Living skills	Maximal level of independence
Monitor changes in tonal states	Teach client to be aware of changes in tone and how to influence it	$\longrightarrow$

$\longrightarrow$, Indicates continuation of same goal.

TYPICAL CLINICAL SIGNS AND PROBLEMS WITH POSSIBLE TREATMENT ALTERNATIVES
Spasticity

Spasticity, a major problem in hemiplegia, has been categorized in at least seven different ways.[36] Regardless of the type, its presence or a sudden increase in its intensity is easily recognized by the therapist and client. If untreated, many secondary problems result, such as joint dysfunction (especially of the hand, fingers, scapula, shoulder, ankle, and forefoot), pain, and asymmetrical weight-bearing patterns.

Although patterns of spasticity are very consistent, different body parts often display varying degrees of spasticity. The hemiplegic hand and fingers may demonstrate more spasticity than the scapula, and the shoulder girdle may demonstrate more spasticity than the pelvic girdle. In treating this increase in tone, it is often easier to achieve success treating the less spastic part first. It will be capable of more voluntary movement, and that movement, along with inhibition of the spasticity, will lead to a decrease in tone in the more spastic muscle groups.

The physical procedures available for the treatment of spasticity include complete elongation of the shortened muscle groups, weight bearing or moving the body on the elongated limb, cooling, vibratory stimulation, and biofeedback. The elongation of the shortened muscle groups at the point of maximally tolerated muscle length has proven effective in inhibiting spasticity.[52] In the client with hemiplegia, elongation of the shortened muscle groups is followed by weight bearing or moving the body as a whole over the elongated limb (Fig. 22-10). The pattern of elongation for an upper extremity that displays spasticity in the scapular downward rotators and adductors, shoulder adductors and internal rotators, elbow flexors, forearm pronators, and wrist and finger flexors is one of scapular protraction and upward rotation, shoulder external rotation and abduction, elbow extension, forearm supination, and wrist and finger extension (Fig. 22-11). Once elongation has been achieved, weight can then be placed on the heel of the hand (Fig. 22-12, *A*) or the hand can be placed in the weight-bearing position, such as against a wall, while the body moves on the arm (Fig. 22-12, *B*). Many of the proprioceptive neuromuscular facilitation (PNF) patterns, which include movements of the body on the limbs, can also be incorporated.[33]

Vibration and other techniques that facilitate the antagonist can be used to inhibit the spastic agonist. The perceptible reduction of spasticity occurs during the vibration,

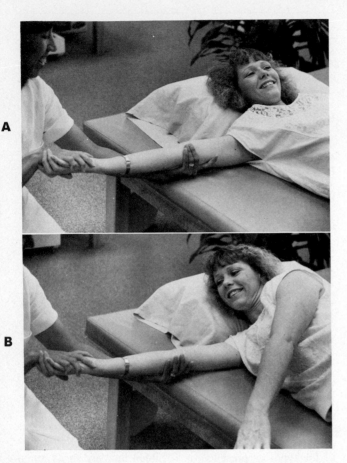

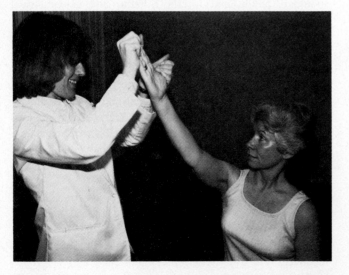

A

B

Fig. 22-10. A, Arm is externally rotated and abducted. **B,** Body moves over the elongated right arm.

Fig. 22-11. Pattern of elongation for an arm that displays spasticity in the scapular downward rotators, shoulder adductors, internal rotators, elbow flexors, and wrist and finger flexors.

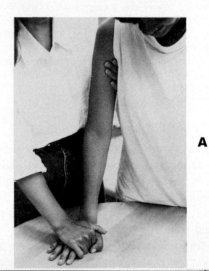

A

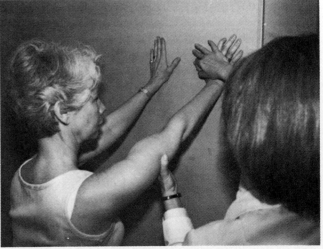

B

Fig. 22-12. A, Weight bearing on an extended right arm. **B,** Weight bearing of the right arm against the wall.

and at that point reeducation of the muscle groups can begin.[7]

Biofeedback can be used to reduce EMG levels in the spastic muscles of clients with hemiplegia. The electrodes are placed over affected muscle groups, and the client's goal is to achieve electrical silence or a 0 reading on the biofeedback equipment during varying environmental and movement situations[73] (see Chapter 26).

Cold has been used historically to temporarily decrease spasticity. The study on the effects of cold on the stretch reflex and H-response on hemiplegic clients revealed that local cooling might decrease, increase, or exert no effect on hemiplegic spasticity.[70] Thus for ice to be a useful tool in treatment of spasticity, careful assessment of the client must first be conducted.

As in biofeedback, many clients can learn to slightly decrease their spasticity through a process of conscious relaxation similar to that taught by Jacobson.[28] This learned ability to change spasticity is often enough to allow the client to position an extremity in a position of weight bearing while performing a functional task. For example, placing the affected arm on the edge of a sink while brushing the teeth enables a better weight shift through the pelvis and both lower extremities (Fig. 22-13).

The temporary decrease of spasticity that occurs with any of these methods does not by itself directly lead to an increase in function. They must be immediately followed by therapeutic exercise to create a learning environment that improves motor performance.[10,62,73]

Loss of mobility—decreasing range of motion

Loss of range of motion can lead to decreased function in clients with hemiplegia. Documentation of affected joints should be followed by an assessment of the active movement present in the involved joint. A loss of active movement at one joint may biomechanically cause a loss of passive movement at another joint.

For example, if assessment reveals a decreasing passive movement in dorsiflexion of the ankle and a loss of pelvic mobility in a posterior direction, resulting in a fixed posture of the pelvis in an anterior tilt, an analysis of the problem may reveal that the position of anterior pelvic tilt causes a shift of weight forward from the heel toward the toe, thus placing the foot in more plantar flexion. If this pelvic posture persists, a decrease in range of motion of dorsiflexion of the ankle will result. To maintain correct ankle range of motion, pelvic mobility and control will need to be established.

While classic "orthopaedic" stretching procedures have been advocated for use in clients with hemiplegia, consideration must be made for the reasons behind the loss of joint range.[46] In hemiplegia slow, maintained stretching or elongation through weight bearing (i.e., functional stretching) in conjunction with the retraining of motor control is more effective than "orthopaedic" stretching in reestablishing joint range and in preventing the future loss of joint range.

> **EXAMPLE:** If a pelvis is anteriorly tilted, the hip flexors may be tight. From an analysis of the development of abnormal tone, we know that the paravertebral musculature on the affected side is often the first to demonstrate high tone. An analysis then reveals that if the paravertebral muscles are tight and if a client with hemiplegia is stood without appropriate support before motor control of the hip extensors and abdominals is sufficient to maintain a neutral pelvic posture, the pelvis will be pulled by the paravertebral muscles and by gravity into an anterior tilt. Stretching the hip flexors will not correct this problem as quickly or as permanently as will supporting the lower extremities and pelvic girdle in a standing position and moving the upper body over the lower body to facilitate abdominal and hip extensor musculature.

Pain

In the client with hemiplegia, pain can be caused by an imbalance of muscles, improper movement patterns, joint dysfunction, improper weight-bearing patterns, and muscle shortening, or it may be of CNS origin. An assessment of the type of pain, the exact anatomical location of the pain, the presence of soft tissue dysfunction, a description of the body position during the active movement that causes pain, or the exact passive movement that causes pain is necessary before treatment planning can begin.

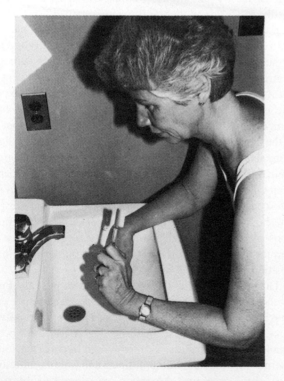

Fig. 22-13. Weight bearing on the affected right side during functional skills.

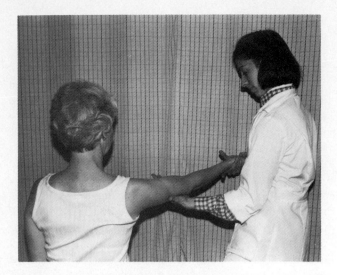

Fig. 22-14. To ensure pain-free movement of the arm, forward flexion must be accompanied by scapula protraction and upward rotation and external rotation of the humerus.

Joint pain. During functional movement, weight-bearing patterns are usually accompanied by normal joint alignment. If, during weight bearing, spasticity is allowed to occur, the spastic pull will stress the joint, the soft tissues, or the tendon and will eventually lead to inflammation. For example, if weight bearing on an extended upper extremity occurs with severe shoulder internal rotation and elbow extension, biceps tendonitis and/or anterior shoulder joint pain can occur. When joints are improperly aligned, passive or active movement of the joint will result in joint or referred pain. This pain is usually sharp.

Pain from muscle imbalance or improper movement patterns is related to biomechanics and joint dysfunction. If, when raising the arm in forward flexion, a sharp pain is reported on the superior portion of the shoulder joint at approximately 60 degrees of forward flexion, the therapist immediately suspects an inability of the scapula to upwardly rotate and protract. If the glenohumeral rhythm is not present above 60 degrees of forward flexion, an impingement of the shoulder capsule between the humerus and scapula occurs and sharp pain results. If pain is present, the therapist should lower the humerus immediately upon complaint of pain, assess the mobility of the scapula, and if this mobility is normal, ask for forward flexion again while passively rotating and protracting the scapula upward and externally rotating the humerus. The movement will then proceed above 60 degrees of forward flexion without pain (Fig. 22-14).

Muscle pain. When a spastic or shortened muscle is slowly stretched, a strong "pulling" type pain is often reported in the region of the muscle belly being stretched. If the amount of stretch is decreased a few degrees, the reported pain subsides.

Shoulder dysfunction

The primary shoulder problems of the person with hemiplegia are subluxation, pain, and a lack of functional movement patterns. To plan treatment programs, an understanding of normal anatomy, biomechanics, and kinesiology must be reviewed in conjunction with the problems that result from CNS damage.[14]

Shoulder subluxation occurs when any of the biomechanical factors contributing to glenohumeral joint stability are interrupted. In persons with hemiplegia, subluxation is related to a change in the angle of the glenoid fossa. In the frontal plane the scapula is normally held at an angle of 40 degrees. When the slope of the glenoid fossa becomes less oblique (and more vertical), the humerus will "slide" down the slope of the fossa and "subluxation" occurs.[6]

This change in obliquity of the glenoid fossa occurs in both the flaccid and spastic stage of hemiplegia. In the flaccid, or low-tone, stage, the scapula, which no longer has stability of its muscular attachments, loses its normal orientation on the thorax and is rotated downward by gravity. Downward rotation occurs as a result of (1) low tone in the rotator cuff and serratus anterior muscles, (2) the depression and downward rotation of the scapula when sitting or standing is allowed without scapular support, and (3) the spinal curvature that occurs with unilateral weight bearing to the sound side. Downward rotation orients the glenoid fossa vertically and the humerus is subluxed inferiorly. This is demonstrated in Fig. 22-15. The client in Fig. 22-16, *A,* has low-tone upper extremity and a downwardly rotated scapula resulting in large subluxation of 2 year duration. In Fig. 22-16, *B,* the scapula is passively rotated upward, and the subluxation is markedly reduced. As subluxation occurs, the shoulder capsule is vulnerable to stretch, especially when the humerus is dependent and resting by the side of the body. In this position, the capsule is taut anteriorly, so any downward distraction of the humerus will place an immediate stretch on the upper part of the capsule. As the humerus is abducted the capsule has more slack anteriorly (Fig. 22-17), thus a greater degree of subluxation in this position is necessary before capsule stretching occurs. The superior portion of the capsule is reinforced by the coracohumeral ligament, which is crucial for shoulder stability. Jensen[30] has discussed the implications of rupture of this ligament as a result of forced abnormal passive motion as a cause of shoulder pain in subluxation.

During the spastic stage, the strong downward pull of the lastissimus dorsi and the active use of shoulder elevators initially cause the glenoid fossa to be vertically oriented and the scapula to begin to elevate on the rib cage. As the humerus postures or moves into hyperextension and internal rotation, the humeral head will sublux anteriorly.

A third type of subluxation, a superior subluxation, occurs if the pattern of active return includes deltoid biceps firing. In these clients the scapula is downwardly ro-

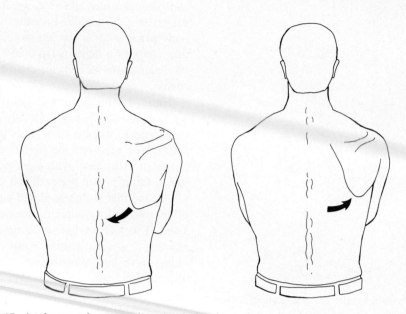

Fig. 22-15. As the scapula rotates downward, the slope of the glenoid fossa becomes less oblique and the humerus "slides" downward.

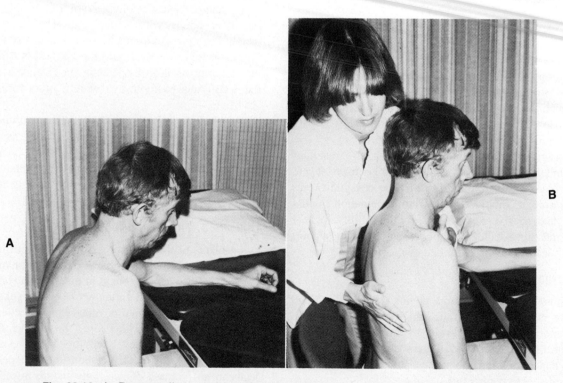

Fig. 22-16. A, Downwardly rotated scapula with a subluxated humerus. **B,** If the scapula is rotated upward to a normally aligned position, the humerus is no longer subluxated.

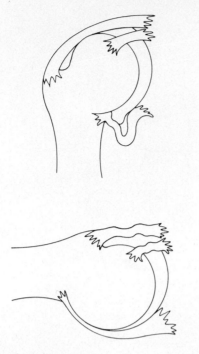

Fig. 22-17. As the humerus abducts, the anterior portion of the shoulder capsule has more slack.

tated and elevated on the rib cage while the humeral head is internally rotated and pulled up under the acromial process.[31,61]

Prevention of subluxation requires (1) proper assessment (low tone versus high tone), (2) appropriate treatment in accordance with assessment, and (3) prevention of shoulder capsule stretch, including support against gravity and positioning to elongate spastic muscles.

Pain occurs in the hemiplegic shoulder as a result of muscle imbalance with loss of joint range from severe long-standing subluxation and from all the possible causes of nonhemiplegic shoulder pain. The combination of loss of active and passive motion, loss of the ability to bear weight, and long-standing subluxation without support eventually leads to what is termed *sympathetic pain*.

Shoulder-hand syndrome

The shoulder-hand syndrome begins with swelling and tenderness of the hand and limited range of finger and shoulder motion. This is followed by a decreased range of movement of the hand and fingers and bone and skin changes, and it culminates with atrophied bone, skin, and muscle and severe contracture.

Not every edematous hemiplegic hand will lead to a shoulder-hand syndrome. Hand edema results from an upper extremity that remains dependent and that does not move for long periods of time. It is essential to teach the person with hemiplegia how to properly care for the hand and to give the responsibility for the care of the hand and

arm to the client. Touching, rubbing, weight bearing, and positioning of the hand increase sensory awareness and begin the process of moving the hand. Interlacing the fingers and palm pressure add phalangeal abduction and metacarpal phalangeal flexion. Pressure of the hand against other body parts, such as the leg or face, or against a firm surface, such as a table or lap board, and the encouragement of bilateral arm movements contributes to the avoidance of edema.

Hand dysfunction. The grasp reflex in the hand normally disappears before voluntary grasp develops. A grasp reflex occurs when a stimulus is placed in the palmar surface of the hand and the fingers close quickly and tightly around it. The client with a grasp reflex requires desensitization through firm pressure and weight bearing.

A hand that is tightly closed can be loosened by proper alignment and by applying pressure on the "heel" of the hand. This can be done on a firm surface through weight bearing or against a softer surface, such as the therapist's shoulder or leg. When opening the thumb, the therapist should place pressure at its base rather than pull from the distal tip of the thumb, which may result in subluxation of the interphalangeal (IP) or metacarpophalangeal (MP) joints. Although the prone position is usually advocated in children to achieve weight bearing through shoulders, elbows, and/or hands, it often is not a comfortable position for older adults with hemiplegia. The same beneficial weightbearing pattern can be achieved in the sitting position by leaning forward onto the elbows and forearms, in the standing position by leaning on extended arms, or in the side-lying position by rotating onto forearms (Fig. 22-18).

To maintain a flexible, open hand and normal joint motion, the importance of weight-bearing patterns through the hand cannot be stressed enough. Pressure on the heel of the hand and maintenance of normal scapulohumeral alignment during upper-extremity weight bearing are keys to successful treatment.

Hip, knee, ankle, and foot problems

Problems of the hip, knee, ankle, and foot in the client with hemiplegia are interrelated. These problems often become evident when the client is placed in a standing position or when he or she attempts to walk, yet these same problems appear minimal or mild when the client is sitting or kneeling. If this is the case, the exaggeration of the problems with higher-level activities is the result of a lack of postural control of the lower trunk and pelvis, which leads to an increase of spasticity in the lower extremity. Because spasticity may be greater in one muscle group than in another, motor control in the client with hemiplegia also varies from muscle group to muscle group. Lack of control and the presence of spasticity in one muscle group leads to abnormal postures in neighboring joints. For example, (1) hip flexion may be the result of an ante-

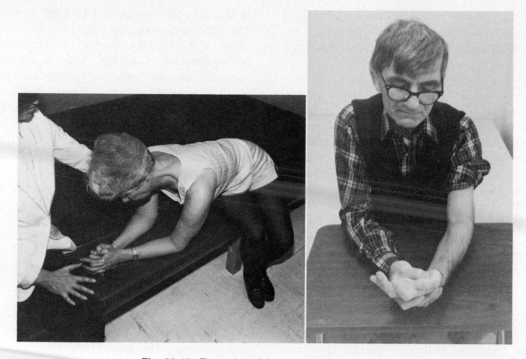

Fig. 22-18. Examples of forearm weight bearing.

riorly tilted pelvis resulting from lack of abdominal control and/or spastic paravertebral muscles; (2) knee flexion may be the compensation to avoid falling forward, if exaggerated anterior pelvic tilt and hip flexion are present; (3) knee hyperextension may result from an excessive anterior tilt of the pelvis with the resulting biomechanical line of gravity falling in front of the knee joint; (4) knee flexion or knee hyperextension may be the compensation for excessive spasticity in the gastrocnemius-soleus muscle group; and (5) ankle plantar flexion can be the result of excessive pelvic lordosis and hip flexion.

Therefore problems of instability should be assessed in light of neighboring compensatory mechanisms before treatment is planned. All too often the excessive knee hyperextension in a person with hemiplegia is blamed on poor knee control. It is usually the result of poor pelvic, hip, and trunk control, spasticity or tightness in the plantar flexors of the ankle, and/or poor ankle and foot control.

Although great emphasis is placed on the ability to dorsiflex the ankle in a client with hemiplegia, the need for the calcaneous to properly bear weight is of greater importance. Proper calcaneal alignment and heel strike allows the ankle to move appropriately. In hemiplegia, in non–weight-bearing situations, the calcaneus frequently is in equino varus, the midfoot supinates, and the forefoot adducts. When the foot makes ground contact, the client has difficulty bearing weight on the heel. The calcaneous remains in equinus and varus while the midfoot pronates in relation to the rearfoot to seek the ground and the forefoot abducts.[60] Both abnormal foot positions must be corrected

before ankle joint range can be assessed. Conventional double upright metal braces, prefabricated or custom-molded polypropylene braces, and inhibitory plaster casts that do not hold forefoot and rearfoot correction will not ameliorate the problems presented by an equinovarus foot. See Chapter 24 for an in-depth discussion of orthotics and their therapeutic implications.

Toe clawing. Toe clawing occurs for two reasons: loss of biomechanical alignment and as part of an equilibrium reaction.

If the calcaneus moves into equinus (because of shortened or spastic gastrocnemius/soleus muscles), the midfoot will shift and the metatarsal heads will become depressed. As the metatarsal heads depress, the phalanges hyperextend proximally and flex distally.[31]

During functional movement, especially during walking, clients with hemiplegia are attempting to move the body's center of gravity over a new base of support. If trunk and pelvic control are not appropriate for the task, the body will recruit an equilibrium reaction and as part of this reaction, the toes will claw.

Problems of blistering and pain in the toes occur in the intermediate and long-term stage of hemiplegia as the result of the toes rubbing on the tops of the shoes and the constant struggle of pushing clawed toes into shoes. In treatment, clawing can be temporarily relieved by realigning the metatarsals and slowly lengthening the shortened long-toe flexor muscles. This often allows a shift of weight from the toes to the heel of the foot, thus allowing a more normal weight-bearing pattern. The problems of pelvic and hip control can then be more easily approached. Inhibition and carryover can be maintained through shoe inserts, toe extensions in polypropylene orthoses, or removable metatarsal pads.

Scoliosis

The appearance of an uncorrectable scoliosis in the sitting position is one of the largest problems of clients with long-standing hemiplegia. Once the person with hemiplegia is placed in a sitting position, the tendency for spinal curves begins as a result of unequal weight distribution, muscle tightness, and rib cage rotation. The presence of the scoliosis will affect the positioning of the scapula and pelvis, which in turn affects the movement possibilities of the upper and lower extremities. Therefore alignment and movement control of the spine and rib cage must be achieved before extremity treatment can be effective.

Gait

The evaluation of gait patterns includes the assessment of the temporal characteristics of each gait cycle, the description of gait deviations, and ideally the assignment of a numerical score representing the efficiency of ambulation.

The temporal characteristics of gait—step time, cycle time, step length, and stride length—can be measured with a piece of chalk and a stopwatch or with more sophisticated equipment such as a gait analyzer.[49,54] These temporal parameters provide an objective measurement of performance and a baseline from which the efficacy of treatment procedures and client progress can be assessed.

Gait deviations in persons with hemiplegia have been described according to their biomechanical and kinesiological abnormalities and in terms of the loss of centrally programmed motor control mechanisms.[34,54] Perry[54] has described common problems of the hemiplegic person's gait as loss of controlled movement into plantar flexion at heel strike, loss of ankle movement from heel strike to midstance (resulting in loss of trunk balance and forward momentum for push off), and loss of the normal combination of movement patterns at the end of stance (hip extension, knee flexion, and ankle extension) and at the end of swing (hip flexion with knee extension and ankle flexion).

Knutsson[34] classified the motor control problems of the hemiplegic gait into three types. Type I is characterized by inappropriate activation of the calf muscles early in the gait cycle with corresponding low muscular activity in anterior compartment muscles. Type II consists of an absence or severe decrease in EMG activity in two or more muscle groups of the involved lower extremity. Type III activation patterns consist of abnormal coactivation of several limb muscles with normal or increased muscular activity levels in the muscle groups of the involved side.

In the Type I activation pattern, the calf musculature is activated before the center of gravity passes over the base of support. This thrusts the tibia backward instead of propelling the body forward in a push-off as normally occurs. The client with hemiplegia compensates for the backward thrust of the tibia by anteriorly tilting the pelvis and/or flexing forward at the hip. Type II activation patterns, markedly decreased muscular activity, result in compensatory mechanisms to gain stability. Type III activation patterns result in a disruption of the sequential flow of motor activity.

The isolation of at least three different motor control problems in the gait of clients with hemiplegia underscores the importance of proper assessment. The major problem is not the same in all clients, therefore retraining programs should be selective to the problem.

The functional ambulation profile (FAP) is a system that attempts to relate the temporal aspects of gait to neuromuscular and cardiovascular functioning and that converts this relationship to a single numerical score.[49,50]

TREATMENT PROCEDURES

The treatment of the deficits in motor control of the person with hemiplegia centers on improvement of function and prevention of greater disability through secondary complications. Much debate exists over the type of treatment that should be used. Two broad and divergent schools of thought exist. Some people believe that hemiplegic clients should be trained to use only their residual motion, and others believe that new learning can be achieved that will provide a more normal foundation on which function can occur. Within the latter school of thought, debate exists over which neurophysiological approach is optimal and whether approaches should or should not be combined. At the present time, none of these questions can or have been objectively answered through well-documented studies. This section does not attempt to answer these controversial questions, but it gives a structure on which each therapist can choose the treatment technique best for him or her. As Mossman[46] so accurately stated, "It is what you do, not what you call it, which matters."

Objectives

Objectives for selective treatment procedures that are based on neurophysiological principles and that are designed to help the client relearn basic postural control and movement patterns include:

1. To reestablish postural control—righting reactions, equilibrium reactions, protective reactions
2. To normalize tactile, proprioceptive, and kinesthetic input
3. To facilitate normal movement patterns within a functional skill
4. To prevent contracture deformity and pain through maintenance of normal joint alignment
5. To inhibit undesired movement patterns

Treatment procedure is divided into two sections. First, procedures and considerations necessary for reestablishing postural control are described. Second, the projections are given for improving selective functional skills.

Reestablishment of postural control

Head, neck, and trunk control. In normal movement, postural control of the head, neck, and trunk frees all extremities for function. A 3-month-old baby, in the prone position, develops the ability to control his or her head and upper trunk and to shift weight from one arm to the other. The skill of shifting and bearing weight over one arm frees the remaining arm for the function of reach, grasp, and release. So too, the person with hemiplegia must develop the ability to control his or her head and trunk so that he or she can shift and bear weight on each side to free an extremity for function.

Along with sensory feedback (tactile, proprioceptive, kinesthetic, visual, and vestibular), movement requires a point of stability or base of support, a point of mobility, and a weight shift. Weight shift, which can be anterior, posterior, lateral, or diagonal, is followed by one or more of the following: righting reactions, equilibrium reactions, protective reactions, or falling. The establishment of head and neck control allows for dissociation of the shoulder and pelvic girdles from the trunk and dissociation of the extremities from the girdles (Fig. 22-19).

Motor skills are learned or relearned through experiencing the movement; the movement must be performed actively.[12] We do not always move the exact same way when performing a functional motor skill, but we always achieve the same purpose. Therefore for the establishment of motor control, the body must be prepared to automatically adjust posture to allow a movement to achieve its purpose.

Treatment should include mobility and active control of straight plane as well as rotational movements. Although

rotation is a combination of anterior or posterior and lateral movement, the therapist need not always wait until anterior, posterior, or lateral control is established before working toward or in a rotational pattern. However, if the spinal vertebrae are not aligned properly, true rotation will not occur.

Head and neck control. Vision, hearing, and labyrinthine influences are essential for normal head control. To establish head and neck control these systems should be incorporated in treatment. It is often necessary to use auditory clues to orient the client to his or her position in space. An auditory stimulus can be presented in midline and, if necessary, the client can be assisted to "find" midline, then allowed to move out of midline to see if he or she can then "find" midline again.

> **EXAMPLE:** "I will help you find the middle. Can you stay here? Now you are falling to the left. I will move you back to the middle, to the right. Can you move back to the middle?" Each time the client is moved out of midline a weight shift will be occurring. This shift can often be reinforced with proprioceptive clues such as deep pressure. Progression from verbal commands to automatic correction of position is desirable.

To establish good head and neck control, axial extension (i.e., a chin tuck), not a forward head, should be facilitated along with upper thoracic extension and normal alignment of the shoulder girdle. Weight bearing through symmetrically positioned arms will help organize the body and orient the head to midline.

Although head and neck control is often treated before trunk control is well established, the trunk must be supported in good alignment before treatment of the head and neck can begin. While children are placed in the prone position for this purpose, the adult with hemiplegia may need alternate positions, for example:

1. The client can be seated on a firm surface (on a mat table or in a wheelchair with a solid seat) with the trunk and upper extremities supported by leaning forward onto a table top or forward onto a wedge or bolster resting on the table (Fig. 22-20, *A*).
2. The therapist can support the client's trunk from the front with the hands controlling the upper trunk and scapula (Fig. 22-20, *B*).
3. The therapist can support the trunk from behind the client (Fig. 22-20, *C*).
4. The client can be placed in the side-lying position with forearm support to one side.

The use of the sitting position requires that the pelvis, hips, and knees be properly aligned and that the feet be able to rest on the floor. If trunk control is not yet established, it is imperative that support be given to the upper extremities, scapula, and upper trunk before facilitation of head and neck control begins.

Trunk control. Trunk movements are encouraged through weight shifts anteriorly, posteriorly, laterally, and

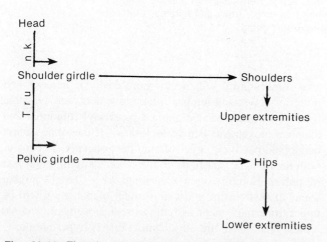

Fig. 22-19. Flowchart establishment of central motor control frees distal components for movement.

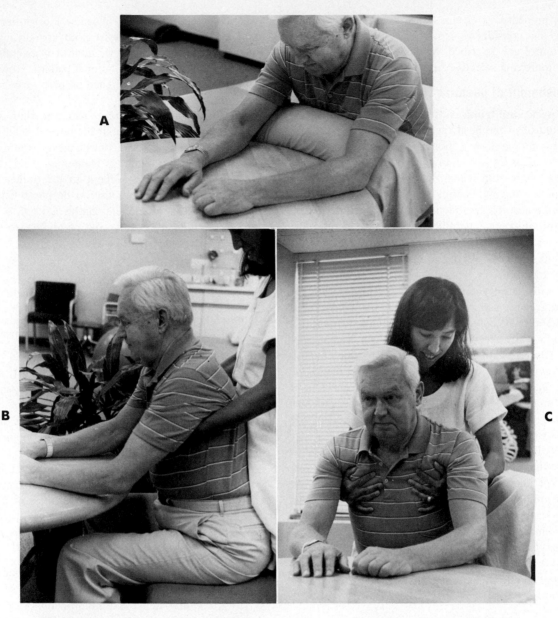

Fig. 22-20. A, Established head and trunk control with support from table and bolster. **B,** Establishing head and trunk control with therapist controlling from upper trunk and scapula. **C,** Establishing head and trunk control with therapist supporting from behind.

diagonally. A gradual lateral weight shift onto the right hip results in an elongation of the right trunk musculature and a shortening of the left trunk musculature (Fig. 22-21).

In hemiplegic clients, this righting response will be impaired on each side, so weight shift and appropriate trunk movements to each side must be included in the treatment process. Before lateral trunk movements can occur, however, the pelvis must be able to be aligned in a neutral position (anterior superior iliac spine and iliac crest in the same plane). If the pelvis is tilted posteriorly or anteriorly, a weight shift will not occur through the hips and the trunk will not be able to respond appropriately. Lateral and diag-

onal trunk control will occur more easily if anterior and posterior pelvic and lumbar spine movements are available first. If the spine can be aligned passively, rotational and diagonal movements can be facilitated. If the spine cannot be aligned passively, true rotation never occurs. In persons with hemiplegia, spasticity in the lower extremity and loss of pelvic mobility often contribute to a "fixed" lumbar spine. If this occurs, most movement of the trunk will be upper trunk movement with the axis of movement centered around T10 or a point on the spine that is hypermobile.

Girdle control. Dissociation of the shoulder and pelvic girdles from the trunk means the ability to separate shoul-

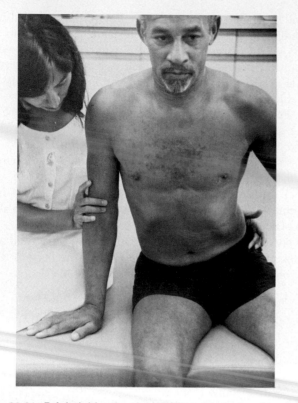

Fig. 22-21. Pelvic initiated weight shift to right to lengthen right trunk musculature.

der and pelvic girdle movements from the trunk. Lack of dissociation results from soft tissue tightness, spasticity, or lack of motor control. After the reasons for lack of dissociation have been assessed, treatment can be chosen appropriately. To dissociate a girdle from the trunk, the therapist can (1) hold or stabilize the trunk through weight bearing and then facilitate movement from the girdle or (2) hold or stabilize the girdle and then facilitate movement from the trunk.

If the scapula will not move on the rib cage, the humerus will not move properly and any passive movement of the humerus will result in pain or discomfort. If the pelvis will not move on the spine, the femur will not move properly in the acetabulum and sitting, standing, and walking will be abnormal.

Extremity control. As in normal development disassociation of the extremities from the girdles occurs through weight bearing as the girdles disassociate from the trunk. The treatment of the hemiplegic arm and leg is made easier by examining this development. As a baby learns to extend the head and neck in the prone position, the scapula and upper extremities move from the position of adduction, downward rotation, hyperextension, and internal rotation to abduction, upward rotation, forward flexion, and external rotation as weight bearing is increased. The adult with hemiplegia whose scapula is downwardly rotated and adducted and whose humerus is hyperextended and inter-

nally rotated can use varying positions of weight bearing and weight shift to facilitate scapular movements on the trunk. Normal scapular movements will allow the humerus to dissociate from the scapula through the facilitation of humeral external rotation and forward flexion.

During weight-bearing treatment, the upper extremity moves toward or into a position of external rotation as the scapula protracts and abducts on the thorax. If during weight bearing with the arms flexed or extended, the shoulder internally rotates or the head of the humerus rolls forward, dissociation will not occur.

Once dissociation begins, normal weight shifting and weight bearing will occur automatically. Then, functional training of the extremities can begin. The therapist will not be training the extremities to move in space through the activity of weight bearing but will be preparing the trunk, girdles, and extremities for functional use.

The extremities participate in both open-ended and close-ended activities and should be specifically trained for each. A closed-ended activity is one where the distal end is fixed to a supporting surface and the body moves across the distal fixed part. This is also referred to as "mobility superimposed on stability" or "mobility in a weight bearing position."[67] The stance phase of gait is an example—the foot is fixed and the body moves over the foot.

An open-ended extremity movement is one in which the extremity moves in space. "Stability superimposed on mobility" or "mobility in a non–weight-bearing position" are synonomous terms. Examples of such movements would be reaching, feeding, bathing, throwing a ball, or the swing phase of gait.[65] When training open-ended extremity movement in clients with hemiplegia, the therapist begins with the arm at or above 90 degrees because in this position the depressors and downward rotators of the scapula and humerus are elongated, allowing optimal position for facilitating the scapula upward-rotators and forward-flexors of the humerus.

During close-ended activities the weight-bearing hand is open and flat. During the reach and grasp of an open-ended activity, the hand displays more of a palmar arch with varying degrees of wrist extension and finger movement.

Functional activities

The goal of all treatment is to restore or optimize function. With the concepts of head and trunk control and extremity dissociation mentioned earlier in mind, treatment procedures to train selected basic functional skills are reviewed.

Bedside care. Although textbooks have provided lists of how to position clients with hemiplegia,[14] these lists are not always applicable. Hemiplegic clients are not all alike, and problems change in the days following the stroke. Some clients need the affected side of the trunk lengthened in bed, others just need the trunk placed in the neutral position, and still others require the upper extremity and shoulder girdle to be positioned in an upward-rotated, forward-flexed, protracted position with the arms overhead supported by a pillow.

Symmetry and midline need to be encouraged and reinforced in the person with hemiplegia. Much of the early intervention can be carried out by the client and family. Family members should be encouraged to sit, visit, talk, feed, and touch the person with the hemiplegia from the client's affected side, unless visual impairment is present. Because family members are often afraid to touch or move the client's affected side, they should be quickly educated to be made a part of the treatment process. The forward and laterally flexed head so commonly seen in the client with hemiplegia can be treated at the bedside initially through proper pillow placement and the facilitation of axial extension (chin tucking). Bilaterality and sensory awareness can be encouraged by bringing both hands to midline and to various body parts, especially the head, face, and mouth. Pressure on the heel of the affected hand will begin to prepare the hand for future weight bearing and eventual function (Fig. 22-22).

The lower extremities can be positioned in many ways with the goals of mirroring functional patterns. Proprioceptive input through the heel of the foot is encouraged during bedside care when hip and knee are held in flexion to prepare the foot for weight bearing in sitting and standing. This flexed position also avoids facilitation of total extension or extensor spasticity. To prepare for ambulation, the lower extremities can be positioned out of total synergistic patterns. For example, position the affected leg in hip extension with knee flexion and ankle dorsiflexion while in the side-lying position (Fig. 22-23).

To avoid later shoulder problems, the therapist can plan bedside treatment that includes scapular positioning as well as scapular facilitation to ensure protraction and upward rotation of the scapula as the humerus is raised above 60 degrees of forward flexion or abduction. The shoulder pain that occurs when the client is lying on the affected side can be relieved immediately by moving the body so that the scapula lies in a normal position on the thorax.

Feeding and swallowing. Symmetry and weight bearing can be encouraged during meals. Before normal head and mouth control and normal feeding can be established, it is necessary to have a degree of trunk and girdle control. Although detailed facilitation and inhibition of oral and neck musculature for feeding and articulated language is a specialty of speech pathologists, the therapist must be able to prepare the trunk and girdles so that feeding and speech is possible. See the following outline for typical head and neck problems and related trunk problems in persons with hemiplegia.

1. Oral problems
   a. Forward head, poor lip closure, loss of saliva and food
   b. Facial asymmetry during function greater than at rest
   c. Inability to swallow
   d. Inability to chew
   e. Inability to lateralize foods
   f. Inability to take liquids from cup or spoon
   g. Poor muscle tone
2. Central problems
   a. Asymmetry of trunk
   b. Poor balance

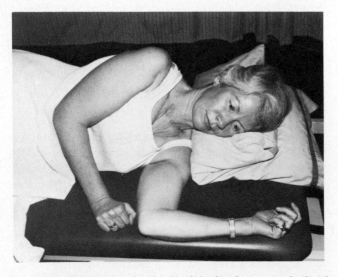

Fig. 22-22. Pressure on the "heel" of the hand prepares the hand for weight bearing and eventual functional tasks.

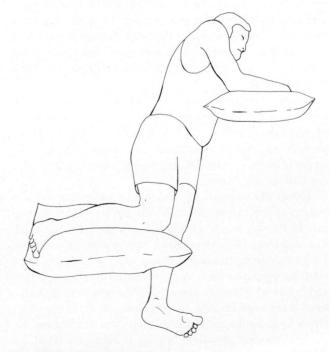

Fig. 22-23. This side-lying position for the right leg mirrors the leg position needed for late stance phase of gait.

   c. Upper body retraction leading to facial asymmetry

   d. Unable to feed self

3. Compensations

   a. Use of gravity—with head and neck extension the food flows down the throat

   b. Chewing on one side only

   c. Using the hand to place food in the mouth

   d. Using the hand to pull food from the cheek

   e. Using thicker food, which is much easier to handle than soft food (soft food is used often)

   f. Labiodental closure versus lip closure

In the majority of cases, swallowing problems are transient in persons with hemiplegia. Following the initial insult and during the flaccid period, many clients exhibit a decreased gag reflex. The assessment of the gag reflex is noted in Chapter 20. Precautions to consider during early recovery include proper trunk, pelvis, and head position before feeding. Liquids, especially water, are often encouraged at this time because they do less damage than nonwater items if they are aspirated to the lung. However, liquids are the hardest for persons with hemiplegia to control because of their thinness and slipperiness. Water, because of its tastelessness, is especially difficult for hemiplegic clients with a decreased gag reflex to control.

The presence of a nasogastric tube will depress and/or diminish the gag reflex. Because the indications for use of a nasogastric tube include an inability to swallow, oral treatment to stimulate the mouth cavity is often indicated when a nasogastric tube is present. To help the person with a decreased but present gag reflex to eat, the therapist should provide a solid surface on which to control the pelvis, trunk, and head. If the person with hemiplegia is eating in bed, the therapist should make sure that the trunk is held over a level pelvis, establish some trunk balance, provide symmetry of the shoulder girdles, and assist with head control, if needed, while providing a diet that will coincide with the hemiplegic person's ability to feed and swallow. Drooling occurs for the following reasons:

1. Poor lip closure as a result of a forward head from lack of trunk control and/or spasticity in cervical paravertebral area

2. Problem number 1 above plus a sensory loss

3. Normal head and mouth control but a primary swallowing problem

Specific feeding programs are noted in Chapters 4 and 20. There are three differences between feeding adults and feeding children. First, when feeding adults it is imperative to remember that someone else's hands in or near the mouth is an invasion of privacy and a very uncomfortable experience. Second, automaticity is a greater factor with adults; it is abnormal for us to chew and swallow on command. Third, adults use many more conscious compensa-

tions than children. Feeding progressions for hemiplegic clients follow the basics as outlined in Chapters 4 and 20. In acute care settings, where liquid diets are often routinely given to persons with hemiplegia, education of hospital staff to the merits of using thicker foods should be considered. Thicker, chopped food is easier to swallow than soft food. Soft food is easier to swallow than liquids. Liquids with distinct taste or texture are easier to swallow than water.

Drooling from the side of the mouth that is paralyzed often presents a problem. The client with hemiplegia may not be able to maintain lip closure, and, in addition, may not feel the saliva running out of the mouth's corner. He or she does not identify a need to swallow. Telling the client to swallow does not treat the problem—it only treats the symptom. If lip closure cannot be maintained as a result of imbalance of muscle tone leading to a forward head, swallowing cannot occur easily. Treating the correct problem, not only the symptom, will result in an automatic improvement of the drooling.

If the client is sitting on a soft mattress with the bed raised to 60 degrees, the pelvis cannot be controlled. This may result in a forward head, poor jaw closure, and thus difficulty in swallowing. Therefore for feeding to be successful and therapeutic, the client needs a firm sitting surface and a neutral pelvic position. If possible, the affected upper extremity should be up on a table in a position to accept weight; it should at least be within the visual field.

Dressing activities require the ability to control the head and trunk against gravity and to shift weight. If these prerequisites are not present, dressing will be stressful, frustrating, and most likely impossible. Assisted dressing should be carried out with as much trunk support as possible. Perceptual problems often prevent success at dressing skills. Thorough understanding of perceptual integration is paramount to understanding development of skill in any complex activity of daily living.

Leisure activities at the bedside throughout the day should be reviewed to establish carryover of treatment principles. Alternate positions for watching television, reading, and resting should be given. If the person with hemiplegia thinks of ways of positioning himself or herself and of moving throughout the day, deformity and pain can be avoided and the repetition necessary for motor learning can be established.

Rolling. When rolling from the supine to the side-lying position, the person with hemiplegia tends to avoid initiating the roll from the involved side. Rolling should be practiced to both sides to promote symmetry and weight bearing on the affected side. Bilateral reaching can be easily incorporated during rolling. This will encourage scapula protraction and will also place the affected arm within the visual field (Fig. 22-22). While lying on the unaffected side, the affected hand can be placed on the bed to encourage weight bearing.

Pillow height affects head position in the side-lying position. If the person with hemiplegia prefers to hold the cervical spine in a position of side bending to the affected side when lying, a high pillow can be placed under the head on the affected side to elongate the shortened muscle groups. Similarly, when positioned on the unaffected side, a low pillow will elongate the shortened muscles.

Facilitating and maintaining trunk rotation while rolling will have a dramatic effect on extremity tone. Rotation within the body axis helps release the extremities' dominant synergistic patterns and free the limbs for more purposeful activities.

Following rolling from the supine to the side-lying position, the function of forearm support on the affected side requires that graduated, appropriate support be given to the weight-bearing scapula, shoulder, and trunk until antigravity control is established (Fig. 22-24). When the affected side is uppermost, the affected upper extremity should be encouraged to move forward or be placed forward so that weight can be placed on the extremity allowing it to function as an assist.

Sitting. The establishment of pelvic control, especially in the anteroposterior plane, is essential for good sitting. The pelvis must be actively controlled in a neutral position for lateral weight shift and appropriate trunk movements to occur. The position and control of the pelvis will influence the position of the lower extremity of the hemiplegic client: if the pelvis is held in a posterior tilt, the lower extremity will tend to abduct, and if the pelvis is held in an anterior tilt, the hemiplegic leg will tend to adduct. While in the sitting position, the hemiplegic client with severe lower-extremity extensor spasticity may demonstrate an anterior tilt of the pelvis and a lower extremity that is pushing into adduction, internal rotation, knee extension,

and plantar flexion. This pushing of the lower extremity is often accompanied by pushing of the entire trunk, usually into the back of the chair or other supporting surface. In treatment, the inhibition of the spasticity, allowing the pelvis to come to a neutral position, and weight bearing and weight shifting to each side will help reestablish control of the sitting posture. When establishing trunk control in the sitting position, the therapist can place the affected foot on the floor in line with, but not in front of, the nonaffected foot so that in weight shift appropriate weight can be accepted and borne through the feet.

The affected upper extremity should not be allowed to hang unsupported or retract severely during sitting activities. A bilateral weight-bearing position for both upper extremities appropriate to the level of the client can be selected and varied during sitting activities. A few ideas include: hands placed on knees, hands fisted or opened down on the chair at the sides of the body, elbows and forearms placed on a lap board or table in front of the client. Care must be taken to keep the scapula in normal alignment during sitting activities.

Transfers. The hemiplegic person should be taught to transfer to all objects (chair, bed, toilet) from each side. This will promote symmetry through weight shift, weight bearing, and rotation to each side and will allow the person to function in any environment regardless of furniture placement.

The pelvis initiates the forward weight shift of a transfer and is accompanied by spinal extension. This same antigravity motor control pattern is present during sit to stand activities. If the shoulders are allowed to initiate the forward weight shift of the transfer, the spine will flex, which is not compatible with the upright posture (Fig. 22-25, *A* and *B*).

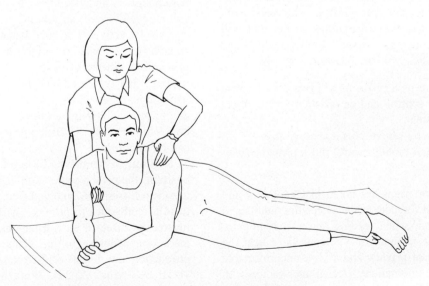

Fig. 22-24. Support is given to the upper trunk to grade the amount of weight taken by the affected right shoulder in the side-lying position.

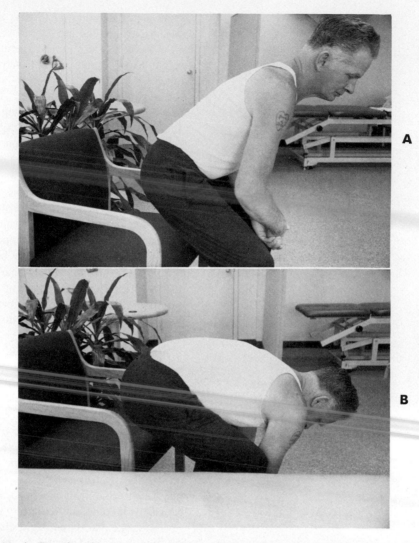

Fig. 22-25. A, Transfer with pelvic initiation and spinal extension. **B,** Transfer with shoulder initiation and spinal flexion.

In treatment, the following points should be considered:

1. Pelvis and trunk movements should be facilitated during the transfer.
2. The upper extremity should not be allowed to hang unsupported.
3. Full standing should not be attempted until pelvic and trunk control is established and until the client can take the "little" steps required to turn the entire body through the transfer.

A partial stand followed by pelvic and lower trunk initiation onto the new supporting surface is necessary in the early stages of recovery (Fig. 22-26).

Transfers to the affected side have the advantage of:

1. Retraining motor control through weight shift and weight bearing to the affected side.
2. Inhibiting the extensor synergy in the lower extremity through the deep pressure obtained by maintain-

ing weight on the affected lower extremity. This can also be accomplished by maintaining some knee flexion to inhibit extension.

3. Directing vision and attention to the hemiplegic side.
4. Protracting and rotating the affected shoulder girdle forward as the upper trunk rotates away from the hemiplegic side during the transfer.

Transfers to the unaffected side have the advantage of being familiar to hospital staff by virtue of the fact that they are the "traditional" textbook way of transferring the person with hemiplegia. Transfers to the affected side are as easy and as safe to teach as transfers to the unaffected side. The inhibition of the extensor thrust in the affected lower extremity and the facilitation of normal movement patterns contribute to the reestablishment of righting and equilibrium reactions. The result is better motor control and balance.

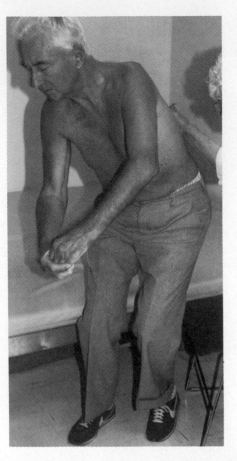

Fig. 22-26. Transfers to the affected side encourage weight bearing onto the leg. This partial stand is followed by pelvic and lower trunk rotation.

Coming to a stand. The ability of the trunk to extend and the pelvis and trunk to flex over the hips (anterior pelvic tilt) is crucial to the function of rising to a stand. Hemiplegic clients often push their trunk backward when trying to stand as a result of a posterior pelvic tilt and the extensor spasticity demonstrated in the lower extremity. If the hemiplegic client pushes back instead of leaning forward and flexing from the hips, tightness of the hips and hamstrings should be assessed.

Along with controlling the trunk in a forward position, weight must be shifted from the pelvis to the feet. This weight bearing through the heel of the affected foot helps inhibit the extensor thrust in the lower extremities and allows retraining of motor control of the knee, hip, and ankle musculature.

The upper extremity should be symmetrically supported during the rise to a stand to take the weight off the trunk and to encourage even weight shift through the lower extremities. Bilateral pushing off from the surface, reaching forward with or without clasped hands, and pushing up with both hands from a table placed in front are possible suggestions.

As a full standing position is approached, the abdominal muscles and the hip extensors need to be facilitated to allow the pelvis to return to a neutral position and to allow weight to be borne appropriately through the lower extremity.

Kneeling to half-kneeling. The process of moving from a kneeling to a half-kneeling position requires the facilitation of or the active control of diagonal trunk patterns. The half-kneeling position is a transitional component of the full stand and should be encouraged to both sides.

When half-kneeling with the unaffected leg forward, the person with hemiplegia will shift his or her weight and bear the majority of weight on the affected side. Hip extension, the most important component of gait for the person with hemiplegia, can easily be facilitated in this position. Weight shift and weight bearing on the affected hip is important for the development of lateral hip control. Half-kneeling with the affected leg forward is a favorable position to facilitate ankle movements and to increase proprioceptive input through the heel.

Standing. Treatment considerations given for the pelvis in preceding sections hold true for pelvic control in standing. With the feet placed in a parallel and even position, weight shift (anterior, posterior, lateral, and diagonal) and weight bearing can begin. This weight shift should be done with the feet parallel and in right step stance and left step stance. The person with hemiplegia will tend to avoid weight bearing onto the affected side especially in standing. The use of external supports is necessary when standing is practiced before good control is established. If trunk and extremity control is poor, as with a severe stroke, the hemiplegic client will use spasticity in the extremities and girdles to "hold" himself or herself in the standing position. To compensate for the lack of central stability in the trunk, the leg will become a rigid pillar. Therefore total inhibition of extensor spasticity in the lower extremity in standing without facilitation of active movement patterns may result in a "collapse" of the lower extremity. The affected foot must be correctly aligned and ankle movement (tibia moving over the fixed foot) must be possible for functional standing to be achieved. It is often necessary to prepare the foot for standing by aligning the foot, facilitating weight transfer through the heel, inhibiting clawing of the toes, and facilitating ankle and forefoot movement. This preparation can be done in the sitting position, the half-kneeling position, or during transfers.

In the standing position, the alignment of the scapula and arm should be maintained, and the upper extremity should be allowed to weight bear when possible (Fig. 22-27) for the purpose of adding stability in the upper trunk while practicing lower trunk and lower extremity movements; this will also prepare the hand for function. Thus guarding the client on the affected side while maintaining the upper extremity in a weight-bearing pattern encourages

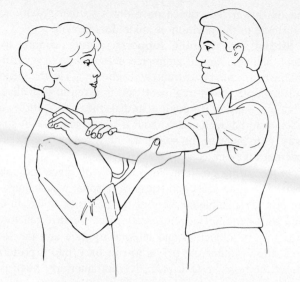

Fig. 22-27. While the client is standing, the upper extremity is allowed to bear weight and lower extremity control is facilitated.

pelvic mobility and appropriate trunk movements while providing inhibition to the spastic upper-extremity patterns.

Gait. If one of the obvious features of walking is its automaticity, gait training should reflect this factor. Before walking is encouraged, the hemiplegic client should have practiced and achieved some control in parallel standing, in step stance, and in unilateral weight bearing on each leg. Lower-extremity positions during walking should be carefully chosen to facilitate weight shift and inhibit spasticity of the trunk and girdles. In the early stages, when walking is being practiced over short distances, common items found in hospitals, such as moveable laundry carts and walkers, allow "reaching" of both upper extremities and allow the upper extremities to be placed in a position that takes the weight of the arm off the trunk and within the visual field. The use of stable objects, such as parallel bars, encourages "pulling" with the upper extremity. This pulling contributes to the spastic flexor pattern in the upper extremity.

Once a particular gait disturbance is identified, specific treatment procedures can be instituted. For example, in a Type I motor control problem with premature activation of the calf muscles, treatment might facilitate forward hip rotation during swing to allow the center of gravity to advance ahead of the foot before the activation of calf muscles pulls the lower leg backward. With a Type II disturbance, training to improve control and power of the leg in standing and walking may be indicated. In a Type III problem, treatment would be directed at facilitation of trunk control. During ambulation, the person with hemiplegia demonstrates an increase in upper-extremity spasticity because of associated reactions, poor trunk control, and

loss of balance. This increase in spasticity hinders the development of arm swing during gait because arm swing is a result of counter-rotational movements between the shoulder and pelvic girdles. This counter rotation within the trunk will not develop when spasticity is present.

When retraining gait in the client with hemiplegia, the therapist should focus on three critical areas: weight acceptance (heel strike to foot flat), double-single limb support (mid-stance to heel off), and limb-length adjustment (swing).

In the weight acceptance phase, the task is weight shifting on a forward diagonal initiated from the pelvis. The heel should strike the ground first, the upper and lower trunk remain aligned, and the hip move from flexion towards extension.

During double-single limb support, the task is shifting weight from the lateral aspect of the heel to the medial aspect of the forefoot. The foot should not supinate excessively, weight must be accepted on the ball of the foot, and appropriate movement components of the hip and knee should be facilitated.

Swing phase of gait requires that the foot "lead" the movement and reach ahead of the body. Prerequisites for swing include: (1) the ability to disassociate (separate) the hip from the pelvis and the pelvis from the rib cage, (2) that the pelvis and lower extremity be in their most posterior position to the trunk for the pendulum action of the leg to perform most efficiently, and (3) that the body continue to move forward in space.

Hand reach, grasp, and release. Treatment of the hand requires normal alignment and reeducation of the wrist, forearm, elbow, and shoulder. Motor reeducation of the hand should be accompanied by tactile, proprioceptive, and visual stimulation. Examples include rubbing or sliding, touching (or pushing the hand into) different surfaces, and encouraging the hand to conform to objects. Grasp is encouraged when carpal, wrist, and forearm alignment can be maintained. Upper-extremity movements should focus on initiation from the hand, especially when the hand is grasping an object. In hemiplegia clients commonly grasp an object and then initiate the movement from the shoulder, which places the hand in a nonfunctional position.

When trunk control is not established and when prolonged sitting is accompanied by an increase in spasticity that results from associated reactions, hand treatment can be performed in the supine or side-lying position. In the supine or side-lying position, the trunk is fully supported with the arm protracted, forward flexed, or abducted, and the scapula is in normal alignment on the thorax.

Treatment of hand function can also begin in sitting with the trunk being supported forward against a high table, with good pelvic and trunk positioning and weight bearing through the elbows and forearms.

If active functional movements of the hand are not possible, treatment should aim at decreasing the associated reactions that occur in the involved upper extremity as a result of one-handed activities. The affected arm and hand can be placed in a weight-bearing position in the visual field, and one-handed activities can be graded to help decrease these undesired associated reactions. These associated reactions often interfere with symmetry and weight bearing. If they persist over long periods of time, the posturing that results may lead to deformity, contracture, and pain.

Equipment

Equipment for persons with CNS dysfunction can be thought of as supports or as an "extra" hand used to allow the client to be more properly aligned or controlled so that he or she can move and function in a more normal or desired way. Too much support or equipment will prevent the person's participation in an activity and will hinder the development of new motor control. Equipment should never be a substitute for treatment and should not be given without first being used during treatment. Ongoing assessment of the appropriateness of the equipment's relation to gains made in therapy must be made so that equipment always contributes to independence and so that it is not a substitute for development of new motor control. Equipment for adults with hemiplegia should be appropriate to the individual and should consist of items commonly found in the individual's environment.

Bedside equipment. When severe spasticity is present, air or water mattresses are used for clients with hemiplegia to provide a movable surface for the facilitation of head and trunk motion.

In acute and rehabilitation settings, pillows, blankets, or towels are used to position the client in bed. With the client in the supine position, the head pillow can be angled so that it slips under the shoulder and scapula to prevent scapular adduction and downward rotation. Towel rolls are used under the greater trochanter to maintain normal alignment of the affected pelvis and lower extremity. If the hip of the hemiplegic client is kept in a neutral position, pressure will not be placed on the lateral malleolus and pressure sores will be avoided.

Foot boards have traditionally been used in the flaccid stage of hemiplegia. A disadvantage of foot boards is that if the foot is firmly placed against the board and spasticity develops, the extension or "pushing" of the lower extremity is increased, facilitating the positive supporting reaction or extension synergy. A pillow placed in front of the foot board gives a soft surface so "pushing" will not be reinforced. The foot board can also be removed as soon as any spasticity develops. As extensor spasticity develops in the lower extremity, loss of ankle range of movement is avoided by changing position frequently, using the sitting position with the feet placed firmly on the floor, and, if possible, lying in the prone position with the knees flexed

and the lower legs raised on pillows so that gravity will contribute to the position of ankle dorsiflexion.

Sitting and standing supports. Sitting, coming to a stand, and standing, if attempted before postural control is established, can be extremely frightening for the person with hemiplegia. In treatment care is given to provide appropriate support through external means to allow the function to be achieved without a severe increase in spasticity. An increase in spasticity may render the desired function impossible.

In the sitting position, support may be given through a chair. The sling seats and backs of hospital wheelchairs do not provide a stable surface for the pelvis or trunk. In clients with hemiplegia, sling seats place the affected lower extremity in adduction and internal rotation and the sling back allows either the pelvis to roll back into a posterior tile or the trunk to lean back over an anteriorly tilted pelvis. Solid seats and backs allow the pelvis, trunk, and extremities to be more normally aligned.

Foam wedges with a thicker edge uppermost can be used in solid chairs to encourage the trunk to remain upright over a neutral pelvis. The therapist can give support to the client's upper body and shoulders by standing in front of the client in the sitting position and placing his or her arms under the axilla and onto the thorax. As the client gains control in the sitting position, support can be gradually withdrawn until only the client's arms are held. Forward sitting can be achieved by having the client with hemiplegia lean against a table. High tables can be used for maximal support, and lower tables can be used as control of sitting improves.

While the client is sitting, lap boards, pillows, and arm rests are used to support the upper extremity. Lap boards and pillows should be used to promote symmetry. The use of a clear plastic lapboard maintains visual body image continuity. This can be an important component of treatment. When the hands are resting at midline, they are in the visual field. The client with hemiplegia should be encouraged to touch and move the affected arm. Arm rests do not offer the advantage of promoting symmetry and, if used, should be placed forward on the wheelchair arm so that the client's upper extremity is not placed in a position of humeral hyperextension, scapular adduction, and/or downward rotation.

Smith offers a review of shoulder slings for hemiplegic clients.[65] Slings should be carefully assessed to see if, following treatment, they "hold" the corrected scapulohumeral position. Slings should not be expected to inhibit spastic muscles or to facilitate the movement necessary to achieve normal alignment of the scapula and humerus.

The ideal shoulder sling is one that maintains the normal angular alignment of the glenoid fossa, decreases the tendency of the humerus to internally rotate, yet allows the upper extremity freedom of movement. In the acute stage,

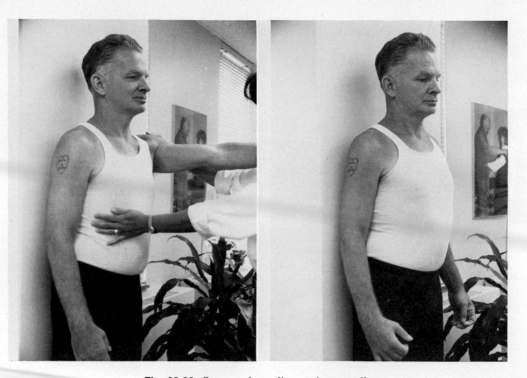

Fig. 22-28. Supported standing against a wall.

if lap boards and pillows are used when the client is seated, slings need only to be used during standing and walking activities when the arm may be dependent.

When the client is coming to a stand, his or her trunk can be supported from under the axilla bilaterally or unilaterally from the affected side. A table, walker, or chairback can be used to control the upper trunk through bilateral arm support as the client practices coming to a stand. Canes or hemi-walkers placed in front of the client provide moderate support through bilateral upper extremity weight bearing during the rise to a stand.

Standing supports for the motor reeducation of dynamic standing should be vertical (i.e., parallel to the body's line of gravity). Supports with forward or backward tilts are only indicated to decrease hip, knee, or ankle contractures. Supported standing is easily achieved through the use of a wall (Fig. 22-28, *A* and *B*). When early standing is attempted, the client's chair can be placed close to the wall so that only a small transfer is necessary before the body is supported.

Activities that can be used in treatment when using this type of support include sliding up and down the wall, moving only the upper body away from the wall, moving only the lower body away from the wall, and moving the entire body away from the wall. Standing forward against a high counter, dresser, or dining room buffet with bilateral upper-extremity weight bearing can also be used as a support.

Equipment used to encourage movement and prevent deformities

Canes. Canes are given to clients with hemiplegia to provide "extra" balance, not as a means to support body weight. Therefore canes should be provided after the ability to shift and bear weight to each side has been established. Four-pointed or "quad" canes are used because they can remain upright and do not wobble when leaned on heavily. However, they foster asymmetry, lack of weight bearing on the affected side, and loss of postural control. Single canes can be modified through the use of elastic bands or wrist loops to eliminate the problem of the cane falling or interfering with use of the unaffected hand.

Braces and shoe modifications. Although the use of knee, ankle, foot orthoses (KAFOs) in hemiplegia is no longer common practice, ankle foot orthoses (AFOs) are frequently used to ensure clearance of the foot in the swing phase of gait and to provide medial-lateral ankle and forefoot stability. Metal, double, upright, short leg braces have the disadvantage of being heavy and of not holding calcaneal-forefoot alignment. Custom-molded AFOs that maintain heel and forefoot alignment are indicated for clients who display a strong pull into inversion, supination, and plantar flexion (Fig. 22-29, *A* and *B*). If a client lacks dorsiflexion, a light prefabricated AFO may be very appropriate. Refer to Chapter 24 for additional discussion.

All AFOs should allow the tibia to move forward over the fixed foot. If normal movement cannot occur passively

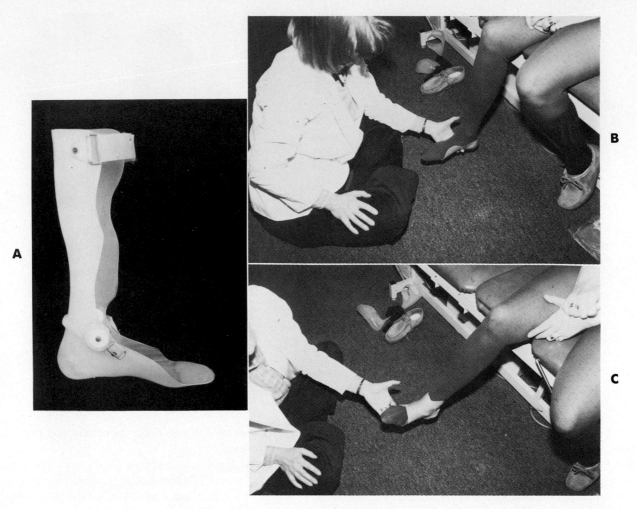

Fig. 22-29. A, Ankle-foot orthosis (AFO) designed to control equinovarus. **B,** University of California at Berkeley Laboratory (UCBL) insert designed to control varus of the forefoot. **C,** An elastic ankle support for minimal foot control.

while the foot is in the orthoses, normal patterns of motor control for ambulation will not be established. Clients should be encouraged to spend time standing without the brace so that dependence on the brace is not established. When possible, short periods of walking without the brace can be practiced. Ace elastic supports can be worn on the ankle to provide some support but less support than provided with the orthoses (Fig. 22-29, *C*). The use of an orthosis can be withheld until good standing is achieved. As motor control of the trunk, hip, knee, and ankle improves, less foot support is appropriate.

Foot control orthoses, such as a University of California at Berkeley Laboratory (UCBL) insert, that maintain alignment of the rearfoot, midfoot, and forefoot are recommended over shoe modifications such as sole or heel wedges. If shoe modifications are attempted, modifications inside the shoe rather than outside offer a better chance of correction.

In the acute stage following a stroke, knee supports are not necessary if trunk, hip, and ankle movements are controlled. However, in the chronic stage, if the knee joint has become weakened or destroyed through inappropriate weight bearing, elastic knee supports or firm knee cages can be used to maintain the knee joint in normal alignment.

Movable surfaces. Movable surfaces such as inflatable balls of varying sizes, large rolls, and castered adjustable stools are used to help increase mobility while postural control is maintained (Fig. 22-30, *A*). To facilitate automatic trunk balance reactions, the client with mild or minimal hemiplegia can sit on a large ball at a table while performing upper-extremity functional activities (Fig. 22-30, *B*).

Large inflatable balls can provide support to the trunk in an all-fours position and to the upper trunk and upper extremities in the kneeling and half-kneeling positions. The use of the large balls helps to facilitate straight plane and diagonal weight shift while incorporating bilateral upper-extremity weight bearing.

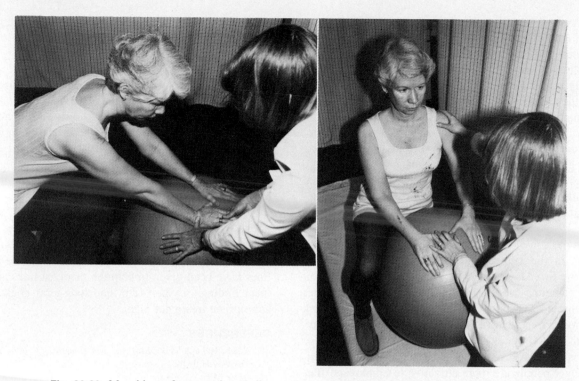

Fig. 22-30. Movable surfaces, such as balls, can be used to encourage dynamic upper extremity weight bearing for the affected right arm.

Hand splints. The practice of splinting the hemiplegic hand is controversial and has undergone change since the introduction of neurophysiological approaches.[51] Controversy exists over whether rigid one-surface dorsal or volar splints facilitate or inhibit spasticity. Hand and wrist splints that are designed to maintain bone alignment and normal length of both flexor and extensor tendons and yet block abnormal muscle pull will decrease spasticity and allow appropriate motor reeducation. One surface dorsal or volar splinting in a functional position does not allow function (reach, grasp, release) to occur because the splint is in the way. Thumb abductor bars or opponens splints often provide some inhibition of flexor spasticity in the hemiplegic hand, yet they have the advantage of allowing functional grasp and release to occur. MacKinnon's splint allows use of functional hand patterns while providing inhibition of flexor spasticity through deep pressure at the metacarpal heads.[40] However, these devices do not provide carpal support or alignment.

Two approaches for casting the hemiplegic ankle and foot and wrist and fingers exist—orthopaedic casting and inhibitory casting. Orthopaedic or static casting takes the joint close to its limit and immobilizes it. Inhibitory or dynamic casting not only places the joint at the end of its limited range, it also provides a weight-bearing surface for movement. Inhibitory casting requires treatment during the period of immobilization, including weight bearing and muscle retraining. Fiberglass plaster is lighter and more appropriate for upper-extremity casting because the weight of regular plaster places a great stress on the hemiplegic shoulder joint. Farber[17] thoroughly discusses the advantages and disadvantages of adaptive equipment as well as a variety of possible alternatives when selecting specific assistive devices and splints.

PSYCHOSOCIAL ASPECTS AND ADJUSTMENTS

The suddenness of a stroke and the dramatic change in motor, sensory, visual, and perceptual performance and feedback may leave the person with hemiplegia confused, disoriented, angry, and fearful. With a stroke, time is not allowed for gradual adjustment to the resulting disability. The usual psychosocial adjustments to disability are compounded in persons with hemiplegia resulting from stroke by the problem of increasing age (see Chapter 7).

The difficulties resulting from deficits in speech, movement, vision, sensation, and perception cause varying degrees of stress and frustration during the performance of functional activity.

Psychosocial adjustments may be more detrimental to long-term stroke survivors than functional disability.[26] Decreased interest in social activity inside and outside the home and decreased interest in hobbies attributable to psychosocial disability hamper the hemiplegic person's return to a normal social life.[35] Feelings of rejection and embarrassment may interfere with the hemiplegic person's interaction with peers or nonpeers outside the home environment. Persons with long-standing hemiplegia often become clinically depressed with symptoms of loss of sleep and appetite, self-blame, and a hopeless outlook. Suicide can result.

Family members and spouses may have difficulty assessing the capabilities of the hemiplegic person and may be overprotective. Overprotection among spouses may be a sign of affection and support or a sign of guilt.[32,48] Long-standing marriages do not tend to dissolve when one member experiences a stroke. However, previous marriage problems and personality traits may become exaggerated as a result of the presence of increased and changing demands and stresses that occur when the person returns home.

A comparison of occupational status of long-term stroke survivors in the United States and Sweden reveals that 40% of the Swedes returned to a form of employment (including part-time work), but none of the United States group returned to work.[19] The scarcity of part-time work and a shorter treatment period dictated by third-party payers in the United States may account for this discrepancy.

Age is a general predictor for return to employment, and younger people are more attractive to employers. Barriers to return to work for the person with hemiplegia include speech, perceptual, and cognitive deficits along with a need for psychosocial support. Architectual barriers can also create severe problems to hemiplegic clients with regard to both work and recreational activities. Stroke clubs, usually organized through hospitals, the Easter Seal Association, or the American Heart Association, provide educational, social, and recreational support for the hemiplegic person and his or her spouse.

The impact of psychosocial disability and the need for its long-term treatment is great. Programs need to be established and continued for years to allow clients and their families to deal with the many problems that result from the stroke.

Sexuality

The majority of persons with hemiplegia experience a decline in sexuality through a decrease in frequency of sexual intercourse without a change in the level of prestroke sexual desire.[20] On return home, the person with hemiplegia faces the uncertainty of sexual skills and the risk of failure. Sexual dysfunction that results from a stroke depends on the amount of cerebral damage, and it includes a decreased ability to achieve erection and ejaculation in men and decreased lubrication in women.[58] The sensory, motor, visual, and emotional disturbances of hemiplegia may cause awkwardness, but these disturbances can be overcome through the education of the spouse in alternate positioning and ways to provide appropriate sensory experiences. The normal factors of aging also interfere with the sexual performance of persons with hemiplegia. The closeness between partners achieved through satisfactory sexual relationship can add to the quality of a hemiplegic person's life.

SUMMARY

Treatment of the person with hemiplegia poses special clinical problems. Although one-sided motor and functional skills may appear to accomplish a "function," such skills will never contribute to the redevelopment of normal postural and movement control. The process of establishing goals and treatment plans for the person with hemiplegia requires a careful assessment of the existing movement patterns.

Active movement patterns, postural control, and functional activities have been reviewed to help the therapist establish a foundation on which an understanding of the hemiplegic person's problems can be established. Guidelines have been given to help the therapist translate assessment findings to short-term and long-term goals and into appropriate treatment plans.

REFERENCES

1. Adams RD and Victor M: Principles of neurology, New York, 1981, McGraw-Hill, Inc.
2. Adler MK and others: Stroke rehabilitation: is age a determinant? J Am Geriatr Soc 28:499, 1980.
3. Anderson TP and others: Stroke rehabilitation: evaluation of its quality by assessing patient outcomes, Arch Phys Med Rehabil 59:170, 1978.
4. Ayres AJ: Sensory integration and learning disorders, Los Angeles, 1979, Western Psychological Services.
5. Bach-y-Rita P: Recovery of functions: theoretical considerations for brain injury rehabilitation, Baltimore, 1980, University Park Press.
6. Basmajian JV: Muscles alive: their functions revealed by electromyography, Baltimore, 1978, The Williams & Wilkins Co.
7. Bishop B: Spasticity: its physiology and management, Phys Ther 57:396, 1977.
8. Bizzi E and Polit A: Characteristics of motor programs underlying movement in monkeys, J Neurophysiol 42:183, 1979.
9. Bjorklund A and others: Regeneration of central neurons as studied in cerebral iris implants. In Scheinberg P, editor: Cerebrovascular disease, Tenth Princeton Conference, New York, 1976, Raven Press.
10. Bobath B: Adult hemiplegia: evaluation and treatment, ed 2, London, 1979, William Heinneman Medical Books.
11. Brodal A: Self-observations and neuroanatomical considerations after a stroke, Brain 96:675, 1973.
12. Brooks VB: Motor programs revisited. In Talbott RE and Humphrey DR, editors: Posture and movement, New York, 1979, Raven Press.
13. Brunnstrom S: Movement therapy in hemiplegia, New York, 1970, Harper & Row, Publishers, Inc.
14. Cailliet R: The shoulder in hemiplegia, Philadelphia, 1980, FA Davis Co.
15. Chine N: Electrophysiological investigation of shoulder subluxation in hemiplegics, Scand J Rehabil Med 13:17, 1981.
16. Easton JKM and others: Intramuscular neurolysis for spasticity in children, Arch Phys Med Rehabil 50:155, 1979.
17. Farber S: Adaptive equipment. In Farber S, editor: Neurorehabilitation: a multisensory approach, Philadelphia, 1981, WB Saunders Co.
18. Fiorentino M Schultz J: NDTA Adult Hemiplegia Course Manual, 1982, Hartford, Connecticut.
19. Fugl-Meyer AR: Post-stroke hemiplegia—occupational status, Scand J Rehabil Med (suppl) 7:167, 1980.

20. Fugl-Meyer AR and Jaaskor L: Post-stroke hemiplegia and sexual intercourse, Scand J Rehabil Med 7(suppl):158, 1980.

21. Fugl-Meyer AR and others: The post-stroke hemiplegic patient: a method for evaluation of physical performance, Scand J Rehabil Med 7:13, 1975.

22. Granger CV and others: Stroke rehabilitation: analysis of repeated Barthel Index measures, Arch Phys Med Rehabil 60:14, 1979.

23. Granit R: Comments. In Granit R, editor: Progress in brain research, Netherlands, 1979, North Holland Biomedical Press.

24. Granit R: Interpretation of suprospinal effects on the gamma system. In Granit R, editor: Progress in brain research, Netherlands, 1979, North Holland Biomedical Press.

25. Gresham GE and others: Epidemiologic profile of long-term stroke disability: the Framingham study, Arch Phys Med Rehabil 60:487, 1979.

26. Gresham GE and others: ADL status in stroke: relative merits of three standard indexes, Arch Phys Med Rehabil 61:355, 1980.

27. Haas AL and others: Respiratory function in hemiplegic patients, Arch Phys Med Rehabil 48:174, 1967.

28. Jacobson E: You must relax, New York, 1962, McGraw-Hill, Inc.

29. Jennett B: Predictors of recovery in evaluation of patients income. In Thompson RA and Green JE, editors: Advances in neurology, ed 22, New York, 1979, Raven Press.

30. Jenson M: The hemiplegic shoulder, Scand J Rehabil Med 7(suppl):113, 1980.

31. Kapandji IA: The physiology of the joints, ed 2, London, 1970, Churchill Livingstone.

32. Kinsella GJ and Duffy FD: Attitudes towards disability expressed by spouses of stroke patients, Scand J Rehabil Med 12:73, 1980.

33. Knott M and Voss DE: Proprioceptive neuromuscular facilitation, New York, 1976, Harper & Row, Publishers, Inc.

34. Knutsson E and Richards C: Different types of disturbed motor control in gait of hemiparetic patients, Brain 102:405, 1979.

35. Labi ML and others: Psychosocial disability in physically restored long-term stroke survivors, Arch Phys Med Rehabil 61:561, 1980.

36. Landau WM: Spasticity: the fable of a neurological demon and the emperor's new therapy, Arch Neurol 31:217, 1974.

37. Lane RE: Facilitation of weight transference in the stroke patient, Physiotherapy 64:260, 1978.

38. Lehmann JF and others: Stroke rehabilitation: outcome and prediction, Arch Phys Med Rehabil 56:383, 1975.

39. Levy DE and others: Prognosis in nontraumatic coma, Ann Int Med 94:293, 1981.

40. MacKinnon F and others: The MacKinnon splint: a functional hand splint, Can J Occup Ther 42:157, 1975.

41. Malkmus D: Levels of cognitive functioning, Ranchos Los Amigos Hospital, Inc.

42. Marshall J: The management of cerebrovascular disease, ed 3, Oxford, 1976, Blackwell Scientific Publications, Ltd.

43. Miller L and Miyamoto A: Computed tomography: its potential as a predistor of functional recovery following stroke, Arch Phys Med Rehabil 60:108, 1979.

44. Moore J: Remarks at Mary Fiorentino Symposium, 1987, Windsor Locks, Connecticut.

45. Moore RY: Response to injury in the mammalian central nervous system. In Scheinberg P, editor: Cerebrovascular disease, Tenth Princeton Conference, New York, 1976, Raven Press.

46. Mossman P: A problem oriented approach to stroke rehabilitation, Springfield, Ill, 1976, Charles C Thomas, Publisher.

47. Mulley G and Espley AJ: Hip fracture after hemiplegia, Postgrad Med J 55:264, 1979.

48. Mykyta LJ and others: Caring for relatives of stroke patients, Age Aging 5:87, 1976.

49. Nelson AJ: Functional ambulation profile, Phys Ther 54:1059, 1974.

50. Nelson AJ: Personal communication, Nov 1981.

51. Neuhaus B and others: A survey of rationales for and against hand splinting in hemiplegia, Am J Occup Ther 35:83, 1981.

52. Odeen I: Reduction of muscular hypertonus by long-term muscle stretch, Scand J Rehabil Med 13:93, 1981.

53. Ostfeld A: A review of stroke epidemiology, Epidemiol Rev 2:136, 1980.

54. Perry J: Clinical gait analyzer, Bull Prosthet Res p. 188, Fall 1974.

55. Petrillo CR and others: Phenol block of the tibial nerve in the hemiplegic patient, Orthopedics 3:871, 1980.

56. Plum F and Caronna JJ: Can one predict outcome of medical coma? In Outcome of severe damage to the central nervous system, Ciba Foundation Symposium 34, Amsterdam, 1975, The Foundation.

57. Primbram KH: Languages of the brain, Englewood Cliffs, vol 5, 1971, Prentice-Hall, Inc.

58. Renshaw DC: Stroke and sex. In Comfort A, editor: Sexual consequences of disability, Philadelphia, 1978, George F Stickley Co.

59. Roland PE: Quantitative assessment of cortical motor dysfunction by measurement of the regional cerebral blood flow, Scand J Rehabil Med 7(suppl):27, 1980.

60. Ryerson S: The foot in hemiplegia. In Hunt G, editor: The foot and ankle in physical therapy, New York, 1987, Churchill Livingstone.

61. Ryerson S and Levit K: The shoulder in hemiplegia. In Donatelli R, editor: The shoulder in physical therapy, New York, 1986, Churchill Livingstone.

62. Sahrmann S and Norton BJ: The relationship of voluntary movement to spasticity in the upper motor neuron syndrome, Ann Neurol 2:460, 1977.

63. Sahs AL and Hartman EC, editors: Fundamentals of stroke care, Washington, DC, 1976, DHEW Publication.

64. Schoenberg BS: Epidemiology of cerebrovascular disease, South Med J 72:31, 1979.

65. Smith RO and Okamoto GA: Checklist for the prescription of slings for the hemiplegia patient, Am J Occup Ther 35:91, 1981.

66. Stern PH and others: Factors influencing stroke rehabilitation, Stroke, 1971.

67. Stockmeyer SA: An interpretation of the approach of Rood to the treatment of neuromuscular dysfunction, Am J Phys Med 46:900, 1967.

68. Taub E: Motor behavior following deafferenation in the motorically mature and developing monkey. In Rerman RM and others, editors: Advances in behavioral biology, New York, 1976, Plenum Publishing Corporation.

69. Teasdale G and Jennett B: Assessment of coma and impaired consciousness: a practical scale, Lancet 2:81, 1974.

70. Urbscheit N and others: Effects of cooling on the ankle jerk and H-response in hemiplegic patients, Phys Ther 51:983, 1971.

71. Wall JC and Ashburn A: Assessment of gait disability in hemiplegics, Scand J Rehabil Med 11:95, 1979.

72. Weinfeld D, editor: The national survey of stroke, Stroke 12(suppl 1):2, 1981.

73. Wolf SL and others: EMG biofeedback in stroke: a 1-year follow-up on the effect of patient characteristics, Arch Phys Med Rehabil 61:351, 1980.

APPENDIX

Audiovisual resources

Inner World of Aphasia—35 minute film
   American Journal of Nursing Film Library
   267 W. 25th Street
   New York, NY 10001
Candidate for Stroke—35 minute film
   American Heart Association

I Had a Stroke—35 minute film
Filmakers Library, Inc.
290 West End Avenue
New York, NY 10023
Living with Stroke
Rehabilitation Research and Training Center
The George Washington University
2300 EYE St., N.W. Suite 714
Washington, D.C. 20037

Evaluation of the Hemiplegic Patient (Sensory/Motor)
Audio-Visual Department
School of Allied Health
University of Maryland
32 Greene Street
Baltimore, MD

Children's book

First One Foot, Then The Other—Tomie de Paola
This book explores the feelings and fears of children to a relative who has had a stroke.

Chapter 23

BRAIN FUNCTION, AGING, AND DEMENTIA

Osa L. Jackson

FRAMEWORK FOR CLINICAL PROBLEM SOLVING
Definition of terms

It was in 37 BC that the Roman poet Virgil described what he saw: "Age carries all things, even the mind, away."[19] The crucial concept for clinical problem solving is not to accept at face value what we see. When a client is observed to have altered brain function, it is necessary to describe the extent and type of the distortion of intellectual capacity and to determine the cause(s) to allow effective treatment and care. There are three major categories of intellectual impairment: retardation, delirium, and dementia. A definition of terms is necessary to ensure that all personnel use the same framework for clinical problem solving.

Retardation. A retarded person has had some degree of mental impairment all his or her life. A retarded person can also develop a delirium or dementia. A delirium or dementia differs from retardation in that there has been a change from what was normal for that person.

Delirium. A delirious person shows a change both in intellectual function *and* in the level of consciousness. The client is less alert than normal and may be confused, disoriented, forgetful, and/or sleepy. Other commonly used terms to describe this condition are "acute brain syndrome" or "reversible brain syndrome." If the underlying medical and emotional problem(s) are treated in a timely fashion, the level of alertness and intellectual functions can return to normal.

Dementia. Dementia is an impairment in some or all aspects of intellectual functioning in a person who is clearly awake. Other terms used to describe this condition are "organic brain syndrome," "senility," "senile dementia," "hardening of the arteries," and "shrinking of the brain." Some diseases that can cause dementia are treatable. In these diseases the distortion of intellectual capacity is reversed when treatment is given and/or the intellectual functioning is prevented from becoming worse. Dementia involves global cognitive impairment affecting memory and at least one of the following:

- Abstract thinking
- Judgment

- Other complex capabilities, such as language use, ability to perform complex physical tasks, ability to recognize objects or people or to construct objects
- Personality[43,55]

Alzheimer's disease. This term is used as a diagnosis when, based on the symptoms of dementia and impaired intellectual functioning, all the other possible causes have been ruled out. It is not possible to ascertain if a client has this disease until an autopsy or brain biopsy has been done. At present there is no known cause or treatment for Alzheimer's disease, but clients and families *can be helped* to cope better with the presenting losses of intellectual functioning.[19] (Refer to Chapter 4).

Demographics

It is estimated today that 1.5 million Americans suffer from severe dementia (incapacitated to the degree that others must care for them continually).[65] It is expected that disorders causing dementia will continue to be a growing public health problem for at least the next 30 years. There are an estimated 5 million persons who are currently suffering from mild or moderate dementia. The actual number of people with severe dementia is expected to increase by 60% by the year 2000. The projected statistics, presuming there are no cures or effective means of preventing the common causes of dementia, are that by the year 2040 there will be five times as many cases of dementia (7.4 million Americans) as there are today. The statistics are important and relate to the increased life expectancy (1900—47.3 years; 1982—74.5 years).[66] The oldest age groups are growing in numbers the most rapidly. The demographics are significant because the prevalence of severe dementia rises from approximately 1% (ages 65 to 74) to 7% (ages 75 to 84) to 25% (over age 85).[24] The large increase in the number of persons over the age of 85 will increase the incidence of dementia.

Framework for assessment and care

There are more than 70 known conditions that can cause dementia.[42] Confusion in the elderly individual can be interpreted as a response of the aging brain to stress, whether somatic or psychological (a demand to adapt to new situations or input) or both. Memory impairment and impairments of abstract thinking or judgment in an elderly individual may be equivalent to convulsions in childhood. As a symptom of acute physical illness in old age, global cognitive impairments are more significant than a rise in temperature or pulse rate, and often it gives useful warning of a more insidious disease.[1] The person and the environment (physical and emotional) need to be systematically evaluated when treating a person with memory impairment and difficulty with abstract thinking, judgment, or language ability.

The discussion of brain function, aging, and dementias will build from the concept that major changes in intellec-

tual capacity are *not* normal in the aging process. For any change, whether it develops slowly over a period of time or happens suddenly, it is essential that efforts be made to diagnose and, where possible, to treat the underlying cause(s) of the delirium or dementia. Even if the cause of the dementia may be untreatable, it is *always* possible to teach the client and the family basic management strategies to make the activities of daily living easier to manage.

The physical and occupational therapist are key parts of the total evaluation, treatment, and ongoing care of the client with delirium and/or dementia. It is important that all care planning be done as a part of a team effort, where the client, the family or significant others, the physician, nurses, social worker, physical therapist, and occupational therapist participate so that a consistency of treatment and approach can be guaranteed.

PHYSIOLOGY OF AGING—RELEVANCE FOR SYMPTOMATOLOGY AND DIAGNOSIS OF DELIRIUM AND DEMENTIAS
The normal brain

The brain of a normal person at age 80 will show some significant changes in physiological function from the brain of a younger person. The changes that will be described make this age group more susceptible to symptoms of confusion, that is, impairment of memory, particularly recent memory, and to a decrease in ability to register, to retain, and to recall current experiences. However, a normal elderly person who is not experiencing severe somatic or emotional stress will show little or *no* functional changes in intellectual capacity because of advanced age. It must also be noted that many persons maintain and/or expand certain parts of their intellectual capacity until the ninth or tenth decades of life.

The following discussion examines many of the variables that need to be considered as a part of the framework for the clinical evaluation of the rehabilitation potential of the person with dementia. The hope is that if the personnel dealing with the aging client are aware of and can therefore compensate for the known vulnerability, the client will have a greater possibility of achieving his or her own potential for self-care and a meaningful existence.

For persons over the age of 80, a slowing down of the natural pace of movement is commonly noted. The slowing down is central to brain function as seen in the slowing down of the electroencephalogram (EEG) rhythms with advanced aging. At the age of 60 the mean frequency of occipital rhythm is 10.3 Hz, and at 80 years of age the mean is 8.7 Hz. The average change is about one cycle per decade in the period of advanced aging.[67] It has been noted that there is a decrease in brain weight with advancing age. For example, the mean weight for women age 21 to 40 is 1260 g; for women over the age of 80 it is 1061 g.[58] The speed of nerve conduction in the elderly can be 10% to 15% slower than it is in younger persons.[10] These physiological changes mean that if the process and structure of evaluation and care of the normal person or the person with dementia focuses on speed of execution or any activities that are timed, *the aged will appear to be less capable than they really are*. It also means that the framework for clinical problem solving will require *more* time in working with persons over the age of 70 than is generally required for the average adult individual.

The function of a normal brain requires a delicate synchronization of a large number of variables. To make normal intellectual function possible, the brain must have (1) no genetic defects; (2) a constant supply of nutrients, both the glucose and amino acid substrates as well as the coenzymes essential for their assimilation and effective use; (3) an unfailing supply of oxygen (implying appropriate blood content, collateral circulation, normal respiratory exchange, and adequate cardiac output); (4) normal blood biochemistry especially involving the water and the electrolytes; (5) normal hepatic and renal function; and (6) freedom from noxious stimuli such as trauma, infection, or toxins. The brain is a physiologically active organ, and it makes heavy demands on the nutrients in the body. For example, the brain represents only 2% of the total body weight, and yet it consumes up to 20% of the oxygen and 65% of the glucose available in the circulation in the entire body.[10] The minimum cardiovascular output required to deliver this is ¾ of a liter per minute, and that is equal to 20% of the total circulation. In light of the high level of nutrient utilization by the brain, it is therefore one of the organs of the body most likely to be affected by infarcts, rapid rises in intracranial pressure, or acute anoxia. The stability of brain physiology is more vulnerable in the elderly because of the normal age-related changes already discussed.

Arndt-Schultz Principle

The physiology of aging causes a change in the body and therefore the brain's ability to respond to stimuli. The Arndt-Schultz Principle summarizes the changes between the younger person and the aged as follows[49]:

1. The elderly require a higher level or a longer period of stimulation before the threshold for initial physiological response is reached.
2. The physiological response in the aged is rarely as big, as visible, or as consistent as is noted in the younger age groups.
3. The only similarity between the response of the young and the elderly to stimuli is that once the threshold is reached, the more stimuli that are provided, the greater is the response.
4. In the aged, on the average, the range of safe therapeutic stimulation is smaller than for the young.

The implication of the Arndt-Schultz Principle for clinical problem solving suggests that the level of stimuli (e.g., heat, cold, sound, light, or emotional stress) needs to be adjusted appropriately to compensate for the altered physiology of the aging client. It is possible that a level of stimulus that is therapeutic for the young may not be so for the older client because it does not reach the threshold for generating a physiological response. It is important to note that when an elderly client does not respond to treatment or presents with an unusual physical response, the question needs to be asked, Is the stimulus too small or too big? Is a modification in the level or timing of stimulation needed because of the unique physiology of aging?

Law of Initial Values

The Law of Initial Values is a physiological principle that states that, with a given intensity of stimulation, the degree of change produced tends to be greater when the initial value of that variable is low. In other words, the higher the initial level of functioning, the smaller is the change that can be produced.[69,70,73] The Law of Initial Values, when defined and applied to younger persons, presumes that homeostasis is at a stable and consistent level. When the law is used to describe the physiological responses in the aged, it cannot be presumed that homeostasis for any physiological variable is predictable or consistent from one person to the next within the 24-hour day. In the young it is possible to define the average times of peak activity for such things as sleeping and wakefulness, as well as intellectual capacity. It is necessary in the clinical assessment of the aged to define the peak times of the day for awareness and intellectual capacity for each individual. It is possible that some clients are best able to participate in learning a new skill in the early morning and some only in the late afternoon.

Biorhythms

The body can be said to have a biological clock because it operates precisely in nearly all physiological functions (e.g., menstruation and pregnancy). Before the evaluation of a geriatric client who presents with dementia or disturbance of intellectual functioning, it is helpful to examine the patient's premorbid biorhythm. Based on the Law of Initial Values, it is likely that each older person will have a unique 24-hour cycle for the various physiological functions, including intellectual activity. Do the policies and procedures of client assessment allow for individual biorhythms? In the care of the aged (alert or with dementia), it is essential to acknowledge (clearly documenting) and then support as much as possible the stability of the client's personal biorhythm. For example, if a woman has worked for 40 years as a night nurse, being primarily active from 11 PM to 7 AM, at what time is it likely that she will be alert and able to participate in a rehabilitation program? Is it possible to let the client choose the best time for treatment, or else, by monitoring the client's behavior, can the staff choose a time for treatment when the client is most alert? For the elderly, and particularly for those who have dementia, the time of assessment and treatment must be noted to maximize the client's potential.

Myths about cognitive changes in aging

In the past 15 years, one concept that has received wide attention is that of crystallized and fluid intelligence.[16] Crystallized intelligence involves the ability to perceive relations, to engage in formal reasoning, and to understand the intellectual and cultural heritage. Crystallized intelligence can be shaped by the environment and attitude of the individual. It is therefore possible that with self-directed learning and education, *there can be an increase in crystallized intelligence as long as a person is alive.* The measurement of crystallized intelligence is usually in the form of culture-specific items such as number facility, verbal comprehension, and general information.

Fluid intelligence is not closely associated with acculturation. It is generally considered to be independent of instruction or environment and depends more upon the genetic endowment of the individual.[56] To test fluid intelligence, the items used include memory span, inductive reasoning, and figural relations, all of which are presumed to be unresponsive to training. Fluid intelligence involves those intellectual functions that are most affected by neurophysiological status, and they are generally assumed to decline with age. *The myth does not hold true.* During middle age, scores for fluid intelligence have been found to be similar to scores in midadolescence.[45]

Botwinick described the classic aging pattern of intelligence.[11] In the adult portion of the life span, two distinct patterns exist: the verbal abilities decline very little, if at all, while the psychomotor abilities decline earlier and to a greater extent. On the Weschsler Adult Intelligence Scale (WAIS), the verbal subtests show virtual stability from age 20 to 60, whereas the motor performance subtests show decline from the late 20s on. The pattern holds for men and women with no variations for race, cultural, or economic standing, or whether they reside in institutions or in their own homes. After age 65 to 70, a decline is noted in both areas, but *it does not affect the person's functional abilities for self-directed behavior.* The variations in scores on the WAIS resulting from aging are of significance for researchers, but they do not or should not lead rehabilitation professionals to automatically view the aged as less viable candidates for rehabilitation. The decline in fluid intelligence with normal aging is offset by the growth in crystallized intelligence for most people. The outcome is that the elderly are as capable as the young to mentally participate in rehabilitation training *if they can control the pace.* The tasks that become most difficult for the aged are those that are fast-paced, unusual, and complex.[45]

The amount of normal decline or change in intellectual function in normal persons over the age of 70 is unclear. The research typically shows a sharp decline, but this may be caused by what has been labeled "terminal drop." This phenomenon, first described by Riegel and Riegel, involves a decline in IQ scores of individuals a few months to a few years before their deaths. The change in intellectual function is thought to result from some predeath changes in brain physiology. It is likely that research studies that show drastic decreases in intellectual function with advanced age have a large percentage of clients who were near death as a part of their sample.[11] If the scores of the clients who are near death are deleted, the research findings have in preliminary studies shown only minor cognitive changes with advancing aging.

Stress and intellectual capacity

Selye[62] defines stress as the nonspecific response of the body to any demand made upon it. All human beings require a certain amount of stress to live and function effectively. When a stressor (stimulus) is applied, the body predictably goes through the three stages of response called the general adaptation syndrome (GAS). The first response is a general alarm reaction, a "fight or flight" response that mobilizes all senses in an effort to make a judgment about the response that is needed. The next stage involves the judgment and selective adaption to the stressor. A decision is made as to which body action is needed, and all other body activities return to homeostasis. If the stimulus continues and goes beyond the therapeutic level, then the body system or part will gradually experience physiological exhaustion. A person in physiological exhaustion is likely to manifest abnormal responses to any new stimulus. The "paradoxical reactions" can result in unusual physiological and/or psychological responses to stimuli (e.g., an erythematous response when an ice pack is applied).

In the process of advanced aging, the body undergoes a series of physiological changes (mentioned previously) that make the older individual less physiologically efficient at responding to stressors (stimuli—physical or psychological). In the elderly the general alarm reaction is poorly mobilized and takes longer to come into effect (Arndt-Schultz Principle). The stage of resistance should yield a series of responses that mean that the body can economize its response to stress. In persons of all ages who are receiving too many different stimuli and for the elderly experiencing normal levels of stimuli, the body becomes less efficient in turning off the general alarm response and replacing it with a more appropriate and limited response. It is possible that stress reactions can elicit global cognitive impairment, including short-term memory loss. Have you ever misplaced your gloves, keys, or purse, or forgotten where you parked the car? (refer to Chapter 4).

The total assessment of an elderly person (oriented or with dementia) needs to include a determination of his or her stress quotient. A person who has experienced a large number of stimuli over a short period of time is likely to manifest many of the symptoms of acute dementia (e.g., inattention to details or loss of short-term memory). The research has quantified various life events and made it possible to predict which clients are at greatest risk of physiological and emotional exhaustion. The elderly, with their numerous chronic problems plus the acute disease under treatment, are likely candidates for experiencing physiological and emotional exhaustion.

The environment and process of rehabilitation care need to be modified to counteract the effect of stress on the intellectual capacity of the older client. It is helpful, as a part of assessment of the elderly (oriented or confused), to calculate the stress quotient. The stress quotient provides a framework within which all other client data can be viewed. If deterioration in intellectual function can be stopped or actually improved through modification of stressors (physical or psychological), it is an efficient and cost-effective part of the total rehabilitation effort.

INTELLECTUAL DECLINE—CHECKING TO IDENTIFY COMMON DISTORTIONS IN BASIC INFORMATION PROCESSING

Each person acts on the data available at the specific moment. When a person is presented with a stimulus, all data (physiological, psychological, sociological, and environmental) are collected, then integrated. Based on the results, a response is decided upon and then acted out. This stimulus-response cycle has four major steps, and at each step there is a possibility for distortion and/or error. In the process of patient assessment, it is necessary to examine at the outset the amount of verbal and written stimuli processed by the client in relation to the amount used as a part of the testing process. With an overview of the client's cognitive capacity, it is possible for the rehabilitation staff to modify the process of evaluation to maximize the client's performance. A basic map of the client's fluid and crystallized intelligence at that moment (time of assessment is documented to allow comparison of cognitive capacity at other times in the 24-hour cycle) provides the clinician with a specific description of what parts of intellectual function appear to be missing and pinpoints those parts of intellectual functioning that are still intact. Based on this approach, it is possible to proceed with the traditional rehabilitation evaluation *in a language that the client is able to understand.*

The Mini-Mental State Examination

The development of the Mini-Mental State Examination (MMS) resulted from a study that noted that 80% of cognitive disorders (loss of one or more of the components of intellectual function) among the elderly were not detected by the general practitioner.[73] The elderly present the rehabilitation team with physiological, psychological, sociological, and environmental needs that are essentially different from those of the general adult population. The professionals on the rehabilitation team (physicians,[20,21] nurses,[15,39] physical therapists,[40,45] and social workers[57,71]) are likely to have had minimal training in gerontology and the special symptoms and needs of the very

old. The MMS provides a screening test for identifying unrecognized cognitive disorders in the elderly.[29] The examination takes only a few minutes to administer, is scored immediately, and can be administered by physicians, nurses, physical therapists, and other personnel on the rehabilitation team. The examination can be used to screen for cognitive dysfunctions, much as a measurement of blood pressure or blood sugar can be used to screen for significant medical disorders.

The MMS for cognitive disorders has been standardized for elderly persons living in the community. The scores on this test correlate significantly with the Wechsler Adult Intelligence Scale and the Wechsler Memory Test and have been shown to be affected by the occurrence of a cerebral lesion as detected by a computed axial tomography (CT) scan.[25,32,64]

The Mini-Mental State Examination (Fig. 23-1) assesses only cognition and does not review other aspects of the traditional mental examination such as mood, delusions, or hallucinations. A score below 24 indicates cognitive dysfunction that is unusual in a normal elderly person. The entire examination grades cognitive performance on a scale from 0 to 30 and takes 10 to 15 minutes to administer. This examination can be used as a springboard for planning how to carry out the traditional rehabilitation evaluation on a client who has some intellectual dysfunction.

A low score on the MMS *does not* (1) signify that the client has a particular brain disease, (2) mean that the cognitive status has been irreversibly impaired, or (3) give any indication of previous mental status before the time of examination. A low score on the MMS indicates the areas of specific cognitive impairment and gives the rehabilitation team data about how to best *communicate* with the client. The MMS can identify if the client is oriented, remembers (short-term), and can read, write, calculate, and see the relationship of one object or figure to another.

A low score on this examination can mean that the client is possibly suffering from the following.[31]

1. A dementia syndrome, a global deterioration of cognitive capacity occurring in clear consciousness
2. Delirium, an alteration in the level of consciousness and the cognitive capacity
3. Mental retardation
4. An amnestic syndrome or Korsakoff's psychosis, which is a deterioration of recent memory out of proportion to other cognitive functions such as language and calculating ability
5. An aphasic disorder, which impairs the client's capacity to understand the questions

"The two common disorders detected by the Mini-Mental State and seen in general practice are dementia and delirium."[32] The data collected by the MMS about the cli-

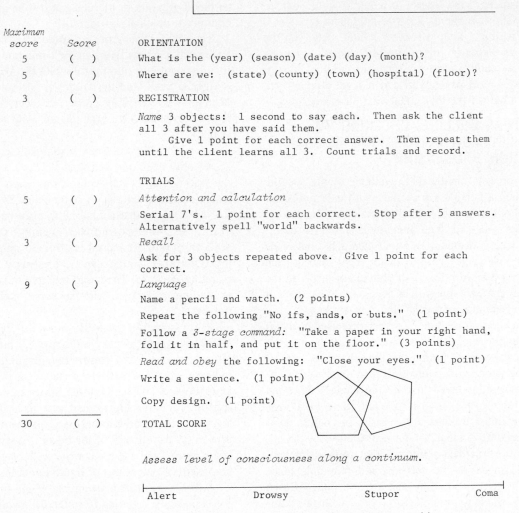

MINI-MENTAL STATE EXAMINATION

Maximum score	*Score*	
5	( )	ORIENTATION
		What is the (year) (season) (date) (day) (month)?
5	( )	Where are we: (state) (county) (town) (hospital) (floor)?
3	( )	REGISTRATION

Name 3 objects: 1 second to say each. Then ask the client all 3 after you have said them.

Give 1 point for each correct answer. Then repeat them until the client learns all 3. Count trials and record.

TRIALS

5	( )	*Attention and calculation*

Serial 7's. 1 point for each correct. Stop after 5 answers. Alternatively spell "world" backwards.

3	( )	*Recall*

Ask for 3 objects repeated above. Give 1 point for each correct.

9	( )	*Language*

Name a pencil and watch. (2 points)

Repeat the following "No ifs, ands, or buts." (1 point)

Follow a *3-stage command:* "Take a paper in your right hand, fold it in half, and put it on the floor." (3 points)

Read and obey the following: "Close your eyes." (1 point)

Write a sentence. (1 point)

Copy design. (1 point)

30	( )	TOTAL SCORE

Assess level of consciousness along a continuum.

Alert	Drowsy	Stupor	Coma

Fig. 23-1. Form used for Mini-Mental State Examination to assess cognition.

ent *allow the clinician to modify rehabilitation evaluation procedures to compensate for any dysfunctions in cognitive capacity.*

Sensory changes with aging

Aging can be defined in terms of adaptation. Aging is the progressive and usually irreversible diminution, with the passage of time, of the ability of an organism or one of its parts to perform efficiently or to adapt to changes in its environment. The consequence of the process is manifested as decreased capacity for function and for withstanding stresses.[30] The rehabilitation evaluation identifies functional problems, and it is necessary to examine the

possibility of contributing sensory losses or disturbances (e.g., vision, hearing, touch, taste, smell, proprioception, and kinesthesia). A partial or total loss of one or more of the normative sensory inputs can result in a disturbance of mental state.

It is accepted that the more sudden the loss of a sensory function, the more difficult is the adaptation to the disability. This is true of any age group but especially of the elderly. Normally adaptation to a sensory loss in one function is accomplished through cross-over to the use of other senses. For example, a young blind client can adapt by using hearing and kinesthesia and usually learns to function well in spite of the loss of visual input. The older the client is when blinded, the more difficulty he or she will have in making adaptive cross-over to other senses. There does come a time in life (different for each individual) when adaptive cross-over from one sense to another is exceedingly difficult, if not impossible, and then behavioral changes occur as a result of the inability to adapt in the new situation. If the disruption of neurosensory input occurs in several channels (e.g., vision, hearing, and touch) and occurs abruptly, there will usually be some temporary and/or permanent abnormal cognitive reaction.

The polio epidemics of the early 1950s demonstrated the interrelationship between sensory input and abnormal behavior. It was observed at that time that clients with anoxic change resulting from poliomyelitis who were placed in tank-type respirators developed intermittent disruptions in mental state. The client's hallucinations or type of delusion have a kind of continuum about them. For example, Dr. Foley describes the case of a 43-year-old woman in a respirator who was unable to move her arms or her legs. She was able to talk and move her eyes and was generally alert. Intermittently, she would vocalize reactions to a hallucination, and later (when alert) she was able to describe the experience in an organized way. In the hallucination she believed herself to be lying in the trunk of a car with her head sticking out the back and the trunk of the car closed down over her chest. She experienced that she was riding around looking for a hospital that would admit her. The dreamlike experience lasted for 1 to 3 hours and was extremely distressing for the client.[30] The analysis of the sensory input received by the client at the time can explain the behavioral response. The woman was in a respirator and was unable to move her arms or legs and unable to touch or move her own body. Because of her muscle weakness, she was denied a sense of bodily contact with herself, and this resulted in a loss of kinesthesia. Vision was restricted because of the shape of the tank-type respirator. The remaining visual field (a large part of it being ceiling) was generally unstimulating. The noise of the respirator and its rhythmical, repetitive movements essentially blanked out all auditory stimulation. By the use of the tank-type respirator, clients were abruptly cut off from a large portion of relevant sensory stimuli. The resulting behavioral change was a predictable response.

An examination of the common sensory changes associated with normal aging,[29,48] the diseases that affect the nervous system and the senses, and the treatment approaches used in the care of the elderly shows clients with exactly the same degree of loss or distortion of significant sensory input. For example, in the past, when a client had cataract surgery, both eyes were covered. It was not uncommon to find that the elderly client would become very agitated and disoriented as a result of this acute blindness. It is significant that a relatively small amount of vision would result in normalization of cognitive function. Another example of a *single* loss of sensory input is the af-

fliction of deafness. The acutely deafened and sometimes the chronically deafened elderly have grave difficulty in relating to the world. It is common for elderly persons who become deaf to experience some episodes of paranoid behavior.

For the average elderly client, there are usually neurosensory changes resulting from normal aging in *more* than one of the senses, and the client usually has several chronic diseases in addition to the acute problem under treatment. The use of medication can also distort kinesthesia and/or retard the activity and movement of the patient. Movement is significant in the maintenance of an efficient nervous system. Anything that denies a person continuing physical movement (e.g., drugs, restraints, or architectural design not adapted to the aged) hastens and extends the difficulty of adapting to advanced age.

It seems clear that movement is necessary for any kind of sensation.[9,27] The psychophysicists have known for a long time that if movement of the eyes does not occur in a proper way, vision becomes ineffective. The same is true to a lesser degree of hearing. If movement does not occur in the course of the hearing process, hearing can become distorted and misrepresented at the central level.

When a client has a distortion in cognitive capacity, a review of neurosensory stimuli (visual, auditory, kinesthetic, gustatory, and olfactory) must be done, as well as a measurement of the capacity to perform these neurological tasks (e.g., visual examination by an ophthalmologist). The normative changes with aging in the neurosensory system have been described at length.[9,29,48] *The challenge in rehabilitation is to design a process and environment of care so that there is compensation/modification that maximizes the ability of the elderly client to adapt to the situation.*

One out of every two blind persons in the United States is over 65.[75] It is possible with environmental adaptation and special measures to organize care to help elderly blind to live independently in the community.[38] The elderly, with their multiple changes in neurosensory input, can benefit from modifications in care, and in some cases this can actually prevent unnecessary disturbance in cognitive status or reverse cognitive distortions already present.

If vision is selected as an example of normative changes in neurosensory input with aging, it is possible to list major structural changes that result in mild to moderate distortion: the lens of the eye yellows and thickens, muscles controlling the eye become weaker, the lens grows unevenly and becomes striated, color perception is altered, and there is slower adaptation to light. With the many types of changes in vision, work has been done to identify the modifications in the environment and process of care necessary to allow the client to function up to his or her maximum potential. For example, the environment would require good lighting; dark, clear print for written instructions in at least the size of large type (example S); low-vision aids (e.g., magnifying glass); verbal orientation by persons accompanying clients in a new environment; consistent furniture placement; explanation when changes occur; clear hallways; an escort when the client is in a new environment (e.g., radiology department); and a systematic storage system for clothes and toilet articles (as the client would naturally have at home).[17,36,37] With modifications in the process and environment of rehabilitation for all major sensory changes associated with normal aging, it is possible for normal and disabled elderly to adapt to changes in their health and functional status.

Older adult learning styles and communication

Learning occurs throughout life. In rehabilitation the client learns new skills of adaptation. The learning process does not change abruptly when an individual reaches old age, but differences in performance have been reported. In light of the many stresses that accompany normal aging, how is it possible to improve the learning efficiency of the older person?

Botwinick[11] notes that learning and performance are not the same. In other words, poor performance on a learning task may mean that insufficient learning has occurred or that the performance does not accurately reflect the extent of learning achieved.[56] If an older client comes for physical therapy and appears unable to follow verbal instructions, it is important to determine how treatment can be modified to facilitate participation by the client.

There are key variables that affect a person's ability to participate in a learning situation: intelligence, skills acquired over the years, and flexibility of learning style. There are also noncognitive factors that can have a strong bearing on an individual's performance. The noncognitive factors include visual and auditory acuity, health status, motivation to learn, level of anxiety, the speed at which stimuli and learning are paced, and the meaningfulness of the items or tasks to be learned.

It is essential that before discontinuing a client from a rehabilitation program because of cognitive and emotional dysfunction a review be made of the common alterations in learning styles seen among the elderly.

Interference. Two major ways exist in which interference can make the learning process less efficient.[23] First, interference can result from a conflict of present knowledge with the new knowledge to be learned. Second, if two learning tasks are undertaken at the same time, they can interfere with each other. Studies show that the elderly have special difficulties if they must concentrate on intake, attention, and retrieval processes at the same time.[23] The implication is that the process and environment of rehabilitation for the elderly and/or confused client must not be cluttered with such things as background noise, other stimuli in the environment, or personal anxiety. When learning a new task, the elderly or confused may require a quiet room with no other stimuli than those offered by the therapist.

Pacing. The pacing of therapeutic intervention is a significant variable in helping an elderly person learn. The elderly (alert or disoriented) perform best if they are given as much time as they need, in other words, when the learning is *self-paced*.[11] The major drawback of fast pacing is that *the elderly would rather choose not to participate than to risk making a mistake*. If extra time is given, it reduces the amount of nonresponse, which is often interpreted as apathy, poor motivation, or confusion.[4] Following individual assessment, the use of group work where concepts can be presented, reviewed, and examined at leisure can reduce the psychological pressure of fast-paced learning. The details of therapy must be carefully planned, including how questions are posed, framing of clear and precise questions in nonmedical language, and, most important, time to respond at a leisurely pace.

Organization. In the learning process, if data are organized in the brain, the retrieval of desired data becomes easier. It is known that older persons are less likely than members of other age groups to spontaneously organize to facilitate learning and later retrieval (memory) of that learning.[5] The elderly who are highly verbal show fewer weaknesses in the ability to organize stimuli. The elderly with poor verbal skills show significant improvement when strategies for organization of data are provided from others (i.e., therapist). Arenberg and Tchabo[5] note that older learners have difficulty in following content because they cannot anticipate what will be taught and do not see the whole that is being presented. It is helpful to organize therapy by beginning with an overview of the entire lesson to be learned in outline form and thereby presenting a conceptual map of the upcoming experience. The use of purposeful organizing can also help to bridge the gap between what the older person knows and the new information or task to be learned. The use of Neurolinguistic Programming (NLP) is especially effective with elderly or confused clients because it builds consciously through language, kinesthesia, and visual input a picture of a new concept from the known and familiar frame of reference.[7]

The implication for older adult learning is that if material is presented in one way and the older person is expected to apply it some other way, this makes for inefficient learning and at times inability to learn. The instruction needs to be provided in the format in which it is to be used—if possible, one piece of new data at a time. A conscious transition needs to be made by the therapist from the client's current frame of reference to the understanding of the new data, and the pace should be set by the client.

There are numerous other strategies for maximizing the efficiency of older adult learners based on awareness of normal age-related changes:

1. Use of mediators—association of word, story, or visual input to help the person to remember.[16]
2. The tasks to be learned need to be meaningful for the client.[14]

3. The more concrete the details of learning can be, the easier it is.[11]

4. Provide a supportive learning environment to prevent the overarousal (as noted by galvanic skin response) that is common among the elderly and that can interfere with efficient learning.[26]

5. Older learners respond better to supportive or neutral feedback and perform worse if feedback is presented in a challenging tone.[61]

6. A rewarding of all responses (although rewarding correct responses more than incorrect responses) can encourage elderly persons to decrease the number of errors by omission, which are often interpreted as apathy or lack of cooperation.[47]

7. A combination of auditory and visual input tends to facilitate the learning process.[4] This is only true if the data presented are similar because variation between the two kinds of messages can result in interference and a decrease in the efficiency of learning.

8. Active learning is known to be more effective. A client who moves the body part to be involved while getting verbal and visual input is likely to be more efficient in mastering the new concept.[56]

9. Design the learning situation so that successful completion of the task is likely.[6] Older people are more likely to focus on errors, which increases anxiety and lowers the self-concept. Worst of all, with all the energy focused on the error, there is a strong chance of repeating the error.

In conclusion, the research presented describes many of the details of the Feldenkrais approach to learning. The Feldenkrais Method has been applied to the needs of the elderly with good results.[28] The foundation principle that learning needs to be pleasurable is especially applicable to disoriented or elderly clients because they are not likely to be as motivated as the young. Despite changes in learning style, the older person (alert or disoriented) can be helped to learn more efficiently through well-planned instruction. The use of techniques to increase learning efficiency for the elderly can decrease the stress that at times may result in emotional or cognitive overload and abnormal cognitive reactions.

Environmental considerations

Hypothermia. The temperature of the living environment must be carefully controlled because aged clients may not perceive that they are chilled and may not experience shivering. For example, an older man comes as an outpatient for physical therapy services and it is winter. The client initially appears confused and drowsy, but after some time indoors, he appears to be alert and able to participate. Accidental hypothermia can happen to an older person at even mildly cold temperatures of 60° F (15.5° C) to 65° F (18.3° C). Accidental hypothermia is a drop in the core body temperature to below 95° F. The following group of clients is especially at risk:

1. Persons over the age of 65
2. Persons showing no signs of shivering or showing pale skin in response to cold
3. Persons taking medications containing phenothiazine (to treat anxiety, depression, nervousness, or nausea)
4. Persons with disorders of the hormone system, especially hypothyroidism
5. Persons with head injuries, strokes, and similar neurological conditions
6. Persons with severe arthritis and Parkinson's disease
7. Persons with atherosclerosis
8. Persons with peripheral vascular disease, chronic ulceration, or amputation

The symptoms can be any one of the following: bloated face, pale and waxy or pinkish skin color, trembling on one side of the body but no shivering, irregular and slowed heartbeat, slurred speech, shallow and very slow breathing, low blood pressure, and drowsiness and confusion. The two principles of treatment are (1) the person will stay chilled unless rewarmed slowly and (2) whatever the apparent severity of the condition, the client should be evaluated by a physician.[76]

If a person is determined to be at risk, specific preventive measures can be taken to prevent unnecessary distortions in cognitive status resulting from accidental hypothermia. First, the room temperature should be set at least to 70° F (21° C). Second, the person should wear adequate clothing: this may include long underwear and undershirt. In addition, good nutrition is a key for these clients' welfare.

It is not unlikely that clients and their families may attempt to save money by lowering their room temperatures and thus inadvertently cause accidental hypothermia. It is also common to find institutions with central air conditioning. This requires special accommodations for the elderly, such as special wings or individual temperature controls in the rooms. The goal is to avoid accidental hypothermia and the potential distortion in cognitive function that can result.[76,77]

Transplantation shock. It is known that some elderly function well in a familiar environment only to become completely disoriented and unable to perform their basic activities of daily living if taken out of their own homes. Based on the previous discussions about adaptation and sensory stimuli, the explanation is the inability of the brain to make sense out of a large volume of stimuli. If a client was alert before admission to an institution and then becomes confused, only by placing the client back in a familiar environment with supervision for 3 to 7 days will it is possible to determine if the distortion in cognitive function is related to the withdrawal from the stable, known environment. All moves by a client from one hospital room to another or from one institution to another must be carefully planned. If a move is anticipated, the client should be involved in the decision making and, if possible, have a chance for a trial visit or two before the actual move. The client should also be informed well in advance. The precautions mentioned can help the client who is at risk of becoming confused because of transplantation shock to make a move and remain able to function maximally.

Emotional capacity to participate in a learning task

Many elderly persons who come for physical therapy are in emotional overload as evidenced by mild confusion, a withdrawn and apparently uncooperative attitude, or overt confusion. A person who is at or near the point of emotional overload needs to be evaluated as to his or her ability to participate in learning tasks that require active input. If the client is found to be in an emotional overload, other forms of therapeutic intervention can be found that allow the client to be a passive recipient. These types of therapeutic intervention, including massage, connective tissue massage, heat, and Feldenkrais Functional Integration, can hopefully promote a relaxation response, lowering the anxiety level and thereby preparing the client to participate in more physically active types of therapeutic exercise. If they are asked directly, most clients will state openly whether they feel able to actively participate. If for any reason the client is not able or willing to state his or her feelings, it is still possible to evaluate the client's ability to participate.

If it is possible to get a client's cooperation, the following movements can be attempted and then evaluated. (These should be used only if no active diseases involving the eyes are present and there is no pain involved in doing the movements.)

1. Close your eyes.
2. Close your eyes and keep them closed for 30 seconds; for 1 minute.
3. Close eyes; move eyes to the right and left slowly (slow movements with control is the goal).
4. Close eyes; move eyes in diagonals, right and up, then left and down; then left and up, right and down.

If a client is unable to perform the movement, feels it requires much effort, or feels it is uncomfortable, this indicates a level of tension that is in excess of what is appropriate for learning. For a client with severe tension, it is necessary to use passive therapeutic procedures. If a person can *comfortably* execute the movements, it indicates that the CNS and the body are able to receive and integrate data and act with ease. It is only possible for the individual to learn when in this state, if the learning requires active participation on the part of the client.

Distortions in intellectual and emotional capacity to receive input, integrate input, and then act on the input affect a person's ability to participate in a learning task. The previous section has pinpointed the most common sources of distortion in information processing that are external to the client and therefore under the direct control of the rehabilitation team. *It is possible for the rehabilitation team to make the choice to acknowledge the common age-related changes and common sources of stress response in the elderly and then to design a process and environment of care that maximizes the elderly client's potential.*

DELIRIUM/ACUTE DEMENTIA: EVALUATION AND TREATMENT

Prevention is the primary focus in the care of the elderly and in preventing unnecessary stress and cognitive dysfunction. The *external* environment and process of care must be carefully designed if they are not to present barriers to the client's ability to function. The following discussion focuses on the client's *internal* environment (physiological/psychological and pathological causes) and presumes that all unnecessary external environmental stressors have been removed. The acute brain syndrome (also called reversible brain syndrome) comes on suddenly over a period of hours, days, or weeks and causes the client to be less alert than normal, confused, disoriented, forgetful (especially of recent events), labile in mood, and/or to have poor judgment.

The establishment of a diagnosis is the key to effective care. The first step is to examine the development of the abnormal cognitive state. Were there precipitating factors—emotional and/or physical? What were the vital signs, intake and output, bowel function, and report of falls during the time that the abnormal cognitive response began? Has there been long-standing use of medications and/or an alteration in medications used?

Medications are prime offenders as causative agents of acute delirium or dementia. The range of medications the patient is taking should be scrutinized. If it is not 100% certain that medications are *not* a possible contributing cause of the acute confusion, a medication holiday should be attempted. A medication holiday involves the withdrawal of all but life-giving medications for a minimum of a 24-hour period to note the physical and cognitive response.

Many elderly are taking medications that have confusion as an unwanted side effect (digitalis, antiparkinsonian drugs [L-dopa; trihexyphenidyl], tricyclic antidepressants, hypotensive agents [especially when combined with thiazide diuretics]). It is also possible for many medications to cause confusion if the person experiences an allergic response to the drug. For these reasons a medication holiday of longer than 24 hours may be needed in some cases before a change can be noted.[50]

In self-administration of medications as well as when they are administered by professionals in an institutional setting, an error rate exists that can be as high as 50%.[50] The interaction between multiple medications is another concern as well as the interaction between food and medication. The interactions can distort the pharmacological effect of the medication. For example:

1. Demeclocycline may react with milk and food high in iron or vitamins fortified with iron.
2. Digoxin (Lanoxin, Vanoxin) may react with prune juice, bran cereals, and other foods high in fiber.
3. Erythromycin (E-Mycin, Ilotycin, Robimycin) may react with acidic fruit juices, syrups, and soft drinks.
4. Acetaminophen (Datril, Nebs, Tempra, Tylenol, Valadol) may react with crackers, dates, jelly, or other carbohydrates and may markedly increase the time it takes for the drug to act as an analgesic.

The examples listed were chosen because crackers, fruit juice, bran cereals, and soft drinks are a common part of most elderly persons' diets.

In evaluating the disoriented client, an examination is also needed of the pharmacokinetics of the medications taken by the client. The rehabilitation team caring for the elderly needs the input of a clinically oriented pharmacist who can help the team focus on such concepts as biological half-life, clearance, bioavailability of drugs, and time course of drug concentration in plasma as a function of dose and frequency.[35] There are normative changes in kidney and liver function with advanced aging, and these affect the distribution and elimination of medication in the body. The dose and/or frequency of administration of medication can be contributing factors to a confusional state. Each member of the rehabilitation team needs to document the client's ability to participate in learning tasks and the time the assessment was done because timing of medication administration can affect performance. The monitoring of the impact of pharmaceutical intervention on the client involves all disciplines.

Fecal impaction is another common cause of acute dementia in the elderly. A fecal impaction may be revealed by a simple rectal examination. Other common causes of delirium/acute dementia include distended bladder caused by prostatic enlargement, with or without urinary tract infection, and dehydration (common age-related change in the thirst reflex). It is estimated that about one half of the causes of acute dementia in the elderly result from extracerebral causes. The most common of these are cardiac problems (alteration in blood pressure because of medication, onset of arrhythmia, myocardial infarction, or congestive heart failure); metabolic disturbances (delirium tremens, diabetes mellitus, myxedema, hyperthyroidism, renal failure/uremia), hematological problems (anemia—iron deficiency or macrocytic anemias); and pneumonia. Brocklehurst[13] describes a toxic confusional state that may be unrelated to the extent of the pneumonia and may occur in acute bronchitis or bronchiolitis without radiological evidence of parenchymal involvement. The syndrome manifests itself in clients with or without a previous history of intellectual dysfunction and usually disappears with treatment of the infection. It is noted that some permanent residual disability is not unusual.

The key to care of the client with dementia is definition of an accurate diagnosis, and this involves a team assessment based on an awareness of normative aging responses to pathological conditions. For example, Rodstein notes that it is common that myocardial infarction in the elderly can appear painlessly with the only symptom being dementia.[18] Diabetes is common among the elderly and it is estimated that 9% have undiagnosed diabetes.[19] A vitamin B_{12} deficiency can also manifest as confusion.

About one third of all cases of acute dementia are related primarily to cerebral causes. Cerebrovascular accident (stroke caused by embolism or thrombosis) is the most common cause of acute confusion related to the CNS. In the elderly it is not uncommon to have confusion as the only symptom of a cerebrovascular accident or have it as one of the several symptoms (paralysis, dysarthria, or aphasia). The confusion following a cerebrovascular accident is usually temporary and requires that the rehabilitation team evaluate the client's remaining cognitive capacity and build a program of care around those abilities. A program of therapeutic intervention, which allows the client to be a passive recipient for 1 to 3 months, can yield good therapeutic results and also prevent unnecessary secondary deconditioning until part or all of the client's cognitive capacity returns.[59]

Acute dementia is common in the elderly as a response to anesthesia. Orientation to time, environment, and people in the near proximity is generally needed. A loss of awareness of how long the confusion has existed can be distressing as the recovery of cognitive function begins, and having concrete input can be helpful. For example, after surgery an elderly man is sure he has been confused for 5 years. He can be helped to grasp that it has only been 5 weeks by having a visit from a grandchild, niece, or neighbor who is still growing. This would show that only 5 weeks had passed because the growth of the child would be obvious if it had indeed been 5 years.

Many causes of acute delirium/dementia are treatable, and if diagnosis and care are provided in a timely fashion (within 3 months), it is likely that the client can regain full command of his or her cognitive processes. Three months is mentioned as the cut-off point because it has been noted that an institutional stay beyond that time is likely to result in learned dependency, which makes return to independent living difficult.[63]

Depression is the most common cause of pseudodementia in the elderly.[63] It has been noted by some reports that as many as 31% of those thought to have dementia have depression instead.[60] Depression can result in cognitive changes affecting immediate recall, attention, and ability to perform basic activities of daily living. Depression is a treatable problem and diagnosis is the key. The decrease in activity level and movement associated with depression can result in many secondary complications. Treatment of depression generally involves pharmacotherapy, psychotherapy, and environmental manipulation, which can require support from the entire rehabilitation team. Again, in treatment of the client with depression, therapeutic techniques that promote a relaxation response and a decrease in anxiety level (massage, heat, or Feldenkrais Functional Integration) can help bring the client to the point where it is possible to involve in aerobic training, which is known to have a beneficial effect. All aerobic training for the elderly should begin with a stress test, modified as necessary to determine the client's safe exercise target heart rate. The modifications most frequently required are that the upper extremities are used to achieve the training effect because the lower-extremity function may be limited and major activities of daily living do involve the upper extremities.

The treatment of the elderly who are experiencing acute dementia consists of treating the underlying cause or causes if possible. A close working relationship is needed between physicians as well as between the other members of the rehabilitation team. During the time when a diagnosis has not been defined, the client should receive the same emotional and physical support as a client with chronic dementia or Alzheimer's disease. The place to begin is to ascertain the extent and types of cognitive loss that are present. The client must feel secure and live in an environment that has as few changes as possible and a consistent and stable time schedule for activities.

COURSE OF ILLNESSES IN NON-ACUTE DEMENTIA

The course of a dementing illness will be unique to each individual and will vary based on the contributing cause(s). The basic generalizations that can be made include:[65]

1. Onset is usually noticed by the person with the disorder, family members, friends, or colleagues at work (rather than by a physician).
2. Signs exist of impairment of mental ability (usually memory loss, poor judgment, or incompetence at work). The patient can often succeed at hiding his or her symptoms for a period of time.
3. A physician will usually be consulted at some point and currently, with a thorough history and physical, an estimated 80% accuracy in diagnosis is achieved. It can be noted that using a battery of psychological and laboratory tests and by radiographic examination, the accuracy of diagnosis can be near 90%.[42]
4. Once the diagnostic process is complete, treatment can be started. Medications can assist removing underlying causes, but if it is determined to be a progressively deteriorating disorder, medication may only be able to slow down the process. The focus of the medical management for the progressive disorders is family education—training caregivers to adapt to the patient, simplifying the individual's living space, and referring relatives to family support services.[68,74]
5. Diagnosis and treatment of acute other illnesses can continue for several years. Many dementing conditions can last up to a decade. A recent study found that the average duration of illness from first onset of symptoms to death was 8.1 years for Alzheimer's disease and 6.7 years for multi-infarct dementia.[8] The duration of dementing illnesses can be unpredictable and, in some unusual cases, can last up to 25 years.

Alzheimer's disease as well as other dementing illnesses can be clinically described with the use of staging instruments. The use of staging instruments to describe the discrete and reliable stages of the disease has several advantages:

1. They enable the family to plan ahead for the individual's needs
2. They help the family prepare themselves for the process of interacting with the patient
3. They make it possible to plan for the appropriate levels of services as an individual's abilities decline (see Table 23-1 for a sample of a staging tool)

The evaluation of the client will involve a description of the behavior as well as an assessment of the client's mental state. The client with dementia can manifest a variety of psychiatric symptoms, including mood disturbance, delusion, hallucination, catastrophic reactions, perseveration, and impersistence.[52] The pattern of onset and the types of psychiatric symptoms are often directly related to the underlying pathological condition. Clients with a slowly progressing course are likely to be suffering from a degenerative problem affecting the CNS, such as Alzheimer's disease or a tumor. Clients who have a step-wise loss of function and periods of slight improvement are apt to be suffering from cerebral vascular dysfunction. The most common causes of dementia are as shown in the box below. In 1907 Alzheimer[32] described a 54-year-old woman who developed morbid jealousy, which was followed by loss of memory, inability to read and understand, and death 4½ years after onset of the illness. It has been noted that 50% of client evaluations for dementia show that the clients are suffering from Alzheimer's disease.[2] In making the diagnosis of Alzheimer's, all other diseases have been ruled out. The disease can occur any time after the age of

Table 23-1. Clinical dementia rating (CDR) scale

	Healthy CDR 0	Questionable dementia CDR 0.5	Mild dementia CDR 1	Moderate dementia CDR 2	Severe dementia CDR 3
Memory	No memory loss or slight inconsistent forgetfulness	Mild consistent forgetfulness; partial recollection of events; "benign" forgetfulness	Moderate memory loss, more marked for recent events; defect interferes with everyday activities	Severe memory loss; only highly learned material retained; new material rapidly lost	Severe memory loss; only fragments remain
Orientation	Fully oriented		Some difficulty with time relationships; oriented for place and person at examination but may have geographic disorientation	Usually disoriented in time, often to place	Orientation to person only
Judgment and problem-solving	Solves everyday problems well; judgment good in relation to past performance	Only doubtful impairment in solving problems, similarities, differences	Moderate difficulty in handling complex problems; social judgment usually maintained.	Severely impaired in handling problems, similarities, differences; social judgment usually impaired	Unable to make judgments or solve problems
Community affairs	Independent function at usual level in job, shopping, business and financial affairs, volunteer and social groups	Only doubtful or mild impairment in these activities	Unable to function independently at these activities though may still be engaged in some; may still appear normal to casual inspection	No pretense of independent function outside home Appears well enough to be taken to functions outside a family home	Appears too ill to be taken to functions outside a family home
Home and hobbies	Life at home, hobbies, intellectual interests well maintained	Life at home, hobbies, intellectual interests slightly impaired	Mild but definite impairment of function at home; more difficult chores abandoned; more complicated hobbies and interests abandoned	Only simple chores preserved; very restricted interests, poorly sustained	No significant function in home outside of own room
Personal care	Fully capable of self-care		Needs prompting	Requires assistance in dressing, hygiene, keeping of personal effects	Requires much help with personal care; often incontinent

From Hughes CP, Berg L, Donziger WL, et al., New clinical scale for the staging of dementia. Br J Psych 140:556-572, 1982. In Losing a million minds: confronting the tragedy of Alzheimer's disease and dementias, US Congress, Office of Technology Assessment, OTA-BA-323, Washington, DC, April, 1987, US Government Printing Office.

50, but it increases in prevalence rate to 20% in confused clients over the age of 85.[44]

The symptoms of Alzheimer's disease progress in three stages. Stage 1 lasts from 2 to 4 years and involves a functional loss of orientation, memory loss, and lack of spontaneity. The client is generally aware of the losses and is in many cases able to cover up the cognitive losses by talking around the issues. This is the time when the client and family may need to deal with the issue of giving up a job, hobbies, and other types of meaningful activity because of the inability to carry them out independently. The person will begin to lose the ability to handle money and the personal budget, will not be able to drive a car safely, and will lose the ability to tell time. The family or meaningful others may have to come to terms with the question, Can the client live alone? In stage 2 there is progressive memory loss and a variety of other symptoms—aphasia, apraxia, tendency to wander off and lose the way home, repetitive movements (tapping, chewing), increased appetite, constant movement, peculiar wide gait, muscle twitches or jerks, spasms of the diaphragm, and then a decrease in the appetite. There are no remissions. In the final stage, stage 3, the client may become mute, stop eating, appear incontinent (forget where to go to the bathroom), develop seizures, and then die.

STRATEGIES FOR TREATMENT AND CARE OF THE CONFUSED CLIENT AT HOME

Acute delirium/dementia can become chronic dementia if the cause cannot be identified and treated. The change in cognitive function and behavior happens to a person who is a part of a circle of support—friends and family. To develop a reasonable approach to caregiving, the rehabilitation team needs to include the caregivers and client as much as possible. A majority of demented elderly people live with family or friends and not in institutions: What can the rehabilitation team offer the client and caregivers? *The goal of rehabilitation must be redefined to ensure that the client remains safe, independent, and able to perform activities of daily living (ADLs) and instrumental activities of daily living (IADLs) for as long as is reasonable.* The rehabilitation process can begin while the diagnostic work-up is still going on. This can take the form of basic training in the activities of daily living. It also includes caregiver training to care for the client and make needed environmental modifications to make safety for the confused person possible in as open an environment as possible. Once the diagnosis is established, the planning for long-term care at home or in an institution must be carefully made. No matter where the client will be living, the involvement of the caregivers and significant others is crucial. It is necessary to ascertain the emotional and physical resources of the client and family and/or significant others who will be the caretakers. A review of the caretakers' willingness to perform basic tasks or visitation, willingness to be taught needed skills, and the realistic need for respite must be determined[46] (Fig. 23-2). Family training and orientation manuals that deal with all the details of caring for a person with dementia are available.[51,54] The same detailed orientation is needed for institutional staff who are to care for elderly clients with dementia. It is possible, by the structure and process of care, to help the clients to be maximally active in their self-care and to prevent unnecessary anxiety and catastrophic reactions. In the early and middle stages of all dementias, including Alzheimer's disease, physical therapy intervention usually can prolong the ability to move with ease. This is an important concept as indicated by result of a survey completed by caregivers describing the impairments in patients' abilities to perform ADLs and IADLs. The survey described the caregivers' responses to persons with dementias in all

---

Disorders causing or simulating dementia

Disorders causing dementia

A. Degenerative diseases
  1. Alzheimer's disease
  2. Pick's disease
  3. Huntington's disease
  4. Parkinson's disease (not all cases)
  5. ALS (not all cases)
  6. Others
B. Vascular dementia
  1. Multi-infarct dementia
  2. Cortical micro infarcts
  3. Lacunar dementia
  4. Binswanger disease
  5. Others
C. Anoxic dementia
  1. Cardiac arrest
  2. Carbon monoxide poisoning
  3. Others
D. Traumatic dementia
  1. Dementia pugilistica (boxer's dementia)
  2. Head injuries
E. Infectious dementia
  1. AIDS dementia
  2. Creutzfeldt-Jakob's disease
  3. Herpes encephalitis
  4. Bacterial meningitis
  5. Brain abscess
  6. Others
F. Normal pressure
  1. Hydrocephalus
G. Space-occupying lesions
H. Multiple sclerosis (some cases)
I. Autoimmune disorders
J. Toxic dementia (e.g., alcohol, lead, mercury)
K. Other disorders
  1. Heat stroke
  2. Epilepsy (some cases)

Disorders simulating dementia

A. Psychological disorders
  1. Depression
  2. Anxiety
  3. Psychosis
  4. Sensory deprivation
B. Drugs
  1. Sedatives
  2. Hypnotics
  3. Antianxiety agents
  4. Antidepressants
  5. Antidysrhythmics
  6. Antihypertensives
  7. Anticonvulsants
  8. Antipsychotics
  9. Digitalis and derivatives
  10. Drugs with anticholinergic effects
  11. Others (mechanisms unknown)
C. Nutritional disorders
  1. Pellagra (B_6 deficiency)
  2. Thiamine deficiency (Wernicke-Korsakoff's syndrome)
  3. Pernicious anemia
  4. Others
D. Metabolic disorders (usually cause delirium, but can be difficult to differentiate from dementia)
  1. Hyper and hypothyroidism
  2. Hypercalcemia
  3. Hyper and hyponatremia
  4. Hypoglycemia
  5. Kidney failure
  6. Liver failure
  7. Cushing's syndrome
  8. Others

Data compiled from Katzman R, Lasker B, and Bernstein N: Accuracy of diagnosis and consequences of misdiagnosis of disorders causing dementia, Contract report for office of technology assessment, US Congress, 1986; Katzman R: Alzheimers's disease, N Engl J Med 314:964, 1986; and Katzman R: Clinical presentation of the course of Alzheimer's disease: the atypical patient. In Rose CF, editor, Modern approaches to the dementias, Basel, Switzerland, 1985, Kraeger.

Activities of daily living	Needed No Yes	If needed: Willing but needs training	Willing if there is respite	Not able (reason)	Cross-check to plan of care: recommendations

Mobility
  Transferring
  Walking (ambulation)
  Wheeling					

Personal care
  Bathing
  Dressing
  Grooming
  Bowel function
  Bladder function
  Eating/feeding					

Rehabilitation/ home program					

Support
  Housekeeping
  Living space
  Meal preparation
  Shopping
  Transportation
  Other					

Fig. 23-2. Family/significant other assessment form. Cross-check with activities of daily living, and include as part of plan of care.

phases of their illness (see Tables 23-2 to 23-4). A brief cognitive rating scale can also be used to assist the clinicians in obtaining important information regarding the client's mental status[78] (see box on p. 677).

From Tables 23-2 to 23-4 it is important to note that initially physical therapy intervention will potentially be involved with facilitating ease of motor planning (i.e.,

dressing or eating) and planning for compensation for IADL losses (cannot safely do housework or handle money). The ability to walk is lost late in dementia, and other studies report comparable levels of impairment.[22,34]

Physical therapy intervention to assist the client and train the caregiver involves facilitating for ease of movement and motor planning and developing or refining envi-

Table 23-2. Ability of dementia patient to do basic tasks

Task	Percent of total respondents			
	Very well	**Somewhat**	**Not at all**	**No answer**
Walk without assistance	35	26	35	5
Eat without assistance	30	32	34	5
Dress without assistance	14	28	52	5
Perform simple household tasks, such as setting the table or simple home repairs	6	19	69	5
Cope with small sums of money	5	15	73	6

NOTE: This table is percentaged horizontally. Also totals may not add because of rounding.

From Yankelovich, Skelly, and White, Inc: Caregivers of patients with dementia, contract report prepared for the Office of Technology Assessment, Washington, DC, 1986, US Congress.

Table 23-3. Assessment of dementia patient's eating skills

Eating skills	Percentage of total respondents
Eats cleanly, with proper utensils	36
Eats messily	23
Only eats simple solids, like crackers, by self	6
Has to be fed by others	28
Is tube fed	4
No answer	4

From Yankelovich, Skelly, and White, Inc: Caregivers of patients with dementia, contract report prepared for the Office of Technology Assessment, Washington, DC, 1986, US Congress.

Table 23-4. Assessment of dementia patient's toilet skills

Toilet skills	Percentage of total respondents
Independent/fully functional	23
Has occasional accidents/needs some help or reminder	25
Has frequent wet beds or accidents	12
Is doubly incontinent (has bowel and urine accidents)	36
No answer	4

From Yankelovich, Skelly, and White, Inc: Caregivers of patients with dementia, contract report prepared for the Office of Technology Assessment, Washington, DC, 1986, US Congress.

ronmental and cognitive cues to assist in carrying out complex tasks. Ultimately the caregiver will need training in how to move, lift, and otherwise assist the patient.

The cognitive impairment is the limiting factor. Accurate assessment helps the caregiver to provide only the help that is absolutely needed, with patients continuing to perform for themselves as many ADLs as possible; for example, to brush his or her teeth, a patient needs to be able to remember the command, to recognize the toothbrush, and to perform the motor action. The patient may only need the help of someone placing the toothbrush in his or her hand and slowly guiding it to the mouth to be able brush his or her teeth.

The accurate assessment of IADL and ADL has been found to be more reliable than medical diagnosis for predicting the amount of assistance and interaction a person will need in a nursing home. The first goal of rehabilitation for dementia patients is to create an environment (emotional and physical) that is supportive (works actively to compensate for the patients' specific cognitive losses as they gradually occur). The ultimate goal is to help patients to feel that they are capable, so that they will continue to try to do those things for themselves that they safely can do whether they remain in their home or live in an institution.

The Alzheimer's Disease and Related Disorders Association, Inc.* is a resource for professionals and caretakers of confused elderly who are unable to care for themselves. The goals of the association are to support research related to the diagnosis, therapies, causes, and cures for Alzheimer's disease, to aid in organizing family support groups, to educate and assist afflicted families, to sponsor educational programs for professionals and lay persons on the topic of Alzheimer's disease, to advise government agencies of the needs of the afflicted families and to promote federal support of research, and to offer help in any manner to clients and their caretakers to promote the well-being of all involved. Through the efforts of the association, it is hoped that humane care can be provided to the client with dementia throughout the course of the illness. Other models of support groups have been tried in individual communities where spouses have worked to develop ongoing respite care.[12]

The rehabilitation team needs to conduct an inventory of services as a part of their annual review of the quality of care that is provided for dementia patients. A survey of persons caring for patients with dementia listed the following services in their perceived order of importance:[65]

1. A paid companion who can come to the home a few hours each week to give caregivers a rest
2. Assistance in locating people or organizations that provide patient care
3. Assistance in applying for government programs, such as Medicaid, disability insurance, and income support programs
4. A paid companion who can come to the home for overnight care so caregivers can go away for one or more days
5. Personal home care for the individual with dementia, such as bathing, dressing, or feeding in the home
6. Support groups composed of others who are caring for individuals with dementia
7. Special nursing home care programs only for individuals with dementia
8. Short-term respite care in nursing homes or hospitals to take care of individuals with dementia while the caregiver is away
9. Adult day care providing supervision and activities away from the home
10. Visiting nurse services for care at home

*This association is located at 360 N Michigan Avenue, Suite 601, Chicago, IL 60601.

Brief cognitive rating scale

Axis 1: Concentration

1. No objective or subjective evidence of deficit in concentration
2. Subjective decrement in concentration ability
3. Minor signs of poor concentration (e.g., subtraction of serials 7s from 100).
4. Definite concentration deficit for persons of their background (e.g., marked deficit on serial 7s; frequent deficit in subtraction of serial 4s from 40)
5. Marked concentration deficit (e.g., giving months backwards or serials 2s from 20)
6. Forgets the concentration task; frequently begins to count forward when asked to count backwards from 10 by 1s
7. Marked difficulty counting forward to 10 by 1s

Axis II: Recent memory

1. No objective or subjective evidence of deficit in recent memory
2. Subjective impairment only (e.g., forgetting names more than formerly)
3. Deficit in recall of specific events evident upon detailed questioning; no deficit in the recall of major recent events.
4. Cannot recall major events of previous weekend or week; scanty knowledge (not detailed) of current events, favorite TV shows, etc.
5. Unsure of weather; may not know current president or current address
6. Occasional knowledge of some recent events; little or no idea of current address
7. No knowledge of recent events

Axis III: Past memory

1. No subjective or objective impairment in past memory
2. Subjective impairment only; can recall two or more primary school teachers
3. Some gaps in past memory upon detailed questioning; able to recall at least one childhood teacher and/or childhood friend
4. Clear-cut deficit: spouse recalls more of the patient's past than patient; cannot recall childhood friends and/or teachers but knows the names of schools attended; confuses chronology in reciting personal history
5. Major past events sometimes not recalled (e.g., names of schools attended)
6. Some residual memory of past (e.g., may recall country of birth or former occupation; may or may not recall mother's name; may or may not recall father's name)
7. No memory of past (cannot recall country, state, or town of origin; cannot recall names of parents, etc.)

Axis IV: Orientation

1. No deficit in memory for time, place, identity of self or others
2. Subjective impairment only; knows time to nearest hour, location
3. Any mistake in time of 2 hours or more; day of the week of 1 day or more; date of 3 days or more
4. Mistakes in month of 10 days or more; or year of 1 month or more
5. Unsure of month and/or year and/or season; unsure of locale
6. No idea of date; identifies spouse but may not recall name; knows own name
7. Cannot identify spouse; may be unsure of personal identity

Axis V: Functioning and self-care

1. No difficulty, either subjectively or objectively
2. Complains of forgetting location of objects; subjective work difficulties
3. Decreased job functioning evident to co-workers; difficulty in traveling to new locations
4. Decreased ability to perform complex tasks (e.g., planning dinner for guests, handling finances, marketing, etc.)
5. Requires assistance in choosing proper clothing
6. Requires assistance in feeding, and/or toileting, and/or bathing, and/or ambulating
7. Requires constant assistance in all activities of daily life

From Reisberg B, Ferris S, and deLeon MJ: Senile dementia of the Alzheimer's type: diagnostic and differential diagnostic features with special reference to functional assessment staging, Proceedings, Second International Tropon-Bayer Symposium, 1984.

It is important to note that in-home care, information about the availability of services and government programs, and various forms of respite care were also highly ranked in the survey. Overall, caregivers (family and friends) of the dementia patient are often able and willing to provide care for the patient throughout their illness if appropriate professional consultation can help them solve problem situations and if adequate rest time is provided to the caregiver(s).

RESEARCH IN DEMENTIA

It has been determined that dementia is a specific disease. In the last 10 years the following conclusions have been made:[51]

1. Dementia is *not* a natural result of aging.
2. It is caused by specific identifiable diseases.
3. Diagnosis is important in identifying treatable conditions.
4. A proper evaluation is important in the management of contributing diseases that at present are not curable.

Research is underway exploring possible causes of dementia, including work that is examining neurotransmitters, structural brain changes, the role of nutrition, aluminum, viruses, drugs, immunological defects, neuropsychology, and the role of heredity.

SUMMARY

In caring for the client with dementia, the therapist can do much to make the quality of life better for the client and the family.[51] A detailed listing of the "how to" has been described in other texts, and it is anticipated that the details needed to develop an environment and process of care for the confused elderly can be found in those sources.[51,54] Specific examples of direct patient care intervention may include:

1. Use of neurological rehabilitation techniques to decrease the presence of abnormal tone and to increase the ease of movement (i.e., Feldenkrais, NDT, or Brunnstrom)
2. Modifying the process of neurological facilitation to enhance the patient's sense of safety and motivation to care for themselves within the security of a supervised environment
3. Increasing patient coordination (as in feeding or walking)
4. Increasing ease of breathing (to enhance endurance and minimize the related sense of anxiety) if the rib cage is carried with massive muscle tightness
5. Simplifying tasks and performing for patients those tasks that they cannot perform for themselves
6. Teaching specific skills related to moving the patient

(e.g., guarding or dressing when the patient is completely unable to help himself or herself

The Hospital Patients Bill of Rights and the Nursing Home Patients Bill of Rights define the minimum quality of care that is needed for any client. The concepts presented in the two bills apply equally well to the care of the confused client no matter what the setting. The provision of considerate and respectful care for the person afflicted with dementia is possible and necessary. The well-planned and tenderly given care prevents unnecessary distortions in cognitive function that can be induced through fear or overload and thereby maximizes all remaining cognitive function. To use the remaining emotional and cognitive resources, the confused client needs to live in an environment and process of care that is modified to meet the special needs created by dementia. The aging of an individual does not normally involve the development of dementia. It is true that with advanced age there are normal changes that may affect the person's ability to adapt to new situations (need for more time to respond to a situation). Nevertheless, the overall picture for growing older can be a positive and pleasant process because life experience and personal knowledge can usually compensate for the minor losses. If, however, an acute or chronic degenerative dementia occurs, it is considered a pathological condition. Effective and timely assessment and treatment are needed to assure an outcome where the patient feels safe and the caregivers are given the training and support to help the patient to help himself or herself as long as it is safe and functionally possible.

REFERENCES

1. Agate J: The practice of geriatrics, ed 2, London, 1970, William Heinemann Medical Books, Ltd.
2. Allison RS: The senile brain, London, 1962, Edward Arnold, Ltd.
3. American Psychiatric Association: Diagnostic and statistical manual of mental disorders, ed 3, Washington, DC, 1980, The Association.
4. Arenberg D: Concept problem solving in young and old adults, J Gerontol 23:279-282, 1968.
5. Arenberg D and Robertson-Tchabo EA: Learning and aging. In Birren JE and Schaie KW, editors: Handbook of the psychology of aging, New York, 1977, Van Nostrand Reinhold Co.
6. Arenberg D and Robertson-Tchabo EA: The older individual as a learner. In Grabowski SM and Mason WD, editors: Education of the aging, Syracuse, NY, 1976, ERIC Clearinghouse on Adult Education.
7. Bandler R and Grinder J: Frogs into princes, Cupertino, Calif, 1979, Real People Press.
8. Barclay LL and others: Survival in Alzheimer's disease and vascular dementias, Neurology 35:834-840, 1985.
9. Bender MB: The incidence and type of perceptual deficiencies in the aged. In Fields WS, editor: Neurological and sensory disorders in the elderly, New York, 1975, Stratton Intercontinental Medical Book Corp.
10. Birren JE: Handbook of aging and the individual, Chicago, 1973, University of Chicago Press.
11. Botwinick J: Aging and behavior—a comprehensive integration of research findings, New York, 1978, Springer Publishing Co, Inc.
12. Brache CI: The aging client and their family network. In Jackson-

Klykken O, editor: Physical therapy care of the geriatric patient, New York, 1983, Churchill Livingstone, Inc.

13. Brocklehurst JC: Textbook of geriatric medicine and gerontology, ed 2, New York, 1978, Churchill Livingstone, Inc.

14. Calhoun RO and Gounard BR: Meaningfulness, presentation rate, list length and age in elderly adults paired association learning, Educ Gerontol 4:49-56, 1979.

15. Campbell ME: Study of the attitudes of nursing personnel toward the geriatric patient, Nurs Res 20:141-151, March-April, 1971.

16. Canestrari RA Jr: Age changes in acquisition. In Talland GA, editor: Human aging and behavior, New York, 1968, Academic Press, Inc.

17. Carroll K, editor: Human development in aging-compensation for sensory loss, Minneapolis, 1978, Ebenezer Center for Aging and Human Development.

18. Cattell RB: Theory of fluid and crystallized intelligence—a clinical experiment, J Educ Psychol 54:1-22, 1963.

19. Charatan FB: Management of confusion in the elderly, New York, 1979, Roerig.

20. Cherkosky M: Patient services in chronic disease, 73.978, 1958, Public Health Report.

21. Comfort A: Geriatrics—the missing discipline? West J Med 128:257, March 1978.

22. Coons D and others: Final report of projection Alzheimer's disease: subjective experience of families, Ann Arbor, Mich, 1983, Institute of Gerontology.

23. Craik IM: Age differences in human memory. In Birren JE and Schaie KW, editors: Handbook of the psychology of aging, New York, 1977, Van Nostrand Reinhold Co.

24. Cross PS and Gukland BJ: The epidemiology of dementing disorders, Washington DC, 1986, Contract report prepared for the Office of Technology Assessment for the US Congress.

25. DePaulo JR, and Folstein MF: Psychiatric disturbances in neurological patients—detection, recognition and hospital course, Ann Neurol 4:113-116, 1978.

26. Elias MF and Elias PK: Motivation and activity. In Birren JE and Schaie KW, editors: Handbook of the psychology of aging, New York, 1977, Van Nostrand Reinhold Co.

27. Feldenkrais M: Awareness through movement, New York, 1972, Harper & Row, Publishers, Inc.

28. Feldenkrais M: The elder citizen, Feldenkrais Resources, Berkeley, Calif, 1989. (Pamphlet and audio cassette tapes.)

29. Fisch L: Special senses—the aging auditory system. In Brocklehurst JC, editor: Textbook of geriatric medicine and gerontology, New York, 1978, Churchill-Livingstone, Inc.

30. Foley JM: Sensation and behavior. In Fields WS, editor: Neurological and sensory disorders in the elderly, New York, 1975, Stratton Intercontinental Medical Book Corp.

31. Folstein MF and McHugh PR: Phenomenological approach to the treatment of organic psychiatric syndromes. In Wolman B, editor: The therapists' handbook—treatment of mental disorders, New York, 1976, Van Nostrand Reinhold Co.

32. Folstein MF and Rabins PV: Psychiatric evaluation of the elderly patient, Primary Care 6:3, 1979.

33. Folstein MF and others: Mini-Mental State—a practical method for grading the cognitive state of patients for the clinician, J Psychiatr Res 12:189-198, 1975.

34. George LK: The dynamics of caregiver burden. Final report submitted to the Association of Retired Persons—Andrus Foundation, 1984.

35. Gibaldi M and Levy G: Pharmacokinetics in clinical practice, JAMA 4:235, 1976.

36. Gobetz GE: Learning mobility in blind children and the geriatric blind, Cleveland, 1967, Cleveland Society for the Blind.

37. Gobetz GE and others: Home teaching of the geriatric blind, Cleveland, 1969, Cleveland Society for the Blind.

38. Gross AM: Preventing institutionalization of elderly blind, Visual Impairment and Blindness 2:49-53, 1979.

39. Gunter LM: Student attitudes toward geriatric nursing, Nurs Outlook 19:466-469, July 1971.

40. Jackson O: Physical therapy and the geriatric patient—a descriptive study of cross-cultural trends in Denmark and the United States, doctoral dissertation, Ann Arbor, 1979, University of Michigan.

41. Katzman R, Lasker B, and Bernstein N: Accuracy of diagnosis and consequences of misdiagnosis of disorders causing dementia, Contract report for Office of Technology Assessment, US Congress, 1986.

42. Katzman R: Alzheimer's disease, N Engl J Med 314:964-973, 1986.

43. Katzman R: Clinical presentation of the course of Alzheimer's disease: the atypical patient. In Rose CF, editor: Modern Approaches to the Dementias, Part II, Basel, Switzerland, 1985, Kraeger.

44. Kay DWK and others: Old age mental disorders in Newcastle-Upon-Tyne. I A study of prevalence, Br J Psychol 110:146-158, 1964.

45. Knox AB: Adult development and learning, San Francisco, 1977, Jossey-Bass, Inc, Publishers.

46. Lang R and Jackson O: Model demonstration of a comprehensive care system for older people, Project Grant Number 90-A-1618, Administration on Aging, 1980, Washington, DC.

47. Leech S and Witte KL: Paired—associate learning in elderly adults as related to pacing and incentive conditions, Dev Psychol 5:180, 1971.

48. Leighton DA: Special senses—aging of the eye. In Brocklehurst, JC, editor: Textbook of geriatric medicine and gerontology, New York, 1978, Churchill Livingstone, Inc.

49. Licht S: Therapeutic heat and cold, New Haven, Conn, 1960, Elizabeth Licht, Publisher.

50. Linde S: Taking your medicine—what you should know, Family Circle 11:62-64, 1980.

51. Mace N and Rabins P: The 36 hour day—a family guide to caring for persons with Alzheimer's disease, related dementing diseases and memory loss in later life, Baltimore, 1981, The Johns Hopkins University Press.

52. Marsden CD: The diagnosis of dementia. In Isaacs AD and Post F, editors: Studies in geriatric psychology, New York, 1978, John Wiley & Sons, Inc.

53. May BJ: An integrated problem solving curriculum for physical therapists, Washington, DC, 1976, American Physical Therapy Association, Section on Education.

54. McDowell FH, editor: Managing the person with intellectual loss (dementia or Alzheimer's disease) at home, White Plains, NY, 1980, Burke Rehabilitation Center.

55. McKhann G and others: Clinical diagnosis of Alzheimer's disease, Neurology 34:939-944, 1984.

56. Peterson D and Orgren RA: Older adult learning. In Jackson-Klykken O, editor: Physical therapy of the geriatric patient, New York, 1983, Churchill Livingstone, Inc.

57. Pfeiffer E and Busse EW: Mental disorders in later life—affective disorders, paranoid, neurotic and situational reaction. In Busse EW and Pfeiffer E, editors: Mental illness in later life, Washington, DC, 1973, American Psychiatric Association.

58. Reichel W, editor: Clinical aspects of aging, Baltimore, 1978, Williams & Wilkins.

59. Rodstein M: Characteristics of nonfatal myocardial infarction in the aged, Arch Intern Med 98:84-90, 1956.

60. Ron MA and others: Diagnostic accuracy in presenile dementia, Brit J Psych 134:161-168, 1979.

61. Ross E: Effect of challenging and supportive instructions in verbal learning in older persons, J Educ Psychol 59:261-266, 1968.

62. Selye H: Stress without distress, New York, 1974, JB Lippincott Co.

63. Solomon K: The elderly patient. In Spittell JA Jr, editor: Clinical medicine, Hagerstown, Md, 1981, Harper & Row, Publishers, Inc.

64. Tsai L and Tsuang MT: The mini-mental state and computerized tomography, Am J Psychiatry 136:436-439, 1979.

65. US Congress, Office of Technology Assessment: Losing a million minds: confronting the tragedy of Alzheimer's disease and other dementias, OTA-BA-323, Washington, DC, 1987, US Government Printing Office.

66. US Congress, Office of Technology Assessment: Technology and aging in america, OTA-BA-264, Washington, DC, 1985, US Government Printing Office.

67. Wang HS: Special diagnostic procedures—the evaluation of brain impairment. In Pfeiffer E and Busse EW, editors: Mental illness in later life, Washington, DC, 1973, American Psychiatric Association.

68. Whitehouse PJ: Alzheimer's disease, In Johnson RT, editor: Current therapy in neurologic disease, 1985-1986, Philadelphia, 1985, BC Decker.

69. Wilder J: Basimetric approach (Law of Initial Value) to biological rhythms, Ann NY Acad Sci 98(article 4):1211-1220, 1968.

70. Wilder J: Stimulus and response: the law of initial value, Bristol, UK, 1967, John Wright & Sons, Ltd.

71. Wilensk H and Barwack JE: Interest of doctoral students in clinical psychology work with older adults, J Gerontol 21:410, 1966.

72. Williamson J and others: Old people at home—their unreported needs, Lancet 1:1117-1120, 1964.

73. Wolf W, conf editor: Rhythmic functions in the living system, Ann NY Acad Sci 98(article 4):753-1326, 1962.

74. Wonigrad CH and Jarvill LF: Physician management of the demented patient, J Am Geriatr Soc 34:295-308, 1986.

75. Worden H: Aging and blindness, New Outlook for the Blind 70:433-437, 1976.

76. Worden H: A winter hazard for the old and accidental hypothermia, Silver Springs, Md, NIA/Expand Associates.

77. Worden H: Report by the comptroller general to the Congress: Entering a nursing home—costly implication for Medicaid and the elderly, PAD-80-12, Nov 29, 1979, Washington, DC.

78. Yankelovich, Shelley & White, Inc: Caregivers of patients with dementia, Contract report prepared for the Office of Technology Assessment, 1986.

Part Three

SPECIAL TOPICS AND TECHNIQUES FOR THERAPISTS

Chapter 24

DISORDERS IN ORAL, SPEECH, AND LANGUAGE FUNCTIONS

Nina Newlin Simmons

The use of language to reconstruct the past, represent the present, and consider the future has been a most remarkable human accomplishment. The need to communicate is so compelling that sophisticated and complex systems of speech, gesture, writing, and graphics have been developed to relay ideas. Through language we learn about things that we have never experienced and impart our own experiences. Language plays a role in solving problems, expressing feelings, and relating to other human beings.

Language is an organized set of symbols used for communication. Speech is the oral manifestation of language, as writing is the graphic form and sign language is the ges-

tural form. Without a language system speech does not develop. The development of language in turn depends on the ability to organize and symbolize concepts. This cognitive or conceptual development is based on integration and association of sensory experiences learned through interaction with the environment. Obviously speech and language are intimately related and dependent upon sensorimotor development.

The development of language is a complex process. Consider the difficulty of learning a language. Assuming an intact conceptual and cognitive system, one must perceive, retain, and produce a variety of speech sounds requiring precise and coordinated activity of the lips, tongue, palate, larynx, and respiratory system. One must sequence the sounds to form words, remember and order the words in an accepted and meaningful way, use syntax appropriate to the intended meaning, inflect and stress words correctly to portray correct meanings and attitudes, and then monitor the production through sensory channels. The rules of communicating that govern acceptability as a speaker and listener must also be learned. Appropriate speaking distance, cues to turn-taking such as eye and hand movements, and sensitivity to the listener's prior knowledge of the subject are examples of pragmatic rules of communication that are learned through interaction. We develop an appreciation for context and intonation that can indicate meaning beyond the literal spoken words. For example, the same words can be spoken seriously, humorously, or sarcastically.

Communication is accomplished through facial expression, body movement, and gestures. These nonverbal components are of great importance in the communication process. Information about attitudes and feelings is portrayed in posture, gaze, and voice inflection. If oral and written language is disrupted, facial expression and body language may be the only means of communication. On the other hand, individuals with severe neuromuscular problems may be unable to project body language information.

The physical therapist undoubtedly will encounter individuals representing all types and degrees of communication disorders. Any combination of the above described aspects of communication can be disrupted through developmental or acquired disorders. It is imperative that the physical therapist understand not only how to communicate best with these clients but also how physical therapy can assist or detract from the development or restoration of communication. This chapter presents concepts fundamental to understanding speech and language disorders typically seen in the physical therapy clinic. Although communication obviously includes speaking, listening, reading, writing, and even signing, discussions are limited primarily to oral communication or speech. This chapter reviews the sensory and motor systems necessary for normal speech and language development, discusses the characteristics, assessment, and treatment of neurogenic speech and language disorders, and summarizes the role of the physical therapist.

OVERVIEW OF NORMAL ORAL COMMUNICATION
Physical structures

The physical structures used for speech serve the primary survival functions of breathing, food intake, chewing, and swallowing. Speech is a sophisticated volitional function that shares the oral mechanism with these vegetative functions. The physical structures composing the speech mechanism include the lips, tongue, cheeks, jaw, pharynx, larynx, palate, and respiratory system (Fig. 24-1). The muscles of the speech mechanism are controlled at various levels within the nervous system, including lower motor neuron, extrapyramidal, upper motor neuron, and cerebellum.[18,72] At the highest level, cortical control of speech appears to be lateralized to the dominant, usually left, hemisphere of the brain.[62]

The *respiratory system,* consisting of inspiratory and expiratory muscles, is responsible for transfer of air to and from the lungs. Vegetative breathing involves regular cycles of inhalation and exhalation involuntarily controlled at the brainstem level.[21] This automatic activity must be modified for speaking. Breathing for speech requires considerable control and coordination. During speech the inhalation cycle is shortened and the exhalation phase is prolonged as the exhaled air is shaped into sound. The loudness of speech and the length of utterances can be controlled by altering the amount or force of exhaled air.[19]

The *larynx* is a cartilaginous structure at the superior aspect of the trachea that acts as a valve by action of the vo-

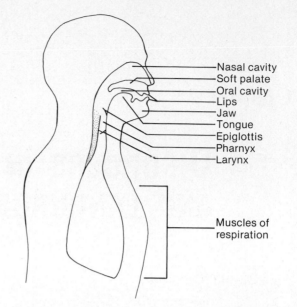

Fig. 24-1. Physical structures of the speech mechanism.

cal folds. The vocal folds remain in an open position to allow passage of air through the larynx during breathing.[32] When swallowing is initiated, the vocal folds close automatically to prevent food from entering the respiratory tract. For speaking the laryngeal valve must be opened, closed, tensed, and relaxed in a finely coordinated fashion to produce the necessary tone for speech.[21] Voice or phonation is produced as the breath stream sets the closed vocal folds into vibration. The pitch of the voice is altered by the tension and length of the folds. Because many speech sounds (such as /s/, /f/, and /p/) do not require voice, rapid opening of the vocal folds must be coordinated with articulation of these sounds, followed by rapid closing for production of voiced sounds (such as /z/, /v/, and /b/).

The *pharynx* is a tube extending from the nasal and oral cavities to the esophagus and larynx.[32] The muscles of the pharynx assist in the transport of food into the esophagus during swallowing. The shape, size, and tension of pharyngeal walls influence the voice quality produced in speaking.

The *palate* consists of the bony hard palate and muscular soft palate, which separate the oral and nasal cavities. During vegetative breathing, the soft palate remains open, allowing air to pass from the pharynx into the nasal passage.[21] As a protective measure during feeding, the soft palate elevates, closing off the nasal passages. All English speech sounds are produced with the soft palate elevated, with the exception of /m/, /n/, and /ng/.

Opening, closing, and lateral movements of the *jaw* allow mastication of food. During speech mandibular opening, closing, and stabilization are rapidly and finely adjusted in the production of speech sounds.[18]

The *cheeks* enclose the oral cavity. The muscles of the cheeks aid the tongue in mixing food with saliva and pushing food onto the teeth during chewing. The cheeks also assist in shaping the oral cavity during speaking.

The *tongue* is made up of intrinsic muscles for altering tongue shape and extrinsic muscles that lift, lower, protrude, and retract the tongue.[18,21] It is capable of an extremely wide variety of complex and fine movements. The tongue moves food in the mouth, mixing it with saliva, placing it for chewing, and finally transporting it to the back of the mouth for swallowing. It also removes food lodged between the teeth and gums. In speech the tongue is responsible for producing speech sounds by rapidly assuming different shapes and contact points in the mouth.

The *lips* form the opening of the mouth cavity. They serve to take food in and retain it within the mouth. The lips open and purse for sucking and close during swallowing. For speech the lips assist in formation of sounds by changing shape and size of the opening.[18,32] The lips, along with the cheeks and eyes, also contribute to communication through facial expressions.

Sensory input for speech production. Speech is not produced or developed solely by movement of the physical structures. Sensory input is responsible for eliciting and maintaining the vegetative responses of sucking, chewing, and swallowing. Sensation produces and maintains a continuous feedback system during production of speech.[32] The sensory systems of primary importance to oral communication include oral sensation, audition, and vision.

Development of oral sensation

The tongue and lips are extremely sensitive to touch, temperature, and pressure to prevent ingestion of inappropriate substances.[32] In addition, texture, size, and position information is required to detect what is in the mouth and where. This provides the lips with feedback to maintain closure and prevent drooling.[51] Sensory input tells the tongue tip where to place material for chewing, when material is too dry and needs moistening, and when food has reached the appropriate consistency for swallowing. Developmentally, these assistive tongue tip motions of feeding promote sensory experience that forms a basis for the selective refined movement of speech. The tip of the tongue is more generously endowed with touch receptors than the back of the tongue or palate.[32,48] The tongue is more sensitive than the lips are. The back of the tongue and posterior walls of the oral cavity respond to pressure that induces swallowing.[51] Pressure at the back of the mouth also elicits the gag reflex. In addition, the tongue is keenly sensitive to taste, especially along the edges[48]: some tastes mobilize the tongue into activity for feeding; others cause a protective response.[48]

Oral sensation is extremely important for speech. Sensory feedback relative to positions and contacts assumed for sound production and pressure of air across structures provides a continuous monitoring and correction loop.[32] It seems that oral sensory function is related to the quality of oral motor proficiency.[58] Neuromotor deficits that change early feeding habits can diminish oral sensory experience and cause impairments in sensorimotor integration. For instance, chewing and swallowing problems of the cerebral-palsied baby may result in continuation of soft or liquid diets, which fail to provide normal sensory variety. Experimental disruption of oral sensation seems to produce deterioration of articulatory proficiency in normal subjects,[32] and poor oral sensory function in cerebral-palsied individuals seems to be associated with defective chewing, drinking, and articulatory ability.[57] Oral sensory deficits have been associated with apraxia of speech[47,55] and dysarthria.[14]

Audition. Audition is possibly the most important sensory component of oral communication. The ravages of disturbed auditory input on speech development are most apparent in the markedly deficient or sometimes nonexistent speech of individuals with profound congenital hearing loss. Auditory input is of extreme importance in learning speech and language and in maintaining adequate speech production. During speech we continuously monitor what we say and how we say it via audition. The smooth flow of speech depends on the auditory system's satisfaction that all is going well. An excellent way of earning respect for auditory monitoring of speech is to speak into a delayed auditory feedback system. These systems, available in many speech clinics, provide several milliseconds of delay between word utterance and hearing that utterance via headphones. The response of most normal speakers is immediate and dramatic difficulty in the fluent production of speech.

In addition to its role in monitoring speech production, audition plays an obvious role in the comprehension of speech. A listener must receive and perceive the sounds in appropriate order, retain the sound sequences for mental processing, and associate meaning to the retained sequences. In addition, undesired sounds (background noise) must be filtered out while desired sounds are localized and processed. Difficulty in auditory sensation, perception of speech sounds, or processing speech for meaning will affect verbal communication.[32]

Vision. Although not primary to monitoring speech production, visual input is important in oral communication. Visual input from the environment provides information on language context, gesture, facial expression, turn-taking cues, and feedback about listener reaction. Seeing a speaker's face also greatly assists in the actual understanding of speech. Information on lip placement and tongue position (lip reading) assists our perception of what is heard. This is apparent at noisy parties when we pay particular attention to watching the speaker's face. Moreover, compensatory production of speech sounds that look wrong but sound exactly like the target sound are often considered error productions. Obviously we see speech as well as hear it.

Development of oral communication. The development of speech and language is a complex process that has been extensively studied and described.[4,8,11,12,23] It is imperative that the physical therapist grasp the process of language and speech development in relation to overall motor development. The acquisition of speech and language is intertwined with the acquisition of motor skills. The physical therapist can play an important role in promoting language and speech development and in reducing the potentially destructive effects of neuromuscular deficits on communication. Too often rehabilitation results in a division of responsibility such that the physical therapist works on motor development and the speech-language pathologist works on language development. In reality, the two develop as an integrated process; treatment should be focused accordingly!

Early oral development. At birth the infant demonstrates the vegetative responses of sucking, swallowing, and breathing that will later be modified for oral communication. The infant's first vocalizations consist of crying in response to discomfort and hunger. Motor responses, including oral behavior, are diffuse and undifferentiated. Yet already the infant is responding to a remarkable range of sensory stimuli that are the building blocks of cognitive and communicative development. For instance, sucking produces tactile stimulation of the mouth, which elicits further sucking. Repetitions of this cycle soon generate integrations in which activity in one modality leads to sensory feedback in another modality.[50]

The motor organization of the speech structures in infancy is similar to the extension-flexion pattern of the extremities.[70] Gently stroking a baby's cheek causes the head to turn toward the stimulus. The jaws open, the lips purse, the tongue protrudes, and sucking begins. An unpleasant stimulus causes the head to turn away, the jaws to close, and the lips and tongue to retract.[21] As the baby matures, the patterned, diffuse oral motions differentiate into an array of movements needed to accommodate solid food.[42] Structural and motor changes in the growing mechanism promote new movements with functional autonomy of structures possible. Although these early developments serve feeding, their importance as the raw material for motor control of speech is obvious.[51] For instance, the lip rounding of sucking can also serve to produce an "oo" sound, while tongue retraction is involved in producing "ah."[21]

Introduction of solid food for chewing and biting provides a similar framework of motor patterns, including lip closure, jaw stabilization, and tongue tip elevation. Speech requires fine control of the lips and tongue tip while reference structures, such as jaw and tongue body, are stabilized. Precursors of these movements are being developed in infancy. With the eruption of the first teeth, the infantile swallow (jaws open and tongue thrust forward) usually begins to give way to an adult swallow (teeth together with tongue retraction). The constant sensory feedback from the changing texture, temperature, and consistency of foods and the oral exploration of objects and body parts and vocalization promote the integration of sensory and motor systems that will ultimately subserve language.

Auditory-vocal development. Although individual timetables of development vary, the infant's use of hearing and vocalization develops in an orderly sequence (Table 24-1). Initially the infant shows a startle response to sudden loud sounds.[70] It has been shown that within the first 2 weeks the child's body movements are synchronized with the pleasant sound of organized adult speech.[13] Babies as young as 1 month old tune in to speech and discriminate between speech and nonspeech sounds.[7] By 2 months the infant ceases body activity to "listen" to interesting sounds. During the second month facial expressions develop. The child begins to associate familiar sights and sounds and to produce sounds of pleasure.[7] Sound localization, tracking, and discrimination become possible as the child develops better head control. The development of head and trunk control also lays the foundation for effective feeding, exploration of the surroundings, and vocalization.[10]

Often the first vocalizations other than crying are sounds produced with the back of the tongue ("goo, goo"), perhaps because myelination of the primary motor cortex proceeds from the back of the mouth to the front.[23] These cooing sounds diversify into a wider variety of sound se-

Table 24-1. Approximate developmental milestones for speech and language[42,51,70]

Age of child	Behavior
0-3 months	Startles to loud noise
	Becomes still with sound of moderate loudness
	Cries and fusses
	Facial expression develops
	Sucking-swallow reflex present
	Tongue-thrust swallow present
3-6 months	Sounds vary and begins to babble; vocal play
	Recognizes familiar persons and objects
	Watches faces; turns to sounds
	Begins intonation patterns
	Early reflexes begin to diminish
6-8 months	Lip and tongue sounds predominate
	Uses voice to influence environment
	Babbling becomes more volitional
8-12 months	Imitates sounds and words
	First word
12 months	Receptive vocabulary increases
	Follows directions
12-24 months	May imitate and echo adult speech
	Uses two to three-word phrases
3 years	Simple sentences and questions

quences called babbling. Initially, choice of sounds is probably biologically dictated by growth of the vocal tract and increases in basic motor control. Infants seem to discover their own sounds and movements and their variations as they move, twist, turn, and breathe. The imitation of these body movements and vocalizations can eventually lead to movements and sounds that serve language. The biologically determined sounds come more and more under self-control.[23]

At this time adults are playing an important role. They imitate the infant's sounds, reinforce productions, and provide models of appropriate intonation patterns. In addition to auditory-vocal stimulation, the infant receives tactile, visual, kinesthetic, and vestibular sensations that contribute to an integrated communication system. The child's movements in space and relationship to objects in space form the basis for mental representations of objects.[7] Children learn that objects that disappear from their zone of vision continue to exist. This mental memory for objects or understanding of object permanence seems important to the development of symbols for objects.[7] The learning of language is closely tied to the learning of the identity of objects, discrimination of object differences, and classification of object similarities. Sensorimotor experience is necessary in the development of these concepts.[1] Objects children see, hear, and manipulate are frequently the ones for which they first learn language symbols,[50] Touch, pressure, and movement during feeding, dressing, and washing form the basis of early perceptual learning and develop the nonverbal framework for interaction.[7] Also, caretakers typically talk to their babies during these activities, instilling the need and pleasure of verbal communication. Exchange of gaze and turn-taking are outgrowths of such interpersonal activities. Children develop a sense of self and body schema and learn to control their environments for their own satisfaction.[3,4]

The child's first means of environmental control (crying) gives way to more sophisticated approaches. Bates and others[3] suggest that functional use of language is a form of tool usage. Initial schemes of tool use (using a stick to obtain another object) precede use of gesture as a tool (pointing to obtain an object), which in turn precedes use of verbalization as a tool (uttering the name of an object to obtain it). Gestures serve an important role in early language learning. Gestures such as showing, giving, eye contact, reaching, and pointing are examples of the capacity for controlling others and a manifestation of emerging communication. During the first year the child begins to use babbling-like sounds with meaningful intonation; these sounds develop as part of the sensorimotor action schemes equivalent to gestures.[3,4]

Around 12 months of age the first real word is often produced.[8] The first words teach us a great deal about the way the child perceives the world. A common attribute of children's first words is that they reflect action (roll, bark, fall). Words for moving, changing, or manipulating objects are learned earlier than names for static objects.[8] Obviously salient sensory stimulation (sight, sound, touch, or movement) dictates early language learning. Impairment in the ability to manipulate objects and receive sensory information about objects has the potential for disrupting language acquisition.[1]

During the first year the child's receptive language and attention span for speech grows steadily. Receptive language exceeds speech production; the child understands more about words than use of words indicates.[8] The child who calls all dogs, horses, cats, pigs, and even birds "doggie" is often swift to point to the horse when asked "Where is the horse?" The child often understands sentences and grammatical constructions before acquiring their productive use.

Developing word production requires increasingly fine motor control. Some children attempt to imitate adult productions. Fortunately, adults seem to intuitively simplify models from which children draw early words. These can be refined as motor control improves.[23] Developing language also requires organization of perceptual experiences. Shape, sound, size, movement, texture, taste, and smell contribute to distinguish concepts.[7] For instance, perception of the particular attributes of dog-ness distinguishes all dogs from cups or cats or objects with different distinct characteristics.

During the second year the child begins to utter words in sequence to represent a chain of events.[7] Later, words are tied into phrases to represent a thought. Early sentences represent action or object relations ("push car" or "mama chair") without descriptors (such as *red* car) or use of adult syntax ("I am *pushing* the *car*" or "*Mama* is sitting on the *chair*").

Receptive vocabulary grows rapidly as does the acquisition of rules of grammar and conversational skills. As the child grows language development is measured by the complexity of syntax, by the clarity of speech production, and by the ability to use language in a variety of ways in different conversational settings.

AN OVERVIEW OF DISORDERS IN ORAL, SPEECH, AND LANGUAGE FUNCTION

Impaired communication can be caused by influences present before, during, or after this developmental process. These influences can be external to the individual, such as poor speech models or environmental deprivation, or internal, such as brain dysfunction, or they may represent an interaction between external and internal factors. A breakdown in any of the processes contributing to oral communication, such as oral motor function, sensory integration, cognition, or language processing, can interfere with speech (Table 24-2). Impaired communication can be classified in a variety of ways depending on the aspect of communication that is deficient (e.g., language, motor

Table 24-2. Primary areas of impairment in neurogenic communication disorders[24,50]

	Primary deficit areas					
Diagnostic label	Receptive and expressive language	Nonverbal intelligence	Hearing	Motor speech production	Interpersonal interaction	Orientation
Developmental aphasia	X	?	—	—	—	—
Acquired aphasia	X	?	—	—	—	—
Apraxia of speech	—	—	—	X	—	—
Dysarthria	—	—	—	X	—	?
Dementia	X	X	—	—	?	?
Mental retardation	X	X	—	—	—	—
Confusion	?	?	—	—	X	?
Schizophrenia	X	?	—	—	X	—
Autism	X	?	—	—	X	—
Rightsided brain damage	—	—	—	—	X	—
Hearing impairment	X	—	X	—	—	—

X, Primary associated deficit; —, not a primary cause; ?, unknown.

speech production, motor speech planning, fluency, or pragmatic skills) or on the cause of the deficit (e.g., neurological deficit, emotional problem, experiential deprivation, sensory deficit, or structural abnormality). Often there are multiple deficits and causes. Such is the case when the primary neuromotor deficit in cerebral palsy causes diminished experiential and sensory input resulting in secondary effects on language.

Acquired versus developmental problems

Although there are many similarities between the acquired and the developmental versions of communication disorders, they cannot be considered synonymous. The failure to develop speech or language must be approached clinically in a very different manner from interference to a fully learned system. Mental and emotional side effects of abnormal development and sudden loss are quite different. The clinician needs to be aware of the developmental level at which communication is arrested and the amount of cognitive and language resources that have been acquired. For instance, the infant demonstrating flaccid weakness of the oral mechanism with diminished ability to suck or swallow has not developed the sensorimotor patterns necessary for speech. Although cortical structures may be unimpaired, the normal learning process may be disrupted by a limited ability to orally explore objects, express pleasure through babbling, or interact normally during feeding. The adult with a similar flaccid weakness of the speech musculature has the benefit of an intact language system, developed cortical association paths, and prior fund of sensory data on which to rely. Because developmental and acquired disorders present different problems, they will be considered separately.

Acquired neurogenic communication disorders

Understanding the communication disorder is of utmost importance in the proper handling of the patient. Disorders of speech, hearing, language, and cognition each require a different approach. Misdiagnosis of the nature of the disorder not only disrupts appropriate interaction and stimulation but also promotes emotional maladjustment and motivational decline. The following section will briefly define and categorize the most typical acquired neurogenic communication disorders.

Motor speech disorders

Dysarthria. The dysarthrias are "a group of speech disorders resulting from disturbances in muscular control—weakness, slowness, or incoordination—of the speech mechanism due to damage to the central or peripheral nervous system or both."[68(p.2)] Dysarthria occurs in children and adults. Although it may coexist with other communication disorders, dysarthria per se has no effect on language, intelligence, or orientation. The causes of dysarthria are varied.[21,68] The speech characteristics of the dysarthric client are a direct reflection of neuromuscular function and neurophysiological status.[21] Just as the physical therapist tests range, speed, and strength of lower-extremity musculature and then observes function through gait, so the speech pathologist tests the range, speed, and strength of the oral musculature and then listens to speech to infer function. Speech symptoms produced by neuromuscular conditions vary considerably from one type of dysarthria to another. Therefore proper identification is imperative to appropriate management. The following dysarthria classification system, developed by Darley and others,[21] relates perceived motor and speech symptoms to underlying neurological processes. Audiotapes depicting the characteristic speech production of each type of motor speech disorder are available to assist in identification (see Appendix).

Flaccid dysarthria. Produced by a lower motor neuron lesion, flaccid dysarthria can affect one or more aspects of the oral motor system, depending on the site and extent of the lesion. Table 24-3 presents the functional relationship

Table 24-3. The relationship of cranial nerves to motor speech production

Nerve	Function for speech	Lower motor neuron lesion effects on speech
Phrenic and spinal intercostal nerves	Control exhaled breath stream	Short phrases Reduced loudness
Trigeminal (V)	Open and close jaw Maintain mouth closure Stabilize jaw for lip and tongue movement	Poor articulation
Facial (VII)	Regulate lip movement for producing sounds	Imprecise articulation of lip sounds
Vagal (X)	Regulate palatal movement for directing air through the mouth or nose	Hypernasality
	Regulate opening and closing of the vocal folds for phonation	Breathy or whispered voice Monotone Short phrases
Hypoglossal (XII)	Regulate tongue movement for producing sounds	Imprecise articulation

of the bulbar nuclei and cranial nerves to speech production and implies location. The neuromuscular conditions associated with this dysarthria are flaccid paralysis or weakness, hypotonicity, and impairment of both voluntary and involuntary movement.[21] Swallowing may be disturbed, and the gag reflex may be impaired or absent.

Spastic dysarthria. Spastic dysarthria is caused by upper motor neuron damage. Because of the bilateral innervation of the speech mechanism above the level of the bulbar system, it has been suggested that bilateral impairment of the corticobulbar tract is required to produce spastic dysarthria.[21] This form of dysarthria (sometimes known as pseudobulbar palsy) affects voluntary movements of the speech mechanism, causing spasticity, weakness, and slowness of movement. A hyperactive gag reflex, sucking reflex, and jaw jerk are often present. Drooling and swallowing difficulty is common because of the slowness and inefficiency of motor mechanisms. A disinhibition of the motor mechanism of crying and laughing is often associated with spastic dysarthria, resulting in what is sometimes called emotional lability, but in fact this is a disinhibited motor reflex. The speech of the client with spastic dysarthria sounds like it is being produced against considerable resistance. The slow, labored articulation and strangled voice quality reflect limited range and spasticity of musculature.

Ataxic dysarthria. Ataxic dysarthria, resulting from cerebellar system dysfunction, is characterized by inaccurate and uncoordinated movement of the speech mechanism.[21] The loss of smooth control results in what has been described as scanning speech: each syllable seems to be given equal stress. The loss of speech rhythm and the equalized pattern is reminiscent of the slow, wide-based gait of the ataxic individual, a step-by-step approach devoid of natural timing. Because of loss of speed and efficiency of movement, there is also an irregular breakdown in articulation of sounds.[21] Moreover, the client has diffi-

culty coordinating rapid articulatory movements with respiration and phonation. The speech of the ataxic client may sound like that of an intoxicated person.

Hypokinetic dysarthria. Hypokinetic dysarthria is seen in disorders of the extrapyramidal system, such as Parkinson's disease. Increased muscle tone, rigidity, and paucity of movement are apparent in the lack of facial expression and limited movement of lips and tongue during speech.[21] The rapid rate of speech, monotone, quiet voice, and imprecise consonant production are probably a reflection of limited range and paucity of movement. Hesitations, inappropriate silences, and then progressive blurring of articulation seem to be the vocal correlate of festination of gait. Palilalia, the repeating of words or syllables, is often present.

Hyperkinetic dysarthria. Hyperkinetic dysarthria is characterized by excess and involuntary movement.[21] Chorea and myoclonus are examples of disorders producing quick, involuntary movements and variable muscle tone, which interfere with the smooth, rapid execution of speech movements. The slow hyperkinesia of athetosis, dyskinesia, or dystonia causes distorted movements and postures, slowed movement, and variable hypertonicity of the speech musculature. The effect on speech depends on the extent and severity of the movement disorder.

Mixed dysarthria. Mixed dysarthria includes characteristics of two or more of the above dysarthrias and is commonly seen in traumatic head injuries, multiple cerebrovascular accidents, amyotrophic lateral sclerosis, and multiple sclerosis. Often one type of dysarthria predominates.

Neurogenic swallowing disorders (dysphagia). The client with dysarthria resulting from weakness, slowness, or incoordination of the oral-pharyngeal motor system commonly has a swallowing disorder, termed dysphagia. Dysphagia can refer to a range of disorders from inefficient handling of food or liquid because of oral motor deficits to severe compromise of nutritional and pulmonary status caused by penetration of food or liquid into the airway (aspiration). The pattern of deficits in swallowing will reflect the neurophysiological cause of the disorder and frequently correlates with observed speech motor symptoms. Signs of oral-stage swallowing problems might include difficulty chewing, maintaining a lip seal, and clearing food or liquid from the spaces in the oral cavity. Signs of aspiration include coughing and choking during meals, excess mucus production, a "wet" voice quality, fever, weight loss, and rejection or spitting out of food. Clients might be unaware of swallowing problems: those with decreased pharyngeal sensation might even aspirate silently[43] with no coughing or outward symptom of laryngeal penetration.

Apraxia of speech. A disruption of speech motor planning caused by brain damage is called apraxia of speech or verbal apraxia.[21] Positioning and sequencing for the voluntary production of sounds is impaired, although there is no significant weakness, slowness, or uncoordination of the speech muscles during automatic activities such as chewing, swallowing, and coughing. Damage to the dominant hemisphere in Broca's area (premotor area) has been associated with this motor programming deficit.[20] Impaired oral sensation is often a correlate of apraxia of speech as well. Because of the proximity of Broca's area to the motor strip, hemiparesis, especially involving the right upper extremity, is often seen.

By definition, the client with pure apraxia of speech shows no decrement in orientation, intelligence, or auditory comprehension; however, apraxia of speech often coexists with aphasia.[21] Inconsistent, variable articulation errors are often preceded by groping movements and struggle behavior. The disability can range in severity from difficulty only on multisyllable tongue twisters to inability to program the mechanism for production of a single syllable or sound. Often the client with apraxia of speech will fluently and accurately produce automatic speech (e.g., cursing or overlearned phrases).

Language disorders: aphasia. Acquired aphasia is an impairment caused by brain damage in the ability to process and/or produce language. Aphasia affects auditory comprehension, reading comprehension, verbal expression, writing, and symbolic gesturing. The disorder is not caused by general intellectual deficits, sensory loss, or motor dysfunction.[68] By definition, aphasia affects both receptive and expressive language, although the degree of involvement in each system can vary.[9] The lesion producing aphasia most often is found in the dominant (usually left) hemisphere of the brain, and the type of behavior varies according to the location and extent of damage.[63] One classification system[28] divides the acquired aphasias into fluent and nonfluent categories depending on the amount and flow of verbal output. The nonfluent client typically struggles to think of words and often uses content words

only ("man uh-uh water uh . . . uh boat"). The fluent aphasic person verbalizes but may substitute words or produce empty speech ("This one here is a snorker for water and I use it over there"). The client with aphasia may or may not be aware of errors, depending on auditory monitoring. The aphasic client is typically not confused or hard-of-hearing. Language is disrupted, not general intelligence. Usually nonlinguistic communication, such as facial expression, turn-taking, and affective tone, is preserved because this aspect of communication seems to be a right hemisphere function. Automatic speech (profanity, greetings, common expressions) may be preserved as well. The aphasic client is alert and oriented, but orientation is often impossible to test in the standard question-answer format.[63] To ensure appropriate management, aphasia must not be confused with dementia, retardation, confusion, or psychotic illness.

Related communication disorders

Dementia. Because cognition and concept development form the infrastructure for language, any factor that hinders cognition will affect speech. Such is the case when speech and language abilities diminish with progressive dementia[5] and organic brain syndrome. The communication deficit is one symptom of a more generalized intellectual deficit.[68] Although the demented client often exhibits aphasic-like language, these symptoms coexist with a variety of behavioral changes not attributable to a language disorder. Aphasia is not an appropriate diagnosis in these cases. Nonverbal performance, orientation, memory, affect, and judgment are impaired. The brain dysfunction causing a generalized deficit is widespread, disseminated, or diffuse, often because of disease (such as Alzheimer's), multiple infarcts, or generalized vascular insufficiency.

Confusion. The language of the confused person is often impaired; however, the disorder is not language specific. The communication reflects "reduced recognition, understanding of and responsiveness to the environment, faulty memory, unclear thinking, and disorientation in time and space. Structured language events are usually normal . . . open-ended language situations elicit irrelevance and confabulation."[68, p.2] Confusion seems to be associated with relatively diffuse brain dysfunction and is frequently a sequela of traumatic head injury.

Traumatic head injury. A traumatic head injury can result in any number of communication deficits depending on the locus and extent of lesion; however, when diffuse injury occurs, the communication disorder is secondary to underlying cognitive disorganization rather than a specific language or speech disorder, such as aphasia or apraxia of speech.[31] In such cases attention, memory, organization, and other cognitive deficits affect both verbal and nonverbal processing. The array of symptoms might include reduced initiation of communication, reduced ability to follow directions, rambling and confabulatory speech, poor organization of thinking reflected in speech and writing, reduced verbal problem solving, poor use of social conversation rules, and inappropriate nonverbal communication.[64]

Schizophrenia. Language disruption is often associated with schizophrenia. Failure to use language interpersonally seems to be the overriding characteristic of schizophrenia. However, irrelevant neologistic output is somewhat reminiscent of fluent aphasia. Because fluent aphasia is often caused by a posterior parietal or temporal lobe brain lesion and may not be associated with hemiplegia, sudden incidence of fluent aphasia may be mistakenly considered a psychiatric problem. The clinician must be careful to avoid misdiagnosis.

Right hemisphere damage. The client with damage to the nondominant (usually right) cerebral hemisphere often shows adequate oral language. However, interactive and affective aspects of communication are disrupted.[20] The client may exhibit a decreased awareness of the rules of communication, such as turn-taking, eye contact, listener sensitivity, and attention to and use of affective cues such as inflection and facial expression. Language is often literal so that humor, sarcasm, metaphors, or implied meanings may be missed.[27] Gardner has described the right-brain–damaged client as "a language machine, a talking computer that decodes literally what is said and gives the most immediate response . . . insensitive to the ideas behind the question, the intentions or implications of the questioner."[26, p. 296]

Developmental neurogenic communication disorders

It is difficult to isolate a single cause-and-effect relationship in developmental problems because the interaction of learning, environment, and CNS dysfunction creates a constantly changing and complicated picture. The learning and behavior deficits found in children with CNS dysfunction encompass a wide range of diagnostic labels, such as developmental language disorder, learning disability, hyperactivity, and developmental delay. The child seen in the speech clinic as exhibiting language disorder may be perceptually impaired to the occupational therapist or tactilely defensive to the physical therapist. The arbitrary fragmentation of development into isolated functions fails to recognize the integrated process of learning. Although the following section will refer to typical diagnostic labels associated with neurogenic communication problems, the therapist should not lose sight of the multiple interacting variables that hinder or facilitate development of the child as a whole. Often the primary problem, such as motor, sensory, cognitive, memory, or attentional deficit, inhibits the language learning process, which is then complicated by emotional overlay, overprotection, and/or maladjustment.

Deficits in motor development. Failure to acquire normal oral motor patterns at any level of development influences speech development. Defective early vegetative function of swallowing, sucking, and chewing may preclude normal speech. Once vegetative motor functions develop, failure to develop voluntary motor control of the speech mechanism hinders speech development. Absence of sensory feedback and sensorimotor integration impedes acquisition of articulation. When speech does not develop normally, negative influences on language, emotion, and affect result.

The most widely recognized childhood neuromotor disorder affecting speech occurs in cerebral palsy. Much has been written about this oral motor dysfunction.[42,51,70] The dysarthrias described in the previous section generally apply to the developmental motor speech disorders of cerebral palsy. However, the sensory, perceptual, or intellectual problems found hinder direct comparison to the acquired dysarthrias. The dysarthrias of cerebral palsy are often mixed, with one condition (e.g., spastic or athetoid) predominating. Compensatory movements, secondary deficits produced by prolonged incorrect postures, sensory deprivation, or lack of experience are potential contributors to the clinical symptoms.

Defective motor planning results in developmental *apraxia of speech*.[47] Children with apraxia of speech show auditory abilities and general cognitive development far superior to verbal expression. The primary disability has been described as a sensorimotor deficit because it is frequently associated with disrupted oral sensation. The child has difficulty producing and ordering the rapid sequential articulatory movements that compose words. The result is often unintelligible speech characterized by omission or substitution of consonant sounds.

Deficits in language development

Developmental language disorder. Developmental language disorder is an impairment in the capacity to process language because of brain dysfunction. There is no apparent oral motor deficit or generalized mental retardation. Yet language development is disturbed. The disturbed development of verbal language is often associated with auditory perception and processing deficits. Nonverbal cognitive development usually far exceeds the development of language, distinguishing this child from the mentally retarded child. The child attempts to communicate and interact through nonverbal channels and is alert to situational cues.

Although the diagnostic distinction is often difficult, a *language delay* can result from a number of causes.[24,56] *Delayed language* is a term used to encompass failure to acquire language normally for a variety of reasons, such as minimal brain dysfunction, hearing loss, emotional disturbance, or experiential deprivation. The term *learning disability* is often associated with language learning disorders. It is important in such cases of neurodevelopmental disorder to avoid focusing on specific labels and view the constellation of symptoms that hinder the learning process.[24] This includes awareness of the interrelated effects of visual, auditory, vestibular, and tactile-kinesthetic systems, motor development, and cognition. Auditory processing, hyperactivity, and tactile defensiveness cannot be pigeonholed into separate categories for treatment.

Mental retardation. Mental retardation reduces the capacity for verbal as well as nonverbal intelligence. Because cognition and concept development form the foundation for language, defective cognitive development precludes normal language acquisition. The degree of mental retardation affects the potential for language learning.

Autism. Autism has been associated with disturbed language development as well as disrupted use of pragmatic or interactive skills. The autistic child often demonstrates literal, echolalic, or bizarre language patterns in conjunction with a constellation of behavioral and interpersonal problems. Many fail to develop language and are mistakenly suspected of being hearing impaired early in development.

EVALUATION OF COMMUNICATION
Role of the physical therapist

The physical therapist working with neuropathologies will undoubtedly encounter clients with communication disorders. The physical therapist's role in the evaluation and remediation of these disorders will vary depending on the setting, nature of the disorder, availability and role of speech pathologists, and the individual experience and expertise of the physical therapist. Generally, however, the goals of the physical therapist working with the communication-disordered client are fourfold.

1. The first goal is recognition and identification of the communication problem. Often the physical therapist is the first professional to note speech and language problems and begin the referral process. Awareness of normal communication and development and the effects of disease or injury will assist in the identification process. All too often families, physicians, or health care professionals take a wait-and-see attitude when early intervention could reverse the course of a disorder. Recognition of a problem not only directs attention to needed services but also allows the physical therapist to incorporate appropriate communication-related activities into the program. The clinician should avoid labeling the communication disorder. The physical therapist must recognize the problem, but actual diagnosis of the communication problem should be in the hands of the speech pathologist.

2. The second goal is to determine how to communicate with the client. Assessment procedures, information gathering, and direction giving require communication between the client and the physical therapist. Clinicians must learn how to alter the situation or their own speech to maximize communication and how to best understand the needs of the client. This goal can best be accomplished if there is a complete understanding of the communication disorder. Information provided by the speech pathologist, family, and caregivers, as well as by direct observation, can be of great help in learning to communicate with the individual.

3. The third goal involves determination of the effects of stimulation, movement, and positioning on the communication of the client. This information is helpful in planning a program and can be relayed to the family and other therapists. For instance, the physical therapist who observes the calming effect of a particular form of sensory stimulation on a hyperactive child might relay this information to the teacher or speech pathologist. Based on this information, a treatment schedule may evolve.

4. The fourth goal involves determining how physical therapists can assist in stimulating speech and language. This requires programming prespeech or communication activities into the physical therapy regime and eliminating tasks that might interfere with development of communication. Although the job of the physical therapist is not to remediate the communication disorder per se, the clinician can provide a sound physiological framework for speech production. For instance, the use of an associated movement to increase activity in a hemiplegic client may also increase laryngeal tone. If the client exhibits spastic dysarthria, this increased laryngeal tone can be destructive to speech. On the other hand, such activity with a flaccid dysarthric client might facilitate voicing. Encouraging the aphasic client to communicate by providing a supportive atmosphere and appropriately structuring a natural conversation facilitates language, while asking an aphasic client to name objects in the room is rarely an appropriate activity for the physical therapy clinic. An awareness of tasks that aid communication is imperative in a holistic approach to treatment.

Motor activities make excellent contexts for language stimulation. Children need to experience objects and events referred to by the speech they hear to learn the relationships between sound and meaning.[7] The physical therapist can provide part of this experience in the clinic. Adults and children with neuromuscular impairments need a background of physiological support upon which to build speech. The physical therapist can provide this. Communication is a social function. The physical therapist can reinforce positive attitudes and promote interaction. A facilitatory and supportive environment promotes functional reorganization of a disturbed communication system. The physical therapy clinic can provide an environment conducive to reorganization and integration.

The organization of nervous system function does not take place piecemeal. The overlap of function extends the role of the physical therapist beyond that of a motivator, supporter, and stimulator of communication. The neural processes underlying movement cannot be separated from speech and language. As McDonald Critchly so eloquently stated, "The headstream of language overflows into every possible channel."[15,p.299] The reverse is also true. We speak with our mouths and our bodies.

Unfortunately, speech has been considered a special and separate function by many. However, research and clinical experience suggest that speech is intimately related to the motor system as a whole.[38] Not only is oral-motor function an outgrowth of early vegetative function, but also it seems intricately tied to other motor functions.

It seems to be no coincidence that the cerebral hemisphere that controls speech also usually controls a person's dominant hand. It has been proposed that left-hemispherical specialization for speech is a consequence not so much of an asymmetrical evolution of symbolic functions as it is a consequence of the evolution of certain motor skills that happen to lend themselves readily to communication.[37] In other words, the left hemisphere evolved language not because it gradually became more symbolic or analytical per se but because it became well adapted for some categories of motor activity.[38] There is an obvious relationship between speech and hand use. Babies punctuate crying with hand movements and begin early manual stressing gestures in time with speech.[13] The pairing of verbal and motor output is not random. There seems to be an interconnection between verbal and nonverbal systems. It is difficult for normal speakers to speak with hand movements that are not in synchrony with the rhythm of their speech. Kimura[36] found that gestures occurring during the speech of right handers were associated almost exclusively with the right hand. Such gestures were not observed during humming. Kinsbourne[38] extended this idea to a presumably biologically preprogrammed linkage between language functions and skilled movements of the right side. This is related to an early association between infant vocalizations and body-orienting response. With maturation, speech is detached from overt body orientations. However, the philosophy that language evolves in a motor context and that there is a neurophysiological link between speech and the right extremities cannot be ignored. While evaluating and treating the motor system, the effects on speech and language should be closely monitored. Moreover, specific knowledge of the functioning of the speech mechanism will assist in heightening awareness of the interrelationships of sensorimotor systems.

Communication screening

Evaluation and diagnosis of communication disorders are complicated and time-consuming procedures for which the speech-language pathologist is specially trained. A staggering array of standardized and nonstandardized test materials are available to assess auditory perception, comprehension, reading, memory, verbal expression, verbal problem solving, motor speech, and writing in both children and adults. Results of a complete evaluation form the basis for decisions regarding diagnosis, prognosis, and treatment. This information can be of great value to the physical therapist. Therefore communication with the speech pathologist is necessary. Often, however, the physical therapist must gain preliminary information before a speech evaluation is completed. Therefore familiarity with informal assessment and observation procedures is needed. Assessment of the functional level of communication can be carried out by (1) observing the client communicate, (2) interviewing family or caregivers, (3) reviewing biographical, medical, and historical information, and (4) requiring that the client perform certain screening tasks. The following section presents a variety of areas that influence communicative adequacy. The age, behavior of the client, and cause of the disorder help dictate the type and extent of assessment. Information acquired should be used to assist in the delivery of physical therapy services, not for the diagnosis and treatment of the communication disorder.

Assessment of oral-motor function. Structural and functional integrity of the speech mechanism is obviously required for adequate speech. Requiring speech of a deficient oral-motor mechanism is like requiring walking before adequate strength, movement, or coordination of the trunk and extremities is obtained. The devastating effects of neuromuscular impairment on speech quality and intelligibility are obvious when we hear the severely dysarthric cerebral-palsied individual attempt to squeeze speech from an uncooperative oral mechanism. The speech mechanism should not be overlooked in the physical therapy clinic. Knowledge of the condition of the motor system as a whole is imperative to suitable treatment.

The following section briefly addresses movements necessary for speech production. Although knowledge of the range of movement, strength, and accuracy of muscle groups is of extreme importance, actual muscle testing and grading of movement is not covered because this information is available elsewhere.[17,35]

The child or adult should be assessed both at rest and while engaged in activity. Symmetry of the face and lips, muscle tone, alignment of the teeth and jaws, involuntary or overflow movement, and facial expression should be observed. The oral cavity can be inspected to note the size, shape, and mobility of the tongue and soft palate. Obvious deviations, such as cleft palate, gross malocclusions, tremors, and deformities, are likely to affect speech.

Oral reflexes should be tested and determination made of appropriateness to the individual's age (Table 24-4). Because the motor functions required for sucking, chewing, swallowing, coughing, and breathing are necessary prespeech movements, knowledge of these activities is needed. Questioning the client or family and directly observing breathing, eating, and drinking provide valuable information regarding (1) adequacy of the motor pattern itself, (2) positions assumed during activity, and (3) interference of movement of extremities and reflexes on oral-motor functions.

Often simple vegetative or voluntary movements are

Table 24-4. Normal and pathological oral reflexes[42,51]

Reflex	Normal (approximate ages)	Abnormal
Rooting	Up to 4 months	In adult
Suck-swallow	Up to 5 months	In adult
Bite reflex	Up to 5 months	In adult
Mature swallow	Normal after 1 year	
Gag	Always normal	
Cough	Always normal	
Cephalic		Abnormal
Chew reflex		Abnormal
Jaw jerk		Abnormal

performed adequately, yet movement cannot be combined into smooth, rapid, fine transitions required for speech. Voluntary movements can be tested with and without visual cues using imitation as well as spontaneous production. Observation of facial expression is helpful in determining functional use of patterns also.

Respiration. Vegetative breathing can be observed with the individual in the supine position by looking across the chest. Infants often demonstrate belly breathing, but by 2 years of age most children begin lifting the upper chest during inhalation. Continued belly breathing may indicate that muscles of upper chest and neck are not able to fix the rib cage against pressure created by diaphragm movement.[70] The breathing pattern should be smooth and rhythmical.

Notation of head and sitting balance contributes to information on respiration because both assist with air intake. For instance, sitting in a flexed position may inhibit upper chest movement and initiation of phonation. Proper support and positioning can dramatically alter breathing and speech.

Breath support for speech requires voluntary control and sufficient air capacity to sustain exhalation through a sentence. Voluntary control can be tested in the older child or adult by taking a deep breath and sustaining the outflow of air as long as possible. Any involuntary motion or lack of smoothness should be noted. The same exercise should be repeated as the client moves one arm, then the other, to see if involuntary activity is triggered.

Laryngeal system. Involuntary function can be inferred from the pitch, quality, and loudness of crying or vocalizations. Coughs should be rapid and sufficiently loud to indicate vocal fold activity; a weak or dragged out cough is a sign of laryngeal problems.

Voluntary vocal fold activity can be tested by having the individual sustain a tone (the proverbial "ah") for as long as possible. Phonation for 10 seconds or less is probably inadequate for normal connected speech. The loudness and pitch of the voice should be noted. A whispered or breathy sound suggests inadequate closing of the vocal folds. The ability to rapidly start and stop phonation can

be tested by having the individual produce "ah ah ah . . ." like a machine gun as fast as possible.[70] The ability to alter the length of the vocal folds can be tested by having the client intone "ah" beginning at a low pitch and building to high pitch.

Palate. Involuntary motion of the palate is easily observed by eliciting the gag reflex. Hyperactivity or hypoactivity and symmetry can be noted. Activity for speech is observed by watching the movement of the palate on production of "ah." The head should not be tilted back because gravity would then assist with palatal movement.

Tongue. With the lips held apart, the involuntary motion of the tongue can be observed during eating. Food can be placed at corners of the mouth, on the upper lip, and in between the cheeks and teeth to observe the mobility of the tongue. Drooling or ejection of food from the mouth or presence of a primitive tongue-thrust swallow should be noted.

Voluntary movement can consist of elevation and lateralization of the tongue tip and protrusion and retraction. With the jaw stabilized open, the client should touch the tongue tip behind the upper teeth. Rapid side-to-side and up-and-down movement is requested with notation made of speed, range, and accuracy or any shift into an extensor retraction pattern. The clinician should note if resistance to movement elicits improved function or overflow activity.

Lips. Adequate sucking requires lip closure as well as action of the cheeks. Drooling or difficulty removing food from a spoon may indicate poor lip closure. Lip closure should be maintained for swallowing in an adult swallow. Lip movements tested for speech include retraction, pressing lips together, and lip rounding. Rapid motion is observed by pursing and smiling or by opening and closing as fast as possible.

Assessment of oral sensation. Because no aspect of voluntary motor activity is independent of its sensory component, the integrity of tactile and kinesthetic feedback should be assessed. This can include light touch and pressure to the face, lips, and palate and tongue tip, sides, and body. The clinician should note presence of hypersensitivity or hyposensitivity or elicitation of abnormal reflexes during testing. When drooling persists in spite of ability to achieve lip closure and tongue movement, decreased sensation is suspect. Oral tactile hypersensitivity may result in gagging, choking, or even an extensor thrust of the tongue when something is introduced into the mouth.[70] Often tactile defensiveness is especially noted on stimulation around the mouth.[1]

Oral stereognosis has been tested by use of small plastic shapes attached to a cord.[57] The shapes are placed in the mouth and the client picks an identical shape from an array. Such procedures must be used with extreme caution by trained professionals because of the potential risk of airway obstruction. Taste and temperature sensitivity are often assessed to assist in swallowing programs and neuromuscular facilitation.[48]

Assessment of speech. In addition to evaluating oral-motor and sensory integrity, an impression of the functional use of these structures for speech is important. When the language system is intact yet the neuromotor system fails to sufficiently support speech (as in dysarthria), the output can be described in terms of intelligibility (how easy it is to understand) and perceived characteristics (such as monotone, breathiness, and excessive loudness). The intelligibility gives an overall impression of the individual's ability to use speech to communicate. The perceived characteristics explain what has gone wrong to disrupt speech. The usefulness of this approach to assessment can be understood with the following treatment example. The physical therapist observes a cerebral-palsied client with shallow, uncoordinated breathing patterns, excessive overflow movement, and deviant positioning. The speech pathologist observes unintelligible speech characterized by short phrasing, reduced loudness, imprecise consonants, and variable breakdown. The physical therapist might work on positioning, facilitate breathing, increase isolated muscle control, and diminish overflows. The speech pathologist might build on this improved speech support by focusing on altering phrasing, rate of speech, and articulation of specific sounds to improve intelligibility.

An impression of the function of oral structures for speech can be gained by having the client imitate isolated syllables, words, and sentences and engage in conversation. It is not uncommon to observe minimal difficulty in producing isolated oral movements, such as elevating the tongue while the system is unable to produce the motion rapidly and in coordination with the rest of the speech mechanism. The speech pathologist usually tests motor speech in ascending levels of motor speech difficulty; for instance, the ability to produce vowels (ah), combine vowels and consonants (pa), rapidly sequence syllables (pa-papa . . .), rapidly alternate syllables (pataka . . .), produce simple words (pie, cat), produce multisyllabic words of varying length (cat, catnip, catastrophe), produce sentences, and converse. During these tasks notation is made of the range, speed, and accuracy of movement, the intelligibility of the product, and the perceived characteristics of the output.

Assessment of mental status. The overall approach to understanding a communication disorder requires carefully ruling out possible contributing variables. The problems must be pinpointed to ensure appropriate goal setting and treatment. For instance, the child with a language learning disorder resulting from inability to attend and from hyperactivity might be overstimulated by exaggerated multimodal sensory stimulation, while the child with aphasia may require exaggerated multimodality sensory input. Biographical, medical, and historical information, as well as

observation of specific behaviors, will help delineate the deficits.

Levels of consciousness. Level of alertness can be determined by observing the individual's response to stimuli and his or her interaction with the examiner. Drifting off to sleep, inattention, and decreased awareness of surroundings are typical of the lethargic client.[63] Specific assessment of speech and language skills are not valid in reduced levels of consciousness because communication disturbance varies with level of alertness and awareness.

Attention. The ability to attend to a specific stimulus without distraction should be observed and described. Inattention caused by hyperactivity and distractibility (midbrain lesion) should be distinguished from that caused by indifference, perseveration, or ability (frontal lobe lesion).[63] Inattention confined to specific modalities should be noted also.

Visual and auditory sensitivity. Knowledge of the integrity of vision and audition are prerequisites of communication testing. If the client cannot clearly visualize objects used to elicit speech, then errors may result from vision, not language. Similarly, the client who does not follow a spoken command may be hearing impaired rather than language impaired.

Mood/nonverbal communication. Observation of nonverbal behavior assists greatly in determining the type of communication problem. Use of facial expression, voice tone, gestures, and body position should be noted. Does the individual watch carefully as though searching for information? Does the client appear motivated to communicate? Aphasic adults and children attempt to relate to others nonverbally through gesture and affective tone. Individuals with generalized intellectual deficits often display shallow or flat affect, bland depression, indifference, or general dullness. A discrepancy between the level of nonverbal and verbal development is an extremely important clinical observation.

Orientation. Orientation is classically assessed in adults by asking name, date, and location information. Too often aphasic clients are mistakenly labeled confused because of this kind of testing. Such an assessment of an aphasic person is not valid. Orientation must be observed functionally, and great caution should be used in interpreting observations.

Memory. A variety of types of memory disturbance are associated with neuropathological conditions. Immediate recall is often tested using digit repetition tasks.[63] Remote memory of general knowledge is assessed by asking biographical questions. Prior knowledge of correct information is imperative. The author has been fooled more than once by confused clients who provide beautiful, believable information that is totally confabulated. Tasks that require the client to recall information provided earlier in the session, remember a string of words, or tell what was served for lunch all provide data on memory. However, the client with speech or language problems may be unable to perform such tasks accurately in spite of adequate memory. It might be helpful in such cases to compare responses to nonverbal memory tasks. Informal tests may be performed, such as placing the client's cane or jacket behind a door while the client is looking and noting later if the individual remembers where it is. A more formal method is to hide objects while the client watches, then in several minutes show a duplicate object and see if the client recalls the location of the hidden object. Observation of information that enhances memory should be made using visual, auditory, and tactile input, repetition, or exaggeration of the stimulus. For instance, some clients (and therapists) will be more likely to remember information if they have seen it in writing, had it repeated several times during the session, or have been shown pictorial examples. Auditory-verbal information must not be required during such tasks because this tests the speech or language problem rather than memory.

Nonverbal intelligence. Observation of the way the adult or child relates to the environment, solves problems, or performs nonverbal tasks such as visual matching helps distinguish between specific speech and language problems and more generalized cognitive deficits. Observation of play is very useful in children. Symbolic play is an important prerequisite for language.

Assessment of language

Auditory comprehension. As noted previously, before assessing auditory comprehension the examiner must determine if peripheral hearing is intact. Does the client turn toward an auditory stimulus or startle to loud noises? Is there differential reaction to varying tone of voice? Does the individual respond differently to speech versus environmental sounds (such as sirens or phone ringing)? When an audiological evaluation rules out hearing impairment yet the client fails to follow commands consistently, the clinician should attempt to determine the degree of comprehension problems.

Comprehension should be assessed without requiring verbal responses from the client and with full knowledge of the correct answer. Questions such as "Did you like breakfast?" may elicit socially appropriate "yes" or "no" responses, but the examiner has no way of knowing if they reflect accurate understanding. Typical comprehension testing usually requires pointing to objects named or carrying out simple directions. Responses are often better for whole body or axial commands ("get up"; "sit down") than for distal commands ("point"; "pick up"). If a motor response is facilitated, does the individual respond better to the verbal command? The clinician should be aware of situational or inadvertent gestural cues that may be assisting the client and note if responses are more accurate when visual, tactile, or situational cues are used.

Verbal expression. Areas generally covered in speech and language evaluations by the speech pathologist include verbal repetition of words or phrases of increasing length, describing a picture, naming and describing the function of common objects, reading aloud, answering questions, and completing sentences. The most obvious informal approach to gaining an impression of an individual's language is to engage in conversation. The approach will vary considerably depending on age. The young child rarely responds well to question-answer interaction; engaging the child in play, using parallel talk, or providing a context in which the child needs to speak (e.g., to ask for a toy) are preferable to approaches asking "What is this?" Adults can be asked open-ended questions, such as "What brought you into the hospital?" A general idea of function can be gained from the amount, accuracy, and appropriateness of spontaneous speech and the ability to interact. In addition, the clinician can check serial speech, repetition, and confrontation naming.

A brief screening of gesturing and writing may be helpful if verbal expression is nonfunctional. Language impaired clients rarely write better than they speak. However, if this channel along with gesturing can add information to verbal output, awareness of the skill is helpful.

Motor function and alternate communication systems. The influence on communication of neuromotor dysfunction can range beyond specific speech and language problems. The ability of the individual with nonfunctional speech to adapt to an alternate form of communication, such as a communication board or signing, can dictate the possibility of functional communication. The range, strength, and fine control of, for example, extremities and sitting balance will determine the appropriateness of various alternate communication systems. The physical therapist will need to work closely with the speech pathologist, the occupational therapist, and the family to ensure that an alternative communication system is appropriate physically, mentally, and socially to the individual.

Environmental variables. The physical characteristics of the environment can markedly affect verbal communication.[45] The physical therapist must be acutely aware of the influences of setting upon the interaction with the client. Common sense dictates that anything that hinders normal communication will interfere with disordered communication. Attempting to speak in a noisy, bustling environment can be distracting to anyone. It can be chaotic and overwhelming to the individual with communication problems. The positions of the client and therapist can inhibit or facilitate interaction. Face-to-face, eye-level communication maximizes the client's and the therapist's use of all cues. Nonverbal information, such as gestures, facial expression, and calming voice quality, can assist. Lighting should be adequate to promote visualization of the speaker and the environment. Attitude and motivation can be enhanced by the appearance of the environment and the therapist. For instance, a child who has been poked, probed, and stuck by physicians for the past year may react negatively to anyone in a laboratory coat. An adult who has suffered a stroke may resent being treated with baby toys.

TREATMENT CONSIDERATIONS

The treatment goals of the physical therapist will be to improve the physiological support for speech production, maximize the client's use of existing communication, and reinforce and stimulate the development of a functional communication system. These goals should be incorporated within the context of physical therapy. The physical therapist must not attempt to do speech or language therapy. Rather, a close working relationship with the speech pathologist and occupational therapist will help in defining roles and ensuring unified, holistic treatment. The following section briefly highlights areas of treatment. The purpose is to familiarize the reader with the variety of treatment needs of the speech impaired client, rather than prepare the clinician to implement such treatment. Clinical experience and education will be necessary to fully appreciate the variety and complexity of treatment variables that influence speech and language learning.

Oral-motor dysfunction

Techniques such as inhibiting, resisting, and facilitating movement, positioning, and muscle strengthening are appropriate for the speech mechanism (refer to Chapter 6).[53,54] However, appropriateness of techniques will depend on the specific type of motor dysfunction or dysarthria. Treatment of the speech mechanism will obviously affect feeding and swallowing. In fact, treatment often centers around feeding activities. Awareness of oral-motor dysfunction should not be limited to these activities. However, during all treatment the effects on the speech mechanism should be noted. Overflow of activity to the oral mechanism should be observed when using techniques to facilitate movement elsewhere. The approach to training oral-motor function should take into account the total pattern of the target movement and the concomitant sensory experiences. Learning proceeds best when a trained, isolated movement is incorporated into meaningful activity with appropriate feedback to allow for discrimination and generalization.[2]

Posturing. Exploring postural influences on speech can provide information on needed modifications. To perceive the pattern of a new speech movement, competing feedback from tension and involuntary movement elsewhere in the body must be reduced. Postures will vary depending on the disorder, the target movement, and the needs of the individual. Postures that inhibit reflexes may help the neurologically impaired individual practice movements for speech that might otherwise trigger massive primitive movement patterns. Correct posturing is also important in preventing abnormal development. For example, a persisting asymmetrical tonic neck reflex could cause deviation of the mandible and restrain articulation. Stabilization

techniques may be necessary in extreme cases when overflow movement precludes speech learning.

Vegetative to voluntary activity. Targeting the more primitive movements of sucking, chewing, swallowing, and vegetative breathing allows the establishment of correct prespeech patterns, with the goal of gradually achieving voluntary control. Feedback through all sensory modalities will heighten awareness of the movement and assist in modifying these for speech.

Respiration and phonation. Prolongation and control of respiration can be stimulated to improve phonation and speech phrasing. Assuming an antigravity position, such as sitting, often helps stimulate lung expansion. Rotation within the body axis tends to decrease spasticity and increase respiratory output. For speech purposes, the client who cannot sit alone should be positioned with adequate support to maximize breathing, assist phonation, and allow eye contact. Strengthening the respiratory musculature is accomplished during activities to improve trunk stability, head control, and sitting balance. During such activities, breathing can be facilitated, progressing from passive to resisted motion. Vibration and pressure to the thorax might facilitate phonation as well. Voluntary control can be encouraged by activities such as blowing a match without extinguishing it, blowing a ping pong ball across a table, or taking a deep breath, holding it, and prolonging a sound.

Sucking and swallowing. When vegetative responses are absent or diminished, facilitatory techniques can often be used to improve function. Effective control of swallowing implies use of the lips, cheeks, tongue, palate, larynx, and respiratory systems. Therefore it is an excellent focus for therapy (refer to Chapter 4). Food is one of the primary facilitators of oral movement because it can stimulate sensations of touch, taste, and temperature, as well as providing visual and olfactory input.

Swallowing is usually approached in a sitting position with the head flexed slightly forward to avoid aspiration. Because aspiration, nutritional imbalance, and negative feelings can be produced by improper techniques, foods, or positions, it is recommended that the clinician become well versed in swallowing therapy[29,41,43,51] and seek assistance from allied professionals specifically trained to conduct videofluoroscopic swallow studies and assess swallow dynamics before initiating this treatment. In conjunction with swallowing therapy or when a full feeding program is not necessary, an array of facilitatory techniques can be used to stimulate the speech mechanism.[53,67,43] Small shapes, strips of cloth, or buttons attached to a cord can be introduced into various parts of the mouth with extreme caution to avoid introducing items into the throat. The stimulation and resistance produced by pulling on the cord might promote activity or increased tone. These movements can be observed and shaped through facilitation techniques. Various tastes can be introduced to elicit responses. Typically, salt mobilizes the tongue, bitter tastes cause protrusion, and sweets elicit retraction.[48]

Lip closure is necessary to prevent drooling and produce sounds.[51] Lip closure can be stimulated by activities such as holding the fingers above and under the lips, stretching the lips and attempting closure against resistance, and placing a button on a string between the lips and teeth and pulling to produce resistance.[51] Shaking the lip sometimes reduces spasticity.[51] Neuromuscular facilitation techniques (e.g., icing or quick brushing) and inhibitory techniques (pressure) can be applied to the lips.[48] Lip closure and rounding can be stimulated by sucking on a gloved finger or through straws of progressively smaller diameter.[53]

Tongue. Tongue movement can be stimulated by passive then resisted motion, quick icing, and stretching.[54] Elevation may be assisted by brushing the ridge behind the teeth and walking down the midline with a tongue blade, then releasing the pressure and elevating the tongue with the blade. The client can be encouraged to lick food from the roof of the mouth, corners of the mouth, or lips after facilitatory activities. A tongue blade can be used for tactile cues, tapping, or sustained pressure as appropriate.

Jaw. Control of jaw stabilization is needed for speech. Using a bite block during tongue and lip exercises will prevent associated jaw movement until isolated tongue and lip movement is achieved. Once this is achieved attention can be directed to the voluntary control of the jaw. Motion can be assisted during chewing movements and the range and rate can be slowly increased.

In cases of pathological bite reflex, pressure at the temporomandibular joint or under the chin might reduce the reflex.[51] Extensor thrust of the jaw often accompanies athetosis, and positioning can often diminish this. Passively opening and closing the jaw while slowly initiating phonation may help disassociate the jaw thrust from voicing.[70]

Treatment considerations in dysarthria

The following section will attempt to orient the reader in a general direction for treatment rather than delineate the treatment of each dysarthria type. The physical therapist is well aware of techniques for physical restoration. Obviously these principles apply to the speech mechanism. In some cases the speech pathologist will prefer doing the physical restoration specific to the speech mechanism. However, the physical therapist might incorporate appropriate treatment tasks into the general therapy regime. The ideal situation involves an overlap of roles because the speech pathologist rarely has the setting or the expertise to explore body position and the physical therapist may need guidance in choice of speech movements relative to difficulty, developmental level, and importance to speech. Obvious precautions should be taken relative to medical diagnoses and to ensure that strengthening and positioning

maintain muscle balance and symmetry. Physical therapy activities must be designed with the purposeful goal of improving the physiological support for verbal communication. The speech pathologist will simultaneously attempt to maximize the client's use of the impaired neuromotor system for speech production. Feedback should be sufficient to allow for generalization. In other words, appropriate sensory input must be given to allow the client to develop an awareness of the movements being facilitated or trained.

The physical management of *flaccid dysarthria* requires increasing muscle tone, strength, and range through facilitation techniques such as brushing, icing, and controlled response elicitation (using taste),[48] or through techniques such as biofeedback.[16] Oral movements can be practiced in positions that allow gravity to assist in the motion (such as producing tongue tip movements with head bent forward or prone), then slowly guiding the tongue tip to work against gravity, then against active resistance. Increased activity of hypotonic speech musculature is observed when clients exert effort elsewhere, as in lifting themselves off a chair, bridging, or sustaining a pushing action with arms against resistance. Vocalizing during such activities sometimes allows the client to learn the feeling of modified tone and may heighten reflexive closure of the vocal folds. Incorporation of such speech activities into general strengthening programs and transfer training can be helpful and efficient.

Muscle strengthening, increasing speed and range of motion, and inhibiting excess tone are the primary targets of treatment in *spastic dysarthria*. Relaxation, slow stroking, and pressure have been recommended as inhibitory techniques[48] as well as exploring effects of postures on muscle tone and speech. Jaw shaking for relaxation and working from the vegetative function of chewing to build volitional motor function has been recommended.[25] Exercises to increase control, such as sustained, relaxed exhalation and voicing, are used. While exercise programs geared to improve speed and range of motion (e.g., repetitive tongue tip elevations) are underway, the speech pathologist often teaches the client to slow down the rate of speech. These procedures are not contradictory. A similar circumstance might be seen when the hemiplegic client is attempting to increase speed and strength of lower-extremity movement yet is required to walk slowly and deliberately to accommodate the remaining neuromotor deficit. Biofeedback is a possible technique for reducing hypertonicity and undesired overflow activity.[52]

The client with *ataxic dysarthria* usually shows improved speech as general stability increases. The primary goal with ataxic speakers is improving the coordination of the speech mechanism. Imposing conscious cortical control over the movements for speech seems to improve the quality and intelligibility of the speech output.

The management of the individual with *hypokinetic dys-*

arthria requires increasing the range of motion and decreasing the excess tone caused by rigidity. Movement seems to increase when the client is asked to exert extra effort. For instance, Parkinson's clients can be asked to take very deep breaths and exaggerate their speech. Using multiple input and output systems often helps, such as touching a colored square each time a word is spoken.[33,46] Movement improves speech and speech improves movement. Therefore gait or exercise activities might logically incorporate speech. Answering a question by saying one word with each step or counting repetitions out loud are examples of this.

The treatment of the client with *hyperkinetic dysarthria* will focus largely on inhibiting involuntary movements that interfere with speech. Postures and positioning will be of utmost importance in eliminating abnormal activity and tone during speech exercises, and stabilization may be necessary when movements of the extremities continually trigger mandible or tongue extension. To isolate tongue and lip movements, the jaw can be stabilized with a bite block. Relaxation and sensory stimulation or biofeedback[22] may be useful in inhibiting excess movement in some cases.

Developmental communication disorders

While the speech pathologist will evaluate and plan actual language remediation, when needed, the physical therapist, other allied health professionals, and family members should assist in language learning. Knowledge of development of communication and learning theory will prepare clinicians for this assistive role.

Several general principles are helpful in approaching language learning. Easy language structures for adults may not be easy language structures for children. Language used with children should be simplified according to developmental levels. The young child is more likely to imitate "Push ball" than "Who is funny?" Therefore simple structures and words geared to the child's functional level can be incorporated into therapy in the form of parallel talk. The therapist describes what is going on ("roll the ball . . . bounce the ball") and reinforces any attempts at communication or imitation by the child. Correcting should be avoided. Rather, positive reinforcement is used to model closer and closer productions. Copying the child immediately after a behavior is produced often encourages increased production. Repetition improves learning. The same words and phrases can be repeated over and over in context by the therapist ("roll ball . . . push ball . . . ball fell down") during routine activities. Providing appropriate speech models and rewarding attempts to repeat or respond are preferable to requiring the child to say "ball." Imitation of speech in the absence of meaningful context is not useful.[7]

The situation and interaction should be structured to motivate communication. Encouraging independence by allowing choices increases a sense of self and desire to control the environment. All forms of communication should be encouraged, such as gestures, facial expression, and eye contact. Songs and rhythm can be combined with movement to tap right hemisphere processing. The therapist should maximize input by combining auditory, gestural, facial, and inflection information.

Learning proceeds best when the sensory input is adequate to build associations. Combining speech with active motion can reinforce concepts. Real objects can be used to provide tactile, visual, and auditory input, such as banging, throwing, or rolling.[8] Assuming various positions in relation to objects assists in integrating experiences while the therapist verbalizes. Young children can be guided into conceptualizing object permanence, and building early symbolic memory with simple hide-and-seek activities. Older children can build concepts of directionality by crawling *into* the box and sitting *on* the box.[7] Motion allows active involvement and often helps focus attention. Therefore activities geared appropriately to the child's developmental level are natural for physical therapy. Treatment should be dynamic, with texture, sight, and sound integrated into motion. Sensory and perceptual integration will promote language learning. Using sand, water, colorful toys, or music can motivate and heighten input.[1]

A note of caution is in order: the clinician must determine which sensory stimulation is consistent with learning and which interferes with learning. Children with auditory or tactile defensiveness may need specific work on reducing this defensiveness. Insufficiently inhibited sensory input in one modality can interrupt learning in another modality.[1] On the other hand, sensory stimuli can facilitate learning in another modality. Such is the case when we remember someone's name (auditory) by remembering a distinctive facial feature (visual). The amount of sensory stimulation can help or hinder language processing also. A listener usually attends more carefully to a question accompanied by a soft touch on the arm; the listener would probably miss the question entirely if simultaneously punched in the arm! Exploring the type and amount of sensory stimulation that facilitates motor and language learning can have far-reaching effects. Ayres[1] has observed that vestibular stimulation contributes to sensory integration, often elicits vocalization, and serves as a precursor to more cognitive approaches to learning.

Constant awareness of the many variables that influence learning must be maintained. Nonverbal information projected by the therapist can influence the child's responses. For instance, a loud voice or a fearful, tense clinician inadvertently might increase hyperactivity in a child. Activities building fine hand control may contribute to motor planning overall. However, speaking during such activities can be an interference unless the speaking activity is expressly geared to mediate motor planning.[39,40,44]

Treatment considerations in confusion and dementia

Frequently the bizarre or tangential verbalizations and apparent learning problems of the confused or demented patient make structured treatment a considerable challenge. In such cases, several general principles for communicating with the individual might prove valuable. First, the goal is rarely to actually "teach" better or more appropriate communication, but rather to provide an atmosphere that lightens the demands on the ravaged "cognitive system" so that the individual can use what cognitive "strengths" remain. For example, providing a predictable structure (treatment at the same time each day with the same activities and instructions) will minimize the demands on memory, allowing the individual to focus mental energy on acquiring the target skill. Also consistency, repetition, and redundancy in verbal and nonverbal communication can facilitate memory and new learning. The tendency to engage in normal "chit chat" with the confused patient during an activity can actually promote increased confusion and agitation; if this appears to be the case, using simple descriptions of what is being done while working with the individual might help inhibit misunderstanding and orient the client to the activity. Spoken instructions or information might be supplemented with simple written instructions to facilitate understanding and attention. Body language and speech tone that is gentle and supportive can also reduce confusion. Overstimulation can occur easily and is frequently evidenced in increased agitation and confused language; reduction in the amount of stimulation might consist of eliminating background noise or eliminating verbal descriptions. In addition, in some cases anticipating clients' needs rather than requiring them to communicate a need can help lighten the demands.

Conversing with the confused or demented client is a true art. Many clinicians feel the need to correct and "teach" the individual by pointing out memory errors or repeatedly "testing" orientation. In fact, this approach serves more to discourage communication than to facilitate it. Reality orientation should be provided in a natural, supportive, conversational manner; orientation information should be given to, rather than requested of, the client. Redirecting is preferable to challenging or calling attention to inappropriate, inaccurate, or tangential verbalization. Topics that the client enjoys and remembers should be encouraged even if they represent remote memories. It is often quite satisfying and reinforcing to the client to talk about the same happy memory every day. Although possibly tedious to the clinician, reinforcement of these lucid memories can form a nonthreatening framework for introducing new information.

Treatment considerations in adult aphasia

The primary goal of the speech pathologist with the aphasic adult is to work toward functional communication. Language training is based on graded levels of difficulty and a variety of specific techniques, such as melodic intonation therapy[61] or visual action therapy.[34] Normal speech and language is rarely achieved in cases of residual aphasia. The goal of the physical therapist is to maximize the client's use of remaining communication ability, provide a motivating and supportive setting to avoid development of maladaptive attitudes, and stimulate the reorganization of physiological processes for language. Because management varies considerably with the type and severity of the aphasia, the physical and occupational therapists will want to work closely with the speech pathologist.

To maximize comprehension in the aphasic adult, certain general principles should be followed. The client's level of auditory comprehension will dictate the alterations needed in communication. One common error seems to be assuming no comprehension and excluding the client from the conversation. Another problem occurs when it is assumed that the client understands everything. Usually this type of client receives visual and inflectional information or responds in a socially appropriate manner with only partial understanding. The therapist must be sure that the client is not receiving faulty or damaging information. Distraction and background noise will interfere with auditory comprehension. This includes conflicting tactile or visual input as well as noise. Asking a client an important question while ranging a painful arm is not conducive to comprehension. Aphasic individuals have difficulty switching tasks. Therefore the therapist must be sure that sufficient time and information (visual, gestural, and auditory) are provided to mark a change in task or topic. Speaking from the front at eye level facilitates comprehension. When important information is given, conversation should be one-on-one. Involving several people, as is done on medical rounds, requires rapid switching, changing speaking distances, and distraction. Gestures, situational cues, visual prompts, voice inflection, and facial expression can enhance or destroy comprehension. The client who hears a loud, clipped "Sit on the mat" may comprehend anger rather than the direction; the client's negative response may appear confused or hostile to the imperceptive clinician. Alerting cues can be used, such as a soft touch, verbalizing the client's name, or using a starter word ("Now . . . push my hand").

Communication should be maintained in a calm, matter-of-fact manner. Sentences should be short and simple; phrasing should allow for processing pauses. The tendency seems to be for people to ask a question, then panic and rephrase, repeat, or answer themselves immediately. Above all, the client should have extra time to listen and to talk. Directions can be formulated to use high-imagery action words, assuming there is right hemisphere processing, and axial commands such as "Pretend you're *swimming*" versus "Move your arms."[69] The organization of proximal versus distal muscle groups seems to have a language correlate. That is, axial commands seem to be easier than distal commands. Altering speech to maximize communication and responsiveness should become a habit. For instance, the following direction could be confusing: "I want you to put your arms over my shoulders and I'm going to lift you up. Then I want you to pivot your feet and we'll lower you onto the mat." This could be rephrased to: "Watch me (gesture) . . . we will *stand up* . . . *turn* . . . and *sit down*" (demonstrate as each verb is said).

Communication is a social, interactive activity. People talk because they have something to say. Unfortunately, many people seem to forget the rules of polite conversation when confronted with a communication-disordered client. Asking an acquaintance "What is my name?" or holding up a banana and asking "What is this?" would be considered bizarre behavior indeed at a dinner party. It is no less inappropriate with an aphasic client. The skill of conversing without making excessive demands enhances the enjoyment of working with aphasic people. Relating an interesting story with questions or comments interspersed or talking about activities without directly requesting a response allows the client to participate when able. Questions can be phrased to allow "yes," "no," or pointing responses. Asking a question that requires a complicated answer and then waiting for a response is insensitive. Instead of asking the client with severe expressive problems "What did you do in Occupational Therapy?" several questions and comments can be used to converse: "Did you go to Occupational Therapy?"; "How *was* OT today?"; "Hard work, I'll bet."; "Did you do some arm work (gesture)?"; "Exercises can be tiring!" Although the details of the questions may not be fully understood, the interaction is reinforcing and social.

Encouraging expressive language should not be restricted to verbal communication. If speech is not available, ask the client to show a response. Upper-extremity gestures sometimes facilitate verbalization. This does not imply that aphasic clients have normal use of pantomime or signs. All channels (writing, speaking, and gesturing) are affected to some degree in aphasia. However, speech pathologists often pair hand movements with verbalization to build verbal expression in nonfluent aphasic clients. Voluntary movement of an extremity promotes neurophysiological reactions in the contralateral cortex.[38] Perhaps activation of the anterior speech areas in the brain is enhanced when neighboring motor and premotor hand areas are activated.

Attempts at speech should not be corrected per se. If the therapist does not understand, an honest statement to that effect or request for repeat is usually best. Sometimes narrowing the field with yes/no questions will help: "Is it about a person? . . . family? . . . your son?" Sometimes tactfully changing the subject avoids frustration when failure continues. When the therapist understands but the utterance was faulty, modeling the correct production unobtrusively is suggested. For example, the client points to the cane and says "My coat"; the therapist might say "OK, here's your cane." Helpful communication strategies are discussed further by Lubinski.[45]

Alternative communication systems

A variety of alternatives to verbal communication are available when speech is not possible.[6,59,65,66] The type and complexity of the system will be dictated by physical, linguistic, and cognitive requirements. The financial situation and attitude of the client will influence the choice also. Systems in popular use include sign languages and communication boards.

Obviously, sign languages require fairly fine control of the upper extremities, although simple systems have been adapted for one-handed use with apraxia of speech.[60] Adequate memory and language is needed to learn the signs. Most sign systems are used by the hearing impaired community. However, the increased use of signs to facilitate language development in autistic, mentally retarded, and aphasic clients[49,60,71] suggests that physical and occupational therapists may be called upon to provide information on praxis and fine hand control as prerequisite to sign usage.

Communication boards—surfaces upon which letters, objects, or actions are represented—range from simple xeroxed alphabet or picture boards to expensive computerized electronic devices.[59,65] The nonverbal client picks out the pictures or words that represent the thought to be communicated. Communication boards can be small, portable lap boards or large systems. A full evaluation by a team of professionals is the best approach because an inappropriate choice is not only a waste of time and money but also an emotionally debilitating experience for the client. The psychologist can determine nonverbal memory, intelligence, emotional maturity, and attitude of the client. The speech pathologist can determine the interactive needs and language capacities. The physical and occupational therapists can determine sitting balance and tolerance, fine and gross motor control, appropriate method of responding (pointing, arm press, head pointer), best positions for responding, placement of the board for maximizing motor function, and fatigability.

Psychosocial implications of communication disorders

As has been mentioned previously, communication is social. However, the reverse is probably more accurate—society is formed through communication. The individual who does not communicate normally is not easily assimilated into society. People tend to feel uncomfortable and avoid communication-impaired individuals. Reactions often reflect prejudices, such as "People who do not speak well are retarded or crazy." Reactions of this kind promote feelings of self-doubt and inadequacy. The need to talk about feelings often goes unfulfilled. In a typical day in a normal person's life, basic needs are communicated quickly and easily. Most speech serves as social, emotional, or intellectual stimulation. The person with a significant communication problem has difficulty communicating even the most basic needs. The result can be embarrassment, discomfort, and humiliation. The enjoyment of expressing one's ideas and opinions and revealing intelligence and emotion is unavailable. If family and friends fail to provide affection and understanding, withdrawal from contact with others often occurs. The result is depression, loneliness, and anxiety.

In many cases the emotional difficulties caused by verbal language problems serve to further reduce the adequacy of communication. Anxiety and stress diminish communicative performance. Reduced communication also affects an individual's ability to participate in school, employment, and social activities. The families of aphasic clients often report that friends and social activities diminish markedly with the onset of aphasia. The communication disorder becomes a family problem and a financial problem. Professionals working with the communication disordered client should take into account these frustrations and fears. Physical therapists can provide a warm, supporting atmosphere, where attempts at communication are welcomed and feelings are accepted. Families can be counseled on the need to develop outside interests, to promote independence, and to foster feelings of self-worth. Communication is maximized when psychosocial difficulties have been minimized.

SUMMARY

Neurological disorders frequently involve deficits in some aspect of communication. Because communication is an integral aspect of behavior and learning, holistic treatment of the neurologically impaired client should include attention to hearing, speech, and language. Understanding communication and its disorders can add an exciting dimension to the practice of physical therapy. It is hoped that this chapter will serve as the scaffolding upon which the clinician can begin to build knowledge through further reading, observation, and interaction with experienced professionals in a team approach to rehabilitation.

REFERENCES

1. Ayres AJ: Sensory integration and learning disorders, Los Angeles, 1973, Western Psychological Services.
2. Basmajian J: Therapeutic exercise, Baltimore, 1978, Williams & Wilkins.
3. Bates E and others: The acquisition of performatives prior to speech, Merrill-Palmer Quart 21:205, 1975.
4. Bates E and others: From gesture to the first word: on cognitive and social prerequisites. In Lewis M and Rosenblum L, editors: Interaction, conversation and the development of language, New York, 1977, John Wiley & Sons, Inc.
5. Bayles K: Language and dementia. In Holland A, editor: Language disorders in adults, San Diego, 1984, College Hill Press.
6. Beukelman DR and Yorkston K: A communication system for the severely dysarthric speaker with an intact language system, J Speech Hear Disord 42:265, 1977.
7. Bloom L and Lahey M: Language development and language disorders, New York, 1978, John Wiley & Sons, Inc.
8. Bowerman M: Words and sentences: uniformity, individual variation and shifts over time in patterns of acquisition. In Minifie FD and Lloyd LL, editors: Communicative and cognitive abilities—early behavioral assessment, Baltimore, 1978, University Park Press.
9. Brookshire RH: An introduction to aphasia, Minneapolis, 1978, BRK Publishers.
10. Carr J and Shepherd R: Physiotherapy in disorders of the brain, London, 1980, William Heinemann Medical Books, Ltd.
11. Clark E: Some aspects of the conceptual basis for first language acquisition. In Schiefelbusch R and Lloyd L, editors: Language perspectives—acquisition, retardation and intervention, Baltimore, 1974, University Park Press.
12. Cohen IB and Salapatek P: Infant perception: from sensation to cognition. Vol 2. Perception of space, speech and sound, New York, 1975, Academic Press, Inc.
13. Condon W and Sander L: Neonate movement is synchronized with adult speech: interactional participation and language acquisition, Science 183:99, 1974.
14. Creech RJ and others: Oral sensation and perception in dysarthric adults, Percept Mot Skills 37:167, 1973.
15. Critchly M: Aphasiology and other aspects of language, London, 1970, Edward Arnold, Ltd.
16. Daniel B: EMG feedback and recovery of facial and speech gestures following neuroanastomosis, J Speech Hear Disord 43:9, 1978.
17. Daniels L and Warthingham C: Muscle testing, Philadelphia, 1980, WB Saunders Co.
18. Daniloff R and others: The physiology of speech and hearing: an introduction, Englewood Cliffs, NJ, 1980, Prentice-Hall, Inc.
19. Darby J: The interaction between speech and disease. In Darby J, editor: Speech evaluation in medicine, New York, 1981, Grune & Stratton, Inc.
20. Darley FL: A retrospective view: aphasia, J Speech Hear Disord 42:161, 1977.
21. Darley FL and others: Motor speech disorders, Philadelphia, 1975, WB Saunders Co.
22. Farrar WB: Using electromyographic biofeedback in treating orofacial dyskinesia, J Prosthet Dent 4:384, 1976.
23. Ferguson C: Learning to pronounce: the earliest stages of phonological development in the child. In Minifie FD and Lloyd LL, editors: Communicative and cognitive abilities—early behavioral assessment, Baltimore, 1978, University Park Press.
24. Flower R: Neurodevelopmental disorders in children. In Darby J, editor: Speech evaluation in medicine, New York, 1981, Grune & Stratton, Inc.
25. Froeschels E: Chewing method as therapy, Arch Otolaryngol 61:427, 1952.
26. Gardner H: The shattered mind, New York, 1974, Random House, Inc.
27. Gardner H and others: Comprehension and appreciation of humorous material following brain damage, Brain 98:399, 1975.
28. Goodglass H and Kaplan E: The assessment of aphasia and related disorders, Philadelphia, 1972, Lea & Febiger.
29. Griffin KM: Swallowing training for dysphagic patients, Arch Phys Med Rehabil 55:467, 1974.
30. Groher M: Dysphagia: diagnosis and management, Boston, 1984, Butterworth Publishers.
31. Hagen C: Language disorders in head trauma. In Holland A, editor: Language disorders in adults, San Diego, 1984, College Hill Press.
32. Hardcastle W: Physiology of speech production, London, 1976, Academic Press, Inc.
33. Helm N: Management of palilalia with a pacing board, J Speech Hear Disord 44:350, 1979.
34. Helm N and Benson F: Visual action therapy for global aphasia, Un-

published paper presented to the Academy of Aphasia, Chicago, 1978.

35. Kendall H and others: Muscles: testing and function, Baltimore, 1971, Williams & Wilkins.
36. Kimura D: Manual activity during speaking. I. Right handers. II. Left handers, Neuropsychologia 11:45, 1973.
37. Kimura D and Archibald Y: Motor functions of the left hemisphere, Brain 97:337, 1974.
38. Kinsbourne M, editor: Asymmetrical function of the brain, Cambridge, England, 1978, Cambridge University Press.
39. Kinsbourne M and Cook J: Generalized and lateralized effects of concurrent verbalization on a unimanual skill, Q J Exp Psychol 23:341, 1971.
40. Kinsbourne M and Murray J: The effect of cerebral dominance on time sharing between speaking and tapping by preschool children, Child Dev 46:240, 1975.
41. Larsen GL: Rehabilitation for dysphagia paralytica, J Speech Hear Disord 37:187, 1972.
42. Levitt S: Treatment of cerebral palsy and motor delay, London, 1977, Blackwell Scientific Publications, Ltd.
43. Logemann J: Evaluation and treatment of swallowing disorders, San Diego, 1983, College Hill Press.
44. Lomas J and Kimura D: Intrahemispheric interaction between speaking and sequential manual activity, Neuropsychologia 14:23, 1976.
45. Lubinski R: Environmental language intervention. In Chapey R, editor: Language intervention strategies in adult aphasia, Baltimore, 1981, Williams & Wilkins.
46. Luria AR: Traumatic aphasia, The Hague, 1970, Mouton Publishers.
47. Macaluso-Haynes S: Developmental apraxia of speech. In Johns D, editor: Clinical management of neurogenic communicative disorders, Boston, 1978, Little, Brown & Co.
48. May A and Hudgens D: Selected proprioceptive neuromuscular facilitation techniques in dysarthria treatment, Unpublished paper presented to the American Speech and Hearing Association Annual Conference, Chicago, 1977.
49. Miller A and Miller EE: Cognitive developmental training with elevated boards and sign language, J Autism Child Schizophr 3:65, 1973.
50. Minifie F and Lloyd L: Communicative and cognitive abilities: early behavioral assessment, Baltimore, 1978, University Park Press.
51. Mueller H: Facilitating feeding and prespeech. In Pearson P and Williams C, editors: Physical therapy services in the developmental disabilities, Springfield, Ill, 1972, Charles C Thomas, Publisher.
52. Netsell R and Cleeland CS: Modification of lip hypertonia in dysarthria using EMG feedback, J Speech Hear Disord 38:131, 1973.
53. Rembisz L and Gribin S: Neuromuscular facilitation therapeutic techniques in treating the dysarthric patient, Exhibit presented at the American Speech and Hearing Association Annual Convention, Washington, DC, 1975.
54. Rembisz L and Gribin S: Neuromuscular facilitation and techniques in treating dysarthria for the cerebral palsied, Exhibit presented at the American Speech and Hearing Association Annual Convention, Chicago, 1977.
55. Rosenbek J and others: Oral sensation and perception in apraxia of speech and aphasia, J Speech Hear Disord 16:22, 1973.
56. Rosenberg S: Disorders of first language development: trends in research and theory. In Gollin E, editor: Malformations in development: biological and psychological sources and consequences, New York, 1984, Academic Press.
57. Rutherford D and McCall G: Testing oral sensation and perception in persons with dysarthria. In Bosma J, editor: Symposium on oral sensation and perception, Springfield, Ill, 1967, Charles C Thomas, Publisher.
58. Scott CM and Ringel RL: The effects of motor and sensory disruption on speech: a description of articulation, J Speech Hear Res 14:819, 1971.
59. Silverman J: Communication for the speechless, Englewood Cliffs, NJ, 1980, Prentice-Hall, Inc.
60. Skelly M: Amer-Ind gestural code based on universal American Indian hand talk, New York, 1979, Elsevier North Holland, Inc.
61. Sparks RW: Melodic intonation therapy. In Chapey R, editor: Language intervention strategies in adult aphasia, Baltimore, 1981, Williams & Wilkins.
62. Springer S and Deutsch G: Left brain, right brain, San Francisco, 1981, WH Freeman & Co, Publishers.
63. Strub RL and Black FW: The mental status examination in neurology, Philadelphia, 1977, FA Davis Co.
64. Szekeres S, Ylvisaker M, and Holland A: Cognitive rehabilitation therapy: a framework for intervention. In Ylvisaker M, editor: Head injury rehabilitation: children and adolescents, San Diego, 1985, College Hill Press.
65. Vanderheiden GC: Non-vocal communication resource book, Baltimore, 1970, University Park Press.
66. Vanderheiden GC and Grilley K: Non-vocal communication techniques and aids for the severely physically handicapped, Baltimore, 1976, University Park Press.
67. Vaughn G and Clark RM: Speech facilitation: extraoral and intraoral stimulation technique for improvement of articulation skills, Springfield, Ill, 1979, Charles C Thomas, Publisher.
68. Wertz RT: Neuropathologies of speech and language. In Johns D, editor: Clinical management of neurogenic communicative disorders, Boston, 1978, Little, Brown & Co.
69. West J: Heightening the action imagery of materials used in aphasia treatment. In Brookshire RH, editor: Clinical aphasiology conference proceedings, Minneapolis, 1978, BRK Publishers.
70. Westlake H and Rutherford D: Speech therapy for the cerebral palsied, Chicago, 1961, National Society for Crippled Children.
71. Wilbur RB: American sign language and sign system, Baltimore, 1970, University Park Press.
72. Zemlin WR: Speech and hearing science, anatomy and physiology, Englewood Cliffs, NJ, 1968, Prentice-Hall, Inc.

ADDITIONAL READINGS

Beasley D and Davis GA: Aging, communication processes and disorders, New York, 1980, Grune & Stratton, Inc.
Bradford L and Hardy W: Hearing and hearing impairment, New York, 1979, Grune & Stratton, Inc.
Leitch S: A child learns to speak, Springfield, Ill, 1977, Charles C Thomas, Publisher.
Simmons-Martin A and Calvert D: Parent-infant intervention; communication disorders, New York, 1979, Grune & Stratton, Inc.
Werner H and Kaplan B: Symbol formation, New York, 1963, John Wiley & Sons, Inc.

APPENDIX
Audiovisual resources

Audio Seminar in Motor Speech Disorders (audio cassettes):

WB Saunders Company
West Washington Square
Philadelphia, PA 19105

Neuromuscular Facilitation Techniques in Treating Dysarthria (slides) and A Feeding Program for the Dysarthric Patient (slides):

Director, Education Department
Children's Specialized Hospital
New Providence Road
Westfield-Mountainside, NJ 07091

Chapter 25

DISORDERS OF THE VISUAL PERCEPTUAL SYSTEM

Mary Jane Bouska, Nancy A. Kauffman, and Steven E. Marcus

Many children and adults with brain dysfunction exhibit some form of visual perceptual disorder. These disorders are common in learning disability, attention deficit disorder, and mental retardation. They often accompany brain lesions resulting from vascular or anoxic conditions such as traumatic head injury, stroke, tumor, and cerebral palsy. Functional sequelae of such deficits can be extremely debilitating. They may include difficulties with reading, writing, drawing, dressing, eating, locating objects, filling out forms, recognizing people, finding one's way within or outside a building, driving, and many other activities essential to daily living.

Unfortunately, these disorders may appear rather subtle in nature. A cursory look at the child in the classroom or the adult on the street may reveal a "normally" functioning individual with no "obvious" disabilities, yet when asked to perform any task requiring visual perceptual processing, the individual is very slow or unable to complete the task. A child in school may be slow in reading and writing and have difficulty with mathematical and spatial concepts and with games and sports. In the rehabilitation hospital a client who has perceptual disorders may also have obvious deficits such as spasticity and paralysis of an arm and leg, aphasia, or gait ataxia. When engaged in physical, occupational, and speech therapy, this client may appear confused and unable to cooperate and learn as efficiently as the rehabilitation team has projected. These individuals are too often labeled "confused," "clumsy," "anxious," "uncooperative," and "unmotivated" by health professionals and educators unaware of the myriad disorders of the visual perceptual system *directly* responsible for such performance inadequacies. The astute clinician is always attuned to the possible presence of visual perceptual disorders in any individual with a diagnosis of central nervous system (CNS) damage. If such damage is suspected, the clinician should screen for specific deficits or refer the client to a team member capable of performing visual and visual perceptual screening, that is, the occupational therapist or psychologist. Any abnormal finding should stimulate further referral for a comprehensive visual or visual perceptual assessment by one or more of the following specialists: a psychologist or an occupational therapist who specializes in these disorders, a neuropsychologist, a neuroophthalmologist, or a developmental or behavioral optometrist.

Within the context of this chapter, perception is defined as the dynamic process of receiving (perceiving) the environment through sensory impulses and translating those impulses into meaning based on a previously developed understanding of that environment. Perception, of course, implies the simultaneous and integrated use of all sensory systems, that is, auditory, tactile, kinesthetic, vestibular, olfactory, and visual. Perception is most efficient when all sensory systems simultaneously contribute as the brain cumulates millisecond-to-millisecond sensory data. Through the process of intermodality association, primary and associative sensory information is exchanged and related among basic sensory regions with the brain. Physiological evidence has indicated that multisensory convergence on single neurons occurs in both the cerebral cortex as well as in subcortical centers.[31] Perception is clearly a complex multisensory phenomenon.

Before evaluation and treatment can be planned, it is essential for the clinician to understand what is required for perception to take place. Gibson and Levin[47] define perception as the continual process of extracting information from stimuli emanating from the objects, places, and events in the world around us. During development this process becomes more refined. It is characterized by increasing specificity of discrimination or *differentiation* as perceptual learning occurs. First, perceptual learning is adaptive to the person's needs—for example, a thirsty person more readily notices the water bottle on the cluttered table. Second, it involves active search behavior. If the water bottle is not readily apparent, it will be searched for. Third, it allows selective ability to extract that information which has utility for decreasing uncertainty. If the water bottle is opaque and of an unfamiliar shape, the thirsty person will selectively perceive the water condensation on the outside of the bottle, revealing its cold liquid contents.

Visual perception should be viewed as one part of the perceptual process. Because the human is so highly visual in orientation to the world, the word *perception* itself is often erroneously associated with vision alone. Although the major focus of this chapter is on disorders within the visual perceptual system, it should remain paramount in the reader's mind that one perceptual system has been "dissected" from the functional perceptual mechanism to delineate disorders within it. (For a discussion of disorders of perceptual systems, see Chapter 11.)

The following example illustrates the interrelationship of visual perception with other sensory channels. If you drop a penny on the kitchen floor, the first perceptual response is most likely a tactile clue that the penny has left your hand. This is followed by an auditory perceptual response as the penny hits the floor. Fairly high-level auditory discrimination is carried out as you instantaneously make spatial judgments as to "where and how" the penny

sounded. That is, did it roll, did it sound near or far when the noise stopped, was there any sound? At this point active visual perception begins as the head and eyes move in various combinations to scan the appropriate part of the environment in search of the penny's perceived location. During the eye movements, information is selectively gathered via the fovea and peripheral visual field. Simultaneously visual-spatial discriminations are made to select the configuration known as "penny" from the spatial background. When you spot the penny, your eye fixates on it; based on visual localization, your head, trunk, and limb movements are synergistically activated to pick up the penny (gross visual-motor coordination). Your eye continues to fixate as your fingers approach the penny to facilitate visual feedback for fine readjustment of finger placement and position (fine visual-motor coordination), and you touch and pick up the penny.

The visual perceptual aspect of task performance requires very specialized abilities,[64] including the ability to:

1. Respond to stimuli incident on all parts of the retina and to adjust focusing for far and near (visual orientation)
2. Accurately move the eyes and head to gather information (oculomotor and vestibuloocular control)
3. Meaningfully interpret the information (visual perceptual ability)
4. Quickly and accurately move a limb in response to a visual cue (visual motor ability)
5. Integrate *1* through *4*

The functional visual perceptual system includes the eye, the oculomotor muscles and pathways, the optic nerve, the optic tract, the occipital cortex, and the associative areas of the cerebral cortex (parietal and temporal lobes). Peripheral or central lesions at any point in this neuraxis can result in visual perceptual deficits.

VISUAL DEVELOPMENT: AN OPTOMETRIC VIEWPOINT

Vision is a cognitive process involving the converting of the raw data of sight into meaningful information. It is the tool that enables us to expand awareness beyond our arms' reach, a vicarious projection of our ability to feel and touch into a limitless conceptual spatial world. Vision is considered the dominant sensory process in humans. During development it becomes integrated with all other sensory and motor processes, including posture and balance. It ranks with speech in complexity and passes through comparable developmental phases.[40,42] Vision needs the stimulation of light to develop and establish the progressive myelination of the optic nerve. Toward the end of the second and beginning of the third month after a baby is born, the structural integrity of three subsystems of the visual process are established: accommodation, oculo-motor, and convergence.[80]

Accommodation: the identification subsystem

Accommodation is the dynamic process by which the crystalline lens of the eye changes shape (curvature) to adjust focus for objects at different distances. This is accomplished by the zonular fibers that are attached to the ciliary muscles (Fig. 25-1). When the eye is at rest or fixed on a distant target, the zonular fibers are tense; this keeps the lens flat (concave). When the eye is fixed on a near target, the ciliary muscles contract, which releases the tension on the zonular fibers and thereby on the lens. This allows the lens to become more convex so that the light is bent to stimulate photoreceptors in the retinal plane. Accommodation is a lenticular-retinal-cortical process used by the organism to obtain clear vision, hence the term *identification subsystem*. The resolving power of the eye as an optical instrument is measured by the smallest visual angle at which two objects can be distinguished separately. This is called the minimum separable distance and is approximately 40 to 60 seconds of arc.[1]

In optical terminology the distance an image may move within the retina and still not produce a perceptible blur is called *the depth of focus*. If an object is moved closer to the eye than the depth of focus permits, the points of light falling on the photoreceptors subtend an arc greater than 60 seconds. To obtain a clear focus under these circum-stances, either the dioptric power of the eye must increase or the eyeball must become longer. It is obvious that the human eye cannot alter its axial length at any given moment; therefore this change of focusing power must take place by changing the dioptric power of the refracting surface. This change, then, is brought about by an automatic altering of the shape of the crystalline lens whenever a change of dioptric power is needed.

Accommodation is a part of the greater visceral nervous system of the body, operating characteristically through smooth muscle and having to do almost exclusively with the internal environment. Visceral muscle action is relatively slow and practically indefatigable. Accommodation changes with the age of the individual, who is assumed to have sufficient accommodative ability when amplitude of accommodation is twice the dioptric working distance.

The act of accommodation is a complex pattern that is made up of many subpatterns: tonic accommodation, aberrational accommodation, convergence accommodation, and psychic accommodation.

Dual innervation of the ciliary muscle occurs through mutually antagonistic sympathetic and parasympathetic nervous systems. It is postulated that negative accommodation is mediated via the sympathetic nervous system and positive accommodation via the parasympathetic nervous system.[1] According to Netter[72] the intrinsic muscles of the eye are innervated mainly through parasympathetic nerves. Sympathetic nerves are distributed only to blood vessels and radial muscles of the iris, which constrict and dilate the pupil. Parasympathetic fibers reach the eye from the ciliary ganglion via the short ciliary nerve. The preganglionic neuron concerned with the parasympathetic innervation of the eye is located in the Edinger-Westphal nucleus, which is incorporated in the nucleus of the oculomotor nerve. This axon reaches the ciliary ganglion through the oculomotor nerve. Postganglionic parasympathetic fibers derived from the ciliary ganglion are distributed to the muscles of the ciliary body and the circular muscles of the iris.

It is our view that parasympathetic stimulation triggers the learning of a spatial range within the object of regard called *the range of positive relative accommodation*. The autonomic system counterpart of the parasympathetic stimulation creates the learning of the spatial range beyond the object of regard called *the range of negative relative accommodation*. This resultant spatial range contributes to our ability to sustain accommodative effort for protracted periods of time at a fixed distance.

Accommodation serves as the physiological component of the greater subprocess of vision called *identification*. Getman[41] states that the normal infant's first manipulative actions are the mouthing acts. At this stage of development the lips and tongue explore and begin the identification of the outside world. Next the mouth and hand combine, and in time, the hand and eye do the manipulating.

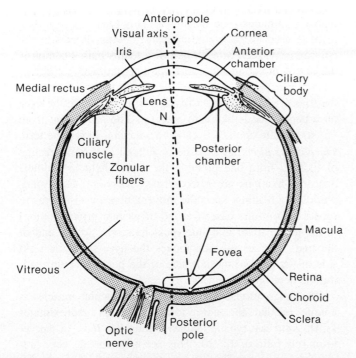

Fig. 25-1. Horizontal section of the eye. (Modified from Wolff E: Anatomy of the eye and orbit, ed 7, London, 1976, HK Lewis & Co, Ltd.)

These basic eye-hand combinations give children confirmation of the direction and spatial results of their own movements. The advancing integrations of visual and tactile inspection and manipulation give them further information on the size, shape, and texture of environmental contents. Through practice they develop recognition of likenesses and differences, and the elaboration of these recognitions allows them to combine, compare, and categorize. As hand-movement patterning produces dexterity and visual recognition of likes and differences expands, the foundations for primitive symbolism are laid. Concurrently, as children develop auditory associations, the visual recognitions and identifications provide them with a primitive visual language relationship. Out of these elaborations of the identification subsystem—which start with mouthing, progress to handling, are elaborated still further into visual recognition, and are finally matched with auditory patterns—comes the basis for symbolic learning.[41]

Oculomotor: the selective attention and information-gathering subsystem

The human eye is one of the most complex motor organs in the body. In fact, the only part of the eye that is sensory in nature is the retina. The retina is anatomically divided into five neural zones, each of which is traceable through the optic nerve and into the different terminal areas of the brain. The first (and major) zone is that of the macular fibers, which consist predominantly of neurons activated by cones. The others consist of each of the four quadrants: superior nasal, superior temporal, inferior nasal, and inferior temporal, which surround the macular area and which are composed predominantly of neurons activated by the rods. The peripheral area of the retina is dense in rods and is specialized for seeing in decreased illumination. The more peripherally the retina is stimulated, the less acute the discrimination becomes. Therefore the blur and its location within the peripheral retinal quadrants tend to inform the central processing mechanism how far off the fovea any particular area of stimulation may be. For example, when visually searching for a ball in the playroom, one moves the eyes until a blurred outline of the ball is seen in, for example, the right inferior temporal field. This blurred image and its location on the retina then lead the next eye movement directly toward the ball for further discrimination by the fovea.

Minkowski[71] states that movements of the eyeballs exist in the fetus, even before the opening of the eyelids. These movements depend on output coming from vestibular centers. During the fifth gestational month myelination of the vestibular central pathways and of posteriolongitudinal fasciculus is already complete. Therefore ocular movements, when produced by vestibular influences (head turning), occur several months earlier than do the ocular movements elicited by light stimulation acting on the retina after birth. The fully developed vestibular-ocular pathways control conjugate eye movements reflexly in response to head movement and position in space. These pathways enable the eyes to remain fixed on a stationary object while the head and body are moving. Functionally, this keeps the fields of vision stable for perceptual interpretation.[49]

Eye movements begin from primary position (midposition) and move to secondary (superior and inferior) to tertiary (oblique) position of gaze within the orbit. The movements of each eye from the primary position into the secondary and tertiary positions of gaze are called *ductions*. The term *versions* is used to describe movements of both eyes in the same direction. Versions are conjunctive movements whereas vergences are disjunctive movements. Each eye is moved by the coordinated actions of the six extraocular muscles (Fig. 25-2). The ocular muscles are striated muscles and are generally considered to be voluntary muscles. The third cranial nerve, the oculomotor nerve, innervates the superior, internal, and inferior recti and the inferior oblique muscle. The fourth cranial nerve, the trochlear nerve, innervates the superior oblique muscle. The sixth cranial nerve, the abducens nerve, innervates the external rectus. The nuclei of all three nerves are adjacent to the medial longitudinal fasciculus.

Two types of eye movements are used to gather information from the environment. These include pursuit eye movements and saccadic fixations. Pursuit eye movements are often termed *tracking*. A pursuit eye movement involves the continued fixation on a moving object, implying a dynamic movement of the eye to keep the image of the object continuously on the fovea. This type of eye movement is used to track continuously moving objects in the environment, such as a fly ball or a tennis ball. Fixation is the act of directing the eye toward a stationary object of regard, causing the image of the object to be centered on the fovea. For example, a fixation is used to hold the eyes on a penny one is about to pick up. The movement from one fixation to another is called a *saccade*, hence the term *saccadic fixations*. A saccade is defined as a rapid change of fixation from one point in the visual field to another. Saccadic fixations are often termed *scanning*. For example, during reading, saccadic movement allows the eyes to progress from one part of a line of written print (fixation) to the next part of that line (next fixation). At the end of the line, a larger saccade moves the eyes from the right side of the page to the left side of the page to begin reading the new line of print.

The innervational control of the extraocular muscles is unique in that the nerve-to-muscle ratio approximates 1:10, whereas typical skeletal muscles have a nerve-to-muscle ratio of 1:120. This accounts for the very precise gradations possible in the motor control of eye movements. Precisely controlled fixation, saccadic movement, and pursuit skills allow humans to effectively gather information and to selectively attend to stimuli.

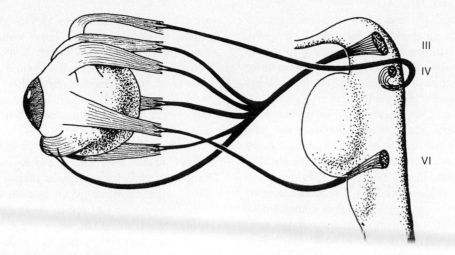

Fig. 25-2. Cranial nerves III, IV, and VI: Oculomotor, troclear, and abducent nerves and their innervation of the extraocular eye muscles. (Courtesy Smith Kline & French Laboratories, Philadelphia, Penn.)

Convergence: the centering spatial localization subsystem

The third primary subsystem of the visual process is convergence, which provides the mechanism for maintaining single vision. The convergence pattern controls the posturing of the eyes in their orbits and the centering of the total organism in its environment. It is controlled by the extraocular striated muscles innervated by the cranial nerves. The convergence pattern is of survival value to the organism since double vision could be catastrophic. Convergence is a complex pattern consisting of several subpatterns: tonic, fusional, accommodative, and psychic convergence. Tonic convergence is the position of the visual axis under conditions of dissociation with far-point fixation. Under these conditions convergence is maximally inhibited. Fusional convergence is the range of permanence in the convergence pattern resulting from a corresponding central representation in each occipital hemisphere. Accommodative convergence is that amount of convergence in action caused by innervation from accommodation. Psychic convergence is that amount of convergence stimulated because of the emotional and psychological reaction of the subject to the surrounding environment.

If an object approaches the observer and attention is demanded, the two eyes will converge on the target so that single vision is maintained. Eventually, the object will approach so close that the observer will no longer be able to maintain singleness of the object. This nearest point of single vision is called the *near point of convergence*. It is analogous to the physiological measurement of accommodative ability called the amplitude of accommodation. To effectively process visual information one must be able to quickly and accurately change alignment or centering from one point in space to another. This convergence-divergence mechanism must be accomplished with speed and accuracy, and a spatial range of convergence and divergence around a fixed point in space is essential for sustained visual attention. As with the accommodative range, the centering range must have latitude and there must be flexibility within this spatial range.

Convergence and accommodation are integrated visual behaviors, the extent and degree of this integration depend on learned relationships existing within the total person. This integration of the two patterns ensures single binocular clear vision for the environmental activities of the organism. When this integration is not adequate for the environmental demand placed on the organism, blurred or double vision will result. The very precise interaction between the autonomic function of accommodation and the skeletal muscle function of convergence creates a high-demand situation for the nervous system; this may account in great part for the many breakdowns seen in visual effectiveness. These breakdowns include blurred vision, double vision, discomfort or fatigue while sustaining visual attention, limited attention span, reductions in comprehension, stress while doing sustained close work, refractive errors, suppressions, and generalized ineffectiveness in visual information processing.

VISUAL PERCEPTUAL DEVELOPMENT

Day by day the developing infant and child learn to extract relevant information from the large number of visual stimuli in their environment. The normally developing child acquires an increased perceptual ability to do three things: (1) recognize and distinguish specific distinctive features (e.g., *b* and *d* are different because of one feature), (2) observe invariant relationships in events that occur repeatedly over time (e.g., a favorite blue ball remains the same even after it has been out of sight for a while and even when distance or partial darkness make it appear smaller or darker), and (3) find a hierarchy of pattern or structure allowing the processing of the largest unit possible for adaptive use during a particular task (e.g., a map of the United States is scanned globally for information about the shape of the country, but subordinate features are scanned for the route of a river or location of a city).[47]

Perceptual learning is self-reinforcing, for humans have an intrinsic motivation to acquire information about their environment. The basis of perceptual learning is the child's own activity as he or she interacts with the physical and social environment. Piaget describes stages that occur in the development of perception.[32,50] Initially, learning occurs in the *sensorimotor stage*, which is dominated by reflex behavior and initial perceptions of the self and environment. These perceptions occur through movement, touch, the vestibular mechanisms and the distance receptors, vision, and audition. During this stage, attention is focused on one feature at a time.

In the *intuitive* or preoperational stage (beginning around age 2), Piaget identifies two thinking errors that may continue as perceptual errors. One is transduction, the kind of reasoning, for example, that leads the child to call all small animals "dog." The other is syncretism, or forming into a global or unanalyzed whole something whose elements are not related operationally. Piaget cites the example of judging similar-sized triangles globally rather than searching for details through exact comparison, such as by superimposing angles and sides to see if they really match exactly. The child at the preoperational stage cannot keep in mind more than one point of view, which may account for difficulty with categorizing, *b* and *d* reversals, and interpreting obliqueness (because of inability to consider both horizontal and vertical features simultaneously). In this stage the child also has difficulty with sequencing perceptual information and with form constancy—or the concept that perceptual units retain their basic characteristics even in different contexts.[32,76]

In the *concrete operations* stage (beginning about age 7), the child's action and early perceptions have become internalized into images or operations that can be grouped, classed, and reversed. The child can increasingly see another's point of view because he or she has become less perceptually self-centered and can organize and order things that are immediately present. This change helps develop correct perceptual orientations of space and time.

In the *formal operations* or propositional thought stage, which begins in adolescence, deductive thinking is possible and the child can combine operations such as classification, seriation, and perceptual correspondence simultaneously.

VISUAL PERCEPTUAL DISORDERS IN CHILDREN

Visual perceptual disorders in children differ in some respects from the types of visual perceptual disorders that occur in adults. Difficulties in children are usually congenital or developmental. Their visual perceptual problems are frequently associated with such diagnoses as learning disability, attention deficit disorder, minimal brain dysfunction, mental retardation, and cerebral palsy. Perceptual deficits also occur more often in children with spina bifida and hydrocephalus than in the normal population.[10,92,93]

In contrast, visual perceptual disorders in adults almost always result from brain lesions acquired from such trauma as stroke, tumor, head injury, or senile dementia. These adult diagnoses result in cortical or subcortical lesions that may be isolated to one hemisphere or one lobe, as in stroke or tumor, or may involve multiple lesion sites, as in head injury or senile dementia. These lesions impinge on a fully developed perceptual system. When stroke, tumor, or head injury occurs in children, it evokes developmental considerations because it interrupts and influences the normal developmental process. Such acquired lesions in children may produce some symptoms quite different from those seen in children with congenital or developmental diagnoses, for example, homonymous hemianopsia.

The first step in the diagnostic workup should be an evaluation of the primary visual system. That is, how efficient is the eye in acquiring visual stimuli for further interpretation by the perceptual brain? Many visual perceptual problems accompany or are worsened by primary visual deficits.

Identification of general visual disorders

Visual screening, referral, and clinical diagnosis. Visual screening consists of a group of basic tests designed to select those individuals who are at high risk for inadequate visual functions. The screening is an extremely gross visual assessment and should not be considered diagnostic. Its purpose is to select those children who should be referred to a qualified vision specialist for a complete diagnostic visual evaluation. The screening should be administered by a therapist or educator familiar with visual and visual perceptual disorders. The initial step in a screening should be a review of a comprehensive list of visual symptoms commonly found in those who demonstrate poor visual performance. The observational checklist in the boxed material on p. 711 is provided as an example.

Positive findings on the checklist may indicate problems with visual acuity, quality of eye movements, accommodation, or convergence. Findings should be reported to the vision specialist. A comprehensive visual screening should include appraisals of acuity of both distance and near vision, convergence near point, horizontal pursuits, distant and near fixations, and stereoscopic visual skills. Both the quantity of the performance and the quality of the response should be recorded. Careful observation of the speed, effort, and accuracy of the child's responses will aid in de-

---

Observational checklist of visual symptoms associated with visual problems

Reading

_____ Comprehension decreases with time
_____ Confusion with similar words or letters
_____ Difficulty maintaining place while reading; omits words
_____ Skips or rereads lines
_____ Uses finger or marker as pointer
_____ Slow or word-by-word reading
_____ Says words aloud or lip reads
_____ Reverses words or letters
_____ Difficulty remembering what has been read
_____ Excessive head turning while reading

Writing and other desk tasks

_____ Difficulty copying from chalkboard or book
_____ Squints or blinks while looking up at chalkboard
_____ Omits or repeats letters, words, or phrase when copying
_____ Poor or slow writing
_____ Reversals persisting in grade 2 or beyond
_____ Weight on the writing arm
_____ Does not use other hand to hold paper
_____ Immature pencil grip
_____ Pure finger movement in writing
_____ Draws with short sketchy lines
_____ Turns paper to draw lines in different directions

Body posture and space awareness

_____ Unusual awkwardness
_____ Frequent tripping or stumbling
_____ Body rigidity while looking at distant objects
_____ Thrusts head forward or backward while looking at distant objects
_____ Confuses right and left directions

Appearance of eyes

_____ Crossed eyes turning in or out
_____ Watering or bloodshot eyes
_____ Red-rimmed, crusted, or swollen lids
_____ Frequent sties

General observations

_____ Holds head too close to material
_____ Gross postural defects while seated at desk
_____ Tilts head so as to use only one eye
_____ Closing or covering an eye
_____ Rubs eyes during or after visual activities
_____ Short attention span for visual activities; restlessness, daydreaming
_____ Frowning, excessive blinking, scowling or squinting during visual activities
_____ Unusual fatigue, tension, or frustration during visual activities
_____ Dislike for tasks requiring sustained visual attention

Questions for children

_____ Does your vision get blurry at any time?
_____ Can you make it clear?
_____ Do you ever see objects double?
_____ Do you have headaches, dizziness, or feel sick to your stomach when you use your eyes, or do you get carsick?
_____ Do letters and lines "run together" or words "jump"?
_____ Do your eyes feel hot or itch?
_____ Does light bother your eyes?
_____ Do you know where to catch a pop-up fly ball, how far to throw a ball, where the ball is going to be?

---

termining the quality of the abnormal or normal visual response.

Visual acuity should be tested for both distance and near vision, as near focusing involves active use of the accommodation and convergence systems. Acuity is usually measured with a Snellen distance chart or near card and recorded in the Snellen fraction 20/− for the right eye, left eye, and both eyes for both tests. The basis for the recorded acuity in the Snellen fraction is the smallest line read. If some items are missed, the line in which over half the letters are read is used, and the number missed in the line is noted after the fraction, such as $20/40^{-3}$. An acuity of 20/20 is normal. An acuity of 20/100 means acuity is decreased so that the child sees at 20 feet what the normal individual would see at 100 feet.[39]

The near point of convergence can be taken with the use of a pencil, a pointer, or a small flashlight. The client is seated comfortably and the fixation target is gradually brought from a position at arm's length toward the child's nose. The target must be in median plane. The eyes must have a downward posture as the target is brought closer, and the examiner observes the movement and positioning of the child's eyes. When the client reports diplopia or when one eye deviates from the fixation target, the distance from the target to the bridge of the nose is recorded. This point represents the near point of convergence (NPC). The normal NPC is approximately 3 inches. Once the near point of convergence is reached, the target should be moved back along the same median plane until the child reports single vision or until both eyes are aligned on the target. When the client breaks fusion but does not report diplopia, the examiner may conclude that the individual is suppressing one eye. The dominant eye is usually the fixating eye; therefore this test is also a test of eye dominance. The NPC does not vary with age; its expected value is constant.

Near-to-far fixations should be done by having the client opposite the examiner but slightly to one side so the child can easily and quickly look over the examiner's shoulder at a distance target. The near fixation target should be held right along the midline and approximately 10 inches from the child. The child should be instructed to look at the distance fixation target on the wall directly ahead. The child continues to look at the distance target until the second command "Now!" when the eyes are to shift as fast as they can to the near target. Most children will demonstrate considerable speed and accuracy in their ability to shift visual attention, especially after one or two trials. Both eyes should fix on each target without additional shifting or further adjustment to get each eye into the proper position.

Horizontal pursuits should be done using a fixation target, starting again 10 to 16 inches from the child's face and along the median plane. The target should be moved in a horizontal plane approximately 12 inches to either side of midline as the child follows the target with both eyes. This should be done for at least 10 complete excursions to the left and 10 complete excursions to the right. The examiner should observe for accuracy of alignment on the moving target, the presence or absence of supportive head movements, and the stress factors involved in accomplishing such a task.

A comprehensive visual screening should include tests in a stereoscope to appraise the quality of fusion (stereopsis). Fusion is defined as the process by which stimuli seen separately by the two eyes are combined, synthesized, and integrated into a unified percept. A stereoscope is an instrument that separates the field of view of the two eyes, either by tubes, a septum, or an arrangement of mirrors, so that only certain portions of stereogram targets viewed through it are seen by one eye and other portions by the other eye to give rise to a combined binocular percept. Keystone visual skills can be obtained from Mast Keystone View Company* and used in an appropriate stereoscope.

Failure on parts of the visual screening along with appropriate symptomatology as demonstrated on the observational checklist should result in a referral to a developmental optometrist† for a complete diagnostic visual evaluation.

A diagnostic visual investigation by a developmental optometrist will begin with a comprehensive history. This history will include information on motor development, visual history, a general medical history, an educational history, and information on social and emotional development. A vital aspect of the optometric evaluation is the visual analysis. This consists of a series of 21 specific tests that probe the dynamics of the accommodative process, the convergence process, and the interaction between the accommodative and convergence mechanisms. Values above or below normal limits may demonstrate a pattern or syndrome. The analytical tools used in investigation of the visual pattern of a client are lenses and prisms. Lenses are used for their specific effect on the accommodative pattern, and prisms are used for their specific effect on the convergence pattern. Another phase of an optometric evaluation consists of a series of tests that will provide additional information about the dynamics of the visual process. These tests include book retinoscopy, bell retinoscopy, objective as well as subjective measurements of oculomotor control, evaluation of accommodative facility, and a series of stereoscopic tests that measure the quality of fusional skills. Special batteries of tests may be used to evaluate strabismus or amblyopia. The final phase of the optometric investigation is the administration of standardized tests to measure central processing skills. These tests measure spatial orientation, visual discriminations and interpretations, intersensory motor matching, visual recall, and visualization.

Vision therapy. The American Optometric Association has defined visual therapy as the art and science of developing visual skills to achieve optimal visual performance and comfort.[3] The goal of therapy is to remediate any visual problems that might be interfering with an individual's ability to fulfill cognitive, physical, or emotional potential.

Skeffington[88] lists the following as the primary goals of a visual training program:

1. To establish good effective unimpeded output in all the measurable and observable visual behavior
2. To develop or produce an adequate full-space awareness
3. To build freedom in all the visual movement patterns
4. To advance and develop any retrogressive or retarded abilities
5. To develop those noninherited abilities demanded by the elaborating cultures

Visual therapy consists of prescribing, in a proper sequence, a set of activities or conditions for learning whose primary purpose is to reeducate visual skills and unify visual functioning with total body action. The primary tools in a visual training program are lenses and prisms. Lenses and prisms act by changing the value and quality of the light gradients as they enter the eye. Changes in input result in changes in output based on previously learned experience. The value of lenses and prisms therefore lies in their ability to alter to varying degrees the motor output of the organism. Lenses primarily alter the output responses of the somatic nervous system. The optometric visual therapy program, then, includes the use of lenses and prisms along with specific instrumentation including Polaroid ac-

*2212 East 12 St., Davenport, Iowa 52803.
†A directory of certified developmental optometrists can be obtained from the College of Optometrists in Vision Development, 353 H Street, Chula Vista, CA 92010.

tivities, anaglyph activities, various stereoscopes, tachisto-scopes, cheiroscopes, saccadic fixators, rotators, prism readers, rotoscopes, perimeters, and many other remedial tools.

It is most important that the optometrist and therapist (physical, occupational, or speech) discuss the optometric findings thoroughly. The therapist should understand how the defined deficits affect function (e.g., gait, sports, reading, calculation). With this understanding, the ingenious therapist can design and select activities that are within the visual capacity of the client. The optometrist and therapist should work together to utilize activities requiring effort at the client's highest visual potential. These activities may be selectively used to enhance visual processing per se. Each member of the rehabilitation team must design individualized treatment programs that incorporate a thorough understanding of each client's visual deficits and their influence on function.

Effective total rehabilitation (learning) in the child and adult with visual deficits is directly related to how well the client can incorporate visual input with other sensory and motor systems. For example, the motor response to catching a ball will be slow or inaccurate if the ball is not seen properly, however, if the ball is brighter or larger and it is seen, the motor response will be quicker and more accurate. Similarly, the therapist treating a gait deviation in a client with visual deficits must understand the specific visual problems of that individual before teaching visual observation to correct the deviation.

Visual perceptual assessment and treatment. Scientific scrutiny of visual perceptual variables as they occur in the normal and dysfunctional brain has been difficult. Research efforts have been directed toward defining features of normal visual perception. Even though high levels of this system have not yet been clearly defined, we do know that sensory systems cumulate stimuli into perceptual constructs that then interact with cognition. We know that complex processing of perception by each sense and the interchange and cumulation among the complex levels of each sense (i.e., synthesis of input from auditory, vestibular, kinesthetic, tactile, olfactory, and visual systems) comprise the process by which humans perceptually contact their world. Historically, further refinement of our knowledge in this area has come from analysis of behavior in individuals with well-defined occipital lesions. Through this method, however, it also became clear that lesions in other perceptual areas of the brain, particularly those involved in multisensory processing (e.g., the parietal lobe), did not always result in well-defined behaviors. In addition, it became clear that multiple lesions (e.g., those occurring after head trauma) demonstrated even more complex and subtle behavioral deficits. In like manner, many subtle diagnoses, such as minimal brain dysfunction or learning disability, represent a whole category of disorders with dysfunctions too complex to define in terms of lesions.

Assessment and remediation are based on acceptance of the following postulates:

1. Because of the complexity of the visual perceptual system and our limited knowledge of it, there are no one system and another (e.g., reading a letter on a Snellen chart requires symbolic interpretation as well as visual perceptual abilities).

2. To effectively define a disordered visual perceptual system, the assessment process must always attempt to separate (or at least consider) variables that may influence sensory perception (i.e., cognitive, language, and social variables). The assessment process must be done in an orderly manner. Primary visual skills (i.e., visual acuity) should be assessed before secondary visual perceptual skills (i.e., visuospatial abilities), and high-level visual tasks that involve cognition (e.g., calculation) should be assessed last. A review of all findings should be used to "diagnose" and design treatment programs.

3. Remediation should also follow an orderly design, from simple visual perceptual acts to more complex tasks. The key to effective learning during the remediation process appears to be related to how the clinician controls the neuropsychological variables, particularly those that are disordered. The perceptual environment must be controlled so that the client can "make sense" of each performance. This process engenders progressive learning of simple to complex constructs and, eventually, concepts. Best of all, it fosters attention and motivation. Clients with poorly defined deficits (because of the complexity of their lesions or superficial assessments) improve least. This is partly a result of the inherent inability to design progressive therapeutic tasks that "make sense" and thereby furnish a learning base on which the client can build. Progressive visual perceptual learning, of course, results in an increased ability to function at higher levels during daily activities, the ultimate goal of all therapy. Learning in the disordered brain should follow the same principles of learning in the normal brain.

4. Remediation of any disordered function in the brain-damaged individual (e.g., gait, coordination, balance, or cognition) will most likely be more effective if the client receives normal visual and visual perceptual input during training. In the normal brain this integration of vision with other brain functions directly influences sensorimotor and cognitive learning. In the client with a disordered visual perceptual system, however, this is not possible. The goal,

then, must become one of manipulating and organizing the visual environment during training so that the client receives as high a level of visual processing as possible. This is defined by Kwatny and Bouska[64] as *visual management during therapeutic activity*. This concept implies that (1) the disordered brain must receive and integrate high-level visual information during learning (visual learning) and (2) the more effectively the brain does this, the better the visual system can compensate for and assist (through visual integration) in central rehabilitation of the disordered function (e.g., gait, language, and cognition).

In summary, the visual system is a powerful therapeutic tool that should be used by all professionals directly involved in rehabilitation of the client with brain dysfunction.

Socialization, language, and attention variables in children. Many children who exhibit perceptual disorders also have serious attentional disorders such as hyperactivity, impulsivity, and short attention span. They may also have language-processing disorders. In addition, their problems with learning may have resulted in a secondary side effect—emotional difficulties related to poor ego strength. These factors must be considered during both evaluation and treatment.

Piaget[50] points out the importance of socialization in the child's learning process. He states that affect and cognition are nondissociable, and in the child's striving for equilibrium or homeostasis, perception, cognition, and affect are all interrelated with attention. It is important, then, that assessment take place under conditions that are as relaxed as possible, with good rapport between the examiner and the child. Remediation should consist of highly motivating and enjoyable activities that are appropriate to the age and intellectual capability of the child.

During the grade school and adolescent years, attention improves as it undergoes several developmental changes. These changes occur spontaneously with perceptual experience and practice, and they include increased ability in the following areas: (1) voluntary control of selective attention, (2) adaptability and flexibility of attention depending on task requirements, (3) ability to plan a strategy that uses attention and scanning skills systematically, and (4) ability to maintain attention over sequences of time, thereby avoiding premature attention closure if feedback suggests that some stimulus elements were missed initially.[35,47]

Children's attention is drawn to stimuli having an optimal degree of novelty. The interest and curiosity of children are most likely to be aroused by moderately complex stimuli. The stimuli must be somewhat different from those previously experienced, but not so discrepant that they are confusing or not perceived at all. Perceptual stimuli that are highly discrepant from current knowledge, by virtue of their overcomplexity or oversimplicity, are considerably less likely to be processed and therefore less effective in promoting learning.[17,35]

Some handicapped children tend to neglect the right or left side of their body and of their surrounding space. They may fail to move toward the neglected side of their body in such gross motor tasks as playing dodge ball or propelling a scooter board. They often do not accurately distinguish touch to that side, or they may fail to visually perceive mathematical problems or reading words on the neglected side of each work sheet or textbook page. During visual perception testing they may fail to pay attention to stimuli on the neglected side of the test booklet. Ayers[8] identified unilateral disregard in some children who show notable right-left asymmetry of attention and competence in the following: moving through space, performing automatic movement responses, developing dominant-assistive hand use, and tracing the long, curvy line on the Southern California Motor Accuracy Test. This syndrome is discussed in detail in the section of this chapter dealing with adults.

Identification of clinical problems associated with visuospatial disorders

Space perception is multifaceted, and handicapped persons may manifest deficits in one, several, or all aspects. There are standardized tests for some spatial competencies; for others an awareness of developmental trends of normal functioning is essential before informal clinical observations can satisfactorily detect inadequacies. Many spatial competencies are associated with functioning of the right cerebral hemisphere, and damage to that area is likely to be accompanied by some form of deficit in space perception.[74] However, it has been established that such deficits also occur frequently in the absence of known hemisphere damage.

Assessment. When the examiner assesses spatial competence in children, evaluation of touch perception and internalized body scheme often gives clues about underlying causative factors that must be dealt with in treatment. Disorders of the vestibular system may also have a causative effect on spatial disorders, and treatment of the vestibular disorder may therefore have a positive effect on the development of spatial competence.[8]

The space visualization portion of the Sensory Integration and Praxis Tests[7] measures one form of visual imagery. This ability to visualize, match, and rotate spatially similar or dissimilar objects can also be measured in children with formboards, puzzles in wooden frames, and simple jigsaw puzzles.

Delays in resolving reversals of *b* and *d* are seen so often in the classroom that they are considered classic examples of deficits involving position in space. Diagnosis of similar confusions among figures, forms, or objects is described in the visual analysis and synthesis section of this chapter. It is important at this point to note that such confusions rarely occur alone; thus training children at a cognitive skill level is rarely sufficient to eliminate the more widespread spatial confusion that usually accompanies these deficits. If they are discrete confusions occurring alone, letter and word reversals (p-q, was-saw) should disappear by about age 7, and inversions (u-n, mom-wow) should be eliminated earlier. Size, length, and shape are spatial concepts that must be developed before mathematics can be learned. These concepts are greatly identifiable by 18-month-old children, who can classify objects as large or small; by age 4 they begin to differentiate middle-sized objects. Ordering or sequencing these objects in a series develops later.[83]

Time perception is closely related to spatial sequencing. Sequencing of events in time, like all spatial concepts, begins with global awareness and proceeds to more and more accurate comparisons. By school age, children should have a good concept of morning, afternoon, and evening. By early grade-school years, they should be able to sequence picture stories (three or four pictures in a set). About the age of 9, they should grasp the measurement of time accurately.

Another spatial ability that proceeds developmentally through the early years is formation of a cognitive map, that is, an internal image of the spatial relationship of distant objects both to oneself and to each other. This skill can be evaluated in the preschool years by asking a child to lead the examiner or "be the navigator" through a route that is either familiar or easily learned. Observations may also be made during imaginative play with transportation vehicles. By about 8 years of age, the child should begin to understand aerial maps—a bird's-eye view.

Auditory localization tasks sometimes give clues to perceptual confusion about relationships within environmental space—for example, instructing the child: "While blindfolded, point to the sound of the little bell ringing." Another clue to spatial confusions can be derived from evaluating a visual imagery task such as: "Pretend you are in your dining room sitting in the armchair. What would you see straight ahead of you?" For this task it is important to be sure the child has sufficient language ability to understand the instructions.

Treatment. If a child's evaluation has suggested that deficits in tactile perception, vestibular functioning, or body scheme underlie or accompany poor space perception, these deficits should be dealt with before improvement in space perception at a more cognitive level can be achieved (see Chapter 11). Sensory integrative therapy by a certified specialist is recommended. The holistic approach of Knickerbocker[63] is also very comprehensive and

useful. Gross motor activities modeled after perceptual-motor programs by Kephart[59] or Cratty's adaptive physical education[26] may also be helpful.

Exploring body-centered space through such programs as those just mentioned helps a child create a cognitive spatial map. To further develop this internal map, games can be designed that require the child to become aware of and remember the location of stationary objects or landmarks within a therapeutic environment (e.g., a desk, a clock, a tree, a building). He or she will first orient to and remember those landmarks that are closest. Sets of landmarks should later be used in a coordinated system of reference points from which generalizations can be made. Eventually, the child should learn to make inferences and to update his or her position with reference to landmarks as movements are made through space. Movement forces the child to apply this landmark reference system to making spatial decisions, which enhances the development of a cognitive spatial map.

Piaget[76] asked children to place objects in matching position on a rotated terrain model and also to reproduce matching models of a village and its environs through object placement and scale-model drawings. Therapists can employ modifications of this technique for children past age 7 or 8, noting Piaget's developmental trends. Maps and floorplans of familiar homes, school, and neighborhood can be used as well as floorplans of key objects placed in a dollhouse or therapy room.

Space visualization or imagery may be enhanced through map and floor plan activities like those mentioned or through the sensory integration technique of following ropes or paths through obstacle courses while blindfolded. In addition, the child can be urged to use language to describe visualized rooms, scenes, or stories.

Sequencing of size and time can be encouraged through play with, respectively, nesting toys[63] and cut-up comic strips that have been placed out of sequence. Formboards, puzzles, pegboards, and parquetry blocks classically have been used to enhance spatial perceptions. Training in spatial concepts prerequisite to developing mathematics skill has been thoroughly presented by Copeland[25] in a program that follows the developmental sequences of Piaget's research.

Elimination of reversals and inversions of letters and words may be enhanced by rigorous training in right and left discrimination on oneself (laterality) and in the environment (directionality).[26,63] Emergence of consistent hand dominance as a reference point is also important. Right-left discrimination must also be accompanied by training specifically to eliminate reversals.[61,63] The classroom teacher should be encouraged to mark as wrong spelling words containing reversals or inversions once a child has passed the mental age at which such errors should have been eliminated.

Identification of clinical problems associated with visuoconstructive disorders

Visuoconstructive ability involves assembling parts to form a whole. Examples include toys that require sequential assembling or building and graphic tasks such as printing and drawing. Performance requires the changing of the spatial relationship of parts to one another in order to form a whole. Developmentally, children first learn to assemble objects that fit into given spaces, such as formboards. Eventually, they learn to assemble new shapes by fitting objects together to form a whole, such as fitted wooden puzzles, jigsaw puzzles, and parquetry blocks.

Assessment. Formboard abilities may be evaluated by the space visualization portion of the Sensory Integration and Praxis Tests.[7] Visuoconstructive performance may be observed during bead stringing while copying a pattern of beads, puzzle assembly, and the reproduction of small block patterns such as the train, bridge, and gate[64] (Fig. 25-3). Ability to produce pegboard designs may also be evaluated. The young child may show great confusion regarding the empty space inherent in pegboard designs. For the preoperational child this task is further complicated by the need to consider the location of peg holes relevant to both vertical and horizontal lines at the same time. The older child, who is beginning to be able to perceive the obliques in designs made of squares slashed diagonally (see Fig. 25-3), may still have difficulty assembling designs made of several of these squares. The child will tend to notice the shape of the colored sections but not of the empty spaces adjoining them.

Graphic copying of forms and letters, as well as creating designs and drawings, are complex visuoconstructive tasks that require competence in many areas of development. Evaluation must consider developmental trends in how children discriminate and perceive objects. For example, children perceive vertical, horizontal, and circular lines and shapes before oblique lines. Development of grasp and release should be thoroughly evaluated (see, for example, Erhardt Developmental Prehension Assessment[33]). Reflex development, head control, equilibrium and oculomotor control are all important for positioning and stabilizing the child for maximum refinement of eye-hand coordination. Muscle tone, sequential movement flow, and tendency to cross the midline are additional considerations, as are cognitive abilities, attention, and motivation. The term *visual perceptual motor integration* represents the use of all of these skills. Evaluation of form and design copying should be thorough enough to determine which area(s) may be influencing faulty performance.

Some formal tests that provide information regarding visual perceptual motor integration ability in children are listed in Table 25-1. It is not uncommon for children to attempt to copy a form, only to notice with frustration that it is not an accurate perceptual match with the stimulus figure.[35] It is sometimes revealing, after all forms have been completed, to ask the child which stimulus figures best match the drawings, an indication of the youngster's ability to discriminate perceptually.

Scribbling, often referred to as the *fundamental graphic act,* occurs spontaneously as early as 12 to 18 months of age. The resulting trace is its own reward and motivates further exploration and feedback regarding the integration of fine motor dexterity and graphic variables. Scribbling/writing improves spontaneously in the preschool years and provides opportunity for noticing and learning distinctive features of shapes and letters.

Ability to copy letters tends to occur more instinctively in children who read early.[47] However, motor practice cannot be assumed to necessarily help the sound/symbol associations required for reading words, a higher-level cognitive function requiring auditory and language processing in addition to perceptual skill. On the other hand, handwriting is often an academic prerequisite for progressing through structured reading programs accompanied by fill-in-the-blank workbooks. Efficient writing, free from strenuous cognitive effort, is also required for spelling, language arts, reports, creative writing, and (in the later grades) rapid note taking and timed tests. Therefore early therapeutic intervention into the daily living skill of handwriting can assist not only this visuoconstructive skill but also academic progress.

Treatment. The child can learn to construct objects within space by first fitting objects into spaces, then assembling new shapes, and later copying designs made of materials the child manipulates. Finally, the child can use

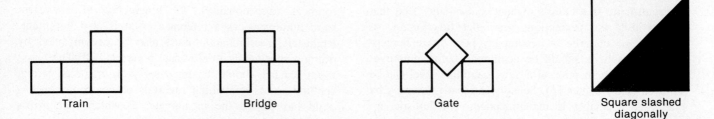

Fig. 25-3. Examples of block patterns for train, bridge, gate, and square slashed diagonally.

Table 25-1. Tests of visual perceptual motor integration ability in children

Test	Ages	Description of task	Comments
Developmental Test of Visual-Motor Integration (K.E. Beery, N. Buktenica) Revised Manual: K.E. Beery Modern Curriculum Press 13900 Prospect Road Cleveland, OH 44136	2-15 years	Copy 24 geometric designs of increasing difficulty. Test ceiling after three consecutive errors.	Simple to administer and score. First several designs are so easy for older children that they encourage carelessness, a detriment in more difficult designs. Age norms for *imitation* of simple designs, a simpler task than copying, are suggested for 1- to 3-year-old children.
Copying portion of Sensory Integration and Praxis Tests (A.J. Ayres) Western Psychological Services 12031 Wilshire Blvd. Los Angeles, CA 90025	4-8 years	Copy designs drawn on grids of dots.	Therapists may become certified to administer, score, and interpret the complete battery of the Sensory Integration and Praxis Tests Design copying is scored for both accuracy and method of drawing.
Motor Accuracy portion of Sensory Integration and Praxis Tests (A.J. Ayres), revised, 1980 Western Psychological Services 12031 Wilshire Blvd. Los Angeles, CA 90025	4-8 years	Trace a long, curvy line that extends on either side of the body. Use preferred, then nonpreferred, hand.	Because this test requires only visual motor integration and eliminates the need for complex visual perception, results may help determine the cause of poor form copying.
Constructional Praxis portion of Sensory Integration and Praxis Tests	4-8 years	Copy two structures made of blocks	Highly motivating test. Shows ability to reproduce simple then complex three-dimensional block buildings.
Fine motor portion of Bruininks-Oseretsky Test of Motor Proficiency	4-14 years	Copy forms, trace inside road cut, manipulate small items, connect lines and tap with pencil.	Test provides three subscores
Goodenough Harris Drawing Test (1963) Harcourt, Brace, Jovanovich, Inc. 757 Third Ave. New York, NY 10017	3-15 years	Draw a picture of a man, a woman, and yourself on a blank page.	This can be scored by detailed method or by general age approximation.
The House-Tree-Person Technique, revised manual (J.N. Bush) Western Psychological Services 12031 Wilshire Blvd. Los Angeles, CA 90025	5 years and older	Draw a picture of a house, a tree, and a person.	This is a nonverbal test of mental ability from which an intelligence score can be computed. Scoring is qualitative and quantitative.
Bender Visual Motor Gestalt Test American Orthopsychiatric Association, Inc. 1790 Broadway New York, NY 10019	4 years and older	Copy designs and pairs of designs.	This test, usually administered by a psychologist, may support the therapist's findings or eliminate the need to further test form copying.
Wechsler Intelligence Scale for Children, revised (1974) Subtests: (1) coding, (2) mazes D. Wechsler Psychological Corp. 757 Third Ave. New York, NY 10017		(1) Reproduce a code of tiny figures (timed). (2) Trace through a labyrinth from start to finish.	This test, administered by a psychologist, may conflict with or support the therapist's findings and give insight into timed performance.
McCarthy Scales of Children's Abilities Subtests: (1) Draw-a-Design, (2) Draw-a-Child D. McCarthy Psychological Corp. 757 Third Ave. New York, NY 10017		Copy forms and draw a picture of a person.	This test, usually administered by a psychologist, may support the therapist's findings or eliminate the need to further test form copying.

objects to copy two-dimensional (and eventually three-dimensional) drawings of the placement of these materials, further enhancing visuoconstruction. Puzzles, blocks, beads, and pegs are appropriate manipulatable materials with which to develop such a sequence.

Ayres[9] encourages children to construct an interesting barrier of large foam shapes with which to collide after descending a ramp on a scooter board. Then the children are asked to reconstruct the barrier exactly according to the previous pattern.

Remediation of form-copying deficits must first deal with gross or fine motor delays or deficits that have been identified through the evaluation process. Neurodevelopmental treatment, sensory integration, or the adaptation process of Gilfoyle and Grady[48] will help structure developmental motor remediation sequences. Another useful tool is the *Visual-Motor Development Remedial Activities*[22], a packaged series of tasks to improve copying, angulation, curves, and sinusoidal skills and writing. (For additional treatment ideas, see Ayres,[8] Erhardt,[33] Gardner,[38] and Knickerbocker.[63])

A clinician who is training a child in making manuscript letters or copying forms (if form copying has been determined to be advisable) must remember normal developmental sequences. Reproduction of vertical and horizontal lines and circles precedes the ability to accurately reproduce intersecting lines, adjacent or overlapping figures, and oblique lines. Practicing new copying tasks by placing toothpicks or sticks to represent lines helps the child who has not quite acquired the motor skill for drawing the same forms. The novice may also benefit from practicing form copying on a chalkboard surface, clay slab, or salt or sand tray. This allows easy erasure without the frustration of smudged or torn paper.

For some children with severely impaired handwriting, improvement does not occur readily following therapeutic measures mentioned above when accompanied by normal special education methods. In that case, specific handwriting intervention by a therapist or specially trained teacher may enormously reduce the frustration that these children experience in school. Emphasis should be placed not only on developing gross and fine motor skills but also on providing auditory cues and visual landmarks to enhance awareness of discriminating features of letters that are the most difficult to form. ("Curve to the top line . . . touch the bottom line . . . go back up the same line to the middle line . . .")

Identification of clinical problems associated with visual analysis and synthesis disorders

Visual analysis is the ability to perceive and analyze distinctive features such as position in space, complex spatial relations, constancy, closure, and configuration. Visual synthesis is the ability to perceive individual features as a unified whole or to place them in a hierarchy of pattern, structure, or sequence.

Assessment. Difficulty with analysis of distinctive features is usually noticed first at school age. At that time a child's difficulty in processing the symbols in reading books becomes apparent. The school psychologist may find evidence of visual perceptual deficits during a battery measuring intelligence. The school therapist may evaluate the child's ability to analyze distinctive features by administering the Motor-Free Visual Perception Test (MVPT),[24] the Test of Visual Perceptual Skills (TVPS),[37] or, if the therapist is trained and certified, the visual perception portion of the Sensory Integration and Praxis Tests.[7]

Cat research and preliminary research on humans suggest that during a critical period of early development, a small amount of visual experience modifies cortical cells so they become selectively sensitive feature detectors. The modification appears to be permanent for a particular type of perceptual feature.[35]

During development, analysis of distinctive features becomes increasingly specific and progressively more differentiated.[47] Even babies less than 2 months of age are capable of form, pattern, and depth perception, although visual acuity, accommodation, and convergence are poor.[35] Methods of testing this discrimination ability in infants must rely on the sequence or duration of apparent or electronically measured visual fixations. Such testing is usually done only in the research laboratory. However, it is easy to evaluate informally a child's interest in and ability to visually follow a moving stimulus even at a very young age. Humans appear to be selectively attentive to perceiving movement, novelty, and contour. This explains babies' early visual preference for the human face. It is now theorized that social attachment to faces develops later.[35] By age 2½ the child begins to be able to perceive and copy simple inch-cube designs, as mentioned previously in the discussion of constructive disorders.

Because of the importance of word and letter discrimination in the life of the early school-age child, it is important for the school therapist to understand developmental trends in letter recognition. In the discrimination of letters, the earliest developmental contrast is in terms of curvature and straightness (O versus □); ability to differentiate intersection at the middle (A versus △) and diagonality (N versus Z) comes later.[47] Letter discrimination progresses spontaneously and is usually complete by the end of first grade. This skill does not include naming the letters, a sound/symbol relationship that develops more slowly. Although more than half of kindergarteners make reversals *(b and d),* only 10% do so by third grade. A reversal is not regarded as an error by a young child, who considers the shape a constant and the directional element irrelevant.[47]

Information processing must become more efficient through increasing ability to detect order and structure.

This efficiency can move toward perceiving the smallest distinction possible, as previously discussed, or identifying the largest units that carry structured information,[47] which involves the process of synthesis and will be considered next.

Evaluation of the *synthesis* aspect of visual perception may include assessment of visuoconstruction, since it requires synthesis of structural information. For example, children who subdivide drawings in form-copying tasks or who fail to make lines in drawings overlap or meet correctly may be demonstrating problems with synthesis. Assessment of spatial competencies includes synthesis. For example, confusion of the sequence of visual perceptual figures in the Visual Sequential Memory subtest of the Illinois Test of Psycholinguistic Abilities (ITPA)[60] may reflect deficits in synthesis of the whole, which may be related to problems in visual memory and sequencing.

The whole/part gestalt aspect of discriminating features may be evaluated through figure-ground and visual closure tests or subtests. The psychologist's findings on certain subtests of the Wechsler Intelligence Scale for Children (WISC)[97] also give important information about synthesis. The most pertinent WISC subtests are picture completion and block design.

Treatment The goal in treatment of visual analysis disorders is to encourage the child to make finer and finer visual discriminations of distinctive features. The goal in treatment of visual synthesis disorders is to encourage the child, when it is appropriate, to be alert to total, whole units of information while retaining the ability to perceive the smallest distinction at will. It includes increased detection of order and structure, foreground and background, whole (closure) and part.

During treatment it is important to present tasks according to the developmental sequence (see the diagnosis section on analysis and synthesis disorders). Visual stimuli presented for discrimination should become increasingly similar or, in the case of figure-ground tasks, increasingly complex but without a major change in difficulty. A major change would discourage the novice from relating the new information to previous experience and thus would discourage generalization. The concept that perceptual prominence enhances attention (i.e., conspicuous features are noticed first) suggests several methods of enhancing discrimination: starting with the maximum contrast and progressing toward resemblances, providing uncluttered examples of the invariant property, and drawing attention to a feature by enhancing the contrast (using such elements as color, size, texture, and verbal discussion).

May[69] determined that children with spastic cerebral palsy, a population that often has difficulty with visual-motor tasks, produced significantly better drawings when the black and white portions of the figure and ground were reversed by using a white pencil on black paper. The normal children in the control group showed no such tendency. Hypothesizing that the white background may have been distracting to the handicapped population, May proposed using a chalkboard for teaching letters (white letters on black) and black paper for visual-motor and projective drawing tests.

As children who are learning analysis and synthesis discrimination approach readiness for new levels (e.g., diagonality and touching and overlapping figures), the new skill should be presented in a wide variety of media (e.g., walking along ropes laid out in designs, finger painting, large chalkboard rhythmic designs, pegboard and pencil copying, and worksheet discrimination tasks). This encourages the child to integrate and generalize the newly acquired information. Tactile perception of increasingly similar objects, angles, or alphabet letters sometimes helps to enhance awareness of their slight differences. The role of writing and copying in helping a child learn to discriminate stimuli visually was previously mentioned as one example of the analysis/synthesis aspect of visuoconstruction tasks.

Commercially available activities for visual analysis include Visual-Perceptual Development Remedial Activities.[23] Also available are supermarket store think-and-do books, educational supply company matching and sorting cards, Ann Arbor Tracking Program,[5] and Fitzhugh Plus Program.[34] The latter two also encourage attention to foreground and background aspects of complex visual stimuli, as do Altair Designs by Holiday.[56] Children can benefit from selecting shapes and patterns in labels on grocery store shelves or correct information from a Kodak film display case or a voting-booth array of levers and candidates' names.

Memory tasks provide one method of encouraging observation of distinctive features once children have passed beginning levels of discrimination. An even more advanced task is the rapid tachistoscopic presentation of visual stimuli. Playing "Concentration" with matched pairs of complex visual perception cards in sets of similarly designed cards is a highly motivating task if presented at the proper level for the child's capability. Reversed designs and closure figures provide the greatest challenge. Getman and others[43] provide a commercially available program for tachistoscopic presentation of carefully sequenced designs.

When providing visual analysis and synthesis remedial activities to children, keep in mind that improvement in these skills is not likely to result in academic improvement unless directly related to letter or word recognition or unless used with pre–reading-level children.

VISUAL PERCEPTUAL DISORDERS IN ADULTS

Adults with brain damage often demonstrate visual perceptual deficits distinct from those observed in children. For the moment it might be helpful to conceptualize visual perceptual disorders as divided into "acquired" and "congenital or developmental" categories. Adult visual perceptual deficits usually result from newly acquired lesions whereas visual perceptual deficits in children are commonly caused by "damage" present since birth or early infancy (congenital or developmental diagnoses) that influences the developing visual perceptual system. In contrast, acquired lesions in adults impinge on a fully developed and normally functioning visual perceptual system. Time of onset, then, in relation to the extent of normal visual perceptual development that has been established, seems to influence the resultant type of visual perceptual deficits. For example, a head injury involving the right parietooccipital area in a 5-year-old (an acquired lesion) may result in some unique disturbances in reading, drawing, and writing development compared to the same lesion in a 50-year-old. Another significant variable in determining type of deficit is extent and location of lesion. Most traumatic or vascular lesions result in hemispheric or lobar damage, for example, discrete lesions as opposed to global inefficiencies as seen in learning disability. This section on adult visual perceptual disorders, then, applies to acquired brain damage; however, information presented here may be applicable to acquired lesions in children that result from stroke, head injury, or encephalitis, particularly if the lesion occurs after some normal visual perceptual function has been established.

The most common conditions resulting in visual perceptual deficits in adults include stroke, head injury, tumor, senile dementia, postsurgical emboli or anoxia to the brain, encephalitis, multiple sclerosis, or any other condition resulting in an anoxic or a chemical destruction of brain tissue. As with children, damage may be present in any part of the visual perceptual apparatus, for example, the eye, the oculomotor pathways (intrinsic and extrinsic muscles of the eye), the optic nerve, the optic tract, the occipital cortex, or the associative areas of the brain (the parietal and temporal lobes). The first step in the diagnostic workup should be an evaluation of the primary visual system, that is, how efficient the eye is in acquiring visual stimuli for further interpretation by the perceptual brain. Many visual perceptual problems are caused or augmented by primary visual deficits. This is particularly true in adults who, because of age and precipitating diagnostic factors, often have premorbid visual conditions such as a cataract or diabetic retinopathy. Any new visual perceptual problems, such as homonymous hemianopsia or problems with visual perceptual interpretation, are augmented by the preexisting visual conditions.

Primary visual disorders

Identification of primary visual disorders: visual screening, referral, and clinical diagnosis. Visual screening is an extremely gross visual assessment and should not be considered diagnostic in any way. It is a method to select those clients with possible disorders of the primary (as opposed to the associative) visual system who require referral to a qualified specialist (ophthalmologist, neuroophthalmologist, or optometrist) for a complete visual evaluation. Visual screening should be carried out only by a therapist knowledgeable in visual and visual perceptual systems and pathology. The screening should include measures of near and distance visual acuity, visual fields, oculomotor alignment (binocularity), range of ocular movement, convergence near point, and gross efficiency of saccades, pursuits, and fixations.

Distance and near acuity should be measured with Snellen distance chart and near card (see the discussion of this procedure in the children's section). Typical reading material, which can be accurately read with various acuities, is listed in Table 25-2 (the "J" or Jeager acuity designation is often used by ophthalmologists to describe acuity[99]). These functional reading translations are valid only if all other visual skills are intact. Problems with fixations, saccades, organized visual exploration, visual spatial integration, or unilateral visual inattention often result in nonfunctional reading in spite of normal acuities.

Reduced acuity for distance or near vision may be caused by premorbid visual conditions, resulting in hyperopia, myopia, presbyopia, astigmatism, opacities in the ocular media (e.g., cataract or corneal scars), glaucoma, or macular disease. Reduced acuity may also result from newly acquired central lesions causing poor fixational skill (inability to place fovea on target), a defect in the visual pathway (e.g., cortical blindness), or cognitive, language, or interpretive deficits.[39] This last category may usually be ruled out by using pictures for testing (Lighthouse Cards for the Blind) or isolating individual letters during testing.

Visual fields should be evaluated by confrontation in both children and adults with acquired lesions. Generally, the examiner holds a 2-mm wand white target and moves it in various directions from the periphery inward along an arc. The client is instructed to continually fixate on a cen-

Table 25-2. Acuity and its relation to reading ability

Snellen fraction	"J"-type designation	Typical reading material
20/20	1+	Near acuity cards
20/25	1	Mail-order catalogs, Bibles
20/30	2	Want ads
20/40	3	Telephone directory
20/50	5	Newspaper print, magazines
20/60-20/70	6-7	Adult textbooks, magazines
20/80-20/130	8-12	Children's books (for ages 7-12), newspaper subheadings
20/170-20/200	14-17	Large-print books, newspaper headlines

tral target such as the examiner's eye or nose and report when the testing wand is first seen. An approximation is noted of the angle of first recognition in four principal meridians—the horizontal, vertical, right oblique, and left oblique—to grossly determine areas of loss in half fields, superior fields, and inferior fields. Common lesions in the visual pathway associated with specific field defects are diagrammed in Fig. 25-4.

Confrontation, however, is a very gross assessment and has been demonstrated to be insensitive, missing as many as half the cases where other methods demonstrate a loss. Glaucous has recommended use of the Keystone Ophthalmic Telebinocular, or the Keystone VS-II Vision Screener for more critical assessment of peripheral points along the horizontal plane. "Depressions" or scotomas (small areas of reduced sensitivity within or outside the central field) are delineated only with a critical peripheral field examination; these areas of loss are often critical to visual function, i.e., a scotoma in the left central field will result in reading errors ("fight will be read as "eight") or in dropping a stitch while knitting.

Oculomotor alignment is measured in the primary position of gaze (looking straight forward) to determine whether the client is using both eyes or has a strabismus. Generally, a penlight is held directly before the client. The examiner notes whether or not the reflection of the source in each eye occupies the same relative corneal position, usually the center of each pupil. If a strabismus is present, the reflection in the nonfixing eye (turned eye) will appear displaced from the position in accordance with the amount and direction of the deviation. If both eyes are not aligned, the client may have one or more of the following symptoms: double vision (diplopia), vertigo, confusion, clumsiness, motion sickness, or poor spatial judgment. Some individuals may have diplopia in some meridians of gaze and not in others. In other words, the oculomotor muscle

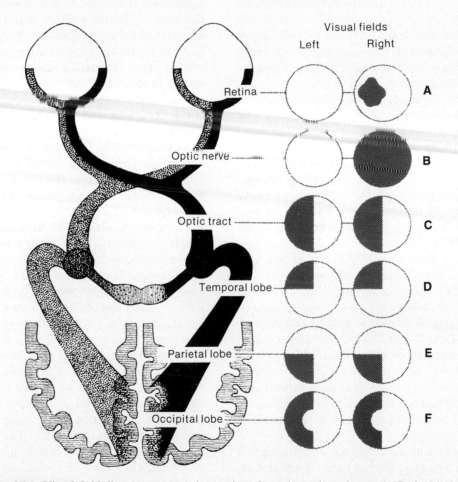

Fig. 25-4. Visual field disturbances at various points along the optic pathway. **A,** Retinal lesion: blind spot in the affected eye. **B,** Optic nerve lesion: partial or complete blindness in that eye. **C,** Optic tract or lateral geniculate lesion: blindness in the opposite half of both visual fields. **D,** Temporal lobe lesion: blindness in the upper quadrants of both visual fields on the side opposite the lesion. **E,** Parietal lobe lesion: contralateral blindness in the corresponding lower quadrants of both eyes. **F,** Occipital lobe lesion: contralateral blindness in the corresponding half of each visual field, but with macular sparing. (Courtesy Smith Kline & French Laboratories, Philadelphia, Penn.)

paresis may be involved only during vertical and not horizontal gaze. These clients complain of double vision only when they look in certain directions. In addition, very mild disorders of ocular paresis may be evident solely when the individual begins to fatigue visually.

The range of motion of the eyes should also be evaluated grossly. Innervation to the oculomotor muscles in one or both eyes may be lost or diminished following head injury or stroke. The client is asked to watch a target (penlight) that is moved slowly and smoothly to the extremes of gaze in all positions. Each of the 12 extraocular muscles has a diagnostic field of gaze. If the target is moved in a large H pattern, each of the muscles can be isolated. Any restrictions in gaze should be noted. (For a discussion of eye movements and information on convergence nearpoint testing, see the discussion on visual screening of children.)

Saccades are measured by asking the client to look rapidly from one object to another. The two objects should be held approximately 6 inches apart, about 12 to 15 inches from the client. Each eye should be tested individually. A light overshoot, undershoot, or refixation of the target may be within normal limits. However, large errors in either direction should be considered abnormal.

The smooth pursuit system is tested by asking the client to follow a target (penlight) that is moving slowly and smoothly across the examinee's field of vision. The target is placed approximately 12 to 16 inches from the client and moved smoothly in a circular path 12 inches in diameter. An inability to maintain smooth pursuit may be associated with lesions of the occipitomesencephalic pathways and result in a pursuit movement supplemented by saccades. This jerky interruption of smooth pursuit is called saccadic pursuit and is considered abnormal.

Fixation ability is tested by asking the client to fix his or her gaze steadily (for a minimum of 5 seconds) first on a near target and then on a distant target (see the section on visual screening of children).

Functional scanning in relation to reading can be measured by the King-Devick Test,[66] which is standardized to age 14. Reading performance of a 14-year-old is considered at an adult level; adult scanning can be compared with these norms. In this test, the three parts become progressively less structured spatially, which consequently requires more spatial control of scanning, e.g., as in reading a bus schedule.

Any visual abnormality noted during visual screening should result in an automatic referral to the vision specialist. The vision specialist should be an individual with interest and experience in evaluating, managing, and treating visual system deficits in brain-damaged individuals. Professionals such as a rehabilitation optometrist,[46] behavioral or developmental optometrist, low vision specialist, neurophthalmologist, or ophthalmologist with special interest in brain-injury rehabilitation may be appropriate. It is ideal if the therapist who did the screening can accompany the client to the ophthalmology or optometry examination. The therapist should alert the vision specialist to specific functional deficits that may be related to visual losses. In addition, the therapist may be able to assist the examiner in dealing with the client's attentional, language, or cognitive deficits during the examination. Both therapist and vision specialist should discuss the findings in relation to management, therapy, and functional implications. Finally, whether or not the client is accompanied to the visual examination, it is imperative that the therapist read and understand the results of the visual consultation.

The visual findings should be understood well enough to define management techniques. For example, an individual with a Snellen acuity of 20/200 in both eyes that cannot be corrected with lenses and who also has a homonymous hemianopsia and unilateral visual inattention should be given special consideration during gait training. If the client is directed to walk toward a target, the therapist must be sure the target is large enough and within the intact visual field. Occupational therapists, neuropsychologists, or psychologists specializing in training visual perception must understand the visual consultation well enough to define treatment techniques. For example, in the example just cited, what type, color, size, and density of targets should be used in facilitating spontaneous visual scanning into the unattended space?

Management and treatment of primary visual disorders. Common primary visual deficits associated with central lesions and their functional symptoms, as well as suggestions for the management and treatment, are listed in Table 25-3.

Decreases in distance or near acuity may result from simple premorbid conditions such as myopia, hyperopia, or presbyopia; such conditions are correctable with appropriate lenses. Premorbid problems with visual acuity because of cataract, glaucoma, diabetic retinopathy, eye injury, or other conditions may not be correctable with lenses. Decreased visual acuity may also be the result of new central lesions. Bilateral lesions in the visual projection cortex may result in cortical blindness and, thereby, a severe bilateral decrease in both distance and near acuity. Near acuity, in particular, may be lost or inconsistent because of problems with accommodation. Internal ophthalmoplegia is a condition in which there is lack of innervation to the third nerve and, thereby, a paralysis of the internal muscles of the eye, that is, the pupils as well as the ciliary muscles. This, of course, affects the accommodation and/or pupillary mechanisms and results in blurred vision under various lighting conditions.

Visual field deficits may include homonymous hemianopsius, quadrantopsias, scotomas (areas of decreased sensitivity), or visual field constrictions (circumferential narrowing of the field). Lesions at or above the superior colliculi usually result in a loss of vertical gaze, also known

Table 25-3. Primary visual deficits associated with central lesions, functional symptoms, management, and treatment

Visual deficit	Functional deficit	Management	Treatment
Decreased visual acuity (distance or near)	Decreased acuity for distance or near tasks (reading)	Provide best lens correction for distance and near	May not be correctable
Inconsistent accommodation	Inconsistent blurred near vision	Ensure appropriate lenses are worn for appropriate activities	
		Determine if bifocal is usable; if not, provide separate lenses for distance and near	
		Enlarge target, control density, use contrast, task lighting	
Cortical blindness	Marked decrease in visual acuity	Evaluated by vision specialist to determine areas and quality of residual vision	Use headlamp to improve visual localization, i.e. functional use of residual vision
	Severe blurring uncorrectable by lenses	Present targets of appropriate size/contrast in best area of visual field	
Visual field deficits include:	Blindness or decreased sensitivity in affected area of visual field	Be aware of normal field position in all meridians of gaze	Scanning training to facilitate compensation
Homonymous hemianopsias		Ask patient to outline working area before beginning task	Training in use of prism
Quadrantanopsias			
Scotomas		Partial press-on FRESNEL prism to facilitate compensation	
Visual field constrictions			
Pupillary reactions	Slow or absent pupillary responses	Sunglasses to control excess brightness	—
Loss of vertical gaze (external ophthalmoplegia)	Inability to move eyes up or down	Raise target or working area to foveal level	—
		Teach patient head movement to compensate	
Conjugate gaze deviation	Inability/difficulty moving eyes from fixed gaze position		—
Lack of convergence	Diplopia or blurred vision for near tasks		Convergence exercises prescribed by vision specialist*
	Decreased depth perception for near tasks		
Oculomotor nerve lesion (strabismus)	Intermittent or consistent diplopia in some or all meridians of gaze	FRESNEL prism to fuse image in select cases	Oculomotor exercises prescribed by vision specialist*
	Loss of depth perception	Occlude deviant eye	
Pathological nystagmus	Movement/blur of image during reading/near activities	Enlarge print/target to decrease blur	—
Poor fixations, saccades or pursuits	Erratic scanning	Decrease density of material	Oculomotor exercises prescribed by vision specialist*
	Unsteady fixation	Isolate targets during evaluation and treatment	Sensory integration activities
			Scanning training
			Use of kinesthetic and tactile systems to lead visual system (eye movements)

© Copyright by Mary Jane Bouska, OTR/L, 1988.

*Treatment methodologies taken from developmental lesions; not validated in adult lesions.

as external ophthalmoplegia. In this condition there is a paralysis of the extraocular muscles that control upward and downward gaze; the individual cannot move the eyes up or down and must, therefore, move the head to change foveal position vertically. This syndrome is often accompanied by the absence of convergence and by abnormal pupillary reactions. A conjugate gaze deviation of the eyes results from a lesion in the cortex or subcortical motor pathway. In this condition the eyes deviate in parallel, and there is no diplopia. The direction in which the eyes turn is dependent on the location and nature of the lesion. Lesions in a single motor nerve to the eyes or its nucleus affect the motions of a single eye and result in misalignment of one eye.[84] This condition, known clinically as strabismus, usually results in diplopia; it is often present following traumatic head injury. Pathological nystagmus may result from lesion of the vestibular system, including its peripheral and central connections, from lesions of the brainstem and cerebellum, from chronic viseral impairment, or from toxic substances. Horizontal nystagmus is most common, although vertical and rotatory forms of nystagmus may also occur.[49] Finally, any disruption in the oculomotor pathways along their circuitous route through subcortical and cortical structures may decrease the quality of saccades, pursuits, and/or fixations. Saccades are mediated by the frontal cortex and the descending frontomesencephalic pathways, and smooth pursuit eye movements are mediated by the cortex of the anterior occipital lobes.[39] Both are susceptible to damage in traumatic head injury.

Treatment of primary visual deficits is usually handled by the vision specialist in coordination with the occupational therapist. Decreased distance or near acuity may be correctable with appropriate lenses. The therapist must ensure that the appropriate lenses are worn. Near lenses inappropriately worn for gait training will automatically *give* the patient a visual deficit. Patients with loss of vertical gaze will be unable to use a bifocal; they must have separate lenses for near activities. If acuity is not correctable with lenses, the therapist should enlarge print/targets, control density, use contrast (yellow on dark background), and always use task lighting. Management of cortical blindness is discussed later in this chapter. With regard to visual field deficits, the therapist should be aware of the normal field in all positions of gaze. In this way, the therapist may dynamically observe whether a patient's error was caused by a scanning omission (not seeing) or by other factors (i.e., perceptual or cognitive). When initiating any activity, the patient should be asked to tactually outline the working area before beginning. Finally, in some cases a partial press-on prism may be applied by a vision specialist at the edge of the field deficit so that when the patient fixes straight forward, the image of the prism is not seen, but when the patient makes a small saccade

toward the visual field cut, he or she gets a blurred image of the environment within the prismatic area. This image then becomes the clue to turn the head and eyes toward the field cut; this increases consistency of compensation. Patients without visual perceptual deficits are the best candidates for this type of prism. It seems to increase perceptual confusion in patients with visual perceptual deficits.

Most evidence supports the view that visual field defects are nontreatable; recovery of the field, if it occurs, is believed to be spontaneous. A recent study, however, showed considerable recovery in hemianoptic individuals.[100] Visual acuity, critical flicker fusion, color perception, and contrast sensitivity improved with a specially designed training program. Even though Balliet and others[11] have reported an inability to duplicate the study, the findings represent some alternative thinking on visual field recovery. In individuals who do not learn to compensate for their field defect by by moving their eyes (i.e., intact visual field) into their lost hemispace, unilateral visual inattention should be considered as an additional disorder. When a patient has lost vertical gaze, the therapist must be sure to raise the working area to the patient's foveal level so that the patient does not have to carry out excessive head movement. This is particularly important in patients with head, postural, and upper-extermity motor deficits. With gaze palsies, material should be presented in the best position for the patient's foveal viewing. Convergence exercises may be prescribed by the vision specialist for a patient with convergence insufficiency. However, such exercises require sustained attention and repetition, which is difficult for some patients. Oculomotor nerve lesions (strabisumus) are generally considered unresponsive to oculomotor therapy in adults;[64] recovery, if it occurs, is considered spontaneous. This is in contrast to developmental strabismus in children, which may respond to oculomotor therapy.

One of the simplest methods for eliminating double vision is to patch an eye. The vision specialist should determine whether or not an eye should be patched, which eye should be patched, and during which activities. In selected cases with very small oculomotor deviations, prisms may be prescribed to decrease diplopia. Surgical intervention may be considered a final method to align the eye and eliminate the double vision. Oculomotor exercises may be recommended or carried out by some vision specialists to help increase the efficiency of saccades, pursuits, fixations, and convergence. Under the guidance of the vision specialist, the therapist responsible for visual perceptual training may incorporate oculomotor exercises within elementary functional activities. Carefully designed visual perceptual programs that require sustained visual attention (i.e., fixation) and organized scanning (i.e., saccades) can enhance oculomotor efficiency.

Visual perceptual dysfunction

This discussion of visual perceptual disorders is divided into a number of categories: unilateral spatial inattention; cortical blindness, defective color perception, and visual agnosia; visuospatial disorders; visuoconstructive disorders; and visual analysis and synthesis disorders. Cortical blindness is a disorder of primary visual input; however, since variations of it may influence perceptual interpretation, it is discussed here. All other disorders listed involve direct problems with the interpretation of visual stimuli. Although each of these terms represents symptoms recognized by many authors, the reader is reminded that there are no clear boundaries between one deficit and another or one system and another. (For a full discussion of the topic, see the introduction on visual perceptual assessment and treatment in children.) Apraxia and body image disorders are not discussed under separate categories because they are not considered "visual" perceptual disorders per se even though their presence may influence and complicate an already dysfunctional visual perceptual system.

Problems of unilateral spatial inattention
Identification of various clinical subproblems

General category. In its purest form, unilateral spatial inattention is defined as a condition in which an individual with normal sensory and motor systems fails to orient toward, respond to, or report stimuli on the side contralateral to the cerebral lesion. Although this condition is not often seen in its pure form, inattention has been documented in persons who demonstrate no accompanying visual field defect (homonymous hemianopsia) or limb sensory or motor loss.[27] In most cases, however, unilateral spatial inattention is not seen alone but is associated with (although not caused by), accompanying sensory and motor defects such as homonymous hemianopsia, decreased tactile, proprioceptive, and stereognostic perception along with paresis or paralysis of the upper limb.

It is easy to become confused by the numerous terms used in the literature, for example, unilateral spatial agnosia, unilateral visual neglect, "fixed" hemianopsia, hemiinattention, or hemiimperception. All terms describe the same deficit. *Unilateral spatial inattention* is used in this chapter because (1) in severe cases the syndrome most likely involves tactile and auditory as well as visual unawareness (i.e., a total spatial unawareness) and (2) the syndrome results in an *involuntary* lack of attention to stimuli contralateral to the lesion whereas the term *neglect* implies a voluntary choice not to respond.

Unilateral spatial inattention occurs most frequently in individuals with diagnoses of cerebrovascular accident, traumatic brain injury, and tumor. Most authors agree that unilateral spatial inattention occurs more often with right hemisphere than with left hemisphere lesions.[20,27,51] This frequency supports theories that the right hemisphere is dominant for visuospatial organization. It is clear, however, that inattention may be present in individuals with left hemisphere lesions. The clinician should remember that even though the chances are statistically less, the client with right hemiplegia may exhibit inattention to right stimuli.

Unilateral spatial inattention has been associated with lesions in both cortical and subcortical structures. It is most commonly seen in inferior parietal lobe lesions[27] but has also been observed in lesions in the dorsolateral frontal lobe, the cingulate gyrus,[53] and in thalamic[96] and putamenal hemorrhage.[55] Finally, lesions in the brainstem reticular formation have induced inattention in cats[81] and monkeys.[96]

Although a number of theories have been postulated regarding the mechanism underlying unilateral spatial inattention, no mechanism has been validly documented in human subjects. The one fact that is clear from all theoretical postulates is that inattention is a hemispheric deficit. LeDoux and Smylie[65] demonstrated this point effectively in an interesting case study of a right-sided lesion. During full visual exposure (bilateral hemispheric) of visual perceptual slides, the individual made visuospatial errors in left space. However, when the same slides were directed only to the right visual field (left hemisphere), performance improved substantially. It is as if the deficient hemisphere fails to receive or orient toward incoming information while the intact receiving hemisphere remains oblivious and goes about its own business. Treatment for inattention is problematic mainly because the mechanisms underlying unilateral spatial inattention are not clearly understood.

Theories on mechanisms underlying unilateral spatial inattention have attempted to explain it as an integrative associative defect as opposed to simply a problem of decreased sensory input. Theories include a unilateral attentional hypothesis suggesting that inattention results from a disruption in the orienting response; that is, the corticolimbic hemisphere is underaroused during bilateral input and therefore stimuli presented to that hemisphere are neglected.[53,54] Another theory is the oculomotor imbalance hypothesis, which suggests that individuals with inattention have a visuospatial disorder worsened by oculomotor imbalance. The hypothesis suggests that the lesion disconnects the frontal eye fields in the damaged hemisphere from their sensory afferent nerves, resulting in an oculomotor imbalance deviating the gaze toward the lesion. This imbalance can be compensated for only momentarily by a voluntary effort to gaze toward the opposite hemispace (i.e., neglected space).[21]

Unilateral spatial inattention with homonymous hemianopsia. Inattention occurs more commonly with visual field defects and is generally worse when the macula is not spared. Individuals with pure hemianopsias are aware of their visual loss and spontaneously learn to compensate by moving their eyes (foveae) toward their lost visual field to expand their visual space and thereby gather information right and left of midline. On visual examination other individuals may demonstrate no visual field defect on unilateral stimulation; however, during bilateral stimulation, they extinguish the target contralateral to their lesion. Other persons may perceive both targets simultaneously, yet when engaged in activity, they may not respond to visual stimuli in one half of visual space contralateral to their lesion. These individuals are unaware of their inattention. Careful observation of their activity reveals a paucity of eye movements into the neglected space. The fovea does not appear to be directed to gather information in this space.

Unilateral visual, auditory, and tactile inattention. Inattention has been described as a multimodal sensory associative disorder involving not only visual but also tactile and auditory unawareness. Clinicians are well aware of the client with left inattention who continues to direct the head and eyes toward the right throughout an entire conversation even though the therapist is standing on the client's left side. When one conceptualizes unilateral spatial inattention as a dynamic decrease or loss of sensory information within one half of the sensory-perceptual sphere (irrespective of hypothetical mechanism), the peculiar behaviors exhibited by these clients are more easily understood.

Unilateral spatial inattention and body image. Body image is often disturbed in individuals with inattention. The defect in these persons is unusual because it affects only that half of the body which is contralateral to the lesion, for example, the left side of the body in right-sided lesions. There appears to be a lack of spatial orientation and attention for one half of intrapersonal space. Those with severe inattention fail to recognize that their affected extremities are their own and function as though they are absent. They may fail to dress one half of their body or attempt to navigate through a door oblivious to the fact that the affected arm may be caught on the doorknob or door frame. In severe cases, individuals may deny their hemiparesis, or they may deny that the extremity belongs to them. This phenomenon is called *anosognosia.*

Behavioral manifestations of unilateral spatial inattention. Persons with inattention orient all their activities toward their "attended" space. The head, eyes, and trunk are rotated toward the side of the lesion during much of the time, including during gait. Careful observation of eye movements (scanning saccades) during activities indicates that all or almost all scanning occurs on only one side of the midline within the attended space; the individual never spontaneously brings the eyes or head past midline into contralateral "unattended" space. Oculomotor examination always shows full extraocular movements and no apraxia for eye movements.

Inattention, as all other perceptual disorders, may be viewed on a scale from mild to severe. Mild cases of inattention may go unrecognized unless behavior is carefully observed. Scanning is symmetrical except during tasks requiring increasingly complex perceptual and cognitive demands. Leicester and co-workers[67] believe that inattention occurs mainly when the individual has a general perceptual problem with the material, that is, some other problem with processing the task. This performance difficulty or stress brings on the additional inattention behavior; for example, neglect for matching auditory letter samples is more common in those with aphasia than in those with right hemisphere involvement without aphasia.

Independence in activities of daily living is often impossible because of inattention to both the intrapersonal and extrapersonal environment. The individual may eat only half of the food on the plate, dress only half the body, shave or apply makeup to only half the face, brush teeth in only half the mouth, read only half the page, fill out only one half a form, miss kitchen utensils, carpentry tools, or items in the store if they are located in the unattended space, collide with obstacles or miss doorways on the unattended side, and when walking or driving a wheelchair, veer toward the attended space rather than navigating in a straight line.

Assessment. Since most tests used to measure cognitive, language, perceptual, and motor skills require symmetrical visual, auditory, and tactile awareness, it is most important to rule out inattention early in the evaluation process of any client with a central lesion. The two most common methods used to distinguish inattention from primary sensory deficits are double simultaneous stimulation testing and assessment of optokinetic nystagmus (OKN) reflexes. Double simultaneous stimuli should be applied in three modalities: auditory, tactile, and visual. Initially, stimuli should be presented to the abnormal side. If primary sensation is impaired (e.g., a visual field loss), one cannot proceed because double simultaneous stimulation testing is invalid in that modality. However, if responsiveness is normal, bilateral simultaneous stimuli should be applied. Unilateral stimuli should be interspersed with bilateral stimuli to ensure valid responses. Lack of awareness (extinction) of stimuli contralateral to the lesion during bilateral stimulation should be noted. Clients with extinction in only one sensory system often do not demonstrate inattention behaviors; however, those with extinction in more than one modality (e.g., tactile and visual) often demonstrate these behaviors. If critical diagnosis of inattention is necessary, the client may be referred for OKN testing.

One of the best evaluation tools is a keen sense of observation. The position of the client's head, eyes, and trunk should be observed at rest and during activity. Persistent deviation toward the lesion may indicate unilateral inattention. The individual should be asked to track a visual target from space ipsilateral to the lesion into contralateral space and maintain fixation there for 5 seconds. The therapist may ask the client to quickly fixate visual targets on command both right and left of midline. Problems with searching for targets in contralateral space should be noted. Some erratic oculomotor searching is normal when making saccades into a hemianoptic field since saccades are centrally preprogrammed by peripheral input. Very slow searching or failure to search should be considered indicative of inattention.

Asymmetries in performance should be noted during spatial tasks. Specific spatial tasks have been designed to detect inattention, including,

1. *Cancellation tasks.* The client may be given a sheet of paper with horizontal lines of numbers or letters and asked to cross out all the *eights* or *A's.*
2. *Crossing out tasks.* In this test, standardized by Albert,[2] the client is asked to cross out diagonal lines drawn at random on an unlined sheet of paper.
3. *Line bisection tasks.* The client is asked to bisect a 4-inch–8-inch line on a piece of paper placed at his or her midline.
4. *Drawing and copying tasks.* The client may be asked to draw or copy a house, clock, or flower or to fill in the numbers of a clock drawn by the examiner. For copying tasks, it is important that the copy be placed in the client's attended space.

Clients with inattention demonstrate one or more of the following behaviors: failure to cancel figures or cross out lines in the unattended space; bisecting the line unequally, placing their mark toward the side of the midline ipsilateral to their lesion; placing their drawing toward the edge of the paper ipsilateral to their lesion rather than in the middle of the page; drawing only the right or left half of the house, flower, or clock; crowding all the numbers of the clock into the right or left half of the clock; or completing numbers on only one half of the clock (Fig. 25-5). When interpreting performance, the examiner is looking specifically for asymmetries in performance. Clients with inattention often have other visual perceptual deficits that result in faulty performance on these tasks; however, these deficits are always symmetrical, that is, evident in any space to which the individual attends.

Asymmetries in performance should be carefully observed during functional activities such as eating, filling out a form, reading, dressing, and maneuvering through the environment. The therapist may note unawareness of doorways and hallways in the unattended space; turns may be made only toward one direction. As a result, these clients lose their way in the hospital or even in the physical therapy clinic. This behavior should be distinguished from a topographical perceptual deficit in which the individual cannot integrate or remember spatial concepts well enough

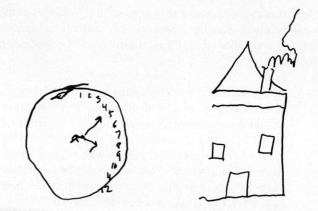

Fig. 25-5 Drawings of a clock and house by a client with a right hemisphere parietal lobe tumor. Note the left unilateral spatial inattention in the drawings.

to find his or her way without getting lost. The Behavioral Inattention Test has recently been published as a standardized measure of functional inattention.[98]

Finally, various studies have shown that inattention may occur during testing that requires visual processing and may therefore invalidate test results.[19,20,44] Unresponsiveness to figures on one side of the page during visual, perceptual, cognitive, or language assessments may be subtle but must be documented to rule out the influence of inattention on raw score; that is, if the patient did not see the entire test display in an item, that test item is invalid. Responses to figures on the right half and left half of the test page should be counted. If the frequency of answers is noticeably less on one half of the page than would normally be expected, one may suspect that inattention may have occurred during testing. This may be used as additional evidence of inattention but, more importantly, this factor should be accounted for when computing test score. Only those test items in which the correct answer was located in the attended space should be scored, that is, only those items in which the correct answer was right of midline in a client with left inattention.

Treatment. As previously stated, the mechanisms underlying unilateral spatial inattention have not been clearly elucidated. This has made treatment rationales difficult. A number of studies, however, have investigated the remediation of unilateral spatial inattention. They have attempted to (1) define effective remediation techniques and (2) measure changes in trained tasks as well as generalization to untrained tasks; that is, does inattention training in one task carry over to other unrelated tasks such as activities of daily living. Treatment techniques used in all of these studies resulted in less inattention in trained tasks.[30,64,89] An overview of these studies suggests that training may decrease inattention, although extent of change and generalization to other tasks may vary widely. Discrepancies in these results may be related to neurological variables in the various client samples, severity of inattention, sample size, or tasks measured. General principles of remediation follow.

1. Effort should be made to increase the client's cognitive awareness of the inattention. The individual should be made keenly aware of what a peripheral visual field loss is and how it is affecting his or her view of the world. The person with normal visual fields but with visual extinction should be treated the same as the individual with an actual visual field loss since the visual experience is similar. Pictures of the visual field deficit may be drawn for illustration. Actual performance examples in the environment should be pointed out to the client to demonstrate the biased field of view.

2. Visual scanning should be emphasized. Initially the client should be made aware of how eye and eye-head movements may be used to compensate for the deficit. The individual should be trained to make progressively larger and quicker pursuits and saccades and longer fixations into the unattended space. Training may be accomplished with interesting targets held by the therapist, for examples, targets secured to the tips of pencils, such as changeable letters, colored lights, or bright small objects. Pursuit or tracking movements of the target leading the eye from attended into unattended space should be stressed first, followed by saccades into the unattended space. Initially, the client may be allowed to move the head during scanning exercises; however, eye movements without head movements should be the major goal. Individuals with inattention often move their head into the unattended space while their eye remains fixed on a target in their attended space (i.e., the visual field remains the same). The client should be taught to independently carry out a daily right-left scanning program with targets appropriately positioned by the therapist. Eventually, these targets can be moved farther into the unattended space.

3. Increased awareness and scanning abilities should be incorporated in increasingly complex visual perceptual and visual motor tasks. Since inattention often increases as task complexity increases, the therapist must select and structure tasks carefully. Examples of simple yet specific scanning tasks might include surveying a room repetitively, rolling toward and touching objects right and left of midline, assembling objects from pieces strewn on a table or the floor, completing an obstacle course, or selecting letters from a page of large print.

4. Scanning should be stressed during functional activities, for example, dressing, shaving, and moving through the environment. The client may be taught to constantly monitor the influence of inattention on functional performance, for example: "When something doesn't make sense, look into the unattended space and it usually will."

5. Diller[29] has designed a number of specific training techniques to decrease inattention during reading and paper and pencil tasks. With a little creativity, these techniques may be applied to other activities. For example, when the client is reading, a visual marker is placed on the extreme edge of the page in unattended space. The individual is instructed not to begin reading until he or she sees the visual marker. The marker is used to "anchor" the client's vision. As inattention decreases, the anchor is faded. Each line may also be numbered and the numbers used to anchor scanning horizontally and vertically. To control impulsiveness, which often accompanies inattention, clients are taught to slow down or pace their performance by incorporating techniques such as reciting the words aloud. Underlining and looping let-

					0	(1)	2	4	5	6	7	8	9	10						
1.	(1)	2	3	5	4	9	7	8	0	6	3	2	10	(1)	2	3	5	4	9	7	1
2.	3	4	9	6	7	10	8	(1)	2	5	0	6	4	9	6	7	10	8	2	8	2
3.	8	0	6	2	(1)	3	5	4	7	9	10	(1)	8	0	6	2	(1)	3	5	7	3
4.	5	7	3	9	6	(1)	2	8	4	10	0	3	5	5	7	3	6	(1)	2	5	4
5.	6	5	(1)	4	2	3	8	10	9	7	9	0	6	5	(1)	4	2	3	8	9	5
6.	4	8	10	0	7	6	9	1	3	2	5	6	3	4	8	10	0	7	6	9	6
7.	9	6	5	3	8	4	2	0	10	1	7	2	4	9	6	5	3	8	2	4	7

Fig. 25-6. Underlining during visual discrimination tasks helps control eye movements (scanning).

ters/words can also be used as a method to slow down impulsive scanning (see Fig. 25-6). Finally, density of stimuli is reduced; decreased density appears to decrease inattention in these tasks.

To stimulate tactile awareness in clients with tactile extinction, Anderson and Choy[4] suggest simulating the affected arm as the individual watches. A rough cloth, vibrator, or the therapist's or client's hand may be used. Eventually, this activity may be done before activities that require spontaneous symmetrical scanning, such as dressing and walking through an obstacle course.

During the early phases of treatment, when inattention is still moderate to severe, the client should be approached from the attended space during treatment for inattention or other deficits such as apraxia, balance, or speech. This ensures that the individual comprehends and views all demonstrations and treatment instructions. Subsequently, as orientation and scanning improve, activities should be moved progressively into the unattended space and the therapist should be positioned in the unattended space during treatment. In the final stages of treatment the client should be able to symmetrically scan regardless of the therapist's position (i.e., the therapist should vary position).

To enhance the integration of scanning behavior during functional tasks such as gait and dressing, the client should be reminded of scanning principles and carried through a series of scanning exercises before initiation of the activity. If inattention reappears during the activity, the therapist should stop and assist the client in becoming *reoriented* before resuming the activity. Inattention results in confusion, and confusion increases inattention. As will be pointed out repeatedly in the following pages, the therapist must control the perceptual environment continuously so that the client is able to sequence bits of information together meaningfully in order to learn or relearn.

Problems of cortical blindness, color imperception, and visual agnosia

Identification of clinical problems

Cortical blindness. Cortical blindness is considered a primary sensory disorder as opposed to a secondary associative disorder. It is discussed here, however, because of the many variations of this lesion that may result in problems with interpretation of visual stimuli. Cortical blindness, also known as central blindness, is a loss of total or almost total vision resulting from bilateral cerebral destruction of the visual projection cortex (Area 17). Similar destruction limited to one hemisphere results in a hemianopsia.[27] The lesion may be ischemic, neoplastic, degenerative, or traumatic in nature. The client may perceive the defect as a "blurring" of vision, a marked decrease in visual acuity, or may be unaware of the complete nature of the disability and even deny it, blaming the problem on glasses that are too weak or a room that is too dark.

Color imperception. Color perception may be impaired in the client with brain damage. This symptom is usually associated with right hemisphere or bilateral lesions.[85] This deficit is different from color agnosia in which there is a problem with naming colors correctly. Clients with defective color perception may see colors as "muddy" or "impure" in hue, or the color of a small target may fade into the background, decreasing the ability to differentiate it from the background.[70,86] Total loss of color (achromatopsia) is rare but can occur.

Visual agnosia. A lesion circumscribed to the visual associative areas (Areas 18 and 19) results in a number of unique visual disorders that are categorized as some form of visual agnosia. Lesions are usually bilateral with combined parietooccipital, occipitotemporal, and callosal lesions. Visual agnosia is defined as a failure to recognize visual stimuli (e.g., objects, faces, letters) even though visual sensory processing, language, and general intellectual functions are preserved at sufficiently high levels.[82] It has also been described as perception without meaning; perception apparently occurs, but the percept seems "disconnected" from previously associated meaning. In this pure form, visual agnosia is a relatively rare syndrome and there is controversy as to whether it is simply an extension of primary visual sensory deficits (variations of cortical blindness) or whether it should be considered as a separate neuropsychological entity.

Three types of agnosia have been recognized: visual, tactile, and auditory. Agnosia is most often modality specific; that is, the individual who cannot recognize the object visually will usually give an immediate and accurate response when touching or hearing the object in use. In visual agnosia, then, poor recognition is limited to the visual sphere.

Visual agnosia is divided into a number of types: visual object agnosia, simultanagnosia, facial agnosia, and color agnosia. These deficits may be seen in isolation or in various combinations, depending on size and location of lesion.

VISUAL OBJECT AGNOSIA. During evaluation for the presence of visual object agnosia, the individual is presented with a number of common objects (e.g., key, comb, brush) and asked to name them. The evaluator may assume that the object is recognized if the client (1) names, describes, or demonstrates the use of the object or (2) selects it from among a group of objects as it is named by the examiner. If the person recognizes (describes or demonstrates) but is unable to name the object, failure is most likely a result of an anomia rather than an agnosic defect. Individuals with real visual agnosia have no concept of what the object is.[82]

SIMULTANAGNOSIA. Along the same vein are visual disorders that constrict or "narrow" the visual field during active perceptual analysis (i.e., when perceptions are tested separately, the visual field is within normal limits). Simultanagnosia is a disorder in which the person actually perceives only one element of an object or picture at a time and is unable to absorb the whole. As the individual concentrates on the visual environment, there is an extreme reduction of visual span. The problem is functionally similar to tubular vision. The narrowing of the functional perceptual field decreases the ability to simultaneously deal with two or more stimuli. It appears as if the person has bilateral visual inattention with macular sparing, although perimetric testing reveals full visual fields. A typical example is the individual whose visual attention is focused on the tip of a cigarette held between his or her lips and fails to perceive a match flame offered several inches away.[52]

FACIAL AGNOSIA. Another special type of agnosia that has been documented is failure to recognize familiar faces. The disorder is also known as *prosopagnosia*. The individual is able to recognize a face as a face but is unable to connect the face and differences in faces with people he or she knows. This person is unable to recognize family members, friends, and hospital staff by face. One must be careful not to confuse this with generalized dementia. There may be categorical recognition problems of items involving special visual experience, for example, recognition of cars, types of trees, and emblems. Facial agnosia is usually seen in combination with a number of other deficits including spatial disorientation, defective color perception, loss of topographical memory, constructional apraxia, and a left upper quadrant visual field loss. These other symptoms are most likely not causative but rather a result of the similar neurological location of these functions.[14]

COLOR AGNOSIA. Finally, the individual may have difficulty recognizing names of colors—that is, an inability to name colors that are shown or to point to the color named by the examiner. This defect is considered agnosic (as opposed to a defect in color perception) because the client is able to recognize all colors in the Ishihara Color Plates[58] and is also able to sort colors by hue. The determining factor here appears to be a problem with visual-verbal association. Color agnosia is most common in left hemisphere lesions and is often accompanied by the syndrome of alexia without agraphia.[82]

Assessment. Cortical blindness and variations of it should be thoroughly assessed by the vision specialist. Assessment for agnosia must be preceded by a thorough visual acuity, visual field, and unilateral visual inattention assessment, since these primary visual sensory and scanning deficits are often mistaken for agnosic performance. Next, basic color perception should be measured using the Ishihara Color Plates and color-sorting or color-matching tasks. Individuals with defective color perception will have difficulty with some visual perceptual tasks since contextual cues related to color and shading are unavailable to them. Agnosia is a valid diagnosis only if (1) the aforementioned primary visual skills are intact and (2) language skills are intact (that is, there should be no word-finding difficulty in spontaneous speech).

Although there are no standardized tests for agnosia, commonly used assessment methods have been included. The presence of simultanagnosia is determined by keen observation of performance that indicates perception limited to single elements within objects, for example, describing only the wheel of a bicycle or, within the environment, describing only one part of a room or an activity.

Object agnosia is tested by placing common real objects (e.g., comb, key, penny, spoon) in front of the client and asking him or her to name or point to the item chosen by the examiner. In pointing and naming tasks, the therapist must be sure that the client is fixating on the appropriate target. This response is considered normal if the object is named correctly, described, or its functional use demonstrated. Abnormal responses will be confabulatory or perserverative, the individual often giving the name of a previous or similar object. Responses may also be completely bizarre and unrelated. The examiner may also present objects at an unusual angle. Abnormal responses will show lack of recognition and/or rotation of the head or body to try to view the object in the "straight on" position. The diagnosis of visual object agnosia is further confirmed if the individual can identify the object by touch or by hearing it in use. Both should be done with vision occluded.

Color agnosia is evaluated by having the client name a color and point to colors named by the examiner. Facial agnosia is evaluated by presenting the individual with photographs of famous world figures, actors, politicians, and family members.[86]

Treatment. There are no reliable studies regarding treatment of cortical blindness, color imperception, or visual agnosia. Treatment principles presented here are based on Bouska's and other clinicians' experience. If cortical blindness or simultanagnosia is suspected, the therapist must first attempt to increase the client's knowledge of foveal versus peripheral vision, that is, where the individual is fixating. A small headlamp attached to the client's forehead may be used under conditions of subdued lighting. This should not be used in a completely darkened room because the client needs to use normal spatial cues from the environment. The movement of the projected light in the environment and kinesthetic input from the neck receptors augment knowledge of where the eye is fixed. To carry out this task, the client must learn to position the eyes in midline of the head. The individual is asked to move the light (his head and eyes) to locate and discriminate fairly large, bright stimuli placed on a plain background (e.g., yellow block on a brown table). As acuity and localization skills improve, stimuli and background should be made smaller and more complex (e.g., paper clip on a printed background or letters printed at different locations on a large page). The client should be encouraged to accurately point to and/or manipulate targets once located with the light or to keep the light on a target as he or she slowly moves the target with one hand. In this mode, the kinesthetic input from the limb can augment visual localization abilities.[64] In patients with color imperception, treatment should initially involve materials/tasks with sharp color contrasts with minimal detail and progress to less contrast (more hues) with more detail.

If the assessment has revealed a narrowing of the perceptual field, treatment should be aimed at progressively increasing the perception of large, bright, peripheral targets. For example, the client may be asked to fixate a centrally placed target while another bright target is brought in slowly from or uncovered in the periphery.[11,100] The individual is encouraged to maintain fixation on the central target while remaining alert for the presence of another target somewhere in the periphery. As the client improves, targets should be smaller, multiple, and exposed for briefer periods. Peripheral targets should always have bright surfaces that reflect light since the peripheral receptors in the retina are mainly rods (light as opposed to color receptors).

The treatment of clients with object agnosia should progress according to the abilities that return first in spontaneous recovery from agnosia. Common real objects should be used before line drawings in treatment. Presentations should be given "straight-on" rather than at an angle or rotated. The client should be asked to point to objects named by the examiner before being asked to name them. Manipulation of the object with simultaneous visual input should be attempted. This may help recognition, or it may simply confuse the client; each case is unique. In general, tactile input with or without simultaneous visual input should be encouraged as a compensation method even though it may not be helpful during treatment sessions.

Color and facial agnosia may be approached by simply drilling the individual with regard to two or three names of colors or names of faces of people important to him or her. The client may be helped to pick out or memorize cues for associating names with faces.[86]

Problems of visuospatial disorder

Identification of clinical problems. Individuals with brain lesions, particularly in the right posterior parietal and occipital areas, may have difficulties with tasks that require a normal concept of space.[27] Disorders of this nature have been termed visuospatial disorders, spatial disorientation, visuospatial agnosia, spatial relations syndrome, and numerous other terms. Visuospatial abilities are complexly interwoven within the performance of many perceptual and cognitive activities such as dressing, building a design, reading, calculating, walking through an aisle, and playing tennis. An attempt is made here, however, to discuss spatial disorders in their purest form—that is, basic disorders—before dealing with visuoconstructive disorders and disorders of analysis and synthesis. Constructional tasks

require spatial planning, a type of planning that involves the building up and breaking down of objects in two and three dimensions. Constructional apraxia is viewed as a particular type of spatial perceptual disorder and will, therefore, be discussed separately under visuoconstructive disorders and disorders of analysis and synthesis. Similarly, although perceptual skills such as figure-ground, form constancy, complex visual discrimination, and figure closure involve spatial concepts, tasks involving these skills often require the intellectual operations of synthesis and deduction. They too will be discussed in the section dealing with analysis and synthesis.

All visuospatial disabilities involve some problem with the apprehension of the spatial relationships between or within objects. Benton[13] has categorized them as the following disabilities:

1. *Inability to localize objects in space, to estimate their size, and to judge their distance from the observer.* The client may be unable to accurately touch an object in space or indicate the position of the object (e.g., above, below, in front of, or behind). Relative localization may be impaired so that the individual may be unable to tell which object is closest to him or her. There may be difficulty determining which of two objects is larger or which line is longer. Holmes[67] reported cases of gross disorder in spatial orientation revealed through walking, with individuals who, even after seeing objects correctly, ran into them. In another example, a man, intending to go toward his bed, would invariably set out in the wrong direction. Difficulty in estimating distances may also extend to judgments of distances of perceived sounds and lead to overly slow and cautious gait or fear of venturing into public areas.

2. *Impaired memory for the location of objects or places,* as in recalling the position of a target previously viewed or the arrangement of furniture in a room. Individuals with this difficulty often lose things because they have no spatial memory to rely on for recall.

3. *Inability to trace a path or follow a route from one place to another.* Persons without this ability, known as topographical orientation, have difficulty understanding and remembering relationships of places to one another so that they may have difficulty finding their way in space, locating the physical therapy clinic in a hospital, locating the housewares department in a store previously familiar to them. Normally functioning individuals often experience mild signs of topographical disorientation. Everyone is familiar with the disoriented feeling of not knowing how to get out of a large department store or losing a sense of direction in a familiar city. Many of the topographical errors made by clients re-

sult from unilateral spatial inattention. For example, someone with left inattention may make only right turns. Topographical disorientation, however, may be seen in a person with no signs of unilateral inattention. This individual will demonstrate route-finding difficulties at certain points and apparently randomly choose a direction.

4. *Problems with reading and counting.* These high-level tasks require directional control of eye movements and organized scanning abilities. Eye movements (saccades) during reading bring a new region of the text on the fovea, the part of the retina where visual acuity is the greatest and clear detail can be obtained from the stimulus. During reading, the line of print that falls on the retina may be divided into three regions: the foveal region, the parafoveal region, and the peripheral region. The foveal region subtends about 1 degree to 2 degrees of visual angle around the reader's fixation point, the parafoveal region subtends about 10 degrees of visual angle around the reader's fixation point, and the peripheral region includes everything on the page beyond the parafoveal region. Parafoveal and peripheral vision contribute spatial information that is used to guide the reader's eye.[79] Visuospatial disorders appear to interfere to varying degrees with the spatial schema of a page of type or numbers and the dynamic organizational scanning that must take place to gather information appropriately. Clients with unilateral spatial inattention will miss words or numbers located on one half of the page. Other spatial problems unrelated to unilateral inattention include skipping individual words within a line or part of a line, skipping lines, repeating lines, "blocking" or the inability to change direction of fixation, particularly at the end of a line, and generally losing the place on the total page. Performance usually deteriorates progressively as the individual continues to read. Eventually, such persons cannot make sense of what they read or, if counting, they complain of being lost or confused. This type of reading or counting disorder has nothing to do with recognition or interpretation of letters or numbers or their spatial configuration; rather it represents a problem with dynamic sequential visuospatial exploration during cognitive processing.

Other visuospatial problems may include loss of depth perception, problems with body schema, and defective judgment of line orientation. There may also be difficulties with discrimination of right and left. Although unilateral spatial inattention is considered a visuospatial disorder by many, it has been discussed separately in this chapter to increase clarity. Problems with judging line orientation (slant) and/or unilateral spatial inattention often interfere with a client's spatial ability to tell time when using a standard watch or clock. Perception of the vertical may also be considered a visuospatial skill. Verticality perception is the interpretation of internal and external cues to maintain body balance. This maintenence is a complex neuromuscular process involving visual, proprioceptive, and vestibular systems. Clients with right lesions, particularly in the parietooccipital region, have more difficulty perceiving verticality than those with left lesions. This may affect posture and ambulation.[28]

Assessment. The client should be asked to accurately touch a number of targets in all parts of the visual field while fixating on a central point. Mislocalization should be noted as well as that part of the visual field in which it occurred. Mislocalization within the central field is infrequent; however, defective localization of stimuli on one or both extramacular fields is more frequently seen.[27] The client should be asked to determine which of a number of small cube blocks (placed perpendicularly in front of him or her) is closest, which is farthest, and which is in the middle. Differences in binocular (stereoscopic) and monocular viewing should be measured in this and other tasks. Impairment in both of these types of depth perception and subsequent inaccuracy in judging distances have been described in individuals with brain injury.[13]

With regard to memory for the location of objects or places, clients should be asked to describe the position of objects in their room from memory. They may also be asked to duplicate from memory the position of two or more targets (on a table or piece of paper) that have been presented for a 5-second period. As the number of targets increases, individuals with short-term memory for spatial localization will begin to make errors in spatial placement. Visual memory per se should be ruled out as a conflicting variable.

Topographical sense is assessed by asking clients to describe a floor plan of the arrangement of rooms in their house or to describe familiar geographical constellations, such as routes, arrangement of streets, or public buildings. Following therapy these persons may also be asked to find their way back to their room after being shown the route several times. Failure suggests a topographical orientation problem. Finally, such a client may be asked to locate states or cities on a large map of the United States. In all of these procedures, the examiner must be sure to separate unilateral spatial inattention errors from topographical errors.

The influence of spatial dysfunction on reading and counting written material may be measured by simply asking the client to read a page of regular newsprint. The examiner should observe performance carefully and document type and frequency of errors. If errors occur, eye movements should be observed to gather additional information. Pages of scanning material (letters or numbers) often give additional information on spatial planning during reading. These are pages of print in which the size and density of the print is controlled. Scanning behavior may be demonstrated by asking the client to circle specific letters. Switching direction in the middle of a line, skipping letters or lines, perseveration, or any other abnormal performance behavior should be noted. Benton's Judgment of Line Orientation Test[15] may be used to document problems with directional orientation of lines. If there is no indication of apraxia, the client may simply be given a ruler and asked to match it to the directional orientation of the examiner's ruler.

Treatment   Treatment for visuospatial deficits should follow basic developmental considerations progressing from simple to more complex tasks. (For additional treatment ideas, see the discussion of visuospatial treatment in children.) As with children, if the evaluation suggests disorders in body scheme, tactile or vestibular input, or right-left discrimination, these should be dealt with first.

Clients who do not know where they are in space need to internalize a spatial understanding before they can make judgments regarding the space around them. In gross motor spatial training, clients can be asked to roll and reach toward various targets. In supine, prone, sitting, and standing, with vision occluded, clients should try to localize tactile stimuli (various body locations touched by the therapist) and auditory stimuli (snapping fingers or ringing bell) presented above, below, behind, in front of, and right and left of their bodies. The individual should state where the stimulus is and then point, roll, crawl, or walk toward it; this verbal, kinesthetic, and vestibular input augments spatial learning. In the occupational therapy kitchen the client, once oriented to the room, may be asked to retrieve one type of object (e.g., cup) from "the top cupboard above your head," from "the bottom cupboard below your waist," from "the table behind you," or from "the drawer on your right or left." These clients may also place objects in various positions within a room. They should then stand in the middle of the room, close their eyes, and from memory visualize, verbalize, and point to where the objects are in relation to themselves. Having localized them, the clients should then walk through the space and retrieve the objects in sequence. Functional carry-over should always be emphasized, such as having individuals remember through visualization where they put their glasses in the living room before they begin searching. Visualization is defined as the internal "seeing" of something that is not present at that moment: a vision without a visual input or internal visual imagery.[36] Visualization (spatial and other) is part of all perceptual tasks and may be used effectively as a treatment strategy. As previously discussed, a small feedback light placed in the middle of the client's forehead can help teach spatial localization through eye-head movements.

More complex spatial skills may be taught by asking

clients to "partition" space and then localize within it. An excellent activity is one in which clients use a yardstick to divide a blackboard into four or more equal parts and then number each section.

Objects may be presented to clients, who must select the largest, the farthest away, or the one placed at an angle; they may be asked to place various objects in certain relationships to each other. As shape, size, and angle begin to "make sense" to these individuals, form boards, simple puzzles, and parquetry blocks may be added to training.

Topographical abilities should improve as clients begin to better conceptualize space; however, they may be trained directly. The therapist may help such clients organize a basic floor plan of their hospital room and the furniture within it while looking at the room. They may then be asked to do this from memory. Activities can progress to drawing plans or larger areas with a number of rooms. These clients should first "navigate" tactually through the area with their finger. Eventually, they should walk or wheel through the route themselves, visualizing and repeating the route until spatial concepts are learned. Imaginary routes may also be taken through maps of cities, states, or countries.

Organized visuospatial exploration (eye movements) during reading or other scanning and cancellation tasks may be taught. Number and letter scanning sheets may be used for such training. Initially, size of numbers and spaces between numbers should be large; this places less stress on visual acuity while training scanning. Before beginning, clients should orient themselves to the page spatially by numbering the right and left edge of each line. These numbers are used as additional spatial localization cues if needed during the scanning task.[29] Clients should then be asked to circle a specific number (or numbers) whenever it occurs. To control erratic or impulsive eye movements, they should be instructed to use a pencil to underline each line and then loop the selected letter as it comes into view Fig. 25-6. They may also be asked to read each letter. Underlining allows the kinesthetic and tactile receptors of the arm to control eye movements; verbalization allows the language and auditory systems to influence eye movements. Visuospatial exploration exercises should progress to large-print magazines, books, or newspapers. The *New York Times* and *Reader's Digest* are both available in large print.

In all training activities it is most important that, before the activity begins, clients fully comprehend the total space in which they will work. It is equally important that they reorient themselves at any point where errors occur. Those who lose their place during reading will eventually lose it again if the therapist simply points to where they should be. Chances are better that they will not lose their place again if they reorient themselves to the page spatially when an error occurs.

Problems of visuoconstructive disorders

Identification of clinical problems. Clients with lesions in either the right or left hemisphere may show problems when trying to "construct." Lesions in the parietal, temporal, occipital, and frontal lobes have been documented in individuals with visuoconstructive disorders.[27,68] The normal ability to construct, also known as visuoconstructive ability and constructional praxis, involves any type of performance in which parts are put together to form a single entity. Examples include assembling blocks to form a design, assembling a puzzle, making a dress, setting a table, or simply drawing four lines to form a square (graphic skills). The skill implies a high level of dynamic, organized, visuoperceptual processing in which (1) the spatial relations are perceived and sequenced well enough among and within the component parts to (2) direct higher-level processing to sequence the perceptual motor actions so that eventually (3) parts are synthesized into a desired whole. Visuoconstructive ability may be compromised if any part of this process is disturbed.

Typical tasks used to measure this ability include building in a vertical direction, building in a horizontal direction, three-dimensional block construction from a model or a picture of a model, or copying line drawings such as house, flower, and geometric designs.[14]

Clients with visuoconstructive deficits, especially those with right lesions, often also have visuospatial deficits. These individuals may rotate the position of a part erroneously, place it in the wrong position, space it too far from another part, be oblivious to perspective or a third dimension, or simply be unable to complete more than two or three steps before becoming entirely confused. This is usually evidence of breakdown because of faulty or inadequate spatial information.

Other clients, usually those with left lesions, have an "executional" or apraxic problem; they seem to have difficulty initiating and conducting the planned sequence of movements necessary to construct the whole. The problem seems to be in planning, arranging, building, or drawing rather than in spatial concepts. This deficit in its purest form is known as constructional apraxia. Constructional apraxia lies clinically outside the category of most other varieties of apraxia and is considered a special kind of "perceptual" apraxia. It occurs frequently in aphasic individuals, and therefore the underlying mechanisms of aphasia and constructional apraxia may be related.[87]

Assessment. Constructional abilities are generally measured through tasks that require (1) copying line drawings such as a house, clock face, flower, or geometric designs (drawing may also be done without copy), (2) copying two-dimensional matchstick designs, (3) building block designs from copy or model, or (4) assembling puzzles. (Table 25-4 lists common tests.) The more complex the picture or design to be copied, the more complex the con-

Table 25-4. Common tests used to assess visuoconstructive skills

Test	Standardization
Drawing picture or shapes with or without copy	Not standardized
Reproducing matchstick designs	Not standardized
Assembling puzzles	Not standardized
The Bender Visual Motor Gestalt Test	Standardized for children only
Kohs' Blocks Test	Standardized for adults
WAIS Block Design Test	Standardized for adults
Benton's Three-Dimensional Constructional Praxis Test	Standardized for adults

structional task. The following are examples of drawing and block construction deficits.

1. Clients may crowd the drawing or design on one side of the page or in one corner of the page or available space on the working surface, usually a result of the influence of unilateral spatial inattention.
2. Lines in drawings may be wavy or broken, too long or short.
3. One line may not meet another accurately or lines may transect each other; in block designs, parts may not be neatly placed but rather may have small gaps.
4. There may be "overdrawing" of angles or parts of the figure because of graphic perseveration (scribble), spatial indecision, or problems with executive planning.
5. Clients may superimpose their copy on the model or superimpose one of their drawings on top of another. In block design construction, they may become confused between the model and their reproduction and use part of the model to complete their design. This has been termed the "closing-in" phenomenon, a failure to distinguish between model and reproduction.[27]
6. Parts of the drawing or design may be reversed. Horizontal reversals are more common than vertical reversals.

A note might be appropriate here regarding dressing apraxia. This problem occurs most frequently with right hemisphere damage. It is considered a "perceptual" apraxia rather than a motor apraxia since the inability to dress is believed to result from body scheme, spatial, and visuoconstructive deficits rather than difficulty in motor execution. Persons with dressing apraxia cannot correctly orient their clothes to their body. They often put clothes on backward or inside out. Failure to dress one side of the body is also often noted and is directly related to unilateral spatial inattention.

Treatment. It must be remembered that both visuoconstructive and visual analysis synthesis skills are often used almost simultaneously during task performance. Thus treatment should not separate the two skills but rather be a precise interrelationship of activities that require finer and finer levels of each facility. For example, arranging an office filing system is both an analytical/synthetical and a visuoconstructive task. The individual must first analyze overall needs and translate them into an imagined visuospatial plan (preliminary synthesis of the whole) that will help organization. Then the organizer begins to use his or her hands to categorize (segment visual space). This building is a visuoconstructive task. Intermittently during building, new ideas of the whole surface, and visuoconstructive tasks change in response to a "better idea" (final synthesis of the whole). Task performance, except for tasks that are rote, usually follows similar perceptual processes. Treatment therefore must be integral. Visuoconstructive skills, however, may be emphasized more than visual analysis and synthesis skills or vice versa.

As previously mentioned, visuoconstructive disorders are thought to result from different underlying problems in different individuals (e.g., visuospatial disorders in persons with right hemisphere lesions and executive, planning, or synthetic disorders in those with left hemisphere lesions). There are few reliable studies on treatment strategies for visuoconstructive disorders. One possible treatment strategy is known as *saturational cuing.*[16] This method involves presenting controlled verbal instruction on task analysis and sequence and presenting cues on spatial boundaries, (cuing is also response related).

If there are problems with planning and sequencing of steps necessary to accomplish a visuoconstructive task, the therapist should begin with simple tasks that require only three to four steps, such as positioning one place setting at a table. The client should discuss the plan and sequence of steps before initiating the activity, while looking at the parts to be used, such as silverware, plate, and glass. These steps may even be written down for additional input. The client should be helped to reorient the plan at any point during task breakdown. Eventually, tasks should increase in complexity (e.g., setting a table for five), and the client should be encouraged to function more independently. Another technique often used by clinicians is known as *backward chaining.* This involves presenting a partially completed task and asking the client to complete the final steps—for example, placing the knife and glass on a partially completed place setting. The perceptual cues of the task already begun appear to stimulate constructional abilities. As the client progresses, he or she should complete more steps.

Treatment for problems with spatial planning during visuoconstructive tasks should begin with simple spatial exercises discussed previously. If problems still exist, the individual may be asked to draw around shapes (blocks) one by one. These shapes should first have been placed in a simple two-dimensional design. The client is then asked to rebuild the design with the shapes alone. Therapy should progress from horizontal to vertical to oblique designs, from two-dimensional to three-dimensional designs, and from tasks with common objects to tasks involving abstract designs. For example, spatial problems with drawing, such as placing windows in a house or numbers on a clock face, are usually a result of underlying spatial disorder. The client should use a ruler or protractor to segment the space and plan placement before drawing. Dot-to-dot tasks may be designed that actually lead and sequence the drawing into a spatial whole. Simple puzzles may also be used to increase visuospatial abilities during visuoconstructive tasks. Finally, if task breakdown results from impulsive visual or motor behavior, these symptoms should be dealt with before further visuoconstructive treatment continues.

Examples of visuoconstructive tasks that may be designed for therapeutic use are:

Setting a table for one to five people
Wrapping a gift
Assembling a piece of woodwork, a toy, a tool, a motor
Changing a tire on a car
Organizing a shelf in a library or a kitchen
Organizing a filing system or cabinet
Putting pieces of a sewing pattern together
Addressing an envelope
Rearranging furniture according to a preset plan
Assembling a craft according to a preset plan
Drawing from memory or copy
Copying two-dimensional block designs
Copying three-dimensional designs with oblique components

The key to effective visuoconstructive learning is, however, not the task itself but rather how carefully the therapist organizes it and monitors performance. Clients with visuoconstructive disorders are often visually or motorically impulsive; they often move or draw parts before analysis has taken place. Once a part is placed inappropriately, it begins to confuse the whole visuoperceptual process. This confusion increases anxiety and contributes to further breakdown in analysis and synthesis. Treatment should be directed at the underlying causes of task breakdown if these can be determined.

Problems of visual analysis and synthesis disorders

Identification of clinical problems. This separate discussion of visual analysis and synthesis is arbitrary. There is never any clear demarcation between the processes of visuospatial orientation, visuoconstruction, and visual analysis and synthesis. Analysis of likes and differences, relationships of parts to one another, and reasoning and deduction occur simultaneously with more basic spatial and constructive percepts. The final visual concept of a task (e.g., what a place setting on a table should look like) is necessary before the task is begun. Similarly, synthesis of one part of a task may be necessary before synthesis of the entire task can occur. For example, the person who is setting a table for four people must be able to conceptualize one place setting before conceptualizing the table with four place settings. Those points during perceptual processing when there is a colligation or blending of discrete impressions into a single perception are known as synthesis. This final stage of coordination and interpretation of sensory data is thought to be deficient in many individuals with perceptual problems. Deficits may be present with either left or right hemisphere damage but are more common and more severe with right lesions.[73,95]

Visual perceptual skills considered to be analytical and synthetic in nature include making fine visual discriminations, particularly in complex configurations; separating figure from background in complex configurations (figure-ground); achieving recognition on the basis of incomplete information (figure closure); and synthesizing disparate elements into a meaningful entity as, for example, conceptualizing parts of a task into a whole.[14]

Assessment. Many tests have been designed to measure the capacity for analysis and synthesis. Test items include complex figures in which small parts of a figure differ from another figure. The client is asked to select the one that is different. Studies have shown that basic discrimination of single attributes of a stimulus such as length, contour, or brightness are intact in many clients.[18,90,91] The problem appears when these individuals are asked to discriminate between more complex configurations with subtle differences. Tests also measure figure-ground ability; the client must select the embedded figure from the background. Functional examples of this problem are the client who cannot find his glasses if they are lying on a figured background, cannot find his white shirt on a white bedspread, and cannot find his wheelchair locks. Figure closure is measured by asking the client to complete an incomplete figure, such as part of the outline of a common shape. Finally, synthesis of parts into a whole, also known as visual organization, is measured by asking the client to conceptualize and organize the whole picture by, for example, looking at separate segments of the picture (such as cup or key) that have been divided and placed in unusual positions. This type of synthesis is necessary for high-level constructional tasks. Table 25-5 outlines examples of tests used to evaluate visual analysis and synthesis.

Treatment. Treatment for deficits in visual analysis and synthesis should follow developmental considerations described in the children's section. Visual discrimination tasks should begin with simple figures and obvious differences in complex figures. Color, size, texture, lighting, and verbal direction may help the client "cue in" on subtle

Table 25-5. Common tests used to assess visual analysis and synthesis

Test	Use
Hooper Visual Organization Test	Standardized for adults
Motor-Free Visual Perception Test	Standardized for adults
Raven's Progressive Matrices	Standardized for adults
The Embedded Figure Test	Standardized for adults
Southern California Figure-Ground Test	Standardized for children only

differences among objects or figures. The therapist should determine the threshold at which the client is capable of discriminating differences and vary the dimension, contrast, and functional activity at this level. For example, if the individual cannot select a can of vegetables from a kitchen shelf stocked with cans of similar size, the therapist may simply change the task to fit that person's level of visual discrimination by removing some of the cans (decreasing the density of the display), replacing some of the cans with boxes of food (increasing the spatial contrast), moving the can to be selected forward or to one edge of the display (decreasing figure-ground difficulty), removing the label from the can (increasing the light and color contrast), or giving cues regarding what to search for (verbal direction). This example is described not as a method of compensation but rather as an approach to be used therapeutically in slowly building the client's visual discrimination abilities. Eventually, high-level visual discrimination skills should be incorporated within tasks requiring three or more steps, such as selecting a can of vegetables, opening the can (which involves selecting the can opener from the utensil drawer), and emptying the vegetables into a specific bowl (which involves selecting the bowl from among other bowls). Visual discrimination and figure-ground skills may appear normal until the client is required to do multiple-step activities, is given time constraints, or becomes anxious or confused. Tabletop games that require high levels of visual discrimination along with cognitive strategies may be therapeutic and motivating. Examples include Monopoly and card games like solitaire. Matching and sorting tasks may also be helpful in enhancing visual discrimination. Examples include matching picture cards or sorting laundry, tools, silverware, or files.

Drawings of figures with subtle differences may also be used for therapy. The client should be encouraged to point to, verbalize, or outline the subtle differences in two or more pictures; this enhances visual attention to detail. If the individual cannot select the discrepant detail(s) among three or more figures, the problem most likely results from an inability to select one feature and compare it with elements in the other figures. This is a fairly high-level skill that requires selective attention and analysis with internal visualization while the individual is still viewing the complete figures. This type of client should practice feature detection and then begin systematic comparisons of likes and differences between two figures, eventually progressing to three or more figures. The therapist may number or outline similar areas of each figure to help the client (1) direct attention to similar areas of all figures and (2) sequence comparisons appropriately. The client should verbalize, draw, or write details concerning similarities and differences in individual aspects of the figures. This enhances visual analysis and also informs the therapist as to how the individual is selecting and comparing features. Eventually, speed should be stressed, the highest level being presentation of tachistoscopic designs.

Visual organization may be emphasized by presenting the client with activities that have multiple parts that must be sequenced together into a whole. Activities involving this type of synthesis are discussed in the preceding section on treatment of visuoconstructive disorders. Figure closure may be emphasized by presenting parts of figures or objects (e.g., half a plate covered by a towel) and asking the client for identification. Figure-closure task difficulty may be increased by placing many objects on a table, some of which partially occlude others. Identification of objects in such a task requires figure closure simultaneous with figure-ground abilities.

Visual analysis and synthesis deficits reflect a disruption in cognitive function with specific regard to visual perceptual features. The affected client may function normally when analytical tasks require another system, for example, language. In others with generalized brain damage (e.g., traumatic head injury and senile dementia), general cognitive analysis and synthesis may be at fault rather than visual analysis. Since most cognitive performance requires visual processing, however, increased ability to analyze and synthesize visual perceptual material often generalizes to an increase in cognitive function.

Perceptual retraining with computers

Over the last 10 years, numerous computer programs have been developed for rehabilitation of brain damage symptoms including cognition (e.g., attention, sequencing, or memory) and perception. Because the computer is so highly visual, it becomes an obvious tool for treatment of visual perceptual dysfunction. Treatment with computers has been coined "computer-assisted therapy." No large treatment studies have yet defined the outcome significance of computer-assisted therapy versus conventional treatment programs. However, reports indicate that computer-assisted therapy is very motivating for patients with poor attention and motivation. Advantages of computer-assisted therapy include control/flexibility of perceptual variables during treatment (e.g., number, size, speed), imme-

diate feedback of performance, and automatic control for learning (i.e., items are repeated if incorrect to facilitate learning). Visual perceptual training with computers should be viewed as one part of a patient's treatment program if used. One should always remember that the computer, monitor, and keyboard are just that: they do not require the many perceptual, vestibular, and motor responses typical of daily performance (e.g., scanning requirements may be bilateral, but they are not global and associated with head movement). A patient's total program may include computer-assisted therapy as an additional tool; however, it should never be substituted for more significant training within the multidimensional environment. Some computer programs for visual perceptual training are listed in the box below.

SUMMARY

Careful organized evaluation should delineate deficits well enough to result in a *visual perceptual function profile* for each client, including both primary and associative visual skills. Clients rarely come with isolated visual perceptual deficits; more often they exhibit a combination of vi-

---

Computer programs for visual perceptual training

Visual Perceptual Diagnostic Testing and Training
   Programs
H. Greenberg and C. Chamoff
Educational Electronic Techniques, Ltd.
1886 Wantagh Avenue
Wantagh, NY 11793

Captain's Log Cognitive Training System
J. Sandford and R. Browne
Computability Corporation
101 Route 46 East
Pine Brook, NJ 07058

Psychological Software Services Programs
Odie Bracey
Psychological Software Services
P.O. Box 29205
Indianapolis, IN 46229

Life Science Associates Programs
R. Gianutsos
Life Science Associates
1 Fenemore Road
Bayport, NY 11705 (Diagnosis and Training)

Cognitive Rehabilitation Series
Hartley Courseware
2023 Aspen Glade
Kingwood, TX 77339

sual perceptual deficits usually interrelated with motor, language, and cognitive dysfunctions. For example, a visual perceptual function profile may reveal a strabismus, left unilateral visual inattention, visuospatial deficits, visuoconstructive deficits, and problems with visual analysis and synthesis—all affecting daily function. Treatment should be organized to progressively build skills emphasizing one component more than another. The goal of treatment is eventual generalization of improvements in individual skills to spontaneous high-level function.

The presentation of information in this chapter represents an attempt to use isolated and mechanistic terms to define a system that is extremely subtle, integrated, and complex. The reader is reminded that much of the normal and abnormal perceptual system has not been well defined. Preliminary studies cited throughout this chapter, however, suggest that disorders may be responsive to management and treatment. Research is needed to standardize evaluation procedures well enough to further define deficits and to investigate the effectiveness of various treatment approaches with varied client populations.

REFERENCES

1. Adler FH: Physiology of the eye, St Louis, 1965, The CV Mosby Co.
2. Albert MA: A simple test of visual neglect, Neurology 23:658, 1973.
3. American Optometric Association: Board of Trustees, policy manual, St Louis, 1966, The Association.
4. Anderson E and Choy E: Parietal lobe syndromes in hemiplegia: a program for treatment, Am J Occup Ther 24:13, 1970.
5. Ann Arbor Tracking Program: Letters and symbols, Naples, Fla, 1975, Ann Arbor Publishers, Inc.
6. Ayres AJ: Sensory integration and learning disorders, Los Angeles, 1973, Western Psychological Services.
7. Ayres AJ: Sensory integration and praxis tests, Los Angeles, 1984, Western Psychological Services.
8. Ayres AJ: The effect of sensory integrative therapy on learning disabled children: final report, Pasadena, 1976, Center for the Study of Sensory Integrative Dysfunction.
9. Ayres AJ: Lecture presented at Occupational Therapy for Sensory Integrative Dysfunction Institute, Cincinnati, June 1981.
10. Badell-Ribera A, Shulman K, and Paddock N: The relationship of nonprogressive hydrocephalus in intellectual functioning in children with spina bifida cystica, Pediatrics 37:787, 1966.
11. Balliet R and others: Rehabilitation of visual function in occipital lobe infarctions, Paper presented at the American Congress of Rehabilitation Medicine and the 43rd Annual Assembly of the American Academy of Physical Medicine and Rehabilitation, San Diego, Nov 1981.
12. Beery KE: Revised administration, scoring, and teaching manual for the Developmental Test of Visual-Motor Integration, Cleveland, 1982, Modern Curriculum Press.
13. Benton A: Disorders of visual perception, disorders of higher nervous activity. In Vinken PJ and Bruyn GW editors: Handbook of clinical neurology, vol 3, Amsterdam, 1975, North-Holland Publishing Co.
14. Benton A: Visuospatial and visuoconstructive disorders. In Heilman K and Valenstein E, editors: Clinical neuropsychology, New York, 1979, Oxford University Press, Inc.
15. Benton A and others: Judgment of Line Orientation Test, Forms H and V, Department of Neurology, University Hospitals, Iowa City, 1975, University of Iowa Press.
16. Ben-Yishay Y and others: Ability to profit from cues as a function of initial competence in normal and brain-injured adults: a replication of previous findings, J Abnorm Psychol 76:378, 1970.
17. Berlyne DE: Conflict arousal and curiosity, New York, 1960, McGraw-Hill, Inc.
18. Bisiach E and others: Hemispheric functional asymmetry in visual discrimination between invariate stimuli: an analysis of sensitivity and response criterion, Neuropsychologia 14:335, 1976.
19. Bouska MJ and Biddle E: The influence of unilateral visual neglect on diagnostic testing, Paper presented at the American Speech, Language and Hearing Association Annual Conference, Atlanta, Nov 1979.
20. Bouska MJ and Kwatny E: Manual for application of the Motor-Free Visual Perception Test to the adult population, Temple University Rehabilitation Research and Training Center No 8, Philadelphia, 1980.
21. Chedru F and others: Visual searching in normal and brain-damaged subjects: contribution to the study of unilateral visual inattention, Cortex 9:94, 1973.
22. Codding KG and Gardner MF: Visual-Motor Development Remedial Activities, San Francisco, 1987, Northern California Medical Services of Children's Hospital of San Francisco.
23. Chow B and Volpe P: Visual-Perceptual Development Remedial Activities, San Francisco, 1987, Northern California Medical Services of Children's Hospital of San Francisco.
24. Colarusso R and Hammill D: The Motor-Free Visual Perception Test, Novato, Calif, 1972, Academic Therapy Publications.
25. Copeland RW: How children learn mathematics: teaching implications of Piaget's research, ed 2, New York, 1974, Macmillan, Inc.
26. Cratty BJ: Developmental sequences of perceptual-motor tasks: movement activities for neurologically handicapped and retarded children and youth, Palo Alto, Calif, 1967, Peek Publications.
27. Critchley M: The parietal lobes, New York, 1966, Hafner Publishing Co.
28. DeCencio DV and others: Verticality perception and ambulation in hemiplegia, Arch Phys Med Rehabil 51:105, 1970.
29. Diller L: The development of a perceptual remediation program in hemiplegia. In Ince L, editor: Behavioral psychology in rehabilitation medicine, Baltimore, 1980, Williams & Wilkins.
30. Diller L and others: Studies in cognition and rehabilitation in hemiplegia, Rehabilitation Monograph No 50, New York, 1974, New York University Press.
31. Eccles JC: Conscious experience and memory. In Eccles JC editor: Brain and conscious experience, New York, 1966, Springer-Verlag, Inc.
32. Elkind D: Children and adolescents, ed 2, New York, 1974, Oxford University Press, Inc.
33. Erhardt RP: Erhardt Developmental Prehension Assessment, Laurel, Md, 1982, RAMSCO Publishing Company.
34. Fitzhugh K and Fitzhugh L: Fitzhugh Plus Program, Galien, Mich, 1976, 1979, and 1980, Allied Educational Press.
35. Flavel JH: Cognitive development, Englewood Cliffs, NJ, 1977, Prentice-Hall, Inc.
36. Forrest EB: Visualization and visual imagery: an overview, J Am Optom Assoc 51:1005, 1980.
37. Gardner MF: Test of Visual-Perceptual Skills, Seattle, 1982, Special Child Publications.
38. Gardner R: The objective diagnosis of minimal brain dysfunction, Cresskill, NJ, 1979, Creative Therapists.
39. Garzia R and Kwatny E: Clinical vision assessment, Temple University Rehabilitation Research and Training Center No 8, Philadelphia, 1980.
40. Gesell A: Vision: its development in the infant and child, New York, 1949, Harper & Row, Publishers, Inc.

41. Getman GN: The visuomotor complex in the acquisition of learning skills. In Helmuth J, editor: Learning disorders, Washington, DC, 1965, Special Child Publications.

42. Getman GN and Bullis G: Developmental vision, Duncan, Okla, 1950-51, Optometric Extension Foundation Papers.

43. Getman GN and others: Developing learning readiness: a visual-motor tactile skills program, New York, 1968, McGraw-Hill, Inc.

44. Gianotti G and Tiacci C: The relationship between disorders of visual perception and unilateral spatial neglect, Neuropsychologia 9:451, 1971.

45. Gianutsos R and Matheson P: The rehabilitation of visual perceptual disorders attributable to brain injury. In Meier M, Benton A, and Diller L, editors: Neuropsychological rehabilitation, New York, 1987, The Guilford Press.

46. Gianutsos R and Ramsey G: Enabling rehabilitation optometrists to help survivors of acquired brain-injury, J Vision Rehabil 2:37, 1988.

47. Gibson EJ and Levin H: The psychology of reading, Cambridge, Mass, 1975, The MIT Press.

48. Gilfoyle EM and others: Children adapt, Thorofare, NJ, 1980, Charles B Slack, Inc.

49. Gilman S and Winans S: Manter and Gatz's essentials of clinical neurology, ed 6, Philadelphia, 1982, FA Davis Co.

50. Ginsberg H and Opper S: Piaget's theory of intellectual development: an introduction, Englewood Cliffs, NJ, 1969, Prentice-Hall, Inc.

51. Hacean H: Aphasic, apraxic and agnosic syndromes in right and left hemisphere lesions, disorders of speech perception and symbolic behavior. In Vinken PJ and Bruyn GW, editors: Handbook of clinical neurology, vol 4, Amsterdam, 1969, North-Holland Publishing Co.

52. Hacean T and de Ajuriaguera J: Balint's syndrome (psychic paralysis of visual fixation) and its minor forms, Brain 77:373, 1954.

53. Heilman K: Neglect and related disorders. In Heilman K and Valenstein E, editors: Clinical neuropsychology, New York, 1979, Oxford University Press, Inc.

54. Heilman K and Valenstein E: Mechanisms underlying hemispatial neglect, Ann Neurol 5:166, 1979.

55. Hein DB and others: Hypertensive putomental hemorrhage, Ann Neurol 1:152, 1977.

56. Holiday E: Altair Designs, New York, 1970, Pantheon Books.

57. Holmes G: Disturbances of visual orientation, Br J Ophthalmol 2:449, 1918.

58. Ishihara color plates, Tokyo, 1977, Kanehara & Co, Ltd.

59. Kephart NC: The slow learner in the classroom, ed 2, Columbus, Ohio, 1971, Charles Merrill Publishing Co.

60. Kirk SA and others: Illinois Test of Psycholinguistic Abilities, Urbana, 1968, University of Illinois Press.

61. Kirshner AJ: Training that makes sense, Novato, Calif, 1972, Academic Therapy Publications.

62. Knabloch H and Pasamanick B, editors: Gesell and Armatruda's developmental diagnosis, ed 3, Hagerstown, Md, 1977, Harper & Row, Publishers, Inc.

63. Knickerbocker BM: A holistic approach to the treatment of learning disorders, Thorofare, NJ, 1980, Charles B Slack, Inc.

64. Kwatny E and Bouska MJ: Visual system disorders and functional correlates: final report, Temple University Rehabilitation Research and Training Center No 8, Philadelphia, 1980.

65. LeDoux JE and Smylie C: Left hemisphere visual processes in a case of right hemisphere symptomatology: implications for theories of cerebral lateralization, Arch Neurol 37:157, 1980.

66. Leiberman S, Cohen A, and Rubin J: NYSOA K-D test, J Am Optom Assocn 54:631, 1983.

67. Leicester J and others: Some determinants of visual neglect, J Neurol Neurosurg Psychiatry 32:580, 1969.

68. Luria AR: Higher cortical functions in man, ed 2, New York, 1980, Basic Books, Inc.

69. May DC: Effects of color reversal of figure-ground drawing materials on drawing performance, Except Child 44:254, 1978.

70. Meadows JC: Disturbed perception of colors associated with localized cerebral lesions, Brain 97:615, 1974.

71. Minkowski M: Sull' evoluzione o la localizzazione delle fuzione nervose, supratutto dei movemento: e dei riflessi nel fetoe nel neonato, Atti del Convento Italoswizzero (Clinica Pediatrica dell' Università di Milano), Bologna, 1948, Editoriale Capelli.

72. Netter FH: The nervous system: The Ciba Collection, Rochester, NY, 1976, The Case-Hoyt Corp.

73. Newcombe F and Russell WR: Dissociated visual perceptual and spatial deficits in focal lesions of the right hemisphere, J Neurol Neurosurg Psychiatry 32:73, 1969.

74. Patterson A and Zangwill O: Disorders of visual space perception associated with lesions of the right cerebral hemisphere, Brain 67:331, 1944.

75. Piaget J: Piaget's theory. In Mussen PH, editor: Carmichael's manual of child psychology, ed 3, New York, 1970, John Wiley & Sons, Inc.

76. Piaget J and Inhelder B: The child's conception of space, New York, 1967, WW Norton Company & Co, Inc.

77. Potegal M: An overview: vestibulo-striated spatial mechanisms, Lecture presented at Neural and Developmental Basis of Spatial Orientation, Teachers College, Columbia University, New York, Nov 1979.

78. Quiros JB and Schranger OL: Neuropsychological fundamentals in learning disabilities, Novato, Calif, 1978, Academic Therapy Publications.

79. Rayner K: Eye movements in reading and information processing, Psychol Bull 85:618, 1978.

80. Redlich F and Bonvicini G: Ueber Mangelnde Wahrnehmung (Autoanasthesie) der Blindkeit Bei Cerebralen Erkrankungen, Neurol Zentralbl 26:945, 1907.

81. Reeves AG and Hagman WS: Behavioral and EEG asymmetry following unilateral lesions of the forebrain and midbrain of cats, Electroencephalog Clin Neurophysiol 30:83, 1971.

82. Rubens A: Agnosia. In Heilman K and Valenstein E, editors: Clinical neuropsychology, New York, 1979, Oxford University Press, Inc.

83. Rudel R: The Oblique mystique: figure perception, Lecture presented at Neural and Developmental Basis of Spatial Orientation Conference, Teachers College, Columbia University, New York, 1979.

84. Scheie HG and Albert DM: Textbook of ophthalmology, ed 9, Philadelphia, 1977, WB Saunders Co.

85. Scotti G and Spinnler H: Colour imperception in unilateral hemisphere-damaged patients, J Nuerol Neurosurg Psychiatry 33:22, 1970.

86. Seiv E and Freishat B: Perceptual dysfunction in the adult stroke patient: a manual for evaluation and treatment, Thorofare, NJ, 1976, Charles B Slack, Inc.

87. Semenza C and others: Analytic and global strategies in copying designs by unilaterally brain-damaged patients, Cortex 14:404, 1978.

88. Skeffington AM: Optometric extension program postgraduate papers, Duncan, Okla, 1969.

89. Stanton K and others: Teaching compensation for left neglect through a language-oriented program, Paper presented at the American Speech, Language and Hearing Association Annual Conference, Atlanta, Nov 1979.

90. Taylor AM and Warrington E: Visual discrimination in patients with localized brain lesions, Cortex 9:82, 1973.

91. Teuber HL and Weinstein S: Ability to discover features after cerebral lesions, Arch Neurol Psychiatry 76:369, 1956.

92. Tew B and Lawrence KM: The effects of hydrocephalus on intelligence, visual perception and school attainments, Dev Med Child Neurol 17:129, 1975.

93. Tew B: Spina bifida children's scores on the Wechsler Intelligence Scale for Children, Percept Mot Skills 44:381, 1977.

94. Trobe JD and others: Confrontation visual field techniques in detection of anterior visual pathway lesions, Ann Neurol 10:28, 1981.

95. Warrington E and James M: An experimental investigation of facial recognition in patients with unilateral lesions, Cortex 3:317, 1967.

96. Watson RT and Heilman RM: Thalamic neglect, Neurology 29:690, 1979.

97. Wechsler D: Wechsler Intelligence Scale for Children (revised), New York, 1979, Psychological Corp.

98. Wilson B, Cockburn J, and Halligan P: Behavioral Inattention Test, Hants, England, 1988, Thames Valley Test Co.

99. Yorkgitis W and Bouska MJ: Unpublished table design within a research and training grant, Temple University Rehabilitation Research and Training Center No 8, Philadelphia, 1979.

100. Zihl J: Blindsight: improvement of visually-guided eye movements by systematic practice in patients with cerebral blindness, Neuropsychologia 43:71, 1980.

ADDITIONAL READINGS

Arnadottir G: Neurobehavioral assessment in adult CNS dysfunction, St Louis, 1989, The CV Mosby Co.

Humphreys G and Riddoch MJ: To see but not to see: a case study of visual agnosia, Hillsdale, 1987, Laurence Erlbaum Assoc, Inc.

Zolton B (editor): Visual system dysfunction, Head Trauma Rehabil, 4(2) (entire issue), June, 1989.

Chapter 26

ELECTRODIAGNOSIS

Katharine B. Robertson

In recent years there has been an increase in the use of electrodiagnostic procedures for client evaluation. This is in part the result of continuous development and improvement of electronic instrumentation, which has made it possible to test the functional status of muscles, nerves, and their interaction with the central nervous system. This permits documentation of how these structures function in health and how they change from the normal state as a result of genetic factors, injury, and disease. Electrodiagnostic evaluations can assist the physician in establishing a client's diagnosis and the therapist in evaluation, program planning, and client management.

Electrical stimulation (ES), nerve conduction velocity (NCV) determination, electromyographic (EMG) studies, F wave and reflex tests, repetitive stimulation studies, somatosensory evoked potential studies (SEPs), and kinesiological electromyography are being performed by physical therapists who have specialized in electrophysiological evaluation. Many texts devoted to electrodiagnosis present both the theory and application of these procedures.[1,2,8,10,14] In this brief introduction only an overview of the subject can be presented.

ELECTRONEUROMYOGRAPHY

Clinical electroneuromyographic (ENMG) studies are used to evaluate the electrical activity arising in nerves, muscles, and the brain in response to electrical stimulation and to observe muscle activity during volitional activities and at rest.[6]

The instrumentation used for clinical electroneuromyography is computer based, and most systems are designed so that peripheral equipment may be added and the unit can be used for multiple functions.[15] Most units have a single input channel; others have multichannel capabilities. In the simplest system, either needle or surface electrodes pick up the electrical activity from the body. This activity is amplified in a series of amplifiers and is displayed on an oscilloscope. It is also sent through an audio system so that the activity recorded can be seen and heard simultaneously. An electrical stimulator is synchronized with the oscilloscope screen to allow recording of evoked responses. In addition, many units include a signal averager that permits enhancement of the electrical signals and supression of the background noise.

The ENMG examination should be done in a quiet and relaxing environment. The procedure should be explained to the client, and he or she should be allowed to see the oscilloscope and the responses if the testing setup will allow this. The client will be assisted psychologically by this and will be able to actively participate in the test process at the appropriate times.

A plan for an ENMG examination is developed from information learned from the client's history, presenting complaints, and physical examination. The physician refers the client with the expectation that the studies will assist in making a diagnosis. Often the referral comes in the form of a question. For example:

1. Is there evidence of bilateral carpal tunnel syndrome?
2. Does this client have evidence of nerve impingement at the L5-S1 level?
3. What muscles remain under voluntary control in this client who has a spinal cord injury?
4. Is there evidence of regeneration in the facial nerve following nerve transplantation in this client with Bell's palsy?

Questions like these allow the electroneuromyographer to plan an appropriate examination. During the examination this plan can be changed whenever information is obtained suggesting that the problem being investigated requires a different focus. Testing should be continued until the question is answered as completely as possible and may require examination of other nerves and muscles adjacent to the area being evaluated, evaluation of the same muscles and nerves on the contralateral side, or use of another type of test.

Training

Post-graduate study is essential for therapists to become electroneuromyographers. An in-depth understanding of traditional, cross-sectional, and surface anatomy is required, as well as extensive knowledge of neurology, neuromuscular physiology, and muscle disease. Expertise in neurological and muscle testing is essential for patient evaluation.[9] In addition, a sufficient background in electronics is required to understand the function and capabilities of the electronic instrumentation and to ensure patient safety. Only when they have this knowledge and expertise are therapists prepared to enter an extended period of clinical training, usually lasting several years, under the supervision of a board certified or licensed clinical electromyographer.

Therapists who do not wish to follow such an extensive program should become familiar with this area of testing and keep current with developments in the field to understand the reports pertaining to the patients they treat.

Nerve conduction techniques

Nerve conduction velocity (NCV) studies are performed on both motor and sensory nerves. Procedures for recording from a large number of nerves are available. The tests are relatively comfortable, noninvasive, and do not require the active participation of the subject. The most commonly tested are the median, ulnar, peroneal, and tibial motor nerves, and the median, ulnar, and sural sensory nerves. Ma and Liveson[11] and Oh[15] have summarized the techniques and normative test data established by a number of prominent electromyographic investigators. This information can serve as a guide in setting up a standardized testing protocol for each ENMG laboratory and in the development of normative data. These data are necessary to en-

sure that test results can be reproduced accurately and that serial tests can be compared.

Clients should be set up for testing in a comfortable position so that the limb to be tested is well supported and relaxed. The procedure should be explained in detail. The client should understand that the stimulation will be momentarily uncomfortable. If the skin is cold (less than 31° C), the limb should be warmed to room temperature as NCVs are decreased at a rate of 1.3 to 2.4 meters per second (m/second) for each drop of 1° C.

Motor nerve conduction. In motor nerve conduction velocity (MNCV) studies, a pair of small disc electrodes are placed on the skin surface over the area to be tested after the skin has been cleaned and its resistance reduced to below 5000 Ω by gently abrading the skin. The electrodes are coupled to the skin with electrode gel. The active electrode (negative) is placed over the motor point of the muscle. The reference electrode (positive) is placed more distally on the tendon of the muscle (Fig. 26-1). A ground electrode is placed between the recording disc electrodes and the stimulating electrode sites. This electrode assists in reducing interference from the artifact created during nerve stimulation if it is placed in this location. It is also essential for patient safety.

The ENMG instrumentation is set up in the NCV motor mode so that the stimulus artifact and evoked response can be seen and stored on the visual display. Markers, which can be moved to indicate the latency intervals on the oscilloscope screen, are available for direct determination of latency measurements. Input from the electrodes is directed so that negative waves appear as an upward deflection on the oscilloscope screen.

The nerve is stimulated in two or more locations along the nerve pathway in areas where the nerve is adjacent to the skin. Stimulation is begun at the distal stimulation site, with the negative stimulus probe placed in the distal position. The stimulus is often applied at a standardized distance, such as 8 cm, from the recording electrode so that the distal latency values can be compared if the test is repeated at a later date. Current from the stimulator is delivered to the nerve by gradually increasing the current flow. The evoked response is observed as it increases in size. When several increases in the output of the stimulator do not cause an increase in the amplitude of the evoked response from the muscle, it is assumed that the nerve is being stimulated supramaximally, and the motor compound muscle action potential (CMAP) is recorded. This CMAP is also called an M wave.

The time interval from the stimulus artifact to the first change in the baseline in the negative direction is then measured and recorded in milliseconds. This latency is called the distal latency (T2 in Fig. 26-1). It includes the time it takes to traverse the nerve, the myoneural junction, and to begin the muscle response.

The stimulator is next moved to a more proximal site,

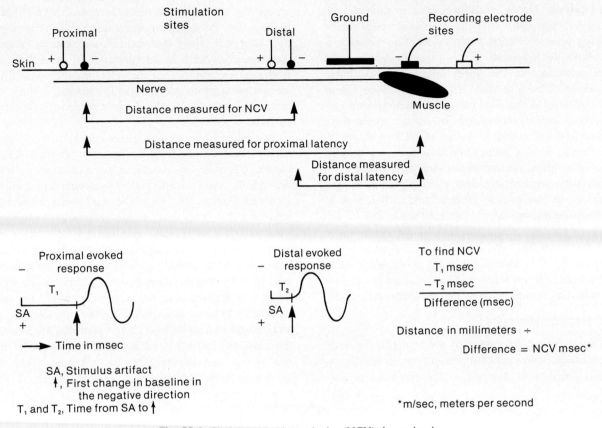

Fig. 26-1 Nerve conduction velocity (NCV) determination

at least 10 cm above the first stimulus site, and the nerve is stimulated again. The evoked response is recorded. The time in milliseconds from the stimulus artifact to the muscle response is measured (T1 in Fig. 26-1). This is called the proximal latency.

To complete the MNCV test the distance between the two negative stimulator probes is measured and recorded in millimeters. Nerve conduction velocity in meters per second can then be computed by subtracting T2 from T1 and dividing this difference into the distance (Fig. 26-1). NCV for more proximal portions of the nerve can be determined by repeating the test sequence on these segments.

Sensory nerve conduction. Sensory nerve action potentials (SNAPs) can be recorded from many superficial sensory nerves. These potentials are small, and their amplitude is measured in microvolts. Often the sensory nerve is associated with the motor nerve over part of its path so that stimulation occurs over a mixed nerve and recording occurs only from the cutaneous nerve. In these instances sensory testing is done after motor NVC testing, because the same stimulation sites can be used for both and the best stimulation sites will have already been determined. For example, a SNAP can be recorded when a stimulus is applied at the wrist over the ulnar nerve and the sensory

evoked response is recorded from the skin at the base of the fifth finger. This is called antidromic conduction. The reverse of this technique, orthodromic conduction, can also be used. Stimuli are applied at the finger and recording of the evoked response is made from paired electrodes placed on the skin along the nerve pathway. Latency values for both techniques are similar.

Paired flexible wire ring electrodes are used for both stimulation and recording from the fingers and toes. When one does orthodromic stimulation, the more proximal ring is active (negative) and the distal electrode is the reference (positive). For the other sensory nerves, stimulation is done with the stimulator probe, and the evoked responses are picked up by disc electrodes. The negative stimulating electrode is always placed closest to the negative recording electrode.

The evoked response resulting from stimulation is a sensory CNAP. The latency of response is usually read from the point of first negative change in baseline. The use of a signal averager, if available, will facilitate this recording. If this portion of the recording is not clear, latency can be read to the peak of the sensory response. NCV in sensory nerves can be determined by dividing the distance by the latency.

Data analysis. Nerve conduction velocity studies, both sensory and motor, can verify the functional status of the nerve being tested. Normal nerve conduction velocity is usually above 40 m/second in the lower extremities and above 50 m/second in the upper extremities. At birth, NCV is about 50% of normal adult values. These values increase gradually as the child matures, reaching adult values between 3 and 5 years of age. In disease states, there may be moderate or severe alteration of NCV parameters. Increases in the sensory latency and slowing of the sensory NCV are most often the first indications of a problem. In some long-term segmentally demyelinating diseases, the NCV may be as low as 6 to 20 m/second. Alterations in the amplitude, duration, rate of rise, and wave form of the evoked response can also give clues to the neurological status of the nerve (Fig. 26-2). When no evoked response can be recorded, it is assumed that the nerve is unable to transmit a signal, either because of interruption of conduction in its myelin sheath or interruption of the entire axon.

Clinical electromyography

Most muscles in the human body are available for study using clinical electromyographic techniques. In needle examinations attention is directed to the electrical activity arising from the muscle fibers at rest, during slight contraction, and during strong contraction. The type of potentials observed, their distribution, and pattern of recruitment are considered in interpretation of the EMG record. It should be emphasized that electromyographic findings are not pathognomonic for specific diseases. None of the potentials observed can be directly related to a specific diagnosis.

In clinical EMG studies, either concentric or monopolar needle electrodes are used for muscle evaluation. The concentric electrode is composed of a fine wire threaded through the shaft of a hypodermic needle and completely insulated from it. The tip of the wire is the active recording electrode. The shaft is the reference electrode. The monopolar needle is made from flexible steel and is coated with a nonconductive material except at its tip. It is used with a second electrode, usually a surface electrode placed near to it on the skin surface. An additional electrode, a ground, is applied near the active electrode. The ground minimizes external interference on the oscilloscope screen and ensures patient safety. These electrodes are attached to the EMG unit, which is set in the EMG mode, and the audio system and loudspeaker are activated. This allows analysis of both the sound and shape of the potentials aris-

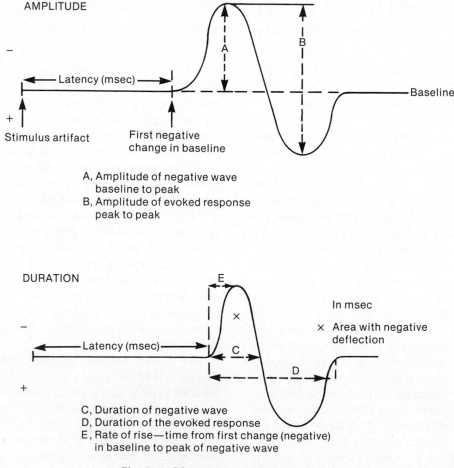

A, Amplitude of negative wave
   baseline to peak
B, Amplitude of evoked response
   peak to peak

C, Duration of negative wave
D, Duration of the evoked response
E, Rate of rise—time from first change (negative)
   in baseline to peak of negative wave

Fig. 26-2. Measurement of evoked responses.

ing from the muscle being examined. During the recording, the sensitivity and sweep speed of the oscilloscope may need frequent adjustment to display the muscle activity appropriately. When a specific sequence of events needs to be evaluated, the activity on the oscilloscope screen can be stopped to allow analysis of the individual potentials.

EMG technique. Clinical electromyography requires patient cooperation. Therefore the client should be told how to respond during the examination. He or she should be warned that the needle will hurt on penetration of the skin, when it is moved, and if the muscle contraction causes the tip to move. The client should be allowed to practice the minimums required when the needle is in place: very slight contraction, muscle relaxation, and strong static contraction against resistance before the needle is placed. This will help the examiner when recording during the test and minimize the client's discomfort.

The muscles examined should be sampled at several depths and in four directions from the point of needle penetration to adequately evaluate the muscle. If there is a question concerning the location of the needle tip, muscle testing of adjacent muscles will assist in making the correct decision concerning the muscle being tested. Two excellent texts by Delagi[5] and Goodgold[7] can assist the examiner with electrode placement.

Because of the discomfort caused by percutaneous electrodes, a team of investigators led by McGill[13] is investigating the use of noninvasive specialized electrodes for EMG. They consist of arrays of very small metal contacts or closely spaced needles that penetrate only the outermost layers of the skin. The signals recorded from the contacts are combined so that superficial motor unit action potentials (MUAPs) are accentuated while the deeper ones are suppressed. This type of electrode would allow greater patient acceptance of the EMG procedure and greater compliance during the testing by both children and adults.

Electromyographic potentials in normal muscle. When a normal muscle is examined at rest, there is no electrical activity; during slight contraction MUAPs are observed. They are activated by the client and are under his or her voluntary control. The MUAP is composed of the summated electrical activity of individual muscle fibers occuring near the tip of the needle and has a biphasic, triphasic, or (rarely) tetraphasic wave form, phases being counted by the number of times the potential crosses the baseline. Normal motor units have a duration from about 2 to 15 milliseconds (msec) and an amplitude from about 200 to 5000 μV. These parameters vary considerably, depending on the individual muscle being evaluated. Small muscles with few muscle fibers per motor unit have potentials with a lower amplitude and shorter duration than muscles that are larger.

When the muscle is examined during a strong contraction, all of the MUAPs occurring in the area lose their individual characteristics and are summated. The resulting activity is called an interference pattern, and its evaluation is quite subjective (Table 26-1).

Interest has recently increased in the development of instrumentation and techniques that will allow more data to be derived from this signal. A method called Automatic Decomposition Electromyography, developed by McGill[12] at Stanford University, allows analysis of individual MUAPs occurring in the interference pattern. It permits evaluation of the amplitude, duration, number of phases, rate of rise, and firing rate of these potentials. It will assist in establishing how normal motor units are recruited for functional activities and will assist in the understanding of how these patterns are changed in pathology.

Electromyographic potentials in pathology. When pathology affects a muscle or the nerve supply to the muscle is partially or completely interrupted, the normal EMG picture may be changed. Traditionally, EMG has been associated only with lower motor neuron and muscular problems. Recently, more interest has been directed to the potential patterns associated with central nervous system pathology. With continued research a greater understanding of the clinical significance of these potentials in relation to a client's diagnosis and prognosis will be possible.

The electromyographic potentials observed in pathological states are summarized in Table 26-1 and are discussed in the following sections.

Table 26-1. Potentials observed during electromyography

	At rest	Slight contraction	Strong contraction
Normal	Silence	Normal MUAPs	Interference
Pathological	Fibrillation	Normal MUAPs	Interference
	Positive sharp waves	Polyphasic MUAPs	Partial interference
	Fasciculation	Low amplitude, short duration	Single MUAPs
	High frequency potentials	MUAPs	Silence
	Waxing and waning	High amplitude, giant MUAPs	
	Constant amplitude		
	Silence		

MUAP, Motor unit action potential.

The muscle at rest

Fibrillation potentials. Fibrillation potentials represent the summated action potentials of single muscle fibers. They have a biphasic or triphasic waveform. The initial phase is in a positive direction, unless the recording is made in the muscle end plate zone. Their duration is from 1 to 4 msec, and their amplitude ranges from 20 to 300 μV. They usually repeat in a regular manner at a rate of 1 to 30 per second. In some instances they have an irregular rhythm or are intermittent.

Fibrillation potentials occur in muscle fibers that have been denervated. These potentials appear from 7 to 35 days after nerve transection or interruption and may continue for many years if reinnervation does not occur. They are seen in numerous neurological disorders, including myelopathies, neuropathies, traumatic nerve injuries, and entrapment syndromes (refer to Chapter 12). Fibrillation potentials have also been observed in clients with myopathies, such as muscular dystrophy, as well as in conditions causing electrolytic imbalance, inflammation, or instability of the muscle membrane.

The incidence of fibrillation potentials in a muscle is variable and is reported by some investigators using a scale from plus one (+1) to plus four (+4). Plus one fibrillation is considered significant and indicates that fibrillation potentials were present at more than three sites in the muscle. Plus four activity designates that marked fibrillation activity was present throughout the entire muscle.

Positive sharp waves. When single muscle fiber action potentials are recorded from an injured portion of a muscle fiber, they take the form of positive sharp waves. These waves are biphasic, with a sharp initial deviation in the positive direction followed by a long-duration negative wave of low amplitude. Their duration is from 10 to 30 msec, and they have an average amplitude of 120 μV. Some investigators consider by these potentials to be a form of fibrillation.

Fasciculation potentials. Fasciculation potentials represent the spontaneous firing of innervated motor units or bundles of muscle fibers. If they occur near the skin surface, they can be recognized by a slight twitch of the skin. They are identified by their random and irregular firing pattern. Their repetition rate varies from many per second to about 1 per minute. These potentials have the appearance of either normal or polyphasic MUAPs. They are observed in normal muscle, especially when the muscle is fatigued, and in many neuromuscular disorders. It is believed that they can be triggered from electrical activity arising from any portion of the neuron, from the anterior horn cell to the terminations of the axon.

High-frequency potentials. High-frequency potentials (HFP) are of two types, a waxing and waning type (myotonic potentials) and a continuous type (repetitive potentials). The former are seen in the myotonias and are re-

markable for their continuous increase and decrease in frequency producing a sound on the loudspeaker like that of a dive bomber. The potentials that make up these trains are biphasic or triphasic and vary in shape and amplitude over time. They are initiated by needle motion, muscle percussion, or voluntary contraction. These high-frequency potentials are also associated with diseases such as hypokalemic and hyperkalemic periodic paralysis and polymyositis.

Repetitive HFP are action potential discharges that occur spontaneously in muscle or on stimulation of the muscle by the needle. They start and stop abruptly, and their amplitude and frequency remain constant. The potentials are often polyphasic. They are seen in clients with diseases like polymyositis and muscular dystrophy.

The muscle during slight contraction. When pathology affects the muscle, normal motor units may continue to be observed. MUAPs that are considered to be abnormal are simply variations from the normal MUAP and are under the voluntary control of the client.

Polyphasic motor unit action potentials. Polyphasic MUAPs have more than five phases. They have a multiphasic appearance because the muscle fibers near the tip of the needle are firing in an asynchronous manner. They may be of short or long duration and may have a wide variation in amplitude. Very complex polyphasic potentials may have as many as 25 phases. They are associated with both neurological and myopathic diseases and are often seen in areas where nerve regeneration is occurring or where regeneration has occurred in the past. They also make up a small percentage of the motor units observed in normal muscles. With increasing age, muscles show a greater and greater percentage of polyphasic potentials.

Low-amplitude short-duration potentials. Potentials with a low amplitude and short duration are associated with both myopathic and neurological disorders. In primary myopathic conditions the potentials are small because of the loss of muscle fibers from the motor unit. At times, so few muscle fibers are activated that the resultant potentials resemble fibrillation potentials. These potentials can be distinguished from fibrillations only because they disappear when the client relaxes the muscle. During reinnervation of muscle, the motor unit may supply only a few muscle fibers. In peripheral neuropathies there may be failure of many of the distal nerve fibers so that the resultant potentials are of low amplitude and short duration. These potentials are very frequently polyphasic because of disorganization of the motor units.

High-amplitude potentials. High-amplitude potentials are associated with nerve regeneration. During the recovery process an axon may send out collateral sprouts and incorporate adjacent denervated muscle fibers into its field of influence. This may increase the total number of muscle fibers in the motor unit, causing it to have a larger than normal amplitude on firing. These potentials do not appear for some time after reinnervation and will not be present immediately after nerve interruption unless there has been a previous problem in the same area. They may have an amplitude of from 5 to over 20 mV. The potentials are often polyphasic and of long duration; others, especially in conditions that have been present for a long time, appear normal in configuration except for their increased amplitude.

Muscles during strong contraction. In disease states, when the muscle is tested against resistance, a complete interference pattern is maintained until the time when so many muscle fibers are lost or isolated from their nerve supply that the density and amplitude of the response is decreased. Evaluation of this decrease is subjective and often requires testing of a normal muscle on the contralateral side for verification. The decrease, when measurable, is called partial interference. If the muscle is markedly denervated, only single motor units may remain, resulting in a pattern of single motor unit action potentials (SMUAPs) of normal or abnormal configuration. The muscle will become electrically silent when the muscle tissue atrophies completely.

In myopathies it may be noticed that minimal effort produces an interference pattern, and individual motor units cannot be recognized. This is because many motor units must be activated and the motor units must fire more rapidly to complete the smallest motion. On strong contraction the amplitude of the interference pattern remains relatively low because of the reduction in the number of muscle fibers participating in the contraction.

Additional studies

There are several other types of evaluative studies that can be used to supplement EMG and NCV studies. All of them give the electroneuromyographer additional data concerning the neuromuscular status of the client.

The F wave. F waves represent the recurrent discharge of alpha motor neurons by impulses travelling antidromically from the site of stimulation and returning orthodromically to the muscle from which the recording occurs. They are late-appearing waves occurring 25 to 50 msec after the M wave on supramaximal stimulation of a motor nerve and are low in amplitude. The F response is usually activated at the distal stimulation site of the median, ulnar, peroneal, or tibial nerves. The stimulator probe is reversed at this site, and a series of about 10 recordings is made. The evoked response is variable and may be blocked. Latency is determined from the start of the evoked response with the shortest latency. The test is often useful in determining the presence of brachial and lumbosacral plexus lesions and in diseases causing proximal slowing of transmission.

The H reflex. The H reflex is a monosynaptic reflex evoked by stimulation of the afferent fibers in a mixed nerve. It is found most easily in the calf muscles in normal subjects. It is also a late-appearing wave that is activated with a minimal stimulus, one with less intensity than that required to evoke the M wave. The H wave reaches its maximal amplitude when the M wave begins and will decrease in amplitude and disappear as the stimulus is increased to supramaximal. The H reflex response is constant in form, and its latency, which is related to the subject's height, is usually less than 35 msec. When the latency is recorded bilaterally, a difference of less than 2 msec in the two latencies is considered normal.[3]

One method of performing the test is to stimulate the tibial nerve at the popliteal fossa and to record from an active recording electrode placed on the leg on a line halfway between the proximal flare of the medial malleolus and the popliteal crease.[3] H reflex testing is most often used in evaluation of suspected S1 conduction lesions.

Repetitive stimulation. Repetitive stimulation studies are used to investigate conditions that affect neuromuscular transmission. These tests require supramaximal stimulation of the muscle tested. To avoid motion artifact, the area being tested must be carefully immobilized, and the stimulating and recording electrodes must be attached firmly to the skin.[15] There are a number of protocols for the stimulation sequence, and the sequence may be changed, depending on the type of transmission defect the client is believed to have. When a normal muscle is stimulated at the rate of 2 or 3 stimuli per second, the evoked responses will remain the same size and amplitude over 5 to 7 responses. When an involved muscle in a myasthenia gravis client is tested in the same way, a gradual decrease will be noticed between the first and last responses. If the same muscle is then exercised and a second train of stimuli are given, there will be moderate facilitation of the evoked responses. Subsequent stimulation at 1, 2, 3, and 4 minutes shows a rapid decrease in the amplitude of the evoked responses. In Eaton-Lambert's syndrome the facilitation component is particularly pronounced following exercise. In other conditions causing transmission defects, the evoked response may decrease immediately following exercise.

Single-fiber electromyography. Single-fiber electromyographic (SFEMG) studies are also used to study fiber density in a motor unit, lower motor neuron disorders, muscular diseases, and myasthenia gravis. These studies are made possible by the use of a special needle that has a recording electrode diameter of only 25 μm and specialized EMG instrumentation that makes it possible to hold one potential stationary and display others that follow it. This setup allows study of the interactions of single muscle fiber action potentials. The relationship of one muscle fiber action potential to an adjacent one in the same motor unit following repetitive stimulation or voluntary contraction is studied. The variability of firing of the second unit in relation to the first potential is measured. This variability is called jitter. In normal muscle, jitter is minimal and the potentials nearly overlap. In myasthenia gravis, the potentials have a much greater temporal dispersion, or the potential may be completely blocked.

Evoked potentials. Three other types of evoked potential studies are in common use today. These are pattern shift visual evoked potentials (PSVEPs), brainstem auditory evoked potentials (BAEPs), and somatosensory evoked potentials (SEPs). These tests allow the examiner to determine sensory function from the periphery to the cerebral cortex. The tests are very sensitive and will show the presence of sensory abnormality early in disease, show where it is located when demyelinating disease is present in the central nervous system, and allow the course of disease to be followed. Normative and pathological data have been documented for each of the tests. This subject has been well presented in texts by Chiappa,[4] Kunimura,[10] Oh,[14] and Wolf.[21]

Pattern shift visual evoked potentials are recorded while the client watches a checkerboard pattern that reverses its squares at a set interval. Brainstem auditory evoked potentials are stimulated by clicks from a square wave generator and are delivered to the ears through shielded headphones. One ear may be tested at a time, or both ears can be stimulated simultaneously. Somatosensory evoked potentials are obtained by stimulating a peripheral nerve such as the median nerve at the wrist.

The evoked potentials are recorded using specialized instrumentation that is able to separate out the evoked responses, following from 200 to 2000 stimuli to the nerve, from the random EEG potentials. Multichannel recorders are required so that several areas along the nerve pathway or over the skull can be monitored. Chiappa[4] feels that at least four channels are essential for this type of testing, with eight being ideal for PSVEPs and SEPs.

Electrodes are placed on the skull according to a standardized pattern for each of the different tests. The 10-20 electrode placement system is used; it is called this because electrode spacing is based on intervals of 10% and 20% of the distance between specified points on the scalp. In SEPs spinal recording electrodes are placed over the appropriate vertebrae. Surface electrodes of the EEG type are used for most of the studies; however, EEG or EMG needles may be required in certain clients.

The evoked responses recorded in each of these tests consist of positive and negative waves that occur at anticipated latencies following the stimulus. The form and shape of the evoked response varies because of many factors, such as electrode location, strength of the stimulus, or type of nerve stimulated. Interpretation of the records has been complicated by the fact that standardized procedures and nomenclature have not been adopted by the investigators.

These tests have expanded our ability to explore central nervous system function. For example, PSVEP studies have been used successfully in investigating optic neuritis and multiple sclerosis. BAEP studies have been used in localizing acoustic neuromas, brainstem tumors, the site of CVAs, and in documenting the presence of demyelinating diseases. SEP studies have also been used in localization of tumors and demyelinating diseases. They have been particularly useful in separating peripheral demyelinating diseases from more proximal ones, often allowing distinction between lesions in the plexus, cauda equina, spinal cord, dorsal column nucleus, medial leminiscus, thalmus, and cortex. They can also provide information concerning the presence and localization and progression of a number of diseases that affect the central nervous system.

Case studies

CASE STUDY 1: NERVE COMPRESSION

A 35-year-old man was referred for ENMG evaluation with a complaint of weakness in the left leg resulting in a "drop foot." The problem had developed gradually over a period of several days, 4 weeks previously. At this time the client had been repairing a roof and had remained in a squatting position for many hours each day.

It was noted that the client walked with a steppage gait and that his left foot slapped on heel contact. Manual muscle testing of the muscles innervated by the left peroneal nerve showed grades in the poor to poor-minus range. All other muscles in the left and right legs were tested and were normal in strength. Knee and ankle reflexes were brisk and equal bilaterally.

NVC of the left peroneal motor nerve was performed. The nerve was stimulated at the ankle, below the fibular head and in the popliteal fossa (Fig. 26-3). The latency from the ankle to the

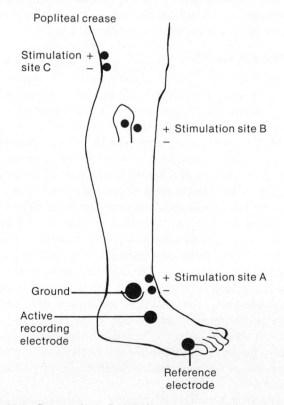

Fig. 26-3. Case study 1. Peroneal nerve motor nerve conduction velocity to the extensor digitorum brevis muscle. An 8 cm distance was used between the active recording electrode and the distal negative stimulating electrode.[1]

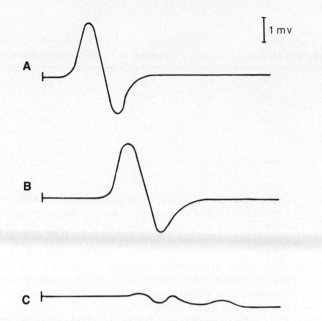

1 mv

A

B

C

Fig. 26-4. Case study 1. Evoked responses, left tibial nerve. **A,** Ankle. **B,** Below fibular head. **C,** Popliteal fossa.

extensor digitorum brevis muscle was 4.8 m/second. The latency from below the fibular head to the ankle was 13.5 m/second. Nerve conduction velocity in this segment was 46 m/second. The evoked responses at these two sites were similar in shape and had an amplitude of 4 mV (Fig. 26-4, *A* and *B*). These values are within the normal range for this nerve. Stimulation at the popliteal fossa resulted in a response that was markedly decreased in amplitude and prolonged in duration (Fig. 26-4, *C*). Conduction velocity in the segment from the popliteal fossa to below the fibular head was 28 m/second. This response is not in the normal range. It was concluded that a de-

creased number of motor units were participating in the response and that the evoked response was slowed in this segment.

Nerve conduction velocity studies of the right peroneal and left tibial nerve were also performed. The evoked responses from each of these nerves exhibited the same amplitude and waveform at each of the stimulation sites. The latency, amplitude, and NCV values were all within normal limits.

Needle examination of the left anterior tibialis, peroneus longus, and extensor digitorum longus muscles showed fibrillation potentials (3+) and positive sharp waves at rest, a few normal motor units on slight contraction, and a very low-level interference pattern or single MUAP pattern on maximal effort. Partial denervation of the muscles in this area had occurred. Muscles not innervated by the common peroneal nerve all showed a normal EMG pattern.

From these tests it could be concluded that the problem was limited to muscles supplied by the left common peroneal nerve, which was probably compressed by the patient while roofing.

CASE STUDY 2: PERIPHERAL NEUROPATHY

A 58-year-old man with a complaint of weakness and decreased sensation in his right leg was referred for ENMG evaluation. The client's symptoms had developed gradually over the past 8 months and he now walked with a drop foot. His physician questioned whether this problem was caused by a mononeuropathy or by a compression of the peroneal nerve at the fibular head. The client was diabetic and was taking anticoagulant medication for a heart condition. Because of the medication, needle evaluation was contraindicated, and studies were limited to nerve conduction velocity determination.

The peroneal and tibial motor nerves and the sural sensory nerves were studied bilaterally (Table 26-2). Nerve conduction velocities in all the motor nerves except the right tibial nerve were slowed. In the right peroneal nerve conduction velocity values were the same across the segment from above and below the fibular head. The distal latencies of the sural nerves were prolonged, and their amplitude was below predicted normal.

Table 26-2. Case study 2: nerve conduction studies

Side	Nerve	Segment	Latency (msec)	Conduction velocity (m/second)	Amplitude	Distance in centimeters from distal stimulus site to active recording electrode
Right	Peroneal motor	Above fibular head	12.6	<u>37</u>	2.0 mV	
		Below fibular head	11.6	<u>38</u>	2.0 mV	
		Ankle	3.7		2.5 mV	8
Left	Peroneal motor	Above fibular head	13.3	<u>37</u>	4.0 mV	
		Ankle	4.4		4.0 mV	8
Right	Tibial motor to the abductor hallucis muscle	Popliteal space	15.6	40	3.5 mV	
		Ankle	<u>6.7</u>		3.5 mV	8
Left	Tibial motor	Popliteal space	15.8*	<u>33</u>	3.2 mV	
		Ankle	4.8*		3.2 mV	8
Right	Sural sensory		<u>7.2</u>+		5 μV	14
Left	Sural sensory		<u>5.3</u>+		8 μV	14

mV, Millivolts; μV, Microvolts; +, Measured to peak of negative wave.
Underlined values are not in the range of predicted normal.
*Double peaked wave at both sites.

Table 26-3. Case study 3: nerve conduction studies

Side	Nerve	Segment	Latency (msec)	Conduction velocity (m/second)	Amplitude (V)	Distance (centimeters)
Left	Peroneal-motor	Fibular head	13.5		4 mV	32
		Ankle	5.4	40	4 mV	8
Left	Sural-sensory	Calf	5.5		12 μV	20
		Ankle	3.3	45	20 μV	10
Left	H wave	Popliteal fossa to	34.1			
Right	H wave	Gastronemius-soleus	34.0			

From this data it was concluded that the client had neither a compression neuropathy nor a mononeuropathy. He had a polyneuropathy. This fact was further documented by additional studies at a later date that showed slowing of nerve conduction and reduced amplitude of the evoked responses in the medial and ulnar motor and sensory nerves. Because the client was a diabetic, it was assumed that this disease was the cause of his problem. Because this assumption does not eliminate the possibility that the polyneuropathy originated from another source, the client should be retested periodically.[19]

CASE STUDY **3**: RADICULOPATHY

A 52-year-old male client was sent for electroneuromyographic evaluation with provisional diagnosis of a disk at the L5, S1 spinal level. Five weeks previously he had suddenly developed a severe burning pain in the left buttock area accompanied by deep aching pain involving the entire left lower extremity. He noted that sitting increased his complaints while prone lying decreased them.

On physical examination it was found that this client had a positive straight leg raising sign on the left with sciatica. Manual muscle testing was equivocal because of apparent pain caused by the testing process. However, the left anterior tibialis muscle seemed to be significantly weaker than the right anterior tibialis.

The client had difficulty doing partial deep knee bends using the left leg and stated that pain was not a factor in his performance. His left knee-jerk was reduced when compared with the right knee-jerk. Ankle-jerks were equal bilaterally. In addition, it was found that there was decrease in sensory perception in the L4-L5 dermatomes on the left. Weakness of the anterior tibialis, decreased response of the patellar reflex, and decreased sensory awareness on the medial side of the leg and foot are associated with problems at the L4 spinal level.

The ENMG evaluation was begun with nerve conduction velocity tests of the left peroneal motor and sural nerves. Latency, amplitude, and velocity values were within normal limits. Then the right and left H waves were recorded. The latency of the left H wave was in the range of predicted normal and was not significantly different from that on the right (Table 26-3).

Needle examination was performed and the data are summarized in Table 26-4. Fibrillation potentials and positive sharp waves were observed in the following muscles on the left side: the vastus lateralis, the rectus femoris, the anterior tibialis, extensor digitorum longus and the L4 lumbar paraspinals. No other spontaneous activity was observed in the remainder of the muscles tested including the paraspinal muscles at L3, L5 and S1. On voluntary activity no abnormal changes were noted in the motor unit action potentials observed in any muscle examined. The interference patterns were complete on strong con-

Table 26-4. Case study 3: electromyographic studies

Side	Muscle	Innervation				Spontaneous activity		Voluntary activity	
		Nerve	Spinal segment			Fibrillation	PSW	MUAP profile	Interference
Left	Vastus lateralis	Femoral	L2 L3	L4		+1	+	Normal	Complete
Left	Rectus femoris	Femoral	L2 L3	L4		+1	+	Normal	Complete
Left	Anterior tibialis	Deep peroneal		L4	L5 S1	+3	+	Normal	Decreased
Left	Extensor digitorum longus	Deep peroneal		L4	L5 S1	+2	+	Normal	Slightly decreased
Left	Peroneus longus	Superficial peroneal		(L4)	L5 S1	0	0	Normal	Slightly decreased
Left	Extensor hallucis longus	Deep peroneal		(L4)	L5 S1	0	0	Normal	Complete
Left	Medial gastrocnemius	Tibial			S1 S2	0	0	Normal	Complete
Left	Biceps femoris (short head)	Sciatic		(L5)	S1 S2	0	0	Normal	Complete
Left	Adductor magnus	Obturator	L2 L3	(L4)		0	0	Normal	Complete
Left	Lumbar paraspinals			L4		+4	+	—	—
Right	Lumbar paraspinals			L4		0	0	—	—
Right	Anterior tibialis	Deep peroneal		L4	L5 S1	0	0	Normal	Complete
Right	Medial gastrocnemius	Tibial			S1 S2	0	0	Normal	Complete
Right	Vastus lateralis	Femoral	L2 L3	L4		0	0	Normal	Complete

PSW, Positive sharp waves.
MUAP, Motor unit action potential.

traction in all but three muscles. These were the left anterior tibialis muscle, which showed a moderate decrease in amplitude, and the left extensor digitorum longus and peroneus longus muscles, which showed a slight decrease in amplitude on strong contraction.

In summary, the nerve conduction velocity studies in this case were normal, ruling out the presence of a segmental demyelinating process. The H reflex test was utilized primarily to rule out S1 nerve root lesion, which it did in this case. The needle examination gave the most helpful data for localization of the lesion. The presence of fibrillation and positive sharp waves in four of the muscles tested showed that axonal demyelination had occurred. The muscles with reduced interference patterns on maximal effort also suggested that a problem was affecting their function. These muscles all share nerve fibers arising from the L4 nerve root. By fitting these observations with the client's complaints, it was concluded that the findings were compatable with a L4 radiculopathy.

CASE STUDY **4**: UPPER MOTOR NEURON LESION

A 31-year-old mother of two suddenly developed a complete right foot drop 7 days before referral for ENMG evaluation. She also complained of a total loss of sensation below her knee. This woman was able to walk with some difficulty wearing a plastic orthosis. Manual muscle testing showed no muscle activity in the muscles below the knee except for the gastrocremius muscles, which had trace activity. The quadriceps, gluteus medius, hip adductors, and hamstring muscles were normal in strength.

Nerve conduction velocity studies of the peroneal and tibial motor nerves bilaterally were within normal limits. Electromyographic examination of the anterior tibialis, extensor digitorum longus and brevis, peroneus longus, and posterior tibialis muscles showed no electrical response. The absence of fibrillation was not significant, as Wallerian degeneration would not have occurred in this time period. On maximal effort a few normal single motor unit potentials were observed in the gastrocnemius muscle on attempted plantar flexion. The vastus medialis, biceps femoris, gluteus medius, adductor longus, and L4, L5, and S1 paraspinal muscles on the right showed a normal response.

The data recorded in this examination did not assist in establishing the cause of the client's problem. It was recommended that she be studied again in 1 month if no explanation for her weakness had been established. In the interim she was diagnosed as having multiple sclerosis on the basis of the results of evoked, potential and magnetic resonance imaging studies. Since this demyelinating disease affects only the central nervous system, no EMG or NCV changes were observed.[6]

CASE STUDY **5**: BRACHIAL PLEXUS INJURY #1

A 78-year-old woman was referred for evaluation of a paralyzed right arm. Ten days earlier she had fallen from an 8-foot ladder onto a washing machine, dislocating her right shoulder. Two hours later the dislocation was reduced at the hospital. It was noted at that time that the dislocation had caused compression of the arterial flow, resulting in ischemia distal to the site.

On preliminary evaluation in the ENMG laboratory it was noted that the client had no sensory awareness or functional control of the arm. She was agitated and very fearful and openly stated that she would commit suicide if her arm did not get better.

Electrical stimulation, with a square wave pulse of 0.1 msec of the median, ulnar, and radial nerves in the region of the elbow resulted in a rapid and brisk response of the muscles distal to the site of stimulation. There was no increase in the threshold of excitability when this muscle response was compared with the response observed on the normal side. The client was reassured by the presence of muscle activity in her forearm and was referred to physical therapy for treatment.

It was decided that this client had a neuropraxic lesion involving all of the muscles below her elbow, because nerve transmission had continued beyond 7 days. Focal compression, such as she had sustained at the plexus level, can cause paranodal intussusception at the nodes of Ranvier.[20] Functional return can be expected approximately 60 days after injury.

Twenty-three days after injury, the first EMG evaluation was performed. Selected muscles innervated by the left median, ulnar, and radial nerves were found to be silent at rest and on attempted motion. These findings were consistent with a neuropraxic lesion. The biceps muscle was also silent at rest. On attempted voluntary motion, a few normal MUAPs were observed. The injury to the musculocutaneous nerve was not complete. The potentials recorded from the three parts of the deltoid were in marked contrast to this. Fibrillation in the +3 or +4 range and positive sharp waves were observed in each muscle, and no activity was observed on attempted motion. The axillary nerve was completely denervated, and recovery could not be predicted at this time.

Fifty-five days after injury a trace of motion was noted in the extensor carpi radialis muscle. Motion returned rapidly in the muscles supplied by the median, ulnar, and radial nerves in the subsequent weeks.

Electromyographic examination on the seventy-third day after injury showed minimal fibrillation in the biceps muscle and a low-level interference pattern. The fibrillation level in the deltoid muscle was also reduced and several low-amplitude, short-duration motor units were observed on attempted voluntary motion, indicating that reinnervation was occurring.

Four months after her injury this client had gained substantial return of hand function. Only slight weakness of the median and ulnar intrinsic muscles remained. On EMG examination the deltoid muscle showed increased numbers of low amplitude potentials on voluntary motion, some with normal configuration and the rest with a polyphasic configuration. All components of the deltiod were graded as poor-minus on muscle testing.

At the end of 8 months many polyphasic and normal MUAPs were present in the deltiod muscle. On maximal effort a complete interference pattern was observed with an amplitude of 2 mV. The client had regained sufficient muscle strength to do all her household activities, including placing light-weight items on overhead shelves. She laughed about her earlier fears and depression and was pleased with her recovery.

CASE STUDY **6**: BRACHIAL PLEXUS INJURY #2

A 45-year-old mechanic was standing in the bed of a pickup truck when it was started unexpectedly. He was thrown over the tailgate and landed on the ground, hitting his left shoulder. After this impact his left arm hung limp at his side, and he could feel nothing in the arm below the shoulder joint.

He was first sent for ENMG examination 3 months after his injury because he had had no return of function. His surgeon was considering exploratory surgery to see if any of the nerves had been severed and were in need of repair.

EMG of the cervical paraspinal muscle showed normal motor unit activity, indicating the injury was more distal than the root level. The muscles tested below this level in the left arm showed nothing but fibrillation potentials, with one exception. In the middle deltoid muscle a few short duration, low amplitude potentials were observed, which were under voluntary control. The surgeon was urged to delay surgery to see if spontaneous recovery occurred.

An EMG examination 1 month later showed motor unit action potentials (MUAPs) under voluntary control in the anterior, middle and posterior deltoid muscles. There were many low amplitude, short duration potentials and a few that were quite polyphasic. This pattern of activity suggested that recovery was occurring and surgery was again deferred.

One month later a greater number of voluntarily activated potentials were observed in the deltoid muscle, including low-amplitude, short-durations polyphasics, and higher amplitude multiphasic potentials; a few normal motor unit potentials were also observed. The biceps muscle showed decreased fibrillation. Surgery was postponed indefinately.

This client was studied monthly for the next 24 months. Each month fibrillation decreased and voluntarily activated potentials appeared at a more distal site. Functional activity appeared first in the shoulder and proceeded distally. Recovery was observed to occur in a manner that coincided with the predicted rate of nerve regrowth following axonotmesis, approximately 2.5 cm/month. This man returned to work 20 months later with the ability to do all the activities he had been able to do before the accident. The last skill to return was the ability to thread a nut on a bolt.

KINESIOLOGIC ELECTROMYOGRAPHY

Kinesiologic electromyography is probably the most underutilized evaluative technique available to physical therapists. It serves as a window through which one can observe muscle function. The electrical activity arising from a single muscle can be studied as it participates in coordinated motor activities, or it can be observed in a single repetitive function under different physiological conditions. More frequently the interaction of a number of muscles are studied simultaneously during both simple and complex motions. The electrical activity recorded does not give information concerning the strength of the muscles or the type of muscle contractions occurring. However, addition of force tranducers and electrogoniometers or some other type of measuring device to the recording system will allow simultaneous documentation of this data. This type of recording can be extremely helpful in evaluation of clients no matter what the cause of their neuromusclar problem might be.

The uses of kinesiologic electromyography are many and varied. Some of the more common clinical uses of these techniques are listed in the boxed material at right. Studies of normal subjects may also be done to determine the interrelationship of the electrical activity of muscles during specific muscle tasks to establish the parameters of normal function. These methods have also been used in training situations to give therapists feedback from their classmates' and clients' muscles as they learn to apply therapeutic procedures.[18]

Instrumentation for kinesiologic electromyography includes surface or internal electrodes, a multichannel amplification and recording system for simultaneous documentation of muscle and other physiological data, and appropri-

---

Uses of kinesiologic electromyography

Kinesiologic electromyographic evaluation can be used:

1. To determine patterns of electrical activity associated with normal or outstanding performance (as in walking or sports activities)
2. To document alteration of muscle function following paralysis, paresis, disease, or aging
3. To study gait, especially in instances where surgery is being considered, to correct imbalance in function
4. To document muscle status in relation to strength, endurance, or maturation to establish the capabilities of the client
5. To establish the most effective exercise program for the client, thereby optimizing the therapeutic results
6. To establish the suitability of biofeedback training for a client by examination with percutaneous electrodes
7. To serve as a means of stimulating clients with motor disorientation by showing them that function is possible in muscles that are not under their voluntary control, since these muscles often come under voluntary control following EMG study
8. To reinforce learning that occurs during the use of proprioceptive neuromuscular facilitation (PNF) and neurodevelopmental therapy (NDT) to allow both the client and the therapist an opportunity to see that they are accomplishing the goals they set for the therapy session
9. To help determine why a client has not benefited from an exercise program or has not reached a rehabilitation goal, by identifying whether or not the client has the muscular ability to do the activity, and by establishing how the muscles work when they are utilized in the activity presented
10. To assist in establishing the effectiveness of braces, splints, prostheses, and other devices used in the rehabilitation process
11. To evaluate the effect of treatment modalities and procedures applied to muscles such as heat, ultrasound, electrical stimulation, traction, vibration, or relaxation
12. To relate muscular activity to energy expenditure and fatigue
13. To determine the results of specific drug therapy on muscle function
14. To select optimal electrode placement sites for clients requiring myoelectrically controlled prostheses, environmental systems, feeders, or wheelchairs
15. To monitor sleep and sleep-related disturbances
16. To establish the capabilities of clients in work environments by studying their muscle activity during specific projects, to determine their limitations and to set up the most efficient work environment

ate devices to document when and how the muscle activity occurs.

Surface electrodes can be used in many applications. Miniature silver–silver chloride electrodes, which float on the skin in a coupling electrode gel, or ultraflexible elastomeric electrodes,[17] which are attached to the skin surface with a nonconductive spray, give the least artifact. These electrodes are applied to carefully cleaned and slightly abraded skin to maximize signal transfer; they are used in pairs placed close together over the muscle being studied and parallel to the muscle fiber direction. A spacing of 1 cm reduces pickup from adjacent muscles. A spacing of 2½ cm is best for pickup for myoelectric control applications.

When small, deep, or weak muscles are evaluated, intramuscular wire electrodes should be used. They should also be used in preliminary studies done before beginning a research study using surface electrodes. If simultaneous recordings from the surface and internal electrodes show the same type of interference pattern from a number of subjects, the use of surface electrodes can be justified. These electrodes are prepared by removing the insulation from about ¼ inch of two fine copper wires. The wires are then inserted through a hypodermic needle and bent backward over its tip. The completed electrode is packaged, autoclaved, and kept sterile until it is used. The needle serves as a vehicle for placement of the wires. When the wires are appropriately placed in the muscle, the needle is removed and the subject can move freely without discomfort. As in all other procedures, a ground electrode is also necessary.

There are a wide variety of commercially available recorders for kinesiology.[2] Multichannel ENMG units, physiological recorders, and telemetry systems are used. They must have the capability to simultaneously record data relating to the event being studied as well as the EMG data. Electrogoniometers, pressure transducers, accelerometers, microswitches, and many other instruments can be used to relate the subject's activity to the muscle performance.

In some applications the goal of the kinesiologic EMG is directed toward assisting the client to gain voluntary control of a specific muscle for a specific activity. In this type of study little preparation is required. For example, a quadraplegic client may be encouraged to bring a specific muscle under his or her own control. By displaying the single motor units or interference activity generated on attempted motion by the client, he or she may be able to learn how to initiate the activity independently and bring in other MUAPs so that useful function of the muscle occurs in an area where none was anticipated. The evaluative sessions could then be turned into muscle feedback sessions repeated several times a day as part of a therapy program.

Other applications of kinesiologic EMG are more similar to research studies and require more extensive planning. To gain the most information in this type of study, the goals for each part of the study should be carefully defined. A written protocol for the study should be developed. It should include a coding system for rapid documentation of the activities observed during the recording session.

Consideration should be given to the instrumentation, equipment, and supplies required and the physical setup of the study. Everything possible should be done to ensure the client's comfort and safety. Then a preliminary run of the study should be done to ensure that the instrumentation has been set up appropriately so that the desired information is adequately displayed. This may involve numerous trials, varying the recording parameters until the desired format for the data is obtained. It is especially important to do trial runs varying the recording speed and vertical sensitivity to be sure that the EMG data are being displayed in the most appropriate way and that no data are being lost. Before the actual study is begun, the client or group of clients to be tested should be informed of the details of the study and told exactly what they are expected to do during the procedure. At the time of recording, all that will remain to be done is to apply the appropriate transducers, direct the client, and monitor the recording.

Many precautions need to be taken in analyzing kinesiologic EMG data. The data should always be viewed in the form in which they were taken from the client before they are averaged, integrated, or altered by a computer program. This will prevent interpretation of artifacts caused by motion artifact, wire sway, poor electrode contact, electrode failure, and extraneous electrical signals, as muscle activity. In the literature emphasis is placed on the sequencing of EMG events and their interrelationships with other muscles and the activity of the client during the recording.[16] Little emphasis is given to the amplitude or shape of the wave envelopes associated with the muscle contraction. The amplitude varies as a result of many factors so that intramuscular and intersubject comparisons based on this aspect of the data must be made with cautious consideration. Usually, amplitude data are reported as a percentage of the interference produced on maximal muscle contraction. This factor does not negate the value of these studies. Attention to the initiation of muscle activity, its variation throughout a movement, its cessation, and its relationship to muscle activity in other areas are important to the understanding of muscle function in both health and disease.

CASE STUDY **7:** HEMIPLEGIC EVALUATION

A group of hemiplegic clients in a rehabilitation center had a common problem that did not seem to be directly related to the cardiovascular accidents (CVA) they had suffered. When they attempted to walk, they fell toward the hemiplegic side and were not able to recover their balance. Manual muscle testing of the abdominal muscles that would prevent this motion suggested that they were too weak to prevent this from happening. Paired surface electrodes were placed on the upper and lower quadrants of the abdomen of each client, and a multichannel EMG unit was set up for recording. Data were collected with the clients in a sitting position while attempting to move from a side-bent position to an upright position. All of the clients had difficulty coming up from the paralyzed side and no problem coming up from the opposite side. The interference patterns observed from the muscles being sampled confirmed that the former motion was difficult for them. Some of the patients were even unable to localize the muscles to initiate the motion. It was noticed that repeated attempts at the righting task resulted in better utilization of these muscles.

To reinforce this evaluation experience, an exercise frame was built that was adjustable in 10 degree increments from 10 to 70 from the vertical position. The clients were given daily muscle feedback training in the frame. The EMG was set up so that they could both see and hear the activity from their muscles while they attempted to straighten up by moving toward the non-paralyzed side. The frame was lowered 10 degrees whenever the client could do 10 successful repetitions of the exercise. All of the clients became safe, independent walkers within 1 to 3 weeks after this program was initiated.

SUMMARY

This brief consideration of electrodiagnosis with emphasis on the use of clinical electroneuromyography and kinesiologic electromyography for evaluation and treatment of clients was presented with selected case studies. This material touches only a tiny segment of the field of electrodiagnosis. Instrumentation for electrodiagnostic recording is being developed rapidly at the present time, allowing more and more to be learned about neuromuscular function. These developments are giving physical therapists an opportunity to expand their knowledge concerning the status of their clients, and with this information they can develop treatment programs that optimize the value of their work. For ideas on treatment procedures following peripheral trauma refer to Chapter 12.

REFERENCES

1. Aminoff MJ: Electrodiagnosis neurology, New York, 1987, Churchill Livingstone Inc.

2. Basmajian JV: Muscles alive, Baltimore, Md, 1985, Williams & Wilkins.

3. Braddom RL and Johnson EW: Standardization of H reflex and diagnostic use in S1 radiculopathy, Arch Phys Med Rehabil 55:161-166, 1974.

4. Chiappa KH: Evoked potentials in clinical medicine, New York, 1983, Raven Press.

5. Delagi EF and others: Anatomic guide for the electromyographer, Springfield, Ill, 1980, Charles C Thomas Publisher.

6. Gilroy J and Holliday P: Basic neurology, New York, 1982, Macmillan Inc.

7. Goodgold J: Anatomical correlates of clinical electromyography, Baltimore, Md, 1983, Williams & Wilkins.

8. Goodgold J and Eberstein A: Electrodiagnosis of neuromuscular diseases, Baltimore, Md, 1983, Williams & Wilkins

9. Hoppenfeld S: Physical examination of the spine and extremities, New York, 1976, Appleton-Century-Crofts.

10. Kimura J: Electromyography: nerve conduction studies, Philadelphia, 1983, FA Davis Co.

11. Ma DM and Liveson JA: Nerve conduction handbook, Philadelphia, 1983, FA Davis Co.

12. McGill KC, Cummins KL, and Dorfman LJ: Automatic decomposition of the clinical electromyogram, IEEE Trans Biomed Eng 32:470-477, 1985.

13. McGill KC and others: Non-invasive electromyography, Palo Alto, Calif, 1988, Rehabilitation Research and Development Center 1988 Progress Report.

14. Oh SJ: Clinical electromyography: nerve conduction studies, Baltimore, Md, 1984, University Park Press.

15. Oh SJ: Electromyography: neuromuscular transmission studies, Baltimore, Md, 1988, Williams & Wilkins.

16. Reiner S: Instrumentation. In Johnson EW, editor: Practical electromyography, Baltimore, Md, 1988, Williams & Wilkins.

17. Robertson K: Electromyographic applications of NASA electrode, Proceedings of the San Diego Biomedical Symposium 12:105-108, 1973.

18. Robertson K and Kent B: Integration of kinesiology and therapeutic exercise using electromyographic techniques, London, 1974, World Confederation for Physical Therapy.

19. Shahani BT: Electromyography in CNS disorders, Boston, 1984, Butterworth Publishers.

20. Spinner M: Injuries to the major branches of peripheral nerves of the forearm, Philadelphia, 1978, WB Saunders Co.

21. Wolf SL: Electrotherapy, New York, 1981, Churchill Livingstone Inc.

Chapter 27

PAIN MANAGEMENT

Linda Mirabelli

OVERVIEW

One of the many challenges facing today's clinician is the treatment of pain. This is a result, in part, of the fact that pain is subjective as well as objective. The underlying physical cause of the pain may readily be identified, but the sensation is open to interpretation and may very well be out of line with the magnitude of the disease. What is excruciating to one individual may be merely uncomfortable to another, and pain tolerances may even vary in intensity within the same individual, depending on any number of external factors. Curing the physical cause may not always bring pain to an end.

There is little agreement on a working definition of pain. It is agreed only that pain is a complex emotional experience and that it is a message from the body meant to draw attention to a harmful or potentially harmful situation. For clinicians, the challenge in pain management comes in identifying and correcting the physical cause for the pain as well as addressing the emotional components.

PAIN THEORIES

How an event comes to be perceived as pain has always fascinated scientists, and historically many have attempted to explain the physical nature of pain by developing "pain theories."

Max von Frey[53] proposed that specific peripheral pain receptors (free nerve endings) project to a cortical pain center (the thalamus) with pain impulses travelling along specific fibers in a specific pathway (A and C fibers travelling in the lateral spinothalamic tracts). His "specificity theory" was the basis for years of nerve sectioning as a treatment for intractable pain, despite the fact that many times the surgical lesions were unsuccessful in abolishing the pain and that occasionally pain actually increased after surgery. This theory did not explain how innocuous stimuli (touch, vibration) could stimulate pain, how pain occurred spontaneously, or how it was referred to unrelated areas of the body. Nor did it account for the interaction between pain and emotions.[40]

Taking the opposite view, Weddel[59] postulated that pain is the result of intense stimulation of nonspecific receptors that produce a specific pattern of impulses that travel along nonspecific fibers to the brain, where their intensity and frequency identify them as pain. This "pattern theory" is no longer accepted, because it is now known that there is receptor-fiber specialization.

As knowledge became more sophisticated, so did the pain theories. Gelhard[15] discusses Goldscheider's hypothesis that pain results from the "summation" of impulses generated from any stimulus, noxious or innocuous. Gelhard himself proposed that any receptor was capable of causing pain if it was stimulated long enough and with enough intensity.

It is now known that there are morphologically distinct nerve endings in the tissues that may cause pain when activated by mechanical or chemical abnormalities. Woven throughout most human tissue is a continuous, three-dimensional plexus of unmyelinated fibers called the *interstitial nociceptor system*. These receptors respond to incision, tearing, laceration, excessive stretching, and compression of the tissues as well as to the accumulation of abnormally high concentrations of chemical substances, including lactic acid, potassium, and histamine.[56]

There is a similar plexus system, called the *perivascular nociceptor system,* in the walls of the peripheral arteries, arterioles, venules, and veins. This system is responsive to the same mechanical and chemical factors, but, in addition, is stimulated by marked constriction or dilation of the vessels.[56]

PAIN PATHWAYS

Information from the nociceptors travels into the dorsal gray matter on A-delta and C fibers, the smallest afferent fibers in the body. Most are less than 5 mm in diameter, and only those with diameters larger than 2 mm are myelinated.

Once in the spinal cord, these primary afferent fibers do one of three things. Some synapse with interneurons that synapse directly with motor nerves and cause reflex movements, for example, withdrawing the hand from a hot object. Others synapse with interneurons that synapse with autonomic fibers from the sympathetic and sacral parasympathetic systems and cause autonomic reflexes. Most, however, synapse with interneurons that travel to the higher centers in the anterolateral tract. Information from primary afferent fibers originating caudal to the pelvis ascends on the contralateral side of the body, whereas information from primary afferent fibers originating cranial to the pelvis remains ipsilateral.[11]

The phenomena of fast and slow pain are the result of the size of the conducting fibers, the number of synapses along the neural pathway, and the brain areas to which the neurons project. Fast pain, the sensation first perceived after injury, travels on large myelinated fibers in a fairly direct route from the dorsal gray matter to the thalamus, through the internal capsule to the postcentral gyrus of the cortex. Fast pain is accurately localized and qualified, and lasts only as long as the duration of the stimulus.[12]

Slow pain travels a more multisynaptic route on slower conducting nonmyelinated fibers. The primary afferents synapse twice in the dorsal gray matter. The second-order neurons then cross the midline and travel in the anterolateral-spinoreticular tracts to the reticular formation, which projects the information to various areas in the midbrain and thalamus. From here it is transmitted to the cortex. Slow pain is poorly localized and outlasts the duration of the stimulus.[12]

The emotional/psychological aspects of pain result, in part, from the various thalamocortical projections that provide the perceptual, affective, memory, and hormonal components of the pain experience. The projections from the thalamus to the postcentral gyrus, previously identified with fast pain, are responsible for the perceptual component. It is from this projection that pain can be localized and qualified as to whether it is pricking, throbbing, burning, and so on.[56]

Projections to the frontal lobes and the limbic system are concerned with the emotional component of pain, specifically with identifying pain as an unpleasant experience. It is this projection that causes pain to "hurt."[56] The limbic system's control over motor control can result in more muscle tone and thus more pain (refer to Chapter 4.)

Pain memory results from projections to the memory storage areas of the temporal lobes. This area also receives input from the limbic and sensory cortical areas mentioned previously. It is from these projections that a memory bank of past painful experiences is developed.[56]

The hormonal response to pain is the result of a noncortical projection, from the thalamus to the hypothalamus, which is responsible for global efferent activity in the autonomic system. It is from this projection that the secretion of sympathetic hormones (i.e., epinephrine) takes place.[56]

PAIN MODULATION

Whether or not stimulation of the nociceptors results in pain depends on a number of modulating factors. The intensity of perceived pain varies considerably, depending on the individual's mood, on the amount of distraction from the pain, and on the positive or negative suggestions of others, as well as on several peripheral and central neurological systems that are capable of modulating transmission at the synapses in the nociceptive pathways.

According to the gate-control theory proposed by Melzak and Wall,[40] presynaptic inhibition in the dorsal gray matter of the spinal cord results in blocking of pain impulses coming from the periphery. Pain fibers enter the spinal cord through the dorsal horn and immediately divide into short ascending and descending branches that synapse with interneurons in the dorsal gray. These interneurons then synapse with neurons that become the lateral spinothalamic tract and transmit impulses to higher brain centers.

The dorsal gray matter has been found to be laminated. Laminae II, III (substantia gelatinosa), and V (transmission "T" cells) have been implicated in pain impulse transmission.

Melzak and Wall's gate control theory states that the T cells must be stimulated for pain to be perceived and that the substantia gelatinosa acts as a gating mechanism that has the capacity of preventing the afferent impulses from reaching the T cells. Input from pressoreceptors and mechanoreceptors travelling on large-diameter A fibers stimulates the substantia gelatinosa; this closes the gate and blocks activation of the T cells. Nociceptive input from small-diameter A-delta and C fibers inhibits the substantia gelatinosa; this opens the gate and allows activation of the T cells. Small fiber input also stimulates the T cells directly. The T cells then convey information to multiple pain centers in the brain, including the cerebrum, the brainstem, the thalamus, and the cortex.

More recently Melzak[39] has added that there is a descending system that also inhibits transmission through the dorsal gray matter. This originates from areas in the brainstem and is activated by intense small fiber activity, so that extreme activity within the pain-conducting system itself also serves to inhibit the transmission of pain impulses.

Although the gate-control theory is widely accepted, it is not without opposition. Opponents note that:[41]

1. It does not clarify the role of the afferent synapses in lamina I, although they have been shown to be receptive to noxious stimuli.
2. It does not account for peripheral blocking mechanisms.
3. It does not explain why patients with thallium-induced polyneuropathy continue to experience pain, although they should not, or why patients with polyneuropathies that destroy large fibers do not have pain, although they should.

As early as 1975[21] naturally occurring substances that possess opiate-like properties, including analgesia, were discovered in the body. Receptors for these endogenous opiates (opioids) are found in high concentrations throughout the CNS, especially in areas associated with nociception and those identified by Melzak and Wall as significant in presynaptic inhibition of pain impulses: the thalamus, limbic system, periaqueductal gray matter, and substantia gelatinosa. Central processing of pain requires multiple neurotransmitter systems, and it is believed that endogenous opiates are neurotransmitters or neuromodulators of pain-related neural impulses.[2]

Endogenous opiates are divided into endorphins, enkephalins, and substance P. Endorphins, long-lasting morphine-like chemicals found primarily in the thalamus, midbrain, pons, medulla, and hypothalamic-pituitary axis, produce analgesia as well as systemic effects on mood and the gastrointestinal, respiratory, and endocrine systems.[2] Endorphin levels in individuals with chronic pain vary depending on whether the pain is of neurogenic, somatoge-

nic, or psychogenic origin.[54] Endorphins are thought to be significant in activating a central regulatory system that originates in the periaqueductal gray matter and inhibits transmission by interneurons in the dorsal gray matter.[2]

Enkephalins mediate a second central pathway in which the descending neurons originate in the reticular formation and inhibit transmission by the interneurons in the dorsal gray matter. This system is enhanced with diversion (including hypnosis) and increased blood concentrations of catecholamines such as epinephrine, norepinephrine, and dopamine.[7]

Depolarization of the secondary neurons in the dorsal gray matter is mediated through release of substance P. Increased mechanoreceptor input inhibits the release of substance P, thereby decreasing pain transmission and perception. There is some conflicting evidence, however, indicating that high concentrations of substance P result in excitation of the afferent neurons, thus facilitating pain transmission.[43]

Although serotonin is not classified as an endogenous opiate, it exerts a profound effect on analgesia and enhances analgesic drug potency. High concentrations of serotonin lead to decreased pain,[35] whereas low concentrations result in depression, sleep disturbances, and increased pain.[51]

There are two cortical modulating systems, both of which can function as either excitatory or inhibitory, depending on the neurons on which they terminate. The direct cortical modulating system originates in the cortex and travels to the dorsal gray matter in the contralateral motor tract. The indirect cortical modulating system originates in the cortex and travels to the dorsal gray matter in the contralateral motor tract. The indirect cortical modulating system is a dual mechanism with neurons from the cortex to the reticular formation and neurons from the limbic system to the midbrain. Since the limbic system deals with affect, changes in mood modify the perception of pain intensity and, thereby, alter the pain threshold.[56]

PAIN PERCEPTION

The physical nature of pain is a product of its site of origin. Pain can arise from the central nervous system (CNS), autonomic nervous system (ANS), and the periphery.

Pain from the CNS

Pain from lesions in the CNS is topographical: the site of the lesion determines the location and character of the symptoms, which can range from paresthesia to pain. The onset is variable, ranging from immediately after the insult to much later, and many times pain is the first indicator of a CNS lesion.[7]

Pain from injury to the dorsal horns is felt ipsilateral to the injury in a pattern corresponding to the nerve root distribution. Injury to the ascending anterolateral tracts results in pain below the level of the lesion on the contralateral side of the body. Pain rising from cortical lesions is referred to regions of the body with the greatest cortical representation, most usually areas of the face, hands, and feet.[7]

Thalamic pain is the classic example of central pain. Although thalamic pain is usually concentrated in the contralateral extremities, any region of the contralateral side of the body can be affected and the pain is frequently migratory. The onset of thalamic pain can be easily elicited by movement, skin contact (even air blowing over the skin), heat, cold, and vibration, but is frequently spontaneous. It may "develop explosively and spread all over the affected side of the body in floods."[11] It is usually unremitting and irreversible.[7]

Pain from the ANS

Pain from lesions in the ANS is quadratic. Sympathetic and parasympathetic fibers travel in the walls of the blood vessels, and since the major vessels serve quadrants of the body, autonomic pain is spread throughout the involved vessel's distribution. Autonomic pain that originates from the sympathetic nervous system is frequently accompanied by other measurable sympathetic disturbances, and because of the sympathetic/parasympathetic connection with emotion, pain originating from the autonomic pathways is far more sensitive to mood changes than is CNS pain.[14] Causalgia and phantom limb pain are examples of ANS pain.

Causalgia is characterized by an intense burning and hyperaesthesia throughout the distribution of an incompletely damaged peripheral nerve that has, most commonly, sustained a penetrating wound. Causalgia usually occurs as healing takes place and is so easily elicited by minor tactile stimulation that the individual refuses to move the affected limb for fear of stimulating the pain. Frequently there are concomitant trophic changes. The skin becomes atrophic and scaly. In the acute stage it will initially be pink, warm, and glossy, then become cyanotic, mottled, and moist. The muscles may atrophy and the bone develop osteoporosis.[6]

Causalgia is thought to result from the development of "false synapses" between the injured autonomic efferent fibers and the afferents, so that the autonomic impulses divert to sensory fibers providing them with continuous autonomic input. The most common treatment for causalgia is sectioning of the involved nerve with variable results.[11]

Phantom limb sensation, the feeling that a missing limb is still intact, commonly occurs after amputation. Phantom limb pain is a burning, squeezing sensation accompanied by "pins and needles" thought to result from the formation of a terminal neuroma from incompletely regenerated nerve fibers and connective tissue at the point of section. This creates an abnormal pattern of afferent impulses that may be accompanied by secondary changes in the CNS,

leading to an interpretation of incoming impulses as having risen from the missing limb.[11] Both phantom limb pain and phantom limb sensation tend to fade in time, and their extinction can be expedited with local percussion or vibration to the stump, as well as other therapeutic modalities, including transcutaneous electric nerve stimulation (TENS) and high-voltage galvanic (HVG) stimulation.

Pain from the periphery

Pain from the periphery results from noxious irritation of the nociceptors. Its character is dependent on the source of the irritation.

Mechanical pain results from deformation of the receptor and is usually sharp in nature. When there is pressure on a neural structure, there may also be paresthesia and "pins and needles." Mechanical pain lasts only as long as the deformation is present and resolves when the deformation is corrected.[36]

Chemical pain occurs when noxious chemical substances occur in quantities sufficient to irritate the nociceptors. Chemical pain is dull and aching and is relieved only when the concentration of chemicals returns to a subthreshold level.[6]

EVALUATION OF THE CLIENT WITH PAIN

Evaluations of the client with pain are very challenging. Because of the subjectivity of pain recall, it is not always possible to clinically reproduce pain matching the quality and intensity of the original sensation: the client is not always accurate in recall of pain experienced a month, or even a week, before, and there is no way to account for the sensory and affective components or the psychological and cultural contributions to the pain experience. Despite this, pain evaluations need to include measurable, reproducible information that identifies the source of the pain, directs the clinician toward appropriate methods of treatment, and assists in establishing attainable goals.

Pain history

Crucial to the evaluation is a comprehensive pain history. It is important to have a standardized format to decrease chances of missing important information and to minimize the possibility that the client might "lead the interview." The following mnemonic device in which the steps in the evaluation are arranged alphabetically, is helpful:

*O*rigin/onset: date and circumstances of the onset of pain. How did the pain start? Gradually or suddenly? Was there a precipitating injury? If so, what was the mechanism of injury?
*P*osition: location of the pain. Have the client demonstrate where the pain is located rather than relying on description.
*P*attern: pattern of the pain. Is the pain constant or pe-

riodic? Does it travel or radiate? Which activities increase it? Which decrease it? Have there been any recent changes in the pattern? Does the client feel that the pain is improving, worsening, or remaining the same?

*Q*uality: characteristics of the pain. Does the client use adjectives indicating mechanical (pressing, bursting, stabbing), chemical (burning), neural (numb, "pins and needles"), or vascular (throbbing) origin?

*Q*uantity: intensity of the pain. Several methods that allow for monitoring change in pain intensity are presented later.

*R*adiation: characteristics of pain radiation. What causes the pain to radiate? Can the radiation be reversed? How?

*S*igns/symptoms: functional and psychological components of the pain. Has the pain resulted in any functional limitations? Does the client's personality contribute to the pain or has the pain caused changes in the client's emotional stability? It may be necessary to interview the client's significant others for an accurate picture.

*T*reatment: previous/current treatment and its effectiveness, including medications and home remedies. It is important also to determine the client's attitude and expectations concerning therapy.

Measuring pain intensity

In the past, attempts to quantify pain have varied from relying on the individual's memory of the pain experience to using external stimuli to reproduce pain of the same intensity. Post hoc questioning[29] has not been found valid for measuring the intensity of chronic pain, which is usually overestimated, but has been of some limited value with acute pain, which is remembered accurately for up to 5 days.

Pain induced by experimental tests utilizing mechanical pressure, temperature, vascular occlusion, and electric stimulation bears little resemblence to the pain produced by disease. In actuality, experimentally induced pain measures only the client's pain threshold and pain ceiling. However, because these parameters are known to change in pathological conditions and to be altered by certain analgesics, they may be of value in monitoring changes in the client's medical condition and assessing the effectiveness of pain medication.[42]

An easy and effective approach to rating pain intensity involves having the client rate the current level of discomfort in one of the following ways (Fig. 27-1):

1. Verbal rating scale: the client rates the pain on a continuum that is subdivided from left to right into gradually increasing pain intensities
2. Visual analogue scale: the client rates the pain on a continuum that has no subdivisions
3. Pain estimate: The client rates the pain on a scale of 0 to 100, where 0 represents a lack of pain and 100 is the most severe pain possible

All of these scales are easy to administer, reliable over time, and sensitive to even the smallest changes in pain intensity when used to measure pain that is present at the time of the evaluation.[26] In the first two scales, measurements can be taken from the left margin to the points marked by the client and a bar or line graft constructed to monitor behavior of the pain. In the third scale the numbers themselves provide the necessary information.

Measuring the character of pain

Clues as to the cause of pain are gathered by examining the characteristics of what the client is experiencing. Pain from muscle, nerve, and the viscera differs in the same way that mechanical and chemical pain are different from each other. It is important to know the cause of pain to treat it as effectively and economically as possible.

One of the leading assessments of pain character is the McGill Pain Questionnaire (MPQ), which involves 20 categories of descriptive words covering the sensory, affective, and evaluative properties of pain. Each word has a

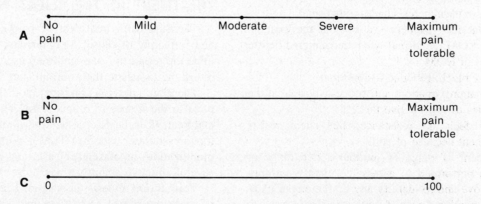

Fig. 27-1. Rating scales for measuring pain intensity. **A,** Verbal rating scale. **B,** Visual analogue scale. **C,** Pain estimate.

numerical value. The client selects the one word in each categoy that best represents his or her immediate pain. If no word in a particular group is suitable, the category is skipped. When completed, the test provides a series of adjectives describing what the client is experiencing as well as a numerical score that can be used to monitor changes in the pain pattern.[37] The MPQ can be completed in 20 minutes. The MPQ has been studied extensively and found valid for chronic and acute pain as well as for a variety of specific pathological states.[5,27,44]

Reliability and validity of this test is based on examiner objectivity. Thus, care must be taken to avoid examiner subjectivity, which may occur if the client is unfamiliar with some of the words and needs them defined during the test.[37]

Examination of the client

The clinical assessment should begin the moment the client enters the door. Clients frequently change posture and affect when they are being formally evaluated, and it is important to gain an accurate view of pain behavior during nonrequested activities to assess the validity of their complaints.

The formal assessment should include the following:

1. Observation of gait and movement patterns, including the use of assistive devices
2. Notation of body type and anomalies
3. Assessment of sitting and standing posture, including both the normal posture and that assumed because of the pain
4. Inspection of the skin for pliability, trophic changes, scar tissue, and other abnormalities
5. Palpation of the soft tissue structures to identify changes in temperature, swelling, tenderness, and areas of discomfort
6. Palpation of the anatomical structures to determine end feel, the sensation felt at the end of the available movement.[9]
   a. Bone-to-bone: hard—normal, for example, at the end range of elbow extension
   b. Spasm: muscular resistance—abnormal
   c. Capsular feel: rubbery—normal at the extreme of full ROM; abnormal when encountered before the end of ROM
   d. Springy block: rebound—abnormal
   e. Tissue approximation: soft tissue—normal at the extremes of full passive flexion
   f. Empty feel: no resistance, but client resists movement because of pain
7. Measurement of range of motion: active range of motion is performed to assess the client's willingness to move and to identify any limitations or painful areas; passive range of motion testing is used to further refine the observations[9]
   a. When active and passive movements are painful and restricted in the same direction and the pain appears at the limit of motion, the problem is arthrogenic
   b. When active and passive movements are painful or restricted in opposite directions, the problem is muscular
   c. When there is relative restriction of passive movement in the capsular pattern, the problem is arthritic
   d. When there is no restriction of passive movement but the client cannot perform the movement actively, the muscle is not functioning, either from intrinsic problems within the muscle or interruption in the neural pathway (central or peripheral)
8. Measurement of muscle strength[9]
   a. When the movement is strong and painful, there is a minor lesion in the muscle or tendon
   b. When the movement is weak and increases the pain, there is a major lesion that needs to be identified with further testing
   c. When the movement is weak but does not increase the pain, there is the possibility of either complete rupture of the muscle or tendon or a neurological disorder
   d. When all resisted movements are painful, the pain may be organic or the patient may be emotionally hypersensitive
   e. If movement is strong and painless, the test is normal
9. Assessment of neurological function including: reflexes, sensation, coordination, and stretch and pressure tests to nerve trunks

The amount of information needed to accurately identify the cause of the client's pain is substantial, and frequently more than one session is needed to perform a full evaluation. It is far better to take several sessions and be accurate than to condense the evaluation into one session and direct treatment at the wrong structures.

TREATMENT OF THE CLIENT WITH PAIN

The successful treatment of pain involves identifying and correcting its cause. As clinicians, we must first determine the reason for pain and then use our clinical skills to return the tissues to their normal state.

There are numerous physical modalities that can be applied to the tissues to relieve pain. These include superficial heat, deep heat, cryotherapy, phonophoresis and iontophoresis, laser therapy, TENS, point stimulation, joint mobilization, myofascial release, and massage, as well as several effective cognitive measures.

This section reviews the physics and physiology of each of these modalities so that we can knowledgeably select the most appropriate when establishing a treatment plan.

The purpose is to provide an understanding of the mechanism of each so that treatment will be based on sound physiological principles.

Thermotherapy

The physiological effects of therapeutic heat and cold applications are frequently reciprocal, although the end product, relief of pain, is often the same. When selecting hot or cold, it is important to understand the mechanism of each so that the appropriate modality is used.

Heat application. The physiological effects of heat depend on the method of application, the depth of penetration, and the rate and magnitude of temperature change.[13] These physiological effects include the following:

1. The cellular metabolic rate increases with rising temperature until an optimal temperature is reached. If the temperature continues to rise, there is a gradual slowing of metabolic activity until cell death results from denaturation of the protein within the tissue.
2. Speed of skeletal muscle contraction increases until the optimal temperature for metabolic processes is reached; then it, too, gradually decreases.
3. Muscle tension declines, probably because chemical energy is released too rapidly to be converted into mechanical energy.
4. Local blood flow increases. If the area remains below core temperature, increased blood flow results in a transfer of heat from the core. If the area becomes warmer than the core, heat is carried centrally.
5. Capillary permeability, capillary hydrostatic pressure, and capillary filtration rate all increase. There is an escape of protein into the interstitial space, leading to edema.
6. Anastomoses that connect arterioles to venules open and blood is shunted past the capillaries. Because venules are longer than capillaries, blood remains in the area longer, allowing greater time for heat transfer to the tissues.
7. Muscle spasms decrease as a result of decreased activity in gamma motor efferents and decreased muscle spindle excitability.
8. Pain decreases. Ischemic pain is relieved by the influx of oxygen-rich blood into the dilated vessels and muscle tension pain is decreased by interruption of the pain/spasm cycle.

Because of these effects there are several precautions when using heat as a modality. Heat should be used with caution in very young and elderly individuals because of their inability to thermoregulate adequately. Heat should also be used with caution in individuals with impaired circulation, diminished sensation, or inadequate cardiac or respiratory reserves. Heat application is contraindicated during acute thrombophlebitis because of the increased risk of emboli. It is also contraindicated over a malignancy because the increased blood flow could nourish the tumor and increase the chance of metastases. Heat should not be used where there is hemorrhage or recent trauma.[52]

Heat can be applied by conduction, convection, and radiation. Heat transfer by conduction involves the exchange of heat down a temperature gradient by two objects that are in contact. Heat transferred from one object is dispersed into another at a rate dependent on the thermal conductivity of the objects, the temperature gradients, and the quantity of blood flow (if the object is living tissue). When heat is transferred faster than it can be dissipated, there is a temperature rise in the receiving object, a decrease in the temperature gradient, and a subsequent slowing of the rate of exchange. Eventually, a state of equilibrium is reached and heat exchange stops.[13]

The depth of penetration with conductive heating is usually 1 cm or less.[13] Moist heat packs and paraffin are examples of conductive heating.

In convective heating heat is transferred through the flow of hot fluid. Fluid density decreases as its temperature increases, making warm fluids lighter than cool fluids. Warm fluids rise, cooling as they move upward. Cool fluids sink, warming as they move downward. Heat is exchanged when the moving molecules collide. Objects in the fluid also exchange heat as they come in contact with the moving molecules.[13] Convective heating, like conductive heating, is superficial. Therapeutic convective heating takes place during hydrotherapy. Objects that are warmed by the energy are heated by radiation.[13] Molecules with a temperature greater than absolute zero are in an excited state and emit energy, thus creating radiant heat.

Radiant heat can be superficial, as with infrared and ultraviolet, or deep, as with diathermy and microtherm. Shortwave diathermy involves making the individual part of a circuit that conducts alternating current from a generator, through a capacitor, through the individual to another capacitor, then back to the generator. The systemic ions create friction as they attempt to line up with the continuously reversing polarity, resulting in an increase in tissue temperature deep within the body.

Current density and, therefore, the magnitude of the temperature increase is dependent on placement of the capacitor. When the capacitor is remote, there is minimal surface heating with a homogenous temperature increase in the deep tissues. When the capacitor is close to the body, there is a greater temperature increase along the current pathway and at the body's surface. Diathermy is indicated where diffuse heating is desired.

In contrast, microtherm converts electrical energy into electromagnetic energy that can be focused on the tissue of choice. Increased temperature results when the electromagnetic waves are absorbed by the tissues. Microwave is far more exact than diathermy and is indicated where heating of individual deep structures is desired.

Deep heating can also be accomplished through the use of ultrasound. Unlike the transverse waves of electromagnetic radiation, the ultrasound wave is longitudinal, with alternating areas of compression and expansion that move forward then backward along the line of propagation. The wave is repeatedly refracted as it encounters tissues of differing acoustical resistance while traveling through the skin toward the bone. At each tissue interface it changes directions, and energy is transferred to the tissues (Fig. 27-2). The areas between the sound head and the coupling agent and the coupling agent and the skin also constitute interfaces where energy can be lost to the environment.

Ultrasound cannot travel through air; therefore it requires a coupling agent for effective transmission. Reid and Cummings[45] evaluated various coupling agents for their ability to transmit ultrasound while minimizing energy loss and found the following overall transmission levels: Aquasonic Gel—72.60%; glycerol—67.75%; distilled water—59.38%; Cardio-cream—26.60%; mineral oil—19.06%; air—00.00%. In addition, they determined that, as the dosage increased, a greater percentage of ultrasound energy reached the tissues. They concluded that selection of the appropriate coupling agent and dosage both appear to be important in ensuring that maximum energy is transmitted to the tissues.

Most of the therapeutic value of ultrasound comes from its ability to selectively raise tissue temperature at the interfaces without causing substantial change in the surrounding tissues. The amount of heat produced depends directly on the dosage (the amount of energy per unit time). At less than 1.0 W/cm^2 there is a minimal increase in tissue temperature. At 1.5 W/cm^2 the superficial tissues

are heated, and at greater than 2.0 W/cm^2 temperature of the deeper tissues are raised.[33]

Dosage is also instrumental in changing the propagation of impulses originating from peripheral nerves. The number of impulses traveling along the nerve decreases at low dosages, but begins to rise slowly beginning at 1.9 W/cm^2. Sounding of C fibers yields pain relief distal to the point of application, whereas sounding of large-diameter A fibers brings relief of spasm by changing gamma fiber activity, making the muscle fibers less sensitive to stretch.[13] Since it is impossible to selectively treat C or A fibers, ultrasound provides both pain relief and relief from muscle spasm, making it effective in the treatment of peripheral neuropathies, neuroma, herpes zoster, and muscle spasm associated with musculoskeletal pathology, including sprains, strains, and contusions.[49]

Ultrasound decreases joint stiffness by changing the viscoelastic properties of joint fluids from a gel to a sol state. In addition, ultrasound increases the extensibility of tendon as a result of thermal depolymerization of protein.[17] These properties make ultrasound effective for treating conditions such as decreased range of motion accompanying adhesive capsulitis and joint stiffness and swelling found in arthritis.[47] (Refer to Chapter 8 of Gould: *Orthopaedic and Sports Physical Therapy*.)

The chemical effects of ultrasound are related, in part, to its thermal properties. Raising the tissue temperature accelerates the metabolic processes, including increasing enzyme activity, increasing the rate of ion exchange, increasing cell membrane permeability, and increasing the rate and volume of diffusion across cell membranes. Because of these properties ultrasound can be rendered even more effective as a pain reliever with the use of phonophoresis. During the process of phonophoresis the ultrasound wave front is used to drive molecules of a pain-relieving chemical into the tissues. Once subcutaneous, the molecules are broken down into ions and taken up into the cells, where they participate in intracellular chemical reactions (Fig. 27-3).

The following pain-relieving chemicals can be administered with phonophoresis:[24]

1. 5% Lidocaine ointment (Xylocaine) for acute conditions where immediate pain relief is the primary goal
2. 1% Hydrocortisone cream or ointment, where pain is the result of inflammation
3. 10% Salicylate cream or ointment, where a combined analgesic-antiinflammatory agent is needed
4. 1%/4% Iodine/salicylate ointment (Iodex with methyl salicylate), where a sclerolytic agent would enhance the analgesic and antiinflammatory effects of salicylate

Following phonophoresis, measurable quantities of these molecules have been found at tissue depths of up to 2 inches.[17]

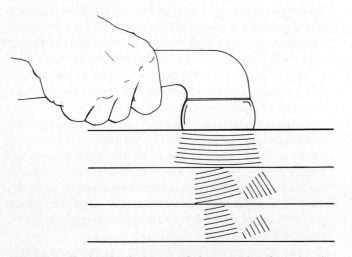

Fig. 27-2. The longitudinal wave of ultrasound is refracted at tissue interfaces where it encounters tissues of differing acoustical resistance. When the wave changes direction, energy is transferred to the tissues, resulting in the production of heat.

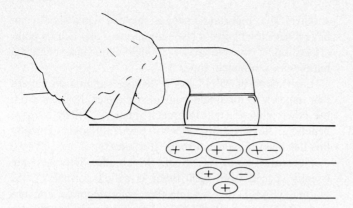

Fig 27-3 Phonophoresis. Molecules of a substance are driven into the tissues by the ultrasound wave front. They are not free for use by the body until they are broken down into chemical ions.

Phonophoresis cannot be performed subaqueously. The dissipation of the wave front by the intervening water reduces the driving forces, and the usual water-soluble ointments are diluted beyond functional levels. For the same reason phonophoresis cannot be administered with solutions. It is advised that a coupling agent be applied over the chemical before the application of ultrasound to prevent the loss of energy and because many of the ointments used in phonophoresis are too viscous for favorable transmission when used alone.[24]

Cryotherapy. The physiological effects of cold make it superior to heat for acute pain from inflammatory conditions, for the period immediately following tissue trauma, and for treating muscle spasm and abnormal tone. These physiological changes include the following:

1. Peripheral nerve conduction velocity in both large myelinated and small unmyelinated fibers decreases 2.4 m/second/° C of cooling; as a result, pain perception and muscle contractability diminish[55]
2. Peripheral receptors become less excitable[55]
3. Muscle spindle responsiveness to stretch decreases; as a result, muscle spasm diminishes[10]
4. Local blood flow first decreases; local edema is decreased, the inflammatory response is diminished, and hemorrhage is minimized; after prolonged cold application, local blood flow increases; known as the "hunting response," this protective mechanism brings core temperature blood to the surface and prevents tissue injury resulting from prolonged exposure[13]
5. Cellular metabolic activities slow; the oxygen requirements of the cell decrease[55]

As with heat, there are several precautions when using cold as a therapeutic modality. Cold application is contraindicated in individuals with Raynaud's phenomenon or cold allergy. It should not be used in individuals with rheumatic disease who, with the application of cold, have increased joint pain and stiffness. It should be used with caution in very young or elderly individuals and those with peripheral vascular disease or other circulatory pathologies.[52]

Cryotherapy is applied in three ways. Convective cooling involves movement of air over the skin (fanning) and is rarely used therapeutically. Evaporative cooling results when a substance applied to the skin uses thermal energy to evaporate, thereby lowering surface temperature. Most commonly, this substance is a vapocoolant spray. Conductive cooling employs local application of cold, either by ice packs, ice massage, or immersion. Cooling is accomplished as heat from the higher temperature object is transferred to the colder object down a temperature gradient. Conductive cooling is the most commonly used form of therapeutic cold application.

Because muscles, tendons, and joints respond differently, the best method of cold application depends on which tissues are causing the pain. Muscle spasm is decreased with cold packs and stretching. Trigger points, irritable foci within muscles, are best treated with vapocoolant spray, deep friction massage, and stretching. Tendonitis responds well to ice massage and exercise. Cold packs are many times the only source of pain relief in acute disk pathology. The inflamed joints of rheumatoid arthritis frequently respond to cold packs or ice massage with decreased inflammation, increased function, and long-lasting pain relief.[33,52]

Transcutaneous electrical nerve stimulation

After Melzack and Wall proposed the gate-control theory of pain modulation in 1965, a dorsal column stimulator (DCS) was developed for individuals with intractable pain. In 1970, while screening surgical candidates to determine their suitability for DCS placement, Shealy[49] discovered that, in many candidates, significant pain relief could be obtained with transcutaneous electrical nerve stimulation (TENS) alone, and Shealy and others began investigating TENS as a viable treatment alternative.

The exact mechanism by which TENS modulates pain still is not known. It appears that, at a high rate, TENS selectively stimulates the low-threshold, large-diameter A-delta fibers resulting in presynaptic inhibition within the dorsal horns[3] either directly via Melzak and Wall's gate, or indirectly through stimulation of the tonic descending pain inhibiting pathways originating in the periaqueductal gray matter and the brainstem.[58] Research has shown that the neurons in the brainstem fire in synchrony with the TENS stimulation frequency,[60] and although the significance of this is not known at this time, it does indicate that the action of high-rate TENS is not limited to the dorsal columns. TENS delivered at a low rate is thought to facilitate elevation of the level of endorphins in the cerebrospinal fluid. Naloxone, a morphine antagonist, reverses the analgesia obtained through low-rate TENS,[1] indicating that at a low rate the action of TENS includes stimulation of the release of endogenous opiates.[54]

Since their origin in 1970, TENS stimulators have undergone considerable evolution and are now miniaturized, portable, solid-state generators that produce a pulsed current. Depending on the sophistication of the stimulator, the parameters of pulse rate (frequency), pulse width, and amperage (intensity) may be adjustable. Although the wave form (shape) is predetermined and usually cannot be changed, the pattern in which the wave is delivered can be manipulated to change the mode of stimulation.

Stimulation at frequencies between one and 250 pulses per second (pps) works to decrease pain. Frequencies between 50 and 100 pps have proven most effective for the majority of individuals receiving high-rate TENS and frequencies between 2 and 3 pps most effective for the majority of individuals receiving low-rate TENS.[35] Stimulation at exactly 2 pps causes an actual increase in the pain threshold.[19] As the frequency is decreased a longer period of time is needed before the onset of relief, but the effects are more long-lasting.[46]

Pulse width duration needs to be appropriate to stimulate the target nerves. Low-threshold fibers are best stimulated at widths between 50 and 100 μ second and high-threshold fibers between 150 and 300 μ second.[35]

Although stimulus amplitude is set to tolerance, it should be sufficient to cause paresthesia throughout the painful area without stimulating muscle contraction during high-rate TENS and strong enough to result in strong, rhythmic muscle contractions during low-rate TENS. Ten to 30 mA is adequate for high-rate TENS while greater than 30 mA is usually necessary during low-rate TENS.[35]

The output from TENS stimulators can be front-end loaded, back-end loaded, or linear. Front-end loaded stimulators provide greater than 50% of their output in the first half of the dial range so that the greatest sensory changes will be perceived during early amplitude adjustments. Back-end loaded stimulators provide greater than 50% of their output in the second half of the dial range. Early dial movements may not produce subjective sensory changes, but small changes late in the dial range can result in a sudden (startling) surge of stimulation. Linear stimulators provide equal degrees of subjective sensory change throughout the entire excursion of the amplitude dial.

Some TENS stimulators maintain constant voltage by varying current intensity, while others maintain constant current intensity by varying voltage. Because they vary the voltage in response to chages in the stimulation area, constant current stimulators appear to deliver more electrical charge to the neurological structures[30] while avoiding focal areas of hyperstimulation (and potential burns) that can occur when electrodes loosen.

Research has shown that there is no ideal waveform, although some individuals respond better to one form than another. The important factor is that the wave should not have a net direct current (DC) component that causes polar effects under the electrodes, which can cause chemical burns with prolonged application.

Each mode of TENS has a distinct stimulation pattern that appears to modulate pain in a manner different from the other modes. Therefore each mode of TENS is more beneficial for a specific type of pain (although clinically this has been proven not to be absolute).[35]

Normal TENS. TENS in which the impulses are equally spaced from each other is called normal TENS. Normal TENS is divided into three subcategories: conventional TENS, low-rate TENS, and brief-intense TENS.

When the impulses are generated at a high rate and relatively narrow width, the stimulation is referred to as conventional TENS. Conventional TENS produces mild to moderate paresthesia without muscle contraction throughout the treatment area. There is a relatively fast onset of relief (seconds to 15 minutes), but the duration of relief after stimulation stops is short-lived (at best up to a few hours). Conventional TENS can be worn continuously, although it is recommended that the stimulator be turned off every hour to reassess if TENS is still needed.[35] Conventional TENS is beneficial for acute pain syndromes, including control of postsurgical incision pain and for anesthesia during childbirth. It is also useful for some deep, achy chronic pain syndromes. The main drawback to conventional TENS is neural accommodation, a decrease in perception of the stimulus that occurs as the nerve becomes less excitable with repeated stimulation. This accommodation can be managed either by frequently adjusting the amplitude or avoided by varying (modulating) the stimulus.

When the impulses are generated at a low rate and a relatively wide pulse width, the stimulation is referred to as low-rate TENS. Low-rate TENS produces strong muscle contractions in the treatment area without the perception of paresthesia. The onset of relief is delayed 20 to 30 minutes, presumably the time it takes to deploy the opiates; however, relief frequently lasts hours or days following treatment. Low-rate TENS is beneficial for chronic pain syndromes[35]; however, it is not always well accepted. To be effective, the intensity of the stimulus must cause strong, rhythmical muscle contractions, which are sometimes greater than what can be tolerated in an already painful area. Modulating the stimulus frequently increases comfort. Because stimulation for periods longer than 1 hour can result in depletion of the body's endorphins, treatment time should be limited to 30- to 45-minute sessions. Sessions can be repeated as pain returns.

Stimulation using high-rate, wide-width impulses is called brief-intense TENS. Brief-intense TENS decreases the conduction velocity of A-delta and C fibers, producing a peripheral blockade to transmission.[35] Brief-intense TENS is beneficial in the clinical setting for use during wound debridement, suture removal, friction massage, joint mobilization, or other painful procedures. Brief-intense TENS should not continue longer than 15 minutes, although sessions can be repeated after a few minutes' rest.

Burst TENS. Stimulation in which the impulses are generated in pulse trains is called burst TENS. The stimulator generates low-rate carrier impulses, each of which contains a series of high-rate pulses. Because burst TENS is a combination of high-rate and low-rate TENS, it provides the benefits of each. The low-rate carrier impulse stimulates endorphin release, and the high-rate pulse trains provide an overlay of paresthesia. The advantage to burst TENS is that muscle contractions occur at a lower, more comfortable amplitude, and accommodation does not occur. Burst TENS is beneficial whenever low-rate TENS cannot be tolerated and conventional TENS is ineffective because of neural accommodation. Treatment time should be limited to 30 to 45 minutes, as with low-rate TENS.[35]

Modulated TENS. Modulating TENS parameters is one way of avoiding the negative aspects of each of the treatment modes. Rate modulation is most beneficial with conventional TENS. By setting the initial pulse rate so that, even with the programed decrement, it will remain within the treatment range, there will be a continuous variation in the impulse rate, and neural accommodation will thereby be avoided.

Modulating the pulse width changes the amount of energy delivered in each impulse. Width modulation is most beneficial with low-rate TENS. By setting the initial pulse width so that, even with the programed decrement, the impulses are wide enough to recruit all motor units, there will be a continuous variation in strength of the muscle contractions with a lesser degree of C fiber recruitment making low-rate TENS more tolerable.

Combined modulation makes strong stimulation more tolerable by alternately recruiting high-threshold and low-threshold fibers while inhibiting accommodation. Because of this, combined modulation is effective with either high-rate or low-rate TENS.

Electrode placement sites have to be carefully selected to ensure that the appropriate nerves are being reached and that there is sufficient current to stimulate them. It must be determined whether the pain originates from the superficial or deep structures, whether it is local, whether it is referred or radiated, and whether it is transmitted by the central or autonomic nervous systems. Superficial pain is usually well localized and nonradiating and occurs almost immediately after the precipitating incident. Deep pain is usually diffuse, difficult to localize, and perceived at areas other than its point of origin (referred or radiated).[35] Pain of CNS vs. ANS origin has previously been discussed.

Electrodes should be the same size. Electrodes with equal surface area will have equal current density beneath them. When electrodes with unequal surface areas are used

in the same circuit, there will be greater density beneath the smaller, creating the potential for skin irritation or burns. Current density varies with the distance between electrodes: the closer the electrodes, the greater the density between them. The depth of current penetration varies with the distance between electrodes: the closer the electrodes, the more superficial the current. Current density decreases as it crosses the body.[35]

Various studies and clinical observations have provided a myriad of choices for electrode placement.[24,34,35,49] Site selection is dependent on the origin of the pain and the mode of stimulation. When using conventional TENS, the best results occur when the area of paresthesia encompasses the pain. The electrodes should be placed around the painful site, with at least one electrode parallel to the involved spinal segment(s). The result of low-rate TENS should be strong, rhythmic muscle contractions in segmentally related myotomes (within or outside of the painful area). Electrodes should be applied over the motor point of the related musculature or over the most superficial point of the mixed or motor nerve(s) serving the muscle(s). Electrode placement during burst TENS depends on which component of the stimulation is being emphasized. If paresthesia is desired the electrodes can be placed as they would be with conventional TENS. If muscle contraction is the goal, the electrode placements used during low-rate TENS can be employed.

Other successful stimulation sites include directly over sensory nerves, linear pathways, acupuncture points, related dermatomes, the nerve plexus, trigger points, the contralateral side of the body (when the client cannot tolerate stimulation to the painful side), the upper cervical spine, or a remote area of the body. Stimulation of the ulnar nerve, for example, has been found to give relief to all areas except the head.[35]

Statistics regarding the efficacy of TENS are impressive. The results of various studies[31,49] report that 80% of all clients with acute pain and 25% to 39% of clients with chronic pain no longer needed pain medication, while another 55% to 60% were able to significantly decrease their need for pain medication. Less than 5% found TENS too uncomfortable to wear,[49] and the single reported side effect was skin irritation at the electrode placement site in 1.6% of all individuals wearing TENS.[5] This is directly attributed to allergy to the adhesive used to attach the electrodes to the skin, to improper electrode attachment, or to infrequent electrode changes.

Although the placebo effect is felt to be of some minimal benefit initially, long-range follow-up over a year showed decrease of its influence. Placebo is of short duration, and the general tendency is a reduction in the amount of stimulation needed with longer periods of relief between stimulation sessions.[31]

The conditions in which TENS has been found to be of the greatest benefit are acute conditions with focal pain, chronic pain syndromes, postoperative incision pain, and during delivery. It has been shown to be least effective with psychogenic pain[32] and pain of central origin.[38]

Iontophoresis

Iontophoresis is a process in which chemical ions are driven through the skin by a small electric current. Ionizable compounds are placed on the skin under an electrode that, when polarized by a direct (galvanic) current, repels the ion of like charge into the tissues. Once subcutaneous, the ions are free to combine with the physiological ions or be transported by the superficial circulation into the systemic blood flow, which carries them to distant areas of the body. In either case, a physiological effect dependent on the characteristics of the ion is obtained (Fig. 27-4).

Ions that are known to be effective analgesics are:[24]

1. 5% Lidocaine ointment (Xylocaine) administered under the positive electrode for an immediate, although short-lived, decrease in pain. Iontophoresis with lidocaine is recommended before range of motion, stretching, and joint mobilization, and when immediate relief of acute pain (as in bursitis) is the object of treatment.
2. 1% to 10% Hydrocortisone administered under the positive electrode for relief of inflammatory pain in conditions such as arthritis, bursitis, or entrapment syndromes. Iontophoresis with hydrocortisone has a delayed onset but a prolonged effect, and it frequently eliminates the underlying cause of pain.
3. 2% Magnesium (from Epsom salts) administered under the positive electrode for relief of pain from muscle spasm or localized ischemia. High levels of extracellular magnesium inhibit muscle contraction, including the smooth muscle found in the walls of the vessels, resulting in localized vasodilation.
4. Iodine (from Iodex ointment) administered under the negative pole for relief of pain caused by adhesions or scar tissue. Iodine "softens" fibrotic, sclerotic tissue, thereby increasing tissue pliability.
5. Salicylate (from Iodex with methyl salicylate) administered under the negative pole for relief of pain from inflammation or tissue congestion. Salicylate is effective for arthritic joint inflammation, myalgia, and entrapment syndromes.
6. 2% Acetic acid administered under the negative pole to dissolve calcium deposits.
7. 2% Lithium chloride or lithium carbonate administered under the positive pole to dissolve gouty tophi. In both acetic acid and lithium iontophoresis, the insoluble radicals in the deposits are replaced by soluble chemical radicals so the deposits can be broken down through natural processes.

The contraindication to the use of any ion is an allergy to that ion. Because most clients will not have had iontophoresis previously, it is important to enquire about experiences that might indicate an allergy. For example, an intolerance for shellfish may be the result of an allergy to iodine, and a poor reaction to dental local anesthesia may indicate a problem with lidocaine.

In addition to the potential for allergic reaction to the ions, skin irritation may occur under the electrodes for several reasons. Because the polarity of the electrodes remains constant throughout the treatment, chemical reactions occur directly below each electrode. The tissue under the positive pole (anode) becomes acidic with the formation of hydrochloric acid, while that under the negative pole (cathode) becomes alkaline with the formation of sodium hydroxide. Either chemical in sufficient quantity can injure the tissues, but irritation and burns most commonly occur under the negative electrode.[24]

Electrical burns can occur when the current density or amplitude exceed safe limits. Iontophoresis is administered using a 5-mA current applied for about 15 minutes with the selected ion source under the like pole electrode. When the procedure is too uncomfortable or when marked skin irritation occurs under the electrodes, the current can be decreased and the treatment time increased. To avoid high current densities between the electrodes (the "edge effect"), the indifferent and active electrodes should be separated by at least the width of one electrode.[24]

The negative electrode should always be the larger of the two, regardless of which is the treating electrode, to decrease current density and a high concentration of polarity-induced chemicals under this more irritating pole. The electrodes, the skin below, and the current setting should be checked every 3 to 5 minutes to prevent skin irritation and chemical burns. Proper aftercare of the skin below the electrodes can further decrease skin irritation. The skin should be massaged with an astringent, a witch hazel solution, or carbolated vasoline, then dusted with cornstarch.[24]

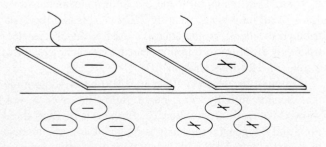

Fig. 27-4. Iontophoresis. Chemical ions are driven into the tissues by a small electrical current. Once subcutaneous they are immediately free to take part in chemical reactions within the body.

Massage

Massage has been recognized as a remedy for pain for at least 3000 years. Evidence of its beneficial effects are first found in ancient Chinese literature, and then in the writings of the Hindus, Persians, Egyptians, and Greeks. Hippocrates advocated massage for sprains and dislocations as well as for constipation.[28]

Massage has both reflex and mechanical effects. Reflex relaxation occurs through changes in muscle tension and circulation brought about by stimulation of the peripheral nerves. Fluid mobilization and intramuscular motion are the result of mechanically compressing and moving the tissues. Massage movements are classified by pressure and the part of the hand that is used.[61]

Stroking involves running the entire hand over large portions of the body. Light stroking involves a very light touch and causes the reflex effects of muscular relaxation and elimination of muscle spasm. Deep stroking, on the other hand, is applied with sufficient pressure to assist in circulation. Both forms of stroking are applied with constant pressure at a constant rate of speed in an even rhythm.

Compression massage, in contrast, is applied with intermittent pressure using lifting, rolling, or pressing movements meant to stretch shortened tissues, loosen adhesions, and assist with circulation. Compression massage is divided into kneading and friction movements. Kneading involves intermittently lifting or compressing a muscle or muscle group so that there is movement within it. Friction massage is performed by using the finger tips to perform circulatory movements that move the superficial tissues over the underlying structures.

Percussion, as it applies to pain management, is performed to stimulate circulation. Hacking involves using the ulnar border of the hand or the fingers to perform a series of brisk, rapid, alternating contacts with the skin. Clapping is done with the palms flat, while cupping is done with the palm formed into a concave surface.

Massage is useful in any condition where pain relief will follow the reduction of swelling or the mobilization of the tissues. These include arthritis, bursitis, neuritis, fibrositis, low-back pain, hemiplegia, paraplegia, quadriplegia, and joint sprains, strains, and contusions. Massage is contraindicated over infected areas, diseased skin, and thrombophlebitic regions.

Myofascial release

Fascia is connective tissue that plays a supportive role within the body. It forms a framework around the viscera, stabilizes articulations, provides a constantly fluctuating biochemical equilibrium to assist in the maintenance of homeostasis in the surrounding tissues, and, in conjunction with muscular activity, assists in the movement of blood and lymph. Fascia contains sensory nerves and tension bands of varying thicknesses.[20]

Ideally, the fascial system is in constant three-dimensional motion: right to left, side to side, and front to back.[20] Under abnormal physical and chemical conditions,

such as faulty muscle activity, alteration in the position or relationship of the bones, altered vertebral mechanics, or unnatural postures, the fascial connective tissue can thicken and shorten, creating hypomobile areas with increased tension[58] that can, because the fascia represents one continuous system, affect movement in remote areas of the body by restricting motion of that fascia. Because the fascia contains sensory nerves, areas of increased tension, sudden tension, or traction are painful.[20]

The goal of myofascial release techniques is to release the built-in imbalances and restrictions within the fascia and to reintegrate the fascial mechanism. The therapist palpates the various tissue layers, beginning with the most superficial and working systematically inward to the deepest, looking for movement restrictions and asymmetry. Areas of altered structure and function are then "normalized" through the systematic application of pressure and stretching applied in specific directions to bring about decreased myofascial tension, myofascial lengthening, and myofascial softening,[58] thereby restoring pain-free motion in normal patterns of movement.

Joint mobilization

There are two forms of movement available to each joint: physiological and accessory. Physiological movement is the gross range of motion (ROM) (defined as flexion, extension, and rotation). Accessory movement is the fine motion that occurs between the surfaces of the opposing bones (defined as distraction, slide, glide, and tilt). Physiological movement can be performed by the individual; accessory movement cannot and requires the application of external force.

Normal accessory movement is necessary for normal physiological movement. When the collagen fibers of the joint capsule become thickened or bound down, accessory movements become restricted, preventing full range of motion. Because the joint capsule is richly innervated, pain is produced when the soft tissue structures are stretched in an attempt to produce full gross movement.[48]

Joint mobilization consists of passive oscillations that allow the collagen fibers to rearrange and loosen, thereby restoring normal accessory movements.[48] In addition, the rhythmic repetition of the motions provides pain relief via the mechanisms specified in the gate-control theory.[40]

The oscillations involved in joint mobilization are graded as follows[34]:

Grade I: small amplitude movements performed at the beginning of the available ROM
Grade II: larger amplitude movements performed further into the available ROM
Grade III: large amplitude movements performed at the end of the available ROM
Grade IV: small amplitude movements performed at the end of the available ROM

Grade V: high-velocity thrust (manipulation) performed at the end of the available ROM

Grades I and II are performed to maintain joint mobility and for pain relief, making them the choice for subacute conditions where pain and potential loss of motion are the primary considerations. Grades III and IV are performed to increase joint mobility and are indicated for chronic conditions where regaining lost motion is the goal. Grade V thrusts are performed to regain full joint mobility.[48]

Joint mobilization is contraindicated with rheumatoid arthritis, bone disease, advanced osteoporosis, pregnancy (pelvic mobilization), as well as in the presence of malignancy, vascular disease, or infection in the area to be mobilized.[34]

Joint mobilization is covered in Chapter 11 of Gould: *Orthopaedic and Sports Physical Therapy* as well as in several excellent texts addressing musculoskeletal disorders.

Point stimulation

The ancient Chinese were the first to become aware of acupuncture points, areas of the skin that become sensitive with internal disease states. Over time they mapped out imaginery lines connecting the points with each other. They believed that energy and nutrients flowed to all parts of the body along these "meridians" and that, when there is disease, the energy flow is interrupted. The most effective sites for treatment, they reasoned, are the acupuncture points.[57]

It is interesting to note that acupuncture points frequently correspond in location to trigger points, tight, elevated bands of tissue that are extremely sensitive when palpated and have a characteristic pattern of radiation to remote regions of the body. Trigger points appear to be areas of "focal irritability" that are myofascial in origin and are usually the site of small aggregations of nerve fibers that produce continuous afferent input when stimulated.

Needling of acupuncture points stimulates the release of endorphins,[57] most probably through the central modulating pathway that originates in the periaqueductal gray matter.[56] Acupressure, finger pressure applied to acupuncture or trigger points, is thought to decrease their sensitivity through the same mechanism. The therapist applies deep pressure in a circular motion to each point for 1 to 5 minutes, until the sensitivity subsides. Pressure must be applied directly to each point for the treatment to be effective. Acupressure can be accompanied by the use of a vapocoolant spray to provide additional sensory stimulation. Acupressure should be followed by full active and passive stretch and rewarming of the muscle in which the trigger point is located.[56]

Sensitive points can also be stimulated using electricity. A point locator is used to identify points along the appropriate meredians that are sensitive to stimulation or more conductive to electricity. Each is then stimulated at the client's level of pain tolerance for 30 to 45 seconds. The points farthest from the site of pain are treated first.

Points that are most sensitive to stimulation are beneficial sites for TENS electrode placement. When point stimulation alone does not provide sufficient pain relief, TENS can be used between sessions for continuous stimulation for more prolonged relief.

Laser

Laser application to painful tissue has been known to bring about an almost immediate relief of spasm. This is thought to be the result of the physiological properties of the laser that allow it to penetrate and be absorbed by human tissue. These properties are as follows:[25]

1. Monochromatism: Light emitted from the laser has a single wavelength.
2. Coherence: Light emitted from the laser has a high degree of order and a fixed phase relationship.
3. Divergence: Light emitted from the laser has a narrow focus and very little divergence.

Once absorbed, laser energy brings about depolarization and repolarization of abnormally contracted tissues, causes reactive vasodilation in arteriolar spasms, and modifies electron excitability in mitochondria leading to changes in metabolic processes.

Kleinkort[25] found the use of lasers on specific acupuncture points effective where there is not anatomical dysfunction at the base of the pain stimuli. He has used it for myofacial syndromes, inflammatory tendonitis, bursitis, localized arthritis, and painful keloids.

Cognitive-behavior methods

Pain perception encompasses not only the sensation of pain but also the emotional state, expectations, personality, and cognitive view of the person experiencing it. Melzak and Wall[40] proposed that pain has three nonphysical components that can be dealt with through cognitive-behavioral means: sensory/discriminative, motivation/affective, and cognitive/evaluative.

Interpretation of sensory input can be modified through hypnosis, biofeedback, and relaxation exercises. Increasing the client's control over the pain addresses the motivational aspect, and changing the client's "self-statements" deals with the cognitive component.[18]

It has been noted that pain is frequently accompanied by stress and tension. The rationale for the techniques that follow is that by decreasing the levels of stress, a decrease in the level of pain can also be expected.[18] The reader is advised to refer to Chapter 4.

Hypnosis

Conscious perception of pain can be altered significantly through the use of hypnosis. After teaching the client to achieve deep relaxation, the hypnotherapist attempts to direct attention away from the pain to something that is imagined or intensified by concentrating on it, for example, a pain-free state. Intense concentration causes the pain to cease to exist in the conscious mind by directing attention away from the sensory input related to it. This has two important consequences. First, hypnosis can be used to ascertain the subconscious reasons for psychosomatic pain and can thereby be significant in its treatment; second, because time is without structure, when hypnotized the client can experience a lengthy reprieve from pain, during which purposeful activity can be carried out.[16]

Neurophysiological data are accumulating that suggest that the hypnotic state enhances the descending reticular central modulating system by facilitating the release of opioids. If this is true, the client can be taught to perform daily self-hypnosis as a means of maintaining increasing levels of the chemicals and thereby obtain continuous pain relief.

Biofeedback. Biofeedback is a training process in which the client becomes aware of and learns to selectively change physiological processes with the aid of an external monitor. It has the following three characteristics[22]:

1. Continuous monitoring of the physiological response
2. Continuous feedback of changes in the response either by a light, sound, or gauge
3. Motivation on the part of the client to change the response

During biofeedback, an instrument that measures a body function such as pulse rate, skin temperature, or muscle tension is placed on the body of the person being treated. The machine provides an initial readout. The client is instructed on how to change the monitored process, and as change occurs, the machine "feeds back" information. With practice, the client learns to control the process without needing an assist from the biofeedback instrument.

Biofeedback is proving to be an effective pain management tool with tension headaches, muscle spasms, and other dysfunctions that lead to chronic pain. The client is taught to recognize and modify increased tension as well as changes in pulse rate, blood pressure, skin temperature, and electromyography (EMG) and electroencephalography (EEG) readings.[22]

Relaxation exercises. Relaxation exercises, which involve volitionally tensing then relaxing muscles, help the individual become aware of what tension feels like so that it can be recognized and eliminated. With proper technique muscles relax, heart rate decreases, respiratory rate slows, skin temperature increases (evidence of parasympathetic dominance), stomach acid production decreases, deep tendon reflexes slow, and the individual experiences a sense of well-being.[8]

Pain relief through relaxation is thought to occur in several ways. First, normal blood flow to the muscles is reestablished and there is a rise in oxygen delivery to the tissues. Second, the individual is able to return to a normal or as close to normal as possible pattern of activity. Self-control of tension and anxiety appear to give the individual a feeling of control over the pain, thus alleviating depression, which can, itself, contribute to the perception of pain.[8]

Operant conditioning. The client with chronic pain frequently develops a pain-supporting behavior because it brings increased attention, because it allows avoidance of distasteful activities, and because well behaviors are frequently regarded negatively. In many instances nonspecific feelings are labeled as pain for this reason. Thus many clients have learned the reward of pain expression and continue to experience pain only because there are more positive than negative reinforcing factors.[18]

The aim of operant conditioning is to change what the client sees as a positive reward. The client is taught to visualize, for example, a painfree state, one in which there is control over pain. The client is taught that this is the desired, achievable state. By learning to challenge what they say to themselves, clients can be taught to revise their "self-statements" and their goals and to gain control over stress, tension, and pain.[18]

Cognitive-behavioral approaches to pain management have two main goals. The first goal is to teach the client to control and not be controlled by pain. The second goal is to reinforce well behavior while not rewarding pain behavior.[18] Used in conjunction with other modalities necessary for immediate relief, these approaches can play a significant role in long-term management and should not be overlooked when seeking a viable pain management alternative.

CLINICAL EXAMPLES

The following clinical examples demonstrate a problem-solving approach to the treatment of pain.

CASE STUDY: MRS. R.

A 68-year-old female inpatient with a stable compression fracture of the body of T7 is referred to physical therapy for "evaluation and pain control." She reports that the fracture occurred when she fell in the bathtub 3 weeks previously and that her physician had been treating her at home with heat, analgesics, and bedrest; there was no significant decrease in pain. She was admitted to the hospital for more aggressive treatment.

The client describes her pain as a constant dull ache and rates the intensity as "75" on a scale of 1 to 100. The pain is localized to the middorsal spine. It is more intense when the client is upright and relieved slightly when she is supine.

On evaluation, the client is found to have a moderate dorsal kyphosis that is the result of an earlier compression fractures resulting from osteoporosis. There is spasm in the paravertebral dorsal musculature bilaterally, and several trigger points can be located within the back extensors. Palpation of the spine of T7 is exquisitely painful and causes increased spasm in the surrounding musculature. There are no neurological deficits in the trunk or extremities.

The client has previously been fitted with and wears a custom orthosis to stabilize her spine and minimize progression of the kyphosis.

The initial focus of physical therapy for this client is to alleviate her acute pain. Moist heat and phonophoresis with salicylate used in combination twice a day will yield both pain relief and decreased spasm. This can be followed by gentle massage to further induce muscular relaxation. The client should be instructed in proper bed posture that is comfortable and that will maintain the spine as straight as possible.

As the pain and spasm subside and as the client becomes more mobile, she should be evaluated for and receive instruction in proper body mechanics during bed mobility, sitting, transfers, and ambulation. Acupressure can be introduced to treat sensitive trigger points. Strengthening exercises for the back extensors can be initiated with the physician's approval.

As the date of discharge approaches, a home program for pain management needs to be established. If there is still significant pain, the client could be fitted with a TENS unit. Arrangements could be made for her to obtain a moist heating pad for home use. She should be instructed in both a home exercise program to increase strength in her back musculature and in joint preservation measures to minimize further stresses on her spine. The client should return home with an understanding of her injury, with a comprehensive plan for pain management, and with a knowledge of how to lessen the chances of further injury.

CASE STUDY: MRS. L.

A 25-year-old female outpatient with a 5-year history of rheumatoid arthritis is referred to physical therapy for "evaluation and treatment of painful, swollen wrists." The arthritis has been maintained in a chronic state for 2 years with medication and it is felt that this inflammation most probably is the result of isolated trauma rather than a generalized flareup.

Examination of the wrists reveals them to be red, warm, and swollen. Range of motion is limited by about 50% in both flexion and extension. The client reports that movement of the wrists and palation of the soft tissue structures is extremely painful. She rates the pain at "90" on a scale of 1 to 100.

The pain this client is experiencing is the result of inflammation. Therefore treatment should be directed at alleviating the inflammation, which will, in turn, bring about pain relief. Double iontophoresis with one electrode on each wrist can be used to introduce antiinflammatory agents locally into the wrists. Hydrocortisone can be introduced through the positive electrode and salicylate can be introduced through the negative electrode. Since salicylate is also an analgesic, the electrodes can be reversed in each treatment session to provide both wrists with antiinflammatory and analgesic medication.

Following each treatment, the joints should be taken through one full range of motion. Between treatments, the acutely inflamed joints should be immobilized in resting splints. As the inflammation subsides, less time can be spent in the splints and first active, then gentle, resisted exercises can be added to the program. The client should be instructed in joint preservation methods to minimize stress and prolong functional use of her wrists.

CASE STUDY: MR. W.

A 36-year-old paramedic is referred to physical therapy for "evaluation and treatment of left shoulder and arm pain" that developed 3 weeks after he completed therapy for a traction injury to the long head of the biceps tendon in the same shoulder. The original injury occurred while he was lifting an injured person from a wrecked car.

He reports persistent burning pain that developed gradually in the shoulder and is now beginning to affect his hand as well. He states the pain can become so severe that he is reluctant to move the arm for fear of provoking "an episode." He grades the pain as 75 at best and 110 (on a scale of 1 to 100) at worst. He cannot work because of the pain, and he is becoming increasingly anxious about his finances.

While this client waited for therapy, he was observed to cradle his left arm against his body. He used his right arm to open the door, hold a magazine, and assist in standing up from a deep chair.

Evaluation of the left shoulder reveals restricted ROM and diffuse tenderness to palpation that he cannot localize to any individual structure. Examination of the hand reveals mild swelling in the fingers, erythema, and glossy skin. With finger extension he reports that there is a tightness in his palm that is "drawing the fingers into the middle."

This client is developing reflex sympathetic dystrophy (RSD) in the left upper extremity, and treatment must be directed at providing pain relief and preventing further loss of ROM. Prolonged immobilization with this condition leads to fibrosis, articular changes, loss of subcutaneous tissue, and osteoporosis.

This client may benefit from TENS in the conventional mode to provide paresthesia through the painful area. As his pain becomes less severe, low-rate TENS can be instituted to decrease wearing time and to facilitate circulation via the pumping action of the associated muscle contractions.

ROM exercises should be instituted immediately. However, because this client is reluctant to move his arm, movement can be performed using joint mobilization to stretch the capsular structures that are becoming restricted and myofascial release techniques to regain fascial balance in the shoulder complex as well as the entire left upper extremity. Mr. W. may find these procedures more comfortable if they are preceded by the application of cool (not cold) packs. As quickly as possible, an active exercise program emphasizing ROM and stretching should be instituted.

Mr. W.'s anxiety is typical in individuals with RSD, and it is thought to contribute to his physical symptoms. It is important, in treating this condition, to be sympathetic and supportive, but also to reinforce the need for early movement of the extremity to avoid permanent disability. He may also benefit from instruction in several relaxation techniques that he can use to counter the effects of his anxiety concerning his job.

REFERENCES

1. Abram S and others: Failure of naloxone to reverse analgesia from transcutaneous electrical nerve stimulation in patients with chronic pain, Anesth Analg 60:81, Feb 1981.
2. Adler M: Endorphins, enkephalins, and neurotransmitters, Med Times 110:32, June 1982.
3. Bromage RR: Nerve physiology and control of pain, Orthop Clin North Am 4:897, 1976.
4. Burton C: Transcutaneous electrical nerve stimulation to relieve pain, Postgrad Med 59:105, 1976.
5. Byrne M and others: Cross-validation of the factor structure of the McGill pain questionnaire, Pain 13:193, 1982.
6. Cash J: Neurology for physiotherapists, London, 1977, Faber & Faber.
7. Cassini V and Pagne CA: Central pain: a neurosurgical survey, Cambridge, Mass, 1969, Harvard University Press.
8. Chapman SL and Shealy CN: Relaxation techniques to control pain. In Brena SF, editor: Chronic pain: America's hidden epidemic, New York, 1978, Atheneum Publishers.
9. Cyriax J: Textbook of orthopaedic medicine, ed 7, London, 1978, Bailliere Tindall.

10. Eldred E and others: The effect of cooling on mammalian muscle spindles, Exp Neurol 2:144, 1960.

11. Evans JH: Neurology and neurological aspects of pain. In Swerdlow M, editor: Relief of intractable pain: monographs in anesthesiology, vol 1, New York, 1974, Excerpta Medica.

12. Felton DL and Felton SY: A regional and systemic overview of functional neuroanatomy. In Farber SD, editor: Neurorehabilitation: a multisensory approach, Philadelphia, 1982, WB Saunders Co.

13. Fischer E and Solomon S: Physiological responses to heat and cold. In Licht S, editor: Therapeutic heat and cold, Baltimore, Md, 1972, Waverly Press Inc.

14. Gandhavadi B and others: Autonomic pain: features and methods of assessment, Postgrad Med 71;85, Jan 1982.

15. Gelhard FA: The human senses, New York, 1953, John S Wiley & Sons.

16. Gorsky BH: Pain origin and treatment: discussions in patient management, New Hyde Park, NY, 1982, Medical Examination Publishing Co Inc.

17. Griffin JE: Physiological effects of ultrasonic energy as it is used clinically, Phys Ther 46:18, Jan 1966.

18. Grzesiak RC: Cognitive and behavioral approaches to management of chronic pain, NY State J Med 82:30, 1982.

19. Holmgren E: Increase in pain threshold as a function of conditioning electrical stimulation, Am J Clin Med 3:133, 1975.

20. Hubbard RP: Mechanical behavior of connective tissue, handout material from seminar entitled Myofascial Release Concepts, Palpatory and Treatment Skills, September, 1986, East Lansing, Mich.

21. Hughes J and others: Identification of two related pentapeptides from the brain with potent opiate agonist activity, Nature 258:577, 1975.

22. Isele FW, Biofeedback and hypnosis in the management of pain, NY State J Med 82:38, 1982.

23. Jacob J: Inflammation revisited: inflammatory pain and mode of action of analgesics, Agents and Actions, vol II;634, 1981.

24. Kahn J: Principles and practice of electrotherapy, New York, 1987, Churchill Livingstone.

25. Kleinkort JA: The cold laser, Clin Man 2(4):30, 1982.

26. Kremer E and others: Measurement of pain: patient preference does not confound pain measurement, Pain 10:241, 1981.

27. Kremer E and others: Pain measurement: the affective dimensional measure of the McGill pain questionnaire with a cancer pain population, Pain 12:153, 1982.

28. Krusen F and others: Handbook of physical medicine and rehabilitation, Philadelphia, 1971, WB Saunders Co.

29. Linton SJ and Melin L: The accuracy of remembering chronic pain, Pain 13:281, 1982.

30. Linzen M and Long D: Transcutaneous neural stimulation for relief of pain, IEEE Trans Biomed Eng 23:341, July 1976.

31. Long D: Cutaneous afferent stimulation for relief of chronic pain, Clin Neurosurg 21:257, 1974.

32. Long D: The comparative efficacy of drugs vs. electrical modulation in the management of chronic pain, current concepts in the management of chronic pain, Miami, 1977, Symposia Specialists.

33. Madsen PW and Gersten JW: The effect of ultrasound on conduction velocity of peripheral nerve, Arch Phys Med Rehabil 42:645, 1961.

34. Maitland G: Peripheral manipulation, Ontario, 1976, Butterworth & Scarborough.

35. Mannheimer JS and Lampe GN: Clinical transcutaneous electrical nerve stimulation, Philadelphia, 1984, FA Davis Co.

36. McKenzie RA: The lumbar spine, Waikanae, New Zealand, 1983, Spinal Publications.

37. Melzak R: The McGill pain questionnaire: major properties and scoring methods, Pain 1:277, 1975.

38. Melzak R: Prolonged relief of pain by brief, intense transcutaneous somatic stimulation, Pain 1:357, 1975.

39. Melzak R: The gate control theory revisited: current concepts in the management of chronic pain, Miami, 1977, Symposia Specialties.

40. Melzak R and Wall P: Pain mechanisms: a new theory, Science 150:971, Nov 1969.

41. Nathan PW: The gate control theory of pain: a critical review, Brain 99:123, 1976.

42. O'Driscoll SL and Jayson MIV: The clinical significance of pain threshold measurements, Rheumatol Rehabil 21:31, 1982.

43. Piercey MF and Folkers K: Sensory and motor functions of spinal cord substance P, Science 214:1361, Dec 1981.

44. Reading A: A comparison of the McGill pain questionnaire in chronic and acute pain, Pain 13:185, 1982.

45. Reid DS and Cummings GE: Factors in selecting the dosage of ultrasound with particular reference to the use of various coupling agents, Physiotherapy 25:5, March 1973.

46. Richard RL: Causalgia: a centennial review, Arch Neurol 16:339, 1967.

47. Roubal PJ: Ultrasound: clinical observations, Technic Journal, Oct 1977.

48. Saunders H: Evaluation, treatment, and prevention of musculoskeletal disorders, Eden Prairie, Minn, 1985, self-published.

49. Shealy C: Transcutaneous electroanalgesia, Surg Forum 23:419, 1973.

50. Shealy C and Mauer D: Transcutaneous nerve stimulation for control of pain, Surg Neurol 2:45, 1974.

51. Shealy C and others: Effects of transcranial neurostimulation upon mood and serotonin production: a preliminary report, Pain 1:13, 1979.

52. Sherman M: Which treatment to recommend? hot or cold, Am Pharm 20:46, Aug 1980.

53. Sinclair D: Cutaneous sensation, New York, 1967, Oxford University Press.

54. Sjolund B and Eriksson M: Electro-acupuncture and endogenous morphines, Lancet 2:1085, 1976.

55. Stillwell GK: Therapeutic heat and cold. In Krusen FH and others, editors: Handbook of physical medicine and rehabilitation, Philadelphia, 1971, WB Saunders Co.

56. Swerdlow M: The therapy of pain, Philadelphia, 1981, JB Lippincott Co.

57. Tappan FM: Healing massage techniques: a study of eastern and western methods, Reston, Va, 1978, Reston Publishing Co, Inc.

58. Ward C: The myofascial release concept, handout material from course entitled Myofascial Release Concepts, Palpatory and Treatment Skills, September, 1986, East Lansing, Mich.

59. Weddel G: Somesthesis and the chemical senses, Ann Rev Psychol 6:119, 1955.

60. Wolf S: Perspectives on central nervous system responsiveness to transcutaneous electrical nerve stimulation, Phys Ther 58:1443, Dec 1978.

61. Wood E: Beard's Massage, Philadelphia, 1974, WB Saunders Co.

ADDITIONAL READINGS

Barron DH and Matthews BHC: Intermittent conduction in the spinal cord, J Physiol 85:73, 1935.

Bowsher D: Pain pathways and mechanisms, Anaesthesia 33:935, 1978.

Head H: Studies in neurology, London, 1920, Oxford University Press, Inc.

Noordenboos W: Pain, Amsterdam, 1959, Elsevier Science Publishers.

Weddell G and others: Nerve endings in mammalian skin, Biol Review 30:159, 1955.

Chapter 28

THERAPEUTIC APPLICATION OF ORTHOTICS

Steven R. Huber

OVERVIEW

This chapter attempts to eliminate the "either or" philosophy of therapeutic exercise and orthotic treatment, and introduces the reader to concepts that demonstrate the mutually beneficial relationship between therapeutic exercise and orthotic intervention when treating the neurologically impaired client.

Orthotic treatment can be defined as the application of an external force(s) generated by an appliance worn by a client. These forces, although biomechanically designed, have significant neurological implications related to the input that they provide to the CNS. A well thought out, carefully designed, and properly fitting orthosis often enhances therapeutic treatment. It is the author's philosophy that an orthosis can be used as an adjunct to a sound therapeutic exercise program to hasten the desired result of the client's treatment program, but orthotic intervention should never be viewed as a replacement for a sound therapeutic exercise program. To presume that an orthosis can replace the techniques used by a highly skilled therapist is naive at best.

Therapists spend relatively short periods of time with each client; if the client wears an orthosis that successfully duplicates (in part) the support, assist, or CNS input given during a therapeutic exercise session, the client's treatment time is increased by the number of hours he or she uses the orthosis. Realistically, the CNS input offered by an orthosis may be inferior to that offered by the therapist, yet for some CNS inputs, for example, prolonged stretch, an orthosis can be more effective than a therapist.

Viewing orthotic intervention as a CNS input requires that it also be viewed as a positive dynamic process when it is applied in a logical manner to obtain a desired result. However, orthotic intervention applied in a careless manner, applied after a less than thorough evaluation, or applied without a specific result in mind can harm the client. It can also negate the effects of a sound therapeutic exercise program. The orthotic treatment and the therapeutic exercise program must address the same or related problems and be directed at the same result, both biomechani-

773

cally and neurologically. As with any treatment designed to have impact on the CNS, orthotic treatment should be closely monitored to ensure the desirability of the input being provided.

To integrate orthotic management with therapeutic exercise, one can use the following sequential thought process. During any therapeutic evaluation, specific clinical findings are discovered indicating a functional result that is other than normal. The therapist evaluates this result and establishes a functional goal that relates specifically to some activity of daily living. To obtain the functional goal, there are biomechanical options (applications of an external force), and each has a neurological consequence; some consequences are desirable, others are not. In planning the therapeutic integration of orthotics, the therapist must clearly understand the neurological consequence of each biomechanical application. The following example may clarify this further:

> A patient in your facility has a simple clinical finding of weak dorsiflexors. The functional result is the inability to clear the foot during the swing phase of gait. The functional goal is to provide the patient with the ability to clear the foot during the swing phase. The biomechanical options include increasing hip flexion, increasing knee flexion, stopping plantar flexion, increasing dorsiflexion, shortening the relative length of the extremity, positioning the foot in maximum equinus during stance phase to avoid toe stubbing during swing phase, and a number of others. Each option can be accomplished biomechanically; however, each has a significant neurological consequence that should be investigated.

When considering the time constraints placed on a therapist in a clinic or private practice setting or the financial restraints placed on most clients, it seems reasonable to seek out systems that can enhance the effects of individual treatment sessions. Realistically, changing reimbursement guidelines for health care institutions and use of review guidelines necessitate that the practicing therapist evaluate and treat clients in a compressed time frame. The client with a cerebrovascular accident (CVA), who will be discharged from a hospital in 10 days, and who does not have available a rehabilitation setting is a poor candidate for 10 days of mat work in preparation for standing and transfers. Selecting an orthosis that enhances the client's mat and exercise program while encouraging function seems a satisfactory alternative to discharging a person unprepared to perform minimal motoric skills. The client who is unprepared for function and who is not protected orthotically may have an increased tendency to develop poor motor skill habits based on inaccurate sensorimotor input.

The use of a carefully selected and properly fitting orthosis allows the physical or occupational therapist increased flexibility when treating the client, and can, in fact, act as an additional pair of hands. Imagine a therapist working with a client on pelvic and trunk stability in the standing position while trying to control calcaneal valgus and plantar flexion of the foot, which is creating genu valgus and genu recurvatum at the knee. An ankle foot ortho-

sis (AFO) that is properly aligned will free the therapist's hands to introduce approximation and/or flexion into the client's system as needed.

There are specific considerations that the therapist must be aware of when orthotically treating a client whose primary disorder is of a neurological nature. These differ significantly from the considerations on which the therapist bases orthotic treatment for the orthopaedically impaired client. A partial listing of considerations includes exteroceptive and proprioceptive input. These are discussed in detail later in the chapter.

BASIC CONCEPTS INVOLVED IN ORTHOTICS
Interim care versus definitive care

Orthotic treatment can be categorized in many ways; two major categories are interim care or definitive care. Interim orthotic care is accomplished by using an orthosis that allows variability without major reconstruction of the orthosis. Interim care is seldom maximally cosmetic or the lightest weight option available. Interim orthotics may require more maintenance than definitive orthotics, but they are more valuable to the therapist working with a client with a dynamic, changing neuromuscular system. An example of interim orthotics would be the use of a metal AFO with a solid stirrup and a double-action ankle joint. This device allows the treating therapist a large variation of ankle joint options, ranging from a locked ankle to a plantar flexion assist to a dorsiflexion assist. As long as a client demonstrates neuromuscular changes, such as gains or losses in strength, gains or losses in range of motion, or sensory or tonal changes, the orthotic treatment of choice should allow the treating therapist, after recognizing these changes, to accommodate them easily.

Definitive orthotic care, in contrast, should be considered when the client no longer demonstrates neuromuscular change and when the client requires an assistive device for safe, maximally independent functioning. The definitive orthosis should be designed and fabricated to be maximally cosmetic for the client. It should be constructed of the lightest weight yet most durable materials to make it energy efficient while requiring little if any maintenance. For example, a definitive orthosis for a client with extension dominance in the right lower extremity that has responded only partially to therapeutic exercise could be a 4 mm thickness, flesh-colored, polypropylene AFO casted with a solid ankle set in a few degrees of dorsiflexion. The most definitive treatment for this client may be a well-placed, purposely induced contracture—this is definitive but difficult to control.

Dynamic treatment versus static treatment

Along with interim or definitive care, the treating therapist must also choose dynamic or static orthotic treatment. Analysis of a client's gait may reveal talipes equino valgus during swing phase, the inability to clear the toe during the non–weight-bearing phase of gait. This clinical situation can be treated in a number of ways: (1) a metal spring-loaded dorsiflexion assist, (2) a plastic AFO casted into dorsiflexion, (3) a plastic or metal orthosis designed to stop plantar flexion from occurring, or (4) a metal orthosis stopping plantar flexion at 5 degrees to allow foot flat and providing the option for 15 degrees of dorsiflexion to encourage smooth roll over. Any of the alternatives may be quite appropriate when used under the correct neurological/musculoskeletal circumstances. Options one and four above are clearly dynamic, and option three is static. Option two may be dynamic or static, depending on the configuration of the trim lines about the medial and lateral malleoli.

Protection

An important concept involved with the therapeutic application of orthotics is that of protection. Orthoses can be used quite effectively to protect muscles, ligaments, bony structures, and nervous tissue during periods in which they are changing status and during periods when the systems are stable. A child who is developmentally trained on a severely valgus foot is, in fact, being encouraged into a position of genu valgus and often acquires knee flexion and equinus of the foot secondarily. Yet, that same child, when fitted with shoe inserts that prevent valgus and when provided with therapeutic exercise, can assume postures of lower-extremity abduction and external rotation. Facilitating movement, posture, or tone on a poorly aligned base causes increased ligamentous and muscular damage and inhibits the effects of the therapeutic program. Orthotic treatment can be very effective in protecting the painful muscles of a client recovering from Guillain-Barré syndrome.

Prevention, facilitation, and inhibition

Along with the need for protection goes the opportunity for prevention of deformity or the development of pathological motor habits that result from various combinations of muscle weakness and modified proprioceptive inputs. The developing child or the adult hemiplegic client who is allowed to bear weight on a hyperextended knee soon learns to lock the knee to bear weight. The locking pattern, along with a weak gastrocnemius soleus complex and a forward trunk as a result of weak hip extensors, results in stretching of the posterior capsule. The stretched capsule, abnormal weight-bearing forces, muscle weakness, and distorted sensation result in recurvatum deformity at the knee. Faulty proprioception and weak musculature may result in serious deformities, which appear as orthopaedic deviations but are in reality neurologically based. A simple AFO with a plantar flexion stop can be used to protect the joint and prevent the deformity. This same orthosis can be used as a sensory training device, which is discussed later in this chapter.

When determining the need for orthotic intervention, a skilled therapist should determine whether he or she desires the orthosis to facilitate or inhibit certain muscle groups, sensory inputs, or postural patterns. After determining the desired function of the orthosis, the therapist, in discussion with the fabricating orthotist, can develop a mechanically feasible yet sufficiently effective orthosis that will inhibit or facilitate as desired. Simple examples include shaping a ridge into the cast for an AFO, which when fabricated will apply deep pressure to Achilles tendon to inhibit plantar flexion or adding a plantar flexion spring assist to an orthosis used by a client with weak dorsiflexors. At each non–weight-bearing phase of gait on the affected extremity, the client's dorsiflexors are given a quick stretch by the antagonistic spring assist. The developing child who postures in flexion can be facilitated toward extension by introducing extension into the CNS. This is easily accomplished by preventing, through the use of a dorsiflexion stop, excessive forward rotation of the tibia on the talus. Although this is a biomechanical answer to excessive knee flexion orthopaedically, it is a sensory/proprioceptive input to the neurologically impaired client that results in increased extensor tone throughout the body.

Sensory training

Using orthotic treatment to enhance sensory training can be very interesting as well as effective. This technique challenges the thought processes of both the therapist, who determines the desired input, and the orthotist, who must fabricate the orthosis using biomechanical principles and sensory inputs requested by the therapist.

Consider these clinical situations. A 7-year-old child is unable to assume the vertical position because of multiple problems, including poor foot and leg alignment; the client exhibit tactile defensiveness in the clinic. His therapeutic exercise program may include over-ball activities and kneeling activities, both with deep pressure handling techniques. In preparation for vertical positioning, this child may be fitted with valgus corrective shoe inserts that will reinforce good base alignment. Additionally, textured strips can be placed in the inserts to enhance the child's sensory retraining program. Starting with coarse strips and progressing to finer fabrics and smaller strips will, along with the deep pressure from weight bearing, help to desensitize the child's feet.

In the next situation, a client with multiple sclerosis with a proprioceptive deficit at the knee that alters her ability to bear weight on extended knees can be fit with AFOs that allow 10 degrees of dorsiflexion and 10 degrees of plantar flexion. By placing stops at the ends of this 20 degrees of available range, the client has standing security and is able to safely practice knee control in weight bearing. The orthosis will abruptly stop knee flexion or recurvatum when the tibia has rotated 10 degrees anterior or 10 degrees posterior from vertical. When the movement stops, the client receives kinesthetic, tactile, and possibly auditory input. The author refers to this technique as "banging."

Alignment

As discussed in the evaluation section of this chapter, orthotic selection, whether neurologically, orthopaedically, or jointly based, must consider flexible versus fixed deformities. In most cases, early intervention will render most deformities flexible. This is especially true with neurologically induced mechanical abnormalities.

If a deformity or abnormal alignment is flexible, it should be corrected to normal alignment, thus allowing ligaments, muscles, and bones to develop anatomical normalcy. If, on the other hand, the deformity is rigid, it should be supported to minimize stress on the involved, adjacent, or related structures.

A flexible pes planus can be corrected by returning the calcaneus to its proper vertical alignment, thus elevating the longitudinal arch of the foot. A fixed painful pes planus can be supported with a properly fitting scaphoid pad.

When orthotic treatment is considered as an adjunct to the therapeutic exercise program for a neurologically impaired client, it is imperative that the concepts of body alignment be considered. To ensure that the orthotic treatment is enhancing the program and that it is in fact facilitating rather than inhibiting progress toward normalcy, normal body alignment must be understood. This is especially true in the trunk and lower extremities. The normal curves of the spine are (1) cervical lordosis from the apex of the odontoid process to T2, (2) thoracic kyphosis from T2 to the middle of T12, (3) lumbar lordosis from the middle of T12 to the sacrovertebral articulation, and (4) sacral kyphosis.[3] These curves become significant as spinal orthotics and the impact that orthotic treatment of one spinal segment has on another segment is discussed.

The hip joint, because it is a ball-and-socket joint, presents no particular alignment difficulty as related to therapeutic exercise and is placed 6 mm anterior and superior to the proximal tip of the greater trochanter. The knee joint is more difficult to manage because of its polycentric nature. As the client walks, the femur flexes in relation to the tibia and rotates externally approximately 10 degrees about its long axis. The flexion and rotation is certainly a consideration when aligning anatomical and mechanical joints since improper joint placement can provide the neurologically impaired client with inaccurate sensory input.

Because of its complex nature and progressive development, the rotation of the ankle joint mortice is most important. At birth the ankle joint mortice is rotated approximately 2 degrees externally in relation to the knee axis. By age 7, when the child has been upright with a sufficiently narrowed base of support for some time, the mortice is rotated 20 to 30 degrees externally in relation to the knee axis. This rotation allows the center of gravity to progress smoothly during gait. The ankle joint mortice is not perpendicular to the line of progression during gait, but it is parallel to the movement of the center of gravity from heelstrike to midstance. The final alignment in the lower extremity is that of the foot. The long axis of the foot is generally rotated externally, approximately 15 degrees from the line of progression.[1]

Maintenance

During each therapeutic exercise session, specific activities are aimed at a desired end result. It is important that the gains obtained during a specific session be maintained between sessions. The importance of this cannot be overlooked. When trying to increase range of motion, a gain of 10 degrees obtained during a treatment session can easily be lost by the next treatment session. A pattern that is beginning to be functional can be negated if not properly reinforced. The therapist can control hip internal rotation or scapular elevation with his or her hands for the length of a treatment session. An orthosis can reinforce correct patterns until the client's next session.

The client who is no longer changing neurologically or musculoskeletally may have reached his or her maximal potential for function. However, that limit may be stretched with some external orthotic device. This is a common situation for the client with multiple sclerosis. A client who might be wheelchair bound as a result of the excessive energy required to ambulate against severe lower-extremity extensor tone can be functionally ambulatory by wearing orthoses that inhibit some of the extensor tone while leaving enough for weight support during gait.

EVALUATION

Material in this section discusses general areas of consideration when evaluating a client for orthotic intervention. Following the general discussion are specifics related to evaluation of the trunk, upper extremity, and lower extremity.

Range of motion and power

A thorough examination of the passive range of motion available to the therapist will provide the therapist with a foundation on which to place information gathered during the evaluation. The passive range evaluation tells the therapist the exact available arc of motion on which external forces can be applied.

Having determined the available range, a determination of power must be made. In an orthotic evaluation, the determination of power is neither a manual muscle test nor a specific test, such as dynometry. It is a more general assessment of the client's ability to move a particular joint through a functional range of motion during a specific activity. A muscle grade of fair minus or fair plus in the gastrocnemius muscle or a power grasp of 4 lb will tell the therapist little related to the specific need for orthotic intervention. Specific muscle grades and force values are, however, invaluable when determining the effectiveness of a therapeutic exercise program. Useful information related to power can be obtained by viewing a function and analyzing the reason for deviations from normal in relation to sufficient or insufficient activity in muscle groups performing the function.

For example, consider the client who has good grasp and full passive range but is unable to feed himself or herself. The important facts to determine here are: (1) is there insufficient flexor activity at the elbow? and (2) is there too much extensor activity about the elbow? Answers to these questions will guide the therapist in the direction of appropriate orthotic intervention. A fair muscle grade assigned to the biceps is less useful information. Concurrent with determining the power, the therapist must determine the source of that power. Is it synergy, isolated muscle strength, or reflex? A flexion/extension synergy in the lower extremity that is slightly modified by orthotic intervention can result in an energy efficient, cosmetic gait.

Sensation

When evaluating tactile sensation, it is useful to categorize findings as normal, hyperesthetic, paresthetic, or anesthetic. These categorizations will aide the therapist in determining materials from which the orthosis will be fabricated and may influence the structural design of the orthosis. Standard configurations can be altered to avoid surface areas where tactile input is perceived as discomfort.

Proprioceptive testing produces the most reliable results, in terms of orthotic application, when it is performed with the tested joint in a functional position under the influence of gravity. For example, the sitting position is preferable to the supine position when testing the upper extremity, and standing is preferable to sitting when testing the lower extremity. In these positions, joints and ligaments can be tested in their more normal environment for function.

Tone and reflexology

Muscle tone and reflexology are evaluated hand in hand. The therapist needs to determine base tone, fluctuations in that base tone, and causes of the fluctuations if present. Tone is also examined in positions of function. If it appears that a reflex is either inhibiting or facilitating function, further testing should be done using standard test positions. The neurologically impaired child who uses an asymmetrical tonic neck reflex to provide the tonal changes for ambulation may be unable to ambulate if the reflex is completely inhibited. During this child's therapeutic exercise program, an array of neurophysiologically based techniques could be used to integrate the reflex. A cervical orthosis designed to limit excessive head rotation—hence altering, but not eliminating, the child's mobility—can act to reinforce those techniques used in the therapeutic exercise program.

A child with low tone who demonstrates excessive head, trunk, and lower-extremity flexion when vertical can be gradually facilitated toward extension with the use of AFOs and a neurophysiologically sound therapeutic exercise program.

Skin integrity

Before completing the orthotic evaluation, skin integrity is examined. Clients seen following trauma with multiple injuries often have interruptions in the skin that may have impact on the structural design of an orthosis. Special attention should be paid to the feet of an ambulatory, neurologically impaired child or adult. Bearing weight on an unprotected or poorly aligned foot can result in ulcerations of the navicular and metatarsal heads.

The trunk

When evaluating the neurologically impaired client, the first questions that come to mind are: "What forces can an orthosis apply that will help reinforce the client's treatment program?" and "What patterns or postures are inhibiting the client's progress?" This is especially true when evaluating the client's trunk. Is it realistic to expect 1 hour of therapeutic exercise to improve a client's head control if the client, when seated, has the head flexed forward? The same client may lie supine in bed with a large pillow holding the head in flexion. It will be difficult for the 1 hour of cervical extension, approximation, and cocontraction training to counteract 23 hours of flexion. The cervical musculature, in this case, must surely be biased incorrectly.

Begin the evaluation of the cervical spine by a simple observation of the posture noted when you first see the client. Is the head stationary or mobile? This is a certain clue to the need for stability or mobility. Is the head centered over the body? Are the eyes directed forward? Is the client able to move on command? Is the skin intact? Does movement of the head alter tone in other parts of the body? Are reflexes such as asymmetrical tonic neck reflex (ATNR), symmetrical tonic neck reflex (STNR), neck righting, or optic righting present? Is there visable asymmetry of the face or upper chest secondary to tonal imbalances? See the following evaluation for an example:

1. Describe the client's initial posture. The client is in a wheelchair, the arms are supported, the feet are on footplates, the trunk is stable, and the head is dropped forward with the mandible on the sternum.
2. Is the client's head stationary or mobile? Stationary.
3. Is the client's head centered? No, it is tipped to the right.
4. Are the client's eyes forward? No, they are downcast.
5. Is the client able to move on command? Yes, but the head flops from flexion with rotation to hyperextension.
6. Does movement alter tone? No.
7. Are reflexes detectable? No.

8. Is there visible asymmetry? Slight, the mandible deviates to the left.

Having gathered the previous information, goals are determined and a treatment plan established. If the immediate goal is the development of head control in the sitting position to improve visual input, encourage more normal body tone and work toward advanced mobility training. The therapeutic program may include passive positioning and facilitation to the cervical extensors through techniques such as tapping, brushing, quick icing, reverse tapping or vibration. To increase stability the therapist may use approximation and attempt to decrease the large arc of motion noted in the evaluation. Prolonged positioning in flexion should be avoided as well.

A program of "cervical stability in neutral training" will be enhanced by the application of the anterior section of a commercially available cervical orthosis, such as a Philadelphia collar. Attaching the orthosis to axillary loops or a figure-of-eight harness will prevent excessive forward flexion, prevent prolonged periods of flexion, and will act as a kinesthetic reminder. When the client, at times, simply rests into the collar, the cervical extensors are being protected from overstretching. Should the extension component of movement remain a problem, the posterior section of the orthosis can be loosly applied in the same manner to prevent excessive extension.

This example is in no manner advocating the use of a tightly applied, mobility-eliminating cervical orthosis. On the contrary, it suggests the use of an orthosis that limits or controls excessive movement and that is designed to reinforce a therapeutic principle.

The three most common situations of the cervical spine where orthotics can be beneficial to the neurologically impaired client in the author's experience are poor anteroposterior head control, tonal or postural torticollis, and excessive cervical mobility.

The thoracic spine, by nature of its anatomical configuration, is less suited for problems of excessive mobility than is the cervical spine. It is, as well, less suited for simple evaluation. In the neurologically impaired client, an x-ray examination is invaluable when dealing with the common problem of excessive curves of the thoracic spine. The radiogram provides information as to the vertebral status, and the evaluating therapist must determine the flexibility or rigidity of any pathological curves. The therapist again looks at range of motion. Is there too much or too little movement, or is it simply misdirected? What is the muscular power available? What is the source? Is the tone of the trunk symmetrical? Is it high, low, or fluxuating? Is the sensory system intact or interpreting inadequately? What does the skin look like, and how does it feel? Is it fragile or thick, cold or warm, clear or erupted, dry or moist, or shiny? This information will assist in determining the amount of corrective force that can be applied to the skin. Finally, are there specific reflexes that seem apparent, such as the ATNR or head on body righting?

It is important to realize that in most cases of orthotic treatment of the thoracic spine in the neurologically impaired client the goal is increased stability. Stabilizing against asymmetrical or rotary based reflexes may appear to increase the intensity of the reflex. A child who demonstrates a strong neck on body righting reflex may be hindered by an orthosis that stabilizes the thoracic spine, thus causing the spine to move as a unit. The nonstabilized spine is capable of absorbing rotation at various levels of the spine, not only at the ends of the stabilized sections. Few clients with neurological disability require orthotic treatment of the thoracic spine for any reason other than scoliosis. These clients may be treated in the conventional scoliosis systems, or they may benefit from an orthosis that is less conventional and employs more concepts based in neurophysiology than in pure biomechanics. This is accomplished by inserting flexible panels or by designing corrective pads that create greater sensory inputs. Kyphotic or lordotic curves in the thoracic spine of a neurologically impaired client can often be sufficiently influenced by altering the cervical or lumbar spine.

When evaluating the lumbosacral spine, it is important to evaluate the client in positions of function. In this area, as in the cervical area, the key will be the relationship of stability to mobility. Is there too much mobility? In what direction or directions does the client's spine appear rigid? In what position? Does the spinal alignment look the same regardless of whether the client is in the supine, prone, sitting, or standing position? What is the power of the flexors, extensors, and rotators? What is the power source? Is the muscular tone constant? What is the nature of the skin? Does the lumbosacral area appear affected by specific reflexes?

The available passive range of motion is the major factor influencing the speed with which orthotic treatment will alter the lumbosacral spine in a neurologically impaired client. If the spine is "locked," orthotic treatment may compound the difficulties by reinforcing stability or the results may appear much more slowly. External forces applied to the lumbosacral spine can generally do one of three things. They may (1) support or hold an existing posture, (2) decrease a lordosis by bridging its apex, placing forces above and below the apex of the curve, or (3) increase a lordosis by placing the major force at the apex of the curve or existing kyphosis. The most significant fact about orthotic treatment of the lumbosacral spine is that forces applied to the lumbosacral spine often have striking effects on the thoracic and cervical spine.

Increasing the lumbar lordosis of a client in the sitting or standing position will generally result in a decreased thoracic kyphosis and an increased cervical lordosis. Increasing the lumbar lordosis with a lumbosacral corset containing rigid stays contoured into extension will often alter the sitting posture of a child who maintains a posterior pelvis. Likewise, a child who maintains an anterior pelvis can be encouraged to rock posteriorly by wearing a corset with stays that bridge the lumbar curve.

When using a spinal orthosis to enhance an established therapeutic exercise program, the treating therapist must be aware of the phenomenon of diaphragmatic alienation. Diaphragmatic alienation occurs when a spinal support is applied in a manner that impedes the downward excursion of the diaphragm during inhalation. The diaphragm, if continually limited in its excursion, loses stretch sensitivity in the shortened range.

The upper extremity

When considering the upper extremity and possibilities for therapeutic orthotics, the evaluators must separate themselves from conventional rationales for uses of orthotic treatment.

The upper extremity is frequently splinted by occupational therapists, physical therapists, and orthotists to allow improved function while the client is wearing the device. Clients may require multiple splints to perform a variety of tasks. This is, in the author's perception, conventional orthotic care of the upper extremity. Conventional orthotic care is often quite helpful and may be the factor that has the most impact on the client's ability to perform activities of daily living. In many cases conventional orthotic care is the best option; in some cases it is not. These concepts attempt to reinforce the use of orthoses as an adjunct to or as an enhancer of the therapeutic program that is aimed at more normal function with minimal extraneous apparatus. Part of upper-extremity orthotic training needs to address the activities for which the orthosis must be worn and those activities for which it should be removed. The goal of a therapeutic orthotic program is to minimize the client's dependence on a device. There is a fine balance between using an orthosis for training muscles, altering tone, or maintaining status between treatment sessions and learning a splinter skill while wearing an orthosis. Although the latter addresses the immediate tasks at hand, the former will have a greater impact on the long-term activities of a client.

The same areas addressed in the spinal evaluation—passive range, power, sensation, tone, skin integrity, reflexology—need to be addressed when dealing with the upper extremity. Although the client's visual status is crucial in conventional orthotic management of the upper extremity, it is less important when using concepts of therapeutic orthotics. Training a client how to perform a task with a conventional upper-extremity orthosis generally requires the client to visually attend to the task. When using therapeutic orthotics, the therapist is attempting to have impact on the client's CNS and indirectly on the ability to perform a task.

The passive range of motion of the upper extremity should be evaluated in positions of function such as the sitting or standing positions. Information that is gathered with the client in the supine position will be of little transferable value as related to purposeful movement. Can the client's arm be moved forward and horizontal to the floor? Can the shoulder be fully flexed? Can the client's arm be externally rotated and abducted to 90 degrees? What is the passive range available for internal rotation? How much motion can passively occur at the elbow, forearm, wrist, and fingers?

How much power is available, and from what source is the power derived? For example, a client is able to flex the elbow against gravity to eat finger foods independently, but only by using a mass pattern that includes excessive scapular retraction and elevation. When the scapula is stabilized during a treatment session, the client is able to work through the mass pattern and obtain smoother movement. Is it reasonable to use a chest strap with an anteroposterior shoulder strap to stabilize the scapula and act as a kinesthetic reminder to inhibit scapular retraction and elevation? The orthosis (externally applied forces) will enhance the existing treatment program by inhibiting the mass pattern that the client would use three times a day at meal periods. Collectively, those meal periods may represent more time than the therapist spends during the therapeutic exercise program inhibiting the pattern.

The client's sensation, both tactile and proprioceptive, should be evaluated in terms of normal, hypesthesia, parasthesia, or anesthesia. Areas noted to be hypesthetic or parasthetic may, when orthotic forces are applied to them, amplify abnormal neuromuscular responses. Anesthetic areas should be monitored to minimize or prevent tissue breakdown. Tone is evaluated concurrently with reflexology, as was done in the spinal evaluation and as will be done in the lower-extremity evaluation. Stimulated by head or neck position, recognition of reflexes that alter upper-extremity tone is extremely important when determining therapeutic orthotic intervention. Use of an orthosis designed to stop the right elbow from extending would be inappropriate if used with a client who demonstrated an ATNR to the right. Clearly, in this example, it is not the elbow that requires treatment.

The upper-extremity evaluation is concluded with assessment of the skin integrity, noting such things as limb color, temperature, texture of skin, presence or absence of hair as compared to the opposite limb, and open areas or scars from previous insults.

When the evaluation is completed, the evaluator determines goals and a treatment plan based on neurophysiological techniques. Compression, traction, tapping, resistance to motion, and tracking techniques can all be enhanced by an upper-extremity orthosis. Most techniques can be satisfactorily simulated with either dynamic or static orthotic treatment. The therapist must determine which techniques are to be simulated.

The lower extremity

The lower extremity, because of its primary purpose as a propeller and its need for stability, is an extremely interesting body part to treat with therapeutic orthotics.[2] As a practicing clinician, it is the author's perception that the majority of lower-extremity pathologies can be influenced from below the knee. To encumber a neurologically impaired client with unnecessary orthoses brings to mind the visualization of a cement balloon. For the minority of clients who require orthotic treatment above the knee, a prime consideration must be the weight of the orthosis and the ease of operation. Uncncumbered mobility and adequate stability can be facilitated in the lower extremity by using appropriate orthotic intervention following thorough assessment.

Passive range of motion of the lower extremity may look very different when tested or observed in non–weight-bearing and weight-bearing positions. Leg lengths that appear equal when tested with the client supine or sitting may be grossly different when the client bears weight. Muscle power that previously masked ligamentous laxity may no longer be present in the client who suffers an acquired neurological disability. Valgus or varus deformities at the subtalar joint and valgus, varus, flexion, or recurvatum deformities at the knee can all result in a relative leg length discrepancy. During the evaluation it will be important to note variations in passive range related to positioning with respect to gravity. In some cases, therapeutic orthotic treatment of the lower extremity will require forces that facilitate mobility and forces that facilitate stability.

The alignment of the calcaneus in weight bearing referred to earlier in this chapter is critical when evaluating the lower extremity of a neurologically impaired client. When viewed posteriorly, the triceps surae tendon should appear perpendicular to the supporting surface. Deviations as slight as 5 to 8 degrees appear to allow sufficient sliding of the talus to permit resultant dropping of the longitudinal arch of the foot. A hallux valgus deformity develops secondary to the pes planus. Progressive genu valgus is seen on occasion.

The author's clinical experience has led him to believe that there is a correlation between valgus of the calcaneus and toe walking in some cases, with the toe walking secondary to the valgus. Anatomically, the wedge-shaped talus that sits between the distal ends of the tibia and the fibula and that rests on the calcaneus is at risk when the calcaneus tips into valgus. The medial lip of the talus, when the calcaneus tips, is pressed against the tibia. The child, unknowingly, raises up on the toes, thus placing the foot in relative plantar flexion, changing the alignment of the talus and reducing the talotibial pressure.

Power of movement in the lower extremity will often appear radically different, depending on the position in which it is tested. In the lower extremity, power that is a summation of selected movement, tone, patterns, and re-

flexology, is easily assessed. Yet the sources of that power are difficult, if not impossible, to quantify individually. Fortunately, it is not necessary initially to quantify those individual components. Careful observation of client responses during the initial treatment sessions will allow the therapist to organize the components in terms of greater to lesser influence. This organization will direct the therapist to the body part requiring treatment if it is, in fact, not the lower extremity.

Therapists who evaluate a large number of clients with neurological disability will recognize specific movements in patterns or synergies. Those patterns may be negligible or quite obvious. They may be complete, involving all lower-extremity joints, or incomplete, affecting an individual segment of the limb. Regardless of whether they are complete or incomplete, the patterns need to be controlled, directed, and hopefully totally integrated to allow smooth, safe, energy efficient movement.

Once power has been assessed, testing for sensation, especially for proprioception, must be completed. Testing with the client in a vertical weight-bearing position will provide information that is most easily applied to functional status. If this is not possible, the ankle and foot should be tested if the client is in a sitting position, and the knee and hip should be tested if the client is in the supine position.

At this point, the evaluating therapist should examine the skin integrity; this is discussed earlier in the chapter. When evaluating the skin, the therapist should take special note of the sole of the foot. The skin thickness under the metatarsal heads and particularly the area under the second and third metatarsal heads should be examined closely. If the client's metatarsal arch has dropped, this area may become quite sensitive and may act as a stimulus for tone alteration during weight bearing.

The evaluating therapist has now assessed range, power, tone, reflexology, tactile and proprioceptive status, and skin integrity. Special attention has been paid to the alignment of the foot. Short-term and long-term goals are now established, and a treatment plan is developed. The treatment plan that the therapist designs will determine the appropriate therapeutic application of orthotics. The therapist must determine the neurophysiological impact that the orthosis should produce, and, as examples in the treatment section of this chapter will demonstrate, there are numerous options.

TREATMENT GOALS

The basic philosophy for, concepts of, and evaluation techniques used with the application of therapeutic orthotics have been discussed. Before reviewing multiple treatment examples, the goals related to the therapeutic application of orthotics should be evaluated. These goals can be divided into two sets: those directed at the orthotic treatment and those that may result from proper therapeutic application of the orthoses. The principal goals for using orthotics therapeutically are to reinforce a therapeutic exercise program, to hasten a client's progress toward more normal movement, posture, or tone, and to indirectly improve the client's functional abilities. These goals can be accomplished by attempting the following:

1. Minimize the orthotic treatment. Discuss options with the designing orthotist that keep the design as simple as possible. The simpler the orthosis is, the more controllable it will be. As the orthosis becomes more complex, there is a greater chance to introduce unwanted inputs to the CNS through unplanned or uncontrolled biomechanical forces. Additionally, the therapeutic exercise program will include exercises that reinforce quality movement and promote a decreased dependence on external devices.

2. Provide options for more movement. Attempt designs that eliminate movement only in cases of excessive motion. With almost every client the therapist works to obtain quality, pain-free mobility of some type. Before eliminating motion in a neurologically impaired limb, the therapist must consider the primary and secondary effects of the elimination of motion. In addition to eliminating motion, we may be eliminating potential progress.

   Consider the client who, when initially evaluated after a cerebrovascular accident (CVA), lacks movement distal to the knee. To order a plastic AFO with a rigid ankle designed to eliminate plantar flexion, dorsiflexion, inversion, and eversion for this client is in error. Once applied, the orthosis provides stability but does not provide the option for normal movement. One therapeutic application of orthotic care to CVA clients will be discussed in detail in the treatment section of this chapter.

3. Select orthotic designs that encourage normal movement, tone, or posture and that encourage function. The purpose of the orthosis is to alter movement, tone, or posture and to protect the extremity. The protected, more normalized extremity increases in value to the client as it is used more easily for purposeful activity. Treatments, orthotic or otherwise, that neither directly nor indirectly facilitate function are generally inconsistent with the goal of therapeutic intervention. Normal tone and movement should reinforce function, and function should reinforce normal tone and movement.

4. Develop designs that are energy efficient. When construction of the orthosis is discussed with the orthotist, keep in mind the relative weight of the materials from which the orthosis will be constructed as well as the final alignment. Request materials that are light weight but durable. Material selection is related to the client's height and weight, the expected activity level of the client, and the forces the orthosis is expected to generate. Most importantly, material selection is secondary in importance to the neuromuscular inputs desired. Desiring a dynamic ankle joint but selecting a rigid plastic design because it is lighter negates the original rationale for therapeutic orthotic intervention. Final alignment is of significant importance when attempting to ensure energy efficiency. Malaligned joint surfaces can create friction on joints intended to be freely mobile. The friction will reduce the energy efficiency of the orthosis and, while actually acting as resistance, may strengthen undesired movement patterns.

5. Consider the cost effectiveness of orthotic treatment. As you begin to develop a rationale for orthotic treatment, consider all alternatives. Consider the expected length of time the orthosis will be used and the cost effects of not using orthotic treatment. A client who is ambulatory with an orthosis may be confined to a wheelchair or bed without the orthosis. The cost to heal skin breakdown is significantly greater than the cost of most orthoses. Consider the cost effectiveness of reducing the number of treatment sessions because neuromuscular changes are being maintained orthotically between treatment sessions. With changes maintained, the therapist can concentrate on progressive treatment without having to use valuable time for maintenance activities.

6. Provide the client with the most cosmetically pleasing orthosis. Seek good cosmesis, but not at the expense of desired function. Clients seem to understand that some orthoses are more noticeable than others. When therapists take the time to explain, patients also seem to understand that maximal cosmesis may temporarily be sacrificed to obtain maximal neuromuscular results. When the client's neuromuscular status has stabilized, determination of final maximal cosmesis can be made. An orthosis that was used by a client during periods of neuromuscular change may be replaced by a more cosmetic orthosis when the client's neuromuscular status stabilizes. A client with Guillain-Barré syndrome may begin ambulation with metal orthoses that protect the extremities and that allow variability to accommodate muscle strength changes. If deficits remain, this same client may require plastic orthoses, at some point, after muscular return has plateaued.

7. Attempt to minimize maintenance. Consider the stresses that will be applied to the orthosis in relation to its perceived durability. The proximity of the client to the supplying orthotist should also be considered or at least acknowledged before initiating orthotic evaluation and fitting. When complicated schedules or minor fitting problems cause delays, the client and the client's family deal more realisti-

cally when the procedures have been clearly outlined from the beginning.

TREATMENT EXAMPLES
Hemiplegia

Clients with hemiplegia secondary to CVA are, in many cases, ideal candidates for therapeutic orthotic management. They are also some of the clients who demonstrate the most changing neuromuscular systems. In the author's experience, the CVA client has benefitted greatly from complementary orthotic and therapeutic exercise programs. Brunnstrom[1] has documented six stages of recovery in the lower extremity following CVA. It is the author's belief that specific orthotic ankle joint adjustments exist that maximize function in each stage of recovery while facilitating the next stage of recovery. Although this material refers to clients recovering from CVA and to the stages classified by Brunnstrom, its applicability is far greater. Clients with closed-head injury and clients with multiple sclerosis often appear similar clinically. When treating clients who have changing neuromuscular systems, it is imperative that the therapist be alert to changes. For the orthotic technique described here to be maximally effective, the therapist must, in the concurrent exercise program, facilitate and inhibit tone to correspond with noted changes. The therapeutic exercise program is dynamic and so must be the orthotic treatment.

In dealing with a flaccid lower extremity, the goals of therapeutic exercise are to maintain range of motion, protect joints, and stimulate tone in preparation for function. Orthotic treatment is initiated by fitting the client with a training AFO with a solid stirrup and double-action ankle joint. The double-action ankle joint consists of a metal casing with two channels, one anterior and one posterior to the axis of rotation of the joint. The channels are capped by channel screws that exert forces on the contents of the channels. Springs can be placed in the channels to assist motions, or rods can be placed in the channels to stop motions. A rod placed inside a spring in the channel can act to assist motion in one direction and stop motion in another direction. The training orthosis, readily available in many physical therapy departments, enables the therapist to begin an orthotic program that will, early on, reinforce the therapeutic exercise program. For the client with a flaccid lower extremity, stimulate tone through weight bearing, proprioceptive input from joint approximation, and stimulus to the metatarsal heads by standing the client in an orthosis that protects the ankle and stabilizes the knee in good alignment. This can be accomplished in two ways: (1) an ankle joint fixed in neutral or a few degrees of plantar flexion or (2) a plantar flexion stop and a dorsiflexion assist to a dorsiflexion stop. (NOTE: a fixed joint has no motion and a stop prevents motion in one direction.) When properly adjusted, either option will prevent knee flexion and recurvatum during standing, if the foot is flat on the ground and if the client's trunk is erect or slightly anterior (causing stabilization of the knee biomechanically).

In this situation tone is stimulated in a functional position. With the client in a protected standing position, the therapist can employ neurophysiologically based techniques for increasing tone, such as tapping, icing, vibration, and approximation. Concepts of elongation and foreshortening can also be used to stimulate tone for weight bearing.

When, in the therapeutic exercise sessions, the therapist notes an increase in tone or minimal voluntary movement in synergy, the orthotic treatment changes.

This section discusses the two options available for helping the client with a flaccid lower extremity to a standing position using an AFO. If option one, a fixed ankle, was used, there were rods in both anterior and posterior channels. When the client demonstrates minimal voluntary movement, the anterior channel screw is loosened to allow 3 to 5 degrees of dorsiflexion, but the posterior channel is kept tight to prevent plantar flexion. The small amount of dorsiflexion will begin to reinforce the dorsiflexion component of the lower-extremity synergy, and the plantar flexion stop will prevent development of a strong extensor thrust that promotes recurvatum and posterior capsular damage. The sidebars, metal joints, and a well-fitting shoe will prevent the development of excessive inversion while guiding the foot into dorsiflexion. The small amount of range available is, however, insufficient to allow the weight line to pass posterior to the knee joint and cause buckling during midstance.

If option two—a plantar flexion stop at neutral and a dorsiflexion assist to a dorsiflexion stop—was used, the assist is removed. This orthotic option, through techniques mentioned previously, has been stimulating tone. In addition, each time the spring-loaded dorsiflexion assist has been activated, the plantar flexors have been provided with a quick stretch. Realizing that, more often than not, extensor tone becomes more powerful than flexor tone in the lower extremity, excessive stimulation is unwarranted.

At this point the orthotic treatment that previously consisted of two options has been consolidated. The client is training in a limited-motion orthosis that allows 3 to 5 degrees of dorsiflexion and that is set in neutral for plantar flexion. This permits motion into flexion at the ankle and knee while discouraging plantar flexion, knee hyperextension, and medial lateral instability at the subtalar joint.

As the therapist notes a continued increase in the synergistic movements in the lower extremity, the ankle joint will require altering. When the client has developed mature synergies, especially the extension synergy, the therapist can completely remove the dorsiflexion stop. This is accomplished by removing the rod from the anterior channel. Although the client is now permitted to dorsiflex using the synergy pattern during the swing phase of gait, he or she is not permitted to bear weight on a hyperextended knee resulting from a mature extension synergy. The inversion component of both patterns is inhibited by the tracking of the mechanical joints. The posterior rod must remain rigid to prevent the development of recurvatum until the client begins to demonstrate in the therapeutic exercise program the ability to deviate from the mass patterns. When hamstring control can be elicited to flex the involved knee past 90 degrees in a sitting position, the therapist may begin to gradually loosen the posterior channel screw and permit more plantar flexion to occur. As the hamstring control increases, the plantar flexion range is increased until there is free plantar flexion.

Fig. 28-1 shows a client with recurvatum uncontrolled by an orthosis that allows too much plantar flexion. Fig. 24-2 shows the same client wearing an orthosis with a plantar flexion stop that is effective in decreasing recurvatum at the knee. As this client's kinesthetic sense improves, more plantar flexion will be eliminated. During ambulation with the AFO pictured in Fig. 28-1, the client demonstrated a relative leg length discrepancy. This did not occur with the orthosis in Fig. 28-2.

Even when the client can demonstrate good knee and ankle control in the sagittal plane, there may be medial lateral instability in the coronal plane. This is especially true when the client is ambulatory on uneven terrain. The orthosis, void of channel contents, continues to protect the ankle in the coronal plane while allowing the anterior and posterior leg musculature to be strengthened by uninhibited use.

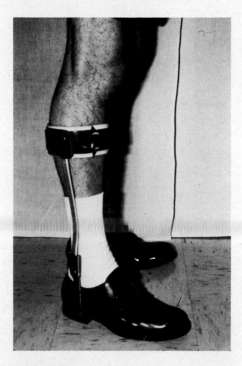

Fig. 28-2. AFO with plantar flexion stop. Recurvation is reduced.

When it is noted that the client is demonstrating voluntary control of the lower extremity and, specifically, dorsiflexion with knee extension, a spring-loaded plantar flexion assist can be created in the orthosis by placing a spring in the anterior channel. This will, at toe off of each step, provide the dorsiflexors of the ankle with a quick stretch to facilitate contraction. Care must be taken to avoid the application of a force so great as to overpower the returning dorsiflexors.

If the client chooses not to wear the orthosis during ambulation once voluntary control is demonstrated, it can be set with a stronger plantar flexion assist and used in a home exercise program for dorsiflexor strengthening.

This particular use of orthotics, although discussed here using the example of hemiplegia, can be applied to other neurologically impaired clients, such as those with head injury, multiple sclerosis, or Guillain-Barré syndrome with slight variations.

Spina bifida

CASE STUDY: KENNY

Kenny, a 4-year-old child with spina bifida and secondary incomplete paralysis below T6, came to Central Maine Medical Center for orthotic evaluation. Kenny's medical history included shunt controlled hydrocephalus and a developing scoliosis. For the purpose of socialization and physiological standing, the child was seen for fabrication of a "functional stander" type orthosis. Passive range of motion evaluation demonstrated that, when the left leg was adducted past 40 degrees of abduction, the pelvis elevated and created a relative 3-inch leg length discrepancy. This directed the evaluators to the hip to determine a hip abduction contracture of 40 degrees.

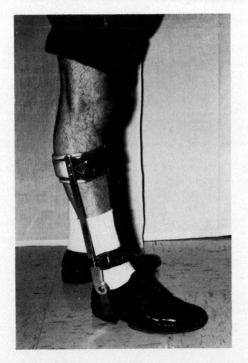

Fig. 28-1. AFO with free plantar flexion. Severe recurvatum resulted in relative leg length discrepancy.

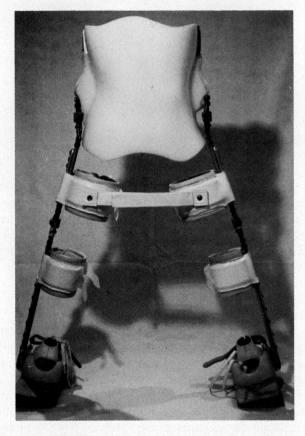

Fig. 28-3. HKAFO with molded body jacket. This orthosis was designed to provide weight bearing and to adjust to eliminate hip abduction contracture.

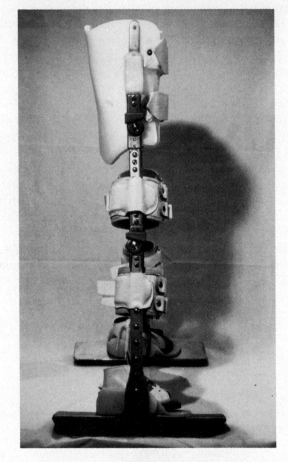

Fig. 28-4. Side view of HKAFO with molded body jacket. Note vertical alignment.

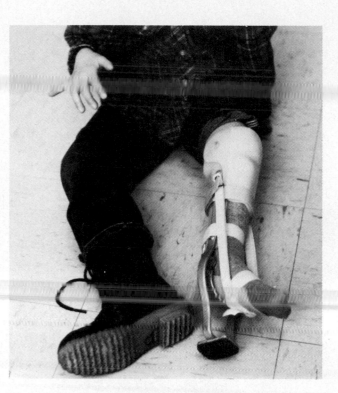

Fig. 28-5. Patellar tendon bearing AFO with polypropelene footplate and adjustable ankle to provide prolonged stretch to posterior leg musculature. Extended bottom equalizes leg length and creates extension force at knee.

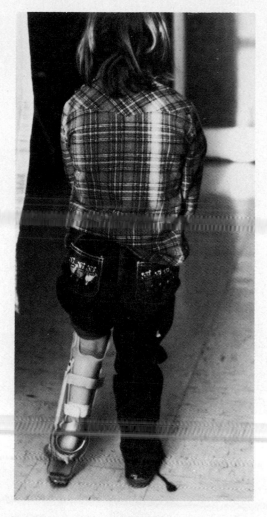

Fig. 28-6. Posterior view of dynamic interim AFO.

Since the child was not a candidate for surgical release because of multiple problems, and since a shoe lift would feed into the hip and spinal problem, an orthosis addressing both problems was designed. The orthosis pictured in Figs. 28-3 and 28-4 resulted. It is designed to allow the child to stand while stabilizing the right hip and creating a prolonged stretch on the left hip abductors. The muscle imbalance and soft tissue contracture must be questioned when there is partial paralysis. The orthosis was adjustable in height to accommodate growth and in abduction range to maintain range gains obtained during therapeutic exercise. Foot wedges were also designed to adjust for proper weight bearing as the legs became positionable in less abduction.

Down's syndrome

CASE STUDY: FRANCINE

This 11-year-old client has a primary diagnosis of Down's syndrome complicated by a right CVA with resultant left hemiplegia has slight hip and knee flexion contractures and a severe equinus deformity. A leg length discrepancy of plus 4 inches has re-

sulted in ambulation on the great toe and first metatarsal head, under which the skin is thickly calloused. A secondary scoliosis is developing and an ATNR is present.

To improve her gait, decrease energy consumption, inhibit the functional scoliosis, and promote normal ranges of motion, the child was fitted with the AFO seen in Figs. 28-5 and 28-6. These photographs were taken during the client's initial fitting.

The child's exercise program is aimed at integrating the reflex and obtaining more normal range of motion for a more energy-efficient gait. Ranges gained during therapeutic exercise will be maintained during functional ambulation. Once range gains have stabilized, appropriate footwear with adequate lifts will be constructed.

Osteogenesis imperfecta

CASE STUDY: PAUL

This child is a 10-year-old male with a primary diagnosis of osteogenesis imperfecta tarda. Of orthopaedic nature, this disease has resulted in over 25 fractures with resultant losses of movement. The child has severe lower-extremity contractures but

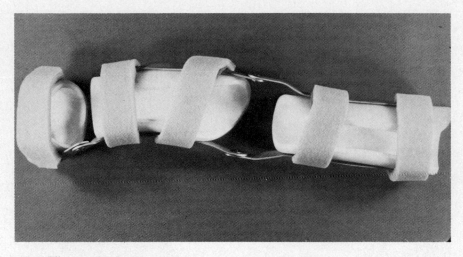

Fig. 28-7. Elbow wrist hand orthosis designed to protect extremity and facilitate movement through traction.

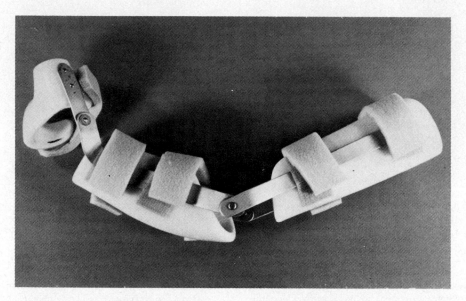

Fig. 28-8. View of ranges available at time of initial fit.

remains ambulatory with a rolling walker. Multiple upper-extremity fractures inhibited safe use of a walker. The child was experiencing less and less kinesthetic sense resulting from limited mobility. The orthosis seen in Figs. 28-7 and 28-8 was designed to protect the limb while creating gentle traction to facilitate movement. Single wrist joint construction was desired for control of weight and control of ulnar drift. The circumferential pressure of the forearm and arm cuffs as useful in creating a sense of security for this child to move without fear of fracturing.

Multiple pathologies
CASE STUDY: MR. P

The orthosis shown in Fig. 28-9 was designed as an interim orthosis for a 67-year-old client with Paget's disease, a CVA, and

third degree burns on the sole and instep of the foot. This demonstrates simple management of multiple pathologies. The client was independently ambulatory with a cane.

AFO for hemiplegia
CASE STUDY: MRS. T

Fig. 28-10 shows the orthosis fabricated for a 64-year-old client to replace a conventional KAFO that the client was fit with after a CVA. Three years following the insult she had equino varus during swing phase, extreme valgus during weight bearing, and genu recurvatum. After the client was fit with a polypropylene AFO with a rigid ankle set in slight dorsiflexion and a valgus corrective flare, her mobility skills improved significantly. The AFO pictured replaced a KAFO with a dorsiflexion assist and a valgus corrective strap.

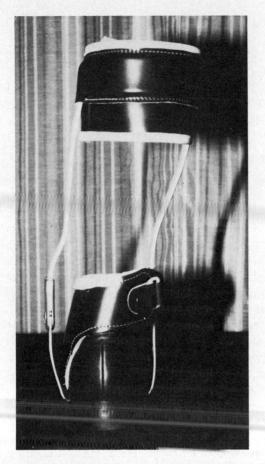

Fig. 28-9. Interim AFO for a client with Paget's disease, cerebrovascular accident, and burns on the foot.

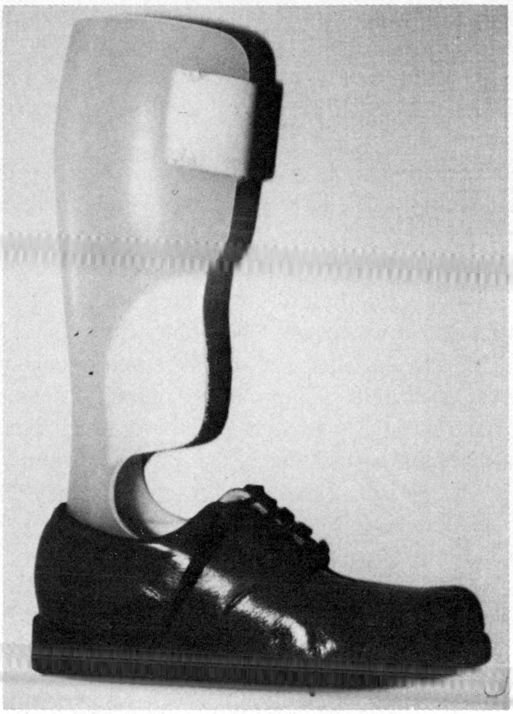

Fig. 28-10. Definitive polypropylene AFO with valgus corrective flare for stabilized client with cerebrovascular accident with valgus on weight bearing and equino varus during swing phase of gait.

IMPRINTING THROUGH CASTING: A NEW TREATMENT CONCEPT

This section describes a technique that incorporates the use of casting with various facilitation and/or inhibition techniques that are applied for a specified time to produce a specific result. It is based on the philosophy that central nervous system learning occurs through consistency of input and repetition. The neurophysiology of the technique is drawn from earlier chapters in this book (see Chapter 6). The basic assumption of the casting concept is that many of the effects of certain facilitation or inhibition techniques can be preserved—or "imprinted"—if the treated limb or body part is set in a cast while the therapeutic procedure is being performed. These techniques may include traction, approximation, rotation, deep tendon pressure, prolonged stretch, the option for movement, single component elimination, foreshortening, or elongation. These techniques are described thoroughly in a number physical therapy sources (refer to Chapters 8 to 23).

Definitions/differentation

Casting can be categorized into the following four types:

1. *Conventional casting* uses material, such as plaster or fiberglass, applied to various body parts to repair osseous or ligamentous tissue. Such casts inhibit motion in the injured part, allowing it to heal. The normal time of cast application is 4 to 6 or more weeks.

2. *Serial casting* uses one or more well-padded plaster or fiberglass casts to increase or occasionally decrease range of motion over a period of time. The body part is taken to the end of the available range, then the area is decreased a few degrees and the cast is applied for 7 to 10 days. At the end of this period, the cast is removed and the process is repeated, with an increase or decrease in the range of motion.

3. *Inhibitory casting* uses casting material applied with specific techniques that attempt to reduce muscle tone and alter range of motion.

4. *Facilitory casting* uses casting materials applied with techniques that increase muscle tone in a specific group and increase or decrease a specific range of motion.

These cast types can be used in an interactive manner. Facilitory and inhibitory techniques, for example, can be used within the same cast. When such techniques are performed repetitively, they move into the category of serial casting.

Facilitory or inhibitory casting techniques, by this author's definition, use casts with minimal padding and for a duration of 48 hours only. The most significant feature of facilitory or inhibitory casting techniques is their subtlety. With minimal padding present, forces must be gentle and pressures on the tissue must be evenly distributed. Use of forces that are too harsh may result in skin breakdown.

If one assumes that imprinting the central nervous system occurs through consistent repetitive input, then facilitation or inhibition techniques that produce desired results during a treatment session can produce dramatic results when applied for prolonged periods of time (48 hours). For a more detailed discussion of this concept, the reader is referred to Chapter 2.

To effectively use facilitory or inhibitory casting techniques, the following procedures must be strictly followed. The patient must be handled before attempting casting so the therapist can clearly identify exactly which techniques elicit a response from the patient's central nervous system. For example, if the person responds to deep tendon pressure, then that technique may well be used in the cast. However, if traction, compression, rotation, or elongation—or any combination of these techniques—seem to have little effect and do not produce a desired outcome, then those techniques will be of little value if applied for the prolonged period of time.

The client to be put in a cast, the family or support system, and any health care provider who will come in contact with the client during the casting period must be well informed regarding specifics of the technique. A well-informed team will undoubtedly enhance the client's chances of having a successful experience with the cast.

The following indications must be clearly defined for those involved in the casting process:

1. Desired increase in range of motion
2. Desired decrease in range of motion
3. Desired increase in muscle tone
4. Desired decrease in muscle tone
5. Desired rebias of muscle spindle
6. Desired provision of a more normal sensory or motor input to elicit a more normal motor response

Contraindications to this technique (in the author's perception) include the following:

1. Uninformed support systems
2. Open wounds
3. Heterotopic bone as evidenced by a solid end feel

Special caution should be taken with a sensory-impaired limb resulting from circulatory problems or diabetes. This is clearly a consideration, although not necessarily a contraindication.

Technique

The casting procedure involves two therapists, one working as the "holder" and the other as the "caster." The two work together to prepare the patient. The therapist who is more skilled in the facilitation or inhibition techniques, or who has a better mastery of the central nervous system techniques, is assigned the task of the holder. The therapist with lesser skills in the facilitation/inhibition arena is given the task of the caster. The caster applies the plaster or fiberglass while the holder facilitates or inhibits those responses previously determined by handling the patient clinically.

Once the roles of holder and caster have been established, the following technique can be performed. A single layer of cotton stockinette is rolled over the extremity to be casted. Enough material is applied to allow a 4- to 6-inch end proximal and distal to the proposed cast trimlines. Cast padding is wrapped circumferentially at the proximal and distal points where the cast is to be terminated. Various pads, such as metatarsal or scaphoid pads or pads that have been cut earlier, are applied in specific areas. One thickness of cast padding is placed over bony prominences. After this, a second layer of stockinette is applied to cover all padding as well as the first layer of stockinette. A length of surgical tubing is now applied to the extremity to make a channel for cast removal. The surgical tubing should extend approximately 3 inches past the point where the cast will end. It is positioned to encourage easy cast removal. Three layers of elastic plaster are now applied distally to proximally, with the caster using no excess tension and simply unrolling the elastic plaster onto the extremity or body part. Ridging or causing a gapping around the tubing must be avoided because this creates a pressure area under the tubing. Once the elastic plaster has been applied, three layers of standard plaster are added for reinforcement. It is crucial that the holder apply the predetermined facilitory or inhibitory technique while the plaster is still wet. Once the casting material has hardened, which usually takes 5 to 8 minutes, the caster turns down the excess length of surgical tubing, turns the excess stockinette back onto the cast, and then tapes the loose ends in place. As a rule, the author pulls an additional piece of stockinette over the entire cast to keep any plaster from scratching or harming the client. If possible, weight bearing on the lower-extremity casts should be avoided for the 48 hours. In addition, the therapist should inspect exposed portions of extremities to ensure that circulation is adequate and swelling has not occurred. If swelling or discoloration becomes a problem, the cast should be removed immediately by simply pulling the surgical tubing from the cast and using cast scissors to cut and remove the cast. As a rule, the author does not use mechanical cast saws, because of the negative auditory and vibratory stimulation to the client. The cast is allowed to remain intact for 48 hours. If no problems have arisen at the end of that time, it is removed and the situation is assessed. If appropriate, a second cast may be applied, but this is generally not necessary. When the cast is removed, appropriate splinting should be provided to avoid loss of the desired result until the client is properly instructed in harnessing the newfound tone, range, or motor response.

Therapists using this technique must take care to avoid the possibility of unwanted motion within the cast. A cast may piston or slide up and down if it is applied to a cylindrical body part with no appropriate purchase. The purchase can be obtained with the elastic plaster by gently molding the plaster to the body part. If the limb is particularly conicular, then harnessing can be wrapped into the cast, such as figure-of-eight harnessing for the shoulder or waist-belt type harnessing for the lower extremity. If the upper extremity is to be casted and the hand allowed to be free, it is crucial the wrist opening be oval and not circular, which allows the extremity to rotate within it. Rotation within the cast will almost certainly cause chafing and skin breakdown. Pressures applied within the cast should be subtle: they should not exceed 4 psi (pounds per square inch).

Again, once the treating therapist has determined those techniques to which the client responds clinically, she or he can determine those which may realistically be incorporated into casting. Having established the techniques and applied the cast (after instructing the client, the family or support system, and the associated health care providers), the therapist must wait the given time period and ensure appropriate follow-up for harnessing the newly accomplished goal.

The limitations of this technique are created by the therapist's understanding of the spectrum of facilitation and inhibition techniques available. Thorough evaluation of the client, appropriate handling, and well-planned application of casts can greatly enhance established therapy treatment programs.

SUMMARY

This material has attempted to describe various concepts and options to be considered when evaluating the neurologically impaired client. Realizing that an orthosis can reinforce sound therapeutic exercise programs and introduce various neurological inputs to the CNS encourages physicians, therapists, and orthotists to add orthotic care to the list of treatments available to the neurologically impaired client.

REFERENCES

1. Brunnstrom S: Movement therapy in hemiplegia, New York, 1970, Harper & Row Publishers.
2. Lehneis HR: Principles of orthotic alignment in the lower extremity. In American Academy of Orthopaedic Surgeons, Instructional course lectures, vol 20, St Louis, 1971, The CV Mosby Co.
3. Pansky B and House E: Review of gross anatomy, New York, 1969, Macmillan, Inc.

ADDITIONAL READINGS

Adams R and Victor M: Principles of neurology, ed 2, New York, 1981, McGraw-Hill Book Co.
American Academy of Orthopaedic Surgeons: Atlas of orthotics: biomechanical principles and application, St Louis, 1975, The CV Mosby Co.
Bobath K and Bobath B: An analysis of the development of standing and walking patterns in patients with cerebral palsy, Physiotherapy June 1962.
Brunnstrom S: Clinical kinesiology, ed 3, Philadelphia, 1972, FA Davis Co.
Carpenter M and Sutin J: Human neuroanatomy, ed 8, Baltimore, 1983, Williams & Wilkins.
Cailliet R: Foot and ankle pain, Philadelphia, 1975, FA Davis Co.
Duncan WR: Tonic reflexes of the foot: their orthopedic significance in normal children and in children with cerebral palsy, J Bone Joint Surg 42A:859, July 1960.
Lehneis H and others: Energy expenditure with advanced lower limb orthoses and with conventional braces, Arch Phys Med Rehabil 57:20, 1976.
Prensky A and Palkes H: Care of the neurologically handicapped child, New York, 1982, Oxford University Press.
Redford J: Orthotics etcetera, ed 2, Baltimore, 1980, Williams & Wilkins.
Salek B: The significance of structural and functional development in the normal foot and therapeutic implications thereof in the child with neuromotor disorder", New York, 1977, Suffolk Rehabilitation Center.

Chapter 29

COLLABORATIVE NURSING THERAPIES FOR CLIENTS WITH NEUROLOGICAL DYSFUNCTION

Marilyn Pires and Margaret Kelly-Hayes

OVERVIEW OF NURSING PRACTICE

Recent medical and technological advances in diagnoses, treatments, and rehabilitation bring to the health professional an ever-expanding population living with chronic illness. The needs of this population have greatly impacted on all health disciplines providing treatment and care, especially nursing.

Nursing addresses itself to a wide range of health-related problems observed in both well and sick persons. It is part of a helping service dedicated to the prevention and treatment of illness. Nurses are directly involved in client care and treatment, and they also provide advice, guidance, and supervision.

Nursing practice includes, but is not limited to, teaching, administration, evaluation of practice, and the execution of prescribed regimens. As early as 1860 Florence Nightingale[11] defined nursing as the everyday practice of providing food, light, bedding, and the interpersonal aspects of understanding the psychosocial needs. She emphasized that nurses help the sick and the well to perform activities that contribute to health and recovery. Today we know nursing as a dynamic profession involved in the promotion of wellness, the prevention of illness, and the rehabilitation of the disabled. Nursing is the diagnosis and treatment of human responses to actual or potential health problems.[18]

Nursing diagnoses

Nurses function from a theoretical framework, based on scientific knowledge, research, and nursing diagnoses. Nursing diagnoses (see Appendix A), as the basis for defining health problems, have evolved over the past several years. Nursing diagnoses, or clinical diagnoses made by nurses, describe health problems that nurses, by virtue of their education and experience, are capable and licensed to treat.[15] The term *diagnosis* refers both to a category name for a health problem and to a process of dealing with the problem. The purpose of nursing diagnosis is to establish a nomenclature for describing nursing approaches and solutions. As in other health disciplines, nursing, through its framework, standardizes the process of collecting data, identifying the nursing needs, planning the nursing action, implementing the plan, and evaluating its effectiveness.

In the medical model the focus of care is on pathology, diagnosis, and treatment. In the nursing model the focus of care is directed toward the human response to personal or environmental stressors, with treatment aimed at the cause of response and the conditions influencing it. For example, a client confined to bed rest can develop a problem with incomplete or infrequent bowel evacuation. The nursing diagnosis category would be constipation. The assessment factors would include premorbid elimination history, evaluation of gastrointestinal pathology, and current nutrition status. Interventions would involve enhancing natural physiological mechanisms, modifying diet, and possibly using cathartics. Nursing diagnosis is the nucleus for focusing client care and assessing real or potential health needs. This is demonstrated later in the chapter.

Setting for nursing practice

Nursing practice takes place in a variety of settings. The setting and the type of health problems dictate the focus of the nursing care and treatment. In the acute care hospital nurses most often provide support and care of those who are rendered dependent by an acute health problem. Nurses monitor critical changes, carry out treatments, and perform techniques to prevent complications secondary to the disease. They participate in the diagnostic workup of clients by assisting in procedures and in client monitoring. Nurses care for the clients undergoing surgical and medical treatment and are involved in discharge coordination. In an illness such as stroke, nurses provide care to support necessary physiological functions during the crisis, participate in the rehabilitation team's efforts to minimize complications, and work collaboratively with team members toward meeting designated rehabilitation goals. It is within the realm of nursing practice to be vigilant in protecting the individual client from the adverse side effects that could result from prescribed treatment such as anticoagulation or bed rest. In the recovery phase of an illness, nurses, in cooperation with other health team members, are responsible for promoting health by assisting the individual in performing activities of daily living and by working with the families in giving guidance and support.

In a rehabilitation center nursing changes its goals from a cure orientation to adaptation. The adaptation process involves redefining and redirecting an individual within the capacity of the disability. Nurses function in the rehabilitation setting by providing direct care and assistance, teaching, and counseling.

In outpatient departments nurses are seen as coordinators, teachers, and health care providers and are often the major link between hospital care and community maintenance programs. Nurses deal with clients on a variety of levels. Their first responsibility is the screening and early detection of potential risk for medical problems. During health assessment screening, the nurse is able to identify those areas for possible intervention. In addition to screening and prevention, nurses are involved on an outpatient basis with the performance of direct client care, such as medication administration or adjustment, education regarding medications, and evaluation of need for intervention by other allied health professionals.

In the community the focus of nursing is primarily on the maintenance of individuals in their own environments by providing whatever support and services are needed to reach this goal. The goal for the majority of chronically ill clients is to maintain themselves in the home setting whenever possible. For example, individuals undergoing treatment for cancer are no longer hospitalized throughout the procedure but can be maintained at home through the resources provided by the community nursing agencies. Nurses in the community see clients for specific technical treatments, such as dressing changes and intravenous therapy. They also perform more subtle interventions, such as helping families to cope with catastrophic illness. The general goal in nursing, whatever the setting, is to facilitate the individual's progress from a dependent to an interdependent and, ultimately, to an independent state.

Rehabilitation nursing

Rehabilitation nursing is a specialty practice within the profession. Rehabilitation nurses diagnose and treat the human responses of individuals and groups to an actual or potential disability that interrupts or alters function and life satisfaction. The goal of rehabilitation nursing is to assist the individual or group in the restoration of maximal health.[14] It is practiced in all health care settings. Under the broad definition of nursing, rehabilitation nursing focuses primarily on a body of knowledge and specialized techniques and processes that address adaptation and restoration of maximum function for those individuals who sustain a disability.

The premise of rehabilitation nursing is that rehabilitation is a process of restoring and maintaining a client at optimal physiological, psychological, vocational, and social functioning. The rehabilitation nurse, like other rehabilitation professionals, adopts a creative, problem-solving approach to disability and establishes a plan of care that encourages active partnership with the client. Interventions are purposeful, pragmatic, and functionally oriented. The goals of rehabilitation nursing are to provide a supportive environment that facilitates independence and to reinforce and integrate teaching that is provided by all disciplines.

The rehabilitation nurse identifies coordination of care among the various rehabilitation team members as a high priority and major responsibility. The goal is to prepare the individual to return to a functional role within the family and community. Assessment of the client is paramount in designing care strategies. The process of providing rehabilitative nursing care requires that the nurse know when to assist the client and when to foster or allow independence toward the achievement of rehabilitation objectives. Rehabilitation nurses view health not merely as an absence of disease symptoms but rather as a unity of all aspects of an individual, including the mind, body, and spirit.

Rehabilitation nurses address two basic concerns: prevention and restoration. Prevention is maintaining function to avoid deterioration of an unafflicted organ or system or further injury to an already affected part. It is a continuous part of care for anyone who has a chronic illness. Restoration, on the other hand, entails using those specific knowledge-based practices that are part of the process of bringing an individual to his or her highest functional potential.

In the selected nursing diagnoses addressed later in this chapter, the specific theory and treatments are defined. Not only is the need for restoration techniques described but also, and equally important, the impact of complications in the entire rehabilitation process is examined. Nurses recognize their responsibility to facilitate clients' attainment of their health goals, to communicate with team members, and to bring together those special services that bring unity to the whole rehabilitation process.

There are several theories on which rehabilitation nurses base their model of practice. One contributor to rehabilitation nursing practice is Dorothea Orem. Orem[16] stated that candidates for nursing treatment are those with deficits between their current or projected capabilities and the qualitative and quantitative demand for care. The reason for the deficit relationship between care capabilities and care demands is the state of health. Other nursing theories believe that nursing should focus on adaptation and the continuous balance between health and illness.

Through a coordinated effort of all members of the rehabilitation team, including nursing, clients can identify the skills necessary to affect change and refocus their potential within their disability. The goal of all health providers should be to maximize the individual's potential through collaboration and clinical actions.

SELECTED NURSING DIAGNOSES: APPLICATION TO NEUROLOGICAL DISORDERS

The ever-expanding population of clients with chronic neurological diseases poses a challenge to health care providers to give appropriate and cost-efficient care. To accomplish this, providers need to work from a knowledge base about the disability involved in specific disorders. In many instances the degree of morbidity is difficult to document because data are not quantitative but are more the client's own perception of the illness. In addition, certain disabilities can be identified as having a detrimental effect on a person's ability to interact within the environment. In evaluating the client's ability to perform, the nurse examines not only the disability but also the environment in which the client is located.

In conjunction with other health care professionals, nurses attempt to identify measures of performance level and functional capacities that can be used as indicators of the appropriateness and effectiveness of the health care provided. The problem of disability is a complex one, with a large number of client disease variables and few widely measured outcomes. There are a number of currently validated functional assessment measurements in use today in

rehabilitation practice.[6] These tools provide a framework for orderly review of those systems important to the fulfillment of social roles and for a satisfactory quality of life. They also provide a taxonomy of functional limitations and abilities related to personal well-being. Functional assessment is made up of three major subdivisions: self-care, mobility, and bowel and bladder function.

A major goal of this chapter is to present selected nursing diagnoses that are applicable to the coordinated care of the client with neurological dysfunction. If the client is to benefit from the total rehabilitation process, it is necessary for therapists to collaborate with rehabilitation nurses in addressing each of these issues. Therapists need to be cognizant of the nursing care plan for each nursing diagnosis to ensure that the plan is integrated into the client's therapeutic day.[15] It is equally necessary for nurses to work collaboratively with the therapists to ensure that the skills the client learns in therapy are integrated into the client's 24-hour activities of daily living.

Under the category of functional limitations, we will address the following areas: neurogenic bladder dysfunction, neurogenic bowel dysfunction, impairment of skin integrity, sexual dysfunction, and self-care deficits.

Altered pattern of urinary elimination: neurogenic bladder dysfunction

Neurogenic bladder dysfunction is a significant consideration in the rehabilitation of the client with neurological disability. No matter how successful the treatment of other neurological dysfunctions, unaddressed continued bladder dysfunction could inhibit the client from reentering the community and/or could contribute to life-threatening complications.

Anatomy and neuroanatomy of the bladder. The bladder functions as a contractile musculomembranous reservoir for urine, which is produced in the kidneys, collected in the kidney pelvis, and passed to the bladder by the ureters. The internal surface of the bladder consists of mucosa. The bladder wall is composed of intricate bundles of smooth muscle fibers arranged in longitudinal, circular, and oblique layers called the detrusor muscle. The detrusor is innervated by parasympathetic nerves. The internal vesical sphincter cannot be considered a true sphincter because it is not a distinct circular band of muscle fibers. The internal "sphincter" is responsible for urinary minute-to-minute continence. This area of the bladder neck is innervated by alpha-sympathetic nerves and is normally in a constant state of alpha-sympathetic tonicity, which is inhibited during micturation. The external urethral sphincter is composed of striated muscle and is under voluntary control. It is innervated by the pudendal somatic nerve. The external sphincter is responsible for preserving continence during periods of increased bladder fullness or during stress.

Neurological control of the bladder is somewhat complicated. Within the CNS areas of the cerebrum, cerebellum, and subcortical nuclei contribute to the act of micturation. It is believed that input from these areas comes together at the pontine mesencephalic reticular formation. The input then travels along the corticoregulatory tract within the reticulospinal tract in the spinal cord and ends at the intermediolateral cell column of the sacral gray matter spinal micturation center. This is the point where higher centers may influence outflow to both parasympathetic bladder innervation and somatic sphincter innervation.[10]

The peripheral nervous system control of the lower urinary tract is more defined. Parasympathetic input to the detrusor arises from parasympathetic outflow of sacral segments 2 through 4 and passes via the pelvic nerve and nervi erigentes to the bladder. The pelvic nerve also carries sensory fibers from the bladder that communicate the sensation of fullness, pain, and temperature.[2] Sympathetic nerves supply the internal sphincter region of the bladder neck. These nerves arise from the thoracolumbar sympathetic outflow of the spinal cord and are carried via the hypogastric and presacral nerves. The somatic motor nerves supply the external sphincter and perineal muscles via the pudendal nerves. These fibers arise from the sacral segments 2 through 4.

Physiology of voiding. The physiology of voiding is basically centered in the simple reflex reaction between the bladder and the spinal cord. The bladder distends to a capacity of approximately 400 ml; at that point sensations of fullness are transmitted to the sacral cord. If voluntary cerebral control is lacking, such as in infants, the efferent side of the reflex arc discharges and spontaneous involuntary voiding occurs. As myelination progresses, cerebral inhibitory function suppresses the sacral reflex, allowing voiding to become a voluntary function. In essence, then, normal micturation is initiated by voluntary suppression of cerebral inhibition.

Classification of neurogenic bladder dysfunction. Classification of neurogenic bladder is based on location of the neurological lesion and its involvement of motor and/or sensory tracts (see Table 29-1). The bladder program initiated must be specific to the type of bladder dysfunction, taking advantage of residual function. For instance, stimulating reflex voiding in a client with a reflex neurogenic bladder can be done by providing sensory stimulation to the S2 through S4 dermatomes.

Management of neurogenic bladder dysfunction. The objectives of a bladder management program should include the following: (1) achievement of balanced bladder functioning so that the bladder consistently empties safely, effectively, and completely; (2) the prevention of complications; (3) achievement of a controlled pattern of elimination; (4) involvement of the least amount of time, expense, and assistance of other people; and (5) active involvement and understanding of the client and family.[5]

The two most common bladder training management programs are a timed voiding program and intermittent catheterization. A timed voiding program is indicated in clients with uninhibited neurogenic bladder or sensory paralytic bladder without residual urine. The goal of this program is to control and/or eventually eliminate urinary incontinence. The program consists of observing for timing of incontinent episodes for 2 to 3 days in order to assess the client's voiding pattern. The post-void residual volume is checked during this period to make certain it is within acceptable limits. The client's fluid intake pattern is then correlated with the voiding pattern. A voiding schedule is then established at periodic intervals. Preferably, the bathroom or the bedside commode should be used for these trials. Men should stand if possible to reinforce their preonset cues for the act of voiding. The scheduled voidings are readjusted as incontinence diminishes. Fluid intake can be titrated with the voiding pattern to further curb incontinence. It is often helpful to restrict fluid late in the evening to control nocturia and enuresis. It is important that the therapist and the nurse communicate and coordinate the client's schedule to facilitate the client getting maximum benefit from both the voiding program and therapy time. The therapist should be aware of the voiding program to (1) assist with the fluid intake schedule, (2) reinforce voiding cues, and (3) avoid client embarrassment resulting from unnecessary incontinence during therapy.

An intermittent catheterization program is indicated in clients with reflex neurogenic bladders or sensory paralytic bladders with residual urine. The goals of an intermittent catheterization program are to (1) ensure bladder emptying on a regular basis to avoid urinary tract infections, (2) establish a pattern of filling and emptying that can stimulate the reflex neurogenic bladder to empty itself, and (3) provide the opportunity to regain as much function as possible by avoiding an indwelling catheter. The program consists of restricting fluid intake to produce urine volumes between 300 and 500 ml per scheduled catheterization. A 24-hour intake of 2000 to 2400 ml will usually provide the appropriate volumes. An initial catheterization schedule of every 4 hours will usually avoid bladder distention. Again, by restricting fluids late in the evening, a catheterization in the middle of the night can be avoided. By keeping a record of urine volumes voided and residual urine volumes, catheterization times can be adjusted. The number of catherizations can be decreased as the residual urine volumes remain consistently below 100 ml, or 10% of bladder capacity. Catheterizations at those specific times can be eliminated or intervals between catheterizations can be expanded to meet the client's needs.

Before each catheterization one of the following bladder stimulation techniques should be utilized depending on the type of neurogenic bladder the client has. Clients with autonomous neurogenic, motor paralytic, and sensory paralytic bladders are candidates for using the Credé maneuver or the Valsalva maneuver as long as they have no docu-

Table 29-1. Classification of neurogenic bladder dysfunction

Bladder function	Level in neuraxis	Possible etiology	Upper motor neuron lesion	Lower motor neuron lesion	Sensory loss	Saddle sensation	Bulbo-cavernous reflex	Bladder behavior	Voiding pattern	Urinary incontinence
Uninhibited neurogenic	Cortical and subcortical	Newborn child, CVA, MS, cerebral arteriosclerosis, brain tumor, pernicious anemia, trauma	+	0	0	Normal	Normal	Capacity: reduced (to 100-400 ml)	Urinary frequency, urgency, nocturia	Present (of the "urge" type)
Reflex neurogenic	Spinal cord above conus medullaris	Trauma, tumor vascular disease, MS, syringomyelia, pernicious anemia	+	0	+	Impaired or absent	Hyperactive	Capacity: reduced (to 50-300 ml) Residual: elevated (to 50-200 ml)	Precipitous, involuntary, infrequent, interrupted and in small amounts	Present, marked (of the reflex type)
Autonomous (nonreflex) neurogenic	Conus medullaris or cauda equina	Spina bifida, myelomeningocele, tumor, postoperative radical pelvic surgery, herniated intervertebral disc	0	+	+	Impaired or absent	Absent	Capacity: normal or elevated (to 400-1000 ml) Residual: normal or elevated (to 0-800 ml)	Infrequent and with straining or compression	Present (may be of the overflow, stress, or continuous type)
Motor paralytic	Anterior horn cells or S2, S3, S4 ventral roots	Poliomyelitis, herniated intervertebral disc, trauma, tumor	0	+	0	Normal	Absent	Capacity: elevated (to 600-1200 ml) Residual: elevated (to 100-500 ml)	Similar to patients with symptoms of "prostatism" strain to void	Occasional (of the overflow type)
Sensory paralytic	S2, S3, S4 dorsal roots or cells of origin or dorsal horns of spinal cord	Diabetes mellitus, tabes dorsalis	0	0	+	Variable	Present	Capacity: elevated (to 800-1500 ml) Residual: elevated (to 200-1000 ml)	Only 1-3 times daily	Occasional (of the overflow type)

Adapted from Staas WE Jr and DeNault PM: Am Fam Physician 7:1, 1973.

mented bladder outlet obstruction, sphincter spasticity, or evidence of reflux. The Credé maneuver consists of placing one hand just below the umbilical area, then placing the other hand on top of it and firmly pressing downward and inward toward the pubic arch. The Valsalva maneuver consists of contracting the abdominal muscles, if possible, and holding one's breath while straining or "bearing down." These two techniques work by increasing intervesical pressure either manually (the Credé maneuver) or muscularly (the Valsalva maneuver) sufficiently to overcome closure of the external sphincter. Clients with a reflex neurogenic bladder are candidates for reflex stimulation techniques. These techniques include tapping over the suprapubic area, stimulation of the perineal area, stroking the medial thigh along the adductor magnus muscle, pinching the abdomen above the inguinal ligaments, pulling the pubic hair, and using the anal stretch maneuver. These techniques work by providing sensory input at the S2, S3, and S4 dermatomes and by triggering facilitation of the voiding reflex.

Intermittent catheterization is usually initiated in the hospital using sterile techniques to minimize the danger of nosocomial infections by virulent organisms. If intermittent catheterization is to be used as the long-term management technique for chronic neurogenic bladder, the client and/or family are often taught clean catheterization technique to be used after discharge. The advantages of clean technique are that it is simple and less expensive.

If the above bladder training techniques are not successful, they can be augmented by pharmacological therapy first and then surgical intervention if complete bladder emptying remains a problem. Some surgeries that might be helpful are a sphincterotomy, an incision into the external urinary sphincter, or a transurethral resection of the bladder neck. Urinary diversion, ileal conduit, or externalizing the ureters to bypass the urinary bladder is not a treatment of choice and should be considered as a last resort only after all other interventions have been tried and/or the client is experiencing severe health-threatening complications.

The goal of a bladder training program is to achieve a safe, catheter-free state while controlling incontinence. This goal is often possible in men with neurogenic bladders, since reflex voiding in reflex neurogenic bladder and a possible overflow incontinence in the autonomous neurogenic bladder can be managed by using an external urine-collection system. The female client, however, has fewer options for dealing with the incontinence that results from successful reflex voiding or overflow. Presently there are several newly designed external urine collection devices for women. None, however, have yet proven to be universally effective. Women will often elect to use either an indwelling catheter if incontinence continues between timed voidings or intermittent catheterization with pharmacological therapy.

There is a medical emergency exclusively associated with spinal cord injuries. This emergency is known as autonomic dysreflexia or hyperreflexia (see Appendix B).

Bowel incontinence: neurogenic bowel dysfunction

Just as neurogenic bladder dysfunction is a significant consideration in the total rehabilitation of the client with neurological disability, neurogenic bowel dysfunction resulting in fecal incontinence can negate all other rehabilitation efforts by keeping the client from reentering the community. Loss of bowel control is an emotionally ladened issue that can potentially prevent the client from participating in the rehabilitation program. Establishing the appropriate bowel program for the client will very often give him or her the confidence needed to take full advantage of the rehabilitation efforts offered by the entire health care team.

Function of the alimentary tract. The function of the alimentary tract is to supply the body with water, electrolytes, and nutrients. The specific functions of the colon are absorption of water and electrolytes from the waste products and the storage of fecal matter until it can be expelled. The proximal half of the colon is concerned principally with absorption and the distal half is concerned with storage. Motor function is divided into tonic contraction of the pyloric, ileocecal, and anal sphincters regulating movement of food within the gut. In addition, it regulates rhythmic contractions to mix the food and peristaltic propulsion to push food through the tract.

The gut is innervated by the intramural plexus beginning in the esophageal wall and extending to the anus. This consists of two layers of neurons: the outer layer (myenteric plexus) and the inner layer (submucosal plexus). The myenteric plexus is mainly motor in function and more extensive than the submucosal plexus, which is mainly sensory. The submucosal plexus receives signals from the gut epithelium and from stretch receptors in the gut wall. Stimulation of the myenteric plexus generally increases the activity of the gut by causing increased tonic contractions or tone of the gut wall, increased intensity of rhythmical contractions, increased rate of rhythmical contractions, and increased velocity of conduction of excitatory waves along the gut wall. The intramural plexus, including both the sensory submucosal plexus and the motor myenteric plexus, is responsible for many of the neurogenic reflexes that occur locally in the gut.[8] Bowel training programs take advantage of these facts by using suppositories to stimulate these nerve endings, which causes an increase in peristalsis.

The gastrointestinal tract has extensive parasympathetic and sympathetic innervation that is capable of altering the overall activity of the entire tract or specific parts of it. Parasympathetic innervation is divided into cranial and sacral divisions. The cranial parasympathetic supply is transmitted almost entirely via the vagus nerve innervating the esophagus and stomach and, to a lesser extent, the small intestine, gall bladder, and proximal colon. The sacral parasympathetic supply originates in S2, S3, and S4 and passes through the nervi erigentes to the distal half of the large intestine. These fibers are especially important in the defecation reflex. The sympathetic supply of the gastrointestinal tract originates between T8 and L3. In most instances stimulation in the sympathetic system inhibits activity in the gastrointestinal tract. In two instances, however, the sympathetic system elicits an excitatory effect on the ileocecal sphincter and the internal anal sphincter. The combined effect of sympathetic stimulation can totally block movement of food through the gastrointestinal tract by inhibition of the gut wall and excitation of two major sphincters. Afferent fibers have their cell bodies in the submucosal plexus and extend to the myenteric plexus. These nerve endings can be stimulated by irritation of the mucosa, excessive distention, and presence of specific chemicals.[8]

Peristalsis is a basic characteristic of all tubular smooth muscle structures. The usual stimulus for peristalsis is distention. As peristaltic waves push food through the gastrointestinal tract, nutrients are absorbed. By the time it reaches the distal portion of the small intestine, only solid waste and water remain. The ileocecal valve is located at the junction between the small intestine and the colon. Its main function is to prevent backflow of fecal contents from the colon to small intestine. Once fecal material reaches the colon, the absorption of water and electrolytes is accomplished by mixing movements of the colon wall called haustrations. As the fecal material becomes more solid in consistency, it is propelled in the distal colon toward the anus by mass movements. These mass movements differ from peristaltic waves higher in the gastrointestinal tract in that they occur only a few times a day. They are most abundant for 15 minutes during the first hour after breakfast, but they do occur after every meal. The mass movements are initiated partially by the gastrocolic and duodenocolic reflexes. These reflexes result from the distention of the stomach and duodenum that accompanies a meal. Mass movements can also be initiated by overdistention of a segment of the colon.[8]

Defecation reflex. When a mass movement forces feces into the rectum, the defecation reflex is initiated and proceeds as follows: distention of the rectal wall initiates afferent signals that spread through the myenteric plexus to initiate reflex peristaltic waves in the descending colon and sigmoid colon, forcing feces toward the rectum. As peristaltic waves approach the anus, the internal anal sphincter is inhibited, causing relaxation. If the external anal sphincter is relaxed, defecation will occur. The external anal sphincter is composed of striated voluntary muscle and is controlled by the somatic nervous system. Voluntary constriction of the external anal sphincter can overcome the defecation reflex, thus giving the individual control over evacuation. The defecation reflex can be enhanced by us-

ing reflexes in the sacral spinal cord. When afferent fibers in the rectum are stimulated, signals are transmitted into the spinal cord and reflexly back to the descending colon, sigmoid colon, rectum, and anus via the parasympathetic nerve fibers in the nervi erigentes. These signals intensify the peristaltic waves, which can be further intensified by performing a Valsalva maneuver.[8] In cooperation with the nurse, the therapist might be very helpful in assessing the client's ability to perform a Valsalva maneuver and teaching and reinforcing the maneuver in therapy.

Classification of bowel dysfunction. The goal of a bowel program is to establish a planned, predictable defecation pattern that is individualized to the client's needs and neurogenic dysfunction. Specifics appear in Table 29-2.

Management of altered elimination patterns. Factors other than the specific neurogenic bowel dysfunction that must be assessed, altered, and/or compensated for include physical exercise; fluid intake, high-fiber foods, and a consistent habit time. An example of a nursing care standard for the person at risk for alteration in fecal elimination pattern is presented in Appendix C.[4] The therapist can contribute greatly to the success of a bowel program by working on improved sitting balance and toilet transfer activities to facilitate the physiologically most optimal position for defecation.

Impaired skin integrity

No other complication of neurological dysfunction is as potentially preventable, as difficult to manage, or as much of a deterent to the rehabilitation of the client and general well-being as loss of skin integrity. The process of skin breakdown is both fast and insidious.[19] All disciplines involved in the care of clients with neurological disability must share in the responsibility of establishing and maintaining a vigilant program to prevent soft tissue damage.

Functions of the skin. Intact skin is the body's first line of defense. The skin protects underlying structures and tissue from loss of water and from the effects of radiant rays and other agents in the environment, and it prevents the entrance of harmful chemicals and organisms. Skin is the body organ in direct contact with the external environment; therefore it is important in the regulation of body temperature. It also contains the afferent receptors for appreciating the sensory modalities of heat, cold, touch, pressure, and pain that assist in the protective function of the skin. Skin is also a secretory organ. The secretion of water by sweat glands aids in temperature regulation, and the sebum secreted by sebaceous glands assists in maintaining suppleness of the skin and its water content.[3]

Pathogenesis of skin breakdown. Any condition that exerts pressure on the skin and thus underlying blood vessels is capable of limiting the capacity to deliver blood. For skin to remain healthy, there must be a free flow of nutrients to the cells and removal of waste products from

Table 29-2. Classification of neurogenic bowel dysfunction

Bowel function	Level in neuraxis	Possible etiology	Upper motor neuron lesion	Lower motor neuron lesion	Sensory loss	Saddle sensation	Bulbocavernous reflex	Fecal incontinence
Uninhibited neurogenic	Cortical and subcortical	CVA, MS, brain tumors, brain trauma	+	0	0	Normal	Normal or increased	Present—associated with sudden urge
Reflex neurogenic	Spinal cord above conus medularis	Trauma, tumor, vascular disease MS, syringomyelia, pernicious anemia	+	0	+	Diminished or absent	Increased	Present—occurs without warning or during reflex
Autonomous (nonreflex) neurogenic	Conus medullaris or cauda equina	Spina bifida, trauma, tumor, intervertebral disc	0	+	+	Diminished or absent	0	Present—may be continuous or may occur during stress
Motor paralytic	Anterior horn cells or S2, S3, S4 roots (ventral)	Poliomyelitis, intervertebral disc, trauma, tumor	0	+	0	Normal	0	Rare, except in widespread disease
Sensory paralytic	S2, S3, S4 roots (dorsal), cells of origin or dorsal horns of spinal cord	Diabetes mellitus, tabes dorsalis	0	0	+	Diminished or absent	Normal, decreased or absent	Rare except in advanced stages

From Staas WE Jr and DeNault PM: Bowel control, Am Fam Physician 7:1, 1973.

the cells. Normal capillary pressure ranges from 16 to 32 mm Hg. When pressure exceeds the level of capillary closure, 30 mm Hg, blood flow is restricted.[3] "Protracted pressure in excess of capillary pressure over bony areas will produce ischemia of skin and underlying tissues. The amount and duration of the pressure exerted are significant determinants of the degree of ischemia and resultant cellular necrosis."[9]

When the pressure over a skin surface exceeds 30 mm Hg, such as between a bony prominence and a mattress or wheelchair cushion, the blood is squeezed out and further blood flow is blocked. This pressure causes the skin under that area to blanch because of ischemic pallor. It is a normal body protective response to increase blood flow to the ischemic area for a short time. After flow has been blocked and the blood returns, the area will turn bright red; this response is known as reactive hyperemia. Reac-

tive hyperemia lasts a few seconds to a few minutes. This reaction provides the client and caregivers with landmarks that can be used to monitor prolonged pressure and thus skin breakdown over vulnerable skin surfaces.[13]

Skin breakdown proceeds through four distinct stages.[12]

Stage I is the least severe stage and is marked by a reddened area of the skin, reactive hyperemia, which is observed for 15 minutes or longer after the pressure has been relieved over the area. In black-skinned clients the skin will have a subtle purplish hue. Beneath the abnormal coloration, the skin will feel warmer and firmer to the touch because of local edema.

Stage II represents deeper involvement and is marked by the presence of blisters or small breaks through the dermis. The abnormal coloration will be more pronounced than in Stage I. Swelling, heat, and firmness in and around the involved area will be present. Pain is associated with

Stage II involvement if the client has intact sensation. Once the skin is broken, the client is susceptible to infection.

Stage III involves the deeper, subcutaneous, fatty tissue layer beneath the dermis. This stage is marked by an opening in the skin. The opening may be covered by a black, leathery crust, eschar. The necrotic tissue below the eschar provides an environment conducive to the growth of bacteria. The wound edges may be discolored, appearing reddened, bluish, or white, and the entire area may feel warmer and firmer to the touch. These signs indicate that edema is present. Edema contributes further to skin breakdown.

Stage IV penetrates through all soft tissue layers between the skin and the bone. After the eschar and necrotic tissue have been removed, it is evident that besides subcutaneous and dermal tissue, muscle and possibly bone have been destroyed. This stage is very often associated with systemic toxicity, dehydration, and anemia. This stage can be life threatening.[13]

Once the skin is broken, the client may require nursing, medical, and possibly surgical treatment depending on the stage. These clients should be referred immediately to appropriate treatment facilities such as their private physician, a follow-up clinic for clients with their particular neurological dysfunction, or, if needed, a hospital emergency room.

It is incumbent on all health care providers to be knowledgeable about pressure and shearing forces as primary factors in the etiology of skin breakdown. Shearing forces are forces that pull tissue rather than press on it. Shearing forces slide one layer of tissue over another. The shearing motion stretches the soft tissue between the bony prominence and the skin, causing some blood vessels to get caught in the stretching. This force can occlude blood flow or tear tissue, causing ischemic damage to the skin.[13] Therapists have an important role to play in minimizing shearing forces by teaching and assisting the client in proper sitting posture, bed mobility, and transfer techniques.

Therapists must also be able to identify secondary factors that contribute to their particular client's risk for loss of skin integrity. Secondary factors include malnutrition, anemia, sepsis, sensory loss, senile dementia or other changes in mental status, paralysis, spasm, and maceration from moisture caused by skin-on-skin contact, sweating, or incontinence.

Therapeutic interventions. Intervention in relation to maintaining skin integrity should revolve around prevention, through action to prevent pressure development and/or to relieve existing pressure. There are many protective devices available that minimize pressure to augment pressure relief maneuvers and position changes, which are the key to prevention of skin breakdown.

The therapist must be cognizant, at every contact with the neurologically disabled client, of the importance of using his or her assessment skills in observing for signs of Stage I skin destruction and taking corrective action as needed. More importantly, however, therapists must teach clients and/or their significant others to be equally vigilant in following a program to maintain skin integrity and be observant for early signs of skin breakdown. An example of nursing management for prevention of skin breakdown and maintenance of skin integrity is presented in Table 29-3.[5]

Sexual dysfunction

Many neurological disorders have a direct effect on the client's potential for sexual functioning. To effectively help the client with these problems, it is necessary to have a basic understanding of normal sexual functioning and the effects that neurological dysfunction may have on it. In addition, all professionals who are involved in the care of clients with neurological dysfunction must consider the elements of body image and self-concept as they might affect the client and or significant other's perception of the client as a sexual being.

Above all, however, each health care provider must examine his or her own comfort level with the many forms of sexual behavior. In addition to behaviors associated with traditional heterosexual patterns, it is important to address one's own feelings about alternative sexual patterns such as homosexuality and masturbation. Each therapist needs to understand his or her own values, attitudes, and skills in the area of sexuality before intervening with clients in regard to their sexuality.

Components of sexuality. "A) Sex (is) a biological drive. B) Sex acts (are) behaviors associated with but not limited to the genitals. This includes such behavior as touching, kissing and feeling, but does not include the person's psychosocial being. C) Sexuality (is) a complex concept involving a combination of sex, sex acts, and a person's psychosocial behavior that is concerned with presentation of self and relationships."[5]

Human sexual response cycle. The same sex response cycle occurs during masturbation and in both homosexual and heterosexual activity.

Male sexual response cycle. "There is only one clearly identified pattern in the male sexual response cycle. Variations are mainly related to duration rather than intensity of the response."[7] The cycle proceeds through the following four phases:

1. Excitement—penile erection; beginning scrotal elevation; increase in muscular tension and cardiopulmonary response.
2. Plateau—blood pressure and heart rate continue to rise.
3. Orgasmic—penile contraction and ejaculation; total body response involving involuntary muscular con-

Table 29-3. Nursing management for prevention of skin breakdown and maintenance of skin integrity

Principle	Nursing assessment	Rationale points of emphasis	Nursing actions	Rationale/points of emphasis
Prevent pressure development/relieve existing pressure	Inspect skin of patient twice daily—while bathing and during afternoon care	If problem areas are identified early, serious skin damage can be avoided	Relieve pressure by: Turning patient at least every 2 hours Teaching patient wheelchair pressure relief (e.g., push-ups and position changes)	Pressure on any area for more than 2 hours leads to ischemia and tissue damage
			Cushion wheelchair and bed surfaces (e.g., eggcrate, water mattress, flotation pads, "bridging" foam cushions)	Helps to distribute pressure and removes pressure from "pressure" points; decrease pressure sore risk by *omitting* pressure Do not use air-inflated rubber rings; this causes significant increase in pressure on all surfaces in contact with the ring
			Reduce shearing force by: Using pull sheets to move patient in bed and to turn	Sheet burns are caused by dragging patient across the bed sheets
			Decrease shearing by using nylon fitted bottom sheets Do not leave patient sitting in Fowler's position more than 2 hours	Patient slides down creating a shearing force and skin trauma
			Teach patient and family routine of skin inspection and care; use mirrors if necessary	Patient/family will be responsible upon discharge; habits taught, practiced, and reinforced may perpetuate
Remove hazards of immobility	Assess extent of patient immobility and sensation impairment	Consider whether the risks of immobility can be reduced by regular therapy	Teach patient about the threats of immobility	Be aware of the patient's level of awareness and education when teaching
			Teach principles and mechanisms of pressure relief Remove hazards until the patient can assume responsibility himself	Teaching must be individualized for each patient

From Core Curriculum Committee: Rehabilitation nursing: concepts and practice—a core curriculum, Evanston, Ill, 1981, Rehabilitation Nursing Institute.

Table 29-3. Nursing management for prevention of skin breakdown and maintenance of skin integrity—cont'd

Principle	Nursing assessment	Rationale points of emphasis	Nursing actions	Rationale/points of emphasis
Recognize neurological, vascular, psychological, and medical threats to skin integrity	Assess influence of these threats, on the patient's physical ability to maintain skin integrity	Pathological states predispose persons to skin breakdown	Perform nursing and medical interventions related to disease Educate the patient about his illness and how it affects physiological and psychological functioning	Teach by demonstration Important to promote and maintain optimal level of wellness to maintain skin integrity
Ensure adequate nutrition	Assess patient's overall nutritional intake Assess deficiencies in diet	Provides a base for developing a balanced, health-promoting diet	Consult with the patient when planning the diet Request dietary consultation when necessary	Basic diet should be high in protein and calories because a negative nitrogen balance will lead to catabolism of muscle and tissue structures
	Assess medical reasons for certain food group considerations	Important for planning diet	Develop a well-balanced diet	Promote nutritious, palatable diet to prevent a negative nitrogen balance
	Assess patient's food preferences	Patients will eat better if they like what they are served	Monitor patient's appetite	
Ensure adequate hydration	Assess patient's skin turgor	Renal and cardiac complications often prohibit increased fluid consumption	Encourage fluids when not contraindicated	Prevent decreased tissue support
	Assess urinary output		Monitor intake and output	Maintain function of multiple organs
	Assess medical problems that would contraindicate increased fluid intake		Offer fluids frequently or according to a therapeutic schedule	
	Assess need for parenteral fluids			
Maintain and promote proper personal hygiene	Evaluate the need for daily baths	Consider age, incontinence, perspiration, circulation	Cleanse patient with appropriate agent (soap) water, lotion	Dry thoroughly Remove all soapy residue Maintain proper skin pH
	Assess need for moisturizer/skin lubricant	Special attention to heels, elbows, and other bony areas	Moisturize/lubricate areas as often as necessary	Avoid the drying affect of alcohol rubs
	Determine potential "trouble spots" for bacterial growth	Beneath breasts, gluteal folds, skin folds from obesity, axilla	Inspect these areas at least bid Cleanse and dry thoroughly Expose to air if possible Apply cornstarch Encourage patient to assess himself	Teach self-hygiene or teach attendant the steps in good hygiene These areas must be kept dry to prevent breakdown; especially difficult to heal
Prevent or manage incontinence	Assess patient's bowel and bladder functions and deficits	Determine need for bowel or bladder program	Carry out bowel and bladder program Check frequently for incontinence Clean thoroughly when incontinent	Reinforce bowel and bladder program learning for patients and/or attendant

tractions; tightening of the rectal sphincter and cardiopulmonary response. Current literature supports the fact that ejaculation and orgasm are two separate occurrences. Orgasm is essentially a cerebral event and ejaculation is a pelvic event.

4. Resolution—final contraction is followed by a refractory period before erection and ejaculation can again occur.[5]

Female sexual response cycle. "The female sexual response cycle is more complicated and less predictable. There are at least three different identified patterns of sexual response in the female with an infinite variety possible in the individual female. Intensity as well as duration of response are factors in the individual female's sexual reaction. The female response is definitely a total body involvement with sexual tensions affecting other than genital organs or structures."[7] Although the timing of progression through each phase may follow three or more different patterns, the female response cycle proceeds through the following four phases:

1. Excitement—breast enlargement, nipple erection, vaginal lubrication, labial and clitoral engorgement; cardiopulmonary response.
2. Plateau—vagina fully expanded; vagina, clitoris, and labia are maximally engorged; cardiopulmonary response is almost maximal.
3. Orgasm—simultaneous contractions involving the uterus; outer portion of the vagina and rectal sphincter accompanied by a total body response.
4. Resolution—involuntary reduction of sexual tension. Unlike men, many women have the potential to be multiorgasmic.[5]

Physiology of the male and female sex act. In the male the degree of erection is proportional to the degree of stimulation. Erection is caused by parasympathetic impulses that pass from the sacral portion of the spinal cord through the nervi erigentes to the penis. Parasympathetic impulses dilate the arteries of the penis and constrict veins, thus allowing arterial blood to flow under high pressure into the erectile tissue of the penis. When sexual stimulation becomes more intense, the reflex centers of the spinal cord begin to emit rhythmical sympathetic impulses, which leave the spinal cord at L1 and L2 and pass to the genital organs through the hypogastric plexus, causing ejaculation. Ejaculation actually can be broken down further. Peristaltic contractions in the ducts of the testes, epididymis, and vas deferens force sperm into the urethra. Simultaneously, rhythmical contractions of the seminal vesicles and the muscular coat of the prostate mix mucus from the urethra with sperm. This constitutes emission. Then rhythmical nerve impulses via the spinal cord and pudendal nerve to the skeletal muscles at the base of the erectile tissue contract, which increases the pressure, resulting in ejaculation.[8]

In the female tumescence of the labia and clitoris occur in much the same manner as penile erection. This engorgement of female erectile tissue is also accompanied by tightening of the introitus. Lubrication occurs when parasympathetic impulses stimulate the Bartholin's glands and increase mucus secretion from the vaginal wall. Again, as sexual stimulation intensifies, reflex centers of the spinal cord emit rhythmical sympathetic impulses that pass to the genital organs through the hypogastric plexus, causing rhythmical contractions of perineal muscles associated with orgasm.[8]

Table 29-4. Neurogenic sexual dysfunction

Level in neuraxis	Possible etiology	Bed mobility	Genital sensation	Sensation in other erogenous zones	Ability to masturbate
Cortical and subcortical	CVA, MS, brain tumors, brain trauma	Altered significantly	Present	Present	Altered
Spinal cord, complete lesion above conus medullaris	Trauma, tumor, vascular disease, MS, syringomyelia, pernicious anemia	Altered significantly	Absent	Present above lesion	Altered
Conus medullaris or cauda equina complete lesion	Spina bifida, trauma, tumor, intervertebral disk	Altered somewhat	Absent	Present above lesion	Altered
Anterior horn cells or S2, S3, S4 ventral roots	Poliomyelitis, intervertebral disk	Altered somewhat	Present	Present	Unchanged
S2, S3, S4 dorsal roots, cells of origin or dorsal horns	Diabetes mellitus, tabes dorsalis	Generally normal	Absent or diminished	Normal or diminished	Unchanged

Some anticipated changes in sexual functioning caused by neurological disorders. Altered self-esteem occurs when changes in body image, self-concept, and behavioral patterns do not match a person's own expectations. Society can also give a person with neurological disability very clear messages about his or her value as a sexual being. Depression decreases libido and can inhibit sexual desire. These, and many more psychosocial concerns, may influence the client's sexual functioning.

It is beyond the scope of this chapter to discuss the myriad of sexual dysfunctions as they correlate to the specific neurological disorders, however, some specific sexual dysfunctions that result from neurological disorders can be briefly enumerated. In males partial or total impotence may result, orgasm may be experienced differently than before onset, and changes in hormonal levels, retrograde ejaculation, and body temperature control may affect fertility. Loss of projectile power during ejaculation may affect the ability to impregnate a partner. In females, changes in sensation may alter the orgasm experience and lubrication may be affected. Usually, however, a woman's fertility is not affected by neurological disorders (see Table 29-4).

Interventions. The goal of rehabilitation in the area of sexuality is to assist clients and their significant others to understand sexual functioning and ways they can take responsibility for their own sexuality. Health care providers must determine for themselves the level at which they want to be involved in intervention for clients with concerns about their sexuality. A helpful model for levels of intervention has been established by Annon.[1] The PLISSIT model conceptualizes levels of intervention beginning with:

P (Permission) This involves being a good listener, being nonjudgmental, and sanctioning the subject of sexuality. It seems this should be the minimum expectation of any professional working with neurologically disabled clients.

LI (Limited Information) This consists of providing information in a variety of forms, such as teaching aids, that relate to the client's specific needs. One must be comfortable with the topic of sexuality and knowledgeable of the content required to give accurate information.

SS (Specific Suggestions) The health care professional actively helps the client and/or significant other set and reach some goals. Generally, some formal continuing education in sexual functioning is necessary to perform at this level.

IT (Intensive Therapy) This consists of an individualized program specifically addressing, in depth, the client's sexual dysfunction. This level requires the skills of health care professionals with extensive formal education in sexuality and sexual dysfunction.

Sexuality is important in the lives of all persons. As such, it is an issue that will concern clients with neurological dysfunction. Sexual concerns should be addressed as openly as any other physiological and psychological concern precipitated by the client's neurological dysfunction.

Self-care deficits

Achievement of independent performance in self-care is one of the most important skills in a client's rehabilitation. Collaboration among the health care providers to help in the mastery of this ability is always a priority. Each disci-

Coitus		Fertility			
Male	**Female**	**Male**	**Female**	**Visible to society**	**Bowel or bladder incontinence**
Altered	Unchanged	Unchanged	Unchanged	Highly	Possible
Altered	Unchanged	Diminished	Unchanged	Highly	Present
Altered	Altered	Diminished	Unchanged	Somewhat	Present
Unchanged	Unchanged	Unchanged	Unchanged	Somewhat	Rare
Altered	Unchanged	Altered	Unchanged	Not generally	Rare

pline may approach it differently, but the goal remains constant.

Self-care is the practice of activities that individuals personally initiate and perform on their own behalf in maintaining health. Self-care is required of each person and, when not maintained, can lead to illness, disease, or death. Nurses at times will manage and maintain care for persons totally incapacitated. At other times they will assist, supervise, or guide the client toward self-care. The individual with neurological disability often requires therapeutic intervention and instruction to reach a maximal level of self-care function.

Dependency in self-care can be viewed as a functional limitation and needs to be assessed along with other problems related to carrying out activities of daily living. In identifying such a deficit, nursing uses two approaches. The first broad level approach is general rehabilitation theory and a second level is that of nursing diagnosis.

Using rehabilitation theory of functional assessment,[6] nurses construct a set of data that profiles the whole person as a means to better understand how the disability affects function. Methodology includes description of abilities and limitations evaluated through performance.

Self-care deficits as conceptualized by nursing diagnosis are divided into four levels: self-feeding, self-bathing, self-dressing, and self-toileting. The major effort in the development of assessment methodology for self-care deficits in nursing has been in judging the effectiveness of nursing care delivered.

Numerical index to measure the degree of functional dependence

0 = Independent; able to perform activity with no one present
1 = Requires use of equipment or device
2 = Requires help from another person for *assistance, supervision,* or *treatment*
3 = Requires help from another person *and* equipment or device
4 = Is dependent, does not participate in activity

Causes for the self-care deficit can include such things as intolerance to activity, pain, neuromuscular-skeletal impairment, musculoskeletal impairment, perceptual and/or cognitive dysfunction, and depression. Within the standard of care for self-care deficits (see Table 29-5), all clients with these deficits have the following scoring. They receive a numerical score defining the level of each deficit. Appropriate nursing intervention is documented in the client's plan of care. Periodic evaluation is used to determine progress of maintenance of a level.

For rehabilitation or long-term clients in chronic care facilities an additional scoring level is added:

2.2 Supervision (may include verbal reinforcement or stand-by assistance)
2.4 Minimal assistance: client does approximately 75% of the work

---

Table 29-5. Sampling from nursing care standard for self-care deficit

Problem	Assessment factors/findings	Nursing interventions
I. Self-feeding deficit (inability to bring food from a receptacle to mouth)	Evidence of pathological condition in the neuromuscular, musculoskeletal systems that involve upper extremity function	Assist, supervise, or teach as indicated Reinforce adaptive equipment Position to facilitate activity
	Perceptual and cognitive intactness	Assist and reinforce steps with the task Supervise for thoroughness Cueing Safety awareness Scanning techniques
II. Self-bathing/hygiene (inability to wash body parts, obtain or get water, and/or regulate temperature and flow)	Pain or discomfort with movement	Medication before activity Application of thermal modifying techniques Appropriate positioning
III. Self-dressing/grooming deficit (inability to dress and undress and maintain appearances)	Role of depression and other psychiatric disorders relating to eating, hygiene, and toileting	Quiet environment One primary assistant involved Reinforcement of positive aspects
IV. Self-toileting deficit (inability to carry out proper toilet hygiene, manipulate clothes, and/or function in environment)	Intolerance to activity (decrease in strength and endurance)	Positioning to minimize energy expenditure Activity pacing Encouraging completion of task
V. Client teaching (inability to learn)	Knowledge level Role of self-care in ability to live independently	Rationale for self-care

2.6 Moderate assistance: client does approximately 50% of the work

2.8 Maximal assistance: client does approximately 25% of the work

Nursing has developed a system for identifying the standards for treating self-care problems. Two primary objectives are to maximize functional ability for independence in self-care and to minimize the need for assistance from resource personnel in the carrying out of personal care.

Expected outcomes are measured according to the changes seen in health patterns and knowledge base. In general, the client and family will do the following:[14]

• Participate in all self-care activities as functionally capable
• Prevent injury
• Integrate new knowledge/skills
• Use adaptive equipment
• Preserve/promote optimal physiological functioning
• Cope with functional deficits
• Maintain positive self-image/self-esteem

Table 29-5 outlines the process of care that nursing uses as a standard in intervening with self-care deficits.

SUMMARY

Clients with neurological disorders can have a number of physical and psychological needs that require intervention from the members of the health teams. In facilitating independence in such critical areas as self-care, mobility, and bowel and bladder function, there can and often is overlap of assistance from the different disciplines. Not only is medicine involved but also nursing, physical therapy, and occupational therapy. For this reason the goals of treatment must always be client oriented and the lines of communication across disciplines be kept open. Establishing and maintaining a therapeutic program through collaboration allows each discipline to understand and complement the work being done by the other involved providers.

Through collaboration among the therapies, we can maximize our impact on the restoration goals and the quality of life issues so often involved in the care of the individual with neurological dysfunction.

REFERENCES

1. Annon JS: The PLISSIT model: a proposed conceptual scheme for the behavioral treatment of sexual problems, J Sex Educ Ther 2:1, 1976.
2. Bors E and Comarr AE: Neurological urology physiology of voiding: its neurological disorders and sequelae, Baltimore, 1971, University Park Press.
3. Briggs E: Care and teaching of maintenance of skin integrity for spinal cord injured, masters thesis, 1968, Boston University.
4. Cannon B: Bowel function. In Martin N and others, editors: Comprehensive rehabilitation nursing, New York, 1981, McGraw-Hill Book Co.

5. Core Curriculum Committee: Rehabilitation nursing: concepts and practice, a core curriculum, Evanston, Ill, 1981, Rehabilitation Nursing Institute.
6. Granger C: Health accounting: functional assessment of the long term patient. In Kottke F, editor: Krusen's handbook of physical medicine and rehabilitation, Philadelphia, 1982, WB Saunders Co.
7. Griggs W: Sexuality. In Martin N and others, editors: Comprehensive rehabilitation nursing, New York, 1981, McGraw-Hill Book Co.
8. Guyton A: Textbook of medical physiology, Philadelphia, 1976, WB Saunders Co.
9. King R: Assessment and management of soft tissue pressure. In Martin N and others, editors: Comprehensive rehabilitation nursing, New York, McGraw-Hill Book Co.
10. Krane RJ: Neurologic disorders of the lower urinary tract. Unpublished paper presented at Boston University School of Medicine, 1980.
11. Leininger M: Nursing and anthropology: two worlds to blend, New York, 1970, John Wiley & Sons, Inc.
12. Meers R: Skin destruction: over-coming the myths, Life Support Nurs 4:6, Sept-Oct 1981.
13. Miller ME and Sach ML: About bedsores: what you need to know to help prevent and treat them, Philadelphia, 1974, JB Lippincott Co.
14. Mumma CM, editor: Rehabilitation nursing: concepts and practice: a core curriculum, ed 2, Evanston, Ill, 1987, Rehabilitation Nursing Institute.
15. North American Nursing Diagnosis Association: Nursing Diagnosis Newsletter, 15:1, 1988.
16. Orem D: Nursing: concepts of practice, New York, 1980, McGraw-Hill Book Co.
17. Staas WE and DeNault PM: Bowel control, Am Fam Physician 7:1, 1973.
18. Task force on the nature and scope of nursing practice and characteristics of specialization in nursing. Nursing: a social policy statement, Kansas City, Mo, 1980, American Nurses Association.
19. Thomas EL: Nursing care of the patient with spinal cord injury. In Pierce DS and Nickel UH, editors: The total care of spinal cord injuries, Boston, 1977, Little, Brown & Co.

ADDITIONAL READINGS

Barrett JE and others: Stroke rehabilitation: analysis of repeated Barthel index measures, Arch Phys Med Rehabil 60:14, Jan 1979.
Berecek KH: Etiology of decubitus ulcers, Nurs Clin North Am 10:157, 1975.
Berecek KH: Treatment of decubitus ulcers, Nurs Clin North Am 10:171, 1975.
Comfort A: Sexual consequences of disability, Philadelphia, 1978, George F Stickley Co.
Emerick CA: Nursing management of the neurogenic bowel, ARN Journal 4:16, Jan-Feb 1979.
Enis J and Sarmiento A: The pathophysiology and management of pressure sores, Orthop Rev 2:26, Oct. 1973.
Feldman RG and others: Clinical assessment of patients with multiple sclerosis. In Feldman RG and others, editors: Spasticity: a disorder of motor control, Chicago, 1980, Year Book Medical Publishers, Inc.
Feustel D: Autonomic dysreflexia, Am J Nurs 76:228, 1976.
Gresham GE and others: ADL status in stroke: relative merits of three standard indexes, Arch Phys Med Rehabil 61:355, Aug. 1980.
Hargast TS: Understanding pressure sores, Rehabil Nurs 6:23, May-June 1981.
Heslinga K and others: Not made of stone: the sexual problems of handicapped people, Springfield, Ill, 1974, Charles C Thomas, Publisher.
Kosiak M: Etiology and pathology of ischemic ulcers, Arch Phys Med Rehabil 40:62, 1959.
Masters WH and Johnson UE: Human sexual response, Boston, 1966, Little, Brown & Co.

Mikulic MA: Treatment of pressure ulcers, ARN Journal 5:21, Sept-Oct 1980.

Rubinault I: Sex, society and the disabled, New York, 1978, Harper & Row, Publishers, Inc.

Shaul S and others: Toward intimacy, ed 2, New York, 1978, Human Sciences Press, Inc.

Taylor AG: Autonomic dysreflexia in spinal cord injury, Nurs Clin North Am 9:717, 1974.

Woods NF: Human sexuality in health and illness, ed 2, St Louis, 1979, The CV Mosby Co.

APPENDIX A

The currently accepted classification of nursing diagnoses* includes the following:

Pattern 1: exchanging

Altered nutrition: more than body requirements
Altered nutrition: less than body requirements
Altered nutrition: potential for more than body requirements
Potential for infection
Potential altered body temperature
Hypothermia
Hyperthermia
Ineffective thermoregulation
Dysreflexia
Constipation
Perceived constipation
Colonic Constipation
Diarrhea
Bowel incontinence
Altered patterns of urinary elimination
Stress incontinence
Reflex incontinence
Urge incontinence
Functional incontinence
Total incontinence
Urinary retention
Altered (specify type) tissue perfusion (renal, cerebral, cardiopulmonary, gastrointestinal, peripheral)
Fluid volume excess
Fluid volume deficit (1)
Fluid volume deficit (2)
Potential fluid volume deficit
Decreased cardiac output
Impaired gas exchange
Ineffective airway clearance
Ineffective breathing pattern
Potential for injury
Potential for suffocation
Potential for poisoning
Potential for trauma
Potential for aspiration
Potential for disuse syndrome
Impaired tissue integrity
Altered oral mucous membrane
Impaired skin integrity
Potential impaired skin integrity

*From North American Nursing Diagnosis Association: Nursing Diagnosis Newsletter 15:1-3, Summer 1988.

Pattern 2: communicating

Impaired verbal communication

Pattern 3: relating

Impaired social interaction
Social isolation
Altered role performance
Altered parenting
Potential altered parenting
Sexual dysfunction
Altered family processes
Parental role conflict
Altered sexuality patterns

Pattern 4: valuing

Spiritual distress (distress of the human spirit)

Pattern 5: choosing

Ineffective individual coping
Impaired adjustment
Defensive coping
Ineffective denial
Ineffective family coping: disabling
Ineffective family coping: compromised
Family coping: potential for growth
Noncompliance (specify)
Decisional conflict (specify)
Health-seeking behaviors (specify)

Pattern 6: moving

Impaired physical mobility
Activity intolerance
Fatigue
Potential activity intolerance
Sleep pattern disturbance
Diversional activity deficit
Impaired home maintenance management
Altered health maintenance
Feeding self-care deficit
Impaired swallowing
Ineffective breastfeeding
Bathing/hygiene self-care deficit
Dressing/grooming self-care deficit
Toileting self-care deficit
Altered growth and development

Pattern 7: perceiving

Body image disturbance
Self-esteem disturbance
Chronic low self-esteem
Situational low self-esteem
Personal identify disturbance
Sensory/perceptual alterations (specify: visual, auditory, kinesthetic, gustatory, tactile, olfactory)
Unilateral neglect
Hopelessness
Powerlessness

Pattern 8: knowing

Knowledge deficit (specify)
Altered thought processes

Pattern 9: feeling

Pain

Chronic pain

Dysfunctional grieving

Anticipatory grieving

Potential for violence: self-directed or directed at others

Post-trauma response

Rape-trauma syndrome

Rape-trauma syndrome: compound reaction

Rape-trauma syndrome: silent reaction

Anxiety

Fear

APPENDIX B
Autonomic dysreflexia

Autonomic dysreflexia is seen in clients with complete spinal cord lesions above T8, those with reflex neurogenic bladder and bowel, and it presents an acute, critical, life-threatening problem. All health care professionals who have contact with this client population should be familiar with this syndrome to assist the client and/or obtain for him or her the proper assistance. Autonomic dysreflexia is an uninhibited reflex response to a noxious stimulus. After the period of spinal shock, reflexes return and tone is recovered in the internal organs. Autonomic dysreflexia then can occur for the first time anywhere from approximately 3 weeks to 6 years after the injury.

The noxious stimulus initiates a reflex action of the autonomic nervous system of total body vasoconstriction which cannot be overcome by the body's normal compensatory mechanisms to vasodilate because the message cannot pass the level of lesion. The message to slow the heart, however, travels via the vagus nerve and continues to cause bradycardia. If not interrupted this cycle can cause either seizures and cerebrovascular accident because of the severe elevation of the blood pressure or cardiac arrest because of continuing bradycardia. The symptoms are as follows: (1) pounding, severe headache caused by increased blood pressure, (2) paroxysmal hypertension with blood pressure as high as 300/180, (3) flushing above the level of injury with pallor below the level, (4) shivering and goose pimples on the skin at first, then profuse sweating above the level of injury, (5) nasal congestion, and (6) fast, pounding pulse, followed by a progressively slowing pulse.

The treatment is as follows: (1) Place the client in the full sitting position, providing the spine is stable, to take advantage of the natural tendency toward orthostatic hypotension. (2) It is also helpful to break ampules of amyl nitrate under the client's nose to further lower the blood pressure while searching for the noxious stimulus. (3) Relieve the noxious stimulus. The bladder should be checked first, since bladder distention or spasm is the most common cause. If there is an indwelling catheter, the tubing and entire drainage system must be checked for kinks. The catheter can be irrigated with no more than 30 ml of normal saline. If it does not irrigate, remove it immediately and recatheterize the client. If a suprapubic catheter is blocked, removing it will be enough to relieve the distention because the urine will drain out of the suprapubic orifice. If there is no catheter in place, the bladder should be palpated and a catheter inserted immediately if it is distended. If the bladder has been eliminated as a cause, the bowel should be checked carefully with minimal stimulation to determine if the rectum is full. If it is, a topical anesthetic ointment should be inserted and gentle digital stimulation done to remove the mass. This will require two people, one to monitor the blood pressure and another to remove the feces. If the bowel and bladder have been eliminated as causes, check for less common stimuli, such as (1) skin irritation, (2) prolonged muscle spasm, (3) pressure sores, (4) constricting clothing or appliances, (5) sudden changes in room temperature, or (6) congested lungs.

If the stimulus cannot be found or relieved and the blood pressure remains elevated for any period of time, a vasodilator may be ordered. If the client is at home when this occurs, he or she must be taken to a local emergency room. When a vasodilator is given and the stimulus removed, the client will have to be watched carefully for rebound hypotension. The normal blood pressure is 90/60 mm Hg, and it will drop even more with a vasodilator on board. It is best to avoid drugs and concentrate on symptomatic relief. Once the client has experienced dysreflexia, he or she is able to identify the headache and direct others in relieving the causal stimulus.

APPENDIX C
Nursing care standard for the person at risk for alternation in fecal elimination patterns

I. Objectives
   A. To achieve a planned defecation pattern to avoid the inconvenience and embarrassment of involuntary evacuation.
   B. To allow people who would normally be restricted from society because of poor or absent bowel control to be socially acceptable.
   C. To prevent skin irritation as a result of incontinence and/or frequent or loose stools.
   D. To prevent impaction.
II. Expected outcomes
   A. Health
      1. The patient is free of fecal incontinence.
      2. The patient is free of skin irritation caused by fecal incontinence and/or frequent or loose stools.
      3. The patient has established an elimination pattern that prevents impaction.
   B. Knowledge
      Patient and/or significant other verbalizes:
      1. An understanding of the normal physiology of fecal elimination.
      2. An understanding of the potential for or cause of alteration in fecal elimination pattern.
      3. Appropriate actions to establish and adjust a regular, predictable fecal elimination pattern.

Process of care

Potential problem	Assessment factors	Nursing interventions
A. Health		

Constipation secondary to neurogenic causes, immobility, altered mental status, narcotic analgesics, other drug treatment regimens, dehydration, dietary alterations, pain, or aging	Premorbid elimination pattern history including
	1. Usual time of elimination
	2. Usual sequence pattern of elimination with activities of daily living
	3. Usual consistency of stool
	4. Dietary habits
	5. Fluid intake
	6. Use of medication or food to promote bowel response
	7. Use of enemas
	8. Usual amount of exercise or daily activity level
		Establish a bowel program as close to premorbid pattern as possible.
		1. Provide and allow time for bowel program in daily schedule
		2. Provide maximum privacy
		3. Encourage and/or allow patient to respond to the first urge to defecate
		4. Take advantage of natural physiologic mechanisms to aid in defecation:
		  a. Sitting position
		  b. Gastro-colic reflex (after a meal)
		  c. Allow maximum activity as indicated

	Frequency and consistency of stool	Adjust dietary intake when possible. 1. Increase fluid to 3000 ml daily 2. Increase high roughage foods 3. Avoid constipating foods
	Evidence of GI pathology, such as: Obstruction (abdominal cramps, abdominal distention, vomiting, increased bowel sounds, minimal diffuse tenderness) GI bleeding Undiagnosed abdominal pain	Assess for contraindication to use of cathartics.
		Obtain order for and give medications as indicated. 1. Stool softeners 2. Bulk formers 3. Cathartics
Fecal incontinence (involuntary stools) secondary to neurogenic causes	Sensory appreciation of the urge to defecate	Establish a planned defecation pattern (bowel training program) by stimulation of peristalsis at a designated time. Obtain orders for and use gentle stimulation techniques, i.e., 1. Milk of magnesia 8-12 hours before program 2. Glycerine suppository 3. Digital stimulation Repeat above steps for 2 days. If no results in 3 days, move to harsher stimulation techniques, i.e.: 1. Stronger cathartic 2. Dulcolax suppository 3. Manual removal of stool 4. Fleet or tap-water enema
Fecal incontinence secondary to altered mental status	Ability to intellectually appreciate and interpret urge to defecate	Establish a planned defecation pattern to anticipate patient's need to defecate. Offer environmental cues as indicated, i.e.: 1. Use of bathroom rather than bedside commode for bowel program 2. Use of commode rather than bedpan
	Ability to communicate need to defecate due to aphasia, language problems, difficulty understanding hospital routines.	Develop a consistent signal to communicate the need to defecate.

By Marilyn Pires, RN, MS, Clinical Nurse Specialist Rehabilitation. Used with permission, University Hospital Nursing Department of Continuing Education, Boston, 1980.

Process of care—cont'd

Potential problem	Assessment factors	Nursing interventions
A. Health—cont'd		
Fecal incontinence secondary to alteration in mobility	Ability to act independently on the urge to defecate	Offer assistance as indicated, i.e.: 1. Place on bedpan 2. Assist to toilet or commode
Diarrhea secondary to impaction	Signs and symptoms of impaction: lack of formed stool, mucus or liquid stool, hard abdomen, feeling of fullness, presence of hard stool in rectum, presence of stool documented by x-ray films	Do a digital examination of the rectum and check for presence of hard stool (contraindicated in patients with MI and patients with known rectal pathology). If stool is present: 1. Attempt to break up impaction manually 2. Give oil retention enema 3. Follow by oral cathartic Establish a planned bowel program as described above to prevent impaction.
Diarrhea secondary to medication treatment regimen	Side effect of medication or radiation on bowel function	Obtain orders for and give antidiarrheal medication in anticipation of side effects, i.e.: 1. Lactobacillus (Lactinex and yogurt) with antibiotic therapy 2. Medications to decrease peristalsis (Lomotil, paregoric, and DTO) 3. Medications to decrease fluid content of stools (Kaopectate)
Diarrhea secondary to dietary indiscretions	Foods patient found overstimulating to the bowel premorbidly Foods patient found constipating premorbidly Recent dietary history	Identify probable irritating foods. Encourage patient to decrease intake of those foods and increase intake of constipating foods.
Skin irritation secondary to incontinence and frequent or loose stools	Skin integrity	Prevent incontinence. Cleanse perineal skin after each bowel movement. Apply protective ointment (i.e., zinc oxide) or protective skin barriers unless contraindicated (check with Radiation Therapy Department for patients receiving radiation treatments).
B. Patient teaching		
Lack of knowledge concerning fecal elimination patterns	Knowledge level Ability to learn cultural values that might affect ability to adapt to components of a bowel program	Teach patient and/or significant other: 1. Normal physiology of fecal elimination 2. Etiology of alteration in fecal elimination pattern 3. Rationale for measures to regulate fecal elimination pattern 4. To report changes in pattern to physician or nurse
C. Discharge planning		
Dependence in fecal elimination	Knowledge skill of significant other or care provider concerning bowel program Ability of significant other or care provider to physically assist with bowel program	Evaluate care provider's psychomotor skill in performing bowel program by demonstration and return demonstration of bowel program. Refer to VNA for reinforcement of teaching on-going assistance with bowel program.

Chapter 30

THERAPEUTIC RECREATION

Fred Humphrey

The purpose of this chapter is to identify and discuss issues that are basic to the effective use of the activity experience as a tool of developmental growth in the lifestyle of individuals, irrespective of diagnostic category or type of setting. An understanding of the issues identified is critical to the functioning of an effective rehabilitation team as well as to the individual members of disciplines comprising the team. For the interested reader a basic description of the nature and scope of therapeutic recreation services across the spectrum of rehabilitation settings at the present time is readily available in references such as O'Morrow,[15] Kraus,[11] and Gunn and Peterson.[4]

Within the conceptual framework outlined, the following issues are addressed: (1) the functional orientation of the rehabilitation process (illness or wellness); (2) the blending of the direct service and process roles in the delivery of human services; (3) an ecological approach to life-style analysis; (4) a historical perspective on therapeutic recreation—a field of service in the rehabilitation process—and the currently unrealized potential for therapeutic recreation; (5) the "Rusalem Ecological Model" for therapeutic recreation and its implications in the areas of assessment and design of ecologies; and (6) Humphrey's leisure facilitation process model. These issues represent factors that must be present if the potential of the activity experience is to be realized.

FUNCTIONAL ORIENTATION OF THE REHABILITATION PROCESS

Dr. Ernest C. Bruder identified a key issue, which the rehabilitation process has yet to resolve, when he stated:

It is to this faceless generation that the sanity of the insane is desperately needed to illuminate the insanity of the sane. Our mentally ill protest emphatically that they cannot tolerate with decency or self-respect the shame and pretensions that make up so much of our modern living. Perhaps they can help us out of the morass in which so many of us have found ourselves. Our mentally ill are often our profoundest teachers—and as we give them their due rights as our teachers, we help them strengthen their weak self-respect.[2]

Although Bruder addressed his remarks specifically to the emotionally ill, the cliche that questions whether a "glass of water is half full or half empty" represents a critical concept in the rehabilitation process irrespective of the category of impairment.

Illich[10] questioned many of the concepts upon which the rehabilitation process is founded. The sequence outlined by Illich through which the "disabling professions" impact negatively on the individuals they are trying to serve is as follows:

1. In an economy such as is currently found in the United States, where the Gross National Product is skewed toward services in contrast to the production of goods, the client in the rehabilitation process is less a person in *need* than a person who is *needed*.
2. To perpetuate the service economy, the following set of professionalized assumptions of need have been developed:
   a. Client needs have been translated into deficiencies. (Is the glass half full or half empty?)
   b. The perceived deficiency is placed in the client despite overwhelming evidence that individual problems develop in a social-economic-political context.
   c. Professionalized definitions of need and translation of need into a client-centered deficiency have led to an ever-expanding range of specializations. Similar to the table mat at restaurants, which divides the cow into cuts of meat, *the client is understood and processed as a set of manageable parts, each with its own service mechanic.*
3. To complete the disabling process, four professionalized assumptions regarding the remedy to the need further magnify this negative impact:
   a. In the mirror image of the definition of need, the assumption that you (client) are the problem, produces the response, I am the answer. I, the professional, produce. You, the client, consume.
   b. The remedy comes to define the need. If servicers can define the question, they have the power to determine the need of their neighbors *rather than to meet their neighbors' need.*
   c. Once professionals have defined need and remedy, they further compound the disabling impact by coding the problem and solution in language that is totally incomprehensible to citizens.
   d. As the service professions gain the power to unilaterally define need, remedy, and code the service in incomprehensible language, a fourth disabling characteristic develops. It is the capacity of servicers to define the output of their service in accordance with their own satisfaction with the result. This fourth characteristic completes the transformation of the citizen into a critical addict, and perpetuation of this addiction is vital to the survival of the service system.

Whether phrased within the context of recognition of intact strengths[2] or disabling professions,[10] the human services professions must clearly establish a conceptual course based upon either the medical model of illness and deficits or the wellness model of intact strengths. It is not possible for both to function within the same system.

BLENDING OF DIRECT SERVICES AND PROCESS ROLES

A second major issue that human services professions must resolve is the definition and/or clarification of roles. The direct provision of services role is, and will remain, a function of the human services professional, but the allocation of resources to this role must vary among the different service providers as well as vary with the needs of the program participants and societal conditions over a period of time. However, the process or supportive role becomes increasingly important as the participant progresses toward greater independence as well as when society encounters greater financial constraints.

Therapeutic recreation as a *service* refers to the conceptual understandings, leadership approaches, and activity skills that an individual must have to effectively involve a disabled and/or excluded person in a recreation-oriented experience. To fill this direct service role requires a breadth of knowledge across a continuum that includes personality development, group dynamics, medical terminology, impairing conditions, anatomy and kinesiology, leadership approaches, activity analysis, activity skills, activity adaptation, architectural barriers, and many other areas. Individuals currently providing the leadership for therapeutic recreation services may be found in all types of rehabilitation settings and in an increasing range of community agencies.

Therapeutic recreation as a *process* refers to the dynamics of what may be described as the catalyst-facilitator role, the indirect service role, or the enabler role. It appears that, for the immediate future, therapeutic recreators will be neither trained nor hired, if available, in sufficient numbers to provide direct service to the disabled and/or excluded population, which has been estimated by some investigators to be as high as 70 million or 35% of the total population.[15, p. 10] Therapeutic recreation as a *process* refers to the role of the therapeutic recreator in providing assistance and consultation to the health services professions (e.g., medicine, social work, psychology, physical therapy, and occupational therapy), community human services professionals, families, and friends of disabled persons in order that recreation experiences may be included in the developmental life style of the disabled person. The net outcome of the *process* role is increased participation of disabled and/or excluded persons in existing general programs that are not a part of the formalized therapeutic recreation service delivery system.

AN ECOLOGICAL APPROACH TO LIFE-STYLE ANALYSIS

Whether therapeutic recreation or the rehabilitation process as a whole is now viewed in a service role or a process role, the time before the year 2000 will demand that human services function within a framework of life-style analysis. No longer can physical therapy professionals deal exclusively with shoulder mobility, vocational rehabilitation professionals focus solely on job placement, or therapeutic recreation professionals babble about the coming of the Leisure Age. Equally critical, the human services professions must assume an ecological orientation and recognize that the environmental impacts (e.g., social, economic, and political) are as basic to the rehabilitation process and a meaningful life style for the individual as are the specific rehabilitation goals of any discipline or profession.[10]

Macarov has outlined a futuristic scenario in which work will become a significantly decreasing alternative, even for our nonhandicapped population, as we move into the decades of the twenty-first century.[13] Given the economic projections to the year 2000, the reality of work as a life-style component is already a less viable alternative for our disabled citizens. Rapidly increasing amounts of enforced discretionary time must be recognized as a vital issue in life-style planning with disabled persons.

THERAPEUTIC RECREATION
Historical perspectives

To understand that the challenges identified for the human services professions must also be addressed by therapeutic recreation, a historical perspective is most appropriate. To place therapeutic recreation in a valid perspective, it is necessary to review the generic use of activity in the rehabilitation process.

Disease and disability are as old as life itself, and the inclusion of recreation and activities such as music, dance, games, and athletics in the life style of people can be traced to prehistoric artifacts. The earliest historical documents also relate these same activities to people's treatment of various illnesses and disabilities. In this sense, therapeutic recreation can be traced to the earliest recorded civilization.

The late 1700s and early 1800s brought the first evidence of formal inclusion of recreation and work activities in the rehabilitation process, particularly in psychiatric institutions. Dr. Benjamin Rush, the first superintendent of the Pennsylvania Hospital of Philadelphia (1812), Dr. Thomas Eddy, New York Hospital (1815), and Dr. Wyman, McLean Hospital of Waverly, Massachusetts (1822), were the earliest recorded supporters of recreational activities in institutional settings in the United States. Between 1843 and 1848 there were reports describing the extensive recreation programs at Hanwell Asylum in London. Florence Nightingale in her book, *Notes on Nursing* (1873), summarized the commitment she had demonstrated to the provision of recreational activities in military hospitals.[9]

Although the Red Cross has assumed responsibility for recreation programs in military hospitals since the entry of the United States into World War I and the Veterans Administration has supported recreation programs in veterans' hospitals since 1931, the greatest single period of growth in recognition and development of therapeutic recreation programs occurred during World War II and the decade that followed. This effort was led by the Red Cross in military hospitals and the Veterans Administration as it sought to cope effectively with the thousands of veterans admitted to its facilities. The decades of the 1960s and the 1970s saw state institutions serving the emotionally ill and mentally retarded make significant advances in the development of comprehensive rehabilitation programs, and the incorporation of therapeutic recreation as an integral part of this process was increasingly recognized.

The decade of the 1960s also can be identified as the period when community public, private, and voluntary agencies began to recognize a responsibility to serve the discretionary time needs of disabled and excluded populations. The expansion of human services programs during the decade of the 1970s included an ever-increasing recognition of the leisure needs of disabled and excluded populations, to the point where presently few city or county departments of recreation and parks have failed to provide programs for the disabled residing in the community.

In a professional sense the field of therapeutic recreation originated with the creation of the Hospital Recreation Section of the American Recreation Society in 1948. This action reflected the philosophy that the recreation experience was the central focus and that services for the disabled differed only in the area of modifications, not purpose. In 1953 an autonomous group called the National Association of Recreation Therapists (NART) was formed. This group had a strong clinical orientation and viewed the prime purpose of recreation as having therapeutic goals with an actual recreation experience being a secondary outcome. A third group, the Recreation Therapy Section of the American Association for Health, Physical Education and Recreation (currently the American Alliance for Health, Physical Education, Recreation and Dance), was formed in 1952. Although, as its name indicated, this group was also highly clinical in orientation, it never achieved an effective membership total or program effort. Although these groups merged in 1966 to form the National Therapeutic Recreation Society (NTRS) as a branch of the parent National Recreation and Park Association, the philosophical dispute between those who view the recreation experience as the prime objective in therapeutic recreation and those who view therapeutic recreation as a clinical-treatment modality has not been resolved.

Of all the specializations within the broad field of leisure services, therapeutic recreation has made by far the greatest progress in the area of registration, certification, and training. A voluntary registration plan for hospital recreation workers was instituted in 1957, and this plan, with updating, was officially adopted by the National Therapeutic Recreation Society following its formation. Continued refinement led to the establishment of the National Council for Therapeutic Recreation Certification in 1981 as an autonomous body to monitor and further develop the competency evaluation process for practitioners in therapeutic recreation. An accreditation process, under the auspices of the National Recreation and Park Association and the American Alliance for Health, Physical Education, Recreation and Dance, contains specific guidelines that must be met by colleges and universities purporting to offer programs in leisure studies and an option-emphasis in therapeutic recreation at the undergraduate level. Continuing professional development opportunities in the area of therapeutic recreation are extensive and include two national management schools, several regional symposiums, institutes at the annual Congress for Recreation and Parks, and numerous local and state level workshops.

A potential unrealized

The historical evolution of therapeutic recreation provides the basis for its definition as a service germane to the rehabilitation process. As previously indicated, in its earliest form this area of recreation was given the site-specific descriptor of *hospital recreation*. Initially therapeutic recreation had its greatest acceptance in psychiatric hospitals, with use in institutions for the retarded, physical rehabilitation centers, institutions serving the aging, penal and correctional settings, and community settings following in a sequential pattern.

With the medical model as the dominant orientation in almost all hospitals and institutional settings that provided the status base for doing "therapy," it was inevitable that recreation would be caught in the trap of emphasis on illness and treatment. Evolving under these circumstances, recreation was first termed *medical recreation* and later operated under the rubric of *recreation therapy*. With the formation of the National Therapeutic Recreation Society in 1966, the term *therapeutic recreation* has become the commonly accepted descriptor, with the adjective "therapeutic" implying that the recreation experience is the prime concept.

Although the clinical-treatment orientation has reached an apex in therapeutic recreation during the 1980's, as reflected in the formation of the American Therapeutic Recreation Association as a second national professional organization, many question the medical model as an appropriate guide for therapeutic recreation, or human services as a whole, as we approach the twenty-first century. The significant growth during the past decade in community-based therapeutic recreation programs, as well as the appearance of a spectrum of community services for individuals with disabilities, reflects increasing societal emphasis on wellness, intact strengths, prevention rather than treatment (hospitalization), and the economics of health care costs.

Major goals of proponents of this new emphasis are: (1) to provide a life-style laboratory within the confines of the rehabilitation environment in which the participant can practice life-style skills acquired during the rehabilitation process; (2) to provide a reality-oriented evaluation environment in which all members of the human services team can obtain the most valid check on the participants "real world" functional performance; (3) to provide the individual with an assimilative and highly ego-systonic (supportive of self-enhancement) environment as a balance to the accommodative and frequently ego-dystonic (destructive of self-enhancement) demands of the formal rehabilitation process; (4) to assist the individual, through a leisure facilitation component, to develop a life-style process that more effectively identifies and uses a discretionary time component; and, (5) to provide effective leadership during the transition to the community living phase relative to planning for the discretionary time component of the noninstitutional life-style.

THE RUSALEM MODEL: EMPHASIS ON INTACT STRENGTHS OF THE INDIVIDUAL

Although the concept has received minimal attention from therapeutic recreation professionals, Rusalem[16] proposed an alternative to the therapeutic model in therapeutic recreation that embodied the following elements:

1. Assessment of ecologies
2. Ecological design
3. Activities design
4. Implementation
5. Evaluation

This conceptual model holds unlimited potential, not only for the specialization of therapeutic recreation but also for the entire human services delivery system. It provides a conceptual umbrella under which the entire service system can unite. With its emphasis on the intact strengths of the individual, the ecological basis of the Rusalem Model combines the current dichotomies of natural and artificial ecologies (e.g., space, barrier-free design, and environmental issues) and human ecology (e.g., crowding, individual and group interaction patterns, and social and economic issues) into an operational entity that is presently unique among the delivery systems that comprise the human services effort.

The definition of health by the World Health Organization, "Health is a state of complete physical, mental and social well being and not merely the absence of disease or infirmity,"[17] clearly legitimizes the Rusalem Model. Although presented over 35 years ago, this definition reflects clearly today's growing societal emphasis on wellness, holistic health, and prevention.

Although obvious limitations make it impossible to explore the many facets of therapeutic recreation program development, a number of major concepts critical to the activity environment have either common roots throughout the rehabilitation process or demand the understanding of all members of the human services team. In the upcoming sections these concepts are discussed as related to the elements of assessment of ecologies, ecological design, and activities design from the "Rusalem Model."

Assessment and design of ecologies

Ecological or environmental psychology attends to both the human and nonhuman components of the environments (behavior settings) in which people function and is a significant but generally ignored element of the rehabilitation process. As defined, attention to the environmental impacts on behavior is a comprehensive task. Although limited in scope, the following concepts represent examples of the factors that must be considered in both the design and evaluation of activity environments if potential benefits are to accrue to participants in the rehabilitation process.

Perceptual view of behavior

In a basic sense, the perceptual view of behavior states that the nature of an individual's response to possible involvement in any type of experience will depend on his or her individualized perceptions of what the nature of this involvement will be like. Underlying the perceptual view of behavior is the prime assumption that the seeking of self-enhancement is a common behavioral motivator for all people. Thus the reluctant participant or nonparticipant, whom we classify as "unmotivated," is actually highly motivated to retain his or her current level of self-enhancement, since involvement in the activity experience encountered at the moment is viewed (perceived) as holding greater ego-dystonic than ego-syntonic potential. *The common denominator of activity leadership is that we are all leaders using the activity group as the vehicle through which we hope self-enhancing experiences will be achieved as a result of voluntary participation.*

Neutrality of activity

The activity experience, per se, is neutral. Involvement in an activity experience holds as much potential to be detrimental for the participant as it does to be beneficial (self-enhancing). A bowling pin or a chunk of clay has no self-enhancing qualities. The potential benefit to the participant develops out of the *interactions* with the human and nonhuman (e.g., equipment or materials) components of the total environment in which the activity group functions.

Paradox of activity involvement

The paradox of activity involvement may be summarized in the statement that the individual most in need of activity involvement is the individual least able to participate voluntarily. The application of this criterion to an evaluation of our program offerings, whether in a hospital, a nursing home, or the community, prompts the uncontested conclusion that the major emphasis in programming is directed toward the individuals *least* in need of our efforts. This conflict is resolved by classifying the unserved

as *"unmotivated"* and by effectively using this rationalization to clear ourselves of any implication of ineffective leadership or program efforts.

Leadership omnipotence

The conflict between leadership omnipotence and participant needs and interests must be evaluated. The perceptual view of behavior totally invalidates the idea that any leader, regardless of the degree of experience, skill, or sensitivity possessed, can effectively decide *what* activity experience *will be good* for a given individual. The activity involvement process is a two-way street constructed only after both verbal and nonverbal communication and interaction with the potential participant has established the "right-of-way" upon which this two-way street will be built.[6]

Needs-interests conflict

Solution of the dilemma in which there is a conflict between the potential participant's interests (wants) and leader-assumed needs is critical. Contrary to our common approach, the perceptual view of behavior suggests that the more appropriate approach to solving this dilemma is through the participant's *interests (wants)* rather than *needs.*

A classic illustration of this dilemma may be found in the case of a reclusive person who, in picturesque language, indicates to the therapeutic recreation leader (activity leader) that he or she *wants* to be left alone. For example, if a person views (perceives) herself or himself as having three left feet and no rhythmic capabilities, in no sense will he or she volunteer for a dance activity that the person is certain will spotlight her or his incompetencies in the presence of peers. Our frequent approach is to force this person into participation through medical prescription and/or other coercive measures. An approach through the individual's wants would involve a subtle and unobtrusive effort to develop a personal relationship with the individual before making efforts to expose the person directly to the activity environment.

Group readiness

An awareness of the basic subgroups that develop around a confrontation with potential activity involvement is important. The challenge of possible activity involvement, regardless of the functional level or age of the individual, results in any group dividing spontaneously into three subgroups: Group I, the ready participant; Group II, the observer or spectator; and, Group III, the isolate or escapee. Two specific principles that are useful in leadership approaches to this evidence of the varying levels of group readiness are:

1. Every individual naturally fits into each of the three levels of group readiness for a specific list of activi-

ties. No one belongs to Group I for the entire spectrum of activity possibilities.

2. The only appropriate leadership approach to the movement of an individual from Group III to Group I is through a period of involvement at the Group II level. In other words, despite the negative cultural connotation attached to the term "spectatorship," the observer role is a normal and necessary stage in an individual's developmental growth in the area of group readiness.

Group holding power

The holding power of a group essentially rests in the degree to which the group experience meets the goal achievement needs of each member. Individuals voluntarily join a group because they think (perceive) that the group will provide them with a better opportunity to achieve their personal goals than would individual efforts on their parts. An individual will voluntarily remain a member of a group only as long as this thought or perception retains its validity through direct experiences with group efforts. The effectiveness with which recreation leaders meet the issue of divergent goals among the members of an activity group represents a critical issue in terms of their overall effectiveness as leaders. Commonly used techniques that are effective in solving the problem of divergent goals among group members include the establishment of subgroups based on activity interest or skill level, the development of a priority schedule that gives appropriate attention to each goal or interest, and the offering of a variety of activities that encompass the varying goals (interests) that are present among group members.

Anticipation, realization, memories (ARM) of activity experience

Just as group development does not occur as a result of singular efforts by the leader, so also does it not occur as a result of "tunnel vision" on the part of the leader. A "tunnel view" can see nothing but the actual activity experience itself. Groups exist before and after the activity experience, and leader involvement in the "memory" and in the "anticipation" phases of the life style of a group is probably a more significant aspect of group development than the involvement that occurs during the actual activity period (Fig. 30-1).

Leadership process

Leadership that results in group development is a process, not a unilateral effort on the part of an activity leader, and this process is most effectively summarized in the statement by Thomas Jefferson as quoted by Danford and Shirley[3, pp. 128-129]:

We cannot always do what is absolutely best. Those with whom we act, entertaining different views, have the power and

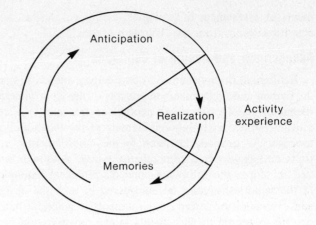

Fig. 30-1. ARM of activity experience. (From Humphrey F and others: Facilitating leisure development for the disabled: a status report on leisure counseling, College Park, Md, 1982, University of Maryland, Department of Recreation.)

the RIGHT of carrying them into practice. TRUTH ADVANCES AND ERROR RECEDES step-by-step only; and to do our fellow men the most good in our power WE MUST LEAD WHERE WE CAN, FOLLOW WHERE WE CANNOT, AND *STILL GO WITH THEM*, WATCHING ALWAYS THE FAVORABLE MOMENT FOR HELPING THEM TO ANOTHER STEP.

The process involves active, willing participation of all group members. The activity should advance the growth of all individuals in a manner reflecting each person's needs and desires and not just that of the activity leader.

Activities design

The design of the activity environment, or for that matter the entire life-style process of people, must be based upon the concept of inclusion versus exclusion. The functional analysis of the environmental interaction process (people and environments) must balance the functional strengths of the individual with the environmental demands required for appropriate involvement in a specific situation. Although every effort is made to increase an individual's functional strengths over time, at any moment when an individual faces an overdemanding environment, exclusion or environmental modification become the only alternatives.

Environmental (activities) design involves an appropriate matching of an individual's functional strengths with an adapted or modified activity or environment so that the probability of a success experience is significantly increased. The concept of inclusion versus exclusion involves identification of the activity and environmental demands inherent in a given situation. Through appropriate adaptation and modification of the activity and the environment so that demands will not overwhelm an individual's functional strengths, the major aspects of exclusion can be eliminated.

The concept of inclusion versus exclusion is far more

functionally realistic than the concept of mainstreaming, which has probably had a more detrimental than beneficial impact on the community placement of disabled children and adults. Mainstreaming, as is true of the great majority of rehabilitation approaches, is heavily oriented to changing people to fit environments instead of changing environments to correspond to the functional strengths of people. Further, mainstreaming is totally unrealistic since "normal" people function in the mainstream only on a selective basis. Examples of activity and/or environmental adaption of "normal" people abound, but the existence of beginner, intermediate, and championship ski slopes or the handicapping system in golf make the point.

Activity analysis involves an identification of the psychomotor, cognitive, and interactive performance requirements of a specific activity. Functional analysis of the individual involves an identification of his or her performance strengths (and limitations) in the three identified behavioral domains. Activity or environmental design involves the skillful matching of the individual's performance strengths with a set of environmental demands that holds high ego-syntonic potential. Although little realized or used, the activity environment offers unlimited potential to the human services team to mix a recipe that is highly appropriate to each individual on a developmental basis.

Obviously, activity and environmental analysis and design are not simplistic in nature. Disciplines such as physical therapy, occupational therapy, and therapeutic recreation have given increased attention to activity analysis over the past 10 years, but efforts have been highly microstructured (activity specific) in nature and have emphasized the psychomotor and cognitive demands of an activity. Little or no attention has been given to the affective and social interactive demands of activity involvement. From the macrostructural perspective, environmental psychology has made significant contributions to the understanding of environmental impacts on behavior.

Although the literature related to activity analysis in therapeutic recreation has expanded significantly in recent years, Berryman and others[1] at New York University have conducted the most research in the area of activity analysis and prescriptive programming in therapeutic recreation. The original intent of the New York University Project was to analyze the psychomotor, cognitive, and affective domains but, as previously identified, the affective-social interaction domain proved to be beyond the scope of the project.

Berryman and others identified 207 factors that were related to activity participation requirements. Further reduction led to the designation of 104 items that were related to type, structure, and requirements of various activities and 103 factors that were related to individual functional issues such as energy cost and social, cognitive, locomotor, and perceptual-motor factors. The 104 factors related to activity type and structure were called *descriptors,* and the 103 items related to individual functional demands were termed *prescriptors.*[1]

Within the *descriptor* category, subcategories were identified such as the number of participants required, activity structure (rules, targets, courts), social structure, formation, levels of participation (individual to team), roles, physical contact, and energy expenditure. The *prescriptor* factors were divided into three major groups identified under the sensory domain, cognitive domain, and perceptual-motor domain. Subcategories under the sensory domain included tactile identification, auditory identification, auditory location, auditory recall, color identification, visual location, and visual recall. Within the cognitive domain, specific categories were symbol matching, symbol identification, structured and unstructured oral communication, and following auditory and visual signals, symbols, and directions. Perceptual-motor subcategories included crossing the midline, directionality, body image, balance manipulation, form perception, throwing, catching, kicking, striking with hand, striking with implement, dribbling, horizontal locomotion, and vertical locomotion.

The New York University Project computerized the activity analysis process so that, based on data provided, an activity prescription for an individual participant could be provided. A unique feature of this project was that the functional analysis of the participants could be conducted in a recreation atmosphere with participants moving from station to station for a series of game-oriented tasks that produced the data base for the activity prescription. However, because of limitations in funding support, a nationwide data bank or the computerized program available to agencies wishing to use this procedure have not been developed.

Leland and Smith[12] provided another unique conceptual approach to activity analysis that they found particularly applicable to working with mentally retarded individuals. They designed an analysis approach that evaluates the degree of structure present in terms of the leadership approach and the materials utilized in the activity environment. The developmental sequence proposed was sequenced from unstructured materials and unstructured leadership through unstructured materials and structured leadership to structured materials and unstructured leadership and finally to structured materials and structured leadership.[12] The rationale supporting this approach is predicated on the assumption that leadership can be more flexible than can materials. The sequential introduction of structure, with leadership structure preceding materials structure and unstructured leadership compensating for materials structure, provides for the developmental growth of the individual.

Humphrey[9] has discussed environmental analysis within the context of inclusion versus exclusion and whether excluding factors are intrinsic to the individual or extrinsically present in society. In conducting an environmental analysis, it is also critical to employ the concept of target populations. As previously discussed, normal people function in the mainstream only on a selective basis, and in analyzing excluded populations it is necessary to focus on a target group. Factors that exclude participation by one individual may be entirely absent in the case of another person. Examples of factors that must be considered in an environmental analysis, from both an intrinsic and an environmental perspective, include skill level, age, sex, race, religion, group readiness level, cognitive level, physiological demands, dress, architectural barriers, schedule of programs, availability of facilities, transportation, leader attitudes and needs, behavioral regulations and requirements in a given setting, activity demands, financial cost, degree of structure, cultural norms, safety factors, rules, available roles, prop availability, and divergent goals. Issues such as age, sex, race, dress, and religion impinge on the cultural norms operating in a given environment and must be considered within this perspective.

THE LEISURE FACILITATION PROCESS: A TOOL FOR ALL HUMAN SERVICES

Despite over 25 years of increased emphasis and growth and thousands of pages of discussion in articles and books,

the issue of leisure facilitation (e.g., leisure counseling, leisure education, avocational counseling, recreation counseling, and retirement leisure planning) remains a controversial subject.[5,8,14] Humphrey and others[8] prepared a diagram (Fig. 30-2) in an effort to provide a comparative frame of reference for the various conceptual orientations to the leisure facilitation process that are currently most prevalent.

A participant-centered ecological orientation to the leisure facilitation process was developed by Humphrey. It placed the highest priority on the behavioral orientation of the leader and identified the major elements of the facilitation process as the ecological world of the leader and participant (client), the interactive readiness level of the leader and participant, nonverbal as well as verbal tools of communication, and the sharing (facilitating) role of leadership (Fig. 30-3).[7]

Participant

This is a participant-centered model, not a counselor-leader–centered model as is true for so much of our leisure counseling efforts at the present time. It is predicated on the well-accepted concept of relating to the individual in terms of his or her present functional strengths and sta-

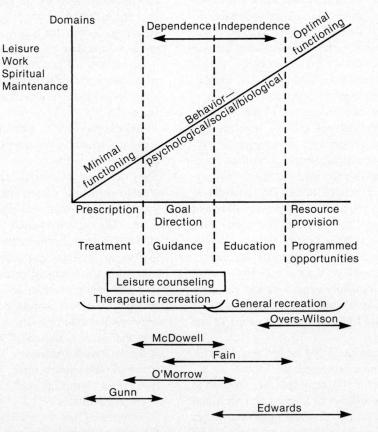

Fig. 30-2. Conceptual model for comparing theoretical orientation in leisure counseling. (From Humphrey F: ARM of the activity experience, Unpublished lecture notes, College Park, Md, 1982, University of Maryland, Department of Recreation.)

tion in life. Analysis of the individuals' functional strengths and the activity-ecological demands to which they are to be exposed is an obvious prerequisite to any intrusive efforts.

In a basic sense, the human services role represents an intrusive act by those involved in the life of others. The leisure facilitation process is no exception, and this represents the prime value clarification issue with which each individual must deal. This premise relates closely to the behavioral orientation criterion. It would seem that the human services professional is in a more solid ethical position when the intrusive effort is directed toward an individual's intact strengths rather than a set of "defined weaknesses" that cannot escape the cultural (ecological) bias of the professional. To relate to an individual in terms of what a culture has arbitrarily defined as "well" and "ill" represents a position of questionable omnipotence from which to start this intrusive leisure facilitation process. Within this limited introduction, the previously identified components of the *leisure facilitation process* will be analyzed:

1. *Ecological world.* The Ecological Model outlined by Rusalem[16] presents a further challenge to the leisure facilitation process in that it is equally critical to consider both the leader's and the participant's relations with the environment (ecological worlds of both leader and participant). Concrete examples in which the ecological world of the leader is not consistent with the ecological world of the participant include referral of a physically impaired person to a program conducted in a facility with extensive architectural barriers or referral of a socially retarded person to a program in which voluntary participation is the only avenue of entry.

2. *Interactive readiness levels.* Interactive readiness is an individual attribute in the same sense as reading readiness. To ignore this fact in developing any process of intrusion is to solicit failure. For example, clients who are shy as well as nonaccepting of their physical disabilities would not be ready to engage in social games that stress their physical limitations.

3. *Vehicle of communication.* To the present, our concept of leisure counseling has been totally predicated on verbal communication and has ignored the rich potential inherent in nonverbal communication. It is ironic that the professionals in the action-oriented disciplines (physical therapy, occupational therapy, therapeutic recreation) have not taken the leadership in demonstrating to all rehabilitation disciplines the value of nonverbal communication. Instead, probably in search of status, we have become clones of the verbal emphasis prevalent in psychiatry, psychology, and social work. The familiar old adage reminds us "A picture is worth a thousand words"; and the statement is equally true in reference to the leisure facilitation process, if we paraphrased it in effect to state "An action is worth a thousand words." Enlargement of our approach beyond the severe limitations enforced by strictly verbal counseling is imperative. That is, the client will nonverbally inform the clinician as to the activities most conducive to his or her needs.

4. *You—the facilitator.* The bottom-line weakness of the "therapist role" is its omnipotence. Failure is the built-in total responsibility of the participant. The facilitator role demands not only a mutual recognition of strengths and weaknesses on the part of both parties but also a mature willingness to use a range of additional facilitation strengths in the long-range process. The facilitator is in no sense the "Master of Ceremonies."

THE FUTURE—WHERE DO WE GO FROM HERE?

The segment of our leisure services delivery system dedicated to the provision of services for excluded populations, both community-based and institutional-based, has been laboring for years to shed the mantle of therapy and concern itself with the intact strengths of people, however limited these strengths may be at a given moment in time. It is generally agreed that the period 1965 to 1975 reflected marked movement away from the highly clinical, therapeutic, illness-oriented approach to the provision of leisure services for excluded populations. The past decade has seen the pendulum swing strongly back to the highly clinical orientation in therapeutic recreation, but, as noted on p. 820, the apex of this swing appears to have passed.

Therapeutic recreation has not led but merely followed the medical-model dominance that has prevailed in human services. Given the statement by former Governor Richard Lamm of Colorado that the United States has the most costly and most inefficient health services system in the

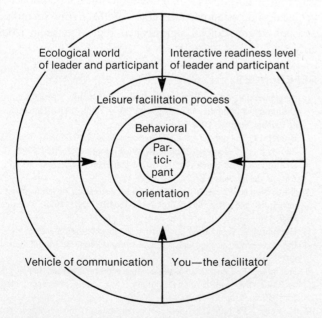

Fig. 30-3. Leisure facilitation process model. (From Humphrey F: The leisure facilitation process, Unpublished lecture notes, College Park, Md, 1982, University of Maryland, Department of Recreation.)

world, it behooves all human services professions to take stock of the major social issues relevant to the 1990s and the twenty-first century. Limitations prevent more than a sketch of selected questions/or examples, such as the following:

- How can human services survive the federal deficit crisis?
- Will the decade ahead produce highly destructive "turf battles" as competition for limited resources embraces not only the traditional human/health services needs but also evolving ones such as AIDS, drug and alcohol addiction, the explosion in the prison population, latch-key children, the unemployed, the homeless, and minorities?
- Are the human service professions reflected in this book germane only to the medical-model orientation and the clinical settings of the 1980s? Or do these professions have the innovative strengths to produce a diversity of roles relevant to the year 2000?
- Are the human/health services professions capable of shedding the reductionist philosophy and developing a conceptual orientation appropriate to evolving patterns of human and health services? The current dispute between the American Medical Association (AMA) and nurses' groups, led by the American Nurses Association, over the AMA proposal to create a new class of health care workers called the "registered care technicians" would indicate a negative response to this question as well as the previous one related to "turf battles."
- Given the evolving demographics, are we prepared to assume a significant role in a society composed of dominant target populations identified as aging, black, Hispanic, and Asian?
- The Department of Defense does not have a monopoly on unethical behavior. State governments are removing the authority to proctor human services from professional societies and establishing governmental units to assume this responsibility. Why? Because the performance of professional societies, led by the medical profession, has been negligent. Are we prepared to make the critical decisions in the area of ethical practices that the next decade will mandate?
- Are we prepared to effectively contribute to the quality-of-life versus length-of-life debate? What is our role in the hospice effort?
- As human/health services professionals, are the efforts and proposals of the "President's Commission on Americans Outdoors" of any concern to us?

To found a leisure facilitation process on a therapeutic or illness orientation presents the strong possibility of a conceptual contradiction. Leisure is a self-generated state of being, and all that people have going for them in this self-generated process are their intact strengths. Thus, to facilitate an individual's independence, the focus must be placed on the person's strength and potential health rather than on the illness that brought the person into the health care environment.

Given the World Health Organization definition of *health* (see p. 814), it seems valid to state that leisure and health share the property of being self-generated to a significant degree. To the degree that this statement is valid, therapeutic recreation and all human/health services professionals share the challenge of mutual resolution of the issues identified if our contribution to and role in a twenty-first–century society is to be worthy of our history.

SUMMARY

In a section entitled "A potential unrealized," five important components of the activity environment were identified (see p. 814). In a comparative sense, to develop, staff, and deliver the activity programs that provide the framework within which the listed goals may be realized is relatively simple. However, these goals can be achieved *only* within the context of an ecological model.

To implement an ecological model—which is based on the intact strengths of the individual and which attends to the issues identified through the concepts of ecological assessment, ecological design, activity analysis, and leisure facilitation—represents a challenge not to therapeutic recreation professionals alone, but to the total human services team. However, the ultimate challenge can be found in our efforts to respond to the issues identified in the section entitled, "The Future—Where Do We go From Here?" Unless we, as the collective of human services professions, can demonstrate levels of innovation and cooperation not yet achieved, effective resolution of the issues identified and our future societal significance appear to be in jeopardy.

REFERENCES

1. Berryman DL and others: Prescriptive therapeutic recreation programming: a computer based system, New York, 1976, Department of Leisure Studies, New York University.
2. Bruder EG: Unpublished inauguration address, President, Association of Mental Hospital Chaplains, Washington, DC, May 1962.
3. Danford HG and Shirley M: Creative leadership in recreation, ed 2, Boston, 1970, Allyn & Bacon, Inc.
4. Gunn SL and Peterson CA: Therapeutic recreation program design: principles and procedures, Englewood Cliffs, NJ, 1978, Prentice-Hall, Inc.
5. Humphrey F: Recreation counseling for the institutional dischargee, Paper presented at the National Recreation Congress, Miami Beach, Oct 1964.
6. Humphrey F: Leadership analysis and activity analysis, Paper presented at the twelfth annual Volunteer Venture Conference, Hartford, Conn, June 1973.
7. Humphrey F: Issues in the leisure facilitation process, Paper presented at the Mid-East Symposium on Therapeutic Recreation, New Carrollton, Md, May 1977.
8. Humphrey F, Kelley JD, and Hamilton EJ, editors: Facilitating leisure development for the disabled: a status report on leisure counsel-

ing, College Park, Md., 1980, Department of Recreation, University of Maryland.

9. Humphrey F: Lecture notes graduate courses, Department of Recreation, College Park, Md., 1988, University of Maryland.

10. Illich I and others: Disabling professions, London, 1977, Marion Boyars, Publishers, Inc.

11. Kraus R: Therapeutic recreation service: principles and practices, Philadelphia, 1978, WB Saunders Co.

12. Leland H and Smith DE: Play therapy with mentally subnormal children, New York, 1968, Grune & Stratton, Inc.

13. Macarov D: Work and welfare: the unholy alliance, Beverly Hills, Calif, 1980, Sage Publications.

14. Olson WH and McCormick JB: Recreational counseling in the psychiatric service of a general hospital, J Nerv Ment Dis 125:237-239, April-June 1957.

15. O'Morrow GS: Therapeutic recreation: a helping profession, ed 2, Reston, Va, 1980, Reston Publishing Co, Inc.

16. Rusalem H: An alternative to the therapeutic model in therapeutic recreation, Therapeutic Recreation Journal, 7(1):8-15, 1973.

17. World Health Organization Constitution: Chronicle of the World Health Organization, 1(3):3, 1947.

ADDITIONAL READINGS

Bezold G, Carlson R, and Peck J: The future of work and health, Dover, Mass, 1986, Auburn House Publishing Co.

Bower C and others: Work in the 21st century, Alexandria, Va, 1984, The American Society for Personnel Administration.

Carter M, Van Andel G, and Robb G: Therapeutic recreation—a practical approach, St Louis, 1985, Times Mirror/Mosby College Publishing.

Didsbury H Jr: The global economy—today, tomorrow and the transition, Bethesda, Md, 1985, World Future Society.

Kennedy D, Austin D, and Smith R: Special recreation: opportunities for persons with disabilities, Philadelphia, 1987, Saunders College Publishing.

Lamm R: Mega-traumas: America at the year 2000, Boston, 1985, Haughton Mifflin Co.

Naisbitt J: Mega trends—ten new directions transforming our lives, New York, 1982, Warner Books.

O'Morrow G and Reynolds R: Problems, issues and concepts in therapeutic recreation, Englewood Cliffs, NJ, 1989, Prentice-Hall Inc.

Schleien S and Ray T: Community recreation and persons with disabilities, Baltimore, 1988, Paul H Brooks Publishing Co.

Sinnott M: Clinical specialization in occupational therapy—a pluralistic view of practice, doctoral dissertation, 1988, University of Maryland.

Sylvester C and others: Philosophy of therapeutic recreation—ideas and issues, Alexandria, Va, 1987, National Recreation and Parks Association.

Therapeutic Recreation Journal (published quarterly), Alexandria, Va, vols 1-22 (1988), National Recreation and Park Association.

Chapter 31

HEALTH EDUCATION: KEY TO AN ENRICHED ENVIRONMENT

Donna El-Din

A conceptual model is presented in Chapter 1 of this text. Umphred states, "The question arises as to why the sequence worked effectively with one therapist one day and not on the next day with the other therapist." Later she notes that "When two people are interacting as in a client-therapist relationship, each person is responding to the moment-to-moment changes occurring within the environment." The author of these phrases has taken a snapshot of the dilemma facing practitioners. If in fact each client has a right to health care, can such care be delivered in the same way by every health care practitioner? Should we, or could we, standardize care?

OVERVIEW

Disability is more likely to be dramatically reduced through preventive programs than advances in biomedical technology. The notion that we should begin here and not after the fact of trauma seems sensible, yet we are faced with innumerable variables of human nature. Decisions made before catastrophic or complex events are often thought to be made on the basis of soft data, whereas the decisions made after catastrophic or complex events appear to be based on logical, hard data. Medicine has been better equipped to deal with the latter.

How would society deal with funding prevention programs over biomedical programs? Whose responsibility is health, anyway? Do people have a right to health? Is there a moral obligation instead to preserve one's own health? How would we measure outcome or progress?

Health is universally revered, and a healthy population ultimately means a productive nation. But can any government or agency, no matter how benevolent or wealthy, promise to deliver health to all people? The term "health" refers to a momentary state. Neither individuals nor societies are stagnant states; they are ever changing. The appropriate time to measure health and to influence the state and the worth of the health of the individual is always the same—the moment of attention to it.

The health of the client changes with changing practitioners, environments, cultures, times of day, and political structures. The client's state of health, from the practitioner's point of view, is influenced by the client's professional education and the person he or she is. The extent to which the client's state of health can be influenced, whether at the prospective or retrospective end of the health continuum, depends on the practitioner and the client's current status. The purpose of the relationship between the practitioner and the client is to share information. It is an opportunity for the client to learn about the practitioner's expectations and for the practitioner to learn about the client's expectations. The learning environment facilitates or inhibits the process.

A number of factors determine the overall situation in which the client and practioner operate. There is the internal environment of the client already alluded to. The lesion is one part of that internal environment. There is the internal environment of the practitioner, whose skills are but one part of his or her internal environment. There is an external environment as interpreted by the client, and an external environment as interpreted by the practitioner. These come together through the learning environment. The principles presented in Chapter 1 deliver a strong message. Individuals need to solve problems and must want to solve the problem given a chance that the solutions will be successful. Unless the task fits the individual's current capability, it will be approached by lower-level problem-solving methods. Learning is taking place in all aspects of the client's and practioner's world, and the client must ultimately take responsibility for the means to solve the problem.

Active participation in life and in relationships promotes learning. Rogers[42] defines significant learning as learning that makes a difference, that affects all parts of a person. We have spoken of a relationship—educational in nature and centered on an individual's health. Additionally, one of the individuals involved in the relationship has knowledge that is to be imparted or skills to be practiced on the other. The relationship "works" if the learning environment facilitates exchange. The concept of equal partners is crucial. The issue and practice of informed consent is not just political or ethical; it is central to client care. Voluntariness has to be practiced by both practitioner and client alike. Each has a moral obligation to facilitate the process of health care within the moment. The Western world of medicine has steadily climbed a mountain toward the peak of excellence in medical technology. Why has it taken us so long to recognize the client's need to assume an equal role or for the practitioner to seek the client's help?

Now we pause to reflect. The pause is thrust upon us by diminishing funds for biomedical research, and equally as much by an honest appraisal by practitioners of the issue of quantity versus quality of life. However, the time allotted allows us to look at other health care systems in the world. As we look down from the peak of Western world medicine, our eyes drift to peaks around us, some at the same level of health care, some higher, and many are peaks of mountains that have stood for centuries. What has brought us to this place and where our journey will lead are questions to be dealt with in coming decades.

MEDICAL MODEL OF HEALTH CARE

The medical model is the dominant model of health care in Western society.[31] It forms the conceptual basis for health care in America. The model assumes that illness has an organic base that can be traced to discrete molecular elements. The origin of disease is found at the molecular level of the individual's tissue. The first step toward alleviating the disease is to identify the pathogen that has invaded the tissue and, after proper identification, to apply appropriate treatment techniques.

It is implicit in the model that specialists who are professionally competent have the sole responsibility for the identification of the cause of the illness and for the judgment as to what constitutes appropriate treatment. The medical knowledge required for these judgments is thought to be the domain of the professional medical specialists and therefore inaccessible to the public.

Western medicine is often viewed as having developed from Greek medicine. The Greeks philosophized that humans and nature were inexplicably intertwined, the mind and the body each influencing the health of the other. Diagnosis and cataloging of diseases became more rational during this period of history, which may be a reason for tracing medicine's beginnings to the Greco-Roman era. However, the theory of the interrelationships of the mind and the body is not true of the present medical model of health care. Disease is now viewed in society as a battle between microbes and humans.

Two developments may be more directly responsible for the establishment of today's model of medical practice. They are the practice of human anatomical dissection and the development of the germ theory of disease. Increasing sophistication in dissection and cellular research formed the basis for scientific medicine as we know it today. The procedure followed is to locate the cells responsible for the disease and eradicate those cells. The health care professional who fails to locate and eradicate the disease is considered by society in general to have failed in his or her responsibility. In the quest to avoid failure, the health care professional therefore welcomes, encourages, and demands technological advances that promise more accurate diagnosis and treatment. Letting nature take its course and allowing the myriad of unmeasurable environmental influences to enter this scientific process is considered a waste of time, money, and resources. The health care professional considers health his or her business only after disease has occurred or stabilized and health has to be restored.[32]

Perhaps the fact that mental illness is now considered a disease in the Western world is further indication of the extent to which medicine focuses on pathology. At any moment a specific pathogen is expected to be found in the tissue of mentally ill patients. Following such an identification, treatment will be possible. Medicine pits technology against nature rather than concentrating on their harmonious coexistence.

Medical science has developed a body of knowledge that the public does not share. It has given the physician and other health professionals, including the therapist, an authority over the public. The knowledge is transmitted from professional to professional in select university settings. The control of the dissemination of knowledge is reinforced by exclusive professional organizations of physicians and other health professionals. The organizations set educational standards for their members, support restricted licensure laws, and enforce a code of ethics. They also monitor, and in some cases control, the practices of groups whose health care activities are related to the particular health profession or impinge on what they consider their particular area of health care.[11]

Health care professionals, on the other hand, are relatively free of control by the public. They have developed a clear professional autonomy over the years. Professionalism has been fostered by rigid admission criteria for students, research-oriented academic departments, and early specialization of practice. The result is that a health care professional who becomes part of such a system embraces its high ideals and then views someone outside the system as having lower status. This approach to professionalism has led to an increasingly narrowed view of dysfunction and its impact on the individual. Such an attitude works against establishing cooperative relationships with the other health professionals who have recently begun to challenge the control that a physician holds over their practices. Extreme professional attitudes that a health care worker may hold regarding the practices of medicine might encourage the professional to see himself or herself as the decision maker in the process of health care. These attitudes would work against the possibility of sharing the role of decision making with the consumer of health care, and they would reflect the model of decision making that was instituted by physicians.[12]

Purtillo and Cassel[38] list three general characteristics of a profession. The first characteristic is that the members claim to have "maximal competence and/or knowledge in a specific area." The second is that a profession "offers a service which is of some significant social value." The third requires that the profession "control its own work": in other words that it have recognized autonomy as a result of its specialized expertise. Physical therapy, for example, is a health profession that has been in existence long enough to see a pattern of professional growth. Physical therapy meets these criteria though it does not have complete autonomy of practice. In most cases, physician's referral is required before a patient can be treated by a physical therapist, but it is not required for patient evaluations in most cases, nor is the actual care monitored on site by the physician.

The health care provided by a physical therapist to the client is based on a medical model. The therapist is trained in medical school environments, licensed by the state following graduation, and has established a national professional organization, the American Physical Therapy Association (APTA).

The APTA[2] accredits physical therapy and physical therapy assistant schools. Individual states license physical therapists, and a physical therapy assistant must, by law, work under the direction of a physical therapist. In the process of this training, a therapist acquires attitudes toward the practice of the profession much like those acquired by a physician. As a result, health professionals continue to seek control of health care through insistence on delivery of health care through the medical model and strengthening of professional organizations. Although the medical model continues to be perpetuated, consumers are now seeking to play a more active role in their health care.

Clients, or consumers of health care, are becoming aware of the impact of medicine's control over their lives. This awareness has been fueled by the price they are paying for that health care. The Surgeon General's report confirms that expenditures for health are increasing.

In addition, preventive care assumes major importance in view of the fact that 75% of all deaths today are the result of degenerative diseases, such as heart disease, cerebrovascular accidents, and cancer. Like other major causes of death, accidents (cited as the most frequent cause of death in persons under age 49) are increasingly linked to life-styles.

The average consumer does not know what medicine can and cannot do for him or her. The physician and patient must therefore be candid with one another. Personal experience with rising hospital costs, depersonalization as a result of technology, and the exposure to national health problems via mass media have encouraged the consumer to take a more active role in his or her health care. Insurance companies also advocate consumer involvement in hope of reducing payments for health care. Levin[25] points out that there is a lot that consumers can do for themselves. Most people can assume responsibility to care for minor health problems. Use of nonpharmaceutical methods to control pain, (e.g., hypnosis, biofeedback, meditation, and acupuncture) are becoming common. The recognition of the value of approaching illnesses in a wholistic approach is receiving increasing attention in society. Treatment of emotional needs as well as physical needs during illness has been advocated as a way to help individuals regain some control over their lives.

WHOLISTIC MODEL

A wholistic model of health care seeks to involve the patient in the process and take the mystery out of health care for the consumer. Successful outcome measures are shifting from the traditional measure of whether the person lives or dies as the outcome indicator of success in health care to the quality of a person's life. The use of the phrase "quality of life" or living implies more than physical health. It implies that the individual is mentally and emotionally healthy as well. It is a holistic (*holos* is the Greek word meaning whole) model of health care that takes the other dimensions of a person's being into consideration regarding health. Hippocrates emphasized treatment of the person as a whole. He emphasized the influence of society and the environment on health. But, as humanity progressed through the ages, the influence of technology and the germ theory of disease moved health care toward a distinct approach based on scientific causation.

A wholistic approach to health care acknowledges that multiple factors are operating in disease, trauma, and aging and that there are many interactions among the factors. Social, emotional, environmental, political, economic, psychological, and cultural factors are all acknowledged to influence health. An approach that takes this perspective centers its philosophy on the individual. The individual with this orientation is less likely to have the physician look only for the chemical basis of his or her difficulty and ignore the psychological factors that may be present.

The wholistic model contains concepts of health care for both the individual and the health care provider. Pelletier[35] mentions six ideas that form the basis for the theory of wholistic health. The first is that all diseases are psychosomatic. All diseases consist of an element that is physical and an element that is emotional or psychological. An individual who is emotionally stressed may trigger onset of disease when infected with a pathogen, whereas another might not. Some stresses can be identified before illness results. Obesity stresses the cardiovascular system. Preventive care that reduces the stress may also reduce chances of illness: this is a prospective outlook on disease. Another concept relates to the importance of people as individuals. An individual exists within the environment in a unique way and responds to stresses in an infinite variety of ways, not in a stereotyped manner. A third concept is that wholistic health care employs not only conventional but also nontraditional methods (such as acupuncture, massage, and biofeedback) to treat disease. It also uses methods that depart from traditional, scientifically proven ones, such as the Eastern practice of meditation, music, and dance. The fourth concept departs from the negative connotation of disease and illness by suggesting that illness may provide an opportunity for an individual to learn more about himself or herself. An individual may use disease as a chance to get to know personal values and look on it as a time to grow and change. The fifth concept is that of keeping human needs central to health care. Humanness is central to the wholistic philosophy; individual needs should determine a course of care. The sixth concept of wholistic care is central to this study. The health professional and the client should interact in a relationship in which each assumes some responsibility for the process of health care and where each respects the other. The traditional approach fosters dependency, with the professional assuming an authoritative role and the client a passive role. An approach that includes the client in the process has the potential to foster an informed, satisfied client who can take more responsibility for his or her health care. A cooperative relationship develops in programs where the client and the health professional, physician, nurse, or physical therapist, for example, form a partnership. A closer relationship between health professionals and clients, one that involves the client in the process, is advocated.

Individuals in health professions internalize values during their training that reinforce the traditional professional attitude alluded to earlier. Many of these values do not support a partnership relationship with the client. Although society is beginning to question the traditional role of the health professional as the expert, the professional training and organizations resist the pressure to change the image. The professions still hold the image of great authority given to them by the public and fostered through increased political activity.

The major purpose of the patient's relationship with the health professional is to exchange information useful to both in the health care of the client. McNerney[31] calls health education of the client the missing link in health care delivery. As the gap grows between technology and the users of that technology, client health education becomes more important than ever. McNerney[31] notes that although health care providers are now making efforts to educate their clients, they are doing so with little consistency, enthusiasm, theoretical base, imagination—and often with little coordination with other services. The health professional continues to receive training and embrace professional organizational membership that places a premium on control of information and control of the decision making. There should be a special effort to introduce health education concepts into the basic educational programs of health care professionals.

When patients are given more information about their illnesses, and retain the information, they express more satisfaction with their caregivers. A study by Bertakis[4] tested the hypothesis that patients with greater understanding and retention of the information given by the physician would be more satisfied with the doctor-patient relationship. The experimental group received feedback and retained 83.5% of the information given them by the doctor. The control group received no feedback and retained 60.5% of the information. Not surprisingly, the experimental group was more satisfied with the doctor-patient relationship.

If the client is to be informed and included in the treatment process, client health education will have to go beyond the present styles of information giving. If the client is to assume some of the responsibility for his or her physical therapy care, the physical therapist will have to facilitate that involvement. The attitude of the physical therapist toward educating clients about their health could affect his or her ability to facilitate client involvement in the care process.

The more the professional sees himself or herself as the

expert, the less likely he or she will be to see the client as capable of responsibility or expertise in the care process. If communication skills and health education were a part of medical school and the other health professional school curricula, perhaps the health care professionals would temper their assumption of the "expert" professional role.

The health care delivery system in America has to serve all of the citizens. That is no easy task. The United States is a society of great pluralism. It is a free society. It is a society that is used to being governed by persuasion, not coercion. Given the variety of economic, political, cultural and religious forces at work in American society, education of the people in regard to their health care is probably the only method that can work in the long run. The future task of health education will be to "cultivate people's sense of responsibility toward their own health and that of the community." Health education is an effective approach with perhaps the most potential to move us toward a concept of preventive care.

Generation of a new model

Carlson[7] thinks that pressure to change to wholistic thinking in medicine continues as a result of a societal change in its perspective of the rights of individuals. A concern to keep the individual central in the care process will continue to grow in response to continued technological growth that threatens to dehumanize care even more. The wholistic model takes into account each person's unique psychosocial, political, economic, environmental, and religious needs as they affect the individual's health.

Engel[12] sees a need to broaden the approach to disease and include the psychosocial aspects without sacrificing the advantages of the biomedicine model. He accepts Von Bertalanffy's theory that all life events are linked to each other in an ascending order of complexity, from molecules to organs to individuals to families to communities, to society to the universe, and that a change in any of these ultimately affects another element of the chain. With this interdependence in mind, a new medical model that has the following characteristics is suggested: (1) a biochemical defect does not have to be present for a human to experience illness; (2) behavioral processes would be related to the biochemical changes; (3) other variables of life would be taken into account as they interact with somatic function; (4) the patient's view of his or her illness would be taken into account; (5) treatment would be directed at the psychosocial aspects of illness as well; and (6) the relationship of the provider and the client would be recognized as it influences the outcome of the disease process.

Fink[14] also views health as a hierarchy of systems and supports a wholistic model of care. He includes the provider and patient relationship as a major variable in health care delivery. Fink envisions a continuum from the point when the patient is a passive recipient of the provider's care to a point where the provider and the patient each contribute to the relationship to the final point of patient self-care.

The unique religious nature of human beings makes health not an end in itself, but an important means to better experience life and allow individuals to accomplish what they strives for. Pastoral counselors who observed patients visiting their physician too late in their illness appealed to the American Medical Association's Committee on Medicine and Religion to use pastoral counseling as a complementary service to the physician, and the first holistic health center was established in 1970. As a result, pastoral counselors met the patient when he or she came in, established a friendly atmosphere, and administered a personal health inventory scale. The patient participates in an internal planning conference, explaining what kind of help he or she wants and participating in selecting alternatives for care.

Life-style/stress

One of the assumptions practitioners of wholistic health commonly make is that a person with a physically or mentally self-abusive life-style is not free of pathology. This statement is made more credible in light of Breslow's findings.[5] Breslow looked at 7000 Californians' health habits of: (1) no smoking; (2) moderate drinking; (3) 7 or 8 hours sleep each night; (4) regular meals with no snacks; (5) breakfast each day; (6) maintenance of normal weight, and (7) regular exercise. He concluded that if a person followed all seven of the habits, his or her health was significantly better than that of a person who followed only six, and so on. He was able to relate the findings with longevity figures to further substantiate his findings.

The most significant cause of all the illness or disorders that cannot be explained at the molecular level is stress. Migraine headache and hypertension have not been found to be convincingly explained by the presence of a pathogen. Rather they develop over a period of time, and stress is thought to play a major role. Selye[46] has done the primary scientific research in this area, and has described a formal syndrome, the General Adaptation Syndrome. It consists of three stages: (1) an alarm reaction when the anterior pituitary gland secretes adrenocorticotrophic hormone, (2) a stage of resistance when physiological secretion ceases, and (3) a stage of exhaustion when the body loses capacity to respond to further stress. If the stage of exhaustion continues, the animal dies. Psychological problems can stress the body. Selye conceptualizes that an organ has a certain capacity for tolerating stress; if this capacity is exceeded, the organism will break down.

In Brown's work[6] with biofeedback, she observed the activity of subconscious action during stress. She reasoned that if subconscious centers are responsible for stress and if stress accounts for a large proportion of illness, an intervention that acts through those centers similar to biofeedback is reasonable. It provides an opportunity for the individual to become aware of his or her internal state and thus to take a first step toward changing it.

Krieger[23] researched the effects of the sensation of touching on decreasing stress. She studied nurses in New York, half of whom used a lot of touching in their patient care and a control group who did not. The patients in the experiment had blood samples drawn before and after treatment. Krieger hypothesized that if touch had an effect, it could be found physiologically in a hemoglobin change in the patient and that the mean hemoglobin values of the experimental group would be higher after treatment. The experimental group did show a significant increase in their hemoglobin mean value, though the increase may only have been part of a larger unidentified response. Kreiger has been the first to define this aspect of human interaction in physiological terms.

Holmes and Rahe[22] hypothesized that an event is probably as stressful as the person perceives it to be. They attempted to quantify events in the social environment that can be classed as stressful, for example, death of a loved one or a change of jobs. The events they chose theoretically required some kind of adaptation by the individual. They listed the events and assigned points for each. It appeared that, when a certain number of such events occurred in a person's life within a prescribed time, that person's chances of becoming physically ill increased.

Friedman and Rosenman[17] classified people who are described as type A and type B. As are hard-driving, aggressive people and Bs are more easy going. They found a significant number of cardiovascular problems occurring in type A people as opposed to type B.

Stein and others[48] reviewed the effect of hypothalamic lesions on the immune processes of the body. The condition of hypothalamus has been identified as a good indicator to the body's reaction to psychosocial stress. They saw corresponding changes in both the autonomic nervous system and in neuroendocrine activity. They recorded further studies to evaluate the immune processes response to stress.

Client participation

Becker and Maiman[3] discussed Rosenstock's Health Belief model as a framework to account for the individual's decision to use preventive services or engage in preventive health behavior. They cite noncompliance with a physician's recommendation in about one third of all patients. Action taken by the individual, according to the model, depends on the individual's perceived susceptibility to the illness, his or her perception of the severity of the illness, the benefits to be gained from taking action, and a "cue" of some sort that triggers action. The cue could be advice from a friend, reading an article about the illness, a television commercial, and so on. In some way, the person is motivated to do something.

Split-brain research, research in the functions of the left and right halves of the brain, seems to be a pertinent area of mind-body research. The left hemisphere of the brain processes experiences in a factual, logical, and analytical way, whereas the right half appears to process the same experiences in the form of images and impressions. The recognition that one half of the brain may be designed to record the impressionistic part of an experience gives further credibility to including the individual's accounts of his feelings and emotions as a part of the input for diagnosis of illness.

Travis[50] considers the responsibility the client takes for his or her own health care to be at the heart of the wholistic health model. Travis is a physician who set up a Wellness Resource Center in California and developed a wellness inventory to assess the individual's present state of health. He recognizes three distinct phases in promoting the health of his client: (1) an assessment (the wellness inventory), (2) education of the client to learn the options available and to participate in choice of treatment, and (3) growth toward wellness. Growth toward wellness includes trying some of the options and reevaluating them after a period of time. He reasons that each person has responsibility for his or her own health and that no one can change anyone unless that person wants to be changed. Wellness is a lifelong process. Travis views health as client-oriented and emphasizes wholistic thinking as opposed to the reductionist thinking of biomedicine.

Two articles that have appeared in reputable medical journals written by patients experiencing a serious illness who have taken responsibility for their own health care. The first article is an account by Norman Cousins[9] Cousins was stricken with ankylosing spondolitis. Bedridden and given 1 chance in 500 to survive, he analyzed his situation. He had been suffering exhaustion, and remembering what he had read about exhaustion and the influence of stress on chemical changes in the glands, he decided that if negative reactions produced stresses, positive ones might halt the process. He had the full support of his doctor. He placed himself in a pleasant environment, reduced his medication, increased his intake of vitamin C, and watched a lot of funny movies to keep his spirits high. He found that the nodules in his hands shrank, he moved with less pain, and he began to walk again. Cousins said that the placebo effect is demonstrated here and that the will to live was translated somehow into a physical reality of healing.

Fiore,[16] a psychologist, wrote of his experience in surviving cancer. He came to a point where he felt that he was taking drugs more to please his oncologist and support a research project than for his own health's sake. He actively sought to regain some control that he felt he had lost by insisting that a hospital tumor board review his case. Because the specialized physician is too busy, he advocated the use of ancillary personnel to provide emotional and psychological support. They can conduct nutrition, fitness, and relaxation classes and help patients communicate their feelings. Fiore encourages patients to become more independent to enhance the quality of their lives. He advocates that patients be viewed as experts about their own feelings.

Three physicians, Glickman, Manson and Ellison,[19] responded with letters to the editor following publication of Fiore's article. Glickman's comment was that a team approach tends to deflect responsibility from the physician who can "best perform those tasks"; Manson thought Fiore was wrong to implicate life-style as responsible for cancer or its cure, and that entering the process as he did is a cause of more harm than help. The last of the three to respond, Ellison, supported Fiore's ideas. He suggested, in particular, that words like "terminal" and phrases like "nothing else can be done" be omitted from conversation between patients and physicians since they form mental images that the patient finds hard to forget or escape from. He supports the active involvement of the patient.

Dubos[10] stated that even though societal and environmental conditions may be harmful to a client in the long run and even though medical experts think they understand and can anticipate what is best for the client, that does not give them the license to decide what is best for the client. The role of medicine, Dubos cautioned, is to help people achieve a healthy state so they can make their own decisions.

Issues

So far, there are no data on comparative studies between the traditional medical model approach to health care and the wholistic model of health care. A few authors have discussed the approaches.[15,33] They list the benefits of a wholistic approach as broadening the perspectives on illness, potentially affecting chronic disease, lowering costs, demystifying health care, making health care more democratic, making clients aware of our current health care delivery system problem, and improving patient-provider relationships. There are limitations of the wholistic approach as well. Limitations include bringing inappropriate areas of living into the health care problem, the fact that people may deal too subjectively with their problems, and that acceptability of the health problem would vary with the social class of the individual.[33] Self-help may ultimately benefit people who already have a better chance for survival. It is also unrealistic to expect changes in health care if societal problems of employment, housing, income, and racism are not dealt with at the same time. The medical profession's power and vested financial interest is one of the societal problems to be dealt with in this context.[15]

Hayes-Bautista and Harveston[20] pointed out that for the person to cooperate and work on the health problem with the provider, the problem does have to be well defined. Many of the daily problems of health care that could respond to wholistic approach are multifaceted and have more than one possible approach or solution. They are often handled at present by community health clinics, which are set up in traditional modes and are not equipped in terms of knowledge, manpower, and resources to deal with health problems in a wholistic way.

Freymann[18] sees a problem getting health care workers excited about preventive care. A successful case of preventive care would mean that no medical action would have to be taken. Clinical medicine involving active intervention, such as surgery, evaluation of complex laboratory tests, and the problem-solving approach to diagnosis, is what excites health care workers today. Freymann ponders the strange logic of traditional medicine, which rewards the specialist who confines his or her practice to a very few and shows little concern for a public health physician whose field is broad and who treats so many. Dramatic traditional medicine does not result in many health benefits for large numbers of people.

McKay[30] asks to what extent health providers are willing to commit themselves to explore and implement alternative forms of health care. The provider-client relationship becomes very important to a successful therapeutic outcome, as does health education and promotion of positive health behaviors. Health providers seem to forget that well-being calls for wellness of the mind, body, and environment. Though they may talk about supporting a focus on health they continue to focus on disease. The training that health providers receive makes disease more interesting than wellness.

Saward and Sorenson[43] make the observation that the mass media has promoted the technology of health care. The consumer thus has a heightened expectation of the quality of care he or she will receive. However, we should avoid excesses in the other extreme. If society adheres to inappropriate life-styles, the health professional cannot turn around and blame the victim for bringing on the illness and absolve himself or herself from responsibility. Wholistic health care carried to an extreme might result in "blaming the victim." Saward and Sorenson see that in the extremes, the medical model and the wholistic model of health care have different objectives, evolve from different historical, philosophical and economic perspectives, and use practitioners with essentially different training and outlook on health care. Perhaps, they suggest, two health care systems should be available to people instead of one.

Szasz and Hollender[49] described five basic relationships between providers and clients on a continuum from a provider-dominated relationship, consistent with the medical model, through a mutual participation relationship, to a relationship where the client accepts the larger share of responsibility, which is consistent with the wholistic model. Whether or not the client takes some responsibility for his or her care depends a great deal on whether the health provider gives some to him or her.

Fink[14] also recognized the importance of the provider-patient relationship and made three points about it. The first is that a relationship between them is given. The second is that what the relationship becomes is mutually agreed upon, consciously or not. Third, whatever the form of the relationship, it should meet the needs and health care requirements of the particular patient.

Trends

Monaco[34] claims that despite the difficulty in identifying all the elements of the wholistic model, the wholistic health advocates are multiplying. They are coming from all walks of life, and their very enthusiasm may produce a rift in the health care field with traditional medicine on one side and wholistic medicine on the other. As the wholistic movement begins to gather data, there will be a more realistic basis for blending the models or for separating them. Monaco thinks it will be the consumer who decides which it will be. Masi[28] sees the technological gains of the past 25 years slowing and biomedical research retrenching. He urges that research in the human sciences be promoted to a point of excellence. Strong support will come from the younger generation with its natural optimism and differing points of view.

One of the issues consumers and society will have to deal with is that standards of care have been traditionally linked to licensure. Wholistic health practitioners are usually unlicensed, and many physicians avoid associating with them in order to protect their image. Yahn[51] urges that standards of care be part of the future for wholistic practitioners and that regulations be set for direction.

Health education has been mentioned by nearly all of the proponents of wholistic care. Sechrist[45] cautioned the health educator not to get on the bandwagon. He feels that wholistic health care's education goals are still very nebulous. To prove its value, health education should address more well-defined problems. Though the wholistic health care goals are in tune with health education, joining the trend might result in disruption within the field just as it is beginning to establish an identity.

Which model will result in better health care? McDermott[29] advocates regularly identifying the variables in whichever model is used, measuring their effect, and taking corrective actions necessary to assure quality care. An important corrective action he suggests is to educate the health provider at the level of the school curriculum. Two major variables present in every health care setting are the attitudes the provider has toward the practice of his or her profession and the attitudes he or she holds toward educating clients and involving them in the process.

CLIENT HEALTH EDUCATION
Client/provider relationship

The relationship between the provider and the client is a major variable in quality of care in every health-related setting. The extent to which the care given is biomedical or wholistic can be traced to that intimate encounter and the attitudes, values, and beliefs that each of the participants bring to it.

Leopold[24] called the relationship of the therapist and client "the emotional bridge over which the more mechanical forms of treatment are conducted." The psychological makeups of the therapist and of the client have an impact on the relationship that is established. The psychological development of both of them during their growth stages of dependency, aggressiveness, and ability to subordinate personal gratification must be acknowledged as having an effect on the relationship.

The illness or trauma of the client that represents a disintegrating force in his or her life may represent an opportunity for the therapist to grow professionally. The client and the therapist may have different psychological backgrounds, and though the client is usually there because of the medical crisis, the therapist may be there for purposes of personal growth, financial gain, prestige, and unconscious gratification in influencing the lives of others through professional skill.

Awareness of the importance of these factors would enable the therapist to approach the relationship with better understanding.

Pratt[37] recognized the large amount of time a physical therapist spends in face-to-face patient contact. In this respect, the therapist has an advantage over most other health practitioners who see the patient at infrequent intervals and who seldom touch the patient as a physical therapist does. The physical contact itself may provide psychological support and promote a close relationship between the therapist and the patient. It is important then that the physical therapist be aware of the importance of the relationship itself. The therapist's attitudes and values can affect the expectations of patients regarding the outcome of treatment. The patient's expectations can be made realistic if he or she is an active participant in care from the start. Any process that involves personal committment and purports to effect change should focus on the person seeking help. An attitude of acceptance of the patient as an equal in the process may be of healing value by itself.

Ramsden[39] discussed the reality that transference (i.e., the client incorporating some of the therapist's qualities) takes place during physical therapy treatments as it does whenever human contact takes place. Though physical therapy purports to recognize the importance of the whole patient, there is still a major focus on the physical aspect of patient care and little on the psychological aspects. Professional responsibility in physical therapy extends to the development of maximal efficiency in interpersonal communication. Enough is known about the area of communication to teach it to practitioners rather than allowing it to develop by chance.

Conine[8] noted that there are reports that physical therapists spend nearly one quarter of their time with patients listening or talking. However, physical therapists have had little training in listening attentively or tolerating silence in conversation. In their own education they also have had too little experience of being listened to in order to appreciate the importance of doing that for others. If listening to a patient can relieve that patient's anxieties, the patient might be more motivated to channel energy into working to help himself or herself. Conine conjectured that much of the superficial conversation that goes on during treatment sessions may be an attempt on the part of the therapist to avoid release of the patient's deep-seated thoughts. The therapist may not feel capable of dealing with those thoughts. Listening to the patient is particularly important if the therapist wants to understand the patient's needs to formulate treatment programs and instruct the patient.

A role common to all physical therapists is that of educator. Patient education in receiving more emphasis, particularly in areas of chronic disease. Patient education programs have to be evaluated to determine how much this contributes to quality care and cost containment. Rand[40] pointed out how rarely patient education programs are evaluated. She advocated a comprehensive evaluation model including listing of needs, goals, criteria for success, plans, and outcomes. The therapist in an educator's role would want to evaluate the patient education program to see if the objectives were met to establish the worth of the program, and to get information to help with decision making.

The scientific foundation of physical therapy relates movement and exercise to pathological conditions. Hislop[21] describes the major role of the physical therapist as that of a pathokinesiologist. She acknowledges that the interpersonal relationships with patients may characterize a major area of a physical therapist's work, but she cautions that the profession must focus on its scientific role if it wants to survive. Basic and applied scientific research supplied by our own professionals, is necessary. Although she recognizes the humanistic and social responsibility that any profession must have, Hislop stresses our lack of a strong base of scientific knowledge and urges that physical therapists take on the research role to add to our body of scientific knowledge. She adds that science must be balanced with humanistic care and does not believe that a sharper scientific focus would obscure our roles as humanistic care givers.

Long[26] suggests that the consumers become as knowledgeable as possible about their condition, find out the level of the physical therapist's professional education, question the physical therapist about the equipment used, be aware of treatments that go on too long or treatments with little result. He also advocates that consumers ask for detailed instructions and demonstrations, use logic, and practice thinking for themselves.

As the consumer becomes more involved, so should the family. The family is seldom brought into the practice. Sasano and others[44] described a patient program that includes the family. They made some comments relative to physical therapy's inclusion of the family in the care process. Patients were happier with the family involved; the family itself felt less anxious and could be more supportive. All of these factors facilitate the work of the physical therapist. The therapist, however, must be willing to facilitate the family involvement and help them learn to take responsibility for some of the care and decision making. Most health professionals are not conditioned to the patient assuming greater authority. The family cannot take responsibility for the care unless the physical therapist allows the family to assume that role.

Lopopola and others[27] formed a comprehensive care team for arthritic patients. The departments of internal medicine, orthopedics, physical therapy, and occupational therapy worked closely with the patient and family. Intensive training and education was carried out, and a followup program was established. A stated goal was to produce an atmosphere to encourage the patient to take responsibility for his or her care. To compare program effectiveness and cost of care, 20 patients were studied in a conventional way and 20 cared for by the team concept. Results of the program showed that for the group that had been cared for by the team concept: (1) length of stay had shortened; (2) communication between the professional departments involved had improved; (3) program planning had become a team effort and included the patient and the family; and (4) patients felt less confused about their program of care. The authors believed they had found a way to increase quality of care and decrease costs for arthritic patients using a team approach.

A multidisciplinary pain management center was the setting for a program described by Roesch and Ulrich.[41] Physical therapy has traditionally focused on the pain reported by the patient. In this center, the therapists applied behavior modification techniques to attempt to extinguish the patient's pain behavior. Education was carried out including assertiveness training and awareness of the dynamics of the chronic pain syndrome. Physical therapy exercises were done in groups and lectures were conducted on body mechanics, exercise, and gait. Self-motivation was encouraged by giving the patient options to increase activity and participate in establishing a schedule to eliminate assistive devises such as braces. The patient and the family participated in the home program planning. The therapists felt that with this overall approach the patients became less anxious and more knowledgeable and thus less susceptible to reinjury. They encouraged the therapists to create an atmosphere that allows the patient to change and gradually move from a focus on treatment of the pain to a focus on activity in the treatment of chronic pain.

The physical therapist is caught up in the same problems of the health care system as other health professionals. Inflation has caused profit to become a more important motive for setting priorities in our clinics than human considerations. Research is heavily focused on technical procedures, yet the relationship with patients in the care process is vital. Singleton[47] labeled this phenomenon a paradox in physical therapy. Despite the commitment to humanistic service on which the profession was founded, the service rendered is mechanistic.

Is the patient approached like a machine? Has scientific technology captured the physical therapist's attention to the extent that he ignores patient care procedures that cannot or have not been scientifically analyzed? Alexander[1] sees the necessity of reorganizing the education and work of the physical therapist to encourage a humanistic approach to care. To what degree, Alexander asks, are we "masters or servants to our patients?" The educational programs could emphasize whole-patient treatment, increase communication skills and interdisciplinary awareness, video-tape students as they interact with others, and encourage role-playing. Finally, he proposes that although restructuring educational experiences is useful, selection procedures also have to be considered.

If medicine succeeds in bringing humanistic medicine into focus and shifting some emphasis from a scientific technology approach, it is conceivable that some people currently suited to practicing physical therapy would find it intolerable to do so in the future.

The community role

Today's complex world of health care goes beyond the one-to-one health care relationship. To achieve quality care for a neurologically disabled individual, the community must be utilized. Prevention of head injuries can be the focus of many community groups. Prevention programs in the community can address both the chemical and mechanical standards of that community's environment. The employers in the area should have safe working environments and programs should exist for stress reduction, counseling, and family-related concerns. Traffic problems, regulations for safe recreational pursuits—everything, in short, that affects our living from day to day—involves our community and that community's willingness to create as hazard-free an environment as possible.

One task of communication is to reduce risk-taking decisions for the client. The responsibility falls first on the shoulders of the health care professional dealing with the patient, but the success of that undertaking is also directly related to the support the client receives from the community in which the client lives. All activities that relate to achieving that end are under consideration for any client, but particularly for the neurologically involved individual whose disability spans the continuum of need for support.

Questions to be considered are: (1) how comprehensive should the services be? (2) how much continuity of service is available? (3) are creative solutions sought to the problems within the community? (4) does a rational planning process exist that gathers input from all citizens and sets priorities? and (5) is there a committment of the community to follow through with the necessary budget support?

Criticisms of community services include lack of committment to such programs, focus on individual problems of the client as opposed to setting broader goals and putting in place programs that benefit many, failure to integrate such services, placing low priority on educating both community lay people and the health care workers in all aspects of the problem, neglecting nontraditional methods of care, and placing low priority on planning and evaluation. The results of research studies that are well controlled and conducted seldom find their way into the publications read or utilized by planners or users of such systems.

Appropriate efforts that could be undertaken by communities to provide support to the neurologically disabled individual include: (1) moving from an emphasis on clinical intervention to a use of community funds for education programs aimed at prevention of, for example accidents and risk-taking behaviors; (2) involving individuals in the community; (3) developing councils of agencies on such matters; (4) sponsoring seminars and workshops for families and peers of clients to help them deal with the stress, anger, and guilt, as well as workshops on care giving and utilizing available resources; (5) clarifying roles of care within the community by making a realistic master plan for the care within the community; (6) educating and training those people who provide the care and not leaving it entirely up to the specific agency or professional group to do it in isolation; (7) bringing in experts in the field to disseminate the latest findings; (8) establishing a reference guide through the library and creating ready access to materials needed by clients and their families; (9) gathering community support for the volunteer services needed by nursing homes in the area and maintaining lines of communication with those homes and the community at large (especially to make clear lines of communication possible in such areas as zoning and housing regulations and transportation within the community); (10) establishing a center in town where clients and/or families can gather, discuss common interests, socialize, and find information, or if such a center cannot be funded, using volunteers trained to man such a center; (11) motivating the leaders of the community to get involved, including the philanthropic and church groups; and (12) as services proliferate, helping the community keep track of them, keeping records becomes increasingly important. Computerization may help coordinate and create access to services. As in all programs run by a collective group, to be successful the group has to want success. Even one well-run service for the client can be a major breakthrough.

A WHOLISTIC APPROACH TO THE NEUROLOGICAL CLIENT

Neurological clients interact with the medical community for short or long periods of time. They present neurological problems of all types that are sudden or insidious in nature. All aspects of human function are represented in the variety of problems. If individual beliefs and values energize and motivate physical behavior, think of the possibilities for stimulating wellness.

Ida Rolf[36] and Moshe Feldenkrais[13] put forth dramatic, new ways of approaching well-being. Research has just begun on naturally occurring opiates within the brain and on the ability to control body functions through sensory feedback. Perhaps the art and science of care are coming closer together. Many areas of therapeutic intervention once ignored by health professionals are watched with more than intellectual curiosity. Flynn[15] states that this new interest quite possibly signals the beginning of a paradigm shift in health care. The shift to a new model should make use of current knowledge, dispose of outdated information, and incorporate new information.

That new information is becoming available. Additionally, some information that has been available is becoming visible.[15] As health care practitioners, our therapeutic choices have widened. Reasons include a heightened awareness of "the Heisenberg Uncertainty Principle," in which Heisenberg hypothesized that if you are specific about the exact location of an electron at any one point of time, you cannot also specify its momentum or velocity. The transfer to therapeutic intervention has been stated in such a way that if you observe or look at an object, that object is changed. It is no longer the object it was before the observation. Thus certain aspects of an object or individual will always remain undefinable. We become part of the person we observe or touch.

Karl H. Pribham, a neurophysiologist, has demonstrated the brain as a holographic model. Dennis Gabor received a Nobel Prize in 1947 for his work in holography, whose idea is that the waveform of light scattered by an object is recorded on a plate as an interference pattern. When the photographic record, hologram, is subjected to a laser beam, the original wave pattern creates a three-dimensional image of the photographed object. A piece of the hologram, when exposed to the laser beam, gives a representation of the whole object. Pribham has proposed, with substantiating evidence, that the brain works that way with long-term memory. The whole of a memory is contained or retrieved from each of millions of fragmented parts. In other words, each of the fragments or parts contains the whole, making it possible, as William Blake wrote, "to see the world in a grain of sand."[15]

It is important to recall that the entire nervous system begins with the formation of one embryonic disc. Each cell is derived from its parent cells in methodical fashion.

Once complete, however, the system attains a complexity of communication that remains little understood. Physical laws have been applied to explain the function. For example, Muller's law of specific energies states that specific sensations are activated by specialized nerve endings for that sensation. The cornea, however, has shown responses of touch, cold, warmth, and pain though only bare nerve endings exist on that surface.

Ilya Prigigine, a physical chemist, proposed a theory of dissipative structures. In general, the theory states that certain fluctuations can be the means used by fluid, self-organizing systems to change. The fluctuations or mechanisms that cause the fluctuation are often a result of altered states of consciousness, such as meditation. These changes in energy fields of neurons have been demonstrated by electroencephalogram. These energy fields create fluctuation in areas of the brain, and the theory states that in this way systems such as the human mind can reorder and reorganize patterns of thinking and feeling. Music, imagery, rhythmic breathing, moving, and relaxation are implicated.[15]

It is beyond the scope of this chapter to begin an exploration of each tool that could be used therapeutically. Some have received more attention than others. A partial list includes biofeedback, acupressure, acupuncture, hypnosis, herbal nutrition, transactional analysis, yoga, Feldenkrais, rolfing, martial arts, occult sciences, transcendental meditation, homeopathic medicine, imaging, awareness of roles of stress, laughter, and relaxation.

The effects of neural activity have been shown to last for tens of minutes through release of synaptic transmitters. Time probably plays a major role in effecting permanent change in the nervous system. The systems mentioned above (i.e., music, breathing, etc.) are potentially reinforcing phenomena with their regular, rhythmical influence. In such cases, perhaps, rhythmic influence over time creates permanent change.

SUMMARY

The responsibility for the well-being of our clients may well rest within our capability more than we know. This chapter has postulated that, with increased understanding of the client-provider relationship and elements of human nature, we can enhance the client's physical function. Quality of life may be influenced as much by programs of prevention within the community as by biomedical research advances day by day. Much of the environment within our reach can be used to create change for the client. The relationships between the client and the health care provider are influential. Patterns of support systems and belief and value systems are also powerful vehicles of change. Perhaps the art and science of health care are moving closer together. The illness-to-wellness continuum is really a circle. One never just backs up or goes forward on the line. One is changed forever from moment to moment. The therapeutic relationship involves two people, changed forever by and within the relationship, circling along the continuum of health, each teaching and each learning.

REFERENCES

1. Alexander DA: Yes, but what about the patient? Physiotherapy 59:391-394, 1973.
2. American Physical Therapy Association: Progress Report 9, July/August, 1980.
3. Becker M and Maiman L: Sociobehavioral determinants of compliance with health and medical care recommendation, Med Care 13:10-24, 1975.
4. Bertakis K: The communication of information from physician to patient: a method for increasing patient practice, J Fam Pract 5:217-222, 1977.
5. Breslow L: A positive strategy for the nation's health, JAMA 242:2093-2095, 1979.
6. Brown BB: Stress and the art of biofeedback, New York, 1977, Harper & Row, Inc.
7. Carlson RJ: Holism and reductionism as perspectives in medicine and patient care, W J MED 131:466-470, Oct, 1979.
8. Conine T: Listening in the helping relationship, Phys Ther 56:159-162, 1976.
9. Cousins N: Anatomy of an illness (as perceived by the patient), N Eng J Med 295:1458-1463, 1976.
10. Dubos R: The state of health and the quality of life, W J Med 25:8-9, 1976.
11. Duffy J: The healers: the rise of the medical establishment, New York, 1976, McGraw-Hill Co.
12. Engel GL: The need for a new medical model: a challenge for biomedicine, Sci 196:129-133, April 1977.
13. Feldenkrais M: Awareness through movement, New York, 1972, Harper & Row, Inc.
14. Fink D: Holistic health: the evolution of western medicine. In Flynn P, editor: The healing continuum, Bowie, Md, 1980, Robert J Bowie Co.
15. Flynn P: Holistic health, Bowie, Md, 1980, Robert J Brady Co, Prentice-Hall Pub. Co.
16. Fiore N: Fighting cancer: one patient's perspective, N Eng J Med 300:284-289, Feb 1979.
17. Friedman M and Rosenman RH: Type A behavior pattern: its association with coronary heart disease, J Clin Res 3:300-312, 1971.
18. Freymann JG: Medicine's great schism, prevention vs. cure: an historical interpretation, Med Care 13:525-536, July 1975.
19. Glickman L, Manson A, and Ellison NM: Letter to the editor, N Eng J Med 12:1219-1220, May 1979.
20. Hayes-Bautista D and Harveston DS: Holistic health care, Soc Pol 7:7-13, March-April 1977.
21. Hislop HJ: The not-so-impossible dream, Phys Ther 55:1069-1080, Oct 1975.
22. Holmes TH and Rahe RH: The social readjustment rating scale, J Psychosom Res 11:213-218, 1967.
23. Kreiger D: Therapeutic touch: the imprimature of nursing, Am J Nurs 75:784-787, May 1975.
24. Leopold RL: Patient-therapist relationship: psychological considerations, Phys Ther 34:8-13, Jan 1954.
25. Levin L: Forces and issues in the revival of interest in self-care impetus for redirection in health, Health Ed Mono 5:115, Summer 1977.
26. Long RW: Physical therapy and the consumer, Health Ed 6:18-21, Nov-Dec 1975.
27. Lopopolo RB and others: Minimal care concept, Phys Ther 58:700-703, June 1978.
28. Masi LA: A wholistic concept of health and illness: a tricentennial goal for medicine and public health, J Chron Dis 31:563-572, 1978.
29. McDermott W: Evaluating the physician and his technology, In Knowles JH, editor: Doing better and feeling worse, New York, 1977, WW Norton Co.
30. McKay S: Holistic health care: challenge to providers, J Allied Hlth, 9:194-201, August 1980.
31. McNerney WJ: The missing link in health services, J Med Ed 50:11-23, Jan 1975.
32. Mechanic D: Medical sociology, New York, 1978, The Free Press.
33. Menke WG: Medical identity: change and conflict in professional roles, J Med Ed 46:58-63, Jan 1971.
34. Monaco AJ: Coming of wholistic medicine, Hosp Top 56:10-11, July-Aug 1978.
35. Pelletier KR: Mind as healer, mind as slayer, New York, 1977, Dell.
36. Pierce R: Rolfing. In Bauman E and others, editors: The holistic health handbook, Berkeley, 1978, And/Or Press.
37. Pratt JW: A psychological view of the physiotherapist's role, Physiotherapy 64:241-242, Aug 1978.
38. Purtillo RB and Cassel CK: Ethical dimensions in the health professions, Philadelphia, 1981, WB Saunders Co.
39. Ramsden EL: Interpersonal communications in physical therapy, Phys Ther 48:1130-1132, Oct 1968.
40. Rand PH: Evaluation of physical therapy education programs, Phys Ther 58:851-856, July 1978.
41. Roesch R and Ulrich D: Physical therapy management in the treatment of chronic pain, Phys Ther 60:53-57, Jan 1980.
42. Rogers C: A humanistic concept of man. In Farsom R, editor: Science and human affairs, Palo Alto, Calif 1965, Science and Behavior Books.
43. Saward E and Sorenson A: The current emphasis on preventive medicine, Sci 200:889-894, May 1978.
44. Sasano E and others: The family in physical therapy, JAPTA 57:153-159, 1977.
45. Sechrist WC: Total wellness and wholistic health—a bandwagon we cannot afford to jump onto!. Hlth Ed 10:27, Sept-Oct 1979.
46. Selye H: The Stress of Life, New York, 1976, McGraw-Hill Co.
47. Singleton M: Profession—a paradox? JAPTA 60:439, 1980.
48. Stein M, Schiavi PC, and Camerino M: Influence of brain and behavior on the immune system, Sci 191:435-440, Feb 1976.
49. Szasz TS and Hollender MH: A contribution to the philosophy of medicine, Arch Int Med 97:585-592, May 1956.
50. Travis JW: Wellness education: a new model for health. In Flynn P, editor: The healing continuum, Bowie, Md, 1980, Robert J Brady Co.
51. Yahn G: The impact of holistic medicine, medical groups and health concepts, JAMA 242:2202-2205, Nov 1979.

ADDITIONAL READINGS

Cai J: Toward a comprehensive evaluation of alternate medicine, Soc Sci Med 25:659-667, 1987.

Coombs R: Mastering medicine: professional socialization in medical school, New York, 1978, The Free Press.

Hancock T: The soft health path: a healthier future for physician? Can Med Assoc J 112:1019, 1982.

Harrison M and Cotanch P: Pain: advances and issues in critical care, Nurs Clin North Am 22:691-697, 1987.

Keller E and Bzdek V: Effects of therapeutic touch on tension headache pain, Nurs Res 35:101-106, 1986.

LaPatria J: Healing: the coming revolution in holistic medicine, New York, 1978, McGraw-Hill.

Pownall M: Holistic nursing: all in the mind's eye, Nurs Times 82:26-27, 1986.

Sarkis J and Skonor M: An analysis of the concept of holism in nursing literature, Holist Nurs Pract 2:61-69, 1987.

Shealy C: Holistic management of chronic pain, Clin Nurs 2:1-8, 1980.

Part Four

STUDY GUIDE

This textbook was designed for students in their latter phases of academic study and for practicing clinicians. Because of that focus a tremendous amount of information and a large number of strategies for clinical performance have been introduced. The study guide was designed to help the reader focus on key concepts presented within each chapter. This guide does not address all issues, concepts, evaluation forms, treatment strategies, or philosophies identified by the authors. Instead, it is a way to help the reader draw out, on initial exposure, those points each author feels are very important to grasp.

There are many learning styles used when presenting the various questions. This variability was encouraged to help the reader process information in a variety of learning styles and modes of thought. Any question can be reformated to help each student learn. All of the authors hope this guide will ease the challenging path the reader assumes when delving into problem solving and the quest toward understanding the human brain.

Study guide questions

Chapter 1

1. List the three major conceptual components identified within the conceptual triad.

2. List the five categories of evaluation forms generally used with neurologically involved clients.

3. **True/False** An individual usually reverts back to a level of motor function that is primitive or familiar when confronted with difficult or new problems.

4. Identify the three general areas addressed within the client profile.

5. **True/False** Visual-analytical problems do not require verbal strategies.

6. List the three general categories of visual-analytical problem solving and sequence them in their hierachical order.

Chapter 2

1. The most basic unit of behavior that a clinician evaluates or observes is the _____?

2. Give examples of positive and negative signs/symptoms of dysfunction in:
   a. homeostasis
   b. posture
   c. goal-oriented movement
   d. higher cortical processing

3. After reading Chapter 6, identify types of therapeutic intervention that could be used to influence the signs and symptoms you listed above.

4. As you read each chapter in the clinical section, identify positive and negative signs and symptoms for that clinical syndrome and the therapeutic approaches that might be used to influence those dysfunctions.

Chapter 3

1. List the two most common types of models used to describe motor control.

2. The tripartate system refers to which three structures within the CNS?

3. **True/False** The primary function of the basal ganglia is to regulate posture with little influence in the control of movement.

4. The cerebellum is involved in:
   a. relative timing of a motor response
   b. force generation of muscle activity
   c. adaptation of motor behavior
   d. all of the above

5. Within the cerebral cortex which four main areas contribute to motor function?
   a.
   b.
   c.
   d.

6. Which motor area plays a key role in both manual and visual exploration of the environment?

7. List the three functional descending systems and their appropriate tracts that regulate movement:
   a.
   b.
   c.

8. **True/False** The corticospinal tract is not necessary for the performance of volitional actions?

9. When discussing a system theory for motor control, certain neurophysiological concepts related to motor function are presented. List three of the four concepts presented.

10. Select one system's concept and discuss the neurophysiological mechanism involved in implementation of this concept.

11. Dynamic postural control is subdivided into two types of movements. Identify and discuss each balance ability.

12. **True/False** All motor programs occur in a proximal to distal synergy pattern.

13. List what are believed to be at least three of the fixed parameters of a motor program.

14. **True/False** Once a motor program is learned, an individual still needs sensory information to execute the activity.

15. **True/False** Sensory conflict can cause an individual to select a wrong motor pattern for the desired response.

Chapter 4

1. **True/False** The limbic system influences both autonomic (visceral) and skeletal muscle responses.

2. The limbic system MOVEs us. Describe the function of each letter in MOVE.

3. **True/False** Without the limbic system a client will not feel a need to act. A response will occur only if it is reflexive.

4. **True/False** An individual who can control his or her feelings of fear and frustration will tend not to become violent.

5. **True/False** Emotions controlled and regulated by the limbic system can drastically affect motor control.

6. List three limbic components or behaviors that may be critical to a successful client/therapist interaction.

7. Discuss the general adaptation syndrome and its cause.

8. In Alzheimer's disease the limbic system is dramatically affected. Discuss the anatomical and clinical problems that a therapist must consider.

9. What is DAI, and why is the limbic system affected?

10. How can a therapist differentiate high tone in a CVA resulting from limbic system versus motor system involvement?

11. What structure would be considered the center of the limbic system?

12. The largest interlinking reciprocal circuit within the limbic system is called _____ .

13. The limbic system is involved in which type of learning: declarative or procedural (underline one).

14. **True/False** Even though the client values the activity, the control over the response is purely motor.

15. To have memory progress from short term to long term, it is necessary to go through one of two structures within the limbic system. List them.

16. Long-term potentiation refers to:
    a. concepts of reverberating circuits
    b. the simplest kind of memory
    c. hippocampal pathways
    d. all of the above

Chapter 5

1. What are the three main phases of prenatal development and what age ranges do they occupy?

2. What are the seven main phases of postnatal development and what are the approximate age ranges that they occupy?

3. The trilaminar embryonic disk is made up of three tissue layers. Name these layers and the body tissues that are derived from them.

4. The peripheral nervous system is derived from which embryonic tissue?

5. What are the nine major events or processes that occur during human nervous system development?

6. How, and from what embryonic tissue, is the neural tube formed?

7. What is the site of initial closure of the neural tube?

8. What are the three primary brain vessicles, how are they formed, and what brain regions (areas) are derived from each?

9. What is the significance of the ventricular layer or zone of the early neural tube?

10. What are the ventricular, intermediate, and marginal zones of the neural tube?

11. The major phase of neuronal proliferation occurs during what age period?

12. What is the significance of the subventricular zone and external granule cell layer?

13. What is the relation among the proliferation of large and small neurons, neurons and glial cells, during early development?

14. Name and describe two processes of neuronal migration?

15. What are the relations between differentiation (or growth) of axons and dendrites?

16. What is the sequence of events involved in forming a synapse in the nervous system?

17. What are the first and last areas of the nervous system to undergo myelination?

18. At what age are the primary and secondary cortical sulci formed?

19. Compare and contrast the alar and basal plates.

Chapter 6

1. Describe the problem-oriented classification system as outlined in the introduction to Chapter 6.

2. Identify the names and functions of the afferent receptors of the muscle spindle. List six techniques that affect the muscle spindle.

3. Contrast the function of the golgi tendon organ (GTO) with the muscle spindle.

4. List the three different types of joints. Outline the names and functions of the four major joint receptors.

5. The exteroceptive system may be considered a dual system. Identify the characteristics of the protopathic and epicritic systems and how they most commonly influence the state of the nervous system.

6. Outline the benefits of brushing and icing. What are the contraindications and precautions of icing as a therapeutic modality?

7. The vestibular system is physiologically divided into the static and kinetic labyrinth. Summarize the anatomical components and most salient effects of each system.

8. Describe the therapeutic benefits of the inverted position to patients with hypertonicity.

9. Why are inhibitory an facilitory techniques aimed at the autonomic nervous system?

10. Suppose that your goal is to normalize muscle tone, and that your patient is towards the sympathetic end of the autonomic nervous system. What are some strategies you can use to achieve a more balanced autonomic response and more normalized muscle tone?

11. The olfactory system has some unique characteristics. Describe how olfactory input can influence neuromuscular responses. How fast does the olfactory system adapt, and how might the therapist control the olfactory stimulus?

12. Why are the olfactory and the gustatory senses related to feeding and prefeeding activities?

13. The visual system has been found to be diffusely related to the motor, autonomic, and limbic (emotional) systems. List some variables that should be controlled during therapeutic intervention.

14. Study Table 6-6. Develop two vertical lists, labeling one "inhibitory" and the other "facilitory." Identify which techniques can be used in both categories. What are the variables that determine whether the technique is facilitory or inhibitory?

15. List some strategies that can be used to modulate a hypersensitive touch system.

16. What is the orthokinetic cuff? Identify the therapeutic benefits of this device.

17. Identify the importance of facial stimulation and the major sensory and motor components of the trigeminal and facial nerves.

18. Describe four different kinds of equipment that promote proprioceptive and vestibular input.

19. Refer to levels of processing on pp. 149 to 154. List the most salient characteristics of the spinal level, lower brainstem level, upper brainstem level, cerebellum, and cortex and basal ganglia.

20. Select a specific neurological problem that affects levels of processing as described in the text. Develop a list of treatment techniques that might benefit your hypothetical patient. Analyze your techniques with respect to their inhibitory and facilitory characteristics.

Chapter 7

1. **True/False** Once adjustment has taken place, the disabled person will not need to deal with adjustment issues again.

2. **True/False** Many authorities feel that there are stages that a disabled person must pass through to reach adjustment.

3. King has stated that there are four components of the adaptive process. Which of the following is NOT one of King's components:
   a. active response
   b. passive acceptance
   c. response organized subcortically
   d. self-reinforcing adaptation

4. The client's adjustment to the disability may be affected by which of the following:
   a. socialization
   b. culture
   c. hand dominance
   d. a and b

5. **True/False** Cognitive age may be a factor in the reaction to loss, because lower age may preclude the ability to abstract and realize the impact of the situation.

6. **True/False** According to Burton, sexuality begins in the first few years of life.

7. According to Burton, which of the following should *not* be a goal of therapy when dealing with a child? Helping him or her:
   a. distinguish between therapeutic and sensual touch
   b. establish ownership of the body
   c. learn that the therapist knows best and the client should submit
   d. that the "new body" is acceptable and good

8. **True/False** Adaptive devices and sexual aids may be used with disabled adults.

9. **True/False** Men and women cannot have sexual intercourse with indwelling catheters.

10. According to Burton, the therapist should ask some basic questions when working with a client to better understand goals of therapy. Which of the following is *not* one of the questions:
    a. why is this person disabled?
    b. what are his or her good points?
    c. what will this person do for enjoyment?
    d. how will this person bring others enjoyment?

11. **True/False** In the context of therapy, client responsibility and independence can be fostered by giving the client choices.

12. **True/False** According to this chapter, if the client does not adjust to his or her new body and change his or her body image and self-expectations, life will be impoverished for that individual.

13. **True/False** Burton feels that problem solving can be encouraged in clients and families by using slides or pictures to analyze potential architectural barriers.

14. **True/False** Sexuality is not representative of how the person feels about his or her adequacy as a person.

Chapter 8

1. Why is the term "infant stimulation" inappropriate for neonatal therapy practice? Why is infant stimulation incompatible with a biobehavioral theoretical framework composed of a pathokinesiology model and a synactive model of infant behavioral organization?

2. What are the educational requirements for a therapist to work in a NICU? Why are therapists without precepted NICU training placing themselves in medical-legal jeopardy by answering NICU consultations?

3. What are the risks of neonatal therapy and which risk management plans should be designed to decrease physiological and musculoskeletal risk to the infant, medical-legal risk to the therapist, and quality assurance risk to the hospital?

4. What is the most common form of cerebral palsy associated with a preterm birth? What neuropathological factors contribute to this form of CP?

5. What assessment instruments would you choose for the preterm infant versus the full-term infant in the neonatal period?

6. Why may the newborn infant's neurological assessment results be unreliable and show variation on retest the next day?

7. What high-risk profiles of neuromotor and behavioral signs are worrisome and are probable indicators for neonatal therapy intervention?

8. What timing considerations are critical to safe and effective practice by a therapist in a NICU?

9. What are the common postures of prematurity? What positioning strategy could be applied to each abnormal posture?

10. What are the physiological risks and the therapeutic benefits associated with neonatal hydrotherapy?

11. Describe the neonatal therapist's role in facilitating hope and empowerment in parents? Which interactive styles and teaching strategies are empowering or depowering to parents? What responsibilities do therapists, as humanistic health care professionals, have in fostering hope in clients?

12. What are the three primary objectives of regular follow-up of at-risk infants following discharge from the hospital? Indicate clinical reasons to support each objective and the role of the physical therapist in accomplishing each objective.

13. Describe a model follow-up clinic that would serve a facility or geographical region familiar to you. Include discussion of the following factors: (1) professional disciplines involved; (2) schedule of clinic visits according to age of child; (3) examinations to be performed at each visit; (4) follow-up/referral protocol for infants with neuromotor abnormalities.

14. Discuss the relevance of *age correction* to the developmental follow-up of premature infants.
    a. State two factors to consider in the decision of whether to correct, how much to correct, and for how long.
    b. Explain how age correction would influence your interpretation of a premature infant's results on a developmental evaluation.

15. Four months has been identified as an optimal age for routine assessment of high-risk infants.
    a. State three benefits or advantages of assessment performed at this age.
    b. State two disadvantages of assessment at 4 months.
    c. Provide clinical examples of situations in which an at-risk infant should be evaluated (1) earlier than 4 months, and (2) later than 4 months.

16. Describe the difference between infant assessments based on either neurological examination or developmental evaluation. Give examples of each type of assessment. List three factors that would influence your choice of assessment in a given clinical situation and describe how each would affect your decision.

17. A physical therapist in a follow-up clinic evaluates a high-risk infant using an assessment tool with a high *sensitivity* rate. The infant's performance is in the normal range of scores. What feedback can the therapist provide the parents regarding developmental expectations for the baby?

18. A physical therapist in a follow-up clinic evaluates a high-risk infant using an assessment instrument with a moderate *specificity* rate. The infant's test score is in the "risk" range, indicating that the infant's performance is deviant and suggestive of abnormality.
    a. What feedback can the therapist provide the parents regarding developmental expectations for the baby?
    b. List three clinical reasons that might account for the infant's abnormal performance other than cerebral palsy?

19. Specific neuromotor clinical signs, such as neck extensor hypertonia, are reported to be significantly related to cerebral palsy.
    a. State three additional factors to be considered in the interpretation of the clinical significance of these signs when observed during the examination of an infant.
    b. Describe an appropriate approach to the clinical management of a high-risk infant who demonstrates one or more of these clinical signs on examination.

Chapter 9

1. What characteristics of cerebral palsy may cause it to be confused with a "progressive disorder"?

2. What are the structural interferences that may influence the development of cerebral palsy characteristics?

3. How is development generally affected by a diagnosis of cerebral palsy?

4. Suggest three issues in the problem of diagnosis and discuss them in relation to the reaction of the family unit.

5. Discuss the relationship of parent expectation to the child's developmental responses with consideration of psychosocial factors.

6. What is the practical result of spasticity or high tone?

7. How does athetosis affect physical control?

8. What is the significance of hypotonicity findings?

9. Which aspects of assessment are completed before the therapist begins direct handling?

10. Discuss the similarities and differences between the child's ability to sustain a position when placed and the ability to assume a position.

11. Describe the dynamic interaction between reflexive reactions and functional movement.

12. What is the role of compensatory movement patterns in planning intervention?

13. How can the therapist and orthopedist interact in a productive way?

14. How do we know what will happen if children with a diagnosis of cerebral palsy are not given direct therapeutic handling and positioning?

15. Discuss the significance of "eclectic" treatment and how a young therapist might arrive at that level of expertise.

16. Discuss characteristics of spasticity that influence planning of dynamic therapy sessions.

17. Why is somewhat intense or prolonged input sometimes appropriate for the child with cerebral palsy?

18. What is the role of "reassessment" in the direct treatment situation?

19. Discuss the ways in which knowledge of normal development is used by the therapist in direct treatment.

20. Describe the major focus of treatment of the hemiplegic child.

21. What factors influence decision making with regard to special equipment for the home?

22. In what ways can the therapist provide input for the child who does not have access to individual therapy sessions?

Chapter 10

1. Identify two categories of genetic disorders.

2. List three modes of inheritance for specific gene defects.

3. Describe the risk of atlanto-axial dislocation associated with Down's Syndrome.

4. Differentiate trisomy 21, trisomy 18, and trisomy 13 with regard to incidence and to the severity and multiplicity of associated handicaps.

5. List the three characteristics of the triad associated with the complete syndrome of osteogenesis imperfecta.

6. List the three characteristics of the triad associated with tuberous sclerosis.

7. Describe why it is important for physical therapists to monitor postural alignment in children with neurofibromatosis.

8. Identify four clinical characteristics of Werdnig-Hoffman's disease.

9. Describe the five steps involved in the problem-oriented approach as outlined by Campbell.

10. List the components of an Individual Education Program (IEP) as defined in PL 94-142.

11. Define an "integrated therapy model" as described by Sternat and colleagues.

12. List two potential benefits associated with an integrated therapy model.

13. List two feeding problems commonly associated with hypotonicity and two feeding problems associated with hypertonicity.

14. Describe two specific therapy techniques aimed at normalizing tone in the child with hypertonicity.

15. Describe two specific therapy techniques aimed at normalizing tone in the child with hypotonicity.

16. Identify two techniques for therapeutic management of hyperextensible joints.

17. Discuss the use of adaptive equipment and mobility devices for children with genetic disorders.

18. Describe the grief process associated with the birth of a child with an obvious genetic disorder.

19. Identify two medical procedures for prenatal diagnosis of some genetic disorders.

20. List two reference texts published during the 1980s that provide additional information about genetic disorders.

Chapter 11*

1. What are the 10 clinical characteristics associated with learning disabilities?

2. Define learning disabilities. What makes the ACLD definition unique? In what ways do educators and medical professionals differ in their definition?

3. List five brain dysfunction theories and name the hypothesized deficit areas associated with each.

4. Listed on p. 289 are the many professionals involved in the assessment and treatment of a child with learning disabilities. What is the major role of the occupa-

tional therapist and physical therapist with this child? How do the roles of the occupational therapist, physical therapist, and physical education teacher differ?

5. What are the prevailing social-emotional problems for children with learning disabilities?

6. What are the two schools of thought regarding the need for territory of professional disciplines in relation to treating learning disabilities?

7. What is the relationship between motor dysfunction and minimal brain dysfunction?

8. What percentage of children with learning disabilities have a motor coordination deficit?

9. What are soft neurological signs? What do they mean? List 10 signs.

10. How do the motor problems of a learning disabled child affect ADL, school, and play behavior?

11. List the four areas occupational therapists and physical therapists assess with relation to postural control and motor performance. Describe the evaluation commonly used in each area.

12. What is the difference between the primitive postural reflexes and motor performance of a learning disabled child?

13. Give 10 examples of long-term goals for improving motor coordination in a child with learning disabilities.

14. When considering remediation, a critical question to ask is whether to attempt improving brain function or increase the child's perceptual, motor, and cognitive skills. Describe the pros and cons for each type of approach.

15. What is the underlying premise of a perceptual-motor theorist in regards to remediation?

16. Describe Ayres' sensory integration theory. Upon which premises is the theory based? How does Ayres' theory differ from neurodevelopmental theory?

17. List the five types of disorders that Ayres has found to be characteristic of children with learning disabilities.

18. Define developmental dyspraxia. What three components need to be integrated for motor planning?

19. What are the five general steps in sensory integration procedures?

20. Describe the basis for neurodevelopmental treatment. How does sensorimotor theory relate to sensory integration and neurodevelopmental treatment?

*The author gratefully acknowledges the contribution of Liz Etheridge, who assisted in the development of the questions for Chapter 11.

21. How has the establishment of the Education for All Handicapped Act (PL 94-142) affected the treatment approach of children with learning disabilities?

22. Why do most learning disabled children have a poor self-image? Describe how it is manifested.

23. How do learning disabilities affect adolescents? Adults? Are learning disabilities outgrown? What age is the best time to treat learning disability problems? Why?

Chapter 12

1. According to Schaumberg's anatomical classification of peripheral nerve injury, Class I injuries would be analogous to:
   a. neuropraxia
   b. axonotmesis
   c. neurotmesis

2. Class III injuries (neurotmesis) are less likely to result in full recovery of function because of:
   a. damage to the axon only
   b. damage to the axon as well as the surrounding connective tissue structures

3. Wallerian degeneration refers to:
   a. changes in the nerve distal to the site of injury
   b. changes at the site of the injury only
   c. change in the nerve proximal to the site of injury
   d. changes both distal and proximal to the site of injury

4. The Schwann cell:
   a. ceases function at the time of and after nerve injury
   b. functions in such a way as to actually guide regeneration of the axon (axonal sprouts) after injury

5. Class I injuries (neuropraxia) result from focal compression and cause symptoms that are:
   a. irreversible
   b. transient and reversible
   c. unaffected by ischemic changes in the nerve

6. The success of a nerve suture procedure is affected by:
   a. location of the injury (i.e., proximal versus distal)
   b. delay time from the initial injury
   c. the age of the patient
   d. all of the above are important considerations

7. **True/False** With regard to surgical repair of severed peripheral nerves, both nerve suture and nerve graft procedures appear to be equally successful.

8. Small diameter fibers are more resistant to compression injury than large diameter fiber. All of the following sensations may be absent with a compression injury, but which one(s) indicate(s) pathology in the small diameter fibers and thus a more severe injury?
   a. proprioception
   b. stereognosis
   c. temperature
   d. a and b only

9. **True/False** The only function of Manual Muscle Testing is to determine the location and presence/absence of muscular strength.

10. Soft tissue palpation may be done to assess:
    a. arterial pulses
    b. mobility of soft tissues
    c. skin fat folds
    d. a and b only
    e. a, b and c

11. Traumatic peripheral nerve injuries can directly result in:
    a. decreased sensation (negative phenomena)
    b. increased sensation (positive phenomena)
    c. weakness/paralysis of denervated muscle
    d. a and c only
    e. a, b and c

12. Traumatic peripheral nerve injuries can indirectly result in:
    a. changes in bone structure
    b. joint weakness and instability
    c. vasomotor paralysis
    d. a and b only
    e. a, b and c

13. Physical therapy treatment of traumatic peripheral nerve injuries should focus on:
    a. the nerve injury per se
    b. anticipating changes secondary to the nerve injury
    c. use of muscle stimulation to regain strength
    d. problems secondary to sensory deficits and limb neglect

Chapter 13

1. Traumatic head injuries that occur distant from the part of the brain sustaining the blow are described as:
   a. acceleration injuries
   b. coup injuries
   c. decelerating injuries
   d. contrecoup injuries
   e. shearing injuries

2. List two types of traumatic head injuries, *other than* closed head injuries.
   a.
   b.

3. List three forms of specific *primary* brain damage that can occur with *closed head injury*.
   a.
   b.
   c.

4. Describe the clinical manifestations of each of the following terms:
   a. coma
   b. obtundity
   c. delirium

5. A term "decerebrate" is sometimes used to describe motor abnormalities that are clinically manifested as:
   a. flexion of upper extremities, extension of lower extremities, and intact righting reflexes
   b. extension of neck, back, upper and lower extremities, wrists flexed, and no righting reflexes
   c. extension of neck, back, upper extremities, flexion of lower extremities and wrists, and intact stretch reflexes
   d. extension of neck, back, upper extremities and lower extremities, wrists flexed, and no stretch reflexes

6. Match the column of diagnostic and/or monitoring procedures (right) with the appropriate description of the procedure (left). No answer may be used more than once.

____ designed to assess and monitor level of consciousness	a. CT scanning
	b. Glasgow Coma Scale
____ permits visualization of intracranial structures	c. Electroencephalography
____ measures changes in electrocerebral potentials that occur in response to specific stimuli	d. Evoked potentials

7. List three possible *sequelae* (*not* complications) of brain injury in each category indicated below:
   Physical
   a.
   b.
   c.
   Cognitive
   a.
   b.
   c.
   Behavioral
   a.
   b.
   c.

8. Posttraumatic amnesia is best defined as the:
   a. loss of the ability to recall events that have occurred during the time period immediately preceding brain injury
   b. inability to form new memory because of decreased attention or inaccurate perception following brain injury
   c. time lapse between the accident and the point at which the functions concerned with memory are restored
   d. loss of the capacity for transferring short-term memory into long-term memory following brain trauma
   e. inability to retain sensory signals in the sensory areas of the brain for a very short interval of time following the sensory experience

9. You have a referral to treat a brain-injured client in ICU.
   a. Name one activity you will want to do before entering the client's room.
   b. After your evaluation and treatment, but before leaving the client's room, what two things will you want to do for the client?

10. You receive a referral to evaluate and treat a client with a traumatic head injury. Thoroughly categorize and outline the content of your plan for evaluating this client (use moderate detail, that is, give the major categories and important subcategories of your evaluation plan specific to the diagnosis given).

11. Indicate two parameters that a therapist cannot test or evaluate by customary methods if the client is unconscious, and describe an alternative testing method for each:

Parameter	*Alternative*
a.	a.
b.	b.

12. Explain what is meant by *controlled* movement or function, and explain the significance of *controlled* movement in evaluation.

13. List three problems or functional deficits in three *different* body systems that are sometimes associated with traumatic head injuries, and indicate if and how therapy may be helpful with each of these complications.

Functional deficits/problems	*Therapy*
a.	a.
b.	b.
c.	c.

14. Discuss three general problems encountered in trying to predict outcome in a client with a traumatic head injury.

15. Based on the following data, fill in the requested information on the blanks provided. Include a *physical and cognitive problem treatable by the therapist* in developing your treatment plan *(be specific, but concise).*

B.W. is a 24-year-old, 6'4", 195 lb medical student living at home with his parents and sister. He was involved in a motor vehicle accident on 7/5 and sustained a closed head injury, right occipital scalp laceration, and multiple arm and hand lacerations. His past history is noncontributory, and he was in good health. P.T. initiated treatment in ICU on 7/17. Client exhibited no response to verbal stimuli; eyes partially open with some inconsistent tracking; supine decerebrate posturing; markedly increased flexor tone bilateral upper extremities; severe extensor spasticity BLEs; 20-degree flexion contracture right elbow; heel cords extremely tight with no passive dorsiflexion possible; responded to noxious stimuli with random movements of upper extremities and moaning; no purposeful movements. Client has a nasogastric tube, IV in the left arm, cardiac monitor, tracheotomy with oxygen, and a urinary catheter.

Positive preinjury prognostic indicators
1.
2.
Positive postinjury prognostic indicators
1.
2.

Client problems (prioritize)	STG	Specific Rx (example)	Re-evaluation	Education (what and whom)
1.				
2.				
3.				

16. Your 17-year-old male head-injured client is at level IV on the Rancho Cognitive scale: confused agitated. He is in a heightened state of activity with severely decreased ability to process information; he is detached from the present and responds primarily to his own internal confusion. He has moderately high tone. Comment *very briefly* on the *general* way you would deal with this client (given his cognitive level) in regard to each of the following areas:
a. Treatment environment
b. Motivation
c. Type of commands used
d. General type of stimuli used
e. Tasks given
f. Amount you will touch this client
g. Length of treatment session

17. In relation to balance mechanisms, define and discuss the following terms:
a. "pattern generator"
b. "ankle strategies"
c. "hip strategies"
d. "postural sway"

18. Your client is an ambulatory, 20-year-old out-patient who comes to your clinic 3 days per week primarily to improve her gait and balance reactions. Her tone, strength, and selective movements are nearly normal. From your examination and assessment, you identify a need to refine the vestibular and visual input in her balance reactions:
a. Select and describe an activity appropriate for this client
b. Describe a progression of this activity to begin as the client's balance reactions improve

19. Select one common behavioral problem frequently encountered in the later recovery stages, and discuss general treatment strategies for the problem you have selected.
a. Behavioral problem
b. Possible treatment strategies

20. How do *you personally* define "quality of life"? What do *you* value most? How will you reconcile differences in your values if they differ from those of the client and client's family?

Chapter 14

1. The most common form of spina bifida is:

_____.

2. The most common level for myelomeningocele is:

_____.

3. Orthopedic deformities are common with myelomeningocele. Name three types of deformities and discuss generally why they occur.

4. What is the percentage of children with myelomeningocele who also have hydrocephalus? What effect does hydrocephalus have on intellectual potential?

5. The two most common types of shunts are:
a.
b.

6. Describe clean intermittent catherization. Why is it superior to the Crede method of bladder emptying?

7. Describe various methods for stimulating movement in infants with myelomeningocele; describe how muscle strength would be graded.

8. Name and briefly describe two developmental evaluations that would be appropriate from birth to 2 years of age.

9. Discuss the importance of early weight bearing and ways it might be achieved in Stage 3, infant to toddler.

10. In stages 2 through 4, describe ways to work on increasing head and trunk righting abilities.

11. Discuss the factors that help determine ambulatory status in the adolescent spinal cord–injured child.

12. Describe some of the psychological problems encountered by the spinal cord–injured child.

Chapter 15

1. **True/False**   Degenerative arthritis is seen more often as a long-term complication in quadriplegia than in paraplegia.

2. **True/False**   Full-finger long flexor motion is essential for the quadriplegic patient who has remaining active wrist extension, but no active motion distally.

3. **True/False**   Determination of a spinal cord–injured patient's developing a pressure sore can initially always be identified by redness and the color of the skin.

4. **True/False**   Spinal cord injured clients with lesions above T12 have impaired temperature regulation, especially during the acute stages of recovery.

5. **True/False**   The two primary problems with respiration experienced by the person with a spinal cord injury are a decreased inspiratory ventilation and a decreased expiratory pressure.

6. **True/False**   Glossopharyngeal breathing (GPB) can increase a spinal cord–injured client's vital capacity by as much as 1000 ml.

7. **True/False**   In spinal cord injury, more energy is required to ambulate with KAFOs than RGOs.

8. Elastic abdominal supports to improve diaphragm function in spinal cord injury should extend from the sixth rib to the iliac crest.

Chapter 16

1. Describe how observation of the client's current functional status can be used to shape the evaluation process.

2. Identify the components of the evaluation process.

3. Discuss the components to be considered in the evaluation of the vital function/autonomic nervous system status. How is this information used throughout the intervention process?

4. Why should therapists incorporate an evaluation of the level of consciousness into the intervention process?

5. Discuss the components of the evaluation of the sensory channels and provide examples on how the information derived influences the intervention process.

6. List the information that can be gathered as the client moves through the sequence of developmental postures. How is each item of information used in formulating the intervention plan?

7. Discuss the components involved in the process of establishing goals, including the concepts of a problem list, asset list, long-term goals, and short-term goals.

8. Write a short-term goal relating to mastery of functional activities in sitting.

9. List the general intervention goals for the intervention process. How is the statement of these goals different from the statement of a long-term goal for a particular client?

10. Discuss the types of sensory input that can be used to promote an alerting response in a client with a decreased level of consciousness. What precautions should be kept in mind when using arousal stimuli?

11. Discuss the influence of the client's postural set on the achievement of each of the other intervention goals.

12. How does movement through developmental sequence activities address dysfunctions in perceptual integration?

13. Discuss how the presence of the normal postural reflex mechanism underpins progression of an individual through developmental sequence activities.

14. Discuss the interrelationship of the intervention goals of enhancing progression through the developmental sequence activities and promoting optimalization of movement patterns.

15. Discuss each of the following concepts in terms of achieving optimal movement patterns: mobility patterns, stability patterns, different types of contractions, reversibility of movement patterns, sequencing of movements, incoordination.

16. Describe several examples of intervention techniques physical therapists can incorporate into their interactions with the client that will promote optimalization of the client's psychosocial and cognitive responses.

Chapter 17
Part I Poliomyelitis

1. Most people ingest the poliomyelitis virus but few develop muscle paresis or paralysis. List four ways that immunity can be acquired by the body.

2. When the poliomyelitis virus crosses the blood-brain barrier, the virus selectively attacks almost all the motor neurons of the CNS (96%). After the 2-week febrile illness these neurons have been found to be histologically _____ or _____ .

3. Describe four physiological processes whereby partially denervated muscles gain strength during the convalescent and rehabilitation phases of poliomyelitis.

4. When a manual muscle test grade of 4, G or Good (+ to −) is found in a muscle after polio, it can be estimated that this muscle has what percentage of its anterior horn cells?
   a. 0% to 10%
   b. 10% to 30%
   c. 30% to 50%
   d. 60% to 90%

5. Functional compensation for the flaccid paralysis of poliomyelitis frequently includes long-term reliance on ligaments for stability, and use of muscles at abnormally high levels of their capacity. What are the long-term consequences of these compensations?

6. The pathological lesion in the postpolio syndrome is considered to involve the giant motor units. Briefly describe three predominant theories on the cause.

7. List the specific musculoskeletal objectives in the management of the postpolio client.

8. Differentiate the muscle pain of postpolio syndrome from pain resulting from joint trauma.

9. Describe five methods for decreasing the workload of muscles without decreasing function.

10. Fifty percent of ambulatory postpolio clients walk in a forward lean posture. Give a specific example of why they do this, what problem the forward lean causes, and how the posture can be safely corrected.

11. When new weakness and fatigue appears, many polio survivors increase exercise programs and physical activities only to find that this causes further fatigue, weakness, pain, or fasciculations. What is the physiological explanation for this response to exercise?

Part II (Human immunodeficiency virus illness)

1. Do the terms HIV illness and AIDS mean the same thing?

2. What is the difference between an antigen and an antibody?

3. If antibodies for HIV can be found in the blood (*see* seropositive), then why does the disease progress?

4. Why are the opportunistic diseases of HIV illness uncommon in people without HIV infections?

5. **True/False** The development of hemiparesis in a person with HIV illness, in the absence of other neurological symptoms, invariably means that a primary viral disease is developing.

6. **True/False** The main distinction between primary and secondary neurological illness in HIV illness is that the primary illness is caused by the direct attack of HIV on CNS tissue and the secondary illness is a result of an opportunistic organism or neoplasm.

7. Why is the development of treatments against HIV so complicated and difficult?

8. Name two significant differences between the evaluation and treatment model for HIV illness and that for other progressive diseases with neurological complications.

9. If your patient complained of being "clumsy" and of losing his or her balance, what subsystem of the CNS would you suspect may be at risk?

10. Is it true that the rehabilitation of cognitive/perceptual deficits in HIV illness focuses on careful retraining in areas of loss?

11. What benefit can a person with HIV illness derive from retraining in avocational pursuits? Is there a type of HIV client for whom this is more critical?

12. What are the three known modalities for transmitting the virus?

13. Are special infection control precautions recommended for dealing with high-risk clients?

Chapter 18

1. To what does the term "sclerosis" refer in multiple sclerosis?

2. What clues have epidemiological studies given to uncovering the cause of MS?

3. What are the three patterns the clinical course of MS may take?

4. Why is MS difficult to diagnose?

5. Of what use is MRI in diagnosing MS?

6. Name three clinical factors that impact on the emotional response of persons diagnosed with MS.

7. What are some of the "secondary" symptoms associated with inactivity experienced by some persons with MS?

8. Name two drugs frequently used to manage spasticity in MS.

9. What is the action of 4-aminopyridine in treating MS?

10. Name two immunosuppressant therapies under study in MS.

11. What is the minimal record of disability?

12. What does a rating of Kurtzke 5 indicate?

13. Why is frequent reassessment and goal setting vital to MS rehabilitation?

14. How would the therapist treat spasticity in the MS client?

15. How is cerebellar dysfunction approached?

16. To what might pain be related in MS?

17. How does MS fatigue factor in therapy?

18. What are the most frequent cognitive changes seen in MS?

19. Why is it useful for a person with MS to have a neuropsychological evaluation?

Chapter 19

1. The circuitry of the basal ganglia can be summarized in terms of internal and external loops. Describe these and try to determine the functional role of each loop.

2. Diseases of the basal ganglia have some common symptoms. Knowledge of the physiology of the basal ganglia may assist in explaining the movement disturbances. Try to list the symptoms and then relate them to physiological studies.

3. Some patients with basal ganglia disease also suffer perceptual deficits. Describe these along with the physiology and how the perceptual problems may affect treatment.

4. One of the greatest advances in medical treatment of neurological disorders emerged with the use of dopamine replacement therapy for Parkinson's disease. Describe the rationale for this treatment.

5. Tardive dyskinesia is a case of external neurotransmitter control gone awry. Explain this. Also explain why decreasing the drug may make the patient's symptoms worsen.

6. One symptom of Parkinson's disease is postural instability. Why must this be assessed without vision?

7. What is usually the cause of death in patients with Parkinson's disease? What must therefore be an important component of treatment?

8. Name two symptoms of Parkinson's disease and for each symptom give two good treatment activities and their rationale.

9. Answer question no. 8 for Huntington's disease.

10. Discuss the ethical problems involved in gene testing for Huntington's disease, including "disclosure."

11. Huntington's disease is a progressive disorder. What can physical therapy really hope to accomplish?

12. Now that an animal model of Parkinson's disease exists, what are two questions you would like to see basic scientists address?

13. Explain the symptoms of alcoholism, based on your knowledge of anatomy and physiology.

14. One of the problems in fetal alcohol syndrome is mental retardation. Explain why this might occur, based on animal research.

15. Explain the DTs of alcoholism in neurophysiological terms.

Chapter 20

1. Explain how the goals for a patient with a brain tumor will differ from those for other patients with CNS disabilities.

2. In what age ranges do most brain tumors occur?

3. Metastases to the brain are:
   a. increasing
   b. decreasing
   c. remaining nearly the same
   Give the rationale for your answer.

4. Briefly describe why use of the term "benign" may be misleading when applied to brain tumors.

5. List four specific areas that should be included in the neurological evaluation of a patient with a brain tumor.

6. Explain why elevation, bed rest, and elastic stockings are extremely important during the immediate postoperative period following surgery for a tumor.

7. Briefly describe the implication of the need for an "adaptive" or "functional" approach for patients with brain tumors.

8. Identify the four standards of care established by Dietz. Describe an appropriate physical therapy management technique for each category. Do not repeat your techniques.

9. Identify two common side effects of tumor treatment that the patient may experience, and explain the impact each may have on your treatment plan.

10. Select two areas of clinical care that would be appropriate for a patient in a hospice program.

Chapter 21

1. Which of the following movement disorders would not be associated with cerebellar dysfunction?
   a. hypotonicity
   b. asthenia
   c. hypertonicity
   d. ataxia

2. Lack of coordination displayed by individuals with cerebellar lesions has many distinctive traits, especially within the trunk and extremities. List three and describe the motor behaviors.

3. Following general assessment of functional abilities, the specifics of cerebellar movement disorders need evaluation. Describe three of the seven areas needing assessment and discuss at least two tests that focus on the specific problem.

4. Select one goal for treatment, and discuss the procedures and why they have been selected.

Chapter 22

1. The initial site of the development of spasticity is:
   a. the elbow
   b. the wrist and fingers
   c. the shoulder and pelvic girdles
   d. the ankle and foot

2. Shoulder subluxation in hemiplegia is caused by:
   a. weak deltoid muscle
   b. stretch of the supraspinatus ligament
   c. the change in the angulation of the glenoid fossa
   d. spasticity in the latissimus dorsi muscle

3. Sensory disturbances accompanying a stroke result in:
   a. loss of recognition of the affected side
   b. disturbances in sensory feedback
   c. loss of movement coordination
   d. all of the above

4. Initial recovery of function following a stroke is attributed to:
   a. reinnervation
   b. reduction of cerebral edema
   c. improved local vascular flow
   d. remyelination
   e. a and c
   f. a and b
   g. b and c
   h. b and d

5. Common perceptual deficits following a RCVA include:
   a. apraxia and poor judgment
   b. sequencing deficits
   c. poor judgment and short attention span
   d. difficulty initiating tasks

6. **True/False** Postural tone is tone that is high enough to keep the body from collapsing into gravity but low enough to allow the body to move against gravity.

7. **True/False** Postural tone, muscle tone, and spasticity are defined in the same way by therapists.

8. **True/False** Exclusive use of one side of the body for function results in asymmetry, poor balance, and an eventual deterioration of function of the unaffected side.

9. **True/False** Three types of shoulder subluxation exist—anterior, inferior, and superior.

10. Shoulder joint pain is described by the patient as:
    a. sharp
    b. pulling
    c. aching
    d. all of the above

11. **True/False** In clients with hemiplegia, hip, knee, and ankle problems are interrelated.

12. Trunk control can be reeducated through the movement of:
    a. anterior, posterior, and lateral weight shifts
    b. anterior, posterior, lateral, and diagonal weight shifts
    c. lateral and rotational weight shifts
    d. anterior and posterior weight shifts

13. **True/False** Weight-bearing activities allow the extremities to disassociate from the "girdles."

14. **True/False** Transfers should be taught towards the unaffected side only.

Chapter 23

1. Describe the three major categories of global cognitive impairment, retardation, delirium, and dementia. Specifically comment on how these 3 are different clinically.

2. Describe the major goal(s) of intervention by the rehabilitation team, including the physical therapist, for a patient with Alzheimer's disease.

3. Describe the normal age-related changes that can interfere with ease of communication.

4. Discuss the clinical significance of crystallized intelligence with advancing age.

5. Describe the similarities between the stress-related distortions in global cognitive function and dementia and detail the specific clinical strategies to help a client to perform at his or her highest level of ability.

6. Describe a "clinical decision-making process" used to identify distortions in basic information processing.

7. Describe the compensations and adaptations that can be made for normal sensory losses with advanced age.

8. Discuss the significance of the therapist being aware of normal changes in older adult learning styles as it relates to organizing physical therapy intervention.

9. Describe specific actions that may be taken by the rehabilitation team to avoid transplantation shock.

10. Discuss how emotional overstimulation can manifest itself in symptoms of mild confusion and describe the clinical interventions the therapist will need to make.

11. Describe the common issues related to medication and cognitive dysfunction. What are the issues that need to be examined to rule out the possibility that medication is not interfering with the patient's psychomotor/cognitive performance?

12. Discuss the clinical course of acute and chronic or nonacute dementia and the primary actions of the rehabilitation team for each patient category.

13. Discuss the options for assisting the dementia patient and the caregiver(s) to provide in-home care if it is desired (general rehabilitation issues and specific physical therapy approaches).

Chapter 24

1. How do oral, auditory, and visual input contribute to speech production?

2. Explain why developmental neuromuscular deficits might interfere with normal language development.

3. Why should the physical therapist have knowledge of normal speech and language development? What are the milestones of normal communication development?

4. Why is familiarity with speech and language diagnosis important to the physical therapist? What are the major neurogenic communication disorders?

5. List and explain the goals of the physical therapist with respect to communication disorders.

6. Provide a brief overview of the areas that might be included in a screening of communication.

7. Are the same physical restoration techniques and oral exercises used for every client with dysarthria? Explain.

8. How can the physical therapist promote communication with the confused patient?

9. Should the physical therapist modify his or her communication patterns to adapt to the communication problems of the client? Provide an explanation in support of your answer.

Chapter 25

1. Visual perceptual deficits result from damage to various structures within the functional visual perceptual system. What anatomical components make up the functional visual perceptual system?

2. List and describe the three subsystems of the visual process.

3. How do visual perceptual disorders in children differ from visual perceptual disorders in adults.

4. The first step in a diagnostic visual perceptual workup should be an evaluation of the primary visual system; this is known as a comprehensive visual screening. Describe this procedure for children.

5. Describe how findings from the vision specialist (developmental optometrist) can be integrated into daily treatment by the physical therapist, occupational therapist, and speech therapist.

6. What does the term "visual management during therapeutic activity" imply? Give three examples.

7. What are three common performance problems that might be reflective of visual spatial deficits in children?

8. Suggest a treatment strategy for each of the visual spatial problems listed above.

9. Printing, handwriting, and form copying are considered visual constructive skills. List some examples of treatment for children with deficits in these areas.

10. Describe the subtle but important difference between treatments for visual analysis and visual synthesis.

11. What should a comprehensive visual screening include when assessing a brain-damaged adult?

12. Any abnormality noted during comprehensive visual screening should result in automatic referral to a vision specialist. What type of vision specialist is most appropriate for evaluating the brain-damaged adult?

13. Describe three primary visual deficits in adults, their functional deficit, and their management.

14. How does unilateral spatial inattention manifest itself in daily function?

15. Describe two treatment strategies for unilateral spatial inattention.

16. Visual agnosia is a disorder of recognition subdivided into a number of types. Describe the four types discussed in this chapter.

17. Describe three functional deficits that might be considered visual/spatial in nature.

18. Describe a treatment activity for:
    a. enhancing an internal spatial understanding
    b. enhancing topographical orientation
    c. enhancing spatial control of eye movements during reading

19. Setting a table and changing a tire are considered visual constructive tasks. Why?

20. What are the two underlying problems thought to be responsible for visual constructive disorders? How should treatment differ for each type?

21. What role can computers play in visual perceptual retraining?

Chapter 26

1. Describe what clinical electroneuromyographic studies evaluate.

2. **True/False** Therapy students should be competent in performance and evaluation of most electromyographic tests before they graduate.

3. Discuss the differences between sensory and motor nerve conduction studies.

4. **True/False** Normal nerve conduction velocity is usually above 40 m/sec, whereas in some chronic demyelinating problems it may drop to as low as 10 m/sec.

5. In clinical EMG studies which statement is false:
    a. either concentric or monopolar needle electrodes can be used.
    b. patient cooperation is required.
    c. clients should not practice the motions required once the needle is in place.
    d. in normal muscle at rest, there is no electrical activity.

6. List three characteristics of nerve potentials that might be seen during electromyography in a pathological state.

7. **True/False** Polyphasic motor unit action potentials are found in normal muscle.

8. Identify one additional type of evaluation procedure that can be used to supplement EMG and MCV studies. Describe either the procedure or the rationale for its use.

9. Kinesiologic electromyography can be used to:
    a. document alteration of muscle function following paralysis
    b. reinforce learning following a therapy session
    c. relate muscular activity to energy expenditure and fatigue
    d. all of the above

Chapter 27

1. Briefly trace pain impulses from the periphery to the brain.

2. Contrast the phenomena of "fast" and "slow" pain.

3. Identify the four thalamocortical projections that account for the emotional/psychological aspects of pain.

4. Identify the cognitive pain-modulating factors.

5. Explain the gate control theory of pain modulation.

6. Identify the criticisms of the gate control theory.

7. Identify the endogenous opiates and explain their role in pain modulation.

8. Explain the differences between CNS, ANS, and peripheral pain and give examples of each.

9. Identify the purpose of the pain evaluation.

10. List the information that should be included in the pain history.

11. Identify three ways to measure pain intensity.

12. Identify a tool with which to measure pain character.

13. Identify the factors to be evaluated during clinical assessment of the client with pain.

14. Explain the significance of six types of end feel.

15. Explain the significance of comparing passive versus active ROM.

16. Explain the significance of muscle strength and pain.

17. Define the factors governing the physiological effects of heat.

18. List the physiological effects of heat and explain how they affect pain.

19. Identify the ways in which heat can be applied during therapeutic procedures.

20. Explain the difference between ultrasound and other forms of therapeutic heating and explain why ultrasound is beneficial in the treatment of pain.

21. Explain phonophoresis and identify four chemicals that can be administered with phonophoresis.

22. Explain the physiological effects of cryotherapy and how they affect pain.

23. Identify the ways cold can be applied during therapeutic procedures.

24. Explain the current theories on the method of action of TENS.

25. Identify five modes of TENS application and explain the applications of each.

26. Discuss electrode placement during TENS.

27. Explain iontophoresis and identify seven chemicals that can be administered using iontophoresis.

28. Contrast iontophoresis with phonophoresis.

29. Explain how joint mobilization affords pain relief.

30. Identify five grades of oscillation used during joint mobilization.

31. Explain how massage affords pain relief.

32. Explain several methods of point stimulation.

33. Identify three nonphysical components of pain and explain four cognitive-behavior techniques that can be used to treat these aspects of pain.

Chapter 28

1. Define orthotic treatment.

2. Discuss orthotic treatment as CNS input.

3. Describe the sequential flow of orthotic application through end result.

4. Differentiate interim from definitive orthotic care.

5. Differentiate dynamic and static orthotic care.

6. Discuss orthotic treatment for facilitation or inhibition purposes by giving patient examples.

7. Describe the technique for using orthotic management for sensory training.

8. Describe alignment of the ankle joint mortice as it relates to fixed and flexible deformities.

9. List six issues for consideration when evaluating the trunk for orthotic intervention.

10. Describe a "cervical stability in neutral training" program.

11. List three common situations of the cervical spine where orthotics may benefit the neurologically impaired client.

12. List three goals that may be accomplished by orthotically applying force to the lumbar spine.

13. Describe positions for evaluation of PROM of the upper extremity when considering orthotic intervention.

14. When establishing treatment goals for use of orthotics, there are at least seven considerations; discuss four.

15. Describe one option for orthotic management of a patient with a hemiparesis as described by Brunnstrom in stage 2.

16. Describe two ways to use an AFO to stimulate lower-extremity extension while avoiding recurvatum in a patient with a low tone lower extremity.

17. List six factors to be evaluated in determining a specific patient's orthotic needs.

18. Discuss the effect of calcaneal malalignment as it relates to the midfoot and forefoot.

19. Describe how an orthosis can be used as home exercise device.

20. Describe how a dynamic or static orthosis is used to maintain gains made in therapy.

Chapter 29

1. List five categories of neurogenic bladder dysfunction.

2. List five categories of neurogenic bowel dysfunction.

3. Identify the risk factors that could potentially lead to skin breakdown.

4. In treating a 16-year-old client with cerebral palsy who has questions about sexuality, what approach can be employed to assist in counseling?

Chapter 30

1. Discuss the following components of the functional orientation concept:
   a. medical model versus wellness model
   b. deficits versus intact strengths
   c. human services professionals as "disablers" or "enablers"
   d. analysis and design of activity participation demands

2. Clearly distinguish between the meaning of a service role and a process role in your professional area of expertise. Are you demeaning your profession if you support an expanded process role function in your area of expertise? What process role areas of expertise do you see as appropriate for your profession to provide other professionals, volunteers, or participants in your programs?

3. Clarify the significant differences between existing approaches to the rehabilitation process and an ecological approach based on life-style analysis.

4. Contrast and compare the historical evaluation of your profession (social work, medicine, physical therapy, occupational therapy) with the historical evaluation of therapeutic recreation. Identify similarities and differences.

5. Is the medical-model orientation appropriate for your profession as we approach the twenty-first century? Are the five elements of a wellness-intact strengths model valid components in the rehabilitation process?

Identify any/all of the five elements that are applicable to your professional role.

6. Is the Rusalem Ecological model an appropriate conceptual basis for the delivery of human services as we approach the twenty-first century? Discuss in a pro/con context. If the model is appropriate, which elements are appropriate for your professional role? Among the members of the human services team (medicine, social work, psychology, nursing, physical therapy, occupational therapy, therapeutic recreation), identify the unique contributions each has to make to each of the five elements of the Rusalem model. How can a delivery service environment be created in which all professions can effectively contribute to each of the elements of the Rusalem model?

7. It has been said that the human services professions could make a far more significant contribution to human growth and development if we ignored people and devoted our total attention to changing human and nonhuman components of the environment. Do you agree or disagree? Support your position on a conceptual and substantive basis.

8. Support or refute the contention, based on the peripheral view of behavior, that no one is unmotivated.

9. The rationale underlying the concepts of neutrality of activity, paradox of activity involvement, and the questioning of leadership omnipotence contradict the prescriptive approach to treatment and rehabilitation. Analyze this dilemma and provide valid support for your analysis.

10. The function of leadership in human services is a highly intrusive act in reference to the life space of individuals whose functional strengths are generally less than the leader's. Analyze the question from Thomas Jefferson in reference to its implications for the intrusive nature of your leadership functions.

11. Does the concept of group readiness have any application to your professional role? Whether your response is "yes" or "no," document your conclusion.

12. Analyze the ARM concept of activity experience from the following perspectives:
    a. apply it to a specific situation encountered in your professional role
    b. select a human services profession with which you work closely and discuss how you think this profession could make effective use of the ARM concept.

13. The statement is made that the concept of inclusion versus exclusion (least restrictive environment) is far more functionally realistic than mainstreaming. Support or reject this statement and provide valid documentation for your position.

14. Select a situation you encounter frequently in your professional role and analyze the situation within the context of an environmental analysis. Form your analysis within the context of inclusion versus exclusion and whether excluding factors are intrinsic to the individual or extrinsically present in society.

15. Distinguish clearly between the terms "leisure counseling" and "leisure facilitation."

16. Does the Leisure Facilitation Process model developed by Humphrey have any application to your interaction role with participants in the rehabilitation process? If yes, apply each of the elements to your interactive role. If no, clearly document why the model elements have no relevance to your interactive role.

17. Within the context of your professional role, respond to the eight societal issues identified on p. 820.

18. Identify and respond to three additional evolving societal issues that face human services professionals as we rapidly approach the twenty-first century.

19. Within the context of your professional role, identify the ways in which your professional role will be different in the year 2010.

Chapter 31

1. Contrast the medical model of health care and the holistic model of health care.

2. Correlate current health care delivery and the development of health care professionals.

3. Define holistic health care.

4. Diagram the relationship between the client and that client's physical and psychological environment.

5. Describe the elements of a strong client/provider relationship.

6. Select a case study and choose an appropriate therapeutic intervention mentioned in this chapter that could positively impact the health care of the client.

7. Use a strong teaching/learning approach with one of your clients and document any change in therapeutic outcome that you observe to be a result of the approach.

8. Create increased community support for clients (e.g., volunteer your expertise, establish a client support legislator).

9. Analyze the effect that today's emphasis on health promotion could have on the health care of the future.

10. Support or refute the use of newer therapeutic interventions in health care.

STUDY GUIDE ANSWERS

Answer	Page found on	Location on page
Chapter 1		
1	p. 5	Fig. 1-1
2	p. 6	Table 1-1
	p. 8	Box
3. True	p. 14	Column one
4. Cognitive Affective Sensorimotor	pp. 20-21	"Problem-solving strategies"
5. False	p. 24	Column 2, paragraph 2
6. Visual recognition Spatial orientation Spatial transformation	pp. 24-25	Column 2, paragraphs 3, 4 through p. 25, column 1, paragraph 1
Chapter 2		
1. Motor unit	pp. 29-30	Last sentence p. 29
2. a.	pp. 32-34	"Homeostasis"
b.	pp. 34-37	"Posture"
c.	pp. 37-39	"Movement"
d.	pp. 39-41	"Higher cortical functions"
3.	Entire chapter	
4.	Entire chapter	
Chapter 3		
1. Hierarchical model	pp. 43-44	
Systems model	pp. 44, 45	
2. Cerebellum	p. 45	
Basal ganglia		
Cerebral cortex		
3. False	p. 45	Column 1, paragraph 3
4. d	p. 45	"Cerebellum"
5. a. Motor cortex	p. 45	Column 2, paragraph 5
b. Pre-motor cortex		
c. Supplementary motor area		
d. Posterior parietal cortex		

Answer	Page found on	Location on page
6. Posterior parietal cortex	p. 46	Column 1, paragraph 5
7. a. Ventromedial system (VMS) (1) Vestibulospinal tract (2) Reticulospinal tract (3) Interstitiospinal tract (4) Tectospinal tract b. Lateral system (LS) (1) Rubrospinal tract (2) Rubrobulbar tract (3) Pontospinal tract c. Corticospinal system (CS) (1) Corticospinal tract (2) Corticobulbar tract	pp. 46-47	"Descending systems"
8. True	p. 47	Column 1, paragraph 2
9. Reciprocity Distributed function Emergent properties Consensus	pp. 47-48	p. 47, column 2, paragraph 2 through p. 48, column 1
10. Reciprocity Distributed function Emergent properties Consensus	pp. 47-48	p. 47, column 2, paragraph 2 through p. 48, column 1
11. Anticipated adjustments made prior to onset of a disrupting force Compensatory control adjustments following an unexpected disrupting force		p. 49, column 1, paragraph 3 through column 2, paragraph 2
12. False	p. 49	Column 2, paragraph 2
13. Sequence or order of muscle activation Duration of muscle activity Force generated by the muscles	pp. 49-50	"Fixed versus relative parameters"

Answer	Page found on	Location on page
14. False	p. 50	Column 2, paragraph 4
15. True	p. 50	Column 2, paragraphs 5, 6

Chapter 4

Answer	Page found on	Location on page
1. True	p. 54	Column 1, paragraph 4
2.	p. 56	Column 1, paragraph 6
3. True	p. 58	Column 1, paragraph 3
4. True	p. 60	Column 2, paragraph 2
5. True	pp. 60-61	p. 60, column 2, paragraph 3 through p. 61, column 1
6. Trust	p. 63	"Trust/ responsibility"
Truth/flexibility	pp. 63-64	"Dedication to reality"
Vulnerability	p. 64	"Vulnerability"
7.	p. 64	Column 2, paragraph 2
8.	p. 65	"Alzheimer's disease"
9.	pp. 65-66	Column 2, paragraph 5
10.	p. 66	Column 2, paragraph 3
11. Hypothalamus	p. 67	Column 2, paragraph 2
12. The fornix	pp. 71-72	Column 2, paragraph 2
13. Declarative	p. 73	Column 1, paragraph 3
14. False	p. 73	Column 1, paragraph 3
15. Amygdaloid system Hippocampal	p. 73	Column 2, paragraph 4
16. d	p. 74	Column 1, paragraph 2
	p. 74	Column 2, paragraph 2
	p. 75	Column 1, paragraph 2

Chapter 5

Answer	Page found on	Location on page
1. Germinal phase (0-2 wks)	p. 80	Column 1, paragraph 3
Embryonic phase (2-8 wks)		
Fetal phase (8-38 wks)		
2.	p. 80 pp. 83-85	Table 5-1 "Postnatal physical development"
3. Ectoderm	p. 80	Column 2, paragraph 2
Endoderm		
Mesoderm		

Answer	Page found on	Location on page
4.	pp. 85-94	"General principles of human nervous system development . . ." through "Normal sequence human nervous system develops . . ."
5.	p. 86	Column 2, paragraphs 2,3
6.	p. 86	Column 2, paragraph 3
7.	p. 87	Column 1, paragraph 2
8.	p. 88	Column 1, paragraphs 2, 3, 4
9.	p. 88	Column 1, paragraphs 2, 3
10.	p. 88	Column 1, paragraph 6
11. a.	p. 88	Column 2, paragraph 3
b.	p. 96	Column 2, paragraphs 1, 2
12.	pp. 88-90	"Cellular proliferation and migration"
13.	p. 89	Column 1, paragraph 3
14.	p. 90	Column 2, paragraph 2
15.	p. 92	Column 1, paragraph 4
16.	pp. 93-94	"Myelination"
17.	p. 95	Column 1, paragraphs 2, 3, 4
18.	p. 95	Column 2, paragraphs 3, 4, 5
19.	p. 96	Column 1, paragraph 2

Chapter 6

Answer	Page found on	Location on page
1. Include description of primary input and four components of the classification system	pp. 111-112	Through column 2, paragraph 1, p. 112
2.	pp. 113-118	"Muscle spindle" through p. 118 column 2, paragraph 3 (summary in Table 4-2)
3.	pp. 113-118	"Muscle spindle"
	pp. 118-119	"The tendon organ"
4.	pp. 119-121	"The joint"
5.	pp. 123-124	"Exteroceptors"
6.	pp. 127-128	"Repetitive icing and brushing," "Prolonged icing," "Neutral warmth," and "Maintained stimulus or pressure"

Answer	Page found on	Location on page
7.	pp. 128-130	"Sensory receptors and physiology"
8.	pp. 132-133	"Total body inhibition followed by selective postural facilitation"
9.	pp. 133-134	"Autonomic nervous system"
10.	pp. 134-135	"Treatment alternatives"
11.	pp. 135-136	"Olfactory system: smell"
12.	pp. 135-137	"Olfactory system: smell," and "Gustatory sense: taste"
13.	pp. 139-140	"Visual system" through p. 140 column 1, paragraph 3
14. This is a synthesis question. Integrate what you have learned so far and some major traits that constitute inhibitory and facility techniques. Are most activities a multimodality synthesis? Or can the degree of the input be controlled by the therapist?	p. 144	Table 6-6
15.	p. 144-145	"Modification of a hypersensitive touch system"
16.	p. 145	"Orthokinetic cuff"
17.	pp. 145-148	"Oral motor facilitation"
18.	p. 148	"Proprioceptive and vestibular input"
19.	pp. 149-154	"Levels of processing" through "Summary"
20. No specific answer		

Chapter 7

Answer	Page found on	Location on page
1. False	p. 163	Column 1, paragraph 1
2. True	pp. 163-166	"Overview" and "Adjustment"
3. b.	pp. 165-166	p. 165, "Active response" through p. 166, column 1, paragraph 1
4. d	pp. 166-167	p. 166, "Awareness of psychological adjustment in the clinic" through p. 167, column 2, paragraph 3
5. True	p. 168	"Cognitive age loss"
6. True	pp. 171-172	"Development of sensuality" and "Pediatric sensuality"

Answer	Page found on	Location on page
7. c	pp. 171-172	"Pediatric sensuality"
8. True	p. 172	"Adult sexuality"
9. False	p. 172	Column 1, paragraph 3
10. a	p. 173	Column 1, paragraphs 1-5
11. True	pp. 173-174	Column 2, paragraphs 2-5
12. True	p. 176	Column 2, paragraph 3
13. True	p. 175	Column 1, paragraph 5, through Column 2, paragraph 2
14. False	pp. 176-177	"Establishment of self-worth and accurate body image"

Chapter 8

Answer	Page found on	Location on page
1.	pp. 196-197	"Level of stimulation"
2.	p. 190	"Educational requirements for therapists"
	p. 197	"Psychological risk management"
3. a. Indications for referral in a formal protocol that has undergone approval by newborn medicine team; quality assurance plan for record reviews, and case reviews (not in chapter); systematically getting approval and precautions for intervening with each infant, at each session working with neonatal nurse who helps monitor infant's tolerance during each session.	p. 191	
b. Specific		
1. Biological risk	p. 191	
2. Established risk	pp. 191-192	
3. Physiological risk	p. 197	
c. Refer to box	p. 191	
4. a. Spastic diplegia	p. 188	"Periventricular leukomalacia"
b. Periventricular leukomalacia, watershed infarct, medial corticospinal tract fibers in periventricular region.		

Answer	Page found on	Location on page		Answer	Page found on	Location on page
5. Full-term: Prechtl, Brazelton, Dubowitz Neurological Assessment. Pre-term: Dubowitz Neurological Assessment, Assessment of Preterm Infant Behavior, Brazelton Scale only if infant currently at 37 weeks gestation. **Dubowitz Calculation of Gestational Age: performed in delivery room or nursery by newborn medicine staff, rarely by neonatal therapists.	pp. 192-196	"Neonatal neurological assessment" through "Summary"		8.	pp. 241-242	Column 2, paragraph 4
				9.	pp. 242-243	"Initial observations"
				10.	p. 243	Column 1, paragraph 3
				11.	pp. 243-244	"Abnormal interferences"
				12.	pp. 244-245	"Primary and compensatory patterns"
				13.	p. 245	Column 2, paragraph 3
				14.	p. 245	Column 2, paragraph 4
				15.	p. 246	Column 1, paragraph 2
6.	p. 196	"Testing variables"		16.	pp. 246-247	"Nature of direct treatment for specific problems"
7.	p. 197-199	"High-risk profiles"				
8.	p. 199	"Timing"				
9.	pp. 200-202	"Positioning"		17.	p. 247	Begin column 1, paragraph 4 through column 2, paragraph 1
10.	pp. 206-209	"Neonatal hydrotherapy"				
11.	p. 210	"Parent teaching"				
	pp. 185-187	"Hope-empowerment model"		18.	p. 247	Column 2, paragraph 2
12.	p. 210	Column 2, paragraph 4		19.	pp. 248-249	Begin column 1, paragraph 2 through p. 249, column 2, paragraph 2
13.	p. 212	"High-risk infant follow-up model"				
14.	pp. 212-213	"Age correction"		20.	p. 249	Column 1, paragraph 2
15.	p. 272	Fig. 8-29				
16.	pp. 215-217	"Neurologic evaluation of the newborn and infant" through "Predictive value of infant assessment tools"		21.	pp. 251-252	"Criteria for equipment recommendations"
				22.	p. 252	"Physical positioning for the child who lacks direct treatment"
17.	pp. 222-223	"Interpretation of infant assessment"				
18.	pp. 220-222	"High-risk clinical signs" Tables 8-12, 8-13				
19.	pp. 223-226	"Intervention"				

Chapter 9

Answer	Page found on	Location on page
1.	p. 238	Column 1, paragraph 3
2.	p. 238	Column 1, paragraph 4
3.	p. 238	Column 2, paragraph 2
4.	pp. 239-240	"Family reactions"
5.	pp. 239-241	"Family reactions" and "Diagnosis and the time of intervention"
6.	p. 241	Column 2, paragraph 2
7.	p. 241	Column 2, paragraph 3

Chapter 10

Answer	Page found on	Location on page
1.	p. 258	Fig. 10-1
2.	p. 258	Fig. 10-1
3.	p. 259	Column 2, paragraph 1
4.	pp. 259-261	"Autosomal trisomies"
5.	p. 262	Column 1, paragraph 4
6.	p. 262	Column 2, paragraph 2
7.	p. 263	Column 2, paragraph 2
8.	p. 264	Column 2, paragraphs 3, 4
9.	p. 268	Column 1, paragraph 2
10.	p. 269	Column 1, paragraph 2
11.	p. 270	Column 2, paragraph 2

Answer	Page found on	Location on page		Answer	Page found on	Location on page
12.	p. 270	Column 2, paragraph 3		17.	p. 302	Column 2, paragraph 3
13.	p. 271	Table 10-2		18.	p. 303	Column 2, paragraphs 5, 6 ("Developmental dyspraxia")
14.	p. 271	Table 10-2				
	pp. 271-272	"Hypertonicity"				
15.	p. 271	Table 10-2		19.	p. 304	Column 2, paragraph 1
	p. 273	"Hypotonicity"				
16.	p. 273	"Hyperextensible joints"		20.	pp. 304-306	"Neurodevelopmental theory of Bobath" and "Sensorimotor therapy"
17.	p. 274	"Adaptive equipment needs"				
18.	p. 276	"Psychosocial aspects of genetic disorders"		21.	pp. 308-309	Begin column 2, paragraph 5 end p. 309, column 1, paragraph 3
19.	p. 276	Column 1, paragraph 6		22.	p. 309	Column 2, paragraph 3
20.	p. 277	Column 2, paragraph 2		23.	pp. 310-312	"Life-span learning disabilities"

Chapter 11

1.	p. 281	"Characteristics," column 2, paragraph 2
2.	pp. 281-282	"Definition"
3.	pp. 284-286	"Brain dysfunction theories"
4.	p. 287	Box
5.	p. 287	Column 2, paragraph 2
6.	p. 288	"Coordinating multiple interventions," column 2, paragraph 2
7.	p. 289	"Terminology"
8.	p. 289	"Incidence"
9.	p. 291	"Neurological approach/soft neurological signs"
10.	pp. 289-290	"Descriptions of motor deficits in the learning-disabled child" and "Descriptive/observational"
11.	pp. 293-294	"Muscle tone," "Integration of primitive postural reflexes," "Vestibular function and equilibrium," and "Posture."
12.	p. 293	"Integration of primitive postural reflexes"
13.	pp. 296-297	See list of 23 goals
14.	p. 297	Column 2, paragraph 3, 4
15.	p. 298	Column 2, paragraph 6
	p. 299	"Perceptual motor theorists"
16.	p. 302	Column 2, paragraph 1

Chapter 12

	Answer	Page found on	Location on page
1.	a	p. 335	Table 12-1
2.	b	p. 335	Table 12-1
3.	a	pp. 335-336	Column 2, paragraph 3
4.	b	p. 336	Column 1, paragraph 2
5.	b	pp. 334-335	Column 2, paragraph 4
6.	d	p. 336	"Surgical repair of peripheral nerve injury"
7.	False	p. 336	"Surgical repair of peripheral nerve injury"
8.	c	p. 338	"Sensory testing"
9.	False	pp. 338-339	"Manual muscle test"
10.	e	p. 339	"Soft tissue palpation"
11.	e	pp. 336-337	"Sensory disturbances"
12.	e	p. 337	"Vasomotor disturbances" "Soft tissue changes" and "Bony changes"
13.	b	p. 339	Column 1, paragraph 3

Chapter 13

1.	p. 348	Column 2, paragraph 1
2.	pp. 348-349	"Types of head injuries"
3.	pp. 348-349	"Closed head injuries"
4.	p. 350	Column 1, paragraph 6
5.	p. 350	Column 2, paragraph 3

Answer	Page found on	Location on page
6.	pp. 351-352	"Diagnostic monitoring procedures and medical management"
7.	pp. 352-353	"Sequelae and complications"
8.	p. 353	Column 1, paragraph 2
9. a.	p. 354	Column 2, paragraph 3
b.	pp. 374-381	"Sensory retraining" thru "The moderately severe flexor spasticity and lethargic responses"
10.	pp. 354-361 p. 355	"Problem-solving approach to evaluation" Box
11.	pp. 355-361	"Subjective data" and "Objective data"
12.	p. 359	Column 1, paragraphs 1, 2
13. Functional deficits	pp. 362-366 p. 367	"Problem identification" Fig. 13-3
Therapy	pp. 370-388	From "Guidelines for treatment" through "A brief review of balance reactions"
14.	p. 363	Column 1, paragraph 2 through column 2, paragraph 3
15. Prognostic indicators	pp. 363-366	Column 2, paragraph 4 through p. 366, column 2, paragraph 3
Problems	pp. 362-363	"Assessment and treatment goals" through column 2, paragraph 3
Goals	pp. 366-367	"General guidelines for establishing goals," "Long-term goals," and "Short-term goals"
Treatment	pp. 367-368	"General treatment procedures" through p. 381, column 2, paragraph 4
Re-evaluation	pp. 355-361	From "Subjective data" through p. 361, column 2, paragraph 3
Education	pp. 367-382	

Answer	Page found on	Location on page
16.	pp. 367-376	From "General treatment procedures" to p. 376, "Early management"
	pp. 383-387	"The client who is hyperactive, confused, and nonaggressive" through "The client who is agitated, confused, hostile, and uncooperative"
17.	pp. 388-389	"A brief review of balance reactions"
18.	pp. 388-390	"A brief review of balance reactions" and "The client who demonstrates movement sequencing latency and unrefined gait and balance reactions"
19.	pp. 390-392	"Strategies to address neurobehavioral and cognitive problems impacting physical management"
20. No specific answer	p. 384	"Quality of life"

Chapter 14

Answer	Page found on	Location on page
1. Myelomeningocele	p. 398	Column 1, paragraph 4
2. Lumbosacral junction	p. 398	Column 1, paragraph 6
3. Scoliosis Kyphosis Subluxed or dislocated hips Club feet	p. 402	Column 1, paragraphs, 4, 5, 6
4. 80% to 90%	p. 402	Column 2, paragraphs 2, 3
5. a. Ventriculoatrial b. Ventriculoperitoneal	p. 404	Fig. 14-4
6.	p. 404	Column 2, paragraph 1
7.	p. 406	Column 1
8.	pp. 408-409	"Developmental/ functional evaluations"
9.	pp. 414-415	p. 414, column 1 through paragraph 1, column 1, p. 415
10.	pp. 411-418	Stage 1-Stage 4
11.	p. 418	Column 2, paragraphs 2, 3, 4, 5
12.	p. 420	Column 2, paragraphs 6, 7

Answer	Page found on	Location on page

Chapter 15

Answer	Page found on	Location on page
1. False	p. 432	"Degenerative joint abnormalities"
2. False	pp. 463-464	Column 2, paragraph 4
3. False	p. 436	Column 1, paragraph 3
	p. 436	Column 2, paragraph 3
	p. 438	"Impaired temperature regulation"
4. False	p. 438	"Impaired temperature regulation"
5. True	pp. 467-468	Column 2, paragraph 6
6. True	p. 468	Column 1, paragraph 2
7. False	pp. 475-476	Column 2, paragraph 2
8. False	p. 468	Column 2, paragraph 3

Chapter 16

Answer	Page found on	Location on page
1.	p. 489	"Observation of current fundamental status"
2.	pp. 488-496	"Evaluation procedures"
	p. 490	Fig. 16-1
3.	p. 489	Column 2, paragraph 3
4.	pp. 490-491	"Evaluation of level of consciousness"
5.	pp. 491-493	"Evaluation of sensory channels"
6.	pp. 493-496	"Evaluation of movement abilities"
7.	p. 496	"Goal setting"
8.	p. 497	Table 16-1
9.	p. 496	Column 2, paragraph 3
10.	p. 496	"Goal setting"
	pp. 497-499	"Promoting homeostasis of ANS and vital functions"
11.	pp. 499-501	"Promoting optimalization of postural set"
12.	pp. 501-502	"Promoting integration of sensory input"
13.	pp. 502-503	"Promoting integration of primitive reflexes to achieve the normal postural reflex mechanism"
14.	p. 503	"Enhancing progression through developmental sequence activities"

Answer	Page found on	Location on page
15.	pp. 503-504	"Promoting normalization of movement patterns"
16.	p. 505	"Promoting optimalization of psychosocial and cognitive responses" (see also Ch. 7)

Chapter 17

Part I (Poliomyelitis)

Answer	Page found on	Location on page
1.	p. 510	Column 1, paragraph 4
2. a.	p. 511	Column 1, paragraph 2
b.	p. 512	Column 2, paragraph 1
3.	p. 511	Column 1, paragraph 4
4.	p. 511	Column 2, paragraph 2
5. a.	pp. 511-512	"Functional compensation"
b.	pp. 514-515	"New muscle weakness," and "Environmental cold intolerance"
6.	p. 512	Column 2, paragraph 1
7.	pp. 513-514	Column 2, paragraph 2
8.	p. 514	"Pain"
9.	pp. 515-516	"Decreasing the work load of muscles" through p. 516, column 1 paragraph 4
10.	pp. 516-517	Column 2, paragraph 4
11.	p. 511	"Physiological processes of recovery of muscle strength"
	p. 517	"Exercise"

Part II (Human immunodeficiency virus illness)

Answer	Page found on	Location on page
1.	p. 518	Column 1, paragraphs 2-5
2.	pp. 518-519	"The immune system"
3.	pp. 519-520	"Pathogenesis of AIDS"
4.	pp. 520-521	"Systemic manifestations"
5. True	pp. 521-522	"Neuropathology"
6. True	pp. 521-522	"Neuropathology," and "Neurological manifestations"
7.	pp. 522-523	"Medical management"

Answer	Page found on	Location on page		Answer	Page found on	Location on page
8.	pp. 523-524	p. 523, column 2, paragraph 6 through p. 524, column 1, paragraphs 1, 2	16.	Spasticity-tendon tightness, paresthesias, tic doloreux, L'hermitte's sign	p. 545	Column 2, paragraph 4
9.	p. 524	Column 2, paragraph 2	17.	Time of day therapy done, number of repetitions in exercising, environment (air-conditioning)	pp. 544-546	"Treatment of sensorimotor dysfunction"
10. False	p. 525	Column 1, paragraph 4				
11.	p. 526	Column 1, paragraph 2	18.	Short-term memory, conceptual reasoning	p. 546	Column 2, paragraph 5
12.	p. 526	Column 1, paragraph 4	19.	Help to develop realistic vocational and personal goals, suggest compensation techniques and therapy, give individual and family insight into extent of illness, clarify misconceptions about attitude and abilities	p. 547	Column 1, paragraph 5
13.	p. 526	Column 2, paragraph 2				

Chapter 18

	Answer	Page found on	Location on page
1.	Sclerotic tissue that replaces damaged myelin	p. 531	Column 2, paragraph 3
2.	Genetic predisposition; viral trigger	pp. 531-534	"Epidemiology"
3.	Exacerbating-remitting Progressive Combination of above	pp. 535-536	"Course and prognosis"
4.	No pathognomic test Early symptoms transient Symptoms not unique	p. 536	Column 1, paragraph 7
5.	Identify small lesions more sensitive than CT scan	p. 536	Column 1, paragraph 7
6.	Unpredictability of course Ambiguity of diagnosis Borderline factor	pp. 536-537	"Psychosocial considerations"
7.		p. 538	Fig. 18-4
8.	Baclofen, diazepam	p. 537	Column 2, paragraph 2
9.	Improved conduction in demyelinated nerves	p. 537	Column 2, paragraph 4
10.	Cyclophosphamide Plasmapheresis	p. 538	Column 2, paragraph 3
11.	Standard assessment tool developed by International Federation of MS Societies	p. 540	Column 1, paragraph 4
12.	Severe disability that prevents working, but client is able to walk unaided	p. 541	Box
13.	Fluctuating course of disease	p. 544	Column 1, paragraph 4
14.	Stretching, ROM, icing, relaxation techniques, positioning, strengthening agonists	p. 544	Column 2, paragraph 2
15.	Strengthening fixation musculature, facilitate contraction, weighting extremities, Frenkel's exercises	p. 545	Column 1, paragraph 3

Chapter 19

	Answer	Page found on	Location on page
1.		p. 554	"Pathways to the motor system";
		p. 553	Fig. 19-2
2.		pp. 554-555	"Physiology"
3.		pp. 557-558	"Perceptual and cognitive functions"
4.		pp. 558-559	"Neurotransmitters motor control"
5.		pp. 573-574	"Etiology"
6.		p. 561	Column 1, paragraph 3
7.		pp. 561-562	"Stages of the disease"
8.		pp. 559-561	"Symptoms"
		pp. 563-568	"Treatment procedures"
9.		pp. 568-569	"Symptoms"
		pp. 571-572	"Treatment procedures"
10.	No reference		
11.		p. 571	"General treatment goals and rationale"
		pp. 571-572	"Treatment procedures"
12.	No reference		
13.		pp. 575-577	"Sign and symptoms of acute alcohol intoxication" and "Signs and symptoms of chronic alcoholism"
14.		pp. 576-577	Column 1, paragraph 2 through p. 577, column 1, paragraph 1
15.		p. 577	Column 1, paragraph 3

Answer	Page found on	Location on page
Chapter 20		
1.	p. 583	Column 1, paragraph 2
2.	p. 584	Column 1, paragraph 3
3. a	p. 585	Column 2, paragraph 2
4.	p. 585	Column 2, paragraph 4
5.	p. 587	Column 2, paragraph 1
6.	pp. 588-589	p. 588, column 2, paragraph 5 through p. 589, column 1, paragraph 1
7.	pp. 592-593	"Appropriate goal setting: adaptive or functional program"
8.	p. 591	"Dietz classification"
9.	p. 592	Column 1, last paragraph
10.	p. 593	Column 1, last paragraph
Chapter 21		
1.	pp. 597-599	"Hypotonicity," "Asthenia," and "Ataxia"
2.	pp. 599-603	"Disturbance of posture and balance"
	pp. 603-605	"Dysmetria"
	p. 605	"Disturbances of gait"
	pp. 605-608	"Movement decomposition"
	p. 606	"Dysdiadochokinesia"
3.	p. 600	Box
4.	pp. 612-615	"Treatment"
Chapter 22		
1. c	p. 624	Column 1, paragraph 2 "The development of spasticity. . ."
2. c	p. 624	Column 2, paragraph 3
3. d	p. 627	Column 1, paragraph 3
4. h	p. 627	"Recovery of motor function"
5. c	p. 631	Box
6. True	p. 632	Column 1, last paragraph
7. False	pp. 632-633	"Tone"
8. True	p. 634	"Functional activities"

Answer	Page found on	Location on page
9. True	pp. 640-642	"Shoulder dysfunction"
10. a	p. 640	"Joint pain"
11. True	pp. 642-644	"Hip, knee, ankle, and foot problems"
12. b	p. 645	Column 1, paragraph 3
13. True	pp. 646-647	"Girdle control"
14. False	p. 650	Column 2, paragraph 3
Chapter 23		
1.	pp. 661-662	"Definition of terms" except Alzheimer's
2.	p. 662	"Alzheimer's disease"
3.	p. 663	"Arndt-Schultz Principle"
4.	p. 664	"Myths about cognitive changes in aging"
5.	pp. 664-665	"Stress and intellectual capacity"
6.	pp. 665-666	"The Mini-Mental State Examination"
7.	pp. 666-668	"Sensory changes with aging"
8.	pp. 668-669	"Older adult learning styles and communication"
9.	pp. 669-670	"Transplantation shock"
10.	p. 670	"Emotional capacity to participate in a learning task"
11.	pp. 670-671	p. 670, column 2, paragraph 3 through p. 671, column 1, paragraph 3
12. Acute	p. 671	Column 2, paragraphs 3, 4, and 5
Nonacute	p. 672	Column 1, paragraph 3 through column 2, paragraph 1
13.	pp. 675-676	p. 675, column 2, paragraph 2 through p. 676, column 1, paragraph 1; p. 676, column 1, paragraph 3 through column 2, paragraph 1; p. 676, column 2 (#1-10)

	Answer	Page found on	Location on page		Answer	Page found on	Location on page
	Chapter 24			5.		p. 694	Column 1, paragraph 5 through column 2, paragraph 3
1.	All provide forms of continuous sensory feedback to help the speaker monitor the accuracy and appropriateness of speech output and correct speech or language production as needed. They also contribute to speech development.	p. 687	"Development of oral sensation," "Audition," "Vision"	6.	The areas that will affect communication and should be briefly reviewed include oral function, oral sensation, motor speech production, mental status, language comprehension and expression, nonverbal communication, and environmental eects on communication.	pp. 695-699	"Communication screening"
2.	Children learn much of their language through sensorimotor experiences with their environment (exploring, manipulating objects). They form concepts and learn symbols (words) by integrating information on touch, taste, sight, movement, and other attributes of objects and activities that contribute to the child's "knowledge of the world" and concept formation frequently occurs with motor impairments.	pp. 688-689	"Auditory-vocal development"	7.	No. The type of dysarthria—flaccid, spastic, ataxic, hyperkinetic, hypokinetic—will dictate the appropriateness of certain techniques. For instance, pushing exercises used with flaccid dysarthria are contraindicated with spastic dysarthria.	pp. 700-701	"Treatment considerations in dysarthria"
3.	The physical therapist working with children is in an excellent position to monitor the development of communication, initiate referral for communication, remediation if needed, and facilitate normal development. For an approximate developmental sequence in normal children, see Table 24-1.	p. 688 pp. 688-689	Table 24-1 "Development of oral communication," "Early oral development," and "Auditory-vocal development"	8.	Reduce the cognitive and communicative demands on the patient by: a. providing a predictable, consistent structure b. using simple directions and repetition c. explaining all activities in simple terms d. avoiding distractions and multiple conflicting inputs e. using redundancy as long as it does not cause overload, such as providing written as well as verbal instructions Give orientation information within the natural structure of communication rather than "testing" memory. Accept and promote lucid recollections. Use redirection to reduce inappropriate behavior.	p. 701	"Developmental communication disorders"
4.	Each type of communication disorder necessitates a different approach to treatment and interaction. Misunderstanding the nature of the disorder can interfere with the interaction between the client and therapist, inadvertently interfere with development or restoration of communication, promote emotional maladjustment, and reduce the client's motivation.	pp. 689-693	"An overview of disorders in oral, speech, and language function" through p. 693, column 1, paragraph 3				

Answer	Page found on	Location on page
9. Yes. Modification of one's own communication pattern can greatly facilitate the communication-disordered client's ability to use any residual communication skills. For example, allowing additional time to respond, simplifying instruction, using gestures and contextual cues, and modifying the content of directions can facilitate comprehension for many aphasic clients.	pp. 702-703	"Treatment considerations in adult aphasia"

Chapter 25

Answer	Page found on	Location on page
1.	p. 706	Column 2, paragraph 3
2. Accommodation	pp. 707-708	"Accommodation: the identification subsystem"
Oculomotor	p. 708	"Oculomotor: the selective attention and information gathering subsystem"
Convergence	p. 709	"Convergence: the centering spatial localization subsystem"
3.	p. 710	"Visual perceptual disorders in children," paragraphs 1 and 2
	pp. 719-720	"Visual perceptual disorders in adults," paragraphs 1 and 2
4.	p. 710	Column 2, paragraph 4
	p. 711	Box
5.	p. 713	Column 1, paragraph 2
6.	pp. 713-714	Column 2, paragraph 4
	p. 723	Table 25-3
7.	p. 714	Column 2, paragraph 4
8.	p. 715	Column 1, paragraph 5
9.	pp. 716-718	p. 716, column 2, paragraph 5 through p. 718, "Treatment"
10.	p. 719	Column 1, paragraph 4
11.	p. 720	Column 1, paragraph 3
12.	p. 722	Column 1, paragraph 7

Answer	Page found on	Location on page
13.	pp. 722-724	p. 722, column 2, paragraph 3 through p. 724, column 1, paragraph 2
	p. 723	Table 25-3
14.	p. 727	Column 1, paragraphs 3 and 4
15.	pp. 727-729	"Treatment"
16.	pp. 729-730	p. 729, column 2, paragraph 4 through p. 730, column 1, paragraph 3
17.	pp. 731-732	"Identification of clinical problems"
18.	p. 733	"Treatment"
19.	p. 734	Column 1, paragraph 1
20.	p. 734	"Identification of clinical problems"
	p. 735	"Treatment"
21.	p. 737	"Perceptual retraining with computers"

Chapter 26

Answer	Page found on	Location on page
1.	p. 741	Column 2, paragraph 1
2. False	p. 742	"Training"
3.	p. 743	"Sensory nerve conduction"
	pp. 742-743	"Motor nerve conduction"
4. True	p. 744	"Data analysis"
5. c—False	p. 745	Column 1, paragraph 2
a—True	p. 744	Column 2, paragraph 2
b—True	p. 745	Column 1, paragraph 2
d—True	p. 745	Column 1, paragraph 5
6.	p. 745	Table 25-1
	pp. 745-747	"Electromyographic potentials in pathology"
7.	p. 746	"Polyphasic motor unit action potentials"
8.	pp. 747-748	"Additional studies"
9.	p. 752	Box

Chapter 27

Answer	Page found on	Location on page
1.	p. 756	"Pain pathways"
2.	p. 756	Column 1, paragraphs 7, 8
3.	p. 756	Column 2, paragraph 2
4.	p. 756	Column 2, paragraph 6

Answer	Page found on	Location on page
5.	p. 756	Column 2, paragraph 7
6.	p. 757	Column 1, paragraph 4
7.	p. 757	Column 1, paragraph 6
8.	pp. 757-758	"Pain perception"
9.	p. 758	Column 2, paragraph 5
10.	pp. 758-759	"Pain history"
11.	p. 759	Column 2, paragraph 2, Fig. 27-1
12.	pp. 759-760	Column 2, paragraph 5
13.	pp. 760	Column 1, paragraph 4
14.	p. 760	Column 1, #6
15.	p. 760	Column 1, #7
16.	p. 760	Column 2, #8
17.	p. 761	Column 1, paragraph 3
18.	p. 761	Column 1, paragraph 3 (#1-8)
19.	p. 761	Column 2, paragraphs 2-5
20.	p. 762	Column 1, paragraph 3 through column 2, paragraph 2
21.	p. 767	Column 2, paragraph 5
22.	p. 763	Column 1, paragraph 2 (#1-5)
23.	p. 763	Column 2, paragraph 2
24.	pp. 763-764	Column 2, paragraph 5
25.	pp. 764-765	"Normal TENS," "Burst TENS," and "Modulated TENS" through column 1, paragraph 5
26.	p. 765	Column 2, paragraph 2
27.	p. 766	Column 1, paragraph 3 (#1-7)
28.	p. 763	Fig. 27-3
	p. 766	Fig. 27-4
29.	p. 767	Column 2, paragraph 4
30.	pp. 767-768	Column 2, paragraph 6
31.	pp. 766-767	"Massage"
32.	p. 768	"Point stimulation"
33.	pp. 768-769	"Cognitive-behavior methods," "Hypnosis"

Chapter 28

Answer	Page found on	Location on page
1.	p. 773	Column 2, paragraph 1
2.	p. 773	Column 2, paragraphs 1-3
3.	p. 774	Column 1, paragraph 2 (include example)
4.	p. 774	Column 2, "Interim care vs. definitive care"
5.	pp. 774-775	"Dynamic treatment vs. static treatment"
6.	p. 775	"Prevention, facilitation, and inhibition"
7.	p. 775	"Sensory training"
8.	p. 776	"Alignment"
9.	pp. 777-778	Column 2, paragraph 4
10.	p. 778	Column 1, paragraph 3
11.	p. 778	Column 1, paragraph 5
12.	p. 778	Column 2, paragraph 4
13.	p. 779	Column 1, paragraph 6
14.	p. 781	Column 1, paragraph 1 (#1-7)
15.	pp. 782-783	"Hemiplegia"
16.	p. 782	Column 2, paragraph 4
17.	p. 780	Column 2, paragraph 5
18.	p. 780	Column 1, paragraph 3
19.	p. 783	Column 2, paragraph 2
20.	p. 776	"Maintenance"

Chapter 29

Answer	Page found on	Location on page
1.	p. 795	Table 29-1
2.	p. 798	Table 29-2
3.	pp. 798-799	p. 798, column 2, paragraph 2 through p. 799, column 1, paragraphs 1-3
4.	p. 803	"Interventions"

Chapter 30

Answer	Page found on	Location on page
1. a, b, c	pp. 811-812	"Functional orientation of the rehabilitation process"
d	pp. 816-818	"Activities design"
2.	p. 812	"Blending of direct services and process roles"
3.	pp. 812-813	"An ecological approach to life-style analysis"
4.	pp. 813-814	"Therapeutic recreation"

Answer	Page found on	Location on page	Answer	Page found on	Location on page
5.	pp. 814-818	"The Rusalem Model" (NOTE: p. 814, column 2, paragraph 2)	16.	pp. 818-820	"The leisure facilitation process: a tool for all human services" and "The future—where do we go from here?"
6.	pp. 814-818	"The Rusalem Model"			
7.	pp. 818-819	"The leisure facilitation process: a tool for all human services"	17.	p. 820	Column 1, paragraph 1 (eight points)
8.	p. 815	"Perceptual view of behavior"	18., 19.	No specific answer	Answers are conceptual and must be thought through by the student
9.	p. 815	"Neutrality of activity," "Paradox of activity involvement," and "Leadership omnipotence"			

Chapter 31

Answer	Page found on	Location on page
10.	p. 816	"Leadership process"
11.	pp. 815-816	"Group readiness"
12.	p. 816	"Anticipation, realization memories (ARM) of activity experience"
	p. 816	Fig. 30-2
13.	pp. 816-818	"Activities design"
14.	pp. 816-818	"Activities design"
15.	p. 818	Column 1, paragraph 2, and column 2, paragraphs 1 and 2, and Fig. 30-2

Answer	Page found on	Location on page
1.	pp. 824-830	"Medical model of health care," and "Wholistic model"
2.	pp. 824-825	"Medical model of health care"
3.	pp. 825-830	"Wholistic model" (also glossary)
4.	p. 826	Column 1, paragraph 2, 3
5.	p. 826	Column 2, paragraph 3
6.-10.	No specific answer	Entire chapter

GLOSSARY

abulia A loss or deficiency of will power.

ACTH (adrenocorticotropic hormone) A hormone released by the adenohypophysis, which stimulates the adrenal cortex to secrete its entire spectrum of hormones. Thought to be immunosuppressive and antiinflammatory in treating multiple sclerosis.

adaptive response An appropriate response to an environmental demand. Adaptive responses require good sensory integration; they also allow the sensory integrative process to progress.

agraphia Loss of ability to write.

alexia Word blindness: inability to recognize or comprehend written or printed words.

Alzheimer's disease A term used as a diagnosis when, based on the symptoms of confusion and impaired intellectual functioning, all other possible causes have been eliminated. It is not possible to ascertain if a client has this disease until an autopsy or brain biopsy has been done. At present, there is no known cause or treatment for Alzheimer's disease, but clients and families *can be helped* to cope better with the presenting losses of intellectual functioning.

amblyopia Dimness of vision not caused by refractive error or organic disease of the eye.

Amigo A scooterlike, battery operated vehicle.

amniocentesis A procedure in which a needle is passed through the mother's abdomen into the amniotic sac of the fetus. Amniotic fluid is withdrawn and analyzed to detect a variety of abnormalities.

angiography The visualization of blood vessels by injection of a nontoxic radiopaque material.

anterograde amnesia The inability to establish new memories.

aphasia An impairment caused by brain damage, which interferes with the ability to process language symbols. It is disproportionate to impairment of other intellectual functions and is not caused by dementia, sensory loss, or motor dysfunction.

apraxia of speech An articulatory disorder resulting from the inability to program the position of speech muscles and the sequence of muscle movements in order to volitionally produce speech. The disorder results from an impairment arising from brain damage.

Arnold-Chiari malformation A deformity in which the medulla and pons are reduced in size, and the cerebellum herniates into the spinal canal.

ASHA American Speech, Language and Hearing Association, which certifies audiologists and speech pathologists with the Certificate of Clinical Competence (CCC).

asthenia Chronic lack of strength and energy.

ataxia Loss of muscular coordination.

ataxia telangiectasia An inherited disorder characterized by progressive ataxia, oculocutaneous dilation of terminal arteries and capillaries, sinopulmonary disease, and abnormal eye movements.

autism A disorder that in childhood is characterized by withdrawal behavior, reduced socialization, perseveration, bizarre behavior, lack of purposeful verbal communication, and echolalia.

autoimmunity Disease in which the body produces a disordered immunological response against its own tissue. Antibodies against normal parts of the body are produced to an extent that causes tissue injury.

automatic speech Words or phrases spoken without voluntary control, such as curse words, expletives, and greetings.

axonotmesis Interruption of the axon with subsequent wallerian degeneration; connective tissue of the nerve, including the Schwann cell basement membrane, remains intact.

babbling A stage in speech development characterized by the production of strings of speech sounds in vocal play.

ballistic movement High-velocity movement, such as a tennis serve or boxer's punch, requiring reciprocal organization of agonistic and antagonistic synergies.

bite reflex This pathological reflex is a swift biting action produced by stimulation of the oral cavity. The bite may be difficult to release in some cases when an object such as a spoon or tongue depressor has been introduced into the mouth.

brain abscess A localized collection of pus in a cavity formed by the disintegration of brain tissue.

cerebellar atrophy (spinocerebellar degeneration) A general term for several familial disorders in which the cerebellum deteriorates.

cerebral evoked potentials (EPs) Study of potentials evoked from the cortex, including *visually evoked potentials* (VEPs) stimulated by light, *auditory evoked potentials* (AEPs) stimulated by sound, and *somatosensory evoked potentials* (SEPs) stimulated by electrical stimulation of the peripheral sensory nerves.

chewing reflex Pathological sign elicited in brain-damaged adults when the mouth is stimulated and repetitive "chewing" motions ensue.

childhood aphasia A disturbance of the capacity to process language resulting from brain dysfunction in childhood.

climbing fibers One of two fiber types carrying input to cerebellar cortex; terminates in 1:1 relationship on a Purkinje cell.

closure Visualization of the whole figure when only a portion is visible.

coma A complete paralysis of cerebral function, a state of unresponsiveness. Clients do not obey commands, speak, or open their eyes.

complex spatial relations Relationship of one figure or part of a figure to another.

computed axial tomography (CT or CAT scan) An x-ray technique designed to show detailed images of structures on separate planes of tissue. When combined these images can often detail multiple sclerosis lesions and other neurological deficits.

concentric contraction Controlled shortening of the muscle.

conceptual disorders A disturbance in thought processes, in cognitive activities, or in the ability to formulate concepts.

configuration Overall shape or enclosure of a figure.

constancy The invariant quality of distinctive features in spite of valuation in location rotation, size, or color.

contrecoup injury Injury to the brain produced distant to the part sustaining the blow.

cortisone, prednisone Synthetic adrenal glucocorticoids, used in multiple sclerosis to reduce edema and other aspects of inflammation. They are immunosuppressive and have also been shown to be useful in improving nerve conduction in demyelinated fibers.

coup injury Injury to the brain at the site of the impact.

cryosurgery Technique of exposing tissues to extreme cold to produce well demarcated areas of cell destruction. The cold is usually produced by use of a probe containing liquid nitrogen. In rare cases, used to destroy thalamic tissue in persons with multiple sclerosis to control severe tremor and other involuntary movements.

decorticate rigidity A term derived from animal transections, sometimes used to describe abnormal posturing in humans, that is characterized by exaggerated flexor responses in the upper extremities and exaggerated extensor responses in the lower extremities. In reporting, it is preferable to describe the posture observed.

Deiter's nucleus One of the vestibular nuclei, also known as the lateral vestibular nuclei; located in the brainstem.

delayed language Failure of language to develop at the expected age because of any number of causes such as hearing loss, emotional disturbance, or brain injury.

delirium A delirious person shows both a change in intellectual function *and* in the level of consciousness. The client is less alert than normal and may be confused, disoriented, forgetful, and/or sleepy. Other commonly used terms to describe this condition are acute brain syndrome or reversible brain syndrome. If the underlying medical or emotional problem(s) are treated in a timely fashion, the level of alertness and intellectual functions will return to normal.

dementia Dementia is an impairment in some or all aspects of intellectual functioning in a person who is clearly awake. Other terms used to describe this condition are organic brain syndrome, senility, senile dementia, hardening of the arteries, and shrinking of the brain. Some diseases that can cause dementia are treatable. In these diseases the distortion of intellectual capacity is reversed when treatment is given and/or the intellectual functioning is prevented from becoming worse.

dentate nucleus One of the deep cerebellar nuclei; found lateral to the emboliform nucleus in man, within the cerebellar hemisphere; receives fibers from the lateral zone of the cerebellar cortex; fibers leave nucleus via brachium conjunctivum; is considered part of the neocerebellum.

developmental dyspraxia A disorder of sensory integration characterized by an impairment in the ability to plan skilled nonhabitual movement.

developmental handling Moving a child through part or all of the developmental sequence to enhance the expression of normal movement patterns (i.e., righting and equilibrium reactions).

dioptric power Unit of measurement of the refractive power of an optic lens.

diplopia double vision

distal sparing The spinal cord below the congenital lesion remains intact. The reflex arc through the spinal cord therefore remains but is unmodified by supraspinal influences. This results in spastic movements distal to the level of the lesion.

ductions Movements of each single eye from the primary position into the secondary or tertiary positions of gaze.

dynamic equilibrium Ability of clients to adjust to displacements of their center of gravity by appropriately changing their base of support.

dysarthria A disorder of articulation resulting from impairment of the central or peripheral nervous system in the control of the muscles of speech—errors in articulation of speech sounds.

dysdiadochokinesia Inability to perform rapidly alternating motion.

dyskinesia A defect in voluntary movements.

dysmetria An inability to position the limbs accurately with respect to another object.

eccentric contraction Controlled lengthening of a muscle.

echolalia Automatic reiteration of words or phrases that have been heard.

ecology Study of the environmental relations of organisms.

ego-dystonic Destructive to self-enhancement.

ego-syntonic Supportive of self-enhancement

electrical stimulation Study of muscle response to electrical currents including reaction of degeneration (RD), rheobase and chronaxie, strength-duration (SD), and galvanic-tetanus ratio tests.

electroencephalography (EEG) Study of the electrical activity of the brain

electroneuromyography (ENMG) The electrical activity of the muscles and their associated motor and sensory nerves.

electronystagmography Study of eye movements to evaluate vestibular function.

electrophoresis The movement of charged particles through the medium in which they are dispersed as a result of changes in electric potential; useful in analysis of protein mixtures because protein particles move with different velocities.

electroretinography Study of the potentials produced by the light-sensitive tissues of the retina.

emboliform nucleus One of the deep cerebellar nuclei in man; receives input from intermediate zone of the cerebellum; involved in control of posture and voluntary movement.

encephalitis Inflammation of the brain tissue.

encephalomeningitis Inflammation of the meninges and the brain substance.

epicritic Pertaining to the somatic sensations of fine discriminative touch, vibration, two-point discrimination, sterognosis, and conscious and unconscious proprioception.

ergotropic Combinations of cortical alpha rhythm, sympathetic nervous system activity, and somatic muscle activation. Activity or work state.

evoked potentials The electrical manifestation of the brain's reception of and response to an external stimulus; a way of measuring efficiency in the CNS.

experimental autoimmune encephalomyelitis (EAE) An induced, laboratory model of multiple sclerosis characterized by inflammation and demyelination.

exteroceptive Receptors activated primarily by stimuli from the external environment.

extrafusal muscle Striated muscle tissue found outside the muscle spindle.

extrinsic ophthalmoplegia Paralysis of the extrinsic ocular muscles.

fastigial nucleus One of the deep cerebellar nuclei; receives input from the medial zone of the cerebellum; involved in the control of equilibrium and posture.

fine motor coordination Motor behaviors involving manipulative, discrete finger movements and eye-hand coordination.

gag reflex Also know as the pharyngeal reflex, this involuntary contraction of the pharynx and elevation of the soft palate is elicited in most normal individuals by touching the pharyngeal wall or back of the tongue.

gaze-evoked nystagmus Abnormal oscillation of the eyes when attempting to fixate gaze on an object.

gestalt Form, space, concept; the configuration of separate units into a pattern that itself seems to function as a unit or a whole.

globose nucleus One of the four deep cerebellar nuclei in man; receives input from intermediate zone of the cerebellar cortex; involved in control of posture and voluntary movement.

gross motor coordination Motor behaviors concerned with posture and locomotion ranging from early developing behaviors to finely tuned balance.

habilitation To supply with the means to develop maximum independence that has never been obtained.

holistic The spiritual dimension of a health care model.

homonymous hemianopsia Loss of the same side of the field of vision in both eyes.

hyperbaric oxygen Oxygen under greater pressure than at normal atmospheric pressure (usually at 1½ to 3 times absolute atmopsheric pressure). Thought to be immunosuppressive in treating multiple sclerosis.

hypermetria Distortion of target-directed voluntary movement, in which the limb moves beyond the target.

hypometria Distortion of target-directed voluntary movement, in which the limb falls short of reaching the target.

hypotonicity Reduced resistance to passive stretch; displayed as inability to hold resting posture against gravity; limp, "floppy" extremities during passive movement.

immunoglobulins Any one of several proteins that are capable of acting as antibodies. May be found in plasma, urine, and cerebrospinal fluid, for example, IgG is an immunoglobulin.

inferior olivary nucleus A large nucleus in the anterolateral medulla; origin of climbing fibers to the cerebellum.

intention tremor An abnormal tremor of 4 to 6 Hz that occurs during voluntary, goal-directed movement.

interferon A protein formed when cells are exposed to viruses. Noninfected cells exposed to interferon are protected against viral infection. Though to be of use in treating multiple sclerosis.

intermediate region of the cerebellum cortex A longitudinal zone of the cerebellar cortex; located on either side of the median zone; involved in the control of posture and voluntary movement; projects to globose and emboliform nucleus in man and the interpositus nucleus in lower animals.

internal ophthalmoplegia Paralysis of the intrinsic muscles of the eye—those of the iris and ciliary body.

interoceptive Receptors activated by stimuli from within visceral tissues and blood vessels.

interpositus nucleus One of the deep cerebellar nuclei in lower animals (globose and emboliform in humans); receives input from intermediate region of the cerebellar cortex; involved in the control of posture and voluntary movement.

intrafusal muscle Striated muscle tissue found within the muscle spindle.

isometric contraction Muscle tension without shortening.

isotonic contraction Contraction associated with shortening or lengthening of the muscle tissue can be either concentric or eccentric.

jaw jerk Closure of the mouth caused by striking the lower jaw while it hangs passively open. This reflex is rare in normal individuals.

kinesiological electromyography Study of the muscle activity produced on motion.

lateralization The tendency for certain processes to be more highly developed on one side of the brain than on the other. In most people, the right hemisphere develops the processes of spatial and musical thoughts and the left hemisphere develops the areas for verbal and logical processes.

lateral region of the cerebellar cortex A longitudinal zone of the cerebellar cortex; located lateral to intermediate zone; comprises bulk of cerebral hemispheres; involved in the control of skilled voluntary movement; receives projection from motor cortex and has output to dentate nucleus.

learning disabilities A disorder in one or more of the basic physiological processes involved in understanding or using spoken or written language. This may be manifested in disorders of listening, thinking, talking, reading, writing, spelling, or doing arithmetic. They include conditions that have been referred to as, for example, perceptual handicaps, brain injury, minimal brain dysfunction, dyslexia, and developmental aphasia. They do not include learning problems that are primarily caused by visual, hearing, or motor handicaps, to mental retardation or emotional disturbance, or to environmental disadvantage.

leptomeningitis Inflammation of the arachnoid and pia mater layers of the meninges. The same condition may be referred to as meningitis.

long-loop stretch reflex Stretch reflex mediated through the brain.

magnetic resonance imaging (MRI) A scanning technique using magnetic fields and radio frequencies to produce a precise image of the body tissue; used for diagnosis and monitoring of disease.

medial zone of cerebellar cortex The longitudinal zone of the cerebellar cortex, which includes the vermis and the flocculonodular lobe; involved in control of equilibrium and posture; projects to fastigial and vestibular nuclei.

meningitis Acute inflammation of the meninges covering the brain and spinal cord.

metencephalon The cephalic part of the rhombencephalon, giving rise to the cerebellum and pons.

minimal brain dysfunction A mild or minimal neurological abnormality that causes learning difficulties in the child with average intelligence.

morphogenesis The morphological transformation including growth, alterations of germinal layers, and differentiation of cells and tissues during development.

mossy fibers One of two fiber types carrying information to the cerebellar cortex.

motor coordination Functions that are traditionally defined as motoric. Includes gross motor, fine motor, and motor planning functions.

motor dysfunction, motor deficit, motor disorder, motor disturbance Generic terms for any type of disorder found in learning disabled children that has a motor component.

motor lag A prolonged latent period between the reception of a stimulus and the initiation of the motor response.

motor planning (praxis) The ability to plan and execute skilled nonhabitual tasks.

movement decomposition Distortion of voluntary movement in which the movement occurs in a distinct sequence of isolated steps, rather than in a normal, smooth, flowing pattern.

movement speed The time elapsed between the initiation of a movement and its completion.

myelencephalon The lower part of the embryonic hindbrain from which the medulla oblongata develops.

myelin A fatlike substance forming the principal component of the sheath of nerve fibers in the CNS.

myelography Radiographical inspection of the spinal cord by use of a radiopaque medium injected into the intrathecal space.

neocerebellum Those parts of the cerebellum that receive input via the corticopontocerebellar pathway.

neologism A new, meaningless word, often spoken by fluent aphasic clients.

neurapraxia Interruption of nerve conduction without loss of continuity of the axon.

neurography Study of the action potentials of nerves.

neurotmesis Damage to the axon and the endoneurial tube with the nerve remaining macroscopically intact, or complete transection of the nerve. Regeneration is less successful than in axonotmesis.

nosocomial Hospital acquired.

nuchal rigidity Reflex spasm of the neck extensor muscles resulting in resistance to cervical flexion.

nystagmus A series of automatic, back-and-forth eye movements. Different conditions produce this reflex. A common way of producing them is by an abrupt stop following a series of rotations of the body. The duration and regularity of postrotary nystagmus are some of the indicators of vestibular system efficiency.

ocular dysmetria The eyes are unable to fix gaze on an object or follow a moving object with accuracy.

oligoclonal banding A process by which cerebrospinal fluid IgG is distributed, following electrophoresis, in discrete bands. Approximately 90% of clients with multiple sclerosis show oligoclonal banding.

oligodendroglia Myelin-producing cells in the CNS.

ophthalmoplegia Paralysis of ocular muscles.

opisthotonus Position of extreme hyperextension of the vertebral column caused by a tetanic spasm of the extensor musculature.

optokinetic nystagmus Nystagmus induced by watching stripes on a drum revolving around one's face.

pachymeningitis Acute inflammation of the dura mater.

papilledema Edema of the optic disc.

parallel talk A form of speech used during play therapy with children in which the clinician verbalizes actions such as what is happening or what the child is doing without requiring "answers" from the child. For instance "I'm making a cake. Mine is good. You're making a cake, too." The clinician often repeats utterances of the child correctly and parallels the child's activities.

paranodal myelin intussusception. The ultrastructural change that occurs at Ranvier's node because of acute focal compression of a nerve, resulting in a neuropraxic lesion.

paraxial Lying near the axis of the body.

pendular knee jerk Upon elicitation of the deep tendon reflex of the knee, the lower leg oscillates briefly like a pendulum after the jerk, instead of returning immediately to resting position.

perceptual-motor The interaction of the various channels of perception with motor activity, including visual, auditory, tactual, and kinesthetic channels.

perceptual-motor match The process of comparing and collating the input data received through the motor system and through perception.

phenol block An injection of phenol (hydroxybenzene) into individual nerves. Used as a topical anesthetic and produces a selective block of these nerves. Sometimes used to control severe spasticity in specific muscle groups.

physiological flexion The excessive amount of flexor tone that is *normally* present at birth because of the existing level of CNS maturation and fetal positioning in utero.

plaque A multiple sclerosis lesion characterized by loss of myelin and hardening of tissue.

plasmapheresis A process by which blood is removed from the client; plasma is discarded and replaced by normal plasma or human albumin. Reconstituted blood is then returned to the client. In treating multiple sclerosis this process is believed to rid the blood of antibodies or substances that are damaging to myelin or that impair nerve conduction.

pneumoencephalogram Radiographical examination of ventricles and subarachnoid spaces of the brain following withdrawal of cerebrospinal fluid and injection of air or gas via lumbar puncture.

polysomnography Study of sleep.

position in space Direction in which figures point, relationship of one body part to another, or the entire body's relationship to objects or others in space.

posttraumatic amnesia The time elapsed between a brain injury and the point at which the functions concerned with memory are determined to have been restored.

postural background movements The subtle, spontaneous body adjustments that make overt movements of the hands easier, for example, reaching for a distant object. These postural adjustments depend on good vestibular and proprioceptive integration.

postural tremor A pathological tremor of 3 to 5 Hz that appears in a limb or the trunk when either is working against the pull of gravity.

pragmatics The study of language as it is used in context.

proprioceptive Receptors that respond to stimuli originating primarily from muscle spindles, Golgi tendon organs, and joints.

protopathic Pertaining to the somatic sensations of fast, localized pain, slow, poorly localized pain, and temperature.

Pro-Ven A processed mixture of cobra, krait, and water moccasin venoms developed by Florida physicians to treat multiple sclerosis. The FDA has banned the sale of Pro-Ven until it is tested for safety and effectiveness.

Purkinje cells Large neurons found in the cerebellar cortex, which provide the only output from the cerebellar cortex after the cortex processes sensory and motor signals from the rest of the nervous system.

rebound phenomenon Inability to stop a resisted muscle contraction, such that movement of the limb occurs when the resistance is unexpectedly withdrawn from the limb.

red nucleus Large, vascular nucleus found in mesencephalon, involved in transmission of cerebellar communications to the motor cortex and thalamus.

reflux Back flow of urine from bladder to ureters.

rehabilitation The restoration of a disabled individual to maximum independence commensurate with his or her limitations.

response speed The time elapsed between presentation of a stimulus and the client's initiation of movement.

retardation A retarded person has had some degree of mental impairment all his or her life. A retarded person can also develop a delirium or dementia. A delirium or dementia differs from retardation in that there has been a change from what was normal for that person.

retrograde amnesia The inability to recall events that have occurred during the period immediately preceding a brain injury.

rooting reflex This normal reflex in infants up to 4 months of age consists of head turning in the direction of the stimulus when the cheek is stroked gently.

saccadic eye movement An extremely fast movement of the eyes, allowing the eyes to accurately fix on a still object in the visual field.

saccadic fixations A rapid change of fixation from one point in a visual field to another.

scanning speech An abnormal pattern of speech characterized by regularly recurring pauses.

sensorimotor therapy Therapy planned to enhance the integration of reflex phenomena and the emergence of voluntary motor behaviors concerned with posture and locomotion.

sensory deprivation An enforced absence of the usual repertoire of sensory stimuli. The continued absence of adequate, normal stimuli can produce severe mental changes, including hallucinations, anxiety, depression, and insanity.

sensory integration The organization of sensory input for use, a perception of the body or environment, an adaptive response, a learning process, or the development of some neural function.

sensory integrative dysfunction A disorder or irregularity in brain function that makes sensory integration difficult. Many, but not all, learning disorders stem from sensory integrative dysfunctions.

sensory integrative therapy Therapy involving sensory stimulation and adaptive responses to it according to a child's neurological needs. Treatment usually involves full body movements that provide vestibular, proprioceptive, and tactile stimulation. It usually does not include desk activities, speech training, reading lessons, or training in specific perceptual or motor skills. The goal is to improve the brain's ability to process and organize sensations.

serial speech Overlearned speech involving a series of words such as counting and reciting the days of the week.

smooth pursuit movement of the eyes When the eyes are following a slowly moving object, they move together at a steady velocity, nor in saccades.

soft neurological signs Mild or slight neurological abnormalities that are difficult to detect.

static equilibrium Ability of an individual to adjust to displacements of his or her center of gravity while maintaining a constant base of support.

stereognosis The ability to recognize the sizes, shapes, and weights of familiar objects without the use of vision.

stereopsis Quality of visual fusion.

strabismus Oculomotor misalignment of one eye.

tactile defensiveness A sensory integrative dysfunction characterized by tactile sensations that cause excessive emotional reactions, hyperactivity, or other behavior problems.

telereceptive The exteroceptors of hearing, sight, and smell that are sensitive to distant stimuli.

tenotomy Surgical section of a tendon used in some cases to treat severe spasticity and contractures.

tongue-thrust swallow An immature form of swallowing in which the tongue is projected forward instead of retracted during swallowing.

topognosis The ability to localize tactile stimuli.

total lymphoid irradiation (TLI) Radiation therapy targeted to the body's lymph nodes; in the treatment of multiple sclerosis, the goal is to suppress immune system functioning (reduce the number of lymphocytes in the blood).

transcutaneous nerve stimulation (TNS) A procedure in which electrodes are placed on the surface of the skin over specific nerves and electrical stimulation is carried out. Stimulation of the CNS in this manner is thought to improve CNS function, reduce spasticity, and control pain.

trophotropic Combination of parasympathetic nervous system activity, somatic muscle relaxation, and cortical beta rhythm synchronization. Resting or sleep state.

truncal ataxia Uncoordinated movement of the trunk.

universal cuff An adaptive device worn on the hand to hold items such as utensils, shaver, or pencil, allowing an individual with weak grasp to participate in self-care activities.

vergences Movements of the two eyes in the opposite direction.

vermis Forms the unpaired medial region of the cerebellum.

versions Movements of the two eyes in the same direction.

vestibular-bilateral disorder A sensory integrative dysfunction characterized by shortened duration nystagmus, poor integration of the two sides of the body and brain, and difficulty in learning to read or compute. The disorder is caused by underreactive vestibular responses.

vestibuloocular reflex A normal reflex in which eye position compensates for movement of the head, induced by excitation of vestibular apparatus.

visual-motor coordination The ability to coordinate vision with the movements of the body or parts of the body.

visual-motor function The ability to draw or copy forms or to perform constructive tasks.

wallerian degeneration The physical and biochemical changes that occur in a nerve because of the loss of axonal continuity following trauma.

wholistic A model or approach to health care that takes into account all internal and external influences during the process.

zero-to-three infant stimulation groups Groups that provide therapeutic services for children from birth to 3 years of age, since this age-group is not yet eligible for public school placement.

INDEX

Page numbers in *italics* indicate boxed material and illustrations.
Page numbers followed by *t* indicate tables.